The GALE
ENCYCLOPEDIA *of*
NURSING AND
ALLIED HEALTH

THIRD EDITION

The GALE
ENCYCLOPEDIA *of*
NURSING AND ALLIED HEALTH

THIRD EDITION

VOLUME

5

P–S

BRIGHAM NARINS, EDITOR

GALE
CENGAGE Learning·

Detroit • New York • San Francisco • New Haven, Conn • Waterville, Maine • London

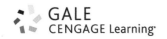

The Gale Encyclopedia of Nursing and Allied Health, Third Edition

Project Editor: Brigham Narins

Editorial: Tara Atterberry, Donna Batten, Laurie Fundukian, Jacqueline Longe, Kristin Key, Kristin Mallegg, Jeffrey Wilson

Product Manager: Kate Hanley

Editorial Support Services: Andrea Lopeman

Indexing Services: Laurie Andriot

Rights Acquisition and Management: Leitha Etheridge-Sims

Composition: Evi Abou-El-Seoud

Manufacturing: Wendy Blurton

Imaging: John Watkins

Product Design: Kristine Julien

© 2013 Gale, Cengage Learning

For product information and technology assistance, contact us at **Gale Customer Support, 1-800-877-4253.** For permission to use material from this text or product, submit all requests online at **www.cengage.com/permissions.** Further permissions questions can be emailed to **permissionrequest@cengage.com**

While every effort has been made to ensure the reliability of the information presented in this publication, Gale, a part of Cengage Learning, does not guarantee the accuracy of the data contained herein. Gale accepts no payment for listing; and inclusion in the publication of any organization, agency, institution, publication, service, or individual does not imply endorsement of the editors or publisher. Errors brought to the attention of the publisher and verified to the satisfaction of the publisher will be corrected in future editions.

LIBRARY OF CONGRESS CATALOGING-IN-PUBLICATION DATA

The Gale encyclopedia of nursing and allied health. / Brigham Narins, editor. 3rd ed.
    p. ; cm.
  Encyclopedia of nursing & allied health
  Gale encyclopedia of nursing and allied health
  Includes bibliographical references and index.
  ISBN 978-1-4144-9888-1 (set : alk. paper) -- ISBN 978-1-4144-9889-8 (v. 1 : alk. paper) -- ISBN 978-1-4144-9890-4 (v. 2 : alk. paper) -- ISBN 978-1-4144-9891-1 (v. 3 : alk. paper) -- ISBN 978-1-4144-9892-8 (v. 4 : alk. paper) -- ISBN 978-1-4144-9893-5 (v. 5 : alk. paper) -- ISBN 978-1-4144-9894-2 (v. 6 : alk. paper) -- ISBN 978-1-4144-9895-9 (e-book)
  I. Narins, Brigham, 1962- II. Title: Encyclopedia of nursing & allied health. III. Title: Gale encyclopedia of nursing and allied health.
  [DNLM: 1. Nursing Care--Encyclopedias--English. 2. Allied Health Personnel--Encyclopedias--English. 3. Nursing--Encyclopedias--English. WY 13]

  610.7303--dc23   2012034778

Gale
27500 Drake Rd.
Farmington Hills, MI, 48331-3535

ISBN-13: 978-1-4144-9888-1 (set)   ISBN-10: 1-4144-9888-8 (set)
ISBN-13: 978-1-4144-9889-8 (vol. 1)   ISBN-10: 1-4144-9889-6 (vol. 1)
ISBN-13: 978-1-4144-9890-4 (vol. 2)   ISBN-10: 1-4144-9890-X (vol. 2)
ISBN-13: 978-1-4144-9891-1 (vol. 3)   ISBN-10: 1-4144-9891-8 (vol. 3)
ISBN-13: 978-1-4144-9892-8 (vol. 4)   ISBN-10: 1-4144-9892-6 (vol. 4)
ISBN-13: 978-1-4144-9893-5 (vol. 5)   ISBN-10: 1-4144-9893-4 (vol. 5)
ISBN-13: 978-1-4144-9894-2 (vol. 6)   ISBN-10: 1-4144-9894-2 (vol. 6)

This title is also available as an e-book.
ISBN-13: 978-1-4144-9895-9   ISBN-10: 1-4144-9895-0
Contact your Gale, a part of Cengage Learning sales representative for ordering information.

Printed in China
1 2 3 4 5 6 7 17 16 15 14 13

CONTENTS

LIST OF ENTRIES

A

Abdomen
Abdominal pain
Abdominal ultrasound
Abortion
Abrasion
Abscess
Acid-base balance
Acid-fast culture and smear
Activities of daily living evaluation
Acupressure
Acupuncture
Administration of medication
Adolescent nutrition
Adrenal gland computed tomography
Adrenal glands
Adrenocortical hormone tests
Adrenomedullary hormone tests
Adult day care
Advance directive
Advanced cardiac life support (ACLS)
Advanced practice nurses
Aerobic training/endurance training
Aerosol drug administration
Aging and the aged
AIDS
AIDS counseling
AIDS tests
Air embolism
Airway management
Alcohol-related neurological disease
Alcoholism
Allergies

Allergy tests
Alternative and complementary medicine
Alzheimer's disease
Ambulatory electrocardiography
Ambulatory surgery centers
American sign language
Americans with Disabilities Act
Amino acid disorders screening
Amniocentesis
Amylase and lipase tests
Anabolic steroids
Anaerobic bacteria culture
Analgesics
Anaphylaxis
Anatomy
Anemias
Anesthesia, general
Anesthesia, local
Anesthesia, topical
Anesthesiology
Aneurysm
Angina
Angiography
Angioplasty
Anorexia nervosa
Antacids
Antepartum testing
Anthrax
Antianxiety drugs
Antiasthmatic drugs
Antibiotics
Antibodies
Anticancer drugs
Anticoagulant and antiplatelet drugs
Antidepressant drugs

Antidiabetic drugs
Antidiuretic hormone (ADH) test
Antifungal drugs, systemic
Antifungal drugs, topical
Antiglobulin tests
Antihistamines
Antihypertensive drugs
Antiparkinson drugs
Antipsychotic drugs
Antiretroviral drugs
Antiseptics
Antiulcer drugs
Antiviral drugs
Anxiety
Apgar testing
Aphasia
Appendicitis
Apraxia
Arrhythmias
Art therapy
Arterial Doppler ultrasound
Arterial insufficiency
Arterial line
Arthrography
Arthroscopy
Artificial organs
Asbestosis
Aseptic technique
Asperger syndrome
Asthma
Astigmatism
Ataxia
Atherosclerosis
Atrial fibrillation and flutter
Attention deficit hyperactivity disorder (ADHD)

Hemorrhoids
Henderson theory of nursing
Hepatitis
Hepatitis virus tests
Herbalism, Western
Hernia
Herniated disk
High-risk pregnancy
Hinge joint
Hip fractures rehabilitation
HIPAA
HIV preventative measures
Hives
Holter monitoring
Home care
Homeopathy
Homosexuality
Hospice
Hospital administration
Hospital-acquired infections
Human anatomy
Human growth and development
Human leukocyte antigen test
Human papilloma virus (HPV)
Human papilloma virus (HPV)
    vaccination
Hydrocephalus
Hydrotherapy
Hyperbaric oxygen therapy
Hypercoagubility tests
Hyperopia
Hypertension
Hyperthermia/hypothermia unit
    management
Hyphema
Hypoglycemia
Hypopituitarism
Hypotension
Hypothermia
Hysterosalpingography
Hysteroscopy

I

Immovable joint
Immune response
Immune system

Immunoassay tests
Immunodeficiency
Immunoelectrophoresis
Immunofixation Electrophoresis
Immunology
Impacted tooth
Impedance plethysmography
Implantable cardioverter-defibrillator
Indium scan
Industrial toxicology
Infant nutrition
Infection
Infection control
Infectious disease
Infectious mononucleosis
Infectious mononucleosis test
Infertility
Influenza
Informed consent
Inheritance, principles of
Integumentary system
Intensive care unit equipment
Internal medicine
Intersex states
Intestinal obstructions
Intestine, large
Intestine, small
Intra-aortic balloon pump
Intradermal injection
Intramuscular injection
Intraoperative care
Intravenous fluid regulation
Intravenous medication
    administration
Intravenous therapy
Intravenous tubing and dressing
    change
Intravenous urography
Intussusception
Iontophoresis
Ipecac
Iron
Iron deficiency anemia
Iron tests
Irritable bowel syndrome
Ischemia
Itching

J

Jaundice
Johnson theory of nursing
Joint fluid analysis
Joint integrity and function
Joint mobilization and manipulation
Journal therapy

K

Kidney failure, acute
Kidney function tests
Kidney radionuclide scan
Kidney stones
Kidney, ureter, and bladder x-ray
    study
Kidneys
King theory of nursing
KOH test

L

Lactation
Lactation consulting
Language acquisition
Language disorders
Laparoscope
Laparoscopy
Laryngoscopy
Laser surgery
Laxatives
Learning theory
Leukemias, acute
Leukemias, chronic
Licensed practical nurse
Life cycle nutrition
Life support
Lipid tests
Lipids
Lipoproteins test
Lithotripsy
Liver
Liver biopsy
Liver cancer
Liver function tests

PLEASE READ—IMPORTANT INFORMATION

The *Gale Encyclopedia of Nursing and Allied Health, Third Edition* is a health reference product designed to inform and educate readers about a wide variety of medical, scientific, theoretical, and practical subjects associated with nursing and health care. Gale, Cengage Learning believes the product to be comprehensive, but not necessarily definitive. It is intended to supplement, not replace, consultation with a physician or other health care practitioner. While Gale, Cengage Learning has made substantial efforts to provide information that is accurate, comprehensive, and up-to-date, Gale, Cengage Learning

makes no representations or warranties of any kind, including without limitation, warranties of merchantability or fitness for a particular purpose, nor does it guarantee the accuracy, comprehensiveness, or timeliness of the information contained in this product. Readers should be aware that the universe of medical knowledge is constantly growing and changing, and that differences of opinion exist among authorities. Readers are also advised to seek professional diagnosis and treatment for any medical condition, and to discuss information obtained from this book with their health care provider.

INTRODUCTION

The Gale Encyclopedia of Nursing & Allied Health, 3rd Edition is a unique and invaluable source of information for the nursing or allied health student. This collection of more than 1,100 entries provides in-depth coverage of specific diseases and disorders, tests and procedures, equipment and tools, body systems, nursing and allied health professions, and contemporary health-care issues. This book is designed to fill a gap between health information designed for laypeople and that intended for medical professionals, which may be too advanced for the beginning student to understand. This encyclopedia employs medical terminology in a judicious, intelligible manner.

SCOPE

The Gale Encyclopedia of Nursing & Allied Health, 3rd Edition covers a wide variety of topics relevant to the nursing or allied health student. Subjects covered include those important to students intending to become registered and licensed practical nurses, nurse anesthetists, nurse practitioners, nurse midwives, biomedical equipment technologists, dental hygienists, dieticians, health care administrators, medical technologists or clinical laboratory scientists, occupational therapists, optometrists, pharmacy technicians, physical therapists, radiologic technologists, and speech-language therapists. The encyclopedia also covers information on related general medical topics, classes of medication, mental health, public health, and human biology. Entries follow a standardized format that provides information at a glance. The standard sections, or rubrics, in each type of entry include:

Diseases/Disorders

- Definition
- Description
- Causes and symptoms
- Diagnosis
- Treatment
- Prognosis
- Health care team roles
- Prevention
- Resources
- Key terms

Tests/Procedures

- Definition
- Purpose
- Precautions
- Description
- Preparation
- Aftercare
- Complications
- Results
- Health care team roles
- Resources
- Key terms

Equipment/Tools

- Definition
- Purpose
- Description
- Operation
- Maintenance
- Health care team roles
- Training
- Resources
- Key terms

Human biology/Body systems

- Definition
- Description
- Function

• Role in human health
• Common diseases and disorders
• Resources
• Key terms

Nursing and allied health professions

• Definition
• Description
• Work settings
• Education and training
• Advanced education and training
• Future outlook
• Resources
• Key terms

Current health issues

• Definition
• Description
• Viewpoints
• Professional implications
• Resources
• Key terms

INCLUSION CRITERIA

A preliminary list of topics was compiled from a wide variety of sources, including nursing and allied health textbooks, general medical encyclopedias, and consumer health guides. The advisory board, composed of advanced practice nurses, allied health professionals, health educators, and medical doctors, evaluated the topics and made suggestions for inclusion. Final selection of topics to include was made by the advisory board in conjunction with the Gale editor.

ABOUT THE CONTRIBUTORS

The essays were compiled by experienced medical writers, including physicians, pharmacists, nurses, and allied health care professionals. The advisers reviewed the completed essays to ensure that they are appropriate, up-to-date, and medically accurate.

HOW TO USE THIS BOOK

The Gale Encyclopedia of Nursing & Allied Health, 3rd Edition has been designed with ready reference in mind.

• Straight **alphabetical arrangement** of topics allows users to locate information quickly.
• **Bold-faced terms** within entries direct the reader to related articles.
• **Cross-references** placed throughout the encyclopedia direct readers from alternate names and related topics to entries.
• A list of **Key Terms** is provided where appropriate to define terms or concepts that may be unfamiliar to the student.
• The **Resources section** directs readers to additional sources of medical information on a topic.
• Valuable **contact information** for medical, nursing, and allied health organizations is included with each entry. An **appendix of organizations** in the back matter contains an extensive list of nursing and allied health associations, agencies, and academies arranged by subject.
• A comprehensive general index guides readers to significant topics mentioned in the text.

GRAPHICS

The Gale Encyclopedia of Nursing & Allied Health, 3rd Edition is enhanced by over 500 color photos, illustrations, and tables.

ACKNOWLEDGMENTS

The editor would like to express appreciation to all of the nursing and allied health professionals who wrote, reviewed, and copyedited entries for *The Gale Encyclopedia of Nursing & Allied Health, 3rd Edition.*

Cover photos were reproduced by the permission of Delmar Publishers, Inc., Custom Medical Photos, and Gale, Cengage Learning.

ADVISORY BOARD

Several experts in the nursing and allied health community provided invaluable assistance in the formulation of this encyclopedia. The advisory board performed a myriad of duties, from defining the scope of coverage to reviewing individual entries for accuracy and accessibility. The editor would like to express appreciation to them for their time and their expert contributions.

Kenneth J. Berniker, MD
Medical writer and editor
El Cerrito, California

Laura J. Cataldo, RN, EdD
Medical writer
Myersville, Maryland

Robert Harr, MS, MT (ASCP)
Associate Professor and Chair
Department of Public and Allied
Health
Bowling Green State University
Bowling Green, Ohio

Amy E. Tyler, PhD
formerly of University of Nebraska
Medical Center
Interlochen, Michigan

CONTRIBUTORS

Margaret Alic, PhD
Eastsound, Washington

Lisa Maria Andres, MS, CGC
San Jose, California

Greg Annussek
New York, New York

Maia Appleby
Boynton Beach, Florida

Bill Asenjo, MS, CRC
Iowa City, Iowa

Paul Arthur
London, England

William Arthur Atkins, PhD
Pekin, Illinois

Howard Baker
North York, Ontario

Laurie Barclay, MD
Tampa, Florida

Julia Barrett
Madison, Wisconsin

Maria Eve Basile, PhD
Roselle, New Jersey

Lori Ann Beck, RN, MSN, FNP-C
Berkley, Michigan

Mary Bekker
Willow Grove, Pennsylvania

Linda K. Bennington, RNC, MSN, CNS
Virginia Beach, Virginia

Abigail V. Berniker, BA
El Cerrito, California

Isaac R. Berniker
Vallejo, California

Kenneth J. Berniker, MD
El Cerrito, California

Mark A. Best
Cleveland Heights, Ohio

Dean Andrew Bielanowski, RN, BNurs (QUT)
Rochedale S., Brisbane, Australia

Carole Birdsall, RNANP, EdD
New York, New York

Bethanne Black
Buford, Georgia

Robert Bockstiegel
Portland, Oregon

Maggie Boleyn, RN, BSN
Oak Park, Michigan

Jack H. Booth, PsyD
Charleston, South Carolina

Barbara Boughton
El Cerrito, California

Patricia L. Bounds, PhD
Zurich, Switzerland

Mary Boyle, PhD, CCC-SLP, BC-NCD
Lincoln Park, New Jersey

Rachael Tripi Brandt, MS
Gettysburg, Pennsylvania

Peggy Elaine Browning
Olney, Texas

Marilyn Butler
Susan Joanne Cadwallader
Cedarburg, Wisconsin

Susan Joanne Cadwallader
Cedarburg, Wisconsin

Rosalyn Carson-DeWitt, MD
Durham, North Carolina

Laura Jean Cataldo, RN, EdD
Myersville, Maryland

Barbara M. Chandler
Sacramento, California

Linda Chrisman
Oakland, California

Rhonda Cloos, RN
Austin, Texas

Angela M. Costello
Northfield, Ohio

David A. Cramer, MD
Chicago, Illinois

L. Lee Culvert
Alna, Massachusetts

Helen Davidson
Chicago, Illinois

Tish Davidson, AM
Fremont, California

Lori De Milto
Sicklerville, New Jersey

Victoria E. DeMoranville
Lakeville, Massachusetts

Janine Diebel, RN
Gaylord, Michigan

Robert Scott Dinsmoor
South Hamilton, Massachusetts

Stephanie Islane Dionne
Ann Arbor, Michigan

Martin W. Dodge, PhD
Inglewood, California

J. Paul Dow, Jr.
Kansas City, Missouri

Douglas Dupler, MA
Boulder, Colorado

Altha Roberts Edgren
St. Paul, Minnesota

Lorraine K. Ehresman
Northfield, Quebec, Canada

Karen Ericson, RN
Estes Park, Colorado

Abraham F. Ettaher, MD
Dearborn, Michigan
L. Fleming Fallon, Jr., MD,
DrPH
Bowling Green, Ohio

Diane Fanucchi-Faulkner,
CMT, CCRA
Oceano, California

Karl Finley
West Bloomfield, Michigan

Janis O. Flores
Sebastopol, Florida

Paula Ford-Martin, MS
Chaplin, Minnesota

Janie F. Franz
Grand Forks, North Dakota

Sallie Boineau Freeman, PhD
Atlanta, Georgia

Rebecca J. Frey, PhD
New Haven, Connecticut

Lisa Frick
Columbia, Missouri

Jason Fryer
San Antonio, Texas

Sandra Galeotti
Sao Paulo, Brazil

Larry Gilman, PhD
Sharon, Vermont

Debra Gordon
Nazareth, Pennsylvania

Lisa M. Gourley
Bowling Green, Ohio

Meghan M. Gourley
Germantown, Maryland

Jill Ilene Granger, MS
Ann Arbor, Michigan

Elliot Greene, MA
Silver Spring, Maryland

Laith Farid Gulli, MD
Lathrup Village, Michigan

Stephen John Hage, AAAS, RT
(R), FAHRA
Chatsworth, California

Maureen Haggerty
Ambler, Pennsylvania

Clare Hanrahan
Asheville, North Carolina

Robert Harr, MS, MT (ASCP)
Bowling Green, Ohio

Daniel J. Harvey
Wilmington, Delaware

Katherine Hauswirth, APRN
Deep River, Connecticut

David L. Helwig
London, Ontario, Canada

Lisette Hilton
Boca Raton, Florida

Fran Hodgkins
Sparks, Maryland

René A. Jackson, RN
Port Charlotte, Florida

Nadine M. Jacobson, RN
Takoma Park, Maryland

Randi B. Jenkins
New York, New York

Michelle L. Johnson, MS, JD
Portland, Oregon

Paul A. Johnson
San Marcos, California

Linda D. Jones, BA, PBT (ASCP)
Asheboro, New York

Crystal Heather Kaczkowski,
MSc
Dorval, Quebec, Canada

Beth Kapes
Bay Village, Ohio

Christine Kuehn Kelly
Havertown, Pennsylvania

Monique Laberge, PhD
Philadelphia, Pennsylvania

Jeffrey P. Larson, RPT
Sabin, Minnesota

Jill S. Lasker
Midlothian, Virginia

Renee Laux, MS
Manlius, New York

Brenda W. Lerner
Montrose, Alabama

Lorraine Lica, PhD
San Diego, California

Peter T. Lin, MD
Foster City, California

Aliene S. Linwood, BSN, RN,
DPA, FACHE
Athens, Ohio

Jacqueline L. Longe
Clearwater, Florida

Jennifer Lee Losey, RN
Madison Heights, Michigan

Nicole Mallory, MS, PA-C
Detroit, Michigan

Warren Maltzman, PhD
Demarest, New Jersey

Liz Marshall
Columbus, Ohio

Mary Elizabeth Martelli, RN,
BS
Sebastian, Florida

Jacqueline N. Martin, MS
Albrightsville, Pennsylvania

Sally C. McFarlane-Parrott
Mason, Michigan

Nancy McKenzie, PhD
Brooklyn, New York

Beverly G. Miller, MT (ASCP)
Charlotte, North Carolina

Christine Miner Minderovic,
BS, RT, RDMS
Ann Arbor, Michigan

Barbara J. Mitchell
Hallstead, Pennsylvania

Mark A. Mitchell, MD
Bothell, Washington

Susan M. Mockus, PhD
Seattle, Washington

Susan J. Montgomery
Milwaukee, Wisconsin

Timothy E. Moore, PhD
Toronto, Ontario, Canada

Alfredo Mori, MB, BS
Oxford, England

Ralph Myerson, MD
Philadelphia, Pennsylvania

Bilal Nasser, MSc
Santo domingo, Dominican
    Republic

Katy Nelson, ND
Marquette, Michigan
David Edward Newton, EdD
Ashland, Oregon

Nancy J. Nordenson
Minneapolis, Minnesota

Erika J. Norris
Oak Harbor, Washington

Debra Novograd, BS, RT (R) (M)
Royal Oak, Michigan

Deborah Nurmi, MS
Atlanta, Georgia

Marianne F. O'Connor, MT, MPH
Farmington Hills, Michigan

Melinda Granger Oberleitner,
RN, DNS, APRN, CNS
Lafayette, Louisiana

Teresa G. Odle, PhD
Albuquerque, New Mexico

Carole Osborne-Sheets
Poway, California

Cindy F. Ovard, RDA
Spring Valley, California

Patience Paradox
Bainbridge Island, Washington

Deborah Eileen Parker, RN
Lakewood, Washington

Genevieve Pham-Kanter
Chicago, Illinois

Jane E. Phillips, PhD
Chapel Hill, North Carolina

Pamella A. Phillips
Bowling Green, Ohio

Deanna Pledge, PhD
Columbia, Missouri

J. Ricker Polsdorfer, MD
Phoenix, Arizona

Elaine R. Proseus, MBA/TM,
BSRT, RT (R)
Farmington Hills, Michigan

Ann Quigley
New York, New York

Robert Ramirez, BS
Stratford, New Jersey

Esther Csapo Rastegari, RN,
BSN, EdM
Holbrook, Massachusetts

Anastasia Marie Raymer, PhD
Norfolk, Virginia

Martha S. Reilly, OD
Madison, Wisconsin

Linda Richards, RD, CHES
Flagstaff, Arizona

Toni Rizzo
Salt Lake City, Utah

Richard Robinson
Tucson, Arizona

Nancy Ross-Flanigan
Belleville, Michigan

Mark Damian Rossi, PhD, PT,
CSCS
Pembroke Pines, Florida

Kausalya Santhanam
Branford, Connecticut

Denise L. Schmutte, PhD
Shoreline, Washington

Joan M. Schonbeck
Marlborough, Massachusetts

Kathleen Scogna
Baltimore, Maryland

Cathy Hester Seckman, RDH
Calcutta, Ohio

Stephanie Dionne Sherk
Ann Arbor, Michigan

Judith Sims
Logan, Utah

Joyce S. Siok, RN
South Windsor, Connecticut

Jennifer E. Sisk, MA
Havertown, Pennsylvania

Patricia Skinner
Amman, Jordan

Genevieve Slomski
New Britain, Connecticut

Bryan Ronain Smith
Cincinnati, Ohio

Allison Joan Spiwak, BS, CCP
Gahanna, Ohio

Lorraine T. Steefel
Morganville, New Jersey

Margaret A. Stockley, RGN
Boxborough, Massachusetts

Dorothy Elinor Stonely
Los Gatos, California

Amy Loerch Strumolo
Bloomfield Hills, Michigan

Liz Swain
San Diego, California

Deanna M. Swartout-Corbeil,
RN
Thompsons Station, Tennessee

Mary Jane Tenerelli, MS
East Northport, New York

Bethany Thivierge
Peggy Campbell Torpey, MPT
Royal Oak, Michigan

Mai Tran, PharmD
Troy, Michigan

Carol A. Turkington
Lancaster, Pennsylvania

Judith Turner, DVM
Sandy, Utah

Samuel D. Uretsky, PharmD
Wantagh, New York

Marianne Vahey, MD
New Haven, Connecticut

James Waun, MD, RPh
East Lansing, Michigan

Michele R. Webb
Overland Park, Kansas

Ellen S. Weber, MSN
Fort Wayne, Indiana

Ken R. Wells
Laguna Hills, California

Barbara Wexler, MPH
Chatsworth, California

Gayle G. Wilkins, RN, BSN, OCN
Willow Park, Texas

Jennifer F. Wilson
Haddonfield, New Jersey

Abby Wojahn, RN, BSN, CCRN
Milwaukee, Wisconsin

Angela Woodward
Madison, Wisconsin

Jennifer Wurges
Rochester Hills, Michigan

Pacemakers

Definition

A pacemaker is an implantable electronic device that delivers electrical stimulation to the **heart** to help regulate its beat.

Purpose

Pacemakers are used to correct abnormal rhythms of the heart, most notably, brachycardia, an abnormally slow heartbeat. Normal heartbeat is 60 to 100 beats per minute (bpm) and brachycardia occurs what that hearbeat falls below 60 bpm. One cause of brachycardia is the failure of the natural pacemaker of the heart, the sinoatrial (SA) node, to function normally. Known as "sick sinus syndrome," this condition results in signals from the node that are too slow or too slow in accelerating to accommodate **exercise** or **stress**. Considered a part of the normal **aging** process, this syndrome results in a heartbeat that is too slow to circulate enough **blood** to meet the needs of the body. Symptoms include fatigue, activity intolerance, or even unconsciousness (also known as **syncope**). Pacemakers cure this condition by providing the needed electrical stimulus when the SA node does not work.

Pacemakers can also be used to treat a condition known as heart block. This problem occurs when the electrical connection between the upper chambers of the heart (atria) and lower chambers of the heart (ventricles) either fails or is significantly slowed. The area of the heart where this signal travels is called the atrio-ventricular (AV) node. The ventricles, without other stimulus, will produce their own beat of about 20 to 40 bpm, which is insufficient to support the body. Accordingly, patients with this problem feel tired and can lose consciousness. A pacemaker can treat this condition by keeping the heart rate within the normal range.

Patients that have brachycardia or heart block are at high risk for developing a tendency to have very fast, very inefficient contractions of the atria known as atrial **defibrillation**. A pacemaker that senses this abnormal rhythm and can switch to a mode of firing that brings it under control has been developed. Once the defibrillation has stopped, the pacemaker automatically switches back to its usual mode of function.

Description

The two main parts of a pacemaker are the pulse generator and the leads. The pulse generator is made of a computer chip, other electronic circuitry, and a lithium battery, all enclosed in a titanium case about the size of three to four stacked fifty-cent pieces. There can be one or two leads that carry the electrical impulse produced by the generator to the heart. The generator works by sensing whether the heart is firing at the right rate and supplying the electrical signal needed to start the heartbeat if it is not. The leads are flexible, double insulated wires that are placed within the heart chambers so that the needed signal is supplied to the area of the heart as needed. The leads can be unipolar, where the implanted tip is the negative pole (the positive is the pacemaker case) or bipolar where both the negative and positive poles are in the tip. Because the electrical signal has to travel across the chest with unipolar leads, pacemakers with leads of this type are more susceptible to outside interference.

If the pacemaker has one lead, it is known as a single chamber pacemaker. The lead can be placed in either the right atrium or the right ventricle. This type of device can be used only if the signal from the SA node or the AV node is the problem, and all other electrical conduction in the patient's heart is working correctly. Patients with this type of pacemaker can sometimes feel an uncomfortable neck throbbing, chest fullness, or faintness when the device fires, a condition known as pacemaker syndrome. Because of this problem, and the general ability to pump a greater volume of blood, some patients are treated with a dual chamber system.

The dual chamber pacemaker has two leads, one that is implanted in the right atrium, and one in the right ventricle. These pacemakers are also called sequentially pacing devices because the electrical signal is produced in a sequence—first to the atrium, then to the ventricle. The signal generators in dual chamber systems evaluate the heart's own electrical production in both chambers and produce their own signal when either or both become inadequate.

A third type of pacemaker is a rate-responsive system. These devices have the ability to sense physical activity and alter the heart rate to accommodate it. The responsiveness of this system results from one or more types of sensors. Some conditions that are sensed include motion, depth and rate of breathing, and blood temperature. As any of these conditions increase, the pacemaker speeds the rate of firing. Rate-responsive pacemakers most closely mimic the way the heart works naturally.

To help treat patients who have **atrial fibrillation**, pacemakers have been developed that can switch the way they work to treat the rapid abnormal heart beat, then return to the normal function.

Operation

Installing a pacemaker is a relatively minor surgical procedure that generally takes about an hour. It is often performed by an electrophysiologist, a specialized cardiologist, or surgeon. Under **local anesthesia**, a small incision is made under the collarbone, then the lead or leads are threaded through the subclavian vein into the heart's right side. Fluroscopy, a type of x ray that involves projecting an image on a fluorescent screen, is used to guide the process and requires the surgeon to wear a lead apron during the procedure. Often, right-handed patients have their pacemaker put in their left side and vice versa to speed return to normal activities.

Once the leads are in place, tests are performed to make sure the placement provides the needed connection for pacing. If the signals from the leads on the heart are too weak, the tip may have been placed in dead heart tissue and may need to be repositioned. The connection can be attached to the surface of the heart by a small corkscrew, known as active fixation, or a tined tip, known as passive fixation. With either passive or active fixation, a layer of fibrin (a blood protein) develops around the lead connection within six weeks of the installation.

Next, the pulse generator is embedded into a pocket under the skin of the chest and the leads are connected.

At this point the pulse generator has to be checked to make sure it is functioning correctly using a pacemaker system analyzer (PSA), a computer which checks the device is working correctly. If all checks out, the skin is sutured in place and a dressing placed over the wound.

Fine tuning of the pacemaker settings occur in the recovery room using a programmer, a special computer equipped with a wand that is placed on the patient's chest over the pacemaker. The programmer and the pacemaker communicate in a method similar to a television remote control. Two important variables in this programming are the pacemaker's capture and sensing. Capture refers to the voltage and pulse width of the electrical signal the device will deliver. The programming is set to ensure that the capture is set high enough that two to three times the threshold (minimum) voltage necessary is delivered, called the margin of safety. However, the capture should not be so high as to unnecessarily drain the battery and require earlier replacement of the device.

Sensing involves the ability of the pacemaker to detect signals coming from the patient's heart and to shut itself off until a predetermined interval passes without a signal. Pacemakers see the heart signals much like an implanted **electrocardiography unit**. Poor sensing is what causes the pacemaker syndrome often seen with single chamber pacemakers. For proper sensing, the leads need to be adjusted so that the intracardial signals are seen at the highest voltage possible. This allows the sensitivity of the pacemaker to be set at a lower level. If the sensitivity has to be turned up too much, chest muscle activity could interfere with the heart signal.

Most patients stay in the hospital for one to two days after implantation, but some can leave the same day.

Safety

Once the pacemaker is installed environmental conditions can affect the functioning of the unit. These include:

• strong electromagnetic fields, such as those used in arc-welding
• contact sports
• shooting a rifle from that shoulder
• cell phones used on that side of the body
• some medical tests such as magnetic resonance imaging (MRI)

Environmental conditions often erroneously thought to affect pacemakers include:

• microwave ovens (The waves affect only old, unshielded pacemakers.)
• airport security (Although metal detector alarms could be set off—patients should carry a card stating they have a pacemaker implanted.)

Maintenance

In general, if the condition of the patient's heart, drug intake, and metabolic condition remain the same, the pacemaker requires only periodic checking every two months or so for battery strength and function. This is done by placing a special device over the pacemaker that allows signals to be sent over the telephone to the doctor, a process called trans-telephonic monitoring.

If changes in medications or physical condition occur, the doctor can adjust the pacemaker settings using a programmer, which involves placing the wand above the pacemaker and remotely changing the internal settings.

Drugs taken by the patient and metabolic conditions affect both capture and sensing thresholds. For example,

drugs such as ephedrine or glucocosteroids cause lower thresholds, while some anti-arrhythmics cause higher thresholds. Hyperoxia (an excess of oxygen in the system) and hypocapnia (a deficiency of carbon dioxide) are two metabolic conditions that can lower thresholds and acidosis (an accumulation of acid in the body) or alkalosis (an accumulation of base in the body) can cause higher thresholds. Reprogramming of the pacemaker can accommodate the new capture and sensing values needed.

When the periodic testing indicates that the battery is getting low, an elective pacemaker replacement operation is scheduled. The entire signal generator is replaced because the batteries are sealed within the case. The leads can often be left in place and reattached to the new generator. Batteries usually last about six to eight years.

Health care team roles

Electrophysiologists are specially trained cardiologists who study and treat problems with the heart conduction system. They are often the type of physician that will implant the pacemaker system and oversee the programming or reprogramming of the device. They are assisted in the operating room by specially trained nurses, who can help with the testing of the pacemaker, and the anesthesiologist, who is responsible for numbing the area of the incision and keeping the patient comfortable. Pacemaker manufacturers often send representatives to be present for the implantation and initial programming.

The maintenance of the pacemaker can be overseen by the electrophysiologist or cardiologist and their staff, which can include specially trained cardiac medical assistants as well as nurses.

Training

The training for pacemakers and their use occurs during medical training (medical or nursing school) and on the job. Physicians, nurses, and other allied health professionals can also receive training in pacemakers as part of their continuing education courses. Such training often focuses on a particular aspect of pacemaker use, such as diagnosing problems in persons having pacemakers implanted, the installation of transient pacing, or the treatment of fibrillation or **heart failure** with pacemakers.

Resources

BOOKS

Barold, S. Serge, R. Stroobandt, and Alfons F. Sinnaeve. *Cardiac Pacemakers and Resynchronization Therapy Step-by-step: An Illustrated Guide*, 2nd ed. Chichester, West Sussex, UK: Wiley-Blackwell, 2010.

Hayes, David L., and Paul A. Friedman. *Cardiac Pacing, Defibrillation and Resynchronization: A Clinical Approach*. Chichester, West Sussex, UK; Hoboken, NJ: Wiley-Blackwell, 2008.

PERIODICALS

Epstein, Andrew E., et al. "ACC/AHA/HRS 2008 Guidelines for Device-Based Therapy of Cardiac Rhythm Abnormalities: A Report of the American College of Cardiology/American Heart Association Task Force on Practice Guidelines (Writing Committee to Revise the ACC/AHA/NASPE 2002 Guideline Update for Implantation of Cardiac Pacemakers and Antiarrhythmia Devices) Developed in Collaboration With the American Association for Thoracic Surgery and Society of Thoracic Surgeons." *Journal of the American College of Cardiology* 51 (2008): 1–62.

Scheibly, Kimberly. "Systematic Assessment of Basic Pacemaker Function." *AACN Advanced Critical Care* 21, 3 (2010): 322–328.

OTHER

Heart Pacemaker. Medline Plus. http://www.nlm.nih.gov/medlineplus/ency/article/007369.htm (accessed April 3, 2012).

Mayo Clinic Staff. *Pacemaker.* http://www.mayoclinic.com/health/pacemaker/MY00276 (accessed April 3, 2012).

ORGANIZATION

American Heart Association. 7272 Greenville Ave., Dallas, TX 75231. (800) 242-8721. Review.personal.info@heart.org. http://www.americanheart.org

Michelle L. Johnson, M.S., J.D.

Packed cell volume *see* **Hematocrit**

Packed red blood cell volume *see* **Hematocrit**

Paillae *see* **Dental anatomy**

Pain

Definition

Pain, medically termed "nociception," is a response to noxious stimuli that is conveyed to the **brain** by sensory **neurons**. The discomfort signals actual or impending injury to the body. However, pain is more than a sensation, or the physical awareness of pain; it also includes perception, the subjective interpretation of the discomfort. Perception gives information on the pain's location, intensity, and something about its nature. The various conscious and unconscious responses to both sensation and perception, including the emotional response, add further definition to the overall concept of pain.

Description

Pain arises from any number of situations. Injury is a major cause, but pain may also arise from an illness. It may accompany a psychological condition, such as depression, or may even occur in the absence of a recognizable trigger.

Acute pain

Acute pain often results from tissue damage, such as a skin burn or broken **bone**, but it may also be a warning of impending damage, such as **angina** or the pain associated with **appendicitis** or the body's attempt to pass a kidney stone. Acute pain is also associated with severe headaches (such as migraines) or muscle cramps. This latter pain usually goes away as the injury heals or the cause of the pain (stimulus) is removed.

To understand acute pain, it is necessary to understand the nerves that support it. Nerve cells, or neurons, perform many functions in the body. Although their general purpose—to provide an interface between the brain and the body—remains constant, their capabilities vary widely. Certain types of neurons are capable of transmitting a pain signal to the brain.

As a group, these pain-sensing neurons are called nociceptors, and virtually every surface and organ of the body is wired with them. The central part of these cells is located in the spine, and they send threadlike projections to every part of the body. Nociceptors are classified according to the stimulus that prompts them to transmit a pain signal. Thermoreceptive nociceptors are stimulated by temperatures that are potentially tissue damaging. Mechanoreceptive nociceptors respond to a pressure stimulus that may cause injury. Polymodal nociceptors are the most sensitive and can respond to temperature and pressure. Polymodal nociceptors also respond to chemicals released by the cells in the area from which the pain originates.

Nerve-cell endings, or receptors, are at the front end of pain sensation. A stimulus at this part of the nociceptor unleashes a cascade of neurotransmitters (chemicals that transmit information within the nervous system) in the spine. Each neurotransmitter has a purpose. For example, substance P relays the pain message to nerves leading to the **spinal cord** and brain. These neurotransmitters may also stimulate nerves leading back to the site of the injury. This response prompts cells in the injured area to release chemicals that not only trigger an **immune response**, but also influence the intensity and duration of the pain.

Chronic and other types of pain

Chronic pain refers to pain that persists after an injury is apparently healed, **cancer** pain, pain related to a persistent or degenerative disease, and long-term pain from an unidentifiable cause. It is estimated that one in three people in the United States will experience chronic pain at some point in their lives. Of these people, approximately 50 million are either partially or completely disabled by the pain and its cause.

Chronic pain may be caused by the body's response to acute pain. In the presence of continued stimulation of nociceptors, changes occur within the nervous system. Changes at the molecular level are dramatic and may include alterations in genetic transcription of neurotransmitters and receptors. These molecular or cellular changes may also occur in the absence of an identifiable cause; one of the frustrating aspects of chronic pain is that the stimulus may be unknown. For example, the stimulus cannot be identified in as many as 85% of individuals suffering lower-back pain.

Other types of pain include allodynia, hyperalgesia, and phantom-limb pain. These pain categories are neuropathic, indicating damage to the nervous system. Allodynia is a feeling of pain in response to a normally harmless stimulus. For example, some individuals who have suffered nerve damage as a result of viral **infection** (like **herpes zoster**) experience unbearable pain from just the light weight of their clothing. Hyperalgesia is

somewhat related to allodynia in that the response to a painful stimulus is extreme. In this case, a mild pain stimulus, such as a pin prick, causes a maximum pain response. Phantom-limb pain occurs after a limb has been amputated; although an individual is missing the limb, the nerve pathways may still perceive pain as originating from the absent extremity, on an intermittent basis.

Causes and symptoms

Pain is the most common symptom of injury and disease, and descriptions can range in intensity from a dull ache to sharp, knifelike or burning pain. Nociceptors have the ability to convey information to the brain that indicates the location, nature, and intensity of the pain. For example, stepping on a nail sends an information-packed message to the brain; the foot has experienced a puncture wound that hurts a lot, at which point (almost simultaneously) the message goes back to the foot and leg to move or change placement immediately, to get away from the stimulus (nail). This has been termed a "knee-jerk reaction."

Pain perception also varies depending on the location of the pain. The kinds of stimuli that cause a pain response on the skin include pricking, cutting, crushing, burning, scraping (skin layers removed), and freezing. These same stimuli would not generate much of a response in the intestine. Intestinal pain arises from stimuli such as swelling, inflammation, distension, and diminished **blood** supply (tissue hypoxia).

Diagnosis

The assessment of pain is subjective and is weighed in relation to other symptoms and individual experiences when trying to determine the source of the pain. An observable injury, such as a broken bone, may be a clear indicator of the type of pain a person is suffering. Determining the specific cause of internal pain is more difficult. Other symptoms, such as **fever** or nausea, help to refine and focus attention to more specific possibilities. In some cases, such as lower-back pain, a specific cause may not be identifiable without image assessment, such as by x ray or CT scan. Diagnosis of the disease or disorder causing a specific pain is further complicated by the fact that pain can be referred, manifesting farther along the pathway than the origin might suggest. For example, pain arising from fluid accumulating at the base of the lung may be referred, with the patient experiencing pain in the shoulder area. In addition, there is the pain (usually muscular) that results from "guarding" against the original pain source. For instance, a rotator-cuff shoulder injury causes acute pain, but it may be associated with muscular pain of the neck and upper back, the result of the body's attempt to either protect itself or get away from sharp pain.

Since pain is a subjective experience, it may be very difficult for the patient to communicate its exact quality and intensity to the nurse or doctor. There are no diagnostic tests that can determine the quality or intensity of an individual's pain. Therefore, a medical examination will include many questions about where the pain is located, its intensity, and its nature (type of pain). Questions are also directed to determining the things that increase or relieve the pain, how long the pain has lasted, and whether there are any variations in it. An individual may be asked to use a pain scale to describe the pain. One such scale assigns a number to the pain intensity; for example, 0 may indicate no pain, and 10 may indicate the worst pain the person has ever experienced. Scales are modified by using faces for infants and children to accommodate their level of comprehension.

Treatment

There are many drugs aimed at preventing or treating pain. Nonopioid **analgesics**, narcotic analgesics, anticonvulsant drugs, and tricyclic antidepressants work by blocking the production, release, or uptake of selected neurotransmitters. Drugs from different classifications may be combined to alleviate specific types of pain.

Nonopioid analgesics include common over-the-counter medications such as aspirin, acetaminophen (Tylenol), and ibuprofen (Advil). These are most often used for minor pain, but there are some prescription-strength medications in this classification. These drugs are called **nonsteroidal anti-inflammatory drugs** (NSAIDS) and relieve pain by reducing inflation.

Narcotic analgesics are available legally only with a prescription and are used for the relief of severe pain, such as postoperative pain from major surgery, or cancer pain. These drugs include codeine, morphine, meperidine, and methadone. Contrary to earlier beliefs, addiction to these medications is not common; people who genuinely need these drugs for pain control typically do not become addicted, because the drugs are usually given for only a short period of time, with the exception of cancer-pain relief.

Anticonvulsants as well as **antidepressant drugs** were initially developed to treat seizures and depression, respectively. However, it was discovered that these drugs also have pain-killing applications. Furthermore, in cases of chronic or extreme pain, it is not unusual for an individual to suffer some degree of depression; therefore, antidepressants may serve a dual role. Commonly prescribed anticonvulsants for pain include phenytoin,

carbamazepine, and clonazepam. Tricyclic antidepressants include doxepin, amitriptyline, and imipramine.

Intractable (unrelenting) pain may be treated by injections directly into or near the main nerve supply that is transmitting the pain signal. One class of medications used in this way is **corticosteroids**. These are powerful anti-inflammatory agents. Pain decreases when the inflammation subsides. In other cases, local anesthetics, such as lidocaine, are used to create a neuromuscular blockade. However, these blockades are for short-term relief only, lasting a few hours, but the result is a break in the pain-response cycle that may have been self-perpetuating. These root blocks may also be useful in determining the site of pain generation. As the underlying mechanisms of pain transmission and perception are uncovered, other pain medications are being developed.

Drugs are not always effective in controlling pain. Surgical methods are used as a last resort if analgesics and local anesthetics fail. The least-destructive surgical procedure involves implanting a device that emits low-level electrical signals. These signals disrupt the nerve and prevent it from transmitting the pain message. However, this method may not completely control pain and is not used frequently. Other surgical techniques involve destroying or severing the nerve (a procedure called a rhizotomy), but the use of this technique is limited by side effects, including residual numbness that may pose a risk for future injury.

Alternative treatment

Both physical and psychological aspects of pain can be dealt with through alternative treatment. Some of the most popular treatment options are **acupressure** and **acupuncture**, massage, **chiropractic** adjustments, and **relaxation** techniques such as **yoga**, hypnosis, and **meditation**. Herbal therapies are gaining increased recognition as viable options. For example, capsaicin, the component that makes cayenne peppers spicy, is used in ointments associated with arthritis; it serves as a counteractive or contradictory pain site—the mind focuses on it, rather than on the joint pain. Contrast **hydrotherapy** can also be very beneficial for pain relief.

Behavioral modification to incorporate a healthier diet and regular **exercise** may be of help. Aside from relieving **stress**, regular exercise has been shown to increase endorphins, pain alleviators that are naturally produced in the body.

Health care team roles

As members of the health care team, **advanced practice nurses** (A.P.N.s), registered nurses (R.N.s), and licensed practical nurses (L.P.N.s) are responsible for assessing the pain response that paints demonstrate, implementing proper pain-medication therapy, assessing the outcomes of pain therapy, documenting the patient's perception of pain severity using a pain scale, as well as describing other pain characteristics and teaching patients pain-management techniques.

Joint Commission on Accreditation of Healthcare Organizations standards

The Joint Commission on Accreditation of Health-care Organizations (JCAHO), which is the accreditating body for all health care facilities, is focusing on auditing health care organizations on their appropriate pain-assessment and pain-management techniques by way of published pain standards. Health care institutions are being held accountable for outcomes of **pain management** according to the standards, and A.P.N.s, R.N.s, and L.P.N.s must be aware of these standards in order to modify practices to meet the new regulations. The 2001 JCAHO standards are:

- to acknowledge that every patient has a right to pain evaluation and pain management
- to evaluate pain in every patient
- to do a thorough examination when the presence of pain has been identified
- to document the examination in a specific format that supports standard reexamination and review
- to establish a customary protocol for observation and management of pain
- to teach practitioners and guarantee health care team proficiency on pain-management standards
- to create guidelines that incorporate adequate dispensing of appropriate medication for pain control
- to create and implement educational materials for pain control to give to patients and families
- to address pain-control measures upon the patient's release from the facility
- to establish tools to evaluate the success of pain management

Assessing characteristics of pain

The health care team must be able to describe the characteristics of pain when identified by the patient. Subjective data should be collected. Information on the following eight variables is essential to get a clear picture of the patient's experience of pain:

- Describe the pain (sharp, dull, aching, stabbing).
- How often (constant or transient—comes and goes).

- Where (point to the exact location, does the pain radiate, or spread)?
- Intensity: Assign a number from 0 (no pain) to 10 (the worst pain you have ever had).
- How long: all the time, or episodes of seconds, minutes, hours?
- Does anything help to relieve the pain (a certain position, medication, ice, or warm compresses)?
- Does anything make it worse (a certain position, exercise)?
- Have you ever experienced this type of pain before?

Importance of pain reassessment

As the R.N. or L.P.N., assessing the outcomes of pain-management therapies is an important part of the health care role. Intravenous medications should provide relief within 10 minutes, intramuscular medications are active within 30 to 40 minutes, and oral medication takes effect within one hour or less. Pain reassessment takes these times into consideration. Reassessment in these

QUESTIONS TO ASK YOUR DOCTOR

- What do you believe is the source of my pain?
- What diagnostic tests are needed for a thorough assessment?
- What treatment options do you recommend for me?
- What kind of changes can I expect to see with the medications you have prescribed for me?
- What are the side effects associated with the medications you have prescribed for me?
- Should I see a specialist? If so, what kind of specialist should I contact?
- What tests or evaluation techniques will you perform to see if treatment has been beneficial for me?
- What changes in my health can I expect to see due to my condition?
- What physical or psychological limitations do you foresee?
- How can my quality of life be improved?
- What symptoms are important enough that I should seek immediate treatment?
- Can you recommend any support groups for me and my family?

time frames allows accurate outcomes evaluation for pain management.

Patient education

Teaching appropriate pain-medication administration as well as informing the patient of ancillary pain-management techniques are important in **patient education**. A person in pain should understand that various medications take time to be absorbed and start working. Also, teaching relaxation techniques, such as meditation, imagery, and aromatherapy, offers measures that complement pain-medication effectiveness and may even reduce the need for medication. Many patients are afraid to take some pain medications, for fear of becoming addicted. Explaining that the appropriate use of the medication, in the dose prescribed and in direct proportion to the level of pain, will avoid the potential for addiction. Health care team members are patient advocates, and they should not allow their patient to suffer.

Prognosis

Successful pain management is dependent on successful identification of the pain's cause. Acute pain will stop when an injury heals or when an underlying condition is treated successfully. Chronic pain is more difficult to treat, and it may take longer to achieve a successful outcome. Some pain is intractable and will require extreme measures for relief.

Prevention

Pain is generally preventable only to the degree that the cause of the pain is preventable; diseases and injuries may be unavoidable. Some injuries, or re-injury, can be avoided. For example, proper muscle use and positioning when lifting heavy objects will prevent back injury. Increased pain, pain from surgery and other medical procedures, and continuing pain may be preventable through appropriate treatments and therapies.

Resources

BOOKS

Gupta, Anita. *Interventional Pain Medicine.* New York, NY: Oxford University Press, 2012.

Pelletier, Kenneth R., MD. *The Best Alternative Medicine* Kindle Edition, Part II, "CAM Therapies for Specific Conditions: Depression." Lady Lake, FL: Fireside, 2010.

Porter, Robert S., ed. *The Merck Manual of Diagnosis and Therapy,* 19th ed. West Point, PA: Merck Sharp & Dohme Corp, 2011.

Zundert, Jan Van., ed., et al. *Evidence-based Interventional Pain Practice: According to Clinical Diagnoses.* Hoboken, NJ: Wiley-Blackwell, 2012.

PERIODICALS

Dahl, J., C. Pasero, and C. Patterson. "Institutionalizing Effective Pain Management Practices: The Implications of the New JCAHO Pain Assessment and Management Standards." Program and Abstracts of the 19th Annual Scientific Meeting of the American Pain Society, November 2-5, 2000, Atlanta, Georgia. Symposium Abstract 302.

McCaffery, Margo. "Overcoming Barriers to Pain Management." Nursing 31 (April 2001): 18.

ORGANIZATIONS

American Association of Neuroscience Nurses. 4700 W. Lake Avenue, Glenview, IL 60025. (888) 557-2266 or (847) 375-4733. http://www.aann.org/.

American Association of Nurse Anesthetists. 222 South Prospect Avenue, Park Ridge, Illinois 60068-4001. (847) 692-7050. http://www.aana.com/Pages/default.aspx.

American Chronic Pain Association (ACPA). P.O. Box 850, Rocklin, CA 95677. Phone: (916) 632-0922. Fax: (916) 632-3208. Tollfree: (800) 533-3231. Email: ACPA@ pacbell.net. http://www.theacpa.org/.

American Pain Society. 4700 West Lake Avenue, Glenview, IL 60025. (847) 375-4715. http://www.ampainsoc.org/.

The Joint Commission. One Renaissance Blvd. Oakbrook Terrace, IL 60181. (630) 792-5942. http://www.jointcommission.org.

Lori Beck
Laura Jean Cataldo, RN, Ed.D.

Pain disorder *see* **Somatoform disorders**

Pain management

Definition

If **pain** can be defined as a highly unpleasant, individualized experience of one of the body's defense mechanisms indicating an injury or problem, pain management encompasses all interventions used to understand and ease pain, and, if possible, to alleviate the cause of the pain.

Purpose

Pain serves to alert us to potential or actual damage to the body. The definition for damage is quite broad; pain can arise from injury as well as disease. After the message is received and interpreted, further pain can be counter-productive. Pain can have a negative impact on a person's quality of life and impede recovery from illness or injury, thus contributing to escalating health care costs. Unrelieved pain can become a syndrome in its own right and cause a downward spiral in a person's health and outlook. Managing pain properly facilitates recovery, prevents additional health complications, and improves an individual's quality of life.

Yet the experiencing of pain is a completely unique occurrence for each person, a complex combination of several factors other than the pain itself. It is influenced by:

• Ethnic and cultural values. In some cultures tolerating pain is related to showing strength and endurance. In others, it is considered punishment for misdeeds.

• Age. The concept that grownups don't cry.

• Anxiety and stress related to being in a strange, fearful place such as a hospital, fear of the unknown consequences of the pain and the condition causing it can all make pain feel more severe.

• Fatigue and depression. It is known that pain in itself can actually cause depression. Fatigue from lack of sleep or the illness itself also contribute to depressed feelings.

Precautions

As noted, the perception of pain is an individual experience. Health care providers play an important role in understanding their patients' pain. All too often, both physicians and nurses have been found to incorrectly assess the severity of pain. A study reported in the *Journal of Advanced Nursing* evaluated nurses' perceptions of a select group of American-born and Mexican-American women patients' pain following **gallbladder** surgery. Objective assessments of each patient's pain showed little difference between the severity for each group. Yet nurses involved in the study consistently rated all patients' pain as less than the patients reported, and with equal consistency, believed that better-educated women born in the United States were suffering more than less educated, Mexican-American women. Nurses from a Northern European background were more apt to minimize the severity of pain than nurses from Eastern and Southern Europe or Africa. Health care staff, and especially nursing staff, need to be aware of how their own background and experience contributes to how they perceive a person's pain.

Description

Before considering pain management, a review of pain definitions and mechanisms may be useful. Pain is the means by which the peripheral nervous system (PNS) warns the **central nervous system** (CNS) of injury or potential injury to the body. The CNS comprises the **brain** and **spinal cord**, and the PNS is composed of the nerves that stem from and lead into the CNS. PNS includes all nerves throughout the body except the brain and spinal cord. Pain is sometimes categorized by its site of origin, either cutaneous (originating in the skin of subcutaneous tissue, such as a shaving nick or paper cut), deep somatic pain (arising from **bone**, ligaments and tendons, nerves or veins and arteries), or visceral (appearing as a result of stimulation of pain receptor nerves around organs such as the brain, **lungs**, or those in the **abdomen**).

A pain message is transmitted to the CNS by special PNS nerve cells called nociceptors. Nociceptors are distributed throughout the body and respond to different stimuli depending on their location. For example, nociceptors that extend from the skin are stimulated by sensations such as pressure, temperature, and chemical changes.

When a nociceptor is stimulated, neurotransmitters are released within the cell. Neurotransmitters are

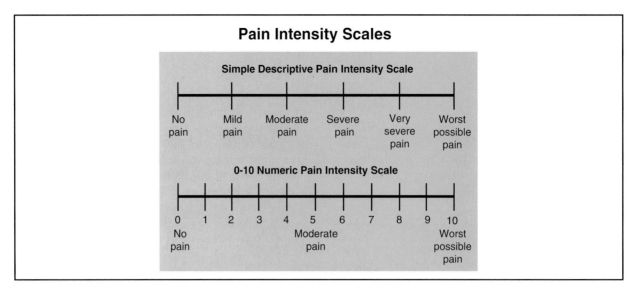

Pain Intensity Scales

Simple Descriptive Pain Intensity Scale

No pain | Mild pain | Moderate pain | Severe pain | Very severe pain | Worst possible pain

0-10 Numeric Pain Intensity Scale

0 No pain | 1 | 2 | 3 | 4 | 5 Moderate pain | 6 | 7 | 8 | 9 | 10 Worst possible pain

(Pain Intensity Scales from Acute Pain Management Guideline Panel. 1992. Acute Pain Management: Operative or Medical Procedures Trauma. Clinical practice guideline. AHCPR Publication No. 92-0033. Rockville, MD: Agency for Health Care Policy and Research.)

chemicals found within the nervous system that facilitate nerve cell communication. The nociceptor transmits its signal to nerve cells within the spinal cord, which conveys the pain message to the thalamus, a specific region in the brain.

Once the brain has received and processed the pain message and coordinated an appropriate response, pain has served its purpose. The body uses natural painkillers, called endorphins, to derail further pain messages from the same source. However, these natural painkillers may not adequately dampen a continuing pain message. Also, depending on how the brain has processed the pain information, certain hormones, such as prostaglandins, may be released. These hormones enhance the pain message and play a role in **immune system** responses to injury, such as inflammation. Certain neurotransmitters, especially substance P and calcitonin gene-related peptide, actively enhance the pain message at the injury site and within the spinal cord.

Pain is generally divided into two additional categories, acute and chronic. Nociceptive pain, or the pain that is transmitted by nociceptors, is typically called acute pain. This kind of pain is associated with injury, headaches, disease, and many other conditions. Response to acute pain is made by the sympathetic nervous system (the nerves responsible for the fight or flight response of the body). It normally resolves once the condition that precipitated it is resolved.

Following some disorders, pain does not resolve. Even after healing or a cure has been achieved, the brain continues to perceive pain. In this situation, the pain may be considered chronic. Chronic pain is within the province of the parasympathetic nervous system, and the changeover occurs as the body attempts to adapt to the pain. The time limit used to define chronic pain typically ranges from three to six months, although some health care professionals prefer a more flexible definition, and consider chronic pain as pain that endures beyond a normal healing time. The pain associated with **cancer**, persistent and degenerative conditions, and neuropathy, or nerve damage, is included in the chronic category. Also, unremitting pain that lacks an identifiable physical cause, such as the majority of cases of low **back pain**, may be considered chronic. The underlying **biochemistry** of chronic pain appears to be different from regular nociceptive pain.

It has been hypothesized that uninterrupted and unrelenting pain can induce changes in the spinal cord. In the past, severing a nerve's connection to the CNS has treated intractable pain. However, the lack of any sensory information being relayed by that nerve can cause pain transmission in the spinal cord to go into overdrive, as evidenced by the **phantom limb** pain experienced by amputees. Evidence is accumulating that unrelenting pain or the complete lack of nerve signals increases the number of pain receptors in the spinal cord. Nerve cells in the spinal cord may also begin secreting pain-amplifying neurotransmitters independent of actual pain signals from the body. Immune chemicals, primarily cytokines, may play a prominent role in such changes.

Managing pain

Considering the different causes and types of pain, as well as its nature and intensity, management can require an interdisciplinary approach. The elements of this approach include treating the underlying cause of pain, pharmacological and nonpharmacological therapies, and some invasive (surgical) procedures.

Treating the cause of pain underpins the idea of managing it. Injuries are repaired, diseases are diagnosed, and certain encounters with pain can be anticipated and treated prophylactically (by prevention). However, there are no guarantees of immediate relief from pain. Recovery can be impeded by pain and quality of life can be damaged. Therefore, pharmacological and other therapies have developed over time to address these aspects of disease and injury.

PHARMACOLOGICAL OPTIONS. General guidelines developed by the World Health Organization (WHO) have been developed for pain management. These guidelines operate upon a three-step ladder approach:

- Mild pain is alleviated with acetaminophen or a non-steroidal anti-inflammatory drug (NSAID). NSAIDs and acetaminophen are available as over-the-counter and prescription medications, and are frequently the initial pharmacological treatment for pain. These drugs can also be used as adjuncts to the other drug therapies that might require a doctor's prescription. NSAIDs include aspirin, ibuprofen (Motrin, Advil, Nuprin), naproxen sodium (Aleve), and ketoprofen (Orudis KT). These drugs are used to treat pain from inflammation and work by blocking production of pain-enhancing neurotransmitters, such as prostaglandins. Acetaminophen is also effective against pain, but its ability to reduce inflammation is limited. NSAIDs and acetaminophen are effective for most forms of acute (sharp, but of a short course) pain.

- Mild to moderate pain is eased with a milder opioid medication plus acetaminophen or NSAIDs. Opioids are both actual opiate drugs such as morphine and codeine, and synthetic drugs based on the structure of opium. This drug class includes drugs such as oxycodon, methadone, and meperidine (Demerol). They provide pain relief by binding to specific opioid receptors in the brain and spinal cord.

- Moderate to severe pain is treated with stronger opioid drugs plus acetaminophen or NSAIDs. Morphine is sometimes referred to as the gold standard of palliative care as it is not expensive, can be given starting with smaller doses and gradually increased, and is highly effective over a long period of time. It can also be given by a number of different routes, including by mouth, rectally, or by injection.

Although **antidepressant drugs** were developed to treat depression, it has been discovered that they are also effective in combating chronic headaches, cancer pain, and pain associated with nerve damage. Antidepressants that have been shown to have analgesic (pain-reducing) properties include amitriptyline (Elavil), trazodone (Desyrel), and imipramine (Tofranil). Anticonvulsant drugs share a similar background with antidepressants. Developed to treat epilepsy, anticonvulsants were found to relieve pain as well. Drugs such as phenytoin (Dilantin) and carbamazepine (Tegretol) are prescribed to treat the pain associated with nerve damage.

Close monitoring of the effects of pain medications is required in order to assure that adequate amounts of medication are given to produce the desired pain relief. When a person is comfortable with a certain dosage of medication, oncologists typically convert to a long-acting version of that medication. Transdermal fentanyl patches (Duragesic) are a common example of a long-acting opioid drug often used for cancer pain management. A patch containing the drug is applied to the skin and continues to deliver the drug to the person for typically three days. Pumps are also available that provide an opioid medication upon demand when the person is experiencing pain. By pressing a button, they can release a set dose of medication into an intravenous solution or an implanted catheter. Another mode of administration involves implanted catheters that deliver pain medication directly to the spinal cord. Delivering drugs in this way can reduce side effects and increase the effectiveness of the drug. Research is underway to develop toxic substances that act selectively on nerve cells that carry pain messages to the brain, killing these selected cells and thus stopping transmission of the pain message.

In 2004, two popular pain medications were taken off the market.Drug maker Merck stopped production of Vioxx (rofecoxib), its arthritis and acute pain medication. The withdrawal was based on three-year data from a prospective, randomized, placebo-controlled clinical trial, the APPROVe (Adenomatous Polyp Prevention on VIOXX) trial. The trial, which was halted, was designed to evaluate the efficacy of Vioxx 25 mg in preventing recurrence of colorectal polyps in patients with a history of colorectal adenomas. In this study, there was an increased relative risk for confirmed cardiovascular events, such as **heart** attack and **stroke**, beginning after 18 months of treatment in the patients taking Vioxx compared to those taking placebo. In 2005, the U.S. Food and Drug Administration (FDA) requested that Pfizer suspend sales of Bextra in the United States. The FDA concluded that there is an increased risk of rare but serious skin reactions associated with Bextra, prescribed to treat arthritis and chronic pain. The FDA is requiring all manufacturers of prescription non-steroidal anti-inflammatory arthritis medicines (NSAIDs), such as Pfizer's Celebrex (celecoxib), to provide additional information about cardiovascular and gastrointestinal risks. The FDA also asked all the manufacturers of over-the-counter NSAIDs to revise their labels to include more information on cardiovascular, gastrointestinal and skin risks.

NONPHARMACOLOGICAL OPTIONS. Pain treatment options that do not use drugs are often used as adjuncts to, rather than replacements for, drug therapy. One of the benefits of non-drug therapies is that an individual can take a more active stance against pain. **Relaxation** techniques, such as **yoga** and **meditation**, are used to focus the brain elsewhere than on the pain, decrease muscle tension and reduce **stress**. Tension and stress can also be reduced through biofeedback, in which an individual consciously attempts to modify skin temperature, muscle tension, **blood pressure**, and heart rate.

Participating in normal activities and exercising can also help control pain levels. Through **physical therapy**, an individual learns beneficial exercises for reducing stress, strengthening muscles, and staying fit. Regular **exercise** has been linked to production of endorphins, the body's natural pain killers.

Acupuncture involves the insertion of small needles into the skin at key points. **Acupressure** uses these same key points, but involves applying pressure rather than inserting needles. Both of these methods may work by prompting the body to release endorphins. Applying heat or being massaged are very relaxing and help reduce stress. Transcutaneous electrical nerve stimulation (TENS) applies a small electric current to certain parts of nerves, potentially interrupting pain signals and inducing release of endorphins. To be effective, use of TENS should be medically supervised.

INVASIVE PROCEDURES. There are three types of invasive procedures that may be used to manage or treat pain: anatomic, augmentative, and ablative. These procedures involve surgery, and certain guidelines should be followed before carrying out a procedure with permanent effects. First, the cause of the pain must be clearly identified. Next, surgery should be done only if noninvasive procedures are ineffective. Third, any psychological issues should be addressed. Finally, there should be a reasonable expectation of success.

Anatomic procedures involve correcting the injury or removing the cause of pain. Relatively common anatomic procedures are decompression surgeries, such as repairing a **herniated disk** in the lower back or relieving the nerve compression related to **carpal tunnel syndrome**. Another anatomic procedure is neurolysis, also called a nerve block, which involves destroying a portion of a peripheral nerve.

Augmentative procedures include electrical stimulation or direct application of drugs to the nerves that are transmitting the pain signals. Electrical stimulation works on the same principle as TENS. In this procedure, instead of applying the current across the skin, electrodes are implanted to stimulate peripheral nerves or nerves in the spinal cord. Augmentative procedures also include implanted drug-delivery systems. In these systems, catheters are implanted in the spine to allow direct delivery of drugs to the CNS.

Ablative procedures are characterized by severing a nerve and disconnecting it from the CNS. However, this method may not address potential alterations within the spinal cord. These changes perpetuate pain messages and do not cease even when the connection between the sensory nerve and the CNS is severed. With growing understanding of neuropathic pain and development of less invasive procedures, ablative procedures are used less frequently. However, they do have applications in select cases of **peripheral neuropathy**, cancer pain, and other disorders.

Preparation

Prior to beginning management, pain is thoroughly evaluated. Pain scales or questionnaires are used to attach an objective measure to a subjective experience. Objective measurements allow health care workers a better understanding of the pain being suffered by the patient. Evaluation also includes physical examinations and diagnostic tests to determine underlying causes. Some evaluations require assessments from several viewpoints, including **neurology**, psychiatry and psychology, and physical therapy. If pain is due to a medical procedure, management consists of anticipating the type and intensity of associated pain and managing it preemptively.

Nurses or physicians often take what is called a pain history. This will help to provide important information that can help health care providers to better manage the patient's pain. A typical pain history includes the following questions:

• Where is the pain located?

• On a scale of 1 to 10, with 1 meaning the least pain, how would the person rate the pain they are experiencing?

• Describe what the pain feels like.

• When did (or does) the pain start?

• How long has the person had it?

• Is the person sometimes free of pain?

• Does the person know of anything that triggers the pain, or makes it worse?

- Does the person have other symptoms (nausea, dizziness, blurred vision, etc.) during or after the pain?
- What pain medications or other measures have the person found to help in easing the pain?
- How does the pain affect the person's ability to carry on normal activities?
- What does it mean to the person that they are experiencing pain?

Aftercare

An assessment by nursing staff as well as other health care providers should be made to determine the effectiveness of the pain management interventions employed. There are objective, measurable signs and symptoms of pain that can be looked for. The goal of good pain management is the absence of these signs:

Signs of acute pain:

- rise in pulse and blood pressure
- more rapid breathing
- perspiring profusely, clammy skin
- taut muscles
- more tense appearance, fast speech, very alert
- unusually pale skin
- pupils of the eye are dilated

Signs of chronic pain:

- lower pulse and blood pressure
- changeable breathing pattern
- skin is warm and dry
- nausea and vomiting
- slow speech in monotone
- inability, or difficulty in getting out of bed and doing activities
- pupils of the eye are constricted

When these signs are absent and the patient appears to be comfortable, health care providers can consider their interventions to have been successful. It is also important to document interventions used, and what ones were successful.

Complications

Owing to toxicity over the long term, some drugs can only be used for acute pain or as adjuncts in chronic pain management. NSAIDs have the well-known side effect of causing gastrointestinal bleeding, and long-term use of acetaminophen has been linked to kidney and **liver** damage. Other drugs, especially narcotics, have serious side effects, such as constipation, drowsiness, and nausea. Serious side effects can also accompany

KEY TERMS

Acute—Referring to pain in response to injury or other stimulus that resolves when the injury heals or the stimulus is removed.

Chronic—Referring to pain that endures beyond the term of an injury or painful stimulus. Can also refer to cancer pain, pain from a chronic or degenerative disease, and pain from an unidentified cause.

CNS or central nervous system—The part of the nervous system that includes the brain and the spinal cord.

Iatrogenic—Resulting from the activity of the physician.

Neuropathy—Nerve damage.

Neurotransmitter—Chemicals within the nervous system that transmit information from or between nerve cells.

Nociceptor—A nerve cell that is capable of sensing pain and transmitting a pain signal.

Nonpharmacological—Referring to therapy that does not involve drugs.

Parasympathetic nervous system—That part of the autonomic nervous system consisting of nerves that arise from the cranial and sacral regions and function in opposition to the sympathetic nervous system.

Pharmacological—Referring to therapy that relies on drugs.

PNS or peripheral nervous system—Nerves that are outside of the brain and spinal cord.

Stimulus—A factor capable of eliciting a response in a nerve.

Sympathetic nervous system—That portion of the autonomic nervous system consisting of nerves that originate in the thoracic and lumbar spinal cord and function in opposition to the parasympathetic nervous system.

pharmacological therapies; mood swings, confusion, bone thinning, cataract formation, increased **blood** pressure, and other problems may discourage or prevent use of some **analgesics**.

Nonpharmacological therapies carry little or no risks. However, it is advised that individuals recovering from serious illness or injury consult with their health care providers or physical therapists before making use of adjunct therapies. Invasive procedures carry risks similar to other surgical procedures, such as **infection**, reaction to anesthesia, iatrogenic (injury as a result of treatment) injury, and failure.

A traditional concern about narcotics use has been the risk of promoting addiction. As narcotic use continues over time, the body becomes accustomed to the drug and adjusts normal functions to accommodate to its presence. Therefore, to elicit the same level of action, it is necessary to increase dosage over time. As dosage increases, an individual may become physically dependent on narcotic drugs.

However, physical dependence is different from psychological addiction. Physical dependence is characterized by discomfort if drug administration suddenly stops, while psychological addiction is characterized by an overpowering craving for the drug for reasons other than pain relief. Psychological addiction is a very real and necessary concern in some instances, but it should not interfere with a genuine need for narcotic pain relief. However, caution must be taken with people with a history of addictive behavior.

Results

Effective application of pain management techniques reduces or eliminates acute or chronic pain. This treatment can improve an individual's quality of life and aid in recovery from injury and disease.

Health care team roles

Physicians, both primary care physicians (PCPs) and surgeons, treat both the conditions causing the pain, and the pain itself. The physician's role as teacher is an important one, alleviating fears about both the patient's condition and the possibility of addiction to narcotics, which is often a fear among patients on narcotic medication. Some physicians specialize in the treatment of pain, and work out of pain clinics.

Registered nurses (RNs) are the professional staff member that will likely spend the most time with the patient, whether the patient is in the hospital or other health care facility, or at home. Gathering the necessary information regarding the person's pain through a pain history, and careful observation and listening can help tremendously in the provision of pain relief. RNs also administer the medications at times, and provide information to the patient about the various medications that may be used, and allay concerns about the use of them.

Licensed practical nurses (LPNs) also spend considerable time with the patient in a health care facility or at home. Like RNs, LPNs administer medications as necessary, and provide information to patients.

Pain clinic staff may be any of the above, or psychologists, social workers, occupational or recreational therapists, or other people with specific training in group therapy, yoga, meditation, or other non-pharmacological means of relieving pain.

Pharmacists fill prescriptions for pain-relieving medications, monitor the use of narcotic medications, and provide information regarding the uses and side-effects of the medications.

QUESTIONS TO ASK YOUR DOCTOR

- What do you believe is the source of my pain?
- What diagnostic tests are needed for a thorough assessment?
- What treatment options do you recommend for me?
- What kind of changes can I expect to see with the medications you have prescribed for me?
- What are the side effects associated with the medications you have prescribed for me?
- Should I see a specialist? If so, what kind of specialist should I contact?
- What tests or evaluation techniques will you perform to see if treatment has been beneficial for me?
- What changes in my health can I expect to see due to my condition?
- What physical or psychological limitations do you foresee?
- How can my quality of life be improved?
- What symptoms are important enough that I should seek immediate treatment?
- Can you recommend any support groups for me and my family?

Resources

BOOKS

Gupta, Anita. *Interventional Pain Medicine.* New York, NY: Oxford University Press, 2012.

Pelletier, Kenneth R., MD. *The Best Alternative Medicine* Kindle Edition, Part II, "CAM Therapies for Specific Conditions: Depression." Lady Lake, FL: Fireside, 2010.

Porter, Robert S., ed. *The Merck Manual of Diagnosis and Therapy*, 19th ed. West Point, PA: Merck Sharp & Dohme Corp, 2011.

Zundert, Jan Van., ed., et al. *Evidence-based Interventional Pain Practice: According to Clinical Diagnoses.* Hoboken, NJ: Wiley-Blackwell, 2012.

PERIODICALS

Armstrong, F. Daniel. "Analgesia for Children with Acute Abdominal Pain: A Cautious Move to Improved Pain Management." Pediatrics (October 2005): 1018-1019.

Bates, Betsy. "Need for Chronic Pain Management is Unmet." Family Practice News (Oct. 15, 2005): 65.

Dieppe, Paul A., and L. Stefan Lohmander. "Pathogenesis and Management of pain in Osteoarthritis."The Lancet (March 12, 2005): 965.

Jancin, Bruce. "Implications of Expected Big Drop in NSAID Use: Cardiovascular Side Effects Likely to Cause Physicians to Seek Other Options for Chronic pain Management."Family Practice News (July 15, 2005): 5.

ORGANIZATIONS

American Association of Neuroscience Nurses. 4700 W. Lake Avenue, Glenview, IL 60025. (888) 557-2266 or (847) 375-4733. http://www.aann.org/.

American Association of Nurse Anesthetists. 222 South Prospect Avenue, Park Ridge, Illinois 60068-4001. (847) 692-7050. http://www.aana.com/Pages/default.aspx.

American Chronic Pain Association (ACPA). P.O. Box 850, Rocklin, CA 95677. Phone: (916) 632-0922. Fax: (916) 632-3208. Tollfree: (800) 533-3231. Email: ACPA@pac-bell.net. http://www.theacpa.org/.

American Pain Society. 4700 West Lake Avenue, Glenview, IL 60025. (847) 375-4715. http://www.ampainsoc.org/.

The Joint Commission. One Renaissance Blvd. Oakbrook Terrace, IL 60181. (630) 792-5942. http://www.jointcommission.org.

Ken R. Wells
Laura Jean Cataldo, RN, Ed.D.

Pain relievers *see* **Analgesics**

Pancreas

Definition

The pancreas is an organ important in digestion and **blood** sugar regulation. It is considered to be part of the gastrointestinal system. The pancreas produces digestive enzymes to be released into the **small intestine** to aid in reducing food particles to basic elements that can be absorbed by the intestine and used by the body. It has another very different function in that it forms insulin, glucagon, and other hormones to be sent into the bloodstream to regulate blood sugar levels and other activities throughout the body.

Description

The pancreas is a pear-shaped organ about 6 in (15 cm) long and located in the middle and back portion of the **abdomen**. It is connected to the first part of the small intestine, the duodenum, and lies behind the **stomach**. The pancreas is made up of glandular tissue, or cells that form substances to be secreted outside of the organ. Glandular tissues can be categorized as endocrine (secreting directly into the bloodstream or lymph) or exocrine (secreting into another organ). The pancreas is both an exocrine and an endocrine organ.

Function

Exocrine secretions

The digestive juices produced by the pancreas are secreted into the duodenum via a Y-shaped duct, at the point where the common bile duct from the **liver** and the pancreatic duct join just before entering the duodenum. In this way, a variety of digestive enzymes (trypsin, chymotrypsin, lipase, and amylase, among others) are delivered into the small intestine to aid in the digestion of **proteins**, fats, and **carbohydrates**. The enzymes are delivered in an inactive form called zymogens. The zymogens are activated by the chemical substances in the small intestine. The digestive enzymes carried into the duodenum are representative of the exocrine function of the pancreas, in which specific substances are made to be passed directly into another organ.

Endocrine secretions

The pancreas is unusual among the body's glands in that it also has a very important endocrine function. Small groups of special cells called islet cells throughout the organ make such hormones as insulin and glucagon, which are critical in regulating blood sugar levels; and vasoactive intestinal peptide, which influences gastrointestinal activity. These hormones are secreted directly into the bloodstream to affect organs all over the body. No organ except the pancreas makes significant amounts of insulin or glucagon, but other tissues do produce vasoactive intestinal peptide. Insulin acts to lower blood sugar levels by allowing the sugar to flow into cells. Glucagon acts to raise blood sugar levels by causing glucose to be released into the circulation from its storage sites. Insulin and glucagon act in an opposite but balanced fashion to keep blood sugar levels stable.

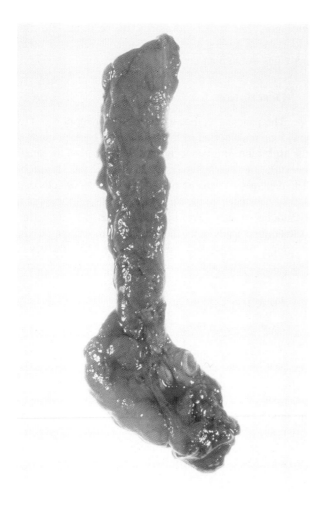

(Pancreas (posterior view), photograph © 1996 Josepj R. Siebert, Ph. Custom Medical Stock Photo, Inc. Reproduced by permission.)

Role in human health

A normal pancreas is important for maintaining good health, preventing malnutrition, and maintaining normal levels of blood sugar. The digestive tract needs the help of the enzymes produced by the pancreas to reduce food particles to their simplest elements, or the nutrients cannot be absorbed. Carbohydrates must be broken down into individual sugar molecules. Proteins must be reduced to simple amino acids. Fats must be broken down into fatty acids. The pancreatic enzymes are important in all these transformations. The basic particles can then easily be transported into the cells that line the intestine, and from there they can be further altered and transported to different tissues in the body as fuel sources and construction materials.

Similarly, the body cannot maintain normal blood sugar levels without the balanced action of insulin and glucagon. Both **hypoglycemia** (low blood sugar) and

hyperglycemia (high blood sugar) cause symptoms and serious health problems.

Common diseases and disorders

Diabetes

Glucose is a simple sugar molecule, but one that is necessary to every type of cell as a major source of energy. Insulin made in the pancreas has a critical role in permitting glucose to enter cells. Without insulin, the cells of the body literally "starve in the midst of plenty," and are unable to make use of sugar in the blood even if blood sugar levels are very high. This condition is called **diabetes mellitus**. Diabetes actually represents a collection of disorders resulting in high blood sugars related to abnormal insulin levels, or abnormalities of the receptor that binds the insulin to allow glucose to enter the cell. Diabetes is quite common in the United States, affecting 1–2% of the general population.

Type 1 diabetes, which is sometimes called insulin-dependent diabetes, is a disease in which a patient must use insulin regularly to avoid serious problems with cells starving for glucose and acidic waste products accumulating in the blood. In this form of diabetes, the pancreas is essentially not producing insulin. Pancreas transplantation is a method of treating type 1 diabetes that has achieved success rates of 80–85% in the past decade, success being defined as the organ recipient's remaining insulin-independent. In type 2 diabetes, or non-insulin-dependent diabetes, blood sugar levels can often be controlled with diet, **exercise**, and medications taken by mouth. In some forms of type 2 diabetes the pancreas is not producing enough insulin; in other cases the receptor that binds insulin is no longer sensitive to it, or too few receptors are made by the cells that need glucose. Sometimes a combination of these problems is present. **Gestational diabetes** mellitus (GDM) is a third type of diabetes, which is a temporary problem with blood sugar levels that exists only during **pregnancy**. Women with GDM, however, need to know they are at increased risk for developing type 2 diabetes.

Pancreatitis

Pancreatitis is a relatively common condition that affects the pancreas. It can occur as an acute (sudden onset) problem or chronic (slow, ongoing) disorder. The common element in both types is inflammation caused by the normal digestive enzymes of the pancreas. In pancreatitis, these secretions act abnormally and start to digest the pancreas itself. Between 50,000 and 80,000

KEY TERMS

Amino acids—The category of molecules used to build proteins.

Diabetes mellitus—A chronic form of diabetes in which insulin does not effectively transport glucose from the bloodstream.

Duodenum—The portion of the small intestine that lies between the stomach and the jejunum. The pancreas empties some of its secretions into the duodenum via a Y-shaped duct.

Endocrine—A type of gland that secretes hormones directly into the blood or lymph.

Enzymes—Complex protein molecules that speed up chemical reactions, or make reactions happen under conditions where they normally would not occur.

Exocrine—A type of gland that secretes its products to an epithelial surface.

Glucagon—A hormone secreted by the pancreas that opposes insulin in the regulation of blood sugar levels.

Insulin—A hormone produced in the islet cells of the pancreas that regulates the metabolism of glucose and other nutrients.

Islet cells—Endocrine cells in the pancreas that are specialized to secrete glucagon or insulin.

Jaundice—A condition in which the skin and whites of the eyes are yellow because of bile products retained in the bloodstream.

Pancreatitis—Inflammation of the pancreas.

Zymogens—Enzyme precursor molecules that may change into enzymes as a result of catalytic change.

people in the United States develop acute pancreatitis every year, usually related to gallstones or alcohol abuse. Most patients recover within a week, but the most severe forms of pancreatitis have a mortality rate of 10%. Chronic pancreatitis is slow and insidious in onset, and so harder to diagnose. Alcohol use is the most common cause of deterioration in pancreatic function over time. Without adequate levels of enzymes and hormones produced by the pancreas, such diseases as diabetes mellitus and malabsorption syndromes will develop. A **malabsorption syndrome** is a condition in which the body is not able to absorb the nutrients it needs from the food it attempts to digest. Vitamin deficiencies, protein malnutrition and problems with frequent, greasy stools may occur.

Complications of pancreatitis include pancreatic necrosis (the death of a significant portion of the cells in the pancreas, putting the patient at risk of bleeding, **infection, shock** and failure of many major organs); pancreatic **abscess** (an infection with a wall of scar tissue around it); and pancreatic pseudocyst (a pocket full of fluid and pancreatic enzymes that may shrink, expand, or rupture). Patients with chronic pancreatitis are also at increased risk of developing **cancer** of the pancreas.

Cancer of the pancreas

Pancreatic cancer is a major cause of death from cancer around the world. Tumors of the pancreas may arise from either endocrine or exocrine cells. Some rare types of pancreatic tumors hypersecrete either glucagon (glucagonomas) or insulin (insulinomas). Cancer of the pancreas is difficult to diagnose in its early stages; about 90% of patients present with **pain, diarrhea**, blood clots, weight loss, or **jaundice** when the cancer has already spread outside the pancreas. As of 2001, about 25,000 people die every year with this disease, and there are few medical interventions to help these patients. Under certain circumstances, **chemotherapy** or surgery to remove part of the pancreas may be attempted. Only 2–5% of patients are alive five years after being diagnosed.

Resources

BOOKS

Gastrointestinal Disorders. in *The Merck Manual of Diagnosis and Therapy*, edited by Mark H. Beers, MD, and Robert Berkow, MD. Whitehouse Station, NJ: Merck Research Laboratories, 2005.

Izenberg, Neil, et al. *Human Disease and Conditions.* New York: Charles Scribner's Sons, 2000.

Tierney, Laurence M., Stephen J. McPhee, and Maxine A. Papadakis. *Current Medical Diagnosis and Treatment 2001.* New York:McGraw-Hill, 2001.

WEBSITE

Pancreas Foundation. http://www.pancreasfoundation.org.

ORGANIZATIONS

American Diabetes Association. 1660 Duke Street, Alexandria, VA 22314. (800) 232-3472.

National Digestive Diseases Information Clearinghouse. 2 Information Way, Bethesda, MD 20892. (301) 654-3810 or (800) 891-5389.

Erika J. Norris

Pancreatitis

Definition

Pancreatitis is an inflammation of the **pancreas**, an organ that is important in digestion. In pancreatitis, normal digestive enzymes act abnormally to break down the pancreas itself.

Description

The pancreas is a complex organ with many critical functions for normal digestion and regulation of **blood** sugar. When inflamed, as in pancreatitis, several potent enzymes are inappropriately activated within the organ itself. In acute pancreatitis, inflammation is sudden and causes symptoms. In almost 90% of acute cases, the symptoms disappear within one week after treatment, and the pancreas returns to its normal function. With chronic pancreatitis, damage to the pancreas occurs over longer periods of time. Symptoms may be persistent or sporadic, as the pancreas is slowly but permanently impaired. More than 90% of pancreatic tissue will be destroyed before serious symptoms begin. Late signs of chronic pancreatitis include **diabetes mellitus** and malabsorption syndromes in which nutrients are poorly absorbed from the digestive tract.

Causes and symptoms

There are a number of causes of acute pancreatitis, the most common of which are gallstones and **alcoholism**. These two diseases are responsible for more than 80% of all hospitalizations for acute pancreatitis. Gallstones may obstruct normal drainage from the pancreas into the **small intestine**, resulting in a backup of normal pancreatic secretions and inflammation of the pancreas until the obstruction is relieved.

The mechanism by which alcohol inflames the pancreas is not well understood. It is thought that alcohol causes **proteins** to collect in the pancreas and results in obstruction and calcification of the organ.

Other factors in the development of acute pancreatitis include:

- certain drugs, including estrogens, sulfonamides, and diuretics
- interferon and ribavirin therapy for chronic hepatitis C infection
- infections
- structural problems of the pancreatic duct and common bile duct
- injury to the abdomen

- abnormally high levels of circulating fats in the bloodstream
- high blood levels of calcium
- complications from kidney failure or transplant
- a hereditary tendency toward pancreatitis
- various forms of vasculitis (inflamed blood vessels)

In pancreatitis, enzymes become prematurely activated so that they actually begin their digestive functions within the pancreas. The pancreas, in essence, begins digesting itself. Digestion of the **blood vessels** in the pancreas results in bleeding. Other active pancreatic chemicals cause blood vessels to become leaky, and fluid begins seeping into the abdominal cavity. The activated enzymes also gain access to the bloodstream through leaky, eroded blood vessels, and begin circulating throughout the body.

Pain is a major symptom in acute pancreatitis, and it is usually quite intense and steady, located in the upper **abdomen**, and radiating to the patient's back. Nausea, **vomiting**, and abdominal swelling are also common symptoms. A patient will often have a slight **fever**, with an increased **heart** rate and low **blood pressure**.

Patients with acute pancreatitis are at risk of complications related to **shock**, a serious syndrome that occurs when the blood pressure is too low to get adequate circulation to critical organs. Without adequate blood pressure, organs are deprived of oxygen, nutrients, and waste removal and may not function well. Kidney, respiratory, and **heart failure** are serious possible outcomes of shock.

Even if shock does not occur, circulating pancreatic enzymes and related toxins can cause damage to the heart, **lungs**, **kidneys**, lining of the gastrointestinal tract, **liver**, eyes, bones, and skin. As the pancreatic enzymes affect blood vessels, the risk of blood clots increases. When blood flow is blocked by clotting, the supply of oxygen is further decreased to various organs and additional damage done.

Other serious complications of acute pancreatitis include pancreatic necrosis, abcess, and pseudocyst formation. Pancreatic necrosis occurs when a significant portion of the pancreas is permanently damaged during an acute attack. Pancreatic necrosis has an increased risk of death and an increased chance of pancreatic **infection**. A pancreatic **abscess** is a local collection of pus that may develop several weeks after the illness subsides. Another late complication of pancreatitis, occurring several weeks after the illness begins, is called a pancreatic pseudocyst, which occurs when dead pancreatic tissue, blood, white blood cells, enzymes, and fluid leaked from the circulatory system accumulate. Pseudocysts cause recurrent abdominal pain and also press on other nearby structures in the gastrointestinal tract, causing disruption of function. Pseudocysts are life threatening when they become infected (abscess) and rupture. Simple rupture of a pseudocyst causes death 14% of the time, but rupture complicated by bleeding causes death 60% of the time.

In severe cases of pancreatitis, called necrotizing pancreatitis, the pancreatic tissue begins to die, and bleeding increases. Due to the bleeding into the abdomen, two distinctive signs may be noted in patients with necrotizing pancreatitis. Turner's sign is a reddish-purple or greenish-brown color to the area between the ribs and the hip (flank). Cullen's sign is a bluish color around the navel.

Alcohol abuse is the cause of tissue damage in 80% of cases of chronic pancreatitis. Tissue damage occurs more slowly, and many digestive functions become disturbed. The quantity of hormones and enzymes normally produced by the pancreas begins to decrease, resulting in the inability to appropriately digest food. Fat digestion, in particular, is impaired. A patient's stools become greasy as fats are passed out of the body. The inability to digest and use proteins results in smaller muscles (wasting) and weakness. The inability to digest and use the nutrients in food leads to malnutrition, vitamin deficiencies, and a generally weakened condition. As the disease progresses, permanent injury to the pancreas can lead to diabetes.

Diagnosis

Diagnosis of pancreatitis, whether acute or chronic, is not simple. History and physical exam are very important, as well as imaging studies and laboratory tests. Levels of amylase and lipase that are three times above the upper limit of normal are predictive of acute pancreatitis. Other abnormalities in the blood may also point to pancreatitis, including increased white blood cells, changes due to dehydration from fluid loss, and abnormalities in the blood concentration of calcium, magnesium, sodium, potassium, bicarbonate, and glucose.

X rays or ultrasound examination of the abdomen may reveal gallstones, possibly responsible for blocking the pancreatic duct. The gastrointestinal tract will show signs of inactivity (ileus) due to the presence of pancreatitis. Chest x rays may reveal abnormalities due to shallow breathing or due to lung complications from the circulating pancreatic enzyme irritants. Computed tomography (CT) scans of the abdomen may reveal the inflammation and fluid accumulation of pancreatitis.

In the case of chronic pancreatitis, lipase and amylase levels will no longer be elevated. However, blood tests will reveal the loss of pancreatic function that occurs over time. Blood sugar (glucose) levels will rise, eventually reaching the levels consistent with diabetes. The levels of various pancreatic enzymes will fall, as the organ is increasingly destroyed and replaced by non-functioning scar tissue. Calcification of the pancreas can also be seen on x rays. Endoscopic retrograde cholangiopancreatography (ERCP) may be used to diagnose chronic pancreatitis in unclear cases. In this procedure, the physician uses a medical instrument fitted with a fiber-optic camera to inspect the pancreas.

Recent developments in understanding of genetics and the role of genetics in susceptibility to pancreatitis may soon lead to use of genetic testing for early diagnosis and prognosis of pancreatitis. The testing can detect abnormalities in trypsin and trypsin inhibitor genes and cystic fibrosis genes.

Treatment

Treatment of acute pancreatitis involves replacing lost fluids intravenously (in a vein). These intravenous (IV) solutions need to contain appropriate amounts of salts, sugars, and sometimes even proteins, in order to correct the patient's disturbances in blood chemistry. Pain is treated with a variety of medications, chiefly meperidine. To decrease pancreatic function, the patient is not allowed to eat. A thin, flexible tube (nasogastric tube) may be inserted through the patient's nose and down into the stomach. The nasogastric tube can empty the stomach of fluid and air that may accumulate due to the inactivity of the gastrointestinal tract.

The patient will need careful monitoring to identify complications that may develop. Infections will require antibiotics through the IV. Severe necrotizing pancreatitis may require surgery to remove part of the dying pancreas, especially if infection has begun. A pancreatic abscess can be drained by a needle inserted through the abdomen and into the collection of pus (percutaneous needle aspiration). An abscess may also require surgical removal. In 25–40% of cases, pancreatic pseudocysts may shrink on their own or continue to expand, requiring needle aspiration or surgery. Surgery may be necessary for the removal of gallstones.

Because chronic pancreatitis often includes repeated flares of acute pancreatitis, the same kinds of basic treatment are necessary. Treatment of chronic pancreatitis caused by alcohol consumption requires that the patient stop drinking alcohol entirely. A low-protein and low-fat diet is prescribed. As chronic pancreatitis continues and insulin levels drop, a patient may require insulin injections to be able to process sugars in the diet. Pancreatic enzymes can be replaced with oral

KEY TERMS

Abscess—A pocket of infection; pus.

Acute—Of short and sharp course; illnesses that appear quickly and can be serious or life-threatening.

Chronic—Of long duration and slow progression; illnesses that develop slowly over time, and do not end.

Diabetes—A disease characterized by an inability to regulate blood sugar levels in the blood.

Endocrine—A system of organs that produces chemicals that go into the bloodstream to affect the function of other organs from a distance.

Enzyme—A chemical that speeds up or makes a particular chemical reaction more efficient.

Exocrine—A system of organs that produces chemicals that go through a duct (or tube) to affect the functioning of other organs.

Gland—A collection of tissue that produces chemicals needed for use outside of the gland itself.

Hormone—A chemical produced in one part of the body that travels to another part of the body in order to exert an effect.

---

medications. As the pancreas is progressively destroyed, some patients stop feeling the abdominal pain that was initially so severe. Others continue to have constant abdominal pain, and may require a surgical procedure for relief.

Prognosis

When necrosis and bleeding are present, as many as 50% of patients with pancreatitis may die. Overall, the mortality rate for patients with mild acute pancreatitis is less than 1%. Those with sever pancreatitis have a mortality rate as high as 25%.

Ranson's criteria can help determine the severity of the disease. The first five categories are evaluated when the patient is admitted to the hospital, including:

• age over 55 years

• blood sugar level over 200 mg/dl

• serum lactic dehydrogenase over 350 IU/L

• AST over 250 μ (a measure of liver function, as well as a gauge of damage to the heart, muscle, brain, and kidney)

• white blood count over 16,000 μL

The following six of Ranson's criteria are reviewed 48 hours after the patient's admission to the hospital, including:

• greater than 10% decrease in hematocrit (a measure of red blood cell volume)

• increase in BUN (blood urea nitrogen, an indicator of kidney function) greater than 5 mg/dL

• blood calcium less than 8 mg/dL

• PaO_2 (a measure of oxygen in the blood) less than 60 mm Hg

• base deficit greater than 4 mEg/L (a measure of change in the normal acidity of the blood)

• fluid sequestration greater than 6 L, or 13 pt (an estimation of the quantity of fluid that has leaked out of the blood circulation and into other body spaces)

Once it is determined how many of Ranson's signs are present in the patient, the physician can better predict the risk of death. A patient with less than three positive Ranson's signs has less than a 5% chance of dying. A patient with three to four positive Ranson's signs has a 15-20% chance of death.

The results of a CT scan can also be used to predict the severity of pancreatitis. Slight swelling of the pancreas indicates mild illness. Significant swelling, especially with evidence of destruction of the pancreas and/or fluid build-up in the abdominal cavity, indicates more severe illness and a worse prognosis.

Health care team roles

The physician will make a full **physical examination** of the patient to determine which tests are necessary. Radiologic technologists will perform imaging studies and clinical laboratory technicians will perform the laboratory tests. Nurses have an active supportive role throughout the patient's illness.

Prevention

Alcoholism is essentially the only preventable cause of pancreatitis. Patients with chronic pancreatitis must stop drinking alcohol entirely. The drugs that may cause pancreatitis should also be avoided when possible.

Resources

BOOKS

Izenberg, Neil, ed. *Human Disease and Conditions.* Charles Scribner's Sons, 2000: 643-644.

Toskes, Phillip P., and Norton J. Greenberger. "Disorders of the Pancreas." In *Harrison's Principles of Internal Medicine,* edited by E. Braunwald, et al. McGraw-Hill, 2001: 1788-1803.

PERIODICALS

Bates, Betty. "Pancreatitis Difficult Etiology Becoming Easier to Pinpoint." *Family Practice News* (March 15, 2005): 72.

Ciombination Therapy for Chronic Hepatitis C May Cause Pancreatitis. *Science Letter* (September 21, 2004): 23.

Genetic Testing May Play Key Role in Management of Pancreatitis. *Genomics & Genetics Weekly* (Deecember 24, 2004): 179.

Managing Acute and Chronic Pancreatitis. *The Practitioner* (October 12, 2005): 672.

Munos, Abilio, and David A. Katerndahl. "Diagnosis and Management of Acute Pancreatitis." *American Family Physician* 62 (July 2000): 164-73.

OTHER

National Institute of Diabetes and Digestive and Kidney Diseases. http://www.niddk.nih.gov/health/digest/pubs/pancreas/pancreas.htm.

The National Pancreas Foundation. http://www.pancreasfoundation.org/diseases.html.

ORGANIZATION

National Digestive Diseases Information Clearinghouse. 2 Information Way, Bethesda, MD 20892-3570.

Erika J. Norris
Teresa G. Odle

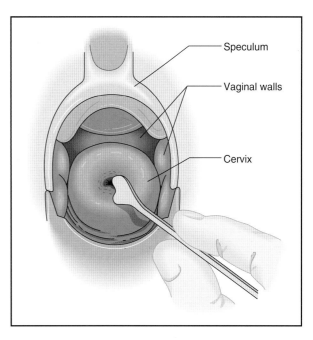

(From Delmar's Medical Terminology Image Library 1st edition by DELMAR. © 1999. Reprinted with permission of Delmar Learning, a division of Thomson Learning:www.thomsonrights.com. Fax 800-730-2215.)

Pap test

Definition

The Pap test (Pap smear) is the microscopic examination of cells scraped from the both the outer cervix (ectocervix) and the cervical canal (endocervix). It is called the "Pap" test after its developer, Dr. George N. Papanicolaou, who described a procedure for staining vaginal and cervical cells that gives clearly defined detail to the nuclear chromatin. Using the Papanicolaou stain, he developed a classification system for abnormal cervical cells. Before the application of the Pap test in the 1940s, cervical **cancer** caused approximately 26,000 deaths in the United States each year. The death rate from cervical cancer since the use of the Pap test has become widely accepted has been reduced by 70%.

Purpose

The Pap test is a screening test used to detect abnormal growth of cervical cells at an early stage, so that if necessary, treatment can be started before the cells become cancerous and invasive. The test helps physicians identify women who are at increased risk of cervical dysplasia (abnormal cells) or cervical cancer. Only an examination of the cervix, and samples of cervical tissue (biopsies) can diagnose precancerous and cancerous changes in the cells that line the uterus, called squamous epithelium.

This microscopic analysis of cells can detect cervical cancer, precancerous changes, inflammation (called vaginitis), infections, and some sexually transmitted diseases (STDs). The Pap test can sometimes detect endometrial (uterine) cancer or ovarian cancer, although it was not designed for this purpose.

Women should begin to have Pap tests at the age of 18 years or whenever they start having sex. Young people are more likely to have multiple sex partners, which increases their risk of certain diseases that can cause cancer, such as human papillomavirus (**HPV**). The American Cancer Society recommends that a Pap test be done annually for two consecutive negative examinations, then repeated once every three years until age 65 for women without symptoms of gynecologic problems. Many other doctors, however, recommend annual Pap tests for all their patients.

Women with certain risk factors should always have yearly tests. Those at highest risk for cervical cancer are women who started having sex before age 18; those with many sex partners (especially if they did not use condoms, which protect against STDs); those who have had STDs such as **genital herpes** or genital warts; and

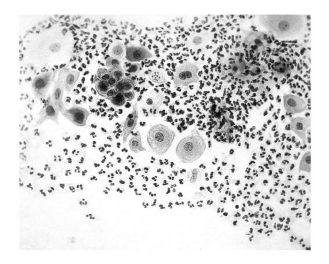

(Stained micrograph of a PAP smear showing normal stellate cells, photograph. AFIP / Science Source.)

those who smoke. Women older than 40 also should have the test yearly, especially in the event of bleeding after **menopause**. Women over age 60 account for 25% of new cases of cervical cancer and 40% of deaths from this disease. Women who have had a hysterectomy (removal of the uterus) may need to have Pap tests, if the surgery was for cancer, or if the cervix was left in place. Pregnant women should have a Pap test as part of their first prenatal examination.

Women who have a positive test result should be retested more frequently. If atypical squamous cells or low-grade lesions are found they should be tested every four to six months until they have three consecutive normal results. The test should be repeated within two to three months if severe inflammation, **infection**, or postmenoposal atrophy is found. If atypical cells or low-grade lesions persist, or high-grade lesions are found, **colposcopy** (examination of the cervix with a magnifying lens) should be performed, and treatment initiated as indicated.

Precautions

The Pap smear is a microscopic evaluation of individual cells, a process that requires interpretation. Differentiation of inflammatory, reactive, and atrophied cells from atypical cells is difficult and cannot always be performed with complete certainty. The test is not 100% sensitive and between 5-10% of cervical abnormalities may be missed. Most false negatives result from poor sample collection (insufficient cervical cells) or poor smear preparation. The finding of abnormal cells on a Pap smear does not mean that the cells were present on previous exams.

The Pap test should be performed in the middle of the menstrual cycle to prevent interference from **blood**. Sexual intercourse, douching, or the use of vaginal suppositories may affect results. Other factors that can affect test results include: water or lubricant on the specimen from the speculum; blood, mucus, or pus on the slide that obstructs the view of epithelial cells; cell damage during collection; and improper slide fixation. An acceptable smear is one that is correctly labeled with the patient's name, age, and last menstrual period; contains squamous cells covering at least 10% of the slide; and demonstrates the presence of cells from the endocervix and transformation zone. The transformation zone is the area where the squamous epithelium of the ectocervix meets the glandular epithelium of the endocervix.

Description

The Pap test is an extremely cost-effective and beneficial test able to detect about 95% of cervical cancer. According to a report published May 16, 2000 in the *Annals of Internal Medicine,* the widespread use of this diagnostic procedure decreased the number of cervical cancers in the United Sates from 14.2 per 100,000 in 1973, to 7.8 per 100,000 in 1994. However, the disease still ranks as the ninth-leading cause of cancer deaths in U.S. women.

During the pelvic examination, an instrument called a speculum is inserted into the vagina to open it. A spatula, (Ayre spatula) that is flat at one end and curved at the other so that its contour complements the ectocervix is used to collect the sample. The spatula is firmly rotated using a circular motion to scrape the cells off the ectocervix. The flat end can be used to pick up cells which have exfoliated from the rear of the vagina. This procedure, called vaginal pool sampling, is recommended for women in menopause and if signs of inflammation are seen. A tiny brush, pointed spatula, or cotton-tipped swab is used to collect cells from the endocervix. These samples can be mixed and spread evenly on a single glass slide, or a slide or slide section can be used for each. The slide should be dipped in 95% alcohol or sprayed with fixative immediately. Though some women find the procedure uncomfortable, it is usually painless and only takes five to 10 minutes.

A new technique called the Thin Prep is being used by some physicians because it is purported to reduce the false negative rate caused by inadequate smear preparation. For the Thin Prep, the sample is placed in a vial containing a preservative solution. The vial is labeled and sent to the laboratory where a processing instrument disrupts the blood cells and mucus and spreads the decontaminated sample in a thin layer over the slide.

Unlike the classical procedure, cells are not left on the collection device. This results in a greater yield of epithelial cells to examine. The staining detail is easier to evaluate because the epithelial cells are not obscured by blood cells or mucus.

Smears are stained with the Papanicolaou stain when they reach the lab. The Pap stain begins with rehydrating the cells in water. The cells are stained with Gill hematoxylin, then dehydrated with 95% ethanol. They are stained with OG-6 followed by EA-65, then fully dehydrated with absolute ethanol. In the last step, they are cleared with xylol, and a coverglass is applied. The entire smear is examined under a **microscope**. In addition to detecting and classifying abnormalities within the squamous epithelium and glandular epithelium, the smears are also examined for the presence of inflammatory cells (polymorphonuclear white cells, lymphocytes, histiocytes), normal vaginal flora (Lactobacilli), coccobacilli (indicative of vaginal infection), trichomonads (vaginal **parasites**), yeast, and cytopathic effects of **viruses** in the epithelial cells.

Squamous epithelial cells from the cervix are evaluated for abnormal intracellular changes that indicate a risk of cancerous transformation. Two systems of classification are widely employed, the CIN (Richart) and Bethesda systems. Both describe a progression of cells from normal to low risk, then to high risk, then to malignant cells. The CIN system uses the term, cervical intraepithelial neoplasia (CIN) to describe premalignant cells. CIN-I is characterized by mild cellular abnormalities (mild dysplasia), CIN-II moderate dysplasia, and CIN-III severe dysplasia. CIN-III includes the presence of immature cells with cancerous features that have not yet invaded the surrounding connective tissue. This is called carcinoma *in situ*. When such cells are found beyond the transformation zone (within the underlying stroma), the lesion is classified as invasive cancer (squamous carcinoma). The CIN classification system classifies cells that are most likely benign (called squamous atypica) and low-risk precancerous cells in the category of CIN-I. In 1989, the Bethesda system was introduced in order to more clearly define the difference between mild dysplasia that is likely to be benign and that which is precancerous. The former comprise a group called ASCUS which stands for atypical squamous cells of undetermined significance. This distinguishes cells that are often reactive from those of the next group, low-grade intraepithelial neoplasia (LSIL) that show precancerous changes, but are at a low risk of transforming into cancerous cells. ASCUS is reserved for cells that cannot be conclusively called benign. Classification of a smear as ASCUS is based upon judgement and depends upon the quality of the smear and the numbers and appearance of atypical cells present. A pap test in which ASCUS is found should be repeated in three to four months, and if ASCUS is detected the second time, the patient should be evaluated by colposcopy and biopsy. Between 19% and 57% of these patients will be reclassified as SIL on the basis of biopsy. The LSIL category is the counterpart of the CIN-I category. The final category of the Bethesda system is high-grade intraepithelial neoplasia (HSIL) which comprises both CIN-II and CIN-III groups including carcinoma *in situ*. Beyond HSIL, the lesion is classified as an invasive squamous cell carcinoma.

In general, cervical cells are classified as ASCUS if the nuclear enlargement is no greater than three-fold the size of the nucleus of a normal intermediate squamous cell, or there is mild hyperchromasia (increased chromatin staining). LSIL cells are superficial or intermediate squamous cells that display a nucleus that is at least three-fold larger than the normal intermediate squamous cell. There is moderate variation in the size and shape of the nucleus. Nuclear hyperchromasia is present either as uniformly granular or smudged chromatin staining. In addition, cells that are associated with infection by HPV have a cytoplasm with hollowed-out cavities. About 80% of cervical cancers are associated with HPV infection. Therefore, these cells, called koilocytes, are classified as LSIL provided that some nuclear abnormality or binucleation is present. HSIL cells are immature squamous cells (smaller cells) with a three-fold or greater nuclear enlargement, an increased nuclear to cytoplasm ratio, severe hyperchromasia with irregular chromatin and nuclear membrane contour. They are usually seen in streaming rows or groups of attached cells.

Preparation

While most women are not routinely advised to make any special preparations for a Pap test, some simple preparations may help to ensure that the results are reliable. Among the measures that may help increase test reliability are:

• Abstain from sexual intercourse 24 hours prior to the test.

• Do not douch 18-72 hours before the test.

• Avoid vaginal creams or medications one week before the test.

If possible, women may want to ensure that their test is performed by an experienced gynecologist and sent to a certified laboratory. Certification requires successful participation in a proficiency testing program approved by the U.S. Department of Health and Human Services. In such a program every cytotechnologist reading pap smears is tested at least once per year and is required to meet specific performance criteria.

Before the exam, the physician will take a complete sexual history to determine a woman's risk status for cervical cancer. Questions may include date and results of the last Pap test, any history of abnormal Pap tests, date of last menstrual period and any irregularity, use of hormones and birth control, family history of gynecologic disorders, and any vaginal symptoms. These topics are relevant to the interpretation of the Pap test, especially if any abnormalities are detected. Immediately before the Pap test, the woman should empty her bladder to avoid discomfort during the procedure.

Aftercare

Harmless cervical bleeding is possible immediately after the test; women may need to use a sanitary napkin. They should also be sure to comply with their doctor's orders for follow-up visits.

Complications

No appreciable health risks are associated with the Pap test. However, abnormal results (whether valid or due to technical error) can cause significant **anxiety**. Women may wish to have their sample retested, either by the same laboratory or via computer-assisted screening. Two re-screening programs approved by the Food and Drug Administration are called Papnet and AutoPap QC.

Results

Normal (negative) results from the laboratory exam mean that no atypical cells were detected, and the cervix is normal. It is important to remember that an abnormal (positive) result does not necessarily indicate cancer. Fully 60-70% of abnormal results resolve by themselves, and only 1% of mild abnormalities ever develop into cancer. Between 19% and 57% of patients with ASCUS will be reclassified as having SIL (mostly LSIL) following biopsy. Approximately 57% of LSIL lesions regress on their own (i.e., return to normal); 32% remain LSIL on retesting, 11% progress to HSIL, and 1% may progress to invasive carcinoma. Approximately 43% of HSIL (CIN-II) lesions regress, 35% remain HSIL on retesting, and 22% progress to CIN-III. Approximately 5% of HSIL (CIN-II) lesions progress to invasive cancer. Approximately 32% of HSIL (CIN-III) lesions regress, up to 55% persist on repeat exam, and more than 12% progress to invasive carcinoma.

Treatment

CHANGES OF UNKNOWN CAUSE (ASCUS OR SQUAMOUS ATYPICA). The most common abnormality (found in 50-60% of abnormal tests) is ASCUS. If squamous atypica is thought to be inflammatory or reactive, this will be noted on the report as well as any evidence of infection (e.g., coccobacilli, yeast, white blood cells) seen on the microscopic exam. These women may be treated for infection and then undergo repeat Pap testing in two to three months. If ASCUS is present without signs of inflammation, re-testing is performed every four to six months for two years or until three consecutive tests are negative. If the lesion persists, or ASCUS is seen twice within a two-year period, colposcopy is recommended.

DYSPLASIA. Typically, dysplasia causes no symptoms, although women may experience abnormal vaginal bleeding. Because dysplasia can be precancerous, it should be treated if it is moderate or severe. Treatment of dysplasia depends on the degree of abnormality. In women with no other risk factors for cervical cancer, mild dysplasia may be simply observed over time with repeat testing, every four to six months as described above. If the lesion persists, colposcopy with biopsy and scraping of the endocervix are often recommended.

The second most common finding (about 30-40% of abnormal tests) is LSIL, which includes mild dysplasia or CIN I and changes caused by HPV. Unlike cancer cells, these cells do not invade normal tissues. Women are most susceptible to mild dysplasia at ages 25-35 years. HSIL (found in 5-10% of abnormal Pap tests) includes moderate to severe dysplasia or carcinoma *in situ* (CIN II or III). The frequency of HSIL is highest at ages 30-40. In women with HSIL lesions, colposcopy, biopsy, and treatment (excision or destruction of the lesion) are performed. In addition to surgical resection (removal), several outpatient techniques are available: conization (removal of a cone-shaped piece of tissue), **laser surgery**, cryotherapy (freezing), electrosurgical cauterization, and radiation. Cure rates are nearly 100% after prompt and appropriate treatment of carcinoma *in situ*. Of course, frequent checkups are then necessary.

In addition to abnormal squamous epithelium, abnormal glandular cells from the endocervix may be found. Atypical glandular cells of undetermined significance (AGUS) is used to designate cells that cannot be classified with certainty as benign, precancerous, or cancerous. AGUS should be investigated further to determine the risk of endometrial carcinoma. Malignant glandular cells may also be found on the Pap smear and may result from cervical or vaginal adenocarcinoma. This cancer is uncommon in women under 40, and most common in women over 50 who have postmenopausal bleeding. Malignant glandular cells are more often recovered from vaginal pool sampling or aspiration than from cervical scraping, and therefore, vaginal cell smears should be made along with cervical smears for women in

KEY TERMS

Carcinoma *in situ*—Precancerous cells that are present only in the ectocervix(i.e., do not extend beyond the basement membrane). The abnormal cells do not extend beyond the transformation zone.

Cervical intraepithelial neoplasia (CIN)—A term used to categorize degrees of dysplasia arising in the cervical epithelium (outer cervix).

Cervix—The opening between the vagina and the uterus, or womb.

Cytology—The study of cells, their origin, structure, function and pathology.

Dysplasia—Abnormal changes in cells.

Human papilloma virus (HPV)—The leading STD in the United States. Various types of HPV are known to cause cancer.

Neoplasia—Abnormal growth of cells, which may lead to a neoplasm, or tumor.

Squamous intraepithelial lesion (SIL)—A term used to categorize the severity of abnormal changes arising in the squamous cells of the cerrvix.

menopause. Hysterectomy is recommended for confirmed cases of endometrial adenocarcinoma.

CANCER. Human papilloma virus (HPV), the most common STD in the United States, may be responsible for many cervical cancers. Cancer may be manifested by unusual vaginal bleeding or discharge, bowel and bladder problems, and **pain**. The peak ages for cervical cancer are between 45 and 55 years. Biopsy is indicated when any abnormal growth is found on the cervix, even if the Pap test is negative.

Invasive cervical cancer is usually treated with surgery or radiation, or both. Most cases of invasive cervical cancer are treated with radical hysterectomy. **Chemotherapy** may be used if the cancer has spread to lymph nodes or other organs. Survival rates at five years after treatment of early invasive cancer are about 90%; rates are below 60% for more severe invasive cancer. That is why prevention, risk reduction, and frequent Pap tests are the best defense for a woman's gynecologic health.

Health care team roles

The slides are prepared by a gynecologist. Cytotechnologists, laboratory professionals who specialize in the study of cells, read the Pap smears looking for abnormal cells. Abnormal findings may be reviewed by the laboratory's pathologist.

Resources

BOOKS

Berek, Jonathan S., Eli Y. Adashi, and Paula A. Hillard. *Novak's Gynecology.* 12th ed. Baltimore: Williams & Wilkins, 1996.

Chernecky, Cynthia C, and Barbara J. Berger. *Laboratory Tests and Diagnostic Procedures.* 3rd ed. Philadelphia, PA: W. B. Saunders Company, 2001.

Illustrated Guide to Diagnostic Tests. 2nd ed. Springhouse, PA: Springhouse Corporation, 1998.

Kee, Joyce LeFever. *Handbook of Laboratory and Diagnostic Tests.* 4th ed. Upper Saddle River, NJ: Prentice Hall, 2001.

Slupik, Ramona I., ed. *American Medical Association Complete Guide to Women's Health.* New York: Random House, 1996.

ORGANIZATIONS

American College of Obstetricians and Gynecologists. 409 12th St. SW, PO Box 96920, Washington, DC 20090-6920. (202) 638-5577. http://www.acog.com.

National Cancer Institute, National Institutes of Health, U.S. Department of Health and Human Services. 9000 Rockville Pike, Bethesda, MD 20892. (301) 496-0265. http://cancernet.nci.nih.gov/.

Victoria E. DeMoranville

Papanicolaou test *see* **Pap test**

Paracentesis

Definition

Paracentesis is a procedure in which excess fluid in the **abdomen** is sampled by aspiration through a needle. The fluid may be called ascites fluid, abdominal fluid, or peritoneal fluid.

Purpose

Paracentesis is commonly performed to identify the cause of newly diagnosed ascites (excess fluid in the abdominal cavity); to diagnose changes in the condition of a patient already known to have ascites; and to relieve pressure from severe distention due to increased fluid in the abdomen. A sample of the fluid withdrawn from the abdominal cavity is nearly always sent for laboratory analysis to determine the presence or absence of **infection**, and/or to learn more about the cause of ascites if necessary. Ascites forms for a variety of reasons, including infection, diseases of various organs, and conditions that result in abnormal **blood** flow. The most common cause in the United States is alcoholic **cirrhosis**.

Precautions

Ascites is difficult to diagnose by physical exam, although with experience health care practitioners can note "shifting dullness" by percussion. Generally at least 500 mL (17 oz) of fluid must accumulate before the effusion is detected by x ray, and 1500 mL (3.2 pt) before ascites is easily detected on physical exam. Ultrasound may be necessary to differentiate ascites from **obesity** and other reasons for abdominal distention. Ultrasound may even be used to guide the needle for paracentesis. When performing this procedure, the physician should observe **universal precautions** for the prevention of transmission of bloodborne pathogens.

Description

Consent should be obtained for the procedure after discussion of the possible complications. The area beneath the umbilicus is cleansed with betadine or other antibacterial solution, and local anesthetic administered. A long thin needle or trochar with a stylet is inserted about 2 in (5 cm) below the umbilicus, and the appropriate amount of fluid withdrawn. Usually a syringe is used, but for large amounts of ascites, polyethylene tubing may be attached to vacuum bottles and the excess fluid aspirated. A minimum of 30 mL (1 oz) of fluid should be collected by sterile technique in two or three sterile syringes. One portion should be transferred to a tube containing EDTA for cell counts and the last syringe should be used to inoculate **blood culture** media. These samples and the remaining fluid should be sent to the laboratory for analysis. If cytologic exam is requested, 100 mL (3.4 oz) of fluid should be submitted to the laboratory.

Cirrhosis of the **liver** and malignant abdominal masses are the two most common causes of ascites. Cirrhosis is usually associated with a transudative fluid, a fluid of low cellularity and protein, while malignancy causes an exudative (inflammatory) fluid of high cellularity and protein. Transudative fluids result from changes in blood flow, and are typically seen in persons with cirrhosis, congestive **heart failure**, and a few other conditions that disrupt normal hemodynamics. An explanation of ascites formation in cirrhosis serves well to explain some principles common to transudative fluid formation. Blood entering the portal vein from the intestines passes through the liver on its way back to the **heart**. When progressive disease such as alcohol damage

or hepatitis destroys enough liver tissue, the scarring that results compresses the hepatic sinusoids and vessels and restricts the blood flow. The blood bypasses the liver and enters the splenic, gastric, and esophageal veins, causing very high hydrostatic pressure. This pressure causes fluid to escape the vessels and enter the abdominal cavity. Slowly the fluid accumulates in the areas with the lowest pressure and the greatest capacity. The free space around abdominal organs receives most of it. This space is called the peritoneal space because it is enclosed by a thin membrane called the peritoneum. The peritoneum wraps around nearly every organ in the abdomen, and lines the entire abdominal cavity, providing many folds and spaces in which fluid can gather. Normally, only 30-50 mL (1–1.7 oz) of fluid is found in the peritoneal cavity. The fluid itself is essentially an ultrafiltrate of plasma. Any condition that causes an increase in peritoneal fluid is called an effusion or ascites. Kidney disease can contribute to this process, since the **kidneys** have a critical role in **fluid balance**. Nephrotic syndrome in particular is associated with ascites formation. In this condition the kidneys lose large amounts of protein into the urine causing a drop in plasma oncotic pressure. Since **proteins** hold fluid in the vascular bed, loss of protein (albumin) causes fluid to enter the tissue spaces. Heart failure also can cause ascites, because decreased cardiac output causes blood to accumulate in the return circulation. The increased venous pressure results in fluid leaking from the circulatory system. First **edema** is noticed in the legs, due to the effect of gravity, then in ascites formation in the abdomen.

Malignancy, infection, **pancreatitis**, bowel obstruction, and several other conditions produce an exudative effusion. These conditions cause inflammation that results in increased blood vessel permeability. The fluid that accumulates typically contains white blood cells and if **cancer** is the cause, malignant cells from the tissue of origin. Malignancy may result from cancerous transformation of the cells that line the peritoneum, called mesothelial cells. Mesotheliomas may be difficult to distinguish from reactive mesothelial cells that occur whenever the lining of the abdomen is traumatized. The two most common metastatic cancers invading the abdomen are ovarian and **breast cancer**, but **lymphoma**, leukemia, lung, and many other cancers can also infiltrate the abdomen. Bacterial peritonitis is an infection of the peritoneum, and is a life-threatening cause of exudative ascites. It can result from intestinal perforation, leakage through a diseased bowel wall, ruptured appendix or gall bladder, or septicemia (infection in the blood). Inflammation of the abdominal wall can also result from blunt trauma, pancreatitis, intestinal obstruction, and other conditions.

Physical characteristics of ascites fluid

Normal ascites fluid is clear and straw colored. Turbid fluid occurs in bacterial peritonitis, malignancy, and pancreatitis. Green fluid occurs when bile is present. This can be caused by a ruptured bowel or perforated bile duct. Bloody fluid occurs in trauma, malignancy, and pancreatitis. Milky fluid contains chyle from the intestinal lymphatics and occurs when lymphatic vessels rupture.

Microscopic analysis

The WBC count is performed using a hemacytometer. Normal fluid has a very low WBC count (less than 300 per microliter) and does not have to be diluted. Counts above 1,000 indicate an exudative process. The differential is performed on a cytocentrifuged sample to concentrate the cells. Macrophages predominate in normal fluid and together with mesothelial cells account for about 70% of the nucleated cell population. Lymphocytes are normally less than 20% and neutrophils less than 10% of nucleated cells. Neutrophils accounting for 50% or 500 per microliter are most often associated with bacterial peritonitis. Lymphocytes will predominate in lymphoma, nephrotic syndrome, and congestive heart failure and may be abundant along with macrophages in **tuberculosis**. Red cell counts are also performed manually. Red cells often enter the fluid during sample collection, a process referred to as a traumatic tap. In this case, the red count will be low, the supernatant fluid will be pale yellow (normal), and the fluid will clear as more is collected. In the absence of a traumatic tap, red blood cells are most often encountered in malignancy and trauma. It is especially important to examine the fluid for the presence of malignant cells. As mentioned, metastatic cancer cells from ovarian and breast cancer are the most commonly seen infiltrates. Malignant mesothelial cells are difficult to distinguish from reactive mesothelial cells. Cytology should be evaluated with both Wright and Papanicilaou stains. Cytochemical tests and flow cytometry may be needed to identify malignant mesothelial cells, leukemic blasts (immature white cells), and lymphoma cells.

Biochemical tests

Chemical tests are performed on ascites fluid by the same methods used for plasma. Total protein, lactate dehydrogenase (LD), and glucose levels should be measured and compared to blood levels. Fluid to serum total protein and LD ratios are used to help distinguish exudative from transudative fluids. The serum albumin minus the fluid albumin is now considered the most sensitive single test to distinguish cirrhosis from malignancy as causes of ascites. Most transudative fluids are associated with cirrhosis and have a difference above 1.1. Most exudative fluids result from malignancy and have a difference less than 1.1. The fluid glucose is normally the same as the plasma glucose. Distinctly lower levels are seen in bacterial peritonitis, peritoneal tuberculosis, and malignancy. Lactate dehydrogenase is increased in bacterial peritonitis and malignant diseases. A fluid:serum ratio of 0.6 or higher has a sensitivity of about 80% in identifying exudative fluids. Amylase is very useful in diagnosing exudates caused by pancreatitis. Levels are usually in excess of three times the upper limit of normal. Fluid amylase testing can detect pancreatitis in approximately 90% of cases, and is also positive in the majority of people with bowel obstruction, proliferation and intestinal cancer. Alkaline phosphatase is elevated in exudates associated with bowel injury, obstruction, and some malignancies such as hepatoma.

Tumor markers may be useful to help distinguish the tissue of origin and to increase the sensitivity of cancer detection. Both carcinoembryonic antigen levels and CA125 levels in abdominal fluid have been found elevated in some persons with malignant infiltration of the abdomen but negative initial cytology. Creatinine may be measured when it is suspected that inadvertent puncture of the urinary bladder occurred during paracentesis. Creatinine in urine is about 100 times higher than in ascites fluid.

Microbiology

Bacterial cultures are usually performed on ascites fluid, but recovery of organisms is low when the fluid is frankly transudative. **Gram stain** detects about 25% of cases of bacterial peritonitis. The sensitivity can be increased by fluorescent microscopy using acridine orange stain. Cultures are positive in about 75% of cases that are eventually documented as infections. Detection of bacterial peritonitis is more sensitive when blood culture bottles containing tryptic soy broth are inoculated immediately after collection of the fluid rather than plating the fluid after transport to the lab. Regardless of the media used, cultures should be performed under both aerobic and anaerobic conditions. Spontaneous bacterial peritonitis that usually occurs in cirrhosis following **sepsis** typically grows a single organism, usually *E. coli* or *Streptococcus pneumoniae*. Peritonitis resulting from bowel sources usually grows several different intestinal organisms.

Preparation

A **hematocrit**, prothrombin time, and platelet count should be obtained within 48 hours of paracentesis. This

KEY TERMS

Ascites—Abnormal quantity of peritoneal fluid, an ultrafiltrate of plasma.

Edema—Fluids that have shifted outside of the circulatory system and are temporarily trapped in soft tissues.

Gram stain—A common laboratory test in which a specimen on a glass slide is subjected to a series of stains and rinses to visualize micro-organisms.

Lymphocyte—A specific type of white blood cell (leukocyte) involved in fighting atypical, fungal and viral infections.

Neutrophil—A specific type of white blood cell (leukocyte) involved in fighting bacterial infections. Also called a polymorphonuclear leukocyte.

will identify which patients may be at risk for bleeding complications, and provide a baseline hematocrit to estimate blood loss should bleeding occur. In addition, blood should be collected for glucose, total protein, lactate dehydrogenase, and albumin at the time of paracentesis. These results are compared to those of ascites fluid as a diagnostic aid. Abdominal girth and **vital signs** should be documented. The patient should be asked to empty his or her bladder, and should be warned about very brief discomfort as the needle goes through the peritoneum, in spite of **local anesthesia**. If very large amounts of peritoneal fluid are to be removed, it may need to be done very slowly to avoid large fluid shifts and a rapid fall in **blood pressure**. In extreme cases, a central venous pressure (CVP) line may need to be placed in order to monitor the patient's fluid status.

Aftercare

Vital signs are documented several times, perhaps even hourly for several hours if a large volume has been removed. The site of needle puncture is covered with a simple sterile dressing, or closed with a stitch if a trochar was used, and the dressing observed for possible continued leakage or bleeding.

Complications

Serious intra-abdominal bleeding is possible, although not very frequent. Puncture of the bladder or bowel are also possible. If good sterile technique is not used, infection could be introduced into the abdomen, resulting in peritonitis.

Results

Results of laboratory tests on ascites fluid are dependent upon the method of analysis used. Most studies are performed with very small sample sizes, and cell counts are performed manually. This results in greater interlaboratory variation in normal ranges than usually is seen for measurements performed on blood. Representative values for commonly measured analytes are shown below:

- Volume: 30-50 mL (1-1.7 oz).
- Color: pale yellow.
- Transparency: clear.
- WBC count: <200 per microliter.
- Total protein: <3.0 g/dL.
- Amylase: 0-130 U/L (similar to plasma for the method used).
- Serum to ascites albumin gradient (serum minus fluid albumin): greater than 1.1 g/dL.
- Fluid: serum LD ratio <0.6.
- Lactic acid: <40 mg/dL.
- Bilirubin: <6.0 mg/dL and serum/fluid ratio below 1.0.

Health care team roles

A physician normally collects the ascites fluid using sterile technique. The physician is usually assisted by a nurse. Nursing staff are responsible for documenting the patient's status before and after the procedure; educating and preparing the patient for the procedure; and observing for complications. Samples must be clearly labeled and sent to the laboratory. Clinical laboratory scientists/medical technologists perform blood counts, biochemical, and microbiological tests. A histologic technician prepares and stains slides for cytological review by a pathologist.

A study in 2004 showed that large-volume paracentesis could be performed safely as an outpatient procedure by gastrointestinal endoscopy assistants, usually licensed practical nurses with special training. The study reported that paracentesis performed in an outpatients setting by these assistants was safe, efficient, and usually completed in two hours. They demonstrated no added risk to patients and said that a major benefit would be significant savings in physician time.

Resources

BOOKS

Glickman, Robert M. "Abdominal Swelling and Ascites." In *Harrison's Principles of Internal Medicine*, edited by Anthony S. Fauci. McGraw-Hill, 1998: 256–257.

Malarkey, Louise M., and Mary Ellen McMorrow. *Nurse's Manual of Laboratory Tests and Diagnostic Procedures*, 2nd ed. W.B. Saunders Company, 2000: 457–461.

Tierney, Lawrence M., Stephen J. McPhee and Maxine A. Papadakis. *Current Medical Diagnosis and Treatment 2001*. Lange Medical Books/McGraw-Hill, 2001: 578–580.

PERIODICAL

Large-volume Paracentesis Can Be Performed Safely as an Outpatient Procedure. *Obesity, Fitness & Wellness Week* (Sept. 11, 2004): 448.

Erika J. Norris
Teresa G. Odle

Paralysis

Definition

Paralysis is defined as complete loss of strength in an affected limb or muscle group.

Description

The chain of nerve cells that runs from the **brain** through the **spinal cord** out to the muscle is called the motor pathway. Normal muscle function requires intact connections all along this motor pathway. Damage at any point reduces the nervous system's ability to control voluntary movements. Incomplete damage may cause **weakness**, also called paresis. Complete loss of communication prevents any willed movement at all. This lack of control is called paralysis. Certain inherited abnormalities in muscle cause periodic paralysis, in which the weakness comes and goes.

The line between weakness and paralysis is not absolute. A condition causing weakness may progress to paralysis. On the other hand, strength may be restored to a paralyzed limb. Nerve regeneration or regrowth is one way that strength can return to a paralyzed muscle. Paralysis almost always causes a change in muscle tone. Paralyzed muscle may be flaccid, flabby, and without appreciable tone, or it may be spastic, tight, and with abnormally high tone that increases when the muscle is moved.

Paralysis may affect an individual muscle, but usually affects an entire body region. The distribution of weakness is an important clue to the location of the nerve damage that is causing the paralysis. Words describing the distribution of paralysis use the suffix *-plegia*, from the Greek word for "stroke." The types of paralysis are classified by region:

- Monoplegia: affecting only one limb.
- Diplegia: affecting the same body region on both sides of the body (for example, both arms or both sides of the face).
- Hemiplegia: affecting one side of the body.
- Paraplegia: affecting both legs and the trunk
- Quadriplegia: affecting all four limbs and the trunk.

Causes and symptoms

Causes

The nerve damage that causes paralysis may be in the brain or spinal cord (the **central nervous system**), or it may be in the nerves outside the spinal cord (the peripheral nervous system). The most common causes of damage to the brain are:

- stroke
- tumor
- trauma (caused by a fall or a blow)
- multiple sclerosis (a disease of that destroys the protective sheath that covers nerve cells)
- cerebral palsy (a condition caused by a defect or injury to the brain that occurs at or shortly after birth)
- metabolic disorder (a disorder that interferes with the body's ability to maintain itself)

Damage to the spinal cord is most often caused by trauma, such as a fall or a car crash. Other conditions that may damage nerves within or immediately adjacent to the spine include:

- tumor
- herniated disk (also called a ruptured or slipped disk)
- spondylosis (a disease that causes stiffness in the joints of the spine)
- rheumatoid arthritis of the spine
- neurodegenerative disease (a disease that damages nerve cells)
- multiple sclerosis

Damage to peripheral nerves may be caused by:

- trauma
- compression or entrapment (such as carpal tunnel syndrome)
- Guillain-Barré syndrome (a disease of the nerves that sometimes follows fever caused by a viral infection or immunization)

- chronic inflammatory demyelinating polyradiculoneuropathy (CIDP) (a condition that causes pain and swelling in the protective sheath that covers nerve cells)
- radiation
- inherited demyelinating disease (a condition that destroys the protective sheath around the nerve cell)
- toxins or poisons

Symptoms

The distribution of paralysis offers important clues to the site of nerve damage. Hemiplegia is almost always caused by brain damage on the side opposite the paralysis, often from a **stroke**. Paraplegia occurs after injury to the lower spinal cord, and quadriplegia occurs after damage to the upper spinal cord at the level of the shoulders or higher (the nerves controlling the arms leave the spine at that level). Diplegia usually indicates brain damage, most often from **cerebral palsy**. Monoplegia may be caused by isolated damage to either the central or the peripheral nervous system. Weakness or paralysis that occurs only in the arms and legs may indicate demyelinating disease. Fluctuating symptoms in different parts of the body may be caused by **multiple sclerosis**.

Sudden paralysis is most often caused by injury or stroke. Spreading paralysis may indicate degenerative disease, inflammatory disease such as Guillain-Barré syndrome or CIDP, metabolic disorders, or inherited demyelinating disease.

Other symptoms often accompany paralysis from any cause. These symptoms may include numbness and tingling, **pain**, changes in **vision**, difficulties with speech, or problems with balance. **Spinal cord injury** often causes loss of function in the bladder, bowel, and sexual organs. High spinal cord injuries may cause difficulties in breathing.

Diagnosis

Careful attention should be paid to any events in the patient's history that might reveal the cause of the paralysis. The examiner should look for incidents such as **falls** or other traumas, exposure to toxins, recent infections or surgery, unexplained **headache**, preexisting metabolic disease, and family history of weakness or other neurologic conditions. A neurologic examination tests strength, **reflexes**, and sensation in the affected and unaffected areas.

Imaging studies, including **computed tomography scans (CT scans)**, **magnetic resonance imaging** (MRI) scans, or **myelography**, may reveal the site of the injury. **Electromyography** and nerve conduction velocity tests are performed to test the function of the muscles and peripheral nerves.

Treatment

The only treatment for paralysis is to treat its underlying cause. The loss of function caused by long-term paralysis can be treated through a comprehensive **rehabilitation** program. Rehabilitation includes:

- Physical therapy. The physical therapist focuses on mobility. Physical therapy helps develop strategies to compensate for paralysis by using those muscles that still have normal function, helps maintain and build any strength and control that remain in the affected muscles, and helps maintain range of motion in the affected limbs to prevent muscles from shortening (contracture) and becoming deformed. If nerve regrowth is expected, physical therapy is used to retrain affected limbs during recovery. A physical therapist also suggests adaptive equipment such as braces, canes, or wheelchairs.

- Occupational therapy. The occupational therapist focuses on daily activities such as eating and bathing. Occupational therapy develops special tools and techniques that permit self-care and suggests ways to modify the home and workplace so that a patient with an impairment may live a normal life.

- Other specialties. The nature of the impairment may mean that the patient needs the services of a respiratory therapist, vocational rehabilitation counselor, social worker, speech-language pathologist, nutritionist, special education teacher, recreation therapist, or clinical psychologist.

Prognosis

The likelihood of recovery from paralysis depends on the cause and how much damage has been done to the nervous system.

Health care team roles

A team of therapists and other health care specialists may be involved in the care of a person with paralysis. A person with paralysis may have difficulty expressing his or her needs. Health care workers should pay particular attention to the individual's emotional and psychological well-being, as well as physical. Particular attention should be paid to providing ongoing **patient education**.

Prevention

Prevention of paralysis depends on prevention of the underlying causes. Risk of stroke can be reduced by controlling high **blood pressure** and **cholesterol** levels. Seatbelts, air bags, and helmets reduce the risk of injury from motor vehicle accidents and falls. Good **prenatal care** can help prevent premature birth, which is a common cause of cerebral palsy.

Resources

BOOKS

Bellenir, Karen, ed. *Brain Disorders Sourcebook: Basic Consumer Health Information.* Detroit: Omnigraphics, 1999.

Fuller, Jill, and Jennifer Schaller-Ayers, ed. *Health Assessment: A Nursing Approach.* 3rd ed. Philadelphia: Lippincott Williams Wilkins, 2000.

Kozier, Barbara, et al., eds. *Fundamentals of Nursing: Concepts, Process, and Practice.* 6th ed. Upper Saddle River, NJ: Prentice Hall Health, 2000.

ORGANIZATIONS

Christopher Reeve Paralysis Foundation. 500 Morris Avenue, Springfield, NJ 07081. (800) 225-0292. http://paralysis. apacure.org.

National Institute of Neurological Disorders and Stroke. NIH Neurological Institute, P.O. Box 5801, Bethesda, MD 20824. (800) 352-9424. http://www.ninds.nih.gov.

Jennifer F. Wilson

Paralysis agitans *see* **Parkinson's disease**

Paramedics *see* **Emergency medical technician**

Paraplegia *see* **Paralysis**

Parasites

Definition

Parasites are organisms that live inside humans or other organisms who act as hosts. They are dependent on their hosts because they are unable to produce food or energy for themselves. Parasites are harmful to humans because they consume needed food, eat away body tissues and cells, and eliminate toxic waste, which makes people sick.

Because of sanitary living conditions in the United States, parasites do not cause widespread life-threatening infections. In other parts of the world, however, parasitic infections are epidemic. They kill and disable millions of people every year. Parasitic **infection** cases in the United States in the 2000s were on the rise, however, due to increased travel to and from underdeveloped countries. In addition, parasitic infections can cause severe infections in **AIDS** patients and other patients with weakened immune systems.

Because parasites can live inside the human body for years without making their presence known, they are more common than one might think. According to one study, approximately half of all Americans have at least one form of parasite. Their presence causes a variety of chronic diseases and conditions such as chronic fatigue, **weakness**, low energy levels, skin rashes, **pain**, constipation, and frequent colds and **influenza**.

Description

There are two types of parasites: large and small. Large parasites such as intestinal worms are easily seen with the naked eye. These are roundworms, flukes, and tapeworms. They usually lay their eggs on the intestinal walls. As they hatch, the young larvae feed on the food in the intestinal tract. Then they grow, reproduce, and start the cycle all over again. They sometimes dig through the digestive tract to get into the bloodstream, muscles, and other organs where they cause even more havoc. These types of parasites often cause malnutrition and anemia because they tend to rob the body of essential nutrients.

Small parasites—mostly protozoa and amoebae— are so tiny that they can only be seen with a **microscope**.

These tiny parasites are even more dangerous to the body than the large ones. Although they usually stay in the intestines, they can migrate virtually anywhere in the body: into the bloodstream, muscles, and even vital organs such as the **brain**, the **lungs**, or the **liver**, where they do substantial damage.

Because parasites are everywhere, it is not difficult to become infected. People can become infested through the following ways:

• being bitten by insects
• walking barefoot
• eating raw or undercooked pork, beef, or fish
• eating contaminated raw fruits and vegetables
• eating foods prepared by infected handlers
• drinking contaminated water
• having contact with infected persons (including sexual contact, kissing, sharing drinks, shaking hands, or sharing toys)
• inhaling dust that contains parasitic eggs or cysts
• playing with or picking up pet litter contaminated with parasitic eggs or cysts

In 2002, the Centers for Disease Control (CDC) announced the first documented cases of transplant patients contracting a dangerous parasitic disease from infection with T. cruzi from organs harvested from a Central American donor. The infection caused Chagas disease, causing two of the three donor recipients to die. The CDC identified two additional cases of Chagas diseased in transplant patients. In one case, reported in 2006, the patient received a **heart** transplant in 2005 and showed symptoms of Chagas in January 2006. The patient was treated medically and recovered. However, he died several months later due to organ rejection. It was found that his donor lived in the United States but had traveled to a portion of Mexico infected with T. cruzi. Another case of Chagas disease was reported in February 2006, one month following a heart transplant. The patient's symptoms disappeared following treatment. He died several months later as a result of cardiac arrest. These represent the fourth and fifth reported cases of Chagas disease caused by T. cruzi. The fact that they occurred in Los Angeles prompted the CDC to encourage physicians in the area to suspect T. cruzi in transplant and transfusion patients, if appropriate symptoms are present.

Causes and symptoms

Risk factors for getting parasitic infections include:

• an immune system weakened by disease or long-term exposure to toxic chemicals or environmental pollution
• prolonged antibiotic use
• alcohol and/or drug abuse
• smoking
• emotional and/or physical stress
• diet high in fat and sugar and low in fiber
• food allergies
• malabsorption syndrome
• obesity

Causes

There are more than 100 types of human parasites. The following describe some of the most common species in the United States.

ARTHROPODS (INSECTS). In the United States, because of high sanitary standards and a temperate climate, parasitic insects do not flourish. Common bugs such as ticks, mites, fleas, lice, and bedbugs may cause intense **itching** in affected areas. They are a nuisance but generally not a major health risk. One exception is the deer tick, which is associated with the debilitating Lyme disease. Other parasites, spread by mosquitoes, cause more serious diseases such as western and eastern equine **encephalitis**, **malaria**, Dengue **fever**, and yellow fever.

INTESTINAL PARASITES. Some of the most common intestinal parasites are:

• Pinworms. This is the most common parasitic infection in the United States. The worm resides in the colon, yet it lays eggs outside the body, usually near the anus, a process that causes severe itching. The disease can be transmitted from one individual to another through dirty hands, clothing, bedclothes, and toys.
• Tapeworms. The two most common tapeworms are *Taenia solium* (pork tapeworm) and *Taenia saginata* (beef tapeworm). *Taenia solium* infestation is caused by eating undercooked pork while *Taenia saginata* (pork tapeworm) infestation is associated with consuming raw beef. Adult tapeworms may become quite big, some as long as 20 feet (6.1 m). Of the two, pork tapeworm is the more harmful. It often causes anemia and weight loss. More seriously, when adult pork tapeworm eggs, excreted in human feces, are ingested by other people (which can happen with poor hygiene and sanitation), the parasitic life cycle that occurs in pigs and cattle takes place in the human host. Once in the human digestive system, the tapeworm eggs, called proglottids, develop into an embryonic form of the parasite called onchospheres that burrow through the intestinal wall and into the bloodstream. From there they migrate into the muscles, eyes, and the brain, a condition called cysticercosis. Cysts in the brain often cause epileptic seizures.

• Protozoa (one-celled organisms) such as *Giardia lamblia, Entamoeba histolytica,* or *Cryptosporidium.* These organisms are some of the most common and infectious parasites in the world. They can be transmitted through contaminated food and water. They can also be spread from one person to another. Protozoa may spread throughout the body, causing abscesses in the lungs, liver, heart, and brain. Cramps, watery diarrhea, abdominal pain, and serious weight loss are common symptoms of Giardia infection. *Entamoeba histolytica* can cause dysentery, a severe form of intestinal infection, as well as liver and lung damage. Cryptosporidia can cause severe diarrhea in AIDS or cancer patients who have weakened immune systems.

According to the Centers for Disease Control and Prevention (CDC), cases of *Cryptospordium* in the United States increased from 3,505 in 2003 to 8,269 cases in 2005. The largest portion of the increase was related to an outbreak in New York that was traced to use of a recreational water fountain. In 2003, 425 cases were linked to unpasteurized apple cider produced from contaminated apples.

CNS PARASITIC INFECTIONS. *Toxoplasma gondii* is the most common parasite that invades the **central nervous system** (CNS). Humans become infected with this organism by eating raw or undercooked meat or by handling infected cat litter, which can contain eggs. Pregnant women who are infected may miscarry or deliver stillborn babies. Infected babies are born with congenital toxoplasmosis and have symptoms that include eye inflammation, blindness, **jaundice**, seizures, abnormally small or large heads, and mental retardation. In people with weakened immune systems, such as AIDS patients, toxoplasmosis can affect the whole body, causing inflammation, convulsions, trembling, **headache**, confusion, **paralysis** in half of the body, or **coma**.

Symptoms

Parasitic infections are difficult to diagnose because many patients exhibit only vague symptoms or no symptoms at all. The following symptoms, however, may indicate parasitic infections:

• Diarrhea with foul-smelling stool that becomes worse in the later part of the day.

• Sudden changes in bowel habits (e.g. constipation that changes to soft and watery stool).

• Constant rumbling and gurgling in the stomach area unrelated to hunger or eating.

• Heartburn or chest pain.

• Flu-like symptoms such as coughing, fever, and nasal congestion.

• Nonspecific food allergies.

• Itching around the nose, ears, and anus, especially at night.

• Losing weight with constant hunger.

Other symptoms of parasitic infections include anemia, **blood** in the stool, bloating, **diarrhea**, gas, loss of appetite, intestinal obstruction, nausea, **vomiting**, sore mouth and gums, excessive nose picking, grinding teeth at night, chronic fatigue, headaches, muscle aches and pains, shortness of breath, skin rashes, depression, and **memory** loss.

Diagnosis

The following tests may be used to help doctors diagnose parasitic infections:

• *Ova and parasite (O & P) test.* Three to six stool samples are collected every one or two days to look for eggs and parasites.

• *Cellophane tape* (applied to the anal area). Ova (eggs) that stick to the tape prove pinworm infestation.

• *Endoscopy.* This procedure is used to obtain samples from the duodenum (the upper part of the small intestine), which are then analyzed for the presence of parasites.

• *Urine sample* and vaginal swab to detect *Trichomonas*, a parasite that causes vaginitis.

• *Blood tests.* High levels of eosinophils (a type of white blood cell) indicate infections. Antibodies against the parasites may also be detected. A study released in 2008 found that blood testing is often necessary to obtain a specific diagnosis. An increase in eosinophils, in particular, is associated with parasitic infections.

• *X ray, MRI, and CT scans.* X rays detect lesions in internal organs. Computed axial tomography (CT) scans and magnetic resonance imaging (MRI) are used to diagnose CNS parasitic infections.

Infected patients who are treated with anti-parasitic drugs or herbal remedies should be retested twice at the end of the treatment program; the two tests should be given one month apart.

Treatment

Alternative therapies for parasitic infections reduce parasitic infections by improving **nutrition** and strengthening the **immune system** through herbal therapy and Ayurvedic medicine. Some herbal remedies are directly anti-parasitic and actually eliminate the organisms that cause disease. Patients taking allopathic anti-parasitic remedies should consult their doctor before using any of these herbs. Care should be taken before giving them to children as they easily **overdose**.

Nutritional therapy

The following dietary changes may help prevent or treat parasitic infections:

- Eating a well-balanced diet with lots of fiber, vegetables, fruits, whole grains, nuts, and seeds. Fiber helps eliminate worms from the intestines; good nutrition improves immune function and protects the body against parasitic invasion.
- Limiting dairy foods, sugar, and fat. Parasites thrive on these foods.
- Avoiding raw or undercooked fish, pork, or beef.
- Take daily multivitamin/mineral supplements to prevent malnutrition and improve immune function.
- Supplementing the diet with probiotics such as *Lactobacillus acidophilus, Bifidobacteria*, and other beneficial intestinal bacteria that cultivate normal intestinal flora and suppress the spreading of parasites.

Herbal therapy

Herbal treatment should be given in combination with supportive dietary treatment and continued until the worms are completely eradicated. The following herbs are helpful in treating parasitic infestations:

- *Melaleuca alternifolia* (tea tree) oil. First discovered by Australian aborigines, tea tree oil has many uses, including treating intestinal parasites, lice, and ticks.
- *Artemisia annua* (wormwood herb) and citrus seed extract. These can be used together to help eliminate intestinal parasites such as *Giardia lamblia*.
- *Berberine-containing herbs*. Berberine is an antimicrobial alkaloid that can prevent parasites from attaching to the intestinal walls of human hosts. One study found that berberine was as effective against amoebal *Giardia lamblia* as metronidazole, the standard treatment. Herbs that contain berberine include goldenseal *(Hydrastis canadensis)*, barberry *(Berberis vulgaris)*, Oregon grape *(Berberis aquifolium)*, and goldthread *(Coptis chinensis)*.

Ayurvedic medicine

Momordica charantia (bitter melon) is a very safe remedy for pinworm infection. The melon is a vegetable shaped like a cucumber with a bitter **taste**. It can be found in most Oriental markets. It should be sliced thinly and eaten raw with other vegetables to reduce its bitter taste. Daily consumption of one to two bitter melons for seven to 10 days can eliminate pinworm infection.

Patients may want to repeat the regimen after several months to prevent reinfection. Chinese herbal combinations also help treat parasitic infections by supporting the gastrointestinal system, stimulating **immune response**, and killing parasites.

Allopathic treatment

Insect infestations

Infestations with lice, ticks, fleas, or bedbugs can be controlled by insecticides and attention to hygiene and household or environmental contact.

Intestinal parasites

Treatment for intestinal parasites usually involves anti-parasitic drugs. Depending on the severity of the condition and the species involved, treatment may include one (or more) of the following drugs: albendazole, furazolidone, iodoquinol, mebendazole, metronidazole, niclosamide, paromomycin, pyrantel pamoate, pyrimethamine, quinacrine, sulfadiazine, or thiabendazole. Nitrazoxinide was approved in 2002 for treatment of *Cryptosporidium* in children ages 1 to 11 years. In 2004, the drug was approved for people older than age 11, including adults. The approval of this drug may have led to a rise in the number of reported cases.

To prevent reinfection and transmission of disease, thorough cleaning of hands, clothes, sheets, and toys is recommended. Treatments should involve all members of the family and repeated treatments may be necessary.

CNS parasitic infections

Babies or AIDS patients with toxoplasmosis are often given spiramycin or sulfadiazine plus pyrimethamine. Treatment may be continued indefinitely for AIDS patients to prevent recurrence.

Expected results

Though parasitic infections are difficult to diagnose, complete recovery from infestation can be achieved with appropriate herbal therapy or anti-parasitic drugs. Because reinfestation is common, multiple treatments may be necessary.

Prevention

The following measures can help prevent parasitic infections:

- Washing hands before eating and after using the restroom.

KEY TERMS

Contaminated—Unclean or infected by contact with or the addition of something.

Eosinophil—A type of white blood cell that increases in number in response to certain medical conditions, such as allergy or parasitic infection.

Infest—To be parasitic in a host.

Intestines—Also called the bowels and divided into the large and small intestine. They extend from the stomach to the anus, where waste products exit the body. The small intestine is about 20 ft (6.1 m) long and the large intestine, about 5 ft (1.5 m) long.

Protozoa—Single-celled microorganisms belonging to the subkingdom Protozoa that are more complex than bacteria. About 30 protozoa cause diseases in humans.

• Wearing gloves when gardening or working with soil or sand because soil can be contaminated with eggs or cysts of parasites.

• For pregnant women, avoiding handling of cat litter.

• Not allowing children to be licked by pets; not allowing children to kiss pets that are not dewormed regularly.

• Washing fresh vegetables carefully. Many people get *Entamoeba histolytica* by eating contaminated raw fruit and vegetables.

• Avoiding eating raw meat, which may contain *Giardia lamblia*.

• Wearing long-sleeved shirts, long pants, and boots when walking in the woods. In addition, spraying insect repellent on clothing to prevent tick bites.

Resources

PERIODICALS

Chagas Disease after Organ Transplantation—Los Angeles, California, 2006. *MMWR Weekly.* 55, no. 29 (July 28, 2006): 798–800.

Page, Kathleen R., and Jonathan Zenilman. "Eosinophilia in a Patient from South America." *Journal of the American Medical Association* 299, no. 4 (January 30, 2008): 437-444.

OTHER

"General Information: Diagnosis of Parasitic Diseases." *Division of Parasitic Diseases: Public Information.* http://www.cdc.gov/ncidod/dpd/public/geninfo_diagnosis_diseases.htm. (February 28, 2008).

"Parasitic Infections." *The Merck Manual of Diagnosis and Therapy.* http://www.merck.com/pubs/mmanual/section13/chapter161/161a.htm. (February 28, 2008).

ORGANIZATIONS

AIDS Treatment Data Network. The NETWORK, 611 Broadway, Suite 613,, New York,, NY 10012. , (212) 260-8868, (800)734-7104., http://www.atdn.org/

Centers for Disease Control and Prevention (CDC). ,International Traveler's Hotline: (404)332-4559. , http://www.cdc.gov/travel/.

Mai Tran
Teresa G. Odle, PhD
Rhonda Cloos, RN

Parasomnia *see* **Sleep disorders**

Parathyroid glands

Definition

The four parathyroid glands are small, light-colored lumps protruding from the surface of the **thyroid gland**. They secrete parathyroid hormone, the most important regulator of **calcium** and **phosphorus** amounts in the body.

Description

The parathyroid glands are located on the thyroid gland, a butterfly-shaped gland found in the neck on both sides of the windpipe. There are then two parathyroid glands on each side of the neck for a total of four. Parathyroid tissue consists of two major cell types: oxyphil cells, whose function is unknown, and chief cells, which produce parathyroid hormone. The structure of a parathyroid gland is very different from that of a thyroid gland. The chief cells that produce parathyroid hormone are arranged in tightly-packed nests around small **blood vessels**, quite unlike the thyroid cells that produce thyroid hormones, which are arranged in spheres (thyroid follicles).

The parathyroid glands secrete parathyroid hormone (PTH), a polypeptide consisting of 84 amino acid residues. A hormone is a chemical messenger of the body, produced and secreted by special glands called exocrine glands. It is released directly into the bloodstream and travels to its target cells, often distant, where it binds to a structure called a receptor, that is found either inside or on the surface of the target cells. Receptors bind a specific hormone and the result is a specific physiologic response, meaning a normal response of the body. The activity of all the hormones or growth factors secreted by endocrine glands and circulating in **blood** is controlled by the

KEY TERMS

Amino acid—A class of organic molecules containing mostly the elements carbon, nitrogen and oxygen, and that combine in linear chains to form polypeptides and proteins. There are 20 naturally-occurring amino acids: alanine, arginine, aspargine, aspartic acid, cysteine, glutamic acid, glutamine, glycine, histidine, isoleucine, leucine, lysine, methionine, phenylalanine, proline, serine, threonine, tryptophan, tyrosine, and valine.

Antagonist—A substance that cancels or counteracts the action of another.

Bone—The hard tissue of the skeleton. Bones mostly consist of calcium carbonate, calcium phosphate, and gelatine.

Bone mineral density—Proper degree of hardness in bones. It is regulated by remodeling, a process that occurs 24 hours a day, seven days a week and involves the continuous breakdown and re-formation of bone.

Calcitonin—A polypeptide hormone produced by the thyroid gland that causes a reduction of calcium levels in the blood. Counteracts PTH.

Endocrine glands—Glands that secrete substances that are released directly into the blood stream and that regulate metabolism and other body functions.

Endocrine system—The system of glands in the body that secrete their hormones directly into the circulatory system.

Extracellular fluid (ECF)—The fluid found outside of the cells and between the cells in body tissues.

Hormone—A naturally occurring substance secreted by specialized cells that affects the metabolism or behavior of other cells possessing receptors for the hormone. Thus, hormones acts like chemical messengers and bind to receptors on target cells.

Metabolism—The sum of all the physical and chemical reactions required to maintain the function of body systems and organs.

Osteoblasts—Cells that are associated with the production of bone as they mature.

Osteoclasts—A large cell with many nuclei associated with the absorption and removal of bone.

Parathyroid hormone (PTH)—Polypeptide hormone consisting of 84 amino acid residues that is secreted by the parathyroid glands. PTH is involved in regulating bone metabolism by controlling calcium and phosphorus levels in the body. Counteracts calcitonin.

Physiologic response—Characteristic of, or conforming to the normal functioning of the body or a tissue or organ.

Receptor—A cell structure, inside or on the surface of cells, that binds a specific hormone and starts a specific physiologic response.

Thyroid gland—A butterfly-shaped endocrine gland located in the neck on both sides of the windpipe. It secretes the hormone thyroxine which controls the rate of metabolism.

exocrine system of the body. PTH finds its major target cells in **bone**, **kidneys**, and the gastrointestinal system.

Function

The function of the parathyroid glands is to secrete parathyroid hormone, which causes the release of the calcium present in bone to extracellular fluid (ECF). The ECF is the fluid found outside cells in all body tissues. PTH does this by activating the production of osteoblasts, special cells of the body involved in the production of bone and slowing down osteoclasts, other specialized cells involved in the removal of bone.

Calcitonin, a hormone produced by the thyroid gland that also regulates ECF calcium levels and serves to counteract the calcium-producing effects of PTH. The adult body contains as much as 1 kg of calcium. Most of this calcium is found in bone and teeth, and less than 1 g is found in the ECF, with 50% in the form of ionized calcium (Ca^{2+}). Both calcitonin and PTH respond to the circulating levels of Ca^{2+}. An increased amount of ECF Ca^{2+} leads to an increased release of calcitonin and a decreased PTH release; similarly, a decreased amount of ECF Ca^{2+} results in a decreased release of calcitonin and an increased PTH release. Overall, calcitonin acts quickly to reduce ECF Ca^{2+} levels, while PTH works more slowly to ensure that adequate Ca^{2+} ECF levels are maintained. PTH action is thus opposed to that of calcitonin.

Three major calcium regulatory processes are affected by PTH:

- Release of calcium from bone: Although the mechanisms remain unclear, it is known that PTH stimulates bone tissue to release calcium into blood.

- Increased calcium absorption in the intestine: Facilitating calcium absorption from the small intestine increases calcium amounts in the blood. PTH also stimulates this process, but indirectly, meaning that it stimulates production of vitamin D in the kidney. Vitamin D in turn facilitates the production of a protein in intestinal cells that binds calcium for its efficient absorption into the blood.

- Suppression of calcium loss in urine: Additionally, PTH slows down the elimination of calcium in urine, thus maintaining calcium levels in blood.

Role in human health

The regulation of ECF calcium levels by PTH is the key for essential body functions such as the transmission of impulses across nerve junctions (synapses), **muscle contraction**, and **blood coagulation**, processes that all require calcium. Calcium imbalance will therefore result in serious adverse health effects.

Another major effect of the calcium regulatory activity of PTH is to play a significant role in bone formation and bone maintenance. Bones are hard because they contain calcium compounds, such as calcium carbonate and calcium phosphate. Thus, they provide a frame to the body for physical support as well as for protection. They also store calcium and phosphorus reserves, the chemicals required for bone growth. Bone formation, or the development of bone mineral density is usually complete around 25-28 years of age. Since bone is a live tissue, just like the other organs of the body, such as the **heart** and kidneys, it maintains its optimal degree of hardness by a very active process, called remodeling. Remodeling occurs 24 hours a day, seven days a week. It involves the continuous breakdown and re-formation of bone to repair any damage that may occur, such as **fractures**, and to maintain the proper levels of calcium in the bone cells.

When the amount of calcium in the ECF falls below normal as a result of the bone remodeling process absorbing it inside the bone cells, the release of PTH then brings it back within the normal range. As calcium amounts increase, the amount of phosphate in blood is also reduced.

Common diseases and disorders

- Primary hyperparathyroidism. The most common disease of parathyroid glands is overactivity, meaning that too much PTH is being produced. Hyperparathyroidism is the result of parathyroid gland disease, which then secretes the hormone in abnormally high amounts. Common symptoms of this disorder are chronic increases of calcium amounts in the blood (hypercalcemia), kidney stones, and decalcification of bone. The major symptom of this condition is decalcification of bone, leading to brittle bones that fracture easily (rubber bones).

- Secondary hyperparathyroidism. In this form of hyperparathyroidism, the condition is due to a disease not directly affecting the parathyroid glands that leads to high levels of PTH. Kidney disease is often associated with this disorder because it reduces the renal excretion of phosphate, causing increased phosphate levels in the blood which then decrease the level of free ionized calcium. In addition, most of the calcium in extracellular fluid is not in the ionized form. Rather, at least 50% of the extracellular fluid calcium is in the non-ionized form bound to proteins and phosphate. Secondary hyperparathyroidism is also due to a poor diet, deficient in calcium or vitamin D, or which is high in phosphorus (found in meat).

- Hypoparathyroidism. Hypoparathyroidism results from inadequate PTH production. It is a rare condition, most commonly caused by damage or removal of the parathyroid glands at the time of parathyroid or thyroid surgery. Typically, it results in decreased concentrations of calcium and increased concentrations of phosphorus in blood. The resulting hypocalcemia often leads to convulsions, and can be life-threatening.

- Parathyroid adenoma. Parathyroid adenoma commonly occurs on only one of the four parathyroids. The condition accounts for 87–93% of all patients diagnosed with primary hyperparathyroidism. The enlarged parathyroid that has the tumor usually secretes all the PTH with the other three glands responding to the high calcium levels caused by the overactive one by becoming dormant. Parathyroid adenoma is very rarely cancerous (less than one in 500), but it slowly damages the body by causing abnormally high level of calcium in the blood.

- Secondary osteoporosis. This bone disorder results from a slight excess of bone removal over bone formation, often the result of prolonged hyperthyroidism.

- Congenital hypoparathyroidism. Individuals with this condition are born without parathyroid tissues. It is due to a genetic disorder resulting in abnormal genes that either encode for abnormal forms of PTH or its receptor, or prevent normal parathyroid gland development before birth.

Resources

BOOKS

Bilezikian, John P., Robert Marcus, and Michael Levine, eds. *The Parathyroids, Second edition.* New York: Academic Press, 2001.

Whitfield, James F., Paul Morley, and Gordon E. Willick. *The Parathyroid Hormone: An Unexpected Bone Builder for Treating Osteoporosis.* Georgetown: Landes Bioscience, 1998.

PERIODICALS

Goltzman, D., and J. H. White, "Developmental and tissue-specific regulation of parathyroid hormone." *Critical Reviews in Eukaryotic Gene Expression* 10 (2000): 135–49.

Weigel, R. J. "Nonoperative management of hyperparathyroidism: present and future." *Current Opinions in Oncology* 13 (January 2001): 33–38.

Whitfield, J., P. Morley, and G. Willick, "The parathyroid hormone, its fragments and analogues-potent bone-builders for treating osteoporosis." *Expert Opinions in Investigative Drugs* 9 (June 2000): 1293–1315.

Monique Laberge, Ph.D.

Parathyroid hormone test

Definition

The parathyroid hormone (PTH) test is a **blood** test performed to determine the serum levels of a hormone secreted by the parathyroid gland. The **parathyroid glands** are small paired glands located near the **thyroid gland** at the base of the neck. Most people have four glands, two on each side of the neck. PTH regulates **calcium** and **phosphorus** levels in the body. It is secreted in response to low blood ionized calcium levels, causing **bone** to release calcium into the blood stream. In addition, it promotes the renal reabsorption of calcium and excretion of phosphorus.

Purpose

The PTH level is measured to evaluate the cause of an abnormal serum or plasma calcium. It is routinely monitored in patients with a kidney disorder called chronic renal failure (CRF). These patients lose calcium via the **kidneys** which stimulates release of PTH. This can lead to bone demineralization. The PTH test is also used to distinguish between primary hyperthyroidism and

malignancies that result in high ionized calcium via secretion of a protein called parathyroid hormone-related protein. This stimulates the PTH receptor of bone causing increased plasma ionized calcium. PTH is also used to distinguish between hypoparathyroidism and a condition called pseudohypoparathyroidism, which results from a poor renal response to the hormone. Persons with primary hypoparathyroidism have a low ionized calcium because the parathyroid glands fail to produce enough PTH. Persons with pseudohypoparathyroidism have a low ioninzed calcium but have a normal or elevated level of PTH.

Description

Measurement of PTH is used for the differential diagnosis of hyperparathyroidism. Primary hyperparathyroidism is most often caused by a benign tumor (adenoma) in one or more of the parathyroid glands. It is rarely caused by parathyroid malignancy. Patients with this condition have high plasma PTH and ionized calcium levels and low plasma inorganic phosphorus. Primary hyperparathyroidism is treated by surgical removal of the tumor(s). The PTH test is used to measure the plasma hormone level during surgery. Complete removal of the tumor is signaled by a return to normal plasma PTH levels.

Secondary hyperparathyroidism is often seen in patients with chronic renal failure (CRF). The kidneys fail to excrete sufficient phosphate and do not reabsorb calcium. The parathyroid gland secretes PTH in an effort to raise the plasma ionized calcium level. Because of the constant stimulation of the parathyroid, CRF patients have high PTH and normal or slightly low calcium levels.

Tertiary hyperparathyroidism occurs when CRF causes proliferation of the parathyroids that does not respond to normal suppression by ionized calcium. Patients with this condition have high plasma PTH and calcium levels and low plasma inorganic phosphorus.

Specific PTH assays

Some PTH is split into peptide fragments by enzymes in the parathyroid gland prior to being released into the blood. Therefore, in addition to intact PTH, three smaller fragments are also present, an amino or N-terminal fragment, a midregion fragment, and a carboxy or C-terminal fragment. Only the intact hormone and fragments containing the amino terminal end of the molecule are physiologically active. A two-site enzyme immunoassay was recently developed to measure PTH.

This method measures only the intact PTH and active fragments and is preferred over other assays that detect the inactive fragments.

Precautions

Drug interactions

Some prescription drugs affect the results of PTH tests. Drugs that *increase* PTH levels include phosphates, anticonvulsants, steroids, isoniazid, lithium, and rifampin. Drugs that *decrease* PTH include cimetidine and propranolol.

Timing

PTH levels are subject to diurnal variation. The plasma level peaks at around 2:00 A.M. and is lowest around 2:00 P.M. Specimens are usually drawn at 8:00 A.M. The laboratory should be notified if the patient works the night shift so that this difference in biological rhythm can be taken into account.

Related blood tests

Due to the relationship between PTH and calcium, ionized calcium and inorganic phosphorus levels should be tested at the same time as PTH. In addition, creatinine and other tests of renal function are helpful in identifying those patients who have secondary hyperparathyroidism caused by renal loss of calcium.

Preparation

The PTH test is performed on a sample of the patient's blood, withdrawn from a vein. The procedure, which is called a venipuncture, takes about five minutes. When performing this procedure, the nurse or phlebotomist should follow **universal precautions** for the prevention of transmission of bloodborne pathogens. The patient should have nothing to eat or drink starting at midnight of the day of the test.

Complications

Risks for this test are minimal, but may include slight bleeding from the puncture site, a small bruise or swelling in the area, or fainting or feeling lightheaded.

Results

Reference ranges for PTH tests vary somewhat depending on the specificity of the **antibodies** used in the assay to detect the hormone. Results should always be interpreted in association with calcium results. The following ranges are typical:

KEY TERMS

Assay—An analysis of the chemical composition or strength of a substance.

Hypercalcemia—Abnormally high levels of blood calcium.

Hyperparathyroidism—Overactivity of the parathyroid glands. Symptoms include generalized aches and pains, depression, and abdominal pain.

Hypoparathyroidism—Insufficient production of parathyroid hormone, which results in low levels of blood calcium.

- intact PTH: 10-65 pg/mL

- PTH N-terminal (includes intact PTH): 8-24 pg/mL

- PTH C-terminal (includes C-terminal, intact PTH, and midmolecule): 50-330 pg/mL.

Abnormally high PTH values may indicate primary, secondary, or tertiary hyperparathyroidism. Causes of secondary hyperparathyroidism include chronic renal failure, **malabsorption syndrome**, and **vitamin D** deficiency. Abnormally low PTH levels indicate primary hypoparathyroidism or hypercalcemia. Primary hypoparathyroidism is less common than hyperthyroidism and may result from surgical removal of the glands (during thyroidectomy) or chronic inflammatory (autoimmune) disease. Malignancies producing parathyroid hormone-related protein are common causes of low PTH induced by high ionized calcium.

Health care team roles

This test is ordered by a physician. The blood sample is collected by a nurse or phlebotomist. PTH levels are usually analyzed by clinical laboratory scientists/medical technologists. If abnormal results occur, the patient is usually referred to an endocrinologist for further evaluation and treatment.

Resources

BOOKS

Jacobs, David S. *Laboratory Test Handbook,* 4th ed. Lexi-Comp Inc., 1996.

Pagana, Kathleen Deska, and Timothy James Pagana, eds. *Mosby's Diagnostic and Laboratory Test Reference.* St. Louis: Mosby-Year Book, Inc., 1998.

Rachael T. Brandt, MS

Parathyroid scan

Definition

A parathyroid scan is sometimes called a parathyroid localization scan or parathyroid scintigraphy. This scan uses radioactive pharmaceuticals that are readily taken up by specific cells in the **parathyroid glands** to obtain an image of the glands. The test is done primarily to detect tumors.

Purpose

The parathyroid glands, embedded in the **thyroid gland** in the neck, but separate from the thyroid in function, control **calcium metabolism** in the body. The parathyroid glands produce parathyroid hormone (PTH). PTH regulates the level of calcium in the **blood**.

Calcium is critical to cellular metabolism, as well as being the main component of bones. If too much PTH is secreted, the bones release calcium into the bloodstream. Over time, the bones become brittle and more likely to break. A person with levels of calcium in the blood that are too high feels tired, run down, irritable, and has difficulty sleeping. Additional signs of too much calcium in the blood are nausea and **vomiting**, frequent urination, **kidney stones**, and **bone pain**. A parathyroid scan is administered when the parathyroid appears to be overactive and a tumor is suspected.

Precautions

A radioactive material is used to obtain the images of the parathyroid glands, therefore patients who are pregnant are cautioned against having this test unless the benefits outweigh the risks. Women who are breast feeding will need to stop for a specified period of time depending on the particular radiopharmaceutical used. People who have had other recent nuclear medicine procedures or an x ray consisting of administration of an intravenous contrast material may need to wait until the earlier radioactive tracers or contrast media have been eliminated from their system in order to obtain accurate results from the parathyroid scan.

Description

Parathyroid scans are typically performed in either in a hospital nuclear medicine department or out-patient **radiology** facility.

A parathyroid scan can be performed using various methods, but are most commonly performed using one of two basic methods. One method uses only one radionuclide whereas the other procedure uses two radionuclides.

In either procedure, the patient is injected intravenously with a radiopharmaceutical that accumulates in certain cells within the parathyroid glands. Initial images are obtained approximately 15 minutes after the injection, and then later, at about three hours. For the procedure using two radiopharmaceuticals, separate images can be obtained simultaneously because the gamma camera has the capability to detect more than one radionuclide at a time. The equipment also has the processing capabilities to subtract one image from another, thus revealing two different sets of images used for comparison

Patients are positioned supine (lying down) under the gamma camera. The camera does not touch, but comes very close to the patient. Each set of pictures takes approximately 30 to 45 minutes.

Preparation

No special preparation is necessary for this test. There is no need to fast or maintain a special diet. The patient should wear comfortable clothing with no metal jewelry around the neck.

Aftercare

The patient should not feel any adverse effects of the test and can resume normal activities immediately.

Complications

There are no known complications associated with this test.

Results

Normal results will show no unusual activity in the parathyroid glands. An increased concentration of radioactive materials in the parathyroid glands suggests excessive activity and the presence of a tumor. False positive results sometimes result from the presence of multinodular goiter, neoplasm, or cysts. False positive tests are tests that interpret the results as abnormal when this is not true. Parathyroid scans are often paired with other imaging studies such as MRI and ultrasound to confirm a diagnosis.

Health care team roles

A parathyroid scan is performed by a nuclear medicine technologist. The technologist is trained to handle radioactive materials, administer the injections, operate the equipment, and process the data. The technologist will obtain any pertinent medical history and explain the test to the patient. The test is interpreted by a doctor who is a radiologist or nuclear medicine specialist. The patient receives the results of the test from their personal physician or the doctor who ordered the test.

Resources

BOOK

Klingensmith III, M.D., Wm. C., Dennis Eshima, Ph.D., and John Goddard, Ph.D. *Nuclear Medicine Procedure Manual 2000-2001.*

PERIODICAL.

Ishibashi, Masatoshi et al. "Comparison of Technetium-99m-MIBI, Technetium 99m-Tetrofosmin, Ultrasound, and MRI for Localization of Abnormal Parathyroid Glands." *The Journal of Nuclear Medicine* (February 1998) 320-324.

OTHER

Parathyroid Function: Normal and Abnormal. http://www.endocrine-surgery.com/function.html.

Christine Miner Minderovic, B.S., R.T., R.D.M.S.

Parentage testing

Definition

In parentage testing, an individual's DNA is used to prove or disprove his or her relatedness to a particular child.

Purpose

Parentage, or paternity, testing may be sought solely for the sake of curiosity, but is most often used to prove or disprove paternity for legal purposes. Legally motivated reasons to seek parentage testing can include contested child support, custody, or visitation rights, immigration status, adoption, and insurance or inheritance claims.

Historically, paternity testing was based on examination of the **blood** groups of the child and putative father, and the test could only exclude the possibility of relatedness when blood groups did not match; matching blood groups could not prove parentage, but only the possibility thereof. Modern testing, based on the examination of DNA, can prove with virtually 100% certainty exclusion of paternity or the probability to a certainty of 99.9% that a given person is the parent of a particular child.

Parentage testing is recommended in adoption cases, as identifying both biological parents can help the adoptive parents judge the possibility that the adopted child will develop certain inheritable medical conditions such as **cystic fibrosis**, or Tay Sachs disease. Further, as the adopted child grows to adulthood, a genetic medical history can prove useful in diagnosis of other conditions such as breast or colon **cancer** or **heart** disease. Also, paternity testing ensures that the true biological father relinquishes parental rights and negates the possibility that the adoption will be contested later.

In the infrequent but dramatic cases of babies being switched at birth, parentage testing allows unequivocal identification of parents. In surrogacy cases, DNA testing can confirm the success of the implantation procedure by verifying the identity of the biological parents.

Precautions

Currently, the vast majority of DNA testing for parentage determination is performed by commercial laboratories that are not associated with a hospital, blood bank, or medical laboratory. The focus of such facilities is often legal rather than medical. Persons seeking testing should be aware that psychological support and **genetic counseling** may be needed following parentage testing to help them deal with the implications of the results.

Many laboratories advertising paternity testing services lack any accreditation. Individuals seeking paternity testing should choose a laboratory that is accredited by the American Association of Blood Banks (AABB), which performs on site laboratory inspections to ensure that the techniques and equipment being used are acceptable and that the methods followed are consistent with the strict national standards established for paternity/parentage testing.

When blood or other body fluid is collected for DNA analysis, **universal precautions** should be observed for the prevention of transmission of bloodborne pathogens.

It is important that the parties seeking parentage testing clearly understand their own motivation for testing. Testing that includes "chain of custody" of the samples to be analyzed—notarized proof of identity of all parties being tested and traceable transport of samples from collection to the testing laboratory—is admissible as evidence in the courtroom, but costlier than testing without chain of custody. However, testing on self-collected samples for curiosity purposes, in which chain of custody protocols are not strictly followed, has no legal standing.

The DNA restriction fragment length polymorphisms (RFLPs) and short tandem repeat (STR) loci that commonly serve as identity markers are noncoding regions (i.e., DNA that is not transcribed into RNA and does not code for **proteins**). As such, the mutation rate in these sections of DNA tends to be higher than in normal genes. Also, the polymerase chain reaction (PCR) used to amplify the STRs is subject to introduction of mutations. These mutation events can complicate the interpretation of results.

Interpretation of parentage testing results are generally based on the assumption that the alleged father is not related to the actual father, which may not be true. Also, extra care is required in the interpretation of results in the case where the mother's DNA is not available for testing.

Description

Modern parentage (paternity) testing is also known as DNA testing, profiling, or fingerprinting. The dramatic evolution of DNA profiling techniques has been in the field of forensic identification, and since 1985, the technologically advanced DNA-based methodology has essentially completely displaced blood-antigen-based paternity investigation.

Restriction fragment length polymorphisms (RFLPs)

One approach to DNA fingerprinting is based on analysis of slight differences between individuals in the sequence of nucleotides, called sequence polymorphisms, in the chromosomal DNA. A sequence change can cause restriction endonucleases, enzymes used to cut the DNA into pieces small enough to analyze, to make fewer cuts in the DNA, leading to DNA fragments of different sizes called restriction fragment length polymorphisms (RFLPs). These RFLPs are well cataloged, and every person will display a given set of them upon analysis. Clusters of RFLPs tend to be consistent within ethic groups. A greater number of matches between individuals indicates a greater probability of relatedness. Each person has RFLPs inherited from both parents, and thus has a unique RFLP "fingerprint."

In a RFLP DNA analysis, 1–5 ml of blood is drawn from which about 100 ng DNA is extracted and treated with a restriction endonuclease. The DNA fragments are separated by electrophoresis on an agar or polyacrylamide gel, denatured and transferred to nitrocellulose paper, and incubated with pieces of radioactively labeled DNA probes complimentary for the RFLPs. The RFLPs that are present in a sample show up as dark bands on X-ray film exposed to the nitrocellulose sheet.

Short tandem repeats (STRs)

The current state-of-the-art approach to DNA profiling is the investigation of short tandem repeat

(STR) loci—short sequences of DNA, normally two to six base pairs that are repeated head to tail numerous times. STRs, also known as microsatellite DNA, are, like RFLPs, well characterized, and each individual carries a distinct set inherited from both parents. STRs are the result of length polymorphisms (inherited differences in the number of these short sequences) as opposed to sequence polymorphisms (inherited differences in the order of bases). The extracted DNA is subjected to amplification in the polymerase chain reaction (PCR), in which fluorescently labeled primer pieces of DNA specific for known STR sequences are incubated with appropriate enzymes and nucleotide building blocks to amplify synthesis of the STR regions of the sample DNA; only the STRs that are present in the sample DNA become amplified. The fluorescently labeled amplified STRs are then separated by gel or capillary electrophoresis, and read by a fluorescence detector. DNA fingerprinting based on STRs has the advantage of being more sensitive than tests based on RFLPs, that is, requiring only 1–5 ng of DNA extracted from a few drops of blood, or from buccal cells collected with a swab from the inside of the cheek. Further, the PCR technique, capillary electrophoresis separation, and fluorescence detection are amenable to automation, leading to faster throughput and less human error.

In 1997, the FBI announced the selection of 13 STR loci to constitute the core of a national DNA profiling database known as CODIS, which has been widely adopted by forensic DNA analysts worldwide. All CODIS STRs are discrete tetrameric repeat sequences that behave according to known principles of population genetics and can be rapidly analyzed with commercially available kits. The CODIS STR set of loci is rapidly becoming the industry standard in paternity testing. A kit that tests the 13 CODIS plus three more STR sites has recently become commercially available.

Testing procedure

The laboratories that perform parentage testing are generally commercial facilities engaged in only parentage testing. The person seeking parentage testing contacts such a laboratory to receive instructions. Generally, the appointment for sample collection is scheduled at a local medical laboratory or clinic contracted by the testing laboratory. At the time of scheduling, the names, addresses, and telephone numbers of all persons to be tested, the date of birth or approximate age of the child(ren) to be tested, the preferred day and time for the sample collection, and the name and contact information of any attorney(s) involved

Amniotic fluid—The watery fluid in the amnion, in which the embryo is suspended; the fluid contains cells of fetal origin.

Buccal—Pertaining to the cheek.

Capillary electrophoresis—A technique for separating biomolecules such as DNA in a fluid-filled thin glass tube on the basis of size and rate of migration in an electric field.

Chorionic villi—Branching outgrowths of the chorion that form the placenta in combination with maternal tissue.

DNA—Deoxyribonucleic acid, a long polymeric biomolecule composed of two self-complementary deoxyribonucleotide strands that adopt a double helical structure and become tightly coiled together with proteins to form chromosomes; DNA is the molecule that stores and transfers the genetic information in virtually all life forms.

Electrophoresis—A technique for separating biomolecules such as DNA in a gel medium on the basis of size and rate of migration in an electric field.

Nucleotide—A biomolecule composed of one of the organic nitrogen-containing bases (adenine, cytosine, guanine, or thymine), a phosphate group, and a pentose sugar that serve as the building blocks of DNA and RNA (in RNA, the thymine base is replaced by uracil).

Polymerase chain reaction (PCR)—A method used in DNA analysis whereby a specific region(s) of the DNA sequence is amplified, allowing rapid DNA analysis.

Polymorphism—The presence of two or more distinct phenotypes in a population due to the expression of different alleles of a given gene.

Restriction endonuclease—Any of a group of enzymes that catalyze the cleavage of DNA molecules at specific sites, used in recombinant DNA technology.

Short tandem repeat—A defined region of DNA, also called microsatellite DNA, containing multiple copies of short sequences of bases repeated a number of times.

is recorded. It is possible to schedule collections for different people in different locations at different times. The samples are all shipped to the testing laboratory to be analyzed simultaneously.

For testing with chain of custody, it is extremely important that everyone being tested is positively identified. For every adult person being tested, the social security number and a picture ID, such as a driver's license, passport, or state identification card, is required and for each child a birth certificate must be provided. Photographs and fingerprints of all persons may be taken at the time of sample collection. Strict chain of custody procedures must be followed, and all information and results are kept strictly confidential and are not released without proper prior authorization.

A small blood sample, usually from a finger prick, is collected from the mother, the child(ren), and alleged father(s). For newborns, the blood sample can be obtained from the umbilical cord at birth, or from a heel prick. Alternatively, cells from the inside of the mouth are collected with a buccal swab. It is also possible to arrange for prenatal testing to be performed on chorionic villi or precultured amniotic fluid cells.

Buccal swabs have become the specimen collection method of choice for DNA testing. The specimen is collected by gently stroking the inner facial cheek with the swab for 30 seconds. It is not necessary to fast before specimen collection, since buccal swab specimens are unaffected by foods, toothpaste, cigarettes, chewing tobacco, lipstick, or bacterial DNA. The collected buccal cells are still usable after years of storage. Buccal samples do not need to be refrigerated nor is immediate shipping to the laboratory required.

To extract DNA from the swab, the head of the swab is transferred to a small plastic tube containing a small amount (0.6 ml) of dilute sodium hydroxide solution (50 mM), and the stick is cut off to allow the tube to be closed (special buccal swabs with ejectable heads have recently become available). The tube is mixed and incubated for five minutes in boiling water, after which the swab head is removed, and a few drops of a buffer (0.06 ml Tris-HCL, pH 8) are added.

For curiosity testing without chain of custody, kits can be obtained for home collection of cheek cells with buccal swabs. The samples are then sent by courier to the testing laboratory.

The fee for testing, with chain of custody, one alleged father and one child, usually with or without the mother, is $400–500, and about $150 is charged for each additional person tested. The level of the fee may also depend on the number of DNA loci or systems probed; generally six to 16 loci are analyzed. Most parentage testing firms require payment of a nonrefundable deposit of $100–150 to initiate the scheduling process; this deposit is applied toward the total fee. Payment may be made by major credit card, certified check, or money order, and is unlikely to be covered by medical insurance. In most cases, the local collection facility additionally charges a specimen collection fee, typically $15–40 per person. The fee for prenatal testing can be substantially higher. Testing without chain of custody can cost $280–400, depending on whether samples are collected at home or by a clinic. Curiosity testing may be performed on samples other than collected blood or buccal cells, such as cigarette butts, chewed gum, bloodstained or semen-stained clothing, used condoms, plucked hair or electric razor debris, or Q-tips containing earwax; additional fees may apply for non-standard samples.

Preparation

No physical preparation is required. For chain of custody testing, identification documents for every person to be tested must be provided at the time of sample collection.

Aftercare

None.

Complications

None.

Results

Results are returned generally after one to two weeks, and are usually not released until all fees have been collected. Many facilities offer express service with shorter turn-around times, but with correspondingly larger fees, for example, up to about $1,500 for results returned within one working day.

The sample from the child(ren) will give rise to banding patterns on the gel or in the electropherogram reflecting bands inherited from each parent. On the basis of the banding pattern, inclusion or exclusion of parentage is decided.

The commercial parentage testing laboratories typically guarantee over 99.9% exclusion and over 99.0% inclusion of paternity. The actual numbers for the state-of-the-art testing protocols are 100% exclusion and 99.99% inclusion of parentage. For analyses in which the mother's DNA is not available for testing, the rates of inclusion can drop dramatically to 80–99% depending on the number of gene loci examined.

Health care team roles

Initial consultations and scheduling of sample collection appointments is carried out by a representative of the commercial parentage testing facility, often by telephone. A nurse, phlebotomist, or laboratory technician collects the samples and verifies documents at the locally contracted clinic or laboratory, and arranges for transport of the samples to the testing facility. At most accredited parentage testing laboratories, the sample analysis is performed by Ph.D. scientists.

Resources

PERIODICALS

Finis, C. J., Ph.D. "Megaplex STR Analysis from a Single Amplification: Validation of the PowerPlex 16 System." *Profiles in DNA* (January 2001): 3-6. *http://www. promega.com.*

Polesky, H. F., M.D. "Impact of Molecular (DNA) Testing on Determination of Parentage." *Archives of Pathology and Laboratory Medicine* 123, no. 11 (1999): 1060-1062.

Thomson, J. A., V. Pilotti, P. Stevens, k. L. Ayres, and P. G. Debenham. "Validation of Short Tandem Repeat Analysis for the Investigation of Cases of Disputed Paternity." *Forensic Science International* 100, no. 1-2 (Mar. 15, 1999): 1-16.

ORGANIZATIONS

DNA Diagnostics Center. 205 Corporate Court, Fairfield, OH 45014. (800) 613-5768. http://www.dnacenter.com/about.html.

DNA Testing Centre, Inc. 1201 W. Airport Fwy. STE 255, Euless, TX 76040. http://www.homedna-test.com.

Genetic Profiles Corporation. 6122 Nancy Ridge Drive,San Diego, CA 92121. (800) 551-7763. http://www.genetic-profiles.com.

GeneTree Inc. 3150 Almaden Expressway #203 San Jose, CA 95118-1253. (408) 723-2670. http://www.genetree.com.

The National HLA Fund, Inc. 909 Oradell Avenue, Oradell, NJ 07649-1924, http://www.nationalhlafund.org.

Patricia L. Bounds, Ph.D.

Parenteral nutrition

Definition

When patients cannot use their gastrointestinal tracts for **nutrition**, parenteral nutrition may be used to maintain or improve the patient's nutritional status. This form of intravenous treatment provides all the nutrients that are delivered to the patient. This treatment may be temporary or long-term.

Purpose

The harmful effects of malnutrition on the overall health of a patient are well documented. Poor nutrition is associated with slowed or impaired recovery from illness and surgery. For wound healing, tissue maintenance, and faster recovery, patients need optimal nutritional intake. When a patient is unable to take in enough food on his own, there are two options. Enteral feeding is preferred because it is less invasive, has a lower risk for **infection**, and is safer than the parenteral method. Though enteral feeding is the preferred route of nutritional intake, parenteral nutrition plays an important role in many clinical situations. Patients who cannot consume enough nutrients on their own, or who cannot eat at all because of an illness, surgery, or an accident, may be fed through an intravenous line.

Precautions

Patients receiving parenteral nutrition need to be monitored closely to ensure that the therapy is providing adequate amounts of fluids, **minerals**, and other nutrients that are needed. Laboratory testing will take place on a regular basis to monitor the patient's status.

Description

Parenteral nutrition, also known as hyperalimentation, is subdivided into two categories: partial parenteral nutrition and total parenteral nutrition. These categories differ by the makeup of the solutions and the site of administration.

Partial parenteral nutrition (PPN) is normally prescribed for patients who can tolerate some oral feedings but cannot ingest adequate amounts of food to meet their nutritional needs. It is usually administered through a peripheral intravenous catheter. Two types of solutions are commonly used in a number of combinations for PPN: lipid emulsions and amino acid-dextrose solutions.

Total parenteral nutrition (TPN) is given when a patient requires an extended period of intensive nutritional support. It is usually administered through a central venous catheter. TPN solutions contain high concentrations of **proteins** and dextrose. Various components like electrolytes, minerals, trace elements, and insulin are added based on the needs of the patient. Total parenteral nutrition provides the calories a patient requires and keeps the body from using protein for energy. TPN is given using an infusion pump.

Both of these types of nutrition may be administered either in a medical facility or in the patient's home. Home parenteral nutrition normally requires a central venous catheter, which must first be inserted in a fully equipped medical facility. After it is inserted, therapy can continue at home.

Preparation

The physician orders the particular PPN or TPN solution as well as any additional nutrients or drugs that should be added. The doctor also specifies the rate at which the solution will be infused. The IV (intravenous) solutions are prepared under the supervision of a doctor, pharmacist, or nurse, using techniques to prevent bacterial contamination.

In the case of home parenteral nutrition, the solution is delivered to the patient's home on a regular basis and should be kept refrigerated. The solution should be allowed to come to room temperature before it is connected to the patient.

Aftercare

Patients who have been receiving parenteral nutrition for more than a few days, and have been given permission to start eating again, should reintroduce foods gradually. This will give the digestive tract time to start functioning again.

Complications

Patients receiving PPN or TPN are at risk for a number of very serious complications. These complications may result from the IV solutions or from the central venous catheter.

Fluid imbalances may occur in patients receiving parenteral nutrition. The extreme hyperosmolarity of the solutions may cause fluid shifts in the body. This hyperosmolarity is caused by the concentrations of dextrose and amino acids. The increased levels of dextrose may cause hyperglycemia, which may in turn cause the dextrose to move into the interstitial spaces into the plasma. This can cause a series of events that may lead to **dehydration** and hypovolemic **shock**. If the patient's **heart** or **kidneys** function poorly, the situation

Parkinson's disease

KEY TERMS

Enteral nutrition—Nutrition provided by introducing nutritional substances into the intestines.

Hyperosmolarity—An increased concentration of osmotically active particles in solution.

may develop into congestive **heart failure** and pulmonary **edema**. The patient should be monitored closely for signs of these complications. Accurate records of intake and output should be maintained, and daily weights recorded. Serum electrolytes and glucose are also monitored.

Another possible complication for those receiving parenteral nutrition is a variety of electrolyte imbalances. Daily serum electrolyte levels are normally ordered to find imbalances. Sodium and potassium imbalances are seen frequently among patients receiving PPN and TPN, especially when insulin is part of the intravenous solution. Hypercalcemia may also occur, although it may be more closely associated with the hazards of immobility than the parenteral therapy itself.

Another complication associated with parenteral nutrition is infection at the site of the central venous catheter. For patients receiving long-term therapy, the risk of infections spreading to the entire body (**sepsis**) is fairly high. Measures should be taken to prevent infections at the catheter site. This includes regular sterile dressing changes, and prompt reporting of any signs of redness, swelling, or drainage.

Results

For those on short-term parenteral therapy, the goal is to provide adequate nutritional supplementation until the patient can transition back to solid foods. Patients receiving long-term therapy should have their nutritional needs met, with a goal of avoiding potential complications.

Health care team roles

A variety of members of the health care team may be involved in the decisions to order parenteral nutrition and in the care required to administer it. These include:

- physicians
- pharmacists
- dieticians
- nurses

Resources

BOOKS

Howard, Lyn. "Enteral and Parenteral Nutrition Therapy." In *Harrison's Principles of Internal Medicine.* 14th ed., Vol. 1. New York: McGraw-Hill, 1998.

Ignatavicius, Donna D., et al. *Medical-Surgical Nursing Across the Health Care Continuum.* Philadelphia: W.B. Saunders Company, 1999.

PERIODICAL

Nguyen, Hung Q., et al. "Internist's Guide to Total Parenteral Nutrition." *Internal Medicine* 21 (April 2000): 37.

Deanna M. Swartout-Corbeil, R.N.

Parkinsonism *see* **Parkinson's disease**

Parkinson's disease

Definition

Parkinson's disease (PD) is a progressive movement disorder marked by tremors, rigidity, slow movements (bradykinesia), and postural instability. It occurs when, for unknown reasons, cells in one of the movement-control centers of the **brain** begin to die.

Description

Usually beginning in a person's late 50s or early 60s, PD causes a progressive decline in movement control, affecting the ability to control initiation, speed, and smoothness of motion. Symptoms of PD are seen in up to 15% of those between the ages 65–74, and almost 30% of those between the ages 75–84.

Genetic profile

Most cases of PD are sporadic. This means that there is a spontaneous and permanent change in nucleotide sequences (the building blocks of genes). Sporadic mutations also involve unknown environmental factors in combination with genetic defects. The abnormal gene (mutated gene) will form an altered end-product or protein. This will cause abnormalities in specific areas of the body where the protein is used. Some evidence suggests that the disease is transmitted by autosomal dominant inheritance. This implies that an affected parent has a 50% chance of transmitting the disease to any child. This type of inheritance is not commonly observed. The most recent evidence links PD with a gene that codes for a protein called alpha-synuclein. Further research is attempting to fully understand the relationship with this protein and nerve cell degeneration.

Demographics

PD affects approximately 500,000 people in the United States, both men and women, with as many as 50,000 new cases being diagnosed each year.

Causes and symptoms

Causes

The immediate cause of PD is degeneration of brain cells in the area known as the substantia nigra, one of the movement control centers of the brain. Damage to this area leads to the cluster of symptoms known as parkinsonism. In PD, degenerating brain cells contain Lewy bodies, which help identify the disease. The cell death leading to parkinsonism may be caused by a number of conditions, including **infection**, trauma, and **poisoning**. Some drugs given for **psychosis**, such as haloperidol (Haldol) or chlorpromazine (Thorazine), may cause parkinsonism. When no cause for nigral cell degeneration can be found, the disorder is called idiopathic parkinsonism, or Parkinson's disease. Parkinsonism may be seen in other degenerative conditions, known as the parkinsonism plus syndromes, such as progressive supranuclear palsy.

The substantia nigra, or black substance, is one of the principal movement control centers in the brain. By releasing the neurotransmitter known as dopamine, it helps to refine movement patterns throughout the body. The dopamine released by nerve cells of the substantia nigra stimulates another brain region, the corpus striatum. Without enough dopamine, the corpus striatum cannot control its target muscles. Ultimately, the movement patterns of walking, writing, reaching for objects, and other basic programs cannot operate properly, and the symptoms of parkinsonism are the result.

There are some known toxins that can cause parkinsonism, most notoriously a chemical called MPTP, found as an impurity in some illegal drugs. Parkinsonian symptoms appear within hours of ingestion and are permanent. MPTP may exert its effects through generation of toxic molecular fragments called free radicals. Reducing free radicals has been a target of several experimental treatments for PD using antioxidants.

It is possible that early exposure to some as-yet-unidentified environmental toxin or virus leads to undetected nigral cell death, and that PD then becomes manifest as normal age-related decline brings the number of functioning nigral cells below the threshold needed for normal movement. It is also possible that, for genetic reasons, some people are simply born with fewer cells in their substantia nigra than others, and develop PD again as a consequence of normal decline.

Symptoms

The identifying symptoms of PD include:

- Tremors, usually beginning in the hands, often occurring on one side before the other. The classic tremor of PD is called a pill-rolling tremor, because the movement resembles rolling a pill between the thumb and forefinger. This tremor occurs at a frequency of about three per second.

- Slow movements (bradykinesia) occur, which may involve slowing down or stopping in the middle of familiar tasks such as walking, eating, or shaving. This may include freezing in place during movements (akinesia).

- Muscle rigidity or stiffness, occurring with jerky movements replacing smooth motion.

- Postural instability or balance difficulty occurs. This may lead to a rapid, shuffling gait (festination) to prevent falling.

- In most cases, there is a typical facial expression called masked face, characterized by little facial expression and decreased eye-blinking.

In addition, a wide range of other symptoms may often be seen, some beginning earlier than others:

- depression

- speech changes, including rapid speech without inflection changes

- problems with sleep, including restlessness and nightmares

- emotional changes, including fear, irritability, and insecurity

- incontinence

- constipation

- handwriting changes, with letters becoming smaller across the page (micrographia)

- progressive problems with intellectual function (dementia)

Diagnosis

The diagnosis of Parkinson disease involves a careful medical history and a neurological exam to look for characteristic symptoms. There are no definitive tests for PD, although a variety of lab tests may be done to rule out other causes of symptoms, especially if only some of the identifying symptoms are present. Tests for other causes of parkinsonism may include brain scans, **blood tests**, **lumbar puncture**, and x rays.

Treatment

There is no cure for Parkinson disease. Most drugs treat only the symptoms of the disease, although one drug, selegiline (Eldepryl), may slow degeneration of the substantia nigra.

Exercise, nutrition, and physical therapy

Regular, moderate **exercise** has been shown to improve motor function without an increase in medication for a person with PD. Exercise helps maintain range of motion in stiff muscles, improve circulation, and stimulate appetite. An exercise program designed by a physical therapist has the best chance of meeting the specific needs of a person with PD. A physical therapist may also suggest strategies for balance compensation and techniques to stimulate movement during slowdowns or freezes.

Good **nutrition** is important to maintenance of general health. A person with PD may lose some interest in food, especially if depressed, and may have nausea from the disease or from medications, especially those known as dopamine agonists. Slow movements may make it difficult to eat quickly, and delayed gastric emptying may lead to a feeling of fullness without having eaten much. Increasing fiber in the diet can improve constipation, soft foods can reduce the amount of needed chewing, and a prokinetic drug such as cisapride (Propulsid) can increase the movement of food through the **digestive system**.

People with PD may need to limit the amount of protein in their diets. The main drug used to treat PD, L-dopa, is an amino acid, and is absorbed by the digestive system by the same transporters that pick up other amino acids broken down from **proteins** in the diet. Limiting protein, under the direction of a physician or nutritionist, can improve the absorption of L-dopa.

No evidence indicates that vitamin or mineral supplements can have any effect on the disease other than in their improvement of general health. No antioxidants used to date have shown promise as a treatment except for selegiline, an MAO-B inhibitor. A large, carefully controlled study of **vitamin E** demonstrated that it could not halt disease progression.

Drugs

The pharmacological treatment of Parkinson disease is complex. While there are a large number of drugs that can be effective, their effectiveness varies among individuals, disease progression, and the length of time the drug has been used. Dose-related side effects may preclude the use of the most effective dose, or require the introduction of a new drug to counteract them. There are five classes of drugs currently used to treat PD.

DRUGS THAT REPLACE DOPAMINE. One drug that helps replace dopamine, levodopa (L-dopa), is the single most effective treatment for the symptoms of PD. L-dopa is a derivative of dopamine, and is converted into dopamine by the brain. It may be started when symptoms begin, or when they become serious enough to interfere with work or daily living.

L-dopa therapy usually remains effective for five years or longer. Following this, many persons develop motor fluctuations, including peak-dose dyskinesias (abnormal movements such as tics, twisting, or restlessness); rapid loss of response after dosing (known as the on-off phenomenon); and unpredictable drug response. Higher doses are usually tried, but may lead to an increase in dyskinesias. In addition, side effects of L-dopa include nausea and **vomiting**, and low **blood pressure** upon standing (orthostatic **hypotension**), which can cause **dizziness**. These effects usually lessen after several weeks of therapy.

ENZYME INHIBITORS. Dopamine is broken down by several enzyme systems in the brain and elsewhere in the body, and blocking these enzymes is a key strategy to prolonging the effect of a dose of dopamine. The two most commonly prescribed forms of L-dopa contain a drug to inhibit the amino acid decarboxylase (an AADC inhibitor), one type of enzyme that breaks down dopamine. These combination drugs are Sinemet (L-dopa plus carbidopa) and Madopar (L-dopa plus benzaseride). Controlled-release formulations also aid in prolonging the effective interval of an L-dopa dose.

The enzyme monoamine oxidase B (MAO-B) inhibitor selegiline may be given as add-on therapy for L-dopa. Research indicates selegiline may have a neuroprotective effect, sparing nigral cells from damage by free radicals. Because of this, and the fact that it has few side effects, it is also frequently prescribed early in the disease before L-dopa is begun. Entacapone (Comtan) and tolcapone (Tasmar), two inhibitors of another enzyme system called catechol-O-methyltransferase (COMT), have recently been approved for use and marketed. They effectively treat PD symptoms with fewer motor fluctuations and decreased daily L-dopa requirements.

DOPAMINE AGONISTS. Dopamine works by stimulating receptors on the surface of corpus striatum cells. Drugs that also stimulate these cells are called dopamine agonists, or DAs. DAs may be used before L-dopa therapy, or added on to avoid requirements for higher

L-dopa doses late in the disease. DAs available in the United States as of 2012, include, pramipexole (Mirapex), cabergoline (Dostinex), ropinirole (Requip), and apomorphine (Apokyn). Other dopamine agonists in use elsewhere include lisuride (Dopergine), intra-duodenal levodopa (Duodopa), rotigotine (Neurpro patch), and apomorphine. Side effects of all the DAs are similar to those of dopamine, plus confusion and hallucinations at higher doses.

ANTICHOLINERGIC DRUGS. Anticholinergics maintain dopamine balance as levels decrease. However, the side effects of anticholinergics (dry mouth, constipation, confusion, and blurred **vision**) are usually too severe in older individuals or in persons with **dementia**. In addition, anticholinergics rarely work for very long. They are often prescribed for younger people who have predominant shaking. Trihexyphenidyl (Artane) is the most commonly prescribed drug.

DRUGS WHOSE MODE OF ACTION IS UNCERTAIN. Amantadine (Symmetrel) is sometimes used as an early therapy before L-dopa is begun, and as an add-on later in the disease. Its anti-parkinsonian effects are mild, and are not seen in many persons. Clozapine (Clozaril) is effective, especially against psychiatric symptoms of late PD, including psychosis and hallucinations.

Surgery

Two surgical procedures are used for treatment of PD that cannot be controlled adequately with drug therapy. In PD, a brain structure called the globus pallidus (GPi) receives excess stimulation from the corpus striatum. In a pallidotomy, the GPi is destroyed by heat that is delivered by long thin needles inserted under anesthesia. Electrical stimulation of the GPi is another way to reduce its action. In this procedure, fine electrodes are inserted to deliver the stimulation, which may be adjusted or turned off as the response dictates. Other regions of the brain may also be stimulated by electrodes inserted elsewhere. In most persons, these procedures lead to significant improvement for some motor symptoms, including peak-dose dyskinesias. This allows a person to receive more L-dopa, since these dyskinesias are usually responsible for any upper limit on the L-dopa dose.

A third procedure, transplant of fetal nigral cells, is still highly experimental. Its benefits to date have been modest, although improvements in technique and surgical candidate selection are likely to increase successful outcomes.

Alternative treatment

Currently, the best treatments for PD involve the use of conventional drugs such as levodopa. Alternative

therapies, including **acupuncture**, massage, and **yoga**, can help relieve some symptoms of the disease and loosen tight muscles. Alternative practitioners have also applied herbal and dietary therapies, including amino acid supplementation, antioxidant (**vitamins** A, C, E, selenium, and **zinc**) therapy, B vitamin supplementation, and **calcium** and **magnesium** supplementation to the treatment of PD. Persons using these therapies in conjunction with conventional drugs should check with their doctor to avoid the possibility of adverse interactions. For example, vitamin B_6 (either as a supplement or from foods such as whole grains, bananas, beef, fish, **liver**, and potatoes) can interfere with the action of L-dopa when the drug is taken without carbidopa.

Prognosis

Despite medical treatment, the symptoms of Parkinson's disease worsen over time, and become less

QUESTIONS TO ASK YOUR DOCTOR

- What are the indications that my loved one may have Parkinson's disease?
- What diagnostic tests are needed for a thorough assessment?
- What treatment options do you recommend?
- What kind of changes can I expect to see with the medications you have prescribed?
- What are the side effects associated with the medications you have prescribed?
- Will medications for Parkinson's disease interact with other medications?
- Should we see a specialist? If so, what kind of specialist should I contact?
- If surgery is needed, what kind of surgical specialist should I contact?
- What tests or evaluation techniques will you perform to see if treatment has been beneficial for my loved one?
- What changes in health can I expect to see as the condition progresses?
- What physical or psychological limitations do you foresee?
- Will physical, occupational, speech, or respiratory therapy benefit my loved one?
- Does having Parkinson's disease put my loved one at risk for other health conditions?
- How can the quality of life of my loved one be improved?
- What research is being done to learn more about Parkinson's disease?
- What symptoms are important enough that we should seek immediate treatment?
- Can you recommend an organization that will provide me with additional information about Parkinson's disease?
- Can you refer me to a qualified person who can make an assessment of my home and recommend changes to make it safer and easier for my loved one to get around?
- Can you recommend any support groups for me and my family?

responsive to drug therapy. Late-stage psychiatric symptoms associated with the disease are often the most troubling. These include difficulty sleeping, nightmares, intellectual impairment (dementia), hallucinations, and loss of contact with reality (psychosis). As of 2012, several clinical trials are underway to explore additional treatment options for Parkinson's disease. Potential participants and individuals who want to learn more about these studies can find information through the PDtrials website at http://www.pdtrials.org/.

Health care team roles

A physician usually makes an initial diagnosis of Parkinson's disease. Treatment is often managed by a family physician or internist. Neurologists may be asked for consultations. Occasionally, neurosurgeons perform surgery in the treatment of parkinsonism. Clinical nutritionists and physical therapists may assist in managing persons with PD. Nurses provide bedside care in the hospital, and administer the frequent patient neurologic evaluations. They also provide patient and family education about the diagnosis and home management.

Prevention

There is no known way to prevent Parkinson's disease.

Resources

BOOKS

Bennett, Robin L. *The Practical Guide to the Genetic Family History,* 2nd ed. New York, NY: Wiley–Blackwell, 2010.

Chaudhuri, Ray, K., and William Ondo. *Movement Disorders in Clinical Practice.* New York, NY: Springer, 2010.

Chou, Kelvin L., Susan Grube., and Paraq Patil. *Deep Brain Stimulation: A New Life for People with Parkinson's, Dystonia and Essential Tremor.* New York, NY: Demos Health, 2012.

Donaldson, Ivan., et al. *Marsden's Book of Movement Disorders,* 2nd ed. New York, NY: Oxford University Press, 2012.

Greenberg, David., Michael Aminoff., and Roger Simon. *Clinical Neurology,* 8th ed. New York, NY: McGraw–Hill Professional, 2012.

Mehrotra, T.N., and Kalyan Bhattacharyya. *Parkinson's disease and Movement Disorders.* New York, NY: Jaypee Import, 2008.

Schaaf, Christian., Johannes Zschocke, and Lorraine Potocki. *Human Genetics: From Molecules to Medicine.* New York, NY: Lippincott Williams&Wilkins, 2011.

Wellstead, Peter., and Mathieu Cloutier, eds. *Systems Biology of Parkinson's.* New York, NY: Springer, 2012.

PERIODICALS

Bogart, Kathleen Rives. "Is apathy a valid and meaningful symptom or syndrome in Parkinsons disease? A critical review." *Health Psychology* 30.4 (2011): 386–400.

"Drugs for treating Parkinson disease." *Nursing* (July 2012): 69.

Dwolatzky, Tzvi. "Cognitive Impairment and Dementia in Parkinson's Disease." *JAMA, The Journal of the American Medical Association* 305.21 (2011): 2232.

Foltynie, T. "Novel treatments for Parkinson's disease." *Journal of Neurology, Neurosurgery and Psychiatry* 82.8 (2011): E2.

"Living with Parkinson's disease involves 'more than motion'." *Journal of Gerontological Nursing* (July 2012): 7.

McKeith, I. "Parkinson's disease and Lewy body disease: the same or different?" *Journal of Neurology, Neurosurgery and Psychiatry* 82.8 (2011): E2.

Mizuno, Yoshikuni. "An update on the management of juvenile and young-onset Parkinson's disease." *Future Neurology* 7.5 (2012): 581.

O'Sullivan, S. "Impulsive and compulsive behaviours in Parkinson's disease." *Journal of Neurology, Neurosurgery and Psychiatry* 82.8 (2011): E2.

Tarsy, Daniel. "Treatment of Parkinson Disease." *JAMA, The Journal of the American Medical Association* 307.21 (2012): 2305.

OTHER

American Academy of Family Physicians. http://www.aafp.org/afp/990415ap/2155.html.

National Institute of Neurological Diseases and Stroke. http://www.ninds.nih.gov/disorders/parkinsons_disease/parkinsons_disease.htm.

National Library of Medicine. http://www.nlm.nih.gov/medlineplus/parkinsonsdisease.html.

Parkinson's Disease Guide. http://www.pdring.com.

PDtrials. http://www.pdtrials.org/.

World Parkinson Disease Association. http://www.wpda.org.

ORGANIZATIONS

American Academy of Neurology. 1080 Montreal Avenue, St. Paul, Minnesota 55116. (651) 695-1940. Fax: (651) 695- 2791. info@aan.org. http://www.aan.com.

American Academy of Physical Medicine and Rehabilitation. 9700 West Bryn Mawr Avenue, Suite 200, Rosemont, PA 60018-5701, (847) 737-6000. http://www.aapmr.org.

American College of Physicians. 190 N. Independence Mall West, Philadelphia, PA 19106-1572. (800) 523-1546. http://www.acponline.org.

American Neurological Association. 5841 Cedar Lake Road, Suite 204, Minneapolis, MN 55416. Telephone: (952) 545- 6284. http://www.aneuroa.org.

American Parkinson Disease Association. Inc. 135 Parkinson Avenue Staten Island, NY 10305. (800) 223-2732. http://www.apdaparkinson.org.

American Physical Therapy Association. 1111 North Fairfax Street, Alexandria, VA 22314-1488. Telephone: (800) 999-APTA (2782) or (703) 684-APTA (2782). TDD: (703) 683-6748. http://www.apta.org.

National Institute of Neurological Disorders and Stroke (NINDS). P.O. Box 5801, Bethesda, MD 20828, (301) 496-5751. TTY: (301) 468-5981, (800) 352-9424. http://www.ninds.nih.gov.

National Institutes of Health (NIH). 9000 Rockville Pike, Bethesda, MD 20892. (301) 496-4000. http://www.nih.gov.

National Institutes of Health Genetic and Rare Diseases Information Center (GARD). PO Box 8126, Gaithersburg, MD 20898-8126. Telephone: (301) 251-4925. Fax: (301) 251-4911. Tollfree phone: (888) 205-2311. http://rarediseases.info.nih.gov/GARD/Default.aspx.

National Parkinson Foundation. 1501 N.W. 9th Avenue / Bob Hope Road, Miami, Florida 33136-1494. (800) 473-4636. http://www.parkinson.org/home.aspx.

Parkinson's Disease Foundation. 1359 Broadway, Suite 1509, New York, NY 10018. (212) 923-4700. http://www.pdf.org.

Parkinson's Disease Society (UK). 215 Vauxhall Bridge Road, London SW1V 1EJ. (020) 7931-8080. http://www.parkinsons.org.uk.

U.S. National Library of Medicine, 8600 Rockville Pike, Bethesda, MD 20894. http://www.nlm.nih.gov/medlineplus/medlineplus.html.

Worldwide Education and Awareness for Movement Disorders. One Gustave L. Levy Place, Box 1052, New York, NY 10029. (800) 437-6683. http://www.wemove.org.

L. Fleming Fallon, Jr., MD, Dr.PH
Laura Jean Cataldo, RN, Ed.D.

Parotid gland scan *see* **Salivary gland scan**

Partial thromboplastin time *see* **Coagulation tests**

Paternity testing *see* **Parentage testing**

Patient-controlled analgesia

Definition

Patient-controlled analgesia (PCA) is a system of providing **pain** medication that allows the patient to self-administer synthetic, opium-like pain-relievers (opioids) on an "as-needed" basis, but only within the limit of a maximum dose every eight (or twelve) hours. A pump-type device delivers the medicine into the veins (intravenously, the commonest of the three methods), under the skin (subcutaneously), or between the dura mater and the **skull** (epidurally). A health care provider programs the device both with the specific dosage to deliver at each request made by the patient and with the total permitted during the time for which the device is set (commonly eight hours, sometimes 12, especially if the health care providers are working 12-hour shifts). Some of these devices are very sophisticated and even monitor themselves and ring an alarm-bell if there is an indication that they might be malfunctioning.

Purpose

The purpose of PCA is improved pain control. PCA allows for immediate delivery of pain medication without the delay that would occur if a nurse, busy with many other patients on the floor, must answer the patient's buzzer or other signal. (It is not as needed if the patient has a full-time, private-duty nurse in the room every minute.) PCA also allows more frequent but smaller doses and thus a more even level of the painkiller in the patient's body. The busy nurse must administer larger doses at one time. Unfortunately, these larger doses peak shortly after administration, often causing undesirable side-effects such as nausea and difficulty in breathing. Their effect often wears off before the next dose is scheduled.

Precautions

Using such a pump requires an understanding of how to work it and the physical strength to do so (usually by pressing a button). Therefore, PCA should not be offered to patients who are confused, unresponsive, or paralyzed. Patients with neurologic disease or head injuries in whom narcotics would mask neurologic changes are not eligible for PCA. Patients with poor kidney or lung function are usually not good candidates for PCA, unless they are monitored very closely.

PCA may be used by children as young as seven years old. It has proven safe and successful in such children in the control of postoperative pain, sickle-cell pain, and pain associated with bone-marrow transplantation.

Whenever opium-like painkillers are administered to the elderly patient, the health care professional must keep several things in mind: older adults may be more susceptible to side effects of narcotics because their **heart**, **liver**, and **kidneys** work less well than when they were younger. The elderly may also clear the narcotic out of their system more slowly. If the pump's timing device is calibrated for the typical younger person's rate of eliminating the drug, the elderly patient, who still has much of an earlier dose in the bloodstream, could accidentally receive an **overdose**. The health care provider should calculate the doses more conservatively for such elderly patients.

Description

PCA uses a computerized pump that delivers a drug in small doses controlled by the patient. The same pump may also be programmed to deliver a large initial dose, or

a steady, even flow of pain medications. The large initial dose or the steady flow is, of course, not patient-controlled analgesic at all, but the same pump can deliver the drug in these two ways when it is not advisable for the patient to control the medication.

The patient presses a button when medication is desired. When this button is pressed, some sound (usually a beep) is heard, indicating that the pump is working properly and that the button was pressed correctly. The nurse should instruct the patient to call a health care provider if the pump doesn't beep (or if its alarm sounds). The painkillers most commonly used in PCA pumps are morphine and meperidine (Demerol). The pump delivers the medication through a plastic tube (the line) and a needle.

The pump may be set to deliver a larger initial dose of the drug (for example, 2 mg of morphine delivered one time only). The health care provider sets the pump to deliver a specified dose on demand with a lock-out time (for example, 1 mg of morphine on demand, but not more frequently than one dose every six minutes). If the patient presses the button before six minutes have elapsed, the pump will not administer the medication. It also generates a record which the health personnel can read to discover that the patient has indeed been pushing the button more frequently than every six minutes. An around-the-clock, even dose may also be set. The practitioner sets a total limit for an hour (or other period) that takes into account the initial dose, the demand doses, and the around-the-clock doses. The pump's computerized controls calculate all these amounts nicely, make a record of the requests it received, of the requests it refused, and even keep inventory and warn the staff when the supply of the drug is getting low.

Here is an example of how a nurse might program the pump. A patient has a prescription for a maximum of 11 mg of morphine an hour. The nurse sets the machine to deliver 1 mg at the beginning of the hour, and 1 mg on demand with a six-minute lock-out. There are 10 six-minute periods in an hour, so the patient could request and receive 10 mg. If he or she pressed the button every three minutes for a total of 20 times, the machine would deliver the same 1 mg every six minutes for the same total of 10 mg as if the patient had conscientiously cooperated with the prescription. The patient who pushed the button only three times for a total of 3 mg would probably be congratulated by the health professionals for being well on the way to recovery and therefore not needing as much pain medication. The nurse might program the machine to give an initial 2 mg, to give 3 additional mg at a steady rate throughout the hour (one twentieth of a mg every minute). That would use up 5 mg of the patient's 11 mg. That in turn leaves 6 mg on demand throughout the hour. There are six 10-minute periods in one hour, so the lock-out time would be 10 minutes.

Preparation

When preparing to initiate PCA, the nurse must assess the patient to determine that PCA is indeed applicable in this case and must then set the total dose and the timings as prescribed by the physician. The small amount of drug prescribed (3,000 doses of 10 mg each weigh less than 1 oz total) would not be sufficient to keep the plastic tube (the line) and the needle through which the drug moves from the pump into patient from clogging and the contents from coagulating. Therefore, the drug must be administered in a solution that will flush out the tube and needle (a flush solution), keep them open, and permit rapid administration The flush solution may also be used if the patient has a reaction to the opioid, to keep the line open for administration of other medication. For example, a patient may have a bad reaction to the painkilling drug and thus need counteractive medication in a great hurry. The flush solution can also help keep the patient from becoming dehydrated. Likewise, many painkillers prescribed (such as morphine sulfate) are solid crystals at room temperature, and hence would have to be dissolved in some fluid in any event.

When entering the settings into the system, the nurse must pay close attention to the physician's orders to ensure that the correct medication is used (there are different painkilling drugs), that the concentration of the drug in the flushing solution is correct, that the dose of the drug itself is correct, that lock-out time is appropriate, and that the total hourly limit is properly entered into the pump's computerized controls. To eliminate the risk of incorrect programming, many institutions have adopted policies that require verification by an RN witness for all programming. That is, everything must be checked by a second nurse, and both must sign the written record.

Another important aspect of PCA is **patient education**. The settings on the PCA pump must be explained to patients so that they understand how and when medications will be available. The nurse should observe the patients as they first start using the button, should ensure that the equipment is functioning properly, and that the patients understand their role in the process and are carrying it out correctly.

Aftercare

While using PCA, patients should be assessed frequently to ensure that they are not being excessively sedated, that they are breathing enough, that the control of their pain remains effective, and that no dangerous side-effects to the medication arise. The nurse must also check regularly to see that the line and needle delivering the drug in the flush solution remain open and thus to enure that the medication is really getting into the patients, not merely into the line, as programmed.

Complications

Problems that may occur with PCA include allergic reactions to the medications and adverse side-effects such as nausea, a dangerous drop in the rate and effectiveness of breathing, and excessive sedation. The device must be monitored frequently to prevent tampering by the patient or family. Many patients would love to change that 10-mg-an-hour maximum to 100. Even sophisticated devices that monitor themselves and sound an alarm when there are indications of something wrong should be checked, since no such machine is perfect. Ineffective pain control must be assessed to determine whether the problem stems from inadequate dosage or from inability, or unwillingness, of the patient to obey the rules.

Results

The goal of patient-controlled analgesia is pain control enhanced by a more stable and constant level of the painkiller in the patient's body than the peaks and valleys often found in the presence of the drug in the body when a nurse administers, for example, only one dose in one hour. PCA also gives the patient some control in an unfamiliar and uncomfortable situation where so much else depends on the actions of others. When administered properly, and with watchful assessment by health care providers, PCA can be a safe alternative to traditional methods of relieving pain.

Interestingly enough, studies have shown that when patients control their painkilling medication, most of them use less pain medication overall than similar patients who have nurse-administered painkillers.

Health care team roles

The nurse has a great responsibility with PCA, first of all to ensure that the pump is set and filled correctly and that the tube or line delivering the medication remains open. While PCA is in use, the nurse has an ongoing responsibility to assess the patient's level of pain, to monitor the patient's **vital signs**, and to check for any indications that the system is not working properly, or that the dose and settings may be inappropriate for the patient.

Patient education

Patient education is an extremely important part of PCA. The patient must be taught about the different settings on the PCA pump. Most pumps lock so that

KEY TERMS

Analgesia—A medicine that relieves pain.

Basal infusion—An around-the-clock, or continuous, even dose of a medication. It is one possible setting on a PCA pump.

Bolus—A large, one-time-only initial dose of medication. A bolus is usually given only when PCA is initiated, but it may also be given if pain is uncontrolled with the basal and on-demand settings.

Demand dose—A dose of painkiller that is given when the patient requests it by pressing a button which activates a pump.

Lock-out time—The minimum amount of time (usually expressed in minutes) after one dose of pain-medication on demand is given before the patient is allowed to receive the next dose on demand.

Opiate—A drug which contains opium or an alkaloid derived from opium.

Opioid—A synthetic drug resembling opium or alkaloids of opium.

Respiratory depression—Decreased rate (number of breaths per minute) and depth (how much air is inhaled with each breath) of breathing It is an undesired side-effect of many opioids. It leads to insufficient oxygen in the body. It can be very severe, even leading to death.

Sedation—A side-effect of many opioids that can range from a feeling of slight tiredness to semiconsciousness.

patients and family members cannot tamper with them. However, patients may need to be reminded that the settings programmed have been determined by their physician to be safe for them and that altering those settings may result in complications. A large, unauthorized overdose could result in death. On the other hand, patients who fear that the pump may give them an overdose should be reassured by information about the lock-out and hour limit settings.

Resources

BOOKS

Lehne, Richard A. *Pharmacology for Nursing Care.* 3rd ed. Philadelphia: W. B. Saunders Company, 1998.

Potter, Patricia A., and Anne G. Perry. *Fundamentals of Nursing Concepts, Process, and Practice.* 4th ed. St. Louis, MO: Mosby, 1997.

PERIODICAL

Eade, Diane M., R.N. "Patient-controlled Analgesia—Eliminating Errors." *Nursing Management* 28, no. 6 (June 1997): 38–40.

ORGANIZATIONS

American Association of Nurse Anesthetists/AANA. 222 South Prospect Avenue, Park Ridge, IL 60068-4001. (847) 692-7050. Fax: (847) 692-6968. info@aana.com. http://www.aana.com.

American Association of Nurse Anesthetists/AANA, Federal Government Affairs Office. 412 1st Street, SE—Suite 12, Washington, DC 20003. (202) 484-8400. Fax: (202) 484-8408. info@aanadc.com.

American Society of Anesthesiologists/ASA. 520 North Northwest Highway, Park Ridge, IL 60068-2573. (847) 825-5586. Fax: (847) 825-1692. mail@asahq.org.

American Society of PeriAnesthesia Nurses/ASPAN. 10 Melrose Avenue, Suite 110, Cherry Hill, NJ 08003-3696. (877) 737-9696 (toll-free). Fax: (856) 616-9601. aspan@aspan.org. http://www.aspan.org.

The National Hospice and Palliative Care Organization/NHPCO. 1700 Diagonal Road, Suite 300, Alexandria, VA 22314. (703) 837-1500. info@nhpco.org.

Jennifer Lee Losey, R.N.

Patient charts *see* **Medical charts**

Patient confidentiality

Definition

Confidentiality is the right of an individual patient to have personal, identifiable medical information kept private; such information should be available only to the physician of record and other health care and insurance personnel as necessary.

Description

Patient confidentiality means that personal and/or medical information given to a health care provider will not be disclosed to others unless the patient has given **informed consent**. This is becoming extremely difficult to ensure in an age of electronic **medical records** and third-party insurance payers.

Viewpoints

Because the disclosure of personal information could cause professional or personal problems, patients rely on physicians to keep their medical information private. It is rare for medical records to remain completely sealed, however. The most benign breach of confidentiality takes place when clinicians share medical information as case studies. When this data is published in professional journals the identity of the patient is never divulged, and all identifying data is either eliminated or changed. If this confidentiality is breached in any way, patients may have the right to sue.

The greatest threat to medical privacy, however, occurs because most medical bills are paid by some form of health insurance, either private or public. This makes it difficult, if not impossible, to keep information truly confidential. Health records are routinely viewed not only by physicians and their staffs, but by insurance companies, **medical laboratories**, **public health** departments, researchers, and many others. If health insurance is provided by an employer, they also may have access to their employees' files.

Professional implications

The American Medical Association (AMA) encourages doctors to guard their patients' privacy despite the widespread use electronic health records. The organization advises its members to get patient consent for any and all releases of medical information, and recommends that all office personnel and consultants be aware of the paramount importance of maintaining confidentiality. Such policies must be in place, especially in care institutions, in order to maintain Joint Commission on Accreditation of Healthcare Organizations (JCAHO) accreditation. Most confidentiality releases identify the types of information that can be released, the people and/or groups that have been permitted access to the information, and limit the length of time for which the release is valid.

Despite these safeguards, unfortunately, patient confidentiality has eroded with the almost-complete dominance of health-maintenance organizations and other types of third-party payers. In light of this, the medical profession must remain constantly vigilant that their patients' right to privacy is upheld. Confidentiality is essential for a good relationship between patient and practitioner, whose duty to keep information private dates from the Hippocratic Oath. If personal information is disseminated without the patient's permission, it can erode confidence in the medical profession and expose health care professionals to legal action.

Physicians are increasingly being sued by patients whose information has been released without their permission, as the following legal cases show. Even though the plaintiffs do not always prevail, the costs of legal action are burdensome to both sides:

• *Estate of Behringer* v. *Princeton Medical Center*, 592 A.2d 1251 (N.J. Super. Ct. Law Div. 1991). The late

KEY TERM

Joint Commission on Accreditation of Healthcare Organizations (JCAHO)—The accrediting organization that evaluates nearly 20,000 U.S. health care organizations and programs. Accreditation is maintained with onsite surveys every three years; laboratories are surveyed every two years.

Behringer, a surgeon who worked at Princeton Medical Center, was diagnosed with and treated for AIDS at the same hospital. Behringer's chart, which included several references to his diagnosis, was kept at the nurses' station on his floor with no special protection. His condition became widely known as a result, and the hospital began requiring his patients to sign a form acknowledging the risk to their health. Ultimately, the doctor's surgical privileges were suspended. Behringer's estate sued the hospital for its failure to take reasonable steps to protect his privacy. The hospital was found to have breached confidentiality by leaving the chart out in the open, but the court said they did not discriminate against Dr. Behringer by requiring his patients' informed consent.

• *Velazquez* v. *St. Clare's Hospital*, (Kings County Supreme Court, New York, 1994). Nydia Velazquez was admitted to St. Clare's Hospital in 1991 after attempting suicide. In 1992, while she was running for election to U.S. House of Representatives, copies of her medical records were faxed anonymously to several newspapers, which ran them in front-page stories. It was never determined whether hospital personnel were responsible for the disclosure. Regardless, Velazquez sued the hospital for breach of contractual and fiduciary duties of confidentiality, for wrongful disclosure, and for negligence in maintenance of the security of her medical records. She won both the seat in Congress and the lawsuit.

• *Doe* v. *Methodist Hospital*, 690 N.E.2d 681 (26 Med. L. Rptr. 1289 (1997)), Hancock County Superior Court, Indiana. According to the filed complaint, Doe, a postal worker who was HIV positive, disclosed his HIV status to paramedics when he was taken to the hospital after a heart attack. The paramedics noted his status on their report, which became part of Doe's medical file. Several coworkers eventually learned of his condition and discussed his HIV status. They were sued, along with the hospital and some of its employees, for invasion of privacy and other wrongful conduct. The court found that Doe's privacy had not been invaded, nor had he been slandered or libeled.

Legal framework

Each state, and the federal government, has enacted laws to protect the confidentiality of health care information generally, with particular attention paid to information about communicable diseases and mental health. For example, through the 1960s substance and alcohol abuse were treated as mental illnesses, with patient confidentiality determined by the laws in each state, since at the time the state was responsible for mental health care and treatment.

In the early 1970s, however, the rising numbers of those needing **substance abuse** treatment came to the attention of the federal government, because drug-related activity, including the treatment for substance abuse, could be the basis for criminal prosecution on a federal level. Congress concluded that this might stop many who needed treatment from seeking it. They enacted a strict confidentiality law to limit disclosure of information that could reveal a patient's identity.

Confusion ensued when practitioners who were treating substance abusers were required to follow two practices for patient confidentiality—one mandated by the state, the other dictated by the federal government. With the varying degrees of protection provided by state mental health laws, the confusion grew further still. While all states specify exceptions to confidentiality, few have spelled out the necessary elements of valid consent for disclosure of mental health information. Some states allow disclosure of the following types of mental health information without client consent:

• disclosures to other treatment providers

• disclosures to health care services payers or other sources of financial assistance to the patient

• disclosures to third parties that the mental health professional feels might be endangered by the patient

• disclosures to researchers

• disclosures to agencies charged with oversight of the health care system or the system's practitioners

• disclosures to families under certain circumstances

• disclosures to law enforcement officials under certain circumstances

• disclosures to public health officials

Providers are increasingly concerned that these exceptions are not addressed uniformly, particularly when providers and payers do business across state lines. This results in open-ended disclosures that specify neither the parties to whom disclosure is to be made nor the specific information allowed to be revealed.

QUESTIONS TO ASK YOUR DOCTOR

• What can I do to protect my privacy and my personal health information?

• What laws do hospitals need to comply with in order to maintain patient confidentiality and protect my health information?

• What steps do you employ in your office to maintain patient confidentiality?

• How have the guidelines and regulations associated with patient confidentiality impacted your delivery of medical care?

The critical nature of confidentiality

Both the ethical and the legal principles of confidentiality are rooted in a set of values regarding the relationship between caregiver and patient. It is essential that a patient trust a caregiver so that a warm and accepting relationship may develop; this is particularly true in a mental health treatment.

Resources

BOOKS

Amatayakul, Margret. *Process Improvement with Electronic Health Records: A Stepwise Approach to Workflow and Process Management.* New York, NY: Productivity Press, 2012.

Beaver, Kevin., and Rebecca Herold. *The Practical Guide to HIPAA Privacy and Security Compliance,* 2nd ed. Boca Raton, FL: Auerbach Publications, 2011.

Carter, Patricia I. *HIPAA Compliance Handbook, 2012.* New York, NY: Aspen Publishers, 2011.

Luepker, Ellen T. *Record Keeping in Psychotherapy and Counseling: Protecting Confidentiality and the Professional Relationship,* 2nd ed. New York, NY: Routledge, 2012.

Moss, Bernard. *Communication Skills in Health and Social Care,* 2nd ed. Thousand Oaks, CA: Sage Publications Ltd, 2012.

Nicholls, Kathy. *Stedman's Guide to the HIPAA Privacy & Security Rules,* 2nd ed. New York, NY: Lippincott Williams &Wilkins, 2011.

OTHER

American Medical Association. "Patient Confidentiality." http://www.ama-assn.org/ama/pub/category/4610.html.

Hall, Christine. "Congress Fights Over Clinton Health ID Number." http://newsmax.com/archives/articles/2001/8/15/155946.shtml.

National Academy of Sciences. "For the Record: Protecting Electronic Health Information." http://www.nap.edu/readingroom/books/for/index.html.

ORGANIZATIONS

American Health Information Management Association (AHIMA). 233 N. Michigan Avenue, 21st Floor, Chicago, IL 60601-5809. Telephone: (312) 233-1100. http://www.ahima.org/Default.aspx.

Healthcare Information and Management Systems (HIMSS). 33 West Monroe Street, Suite 1700, Chicago, IL 60603-5616. Telephone: (312) 664-6143. http://www.himss.org/ASP/index.asp

Jacqueline N. Martin, M.S.
Amy Loerch Strumolo
Laura Jean Cataldo, RN, Ed.D.

Patient education

Definition

Patient education involves helping patients become better informed about their condition, medical procedures, and choices they have regarding treatment. Nurses typically have opportunities to educate patients during bedside conversations or by providing prepared pamphlets or handouts. Patient education is important to enable individuals to better care for themselves and make informed decisions regarding medical care.

Description

Patients acquire information about their condition in a variety of ways: by discussing their condition with health professionals; by reading written materials or watching films made available in hospitals or doctors' offices; through specific health care organizations, such as the American **Cancer** Association; and through drug advertisements on television and in popular magazines. With the explosion of information on the World Wide Web, patients can access a wide range of medical information, from professional medical journals to on-line support and chat groups with a health focus.

Patients may wish to ask their health practitioners questions about **evidence-based practice**, and about prior process and outcomes, in reference to proposed treatment options and their plan of care.

Viewpoints

Being informed about one's health care options is essential to a patient's health and well-being. Especially

with the increase in managed care, in which economics and efficiency is sometimes paramount, patients may be able to obtain better health care if they are knowledgeable and assertive about their needs and wishes. Informed patients may benefit, for example, by realizing they have a choice of a variety of medications, a variety of treatments, and of various lifestyle patterns that may impact or affect their condition.

Professional implications

Professional health care givers have traditionally borne the responsibility for patient education. In recent years, however, patients independently have easy access to a wide range of health information. However, many patients cannot easily obtain information, especially if they are not well educated or are not fluent in English. In addition, many patients may not understand enough about their condition to ask relevant questions. Finally, a significant amount of popular information is inaccurate or publicized for a profit motive rather than for education purposes. Patients may not be able to sort out what is true or what is relevant to their own condition.

Another relatively recent aspect of patient education centers around legal ramifications. When a patient is fully informed about the risks and benefits of a particular procedure or therapeutic approach, the likelihood of a lawsuit resulting from a complication is sharply reduced. A patient must be made aware of risks before accepting treatment.

Nurses play an important role in providing health education. They are often the best sources of information regarding caring for patients, such as learning to breast feed, soothing fussy babies, or staying comfortable in the hospital. They may be more accessible than doctors, both because they may spend more time with patients, and because patients may feel less intimidated by nurses and more comfortable asking questions and sharing fears. It is

QUESTIONS TO ASK YOUR DOCTOR

- What changes in the delivery of patient education have been integrated into your medical practice?

- What research is being done to expand options in receiving patient education?

- How has the enhancement of patient education impacted your delivery of medical care?

important that nurses do not provide information they are unsure about, or falsely reassure patients about their condition.

Resources

BOOKS

Barr, Donald A., MD, Ph.D. *Introduction to U.S. Health Policy: The Organization, Financing, and Delivery of Health Care in America.* 3rd ed., Baltimore, MD: The Johns Hopkins University Press, 2010.

Brown, Sara Jo.*Evidence-Based Nursing: The Research-Practice Connection,* 2nd ed. New York, NY: Jones & Bartlett Learning, 2010.

Carley, Maura Loughlin, MPH, CIC.*Health Insurance: Navigating Traps &Gaps.* Chicago, IL: Ampersand, Inc., 2012.

Melnyk, Bernadette M., and Ellen Fineout-Overholt. *Evidence-Based Practice in Nursing & Healthcare: A Guide to Best Practice,*2nd ed. New York, NY: Lippincott Williams & Wilkins, 2010.

Rubin, Allen., and Jennifer Bellamy. *Practitioner's Guide to Using Research for Evidence-Based Practice,* 2nd ed. New York, NY: Wiley, 2012.

PERIODICALS

Rubsamen, David S. "Calibrate Informed Consent to Suit Patient's Need." Physicians Financial News.

Wofford, James L., M.D., M.S., Dorothy Currin, M. P. H., Robert Michielutte, Ph.D., and Marcia M. Wofford, M.D. The Multi-Media Computer for Low-Literacy Patient Education: A Pilot Project of Cancer Risk Perceptions.

ORGANIZATIONS

Agency for Healthcare Research and Quality, Office of Communications and Knowledge Transfer, 540 Gaither Road, Suite 2000, Rockville, MD 20850. Telephone: (301) 427-1104. http://www.ahrq.gov

Association of State and Territorial Directors of Health Promotion and Public Health Education. 750 First St., NE, Suite 1050, Washington, DC 20002. (202) 312-6460. http://www.astdhpphe.org.

Centers for Disease Control and Prevention (CDC). 1600 Clifton Road, Atlanta, GA 30333. http://www.cdc.gov.

U.S. Department of Health and Human Services (USDHHS), Office of Disease Prevention and Health Promotion. 1101 Wootton Parkway, Suite LL100, Rockville, MD 20852. (240) 453-8280. http://odphp.osophs.dhhs.gov/Default.asp.

ORGANIZATIONS

National Institutes of Health (NIH), 9000 Rockville Pike, Bethesda, MD 20892, (301) 496-4000, http://www.nih.gov/index.html

U.S. National Library of Medicine, 8600 Rockville Pike, Bethesda, MD 20894, http://www.nlm.nih.gov/.

Jacqueline N. Martin, M.S.
Laura Jean Cataldo, RN, Ed.D.

Patient representation

Definition

Patient representation is the involvement of an individual or group to protect the best interests of the patient in the medical system.

Description

Many definitions are offered for patient representation, ranging from one individual acting as a guardian or liaison for an individual patient to organized groups within hospitals and society that campaign for preservation of patient's rights and improved patient safety. Patient representation also may be called patient advocacy.

In the past, patients often followed any advice given by the physician and asked no questions. Many events have changed this way of thinking. Some of the suggested causes for change are managed care, consumers who are more well informed due to available information from the Internet and other sources, and increased concern about medical errors. The 1997 Convention on Human Rights and Biomedicine saw respect for a patient's autonomy as key to supporting patient's human rights within the health care context. In 1999, the Institute of Medicine released a report titled *To Err Is Human: Building a Safer Health Care System.* The report included findings that at least 44,000 people, and as many as 98,000 people, die in hospitals each year as a result of medical errors.

Many health care institutions have created patient representatives to serve as liaisons between patients and family members and the institution's staff. They may help ensure timely investigation of complaints and oversee quality improvement activities. In other institutions, patient representation is considered a new way of thinking as providers are educated on concepts such as "patient-centered care.". Some adopt a "Patient's Bill of Rights," which reminds staff of their responsibilities regarding patient interests and rights. A formal bill of the same name was introduced into the U.S. Senate in 2004 in an attempt to advance rights of enrollees in **managed care plans**. Educating providers about compassionate care, cultural competency, and speaking out for patients has been emphasized more in recent years as part of patient representation.

The 2005 case of Terri Schiavo, in which the woman with **brain** damage had failed to put her wishes concerning end-of-life decisions in writing, led to extended court battles between family members and international attention. It also has increased emphasis on advance directives and durable powers of attorney. When a patient does not express his or her wishes with advance directives, a patient guardian or advocate often is appointed to act on behalf of the patient as an intermediary between health care providers and even family members.

Informed consent is an example of formal, required patient representation. It is a process of informing patients of medical procedure risks.

In the United States and other countries, councils, organizations, and local efforts continue to form to address issues related to patient safety, autonomy, end-of-life matters, and disease-specific advocacy. Whether patient representation is formal, informal, individual or collective, it is an important emerging development in health care.

Viewpoints

Some traditional physicians and those involved in the **medical ethics** debate may argue that physicians still know what is best for the patient and that sometimes it is more kind to withhold information, such as when a patient is dying. However, people involved in advocating for patients believe that while empathy and compassion are important, commitment to the truth is equally important. Proponents of patient advocacy and patient-centered care say that the benefits are numerous to the patient, who will feel empowered. But they say it also benefits the provider to work in cooperation with an informed patient. Patient advocacy may reduce legal risks and litigation, improve job satisfaction for health care professionals, and improve overall quality of medicine.

Professional implications

When an individual health care professional serves in the role of patient representative, he or she often feels "caught in the middle." Being an advocate for patients carries an inherent risk of confronting other parties within a facility or the medical field. For example, a nurse who serves as patient representative in her hospital may have to confront a physician concerning a patient's complaints.

For health care professionals who take a more patient-centered approach, advocating for patients brings many benefits, including job satisfaction and improved patient care. However, the staff member who speaks up about problems within a health care institution that negatively affects one or all patients may feel threatened unless the entire organization adopts a "patient first" attitude. In the broadest sense, patient representation may change how some providers interact with patients, eventually leading to improved patient care, outcomes, and patient safety throughout society as advocacy organizations work as a collective voice to improve the patient experience.

Resources

BOOKS

Allen, James. *Health Law and Medical Ethics.* Upper Saddle River, NJ: Prentice Hall, 2012.

Herring, Jonathan. *Medical Law and Ethics,* 4th ed. New York, NY: Oxford, 2012.

Mason, Diana J., et al.*Policy &Politics in Nursing and Health Care,*6th ed. New York, NY: Saunders, 2011.

Moss, Bernard. *Communication Skills in Health and Social Care,*2nd ed. Thousand Oaks, CA: Sage Publications Ltd, 2012.

Schimpff, Stephen C., MD.*The Future of Health-Care Delivery: Why It Must Change and How It Will Affect You.* Dulles, VA: Potomac Books Inc, 2012.

PERIODICALS

Ashley, Ruthe C. "Why Are Advance Directives Legally Important?" Critical Care Nurse (Aug. 2005):56.

Baldwin, MA. "Patient Advocacy: A Concept Analysis." Nursing Standard (Feb. 5, 2003):33-39.

Church, Elizabeth J. "Patient Advocacy: The Technologist's Role." Radiologic Technology (March/April 2004): 272-292.

Goeltz, Roxanne J. "Be a Partner in Your Health Care." FDA Consumer (May-June 2003):40.

Smith, Alison P. "Patient Advocacy: Roles for Nurses and Leaders." Nursing Economics (March-April 2004):88-90.

Smith, Nick. "GP Business: New Patient Representation Forums Arrive." GP (Dec. 1, 2003):22.

Stein, Patricia. "Pushing Through Barriers to Advocate for a Patient." AORN Journal (Sept. 2004):553-558.

ORGANIZATIONS

Consumers Advancing Patient Safety. 405 N. Wabash Ave., Suite P2W, Chicago, IL 60611. (312) 464-0602. http://www.patientsafety.org.

Institute for Patient–and Family-Centered Care. 6917 Arlington Road, Suite 309, Bethesda, Maryland 20814. (301) 652-0281. http://www.familycenteredcare.org.

National Patient Advocate Foundation, 725 15th St. NW, 10th Floor, Washington, DC 20005. Phone: (202) 347-8009, Fax: (202) 347-5579. http://www.npaf.org .

Teresa G. Odle
Laura Jean Cataldo, RN, Ed.D.

Patient rights

Definition

Patient rights encompass legal and ethical issues in the provider-patient relationship, including the patient's right to privacy, the right to quality medical care without prejudice, the right to make informed decisions about care and treatment options, and the right to refuse treatment.

Purpose

The purpose of delineating patient rights is to ensure the ethical treatment of persons receiving medical or other professional health care services. Without exception, all persons in all settings are entitled to receive ethical treatment.

Description

Many issues comprise the rights of patients in the medical system, including a patient's ability to sue a health plan provider; access to emergency and specialty care, diagnostic testing and prescription medication without prejudice; confidentiality and protection of patient medical information; and continuity of care.

Health care reform led to an emergence of health maintenance organizations (HMOs) and other managed health care plans. The rapid change in medical care moved health care decision making from medical professionals to business entities, a move many consider to be detrimental to the health care industry in general. Establishing a patient's bill of rights has been the response to this concern. The Bipartisan Patient Protection Act of 2001 has been signed into law.

At issue, besides basic rights of care and privacy, is the education of patients concerning what to expect of their health care facility and its providers. These basic rights include the right to:

• participate in the development and implementation in the plan of care

• be treated with respect and dignity

• be informed about condition, treatment options, and the possible results and side effects of treatment

• refuse treatment in accordance with the law, and receive information about the consequences of refusal

• quality health care without discrimination because of race, creed, gender, religion, national origin, or source of payment

• privacy and confidentiality, which includes access to medical records upon request

• personal safety

• know the identity of the person treating the patient, as well as any relationship between professionals and agencies involved in the treatment

• informed consent for all procedures

• information, including the medical records by the patient or by the patient's legally authorized

KEY TERMS

Health Maintenance Organization (HMO)—
A Health Maintenance Organization provides health care coverage to individuals who are enrolled in it. Individuals enroll in an HMO through hospitals, physicians, and other healthcare providers, or through laboratories who have a contract with the HMO.

Joint Commission on Accreditation of Healthcare Organizations (JCAHO)—The accrediting organization that evaluates nearly 20,000 U.S. health care organizations and programs. Accreditation is maintained with onsite surveys every three years; laboratories are surveyed every two years.

QUESTIONS TO ASK YOUR DOCTOR

- What are my rights as a patient?
- What should I do if I feel my rights have been violated?
- What laws do hospitals need to comply with in order to maintain the rights of their patients?
- How have the guidelines and regulations associated with patient rights impacted the delivery of your medical care?
- Does this hospital have an ethics committee?

representative and hospital charges, except for Medicaid and general assistance

- consultation and communication
- complain or compliment without the fear of retaliation or compromise of access or quality of care

Patients are expected to meet a fair share of responsibility by following the plan of care, providing complete and accurate health information, and communicating comprehension of instructions on procedures and treatment. The patient is further responsible for consequences of refusal of treatment, of not following the rules and regulations of a hospital, and of not being considerate of others' rights. The patient is also responsible for providing assurance that financial obligations of care are met.

The American Hospital Association provides an informal bill of rights for patients who are hospitalized. In it, the hospital informs patients that they have the right to refuse any procedure or medication that is prescribed, stating that full information should be provided by the attending physician if the patient has doubt or concerns.

Persons United Limiting Substandards and Errors in Health Care (PULSE), a non-profit organization concerned with **patient education** and improving communication within the health care system, encourages the partnership of health care professionals and patients. A patient who is educated about his or her own medical condition can work together with health care providers regarding treatment decisions.

President Barack Obama signed a law in March, 2010 entitled the 'Patient Protection and Affordable Care Act'. This health care reform legislation will impact patients rights in a number of ways. First, the law will extend health coverage to 32 million Americans who were previously uninsured. This translates to numerous Americans having a voice in their healthcare around such things as healthcare provider, diagnostic tests, and treatment plans. Second, the law will expand scrutiny regarding discriminatory practices from health insurers thereby, aiding in the protection of individuals from such things as condition exclusions, cancelation of coverage, and the establishment of lifetime limits. Third, the law focuses considerable attention to the area of prevention, and extended services for **public health** programs, thus, helping individuals receive attention in their pursuit of wellness in both mental and physical health.

New federal privacy rules, beyond the proposed Patient Bill of Rights, give patients additional control over private medical information. Patients have the right to examine their own **medical records** and to amend them if necessary. In practice, medical personnel have often been reluctant to part with patient records, even to the patients themselves. While health care providers and patients assume that medical records are private, the widespread use of computer transmissions opens the potential for seriously compromising **patient confidentiality**. Regulations recently imposed by the federal government are aimed at protecting patient records by creating limits on the methods in which medical information is shared. Direct authorization from a patient must be gained before information may be released. Criminal and civil penalties may be imposed for a privacy violation. Intentional disclosure of private information can bring a $50,000 fine and one-year prison term. Penalties for selling medical information are higher. Following a two-year implementation period, the rules became enforceable in February 2003.

Viewpoints

Not all individuals or organizations agree with the new regulations. Some complain that they are too restrictive, while others maintain that they are not restrictive enough. The Joint Commission on Accreditation of Healthcare Organizations (JCAHO) cites complexity and cost factors as major problems, and that the full extent of the impact caused by the ruling was not adequately considered when it passed in 2003. The government estimated that it will cost taxpayers $17.6 billion over 10 years to comply with the privacy regulations. Critics of the regulations imply that the cost will be more than triple the estimate, and that billable hours for attorneys specializing in the complexities of the regulations will skyrocket, thus resulting in even higher costs of patient care.

Resources

BOOKS

Allen, James. *Health Law and Medical Ethics.* Upper Saddle River, NJ: Prentice Hall, 2012.

Bondeson, William B., and James W. Jones., eds. The Ethics of Managed Care: Professional Integrity and Patient Rights. New York: Springer, 2010.

Clark, Jean S. The Chapter Leader's Guide to Patient Rights: Practical Insight on Joint Commission Standards.Danvers, MA: HCPro, 2011.

Mason, Diana J., et al.*Policy &Politics in Nursing and Health Care,*6th ed. New York, NY: Saunders, 2011.

Moss, Bernard. *Communication Skills in Health and Social Care,* 2nd ed. Thousand Oaks, CA: Sage Publications Ltd, 2012.

Schimpff, Stephen C., MD. *The Future of Health-Care Delivery: Why It Must Change and How It Will Affect You.* Dulles, VA: Potomac Books Inc, 2012.

PERIODICALS

Ackerman, M. J. "The personal health record." Journal of Medical Practice Management 23, no. 2 (2007): 84–85.

Applebaum, P. S. "Clinical practice. Assessment of patients' competence to consent to treatment." New England Journal of Medicine 357, no. 18 (2007): 1834–1840.

Barash, C. I. "Threats to privacy protection." Science 318, no. 5838 (2007): 913–914.

Campbell, B., H. Thompson, J. Slater, C. Coward, K. Wyatt, and K. Sweeney. "Extracting information from hospital records: what patients think about consent." Quality and Safety in Health Care 16, no. 6 (2007): 404–408.

Haque, O. S., and H. Bursztajn. "Decision-making capacity, memory and informed consent, and judgment at the boundaries of the self." Journal of Clinical Ethics 18, no. 3 (2007): 256–261.

Harris, Steven M. "Patient Privacy Rights Extend Beyond Electronic Records." American Medical News 44, no. 12 (March 26, 2001): 19.

Hussong, Sharon J. "Medical Records and Your Privacy: Developing Federal Legislation to Protect Patient Privacy Rights." American Journal of Law and Medicine 26, no. 4 (Winter 2000): 453.

Mitka, M. "Aiding emergency research aim of report on exceptions to informed consent." Journal of the American Medical Association 298, no. 22 (2007): 2608–2609.

ORGANIZATIONS

American Academy of Family Physicians. 11400 Tomahawk Creek Parkway, Leawood, KS 66211-2672. (913) 906-6000. E-mail: fp@aafp.org. http://www.aafp.org.

American College of Physicians. 190 N Independence Mall West, Philadelphia, PA 19106-1572. (800) 523-1546, x2600, or (215) 351-2600. http://www.acponline.org.

American Medical Association. 515 N. State Street, Chicago, IL 60654. (800) 621-8335. http://www.ama-assn.org.

National Patient Advocate Foundation, 725 15th St. NW, 10th Floor, Washington, DC 20005. Phone: (202) 347-8009, Fax: (202) 347-5579. http://www.npaf.org .

Persons United Limiting Substandards and Errors in Health Care (P.U.L.S.E.). http://www.pulseamerica.org.

L. Fleming Fallon, Jr, MD., DrPH.
Jacqueline N. Martin, M.S.
Laura Jean Cataldo, RN, Ed.D.

PCV *see* **Hematocrit**

Peak acid output *see* **Gastric analysis**

Pediatric assessment tests *see* **Development assessment**

Pediatric nutrition

Definition

Pediatric **nutrition** considers the dietary needs of infants to support growth and development, including changes in organ function and body composition.

Purpose

Decisions parents make about nutrition and feeding their infants have short- and long-term effects on the babies' subsequent growth and development. **Infectious disease** and chronic digestive disease can be reduced with good nutrition choices such as breastfeeding. Breastfed infants have better overall health, so choices about pediatric nutrition are important considerations.

Since the mid-1970s, the prevalence of **obesity** and overweight has increased signicantly in the United States. The prevalence of overweight has tripled among children and adolescents, and almost two out of three adults are either overweight or obese. Obese children are more likely to become obese adults without intervention.

Precautions

Infants consume small amounts of food at a time, but they should not be fed directly from the jar because **bacteria** is introduced into a jar from the babies' mouth. If uneaten food is then put into the refrigerator, bacteria will likely grow and may cause **diarrhea**, **vomiting**, or other signs of food-borne illness. In order to prevent food sensitivities, some foods such as wheat, eggs, and chocolate should be avoided until the child is one year of age.

Ensuring adequate water intake, which can be derived solely through milk, is critical to maintain **electrolyte balance** and therefore the overall health of infants and young children.

Description

Breastfeeding for optimum health

There are several advantages that breastfeeding provides compared to bottle-feeding. Breast milk imparts superior nutritional, immunological, and psychological benefits to infants. Breastfeeding is also much more economical, and no preparation is required. The American Dietetic Association advocates breastfeeding exclusively for four to six months, and breastfeeding with weaning foods for at least 12 months. The American Academy of **Pediatrics** also advocates breastfeeding, stating, "Exclusive breastfeeding is ideal nutrition and sufficient to support optimal growth and development for approximately the first six months after birth … It is recommended that breastfeeding continue for at least 12 months, and thereafter for as long as mutually desired.

Breast milk's nutritional advantages are:

• It provides infants with most of the nutrients they need for growth and is a readily available energy source.

• It contains large amounts of vitamin E, which may help prevent anemia. Additionally, vitamin E is an important antioxidant.

• It is compatible with infants' enzymes.

• Unlike cow's milk, it has an optimum calcium to phosphorus ratio of 2:1.

• Breastfeeding transfers antibodies from mothers to infants.

• All infectious diseases occur less frequently in infants who are breastfed rather than bottle fed.

• It favorably changes the pH of stools and the intestinal flora, thus protecting against bacterial diarrheas.

Formula feeding

There are a number of commercially prepared infant formulas on the market available in powder, concentrated liquid, and pre-diluted liquid forms. The American Academy of Pediatrics advises that whole cow's milk should not be given to a child during the first year of life. It also recommends iron-fortified formula for all infants on formula. Infant formula has more protein and more **iron** than human milk, but lacks **antibodies**.

Introduction of solid foods

The age to start solid foods depends on infants' needs and readiness, but they do not need solid food before six months of age, particularly breastfed infants. Tongue and mouth movement is usually adequate by four months. If infants are force-fed early, some will rebel and develop feeding problems. Weaning of a breastfed infant depends on the preferences and needs of the mother and infant. Weaning gradually over weeks or months is easiest. When the infant is about seven months old, breastfeeding once a day should be replaced by a bottle or cup of modified formula or fruit juice. By 10 months, the infant may be weaned to a cup. Thereafter, one or two feedings daily can be continued until age 18 to 24 months. A full diet of solid foods and fluids by cup should be given to infants who are nursed even longer.

To determine an infant's tolerance, solid foods should be offered by spoon and introduced one flavor at a time. Many commercial baby foods (desserts and soup mixtures, in particular) are high in starch, calories, have no or little vitamin or mineral value, and are high in cellulose, which is poorly digested by infants. Commercial baby foods with high sodium content, more than 200 mg/jar, should be avoided. The daily sodium requirement is 17.6 mg/kilogram. Pureed home foods will suffice. Meat should be preferentially introduced to high-carbohydrate foods; however, because infants often reject meat, it must be introduced patiently and carefully.

To ensure infants eat enough fat when weaning from breast milk or formula, choose whole milk up to two years of age. Two good sources of protein and fat that infants enjoy are peanut butter and cheese. If there are concerns about obesity, lean protein choices provide the fat and protein. Adequate intakes of grains, fruits, and vegetables will ensure that infants receive all the necessary **vitamins** and **minerals**.

Preparation

In order to make appropriate choices about pediatric nutrition, it is important to be aware of the nutritional needs of infants. The following are the recommended vitamin and mineral intakes for infants and young children:

- Vitamin A for infants 0–6 months: 400 micrograms/day (mcg/d); 7–12 months: 500 mcg/d; children 1–3 years: 300 mcg/d.

- Thiamin (vitamin B_1) for infants 0–6 months: 0.2 milligrams/day (mg/d); 7–12 months: 0.3 mg/d; children 1–3 years: 0.5 mg/d.

- Riboflavin (vitamin B_2) for infants 0–6 months: 0.3 mg/d; 7–12 months: 0.4 mg/d; children 1–3 years: 0.5 mg/d.

- Niacin for infants 0–6 months: 2 mg/d; 7–12 months: 4 mg/d; children 1–3 years: 6 mg/d.

- Vitamin B_6 for infants 0–6 months: 0.1 mg/d; 7–12 months: 0.3 mg/d; children 1–3 years: 0.5 mg/d.

- vitamin B_{12} for infants 0–6 months: 0.4 mcg/d; 7–12 months: 0.5 mcg/d; children 1–3 years: 0.9 mcg/d.

- Pantothenic acid for infants 0–6 months: 1.7 mg/d; 7–12 months: 1.8 mg/d; children 1–3 years: 2.0 mg/d.

- Biotin for infants 0–6 months: 5 mcg/d; 7–12 months: 6 mcg/d; children 1–3 years: 8 mcg/d.

- Folate for infants 0–6 months: 65 mcg/d; 7–12 months: 80 mcg/d; children 1–3 years: 150 mcg/d.

- Vitamin C (ascorbic acid) for infants 0–6 months: 40 mg/d; 7–12 months: 50 mg/d; children 1–3 years: 15 mg/d.

- Vitamin D (in the absence of adequate sunlight) for infants 0–6 months: 5 mg/d; 7–12 months: 5 mg/d; children 1–3 years: 5 mg/d.

- Vitamin E for infants 0–6 months: 4 mg/d; 7–12 months: 5 mg/d; children 1–3 years: 6 mg/d.

- Vitamin K for infants 0–6 months: 2.0 mcg/d; 7–12 months: 2.5 mcg/d; children 1–3 years: 30 mcg/d.

- Calcium for infants 0–6 months: 210 mg/d; 7–12 months: 270 mg/d; children 1–3 years: 500 mg/d.

- Phosphorus for infants 0–6 months: 100 mg/d; 7–12 months: 275 mg/d; children 1–3 years: 460 mg/d.

- Magnesium for infants 0–6 months: 30 mg/d; 7–12 months: 75 mg/d; children 1–3 years: 80 mg/d.

- Selenium for infants 0–6 months: 15 mcg/d; 7–12 months: 20 mcg/d; children 1–3 years: 20 mcg/d.

- Zinc for infants 0–6 months: 2 mg/d; 7–12 months: 3 mg/d; children 1–3 years: 3 mg/d.

- Iron for infants 0–6 months: 0.27 mg/d; 7–12 months: 11 mg/d; children 1–3 years: 7 mg/d.

- Breastfed infants need 400 international units (IU) of vitamin D and 0.25 mg of fluoride daily.

The following is the Recommended Dietary Allowance (RDA), (adapted from the Dietary Reference Intakes report) for carbohydrate, protein, and fat intakes for infants and young children:

- Carbohydrate for infants 0–6 months: 60 g/d; 7–12 months: 95 g/d; children 1–3 years: 130 g/d (acceptable range 45-65 g/d); children 4–8 years: 130 g/d (acceptable range 45-65 g/d)

- Protein and amino acids for infants 0–6 months: 9.1 grams per day (g/d) and 7–12 months: 11 g/d based on 1.5 g/kg/day for infants; children 1–3 years: 13 g/d based on 1.1 g/kg/day for children 1-3 y (acceptable range 5-20 g/d). Children 4-13 y: 11 g/d based on 0.85 g/kg/day (acceptable range 10-30 g/d).

- Fat for infants 0–6 months: 31 g/d; 7–12 months: 30 g/d; children 1–3 years: acceptable range 30-40 g/d; children 4–8 years: acceptable range 25-35 g/d The RDAs are set to meet the needs of 97–98% of the population.

Breastfeeding does not require any preparation, but bottle feeding requires some preparation, such as ensuring the milk is the right temperature and the nipples are sterilized, if sterilized disposable nipples are not used.

Complications

Obesity may start with excessive feeding in infancy. If an infant has two obese parents, it is particularly important to monitor and control weight gain as the infant has an 80% chance of becoming obese.

Diarrhea may be caused by conditions such as celiac disease (gluten enteropathy), **cystic fibrosis**, and sugar (lactose) intolerance.

Results

Infants should be closely monitored for proper weight gain to ensure they are receiving adequate nutrition. Resources such as the National Center for Health Statistics growth charts can be used as a guide.

Health care team roles

Breastfeeding education efforts are important steps for health care teams. They should encourage a longer duration of breastfeeding to achieve maximum nutritional benefits for infants. A dietitian can assist in providing advice regarding pediatric nutrition feeding decisions.

Resources

BOOKS

Samour, Patricia Queen, and Kathy King. *Pediatric Nutrition*, 4th edition. Jones & Bartlett Learning, 2010.

Samour, Patricia Queen, and Kathy King. *Essentials of Pediatric Nutrition.* Jones & Bartlett Learning, 2011.

Suskind, David, and Polly Lenssen, eds. *Pediatric Nutrition Handbook.* Wiley-Blackwell, 2011.

PERIODICALS

Krawinkel, Michael B. "Current Challenges in Pediatric Nutrition." *Current Problems in Pediatric and Adolescent Health Care* 41.9 (2011): 234.

Webster, Sandy Todd. "Energy drinks could pose serious risk for youth." *IDEA Fitness Journal* (May 2011): 60.

ORGANIZATIONS

American Dietetic Association. 120 South Riverside Plaza, Suite 2000, Chicago, IL 60606-6995. (800) 877-1600. http://www.eatright.org/.

Food and Nutrition Information Center, Agricultural Research Service, USDA. National Agricultural Library, Room 105, 10301 Baltimore Avenue, Beltsville, MD 20705-2351. (301) 504-5719. Fax: (301) 504-6409. http://www.nal.usda.gov/fnic/. fnic@nal.usda.gov.

International Food Information Council. 1100 Connecticut Avenue, NW, Suite 430, Washington, DC 20036. (202) 296-6540. Fax (202) 296-6547, http://www.ific.org/. Email: foodinfo@ific.org

La Leche League International. 1400 N. Meacham Road, Schaumburg, IL 60168-4079. (847) 519-7730. http://www.lalecheleague.org/.

USDA Food and Nutrition Service. 3101 Park Center Drive, Alexandria, VA 22302 http://www.fns.usda.gov/fns/

U.S. Department of Health and Human Services. 200 Independence Avenue, S.W., Washington, D.C. 20201. (202) 619-0257 or (877) 696-6775. http://www.hhs.gov/

U.S. Department of Health and Human Services, CDC, National Center for Health Statistics, 3311 Toledo Road, Hyattsville, MD, 20782.(866) 441-NCHS (6247). http://www.cdc.gov/nchs/. Email: nchsquery@cdc.gov

U.S. Department of Health and Human Services, Centers for Disease Control and Prevention (CDC). 1600 Clifton Rd, Atlanta, GA 30333. (800) CDC-INFO. http://www.cdc.gov/. Email: cdcinfo@cdc.gov

Women, Infants, and Children. The Food and Nutrition Service Headquarters. 3101 Park Center Drive, Alexandria, VA 22302. (703) 305-2746.

Crystal Heather Kaczkowski, M.Sc.

Pediatric physical therapy
Definition

Pediatric **physical therapy** is concerned with the examination, evaluation, diagnosis, prognosis, and intervention of children, aged birth through adolescence, who are experiencing functional limitations or disability due to trauma, a disorder, or disease process.

Purpose

Pediatric physical therapy is indicated when a child has a pathology or suffers a trauma which results in an impairment leading to the loss of function and/or societal disability. Pathologies may include non-progressive neurological disorders such as **cerebral palsy**, which results from trauma to the **brain** during or shortly after birth. Children born with genetic syndromes, **heart** and/or lung defects, **hydrocephalus**, spina bifida, **fetal alcohol syndrome**, or drug addiction may also be seen by physical therapists.

Pathologies resulting in musculoskeletal impairments include, but are not limited to: juvenile **rheumatoid arthritis**, **hemophilia**, **scoliosis**, peripheral nerve injury, arthrogryposis, osteogenesis imperfecta, and **muscular dystrophy**. Acquired pathologies that may require physical therapy include traumatic brain injury, **spinal cord injury**, and **cancer**.

Pediatric physical therapists are employed in several different settings, including hospitals, outpatient clinics, and school systems. In the hospital, a pediatric physical therapist may work with patients such as those recovering from heart or lung conditions or surgery, burn trauma, orthopedic surgeries, or any number of other conditions. In addition, many neonatal intensive care units (NICUs) also employ physical therapists to evaluate and treat high-risk or **premature infants**. In an outpatient setting, the same children may be seen further along in their recovery. Children with lifelong conditions may be referred to outpatient clinics upon manifestation of secondary impairments. School physical therapists are employed to insure that children with disabilities or developmental difficulties are functioning adequately in their least restrictive environment.

In any case, the goal of treatment is to diminish impairments and functional limitations to prevent or decrease disability. Treatment may be focused on improving developmental tasks, motor planning, manipulation skills, balance, and/or coordination. The affected child may present with difficulties with ambulation, positioning, communication, attention, cognition, and/or motor function. All of these problems need to be addressed, as they can result in the inability to keep up with peers or perform work at school.

Precautions

Upon patient examination, a physical therapist collects the patient's history and does a systems review. The review includes assessment of the cardiovascular, respiratory, integumentary, musculoskeletal, and neuromuscular systems, including cognition. Physical therapists are educated in differential diagnosis for the purpose of identifying problems that are beyond the scope of physical therapy practice or require the attention of another health care professional.

Description

Examination

Determining a child's need for physical therapy requires both qualitative and quantitative measures to gather information. Observation in natural settings, personal and family history, and subjective information from teachers or caregivers are all valuable pieces of the puzzle. A systems review should be performed, as discussed above. Through observation and measurement, active and passive range of motion and strength should be assessed. In addition, equilibrium and righting reactions and persistent abnormal **reflexes** should be noted. Posture and gait observation and assessment are essential for providing recommendations regarding exercises, seating, orthotics, and assistive devices.

Assessment of functional motor ability is often performed using a standardized test. In infants, tests often used include, but are not limited to: Movement Assessment of Infants, Peabody Developmental Motor Scales (PDMS), Test of Infant Motor Performance, Alberta Infant Motor Scale, and Bayley Scales of Infant Development II. Tests for children include the PDMS, Bruininks-Oseretsky Test of Motor Proficiency, and Gross Motor Function Measure. These tests look at the ability to perform tasks such as maintaining a prone position or rolling in infants, to walking a balance beam or throwing a ball in children.

Evaluation, diagnosis, and prognosis

Although a child may have been given a medical diagnosis, the therapist should formulate a physical therapy diagnosis upon evaluation of the examination findings. The physical therapy diagnosis focuses not on the pathology (e.g., hydrocephalus), but rather on the dysfunction(s) toward which the therapist will direct intervention (e.g., decreased balance).

The prognosis encompasses a prediction of the level of function realistically attainable and the time period in which it will be accomplished. The prognosis includes the plan of care, which outlines treatment procedures and frequency, in addition to specifying long-term and short-term goals. In a **rehabilitation** or outpatient clinic setting, goal-setting may be more short-term than in an educational setting, where the tendency is to set yearly goals related to school function.

While goals often encompass the reduction of impairment to prevent functional limitations, reductions of primary impairment can help to prevent secondary impairment as well. For example, a goal focused on reduction of spasticity through proper positioning can help to prevent or diminish the occurrence of muscle shortening and joint contractures.

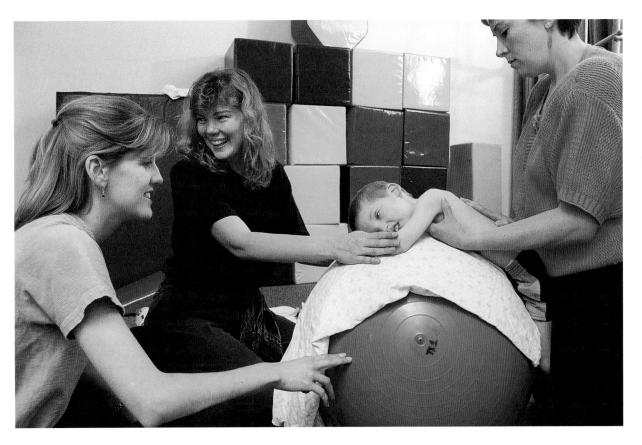

(Physical therapist Beth Fliori Kral massages four-year-old Adam Russell, born with Martsolf syndrome, Huff Center, Thoms Rehabilitation Center, Asheville, North Carolina. © Owen Franken/Corbis)

Intervention

Intervention involves the interaction between therapist and patient. It also includes communication with the family and other professionals as needed, including physicians, nurses, psychologists, occupational therapists, speech and language pathologists, physical therapist assistants, and social workers. In the educational setting, interactions also take place with classroom and physical education teachers, along with paraprofessionals.

Intervention encompasses the coordination and documentation of care, specific treatment procedures, and patient/family education. Physical therapists also must be skilled in recognizing the need to refer a patient back to a physician or recommend the services of other professionals as necessary. The physical therapist usually plays a key role in making recommendations or sometimes participating in the fabrication and fitting of orthoses, walking aids, and wheelchairs. In addition, the physical therapist is instrumental in choosing appropriate adaptive equipment, such as

seating devices or standing frames, for the classroom or home.

Specific treatment procedures are numerous, falling into several categories: functional training for activities of daily living; **therapeutic exercise**; manual techniques such as mobilization and stretching; and therapeutic modalities. **Evidence-based practice** requires the use of recent motor control, motor development and motor learning theories as an umbrella over these treatment procedures. Motor control, development, and learning theories focus on the idea that several factors contribute to emergence of motor behavior. These factors include not only the **central nervous system** (CNS) as the driving force, but also biomechanical, psychological, social, and environmental components. Teaching and practice of skills under these theories is task-oriented and intermittent versus rote and repetitive. Higher-level learning takes place through problem-solving by the child rather than by the therapist's hands-on facilitation. Emphasis has also been placed on the importance of family-centered care, transdisciplinary service, and treatment in natural environments.

Treatment sessions may take place as frequently as once or twice a day in a rehabilitation setting, to once or twice a month in a school setting. Sessions may last 20 minutes to a full hour. Consultation with other professionals also takes place frequently during a patient's length of stay or a student's education.

Re-examination

A physical therapist is continually assessing a child's abilities and adjusting treatment appropriately. Some or all of the same tests and measures used during initial examination may be again used in order to evaluate progress and determine the need to modify, redirect or discontinue treatment.

Aftercare

Aftercare depends upon the setting in which the child has been treated. After a stay in a hospital, a child may be discharged with the recommendation to continue outpatient or school-based physical therapy. Upon discharge in any case, a physical therapist should provide recommendations for exercises or adaptations, if any, which should be continued at school or at home. In addition, a therapist may make suggestions regarding participation in programs such as adaptive sports leagues, therapeutic horseback riding, camps, etc.

Results

Although pediatric physical therapy addresses problems related to a wide variety of pathologies, the common goal usually is that functional activity increases and that disability decreases. In the case of non-progressive disorders, long-term retention of learned skills and the ability to transfer skills to different environments and situations are results of effective physical therapy intervention. In the case of progressive disorders such as muscular dystrophy, maintenance of capabilities and/or slowing of functional losses may be the goal.

Health care team roles

The physical therapist and the physical therapist assistant, under the supervision of the physical therapist, are the direct providers of pediatric physical therapy. There are, however, many other key players. Although

---

KEY TERMS

Evidence-based practice—The process by which health care providers incorporate the best research or evidence into clinical practice in combination with clinical expertise and within the context of patient values.

Motor control—The control of movement and posture.

Motor learning—A set of processes related to practice or experience that results in relatively permanent changes in the ability to produce a skilled action.

Motor planning—The ability to execute skilled nonhabitual tasks.

Neuromuscular re-education—The training of an individual to recover or develop effective sensory and motor strategies for task demands.

---

many states allow direct access to physical therapy, many require a referral from a physician. The physician usually provides the therapist with a prescription for physical therapy that outlines the medical diagnosis, and sometimes, precautions and recommendations. The child's physician and nurses also may provide valuable information regarding past medical history, surgical procedures, and medications.

Occupational therapists, speech and language pathologists, social workers, and psychologists also play important roles in the transdiciplinary provision of services. Physical therapists may work closely with these professionals to combine efforts toward fulfilling a child's maximum potential.

To summarize the various roles of a therapist in pediatric physical therapy, it is necessary to recognize that in addition to the description outlined above, he or she is responsible for consultation, education, critical inquiry, administration, and supervision.

Consultation

There are many facets to the role of consultation. Physical therapists may be called upon to assist other health care professionals in determining whether or not physical therapy services are required for a specific patient, and which types of service are required. In addition, physical therapists may be asked to perform

---

QUESTIONS TO ASK YOUR DOCTOR

- What are the indications that my child may need physical therapy?
- What diagnostic tests are needed for a thorough assessment?
- In what way will physical therapy benefit my child?
- Should we see a specialist? If so, what kind of specialist should I contact?
- What tests or evaluation techniques will you perform to see if physical therapy has been beneficial for my child?
- What physical or psychological limitations do you foresee?
- How can my child's quality of life be improved?
- What symptoms are important enough that I should seek immediate treatment?
- Can you refer me to a qualified person who can make an assessment of my home and recommend changes to make it safer and easier for my child to get around?
- Can you recommend any support groups for me and my family?

activities such as: assessing an environment or program for accessibility; providing opinions or recommendations on adaptations in the classroom, home or recreational arena; and making recommendations for compliance with the Individuals with Disabilities Education Act or the **Americans with Disabilities Act**.

Education

Physical therapists are responsible for educating patients and families, as discussed earlier. This education may include: general information about a disease and course of physical therapy treatment; teaching of home exercises and adaptations; instruction on prevention of secondary impairments; and suggestions for long-term wellness. In addition, pediatric physical therapists may be asked to provide information about disabilities to teachers or students in a school, or provide in-services to physical education teachers about

adaptive sports. Pediatric physical therapists also are responsible for furthering their own education, mentoring future physical therapists and PT assistants, and increasing public awareness of areas in which physical therapists have expertise. The American Physical Therapy Association (APTA) offers a program for specialized certification, which is governed by the American Board of Physical Therapy Specialties (ABPTS) to facilitate the continuing education of physical therapists.

Critical inquiry

Pediatric physical therapists have a responsibility to the profession to critically examine research findings and apply them when appropriate to their daily practice. In addition, physical therapists should look for ways to conduct and/or participate in research to evaluate the effectiveness of interventions and philosophies used in the profession.

Administration and supervision

The pediatric physical therapist must be concerned with administrative activities related to human resources, equipment, finances, and facilities. Supervision of physical therapist assistants, student physical therapists and assistants, and physical therapy aides is often a responsibility. This responsibility may include monitoring quality of care and productivity as well. The physical therapist is directly responsible for the actions of these individuals and therefore should adhere to American Physical Therapy Association guidelines stipulating the levels of supervision required.

Resources

BOOKS

Campbell, Suzann K., Robert J. Palisano, and Margo Orlin. *Physical Therapy for Children,*4th ed. New York, NY: Saunders, 2011.

Danto, Ayelet H., and Michelle Pruzansky. *1001 Pediatric Treatment Activities: Creative Ideas for Therapy Sessions.* Thorofare, NJ: Slack Incorporated, 2011.

Effgen, Susan K. *Meeting the Physical Therapy Needs of Children,*2ndh ed. Philadelphia, PA: F.A. Davis Company, 2012.

PERIODICALS

Hayes, Margo Starks, et. al. "Next Step: A Survey of Pediatric Physical Therapists' Educational Needs and Perceptions of Motor Control, Motor Development, and Motor Learning as They Relate to Services for Children with

Developmental Disabilities." Pediatric Physical Therapy 11. no. 4 (Winter 1999): 64-182.

King, G. A., et. al. "An Evaluation of Functional, School-Based Therapy Services for Children with Special Needs." Physical and Occupational Therapy in Pediatrics 19, no. 2 (1999): 31-52.

ORGANIZATIONS

American Academy of Pediatrics. 141 Northwest Point Boulevard, Elk Grove Village, IL 60007-1098. (847) 434-4000. http://www.aap.org.

American Physical Therapy Association, Section on Pediatrics. 1111 North Fairfax Street, Alexandria, VA 22314-1488. (703) 684-2782. http://www.apta.org.

Peggy Campbell Torpey, MPT
Laura Jean Cataldo, RN, Ed.D.

Pediatric surgery

Definition

Pediatric surgery is a specialized field of surgery for the treatment of conditions that can be surgically corrected in a baby, child, or adolescent.

Purpose

The purpose of pediatric surgery varies with the procedure. In general, the purpose is to surgically correct a congenital condition, disease, traumatic injury, or other disorder in the pediatric patient.

Demographics

Pediatric surgeons provide treatment for young patients—newborns up through late adolescence.

Description

Pediatric surgery is the surgical branch that uses operative techniques to correct certain pediatric conditions (i.e., congenital abnormalities, tumors, chronic diseases, and traumatic injuries). There are different specialties within the field that include:

• pediatric general surgery

• pediatric otolaryngology (ear, nose, and throat)

• pediatric ophthalmology (eye)

• pediatric urology (urogenital system)

• pediatric orthopedic (bone) surgery

• pediatric neurological (brain and spinal cord) surgery

• pediatric plastic (reconstructive and cosmetic) surgery

The American Academy of **Pediatrics** has established specific guidelines for referral to subspecialists. The pediatric patient has special considerations that differentiate him or her, both physically and psychologically, from an adult. A neonate (newborn) poses great challenge in surgical treatment since the tiny structures and immature organ systems may not cope with disease-induced **stress** and the physical demands of a major operative procedure. A newborn infant may still be developing key bodily functions, or may have special requirements. Key areas of concern in the newborn include:

• cardiovascular (heart) system

• thermoregulation (temperature requirements of 73°F [22.8°C]).

• pulmonary (lung) function

• renal (kidney) function

• immature immunity and liver

• special requirements for fluid, electrolyte (necessary elements such as sodium, potassium, and calcium) and nutrition

The pediatric surgeon must take into account the special requirements unique to the young surgical patient. The pediatric surgeon is trained to treat the entire spectrum of surgical illnesses. The following is an overview (with symptoms) of the more common pediatric conditions that require surgery typically performed by the pediatric surgeon.

Alimentary tract obstruction

Obstruction of the alimentary tract (tubes of digestion extending from the mouth to the anus) is characterized by four cardinal symptoms:

• abdominal distention (an abdomen that becomes large and appears swollen)

• bilious vomiting (due to bile in the stomach)

• maternal polyhydramnios (excess amniotic fluid in the amniotic sac, greater than 2,000 ml) before birth

• failure to pass meconium (dark green or black sticky excretion passed via the newborn's rectum) in the first 24 hours of life

ESOPHAGEAL ATRESIA AND TRACHEOESOPHAGEAL FISTULA. This is a congenital deformity of the esophagus (the tube that passes food from the mouth to the **stomach**) does not connect to the stomach. Symptoms include severe respiratory distress (the neonate cannot breathe) and excessive salivation. Other clinical signs include **cyanosis** (bluish discoloration of the skin due to oxygen deprivation), **choking**, and coughing.

KEY TERMS

Atresia—Thinning or narrowing of a body passageway.

Large intestine—The portion of the colon that includes the cecum; ascending, transverse, and descending sigmoid colon; rectum; and anal canal.

Oliguria—Decreased urine production.

Pediatric aged patient—The pediatric aged patient encompasses several periods during development. The first four weeks after birth are callled the neonatal period. The first year after birth is called infancy, and childhood is from 13 months until puberty (between the ages of 12 and 15 years in girls and 13 and 16 years in boys).

Polyp—A tumor mass, generally benign and capable of surgical removal.

Pylorus—The area that controls food passage from the stomach to the first part of the small intestine (duodenum).

Small intestine—The part of the intestines that consists of the duodenum, jejunum, and ileum.

PYLORIC ATRESIA AND RELATED CONDITIONS. Pyloric atresia is a condition that occurs when the pyloric valve, located between the stomach and duodenum, fails to open. Food cannot pass out of the stomach, resulting in **vomiting** clear gastric juice at attempted feedings. Maternal polyhydramnios is present before birth in more than 60% of cases.

Other areas of the colon (duodenum, jejunum, ileum) can be obstructed during development, with symptoms present at birth. Most of these disorders share the four cardinal symptoms of alimentary obstruction.

INTUSSUSCEPTION. **Intussusception** accounts for 50% of intestinal obstruction in patients who are three months to one year of age. Eighty percent of cases are observed by the child's second birthday. The cause of intussusception is not known, and it is more common in males who are well nourished and apparently healthy. The symptoms include a sudden onset of **abdominal pain** characterized by episodic screaming and drawing up of the legs. In 60% of patients, vomiting and **blood** in the stool are common findings (either bright red or occult [hidden] blood). Typically, the bowel movements look like currant jelly, consisting of mucus and blood mixed together. Currant jelly stool is the most common clinical observation for patients with intussusception. During **physical examination**, patients will exhibit abdominal distention, and in 65% of cases there is a sausage-shaped mass that can be felt in the upper right portion of the **abdomen** toward the mid-abdomen. Ultrasound studies are a reliable method of diagnosis.

FAILURE TO PASS MECONIUM. Failure to pass meconium (meconium ileus) is associated with **cystic fibrosis** (a genetic disorder), colonic obstruction (colonic atresia), meconium plug syndrome, and aganglionic megacolon (also called Hirschsprung's disease, a congenital absence of the nerves that provide gastrointestinal tract mobility).

Anorectal anomalies

There are many different types of anorectal anomalies common to male and female neonates, as well as deformities that are gender-specific since involvement of genitalia can occur. The surgery for these cases is complicated, and must be performed by an experienced pediatric surgeon. Complications of these procedures could result in permanent problems.

Necrotizing enterocolitis (NEC)

NEC affects 1–2% of patients admitted to a neonatal intensive care unit. It is a life-threatening illness characterized by abdominal distention, bilious vomiting, lethargy, **fever**, occult (not obvious) or gross (clearly seen) rectal bleeding. Additionally, affected patients may exhibit signs of **hypothermia** (temperature less than 96.5°F or 35.8°C), bradycardia (slow **heart** rate), abdominal mass (felt during palpation), oliguria, **jaundice**, and episodes of breathlessness (apnea). Survival of NEC surgery can be expected for 60–70% of patients.

Abdominal wall defects

Omphalocele is a defect that involves protrusion of abdominal contents into an external sac. This disorder occurs in one per 5,000 births. More than 50% of omphalocele patients have serious genetic deformities involving these body systems: cardiovascular (heart), musculoskeletal (muscle and bones), genitourinary (genital and bladder systems), and central nervous (**brain** and **spinal cord**). The overall survival rate for infants with omphalocele varies, and depends on defect size, other associated genetic abnormalities, and age of newborn. (Many infants with omphalocele are premature.) Approximately 33% of patients with omphaloceles do not survive.

GASTROSCHISIS. Gastroschisis is a defect in the abdominal wall to the side (lateral) of the umbilicus. It usually occurs to the right of an intact normal umbilical cord. The cause is unknown. The bowel protrudes to the outside of the abdomen during intrauterine life (while the embryo is developing inside the uterus). The amniotic fluid has an irritating effect on the exposed bowel, and causes **infection** of the bowels. The problem can be detected by ultrasound studies during **pregnancy**. Some pediatric surgeons and obstetricians recommend **cesarean section** (early elective delivery) to spare bowel trauma. The newborn patients typically require surgery, **tube feedings** for three to four weeks, and hospitalization for several weeks. The current survival rate for infants with gastroschisis is greater than 90%.

Congenital diaphragmatic hernia (CDH)

CDH can be diagnosed by the fourth month of pregnancy via ultrasound studies. Of the infants with congenital diaphragmatic **hernia** (CDH), 44–66% have other congenital abnormalities as a result of developmental malformations. Anatomically, patients with CDH have a defect in development that allows a communication between the chest and abdomen. Through this defect, the abdominal contents enter the lung cavity and interfere with normal lung development. The incidence is approximately one per 2,200 live births, and males are more commonly affected than females. Usually the infants are full-term, and the defect occurs on the left side in the majority—88%—of patients.

Treatment is extensive, and usually requires three major areas:

• stabilization of patient and preoperative preparation

• operative treatment

• postoperative respiratory, metabolic, circulatory and nutritional supportive measures

Postoperatively, the infant is monitored in the neonatal intensive care setting. The postoperative period is more critical if a lung is severely underdeveloped.

Pyloric stenosis (PS)

Pyloric stenosis is an obstruction in the intestine due to a larger-than-normal size of the muscle fibers of the pylorus (lower stomach opening). Pyloric stenosis is a common hereditary condition that affects males more than females, and occurs in one per 750 births. The typical symptoms include a progressive, often projectile, vomiting after attempted feedings. The gastric vomitus (bloody in 80% of patients) usually begins during the second and third week of life, and increases in force and frequency. Typically, the infant fails to gain weight, and the number of bowel movements and rate of urination decreases.

Physical examination is usually helpful in establishing a diagnosis. Palpation of the enlarged muscle fibers can be felt as an olive-shaped mass located along the midline approximately one-third to one-half of the distance from the umbilicus to the xiphoid (end of the breastbone), when the stomach is empty. Careful abdominal examination and palpation can usually identify the pyloric mass in 85% of cases.

Gastroesophageal reflux

Gastroesophageal reflux disease (GERD) is a common disorder in infancy, and usually disappears by the baby's first birthday. The largest group of patients with clinically significant GERD are those who have neurologic impairment. Symptoms often include vomiting, repeated lung infections (from aspirating gastric contents during regurgitation of foodstuffs), and delayed gastric emptying. The success rate with infants who have procedures necessary to correct GERD is over 90%.

Meckel's diverticulum

Meckel's diverticulum occurs in approximately 2% of the U.S. population. The diverticulum is an outgrowth of intestine that is located in a portion of the intestines called the ileum. Symptoms of obstruction are more often observed in infants, and bleeding is more common in patients after age four.

Intestinal polyps

Juvenile polyps are usually present between the ages of four and 14 years, and tend to be inflammatory. The most common symptom of intestinal polyps is rectal bleeding, which is commonly due to a solitary polyp (80% of cases). Diagnosis can be done by proctosigmoidoscopy, which allows visualization of 85% of polyps.

Acute appendicitis

Acute **appendicitis** is a relatively common surgical emergency that is misdiagnosed in 28% of patients due to a broad spectrum of symptoms that can confuse the clinician. The classic clinical symptom of acute appendicitis is the onset of **pain** in the middle region of the abdomen that is followed by anorexia (loss of appetite), nausea, and vomiting. The pain is persistent and radiates to the right lower abdomen, becoming more intense and localized. The physical and abdominal examinations must be carefully and accurately performed. Patients with acute appendicitis usually have an increased white blood cell (cells that fight infection) count.

Once the diagnosis is established, the child is prepared for surgery. Preoperative **antibiotics** are started at least one half-hour before the operation. If the appendix is perforated (ruptured), complications can occur as a result of kidney (renal) failure, seizures due to fever, and gram-negative **sepsis** (an infection that enters the bloodstream and interferes with life-saving chemical reactions). Patients who are very young, or those who were misdiagnosed and incurred long delays in treatment, are susceptible to death.

Inflammatory bowel diseases

Some cases (approximately 25%) of inflammatory bowel disease are found in persons younger than 20 years of age. Two types can occur, **Crohn's disease** and ulcerative **colitis**.

The diagnosis of inflammatory bowel disease is usually based on presenting clinical symptoms, laboratory analysis results, endoscopic appearance, and radiologic findings. Approximately 50–60% of patients have bloody **diarrhea**, severe cramping, abdominal pain, and urgency.

CROHN'S DISEASE. The symptoms of Crohn's disease includes cramping abdominal pain, diarrhea, and strictures (constriction) resulting from bowel obstruction. Removal of diseased portions in children with Crohn's disease may be temporarily beneficial, but recurrence after surgical removal occurs in about 50% of cases within four years. Chronic symptoms may remain into adult life, making long-term follow-up essential.

ULCERATIVE COLITIS. Ulcerative colitis is limited to the colon. A surgical procedure known as colectomy is curative, and indicated for intractable disease (64% of patients). Colectomy is the removal of the entire colon, or the inflamed part of it.

Biliary tract disorders

A variety of biliary tract conditions may be present at birth, some requiring surgical correction.

NEONATAL JAUNDICE. Neonatal jaundice is common, and results from an immature system not capable of some basic biochemical reactions. Food intake can help speed these reactions, which usually resolve the condition within seven to 10 days. Jaundice that persists for over two weeks is abnormal, and could be caused by over 30 possible disorders.

BILIARY ATRESIA. Biliary atresia is a disease that causes inflammation of the ducts within the biliary system, resulting in fibrosis of these ducts. The incidence of biliary atresia is one per 15,000 live births, and is more

WHO PERFORMS THE PROCEDURE AND WHERE IS IT PERFORMED?

Pediatric surgery is performed by a pediatric surgeon who has had five years of general surgery training, along with further specialized instruction and experience, and is certified in pediatric general surgery or in a specific pediatric specialty.

common in females. Time is critical, and most patients must have surgery by two months of life. Approximately 25–30% of patients who receive early operative intervention have long-term successful outcomes. Some patients may require **liver** transplantation, and 85–90% of these patients survive.

CHOLELITHIASIS. Gallbladder obstruction in infants and young children is usually caused by pigmented (colored) stones resulting from blood disorders. Removal of the gallbladder (laparoscopic cholecystectomy) is the treatment of choice.

Trauma

Accidents are the leading cause of death in children between the ages of one and 15 years, and accounts for 50% of all deaths in the pediatric age group. More than half of these deaths are due to motor vehicle accidents, followed by **falls**, bicycle injuries, drowning, **burns**, **child abuse**, and birth trauma. Head trauma is the single most common organ associated with traumatic death. Within recent years, the number of fatalities related to the use of firearms and violence has increased.

More than 20 million children each year sustain injuries requiring treatment. These injuries account for 100,000 cases of permanent pediatric disability. Response to trauma in pediatric patients is significantly different from older patients. Pediatric patients require special attention concerning temperature regulation, blood volume, metabolic rate and requirements, and airway maintenance. Other special pediatric considerations include response to stress, communication difficulties, psychological trauma, a different pediatric trauma score system, smaller airway diameter, and increased risk of aspirating gastric contents (which could cause **pneumonia**). Pediatric trauma patients should have access to appropriate pre-hospital transportation, and must receive medical attention in a

QUESTIONS TO ASK THE DOCTOR

- What are the risks of surgery?
- What is the benefit of the surgery?
- What type of anesthesia will be used?
- How many surgeries of this type has the surgeon performed?
- Is there an alternative to surgery?
- Is a full recovery expected, and if not, what deficits will the child have?
- What should the parents and child do to prepare for surgery?
- What care is needed following the surgery?
- When will the child be able to return to normal activity?

pediatric trauma center capable of providing the complex level of care necessary for serious pediatric trauma situations.

Neck masses

Neck masses during infancy and childhood may be caused by tumors or infections, or they may be congenital. Lymphadenitis is an infection of a lymph node that becomes enlarged and tender. Most cases are resolved by treating the primary source of infection (i.e., middle ear infection and **tonsillitis**). Some inflamed nodes may require an incision and drainage of infection.

Hernias

INGUINAL HERNIA AND HYDROCELE. Inguinal (groin) hernia is the most frequent disorder requiring surgery in the pediatric age group. Clinically, a right-sided inguinal hernia is more common in males (60% of cases), and there is a familial tendency. The incidence is higher in full-term infants (3.5–5%). Full-term infants and older children (without underlying diseases) can receive surgical repair in an outpatient setting. An inguinal hernia may result in herniation of the scrotum, and a communicating hydrocele (hernia with a small connection to the peritoneal cavity).

UMBILICAL HERNIA. Umbilical hernia is a defect of the umbilical ring, and is more common in females and African American children. Spontaneous involution occurs in 80% of cases. Larger defects may be observed

for several years without complications, and their spontaneous resolution is possible. If the umbilical hernia persists, patients may develop feeding intolerance, pain, and local skin breakdown.

Undescended testes

Undescended testes are observed in 1–2% of full-term males. Approximately 30% of preterm males may have an undescended testis. Undescended testis in **premature infants** may descend by the first year of life, and observation is often the treatment during that time.

Tumors

Wilm's tumor (nephroblastoma) is a tumor in the **kidneys** that forms during embryonic development. The tumor is due to a genetic abnormality; and approximately 80% of children are diagnosed between one and five years of age. In about 75–95% of cases, the patient has an abdominal mass that is detected by a parent during bathing. Blood in the urine (hematuria) occurs in 10–15% of cases, and high **blood pressure** (**hypertension**) is present in 20–25% of cases. Hypertension is the result of the tumor compressing the kidney in a specific area, causing it to release a chemical called renin, which elevates blood pressure. During physical examination, the Wilm's tumor is a smooth, round, hard, nontender flank mass. The treatment of Wilm's tumor depends on its stage, and may include surgery, **chemotherapy**, or **radiotherapy**.

Resources

BOOK

Townsend, Courtney. *Sabiston Textbook of Surgery,* 16th ed. St. Louis: W. B. Saunders Company, 2001.

PERIODICALS

Coran, A. "American Academy of Pediatrics: Guidelines for Referral to Pediatric Surgical Specialists." *Pediatrics* 110, no. 1 (July 2002).

Okada P. J., B. Hicks. "Pediatric Surgical Emergencies: Neonatal Surgical Energencies." *Clinical Pediatric Emergency Medicine* 3, no.1 (March 2002:).

ORGANIZATION

The American Pediatric Surgical Association. 60 Revere Drive Suite 500 Northbrook, Il 60062. (847) 480-9576. Fax: (847) 480-9282 E-mail: eapsa@eapsa.org.

Laith Farid Gulli, M.D., M.S.
Nicole Mallory, M.S., PA-C
Abraham F. Ettaher, M.D.
Robert Ramirez, B.S.

Pediatrics

Definition

Pediatrics is a specialized the branch of medicine that cares for children from birth through age 21.

Description

Pediatricians care exclusively for children from infants through young adults. They practice **preventive medicine** in healthy children through well-child checkups to monitor a child's growth and development. They encourage disease prevention directly through immunizations and indirectly through education of both parents and children about maintaining healthy lifestyles.

Pediatricians also diagnose and treat infectious diseases, injuries, congenital and genetic defects, and childhood cancers. They monitor children and adolescents for behavioral and psychiatric problems and developmental delays. They are, by law, required to report any suspected **child abuse** or **neglect**.

As of 2010, about 13% of practicing physicians in the United States were pediatricians. Also, according to the American Academy of Pediatrics, as of 2010, 56% of board certified pediatricians were women, and about 20% of all board certified pediatricians were working part time (defined as 25 hours or less per week). In multiple surveys, pediatric is consistently reported as being in the top five medical specialties in job satisfaction.

The work of a pediatrician is more collaborative than many medical specialties. Pediatricians must work with parents both to maintain the health of the child and to treat disease. Primary care pediatricians are generalists who, when they suspect a problem, will collaborate with the a pediatric subspecialist.

Board certified subspecialties in pediatrics include:

- adolescent medicine
- allergy and immunology
- cardiology
- child abuse
- child and adolescent psychiatry
- critical care
- dermatology
- developmental and behavioral medicine
- emergency medicine
- endocrinology
- gastroenterology
- hematology-oncology
- infectious diseases
- neonatology
- nephrology
- pulmonary medicine
- rheumatology

Registered nurses (RNs) can also specialize in pediatrics and become certified through examination by the Society of Pediatric Nurses. Several different certifications are available including, Certified Pediatric Nurse (CPN) and Pediatric Nurse Practitioner (PNP) and **Clinical Nurse Specialist** (CNS) in Pediatrics.

Origins

For many years, children were treated as miniature adults. However, as physicians acquired a better understanding of the development and functions of the body, they became aware that children responded to drug therapy differently from adults and sometimes needed different treatment or treatment delivered in a different way. The first known Western book on pediatrics was written in Italy in 1472.

Recognition of the special needs of children gave rise to hospitals specifically for treating sick children. The first of these children's hospitals opened in Paris in 1802 and still functions today. By the end of the 1830s, there were children's hospitals in Berlin, Vienna, St. Petersburg, and Wroclaw. The first children's hospital in London was founded in 1852. The first children's hospital in the United States was Children's Hospital of Philadelphia, founded in 1855 and still one of the leading children's hospitals in the country today.

Purpose

The purpose of pediatrics is to keep children healthy, recognize and treat developmental delays and behavioral problems or psychiatric illness, treat acute diseases and injuries, and manage chronic diseases. Pediatricians also educate parents about normal childhood growth and development.

Training and certification

To become a primary care (general) pediatrician in the United States, one must graduate from an accredited medical school, do a one-year internship and a three-year residency, and pass the appropriate examinations. Individuals who have successfully completed the requirements to become a licensed pediatrician can apply to specialty programs for additional certification. The amount of training varies among subspecialties but generally lasts two years. Various programs can reduce the time spent in training for pediatricians who wish to become certified in

KEY TERMS

Hematology—The treatment of diseases and disorders of the blood and blood-forming organs.

Nephrology—The treatment of diseases and disorders of the kidney.

Pulmonary—Of or relating to the lungs.

Rheumatology—The treatment of diseases that affect the bones, muscles, and joints.

more than one area. For example, a four-year residency program allows a physician to become certified in both pediatrics and **internal medicine**.

To remain certified, the pediatrician must accumulate through approved educational activities a specific number of points in 6 core areas every five years and pass a written examination every 10 years.

Registered nurses who wish to be certified as pediatric nurses generally work at a site that serves pediatric patients. After several years of clinical experience, they can take an examination administered by the Society of Pediatric Nurses, and upon passing, become a CPN. Advanced nurse certification for the positions of PNP or CNS requires a master's degree in nursing from an accredited university along with passing a national exam. The master's degree generally takes two years of full-time study.

Resources

BOOKS

American Academy of Pediatrics. *Caring for Your Baby and Young Child: Birth to Age 5*, 5th edition. Bantam, 2009.

Hay, William, and Myron Levin, *Robin Deterding, Mark Abzug. CURRENT Diagnosis and Treatment: Pediatrics*, 21st edition. McGraw-Hill Professional, 2012.

Marcdante, Karen, and Robert M. Kliegman, Richard E. Behrman, Hal B. Jenson. *Nelson Essentials of Pediatrics*, 6th edittion. Saunders, 2010.

PERIODICALS

"DEVELOPMENTAL-BEHAVIORAL PEDIATRICS." *Journal of Paediatrics and Child Health* 47.3 (2011): 156.

McMillan, Julia A. "Pediatrics: it's not just for kids anymore." *Contemporary Pediatrics* (June 2012).

Mele, Cheryl. "Nanotechnology in Pediatrics: Science Fiction or Reality?" *Journal of Pediatric Nursing* 26.4 (2011): 379.

Shalowitz, Madeleine U. "What should be the research agenda for developmental behavioral pediatrics?" *Journal of Developmental & Behavioral Pediatrics* (July-August 2012): 504.

OTHER

What is a Pediatrician? University of Maryland Children's Hospital. March 29, 2012 [accessed August 27, 2012]. http://www.umm.edu/pediatrics/pediatrician.htm

ORGANIZATIONS

American Academy of Child and Adolescent Psychiatry, 3615 Wisconsin Avenue, NW, Washington, DC 20016-3007, (202) 966-7300, Fax: (202) 966-2891, http://www.aacap.org

American Academy of Pediatrics, 141 Northwest Point Boulevard, Elk Grove Village, IL 60007-1098, (847) 434-4000, Fax: (847) 434-8000, http://www.aap.org

American Board of Pediatrics, 11 Silver Cedar Court, Chapel Hill, NC 27514, (919) 929-0461, Fax: (919) 929-9255, abpeds@abpeds.org, https://www.abp.org

Council of Pediatric Subspecialties, 6728 Old McLean Village Drive, Mclean, VA 22101, (703) 556-9222, Fax: (703) 556-8729, info@pedsubs.org, http://www.pedsubs.org

Society of Pediatric Nurses, 7044 S. 13th Street, Oak Creek, WI 53154, (414) 908-4950, http://www.pedsnurses.org.

Tish Davidson, AM

Pedodontics *see* **Dental specialties**

Pelvic ultrasound

Definition

Pelvic ultrasound is a procedure in which high-frequency sound waves are used to create images of the pelvic organs by projecting the sound waves into the pelvis and measuring how the sound waves reflect, or echo, back from the different tissues.

Purpose

Ultrasound is a preferred method of examining the pelvis and functions as an extension of a **physical examination**, particularly for obese patients. It is a common initial step after physical examination when a patient complains of pelvic **pain** or abnormal vaginal bleeding. The procedure is performed routinely during **pregnancy** and examinations to determine the cause of **infertility**. Ultrasound has the ability to detect the size and shape of pelvic organs, such as the bladder, and is useful in evaluating the cause of bladder dysfunction. In women, pelvic ultrasound is used to examine the uterus, ovaries, and vagina. In general, ultrasound can detect inflammation, free fluid, cysts (abnormal fluid-filled spaces), and tumors in the pelvic region.

A primary use of pelvic ultrasound is during pregnancy. In early pregnancy (at about five to seven weeks), ultrasound may determine the size of the uterus or the fetus to confirm the suspected due date, to detect

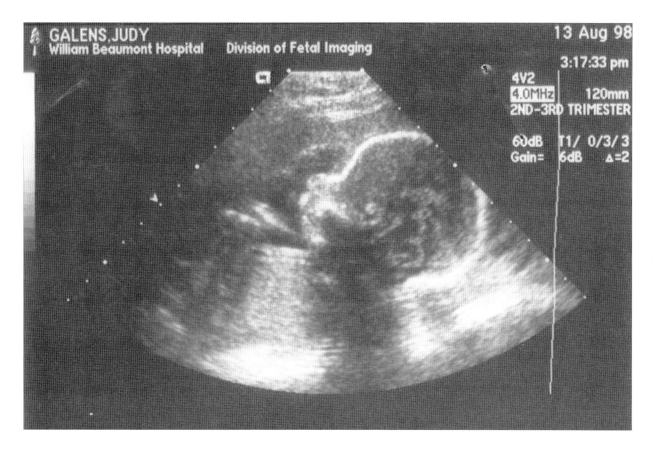

GALENS,JUDY
William Beaumont Hospital   Division of Fetal Imaging

13 Aug 98
3:17:33 pm

4V2
4.0MHz   120mm
2ND-3RD TRIMESTER

60dB   T1/ 0/3/3
Gain=   6dB   Δ=2

(Fetal ultrasound (2nd-3rd trimester), photograph. Brigham Narins. Reproduced by permission.)

multiple fetuses, or to confirm that the fetus is alive (or viable). Ultrasound is particularly useful in distinguishing between intrauterine (within the uterus) and ectopic (outside the uterus) pregnancies. Toward the middle of the pregnancy (at about 16–20 weeks), the procedure can confirm fetal growth, reveal defects in the **anatomy** of the fetus, and check the placenta. Toward the end of pregnancy, it may be used to evaluate fetal size, position, growth, or to check the placenta.

Doctors may use ultrasound to guide the biopsy needle during **amniocentesis** and **chorionic villus sampling**. The imaging allows precise placement of the long needle that is inserted into the patient's **abdomen** to collect cells from the placenta or amniotic fluid.

Precautions

There are no special precautions recommended before an ultrasound examination. Unlike x rays, ultrasound does not produce harmful radiation so it does not pose a risk to the technologist, patient, or a fetus.

Description

Depending on the goal of the procedure, a pelvic ultrasound can also be called a **bladder ultrasound**,

pelvic gynecologic sonogram, or obstetric sonogram. Ultrasound examinations are often done in a doctor's office, clinic, or hospital setting. Typically, the patient will lie on an examination table with the pelvis exposed. Special gel is applied to the area to make sure that there is no air between the hand-held transducer and the skin and to facilitate moving the transducer. The doctor or technologist will move the transducer over the abdomen. The transducer both creates and receives the echos of the high-frequency sound waves (usually in the range of 3.5-10.0 megahertz). An ultrasound scan reveals the shape and densities of organs and tissues. By performing repeated scans over time, much like the frames of a movie, ultrasound can also reveal movement, like the movement of a fetus. This technique is called real-time ultrasound.

Using a computerized tool, called a caliper, the ultrasound technologist can measure various structures shown in the image. For example, the length of the upper thigh **bone** (femur) or the distance between the two sides of the **skull** can indicate the age of the fetus.

Ultrasound technology has been used safely in medical settings for over 30 years, and several significant extensions to the procedure has made it even more useful. A specially designed transducer probe can be placed in the vagina to provide better ultrasound images. This transvaginal or endovaginal scan is particularly useful in early pregnancy or in cases where ectopic pregnancy is suspected. In men, transrectal scans, where the probe is placed in the rectum, are done to check the prostate. Doppler ultrasound has the ability to follow the flow of **blood** through veins and arteries and can be useful in detecting abnormalities such as abnormal blood flow associated with **ovarian torsion**, a twisted blood supply that causes pelvic pain. Color enhancement is particularly useful in Doppler imaging, where shades of red signify flow away from the transducer and shades of blue signify flow toward.

Hysterosonography is another variant ultrasound procedure. It involves the injection of saline solution into the uterus during an endovaginal scan. The saline distends the uterine cavity and simplifies the identification of polyps, fibroids, and tumors. The saline outlines the lesion, making it easier to find and evaluate. Hysterosonography can also be used in the testing of patency (openness) of the fallopian tubes during infertility evaluations.

Preparation

Before undergoing a pelvic ultrasound, the patient may be asked to drink several glasses of water and to avoid urinating for about one hour before the examination. When the bladder is full, it forms a convenient path, called an acoustic window, for the ultrasonic waves. A full bladder is not necessary for an endovaginal examination, sometimes making it a preferred choice for emergency situations. Women usually empty their bladders completely before an endovaginal exam.

Aftercare

For a diagnostic ultrasound, the lubricating gel applied to the abdomen is wiped off at the end of the procedure and the patient can immediately resume normal activities.

Complications

Ultrasound carries with it almost no risk for complications.

Results

A normal scan reveals no abnormalities in the size, shape, or density of the organs being scanned. For a scan taken during pregnancy, a normal scan reveals a viable fetus, of expected size and developmental stage. Although ultrasound is an extremely useful tool, it cannot detect all problems in the pelvic region. If a tumor or other lesion is very small or if it is masked by another structure it may not be detected. When used during pregnancy, patients should be advised that all fetal abnormalities may not be seen with ultrasound. Additionally, the reliability of ultrasound

---

KEY TERMS

Acoustic window—Area through which ultrasound waves move freely.

Amniocentesis—A procedure where a needle is inserted through the pregnant woman's abdomen and into the uterus to draw off some of the amniotic fluid surrounding the fetus.

Chorionic villus sampling—A procedure where a needle is inserted into the placenta to draw off some of the placenta's inner wall cells surrounding the fetus.

Ectopic pregnancy—A pregnancy where the fertilized egg becomes implanted somewhere other than in the uterus; if in a fallopian tube it is called a tubal pregnancy.

Real-time—A type of ultrasound involving the taking of multiple images over time in order to record movement.

Sonographer—A technologist who uses an ultrasound unit to takes ultrasound images of patients.

Transducer—The handheld part of the ultrasound unit that produces the ultrasound waves and receives the ultrasound echos.

Ultrasound—Sound above what can be heard by the human ear, generally above 20,000 Hz (cycles per second).

---

readings can depend on the skill of the technologist or doctor performing the scan.

An abnormal scan may show the presence of inflammation, cysts, tumors, or abnormal blood flow patterns. These results may suggest further diagnostic procedures or surgical or pharmacological treatment. Ultrasound examinations in obstetrics may alter the anticipated due date or detect abnormalities or defects in the fetus. This information may reveal that the fetus cannot survive on its own after birth or that it will require extensive treatment or care. The technologist performing the ultrasound should be sure to consult with a radiologist or other doctor if any questionable results appear.

Health care team roles

Ultrasound units are often run by specially trained ultrasound technologists. These technologists are thoroughly trained in the use of the **ultrasound unit** to produce diagnostically useful images. Nurses aid in patient preparation and education about the procedure. A physician such as a radiologist or gynecologist does the final review and diagnosis based on the results of the ultrasound. The doctor can be present for the exam or may make the final review and diagnosis based on saved images.

Patient education

It is very important that patients understand the limitations of ultrasound, particularly when it is performed during a normal pregnancy. Many fetal malformations are not detectable, or are unreliably detectable, using ultrasound alone. The patient must understand that a normal ultrasound result does not necessarily guarantee that the fetus is normal.

Training

Being hired as an ultrasound technologist to perform pelvic ultrasounds usually involves successful completion of a training program at a two-year college or vocational program. Certification of ultrasound technologists is available through the American Registry of Diagnostic Medical Sonographers as a registered diagnostic medical sonographer (RDMS). Specialty areas within the sonographer credentials that might be useful for performing pelvic ultrasounds include abdomen or obstetrics and gynecology.

Resources

BOOK

Sanders, Roger C. *Clinical Sonography: A Practical Guide.* Boston: Little, Brown and Company, 1998.

ORGANIZATIONS

American Institute of Ultrasound in Medicine. 14750 Sweiter Lane, Suite 100, Laurel, MD 20707-5906. (301) 498-4100. (800) 638-5352. http://www.aium.org.

American Registry of Diagnostic Medical Sonographers (ARDMS). 600 Jefferson Plaza, Suite 360, Rockville, MD 20852-1150. (301) 738-8401. (800) 541-9754. http://www.ardms.org.

Michelle L. Johnson, M.S., J.D.

Percutaneous transhepatic cholangiography

Definition

Percutaneous transhepatic cholangiography (PTHC) is used to identify obstructions that slow or stop the flow of bile from the **liver** to the **digestive system**.

Purpose

PTHC allows doctors to determine what is causing a patient's **jaundice** (an obstructed bile duct or liver disease) and why upper **abdominal pain** continues after **gallbladder** surgery. It is not a first line test due to its invasive nature. PTHC is usually done only after computed tomography or ultrasound tests have been performed, when those tests indicate the need for PTHC to further delineate biliary **anatomy**.

Precautions

Patients should report allergic reactions to:

• anesthetics

• contrast media (dyes) used in radiographic tests

• iodine

• shellfish

PTHC should not be performed on anyone who has:

• cholangitis (inflammation of the bile ducts)

• massive ascites

• a severe allergy to iodine

• a serious uncorrectable or uncontrollable bleeding disorder

Description

The patient lies on a movable x-ray table and is given a local anesthetic. A footrest and shoulder rest prevent the patient from sliding when the position of the table is changed. The patient will be told to hold his or her breath, and a doctor, usually a radiologist, will place a needle into the liver and then inject contrast medium into the liver as the patient exhales.

The patient may feel a twinge when the needle penetrates the liver, a pressure or fullness, or brief discomfort in the upper right side of the back. Hands and feet may become numb during the 30–60 minute procedure.

The x-ray table will be tilted several times during the test, and the patient helped to assume a variety of positions. A special x-ray machine called a **fluoroscope** will track the contrast medium's passage through the bile ducts and show whether the fluid is moving freely or how its passage is obstructed. After the x rays have been taken, the needle is removed.

PTHC costs about $1,600. The test may have to be repeated if the patient moves while x rays are being taken.

Preparation

An intravenous antibiotic may be given every four to six hours during the 24 hours before the test. The patient will be told to fast overnight and may be given a sedative a few minutes before the test begins.

KEY TERMS

Ascites—Abnormal accumulation of fluid in the abdomen.

Bile ducts—Tubes that carry bile, a thick yellowish green fluid that is made by the liver, stored in the gallbladder, and helps the body digest fats.

Fluoroscope—An x-ray machine that projects images of organs.

Granulomatous disease—Disease characterized by the growth of tiny blood vessels and connective tissue, which forms tissues known as granulomas.

Jaundice—Disease that causes bile to accumulate in the blood, causing the skin and whites of the eyes to turn yellow. Obstructive jaundice is caused by blockage of bile ducts. Non-obstructive jaundice is caused by disease or infection of the liver that causes liver dysfunction.

Aftercare

A nurse will monitor the patient's **vital signs** until they return to normal and watch for:

• itching

• flushing

• nausea and vomiting

• sweating

• excessive flow of saliva

• occasional serious allergic reactions to contrast dye

The patient should stay in bed for at least six hours after the test, lying on the right side to prevent bleeding from the injection site. The patient may resume normal eating habits and gradually resume normal activities.

Complications

Septicemia (bloodpoisoning) and bile peritonitis (a potentially fatal **infection** or inflammation of the membrane covering the walls of the **abdomen**) are rare but serious complications of this procedure.

Contrast material occasionally leaks from the liver into the abdomen, and there is a slight risk of bleeding or infection.

Results

Normal x rays show contrast material evenly distributed throughout the bile ducts. **Obesity**, gas, and failure to fast can affect test results.

Enlargement of bile ducts may indicate:

• obstructive or non-obstructive jaundice

• cholelithiasis (gallstones)

• cancer of the bile ducts or pancreas

• hepatitis (inflammation of the liver)

• cirrhosis (chronic liver disease)

• granulomatous disease

Health care team roles

PTHC is performed in a hospital, doctor's office, or outpatient surgical or x-ray facility. The procedure is usually performed by a radiologist, with the assistance of a radiologic technologist.

Resources

OTHER

"Percutaneous Transhepatic Cholangiography." http://207.25.144.143/health/Library/medtests/.

"Percutaneous Transhepatic Cholangiography (PTHC)." http://www.uhs.org/frames/health/test/test3554.htm.

"Percutaneous Transhepatic Cholangiography (PTHC)." McLeod Health Health Information Library. http://www.mcleodhealth.org/library/test/3554/.

Stephen John Hage, AAAS, RT-R, FAHRA

Periapical abscess *see* **Dental abscess**

Pericardial effusion

Definition

A pericardial effusion is a fluid collection that develops between the pericardium, the lining of the **heart**, and the heart itself. Pericardial effusions can be found in up to 20% of **cancer** patients at **autopsy**, but of those, only about 30% would have had symptoms from their effusions.

Description

Most of the organs of the body are covered by thin membranes. The membrane that surrounds the heart is called the pericardium. Normally, only a few milliliters of fluid sit between the pericardium and the muscle of the heart. Any larger, abnormal collection of fluid in that space is called a pericardial effusion.

A pericardial effusion can interfere with the normal contraction and expansion of the heart muscle, which decreases the heart's ability to pump **blood** effectively. A

KEY TERMS

Pericardium—The thin membrane that surrounds the heart.

Sclerosing agents—Drugs that are instilled into parts of the body to deliberately induce scarring.

Tamponade—A medical emergency in which fluid or other substances between the pericardium and heart muscle compress the heart muscle and interfere with the normal pumping of blood.

Thoracoscopy—Chest surgery done with the guidance of special video cameras that permit the surgeon to see inside the chest.

large or rapidly developing effusion can cause a condition called cardiac tamponade. Tamponade is a medical emergency and can be fatal if not diagnosed and treated promptly. Symptoms of tamponade include shortness of breath, rapid pulse, **cough**, and chest discomfort. As tamponade progresses, low **blood pressure** and **shock** develop and cardiac arrest can follow.

A smaller or more slowly developing pericardial effusion also causes chest discomfort. Other symptoms, such as shortness or breath, difficulty swallowing, hoarseness or hiccups result from pressure from the enlarged, fluid-filled pericardium pressing against nearby organs. Although chronic or smaller effusions are not emergencies, they do cause discomfort and can become more serious.

The diagnosis of pericardial effusion is made on the basis of patient history, **physical examination** and appropriate laboratory studies. Heart sounds can be muffled, the veins in the neck engorged and the pulse rapid. A **chest x ray** shows enlargement of the silhouette of the heart. An echocardiogram or cardiac ultrasound will show the fluid surrounding the heart, as will CT and MRI scans.

Causes

A pericardial effusion in a cancer patient is caused either by the disease itself or by the treatment for the disease.

Many cancers can metastasize or spread to the pericardium or the heart itself. They include:

• lung

• breast

• thyroid

• esophagus

• kidney

• pancreas

• endometrium

• larynx

• cervix

• stomach

• mouth

• liver

• ovary

• colon

• prostate

• leukemia

• melanoma

• lymphoma

• sarcoma

• myeloma

The presence of the cancerous cells on the pericardium is an irritant and causes a reactive fluid buildup, much as a blister forms under the skin due to irritation. Some cancers cause less fluid buildup, instead thickening the pericardium and making it less elastic. This can also cause symptoms of tamponade.

Another cause of pericardial effusion in a cancer patient is previous radiation therapy to the chest, especially in the case of **lung cancer** or **lymphoma**. While such effusions are less likely to produce tamponade, it is possible.

Many of the drugs that are used to treat cancer can cause pericardial disease and can thus potentially cause pericardial effusions. Some of the chemotherapeutic drugs that can affect the pericardium are cytarabine, fluorouracil, cyclophosphamide, doxorubicin and daunorubicin. Granulocyte-macrophage colony-stimulating factor (sargramostim), often given to help increase the population of white blood cells during intensive **chemotherapy**, is also a pericardial irritant.

Other causes of pericardial effusions are **heart failure**, **liver** disease, and kidney disease. Any of these can also affect cancer patients.

Treatments

Treatment of pericardial effusion depends on the presence or absence of cardiac tamponade. Tamponade is a medical emergency and symptoms such as **cyanosis**, a blue tinge to the lips and skin, shock, or a change in mental status require urgent drainage of the fluid. This drainage is accomplished with a procedure called **pericardiocentesis**, in which a needle is inserted into the pericardial space and the fluid withdrawn into a large syringe. Chronic effusions can be drained electively, and some need not be drained at all. If a patient's prognosis is poor and the pericardial effusion is not compromising the function of the heart, the risks of a drainage procedure may outweigh its benefits and the effusion may be left alone. Effusions caused by lymphoma often resolve after aggressive chemotherapy and need no further treatment.

Elective drainage of a pericardial effusion is done by one of several surgical procedures. The surgeon might open the chest, make a small incision under the bottom of the breastbone, or use a video-assisted technique called **thoracoscopy**. In addition to permitting drainage of the pericardial fluid, these procedures permit the surgeon to take a pericardial biopsy, which can confirm the diagnosis of metastatic cancer.

Sometimes a catheter is placed in the pericardium and connected to an external drainage system to collect any fluid that might reaccumulate.

Occasionally, sclerosing agents—drugs that cause scarring—are infused into the pericardium through a catheter. These agents, such as tetracycline, minocycline or bleomycin, irritate the pericardium, causing it to thicken and adhere to the heart muscle. This scarring prevents the further accumulation of fluid. Some malignant pericardial effusions resolve after the installation of chemotherapeutic drugs such as thiotepa or platinum directly into the pericardial cavity. Others resolve after radiation therapy directed at the pericardium.

Alternative and complementary therapies

No complementary or alternative treatments are aimed specifically at treating pericardial effusions, but practitioners of **acupressure** and **acupuncture** designate a pressure point for the pericardium at two and a half finger breadths above the wrist crease on the inner aspect of the arm. Acupressure and acupuncture do offer some relief of symptoms to those suffering from shortness of breath and might offer benefit to those with pericardial effusions.

Resources

BOOKS

Moore, Katen, and Libby Schmais. *Living Well with Cancer: A Nurse Tells You Everything You Need to Know About Managing the Side Effects of Your Treatment.* New York: Putnam Publishing Group, 2001.

PERIODICALS

Brigden, M. L. "Hematologic and Oncologic Emergencies. Doing the Most Good in the Least Time." *Postgraduate Medicine* 109, no. 3 (March 2001): 143-6, 151-4, 157-8.

Gibbs, C. R., R. D. Watson, S.P. Singh, and G.Y. Lip. "Management of Pericardial Effusion by Drainage: A Survey of 10 Years' Experience in a City Centre General Hospital Serving a Multiracial Population." *Postgraduate Medicine Journal* 76, no. 902 (December 2000): 809-13.

OTHER

Heart Center Online Home Page [cited June 6, 2009]. http:// www.heartcenteronline.com/ . This web site serves cardiologists and their patients and has sections on pericardiocentesis, pericarditis and tamponade.

Marianne Vahey, M.D.

Pericardiocentesis

Definition

Pericardiocentesis is the removal by needle of pericardial fluid from the sac surrounding the **heart** for diagnostic or therapeutic purposes.

Purpose

The pericardium, the sac (or membrane) that surrounds the heart muscle, normally contains a small amount of fluid that cushions and lubricates the heart as the heart expands and contracts. When too much fluid gathers in the pericardial cavity, the space between the pericardium and the outer layers of the heart, a condition known as **pericardial effusion** occurs. Abnormal amounts of fluid may result from:

- pericarditis (caused by infection, inflammation)
- trauma (producing blood in the pericardial sac)
- surgery or other invasive procedures performed on the heart
- cancer (producing malignant effusions)
- myocardial infarction, congestive heart failure
- renal failure

Possible causes of **pericarditis** include chest trauma, systemic **infection** (bacterial, viral, or fungal), **myocardial infarction** (heart attack), or **tuberculosis**. When pericarditis is suspected, pericardiocentesis may be advisable in order to obtain a fluid sample for laboratory analysis to identify the underlying cause of the condition.

Pericardiocentesis is also used in emergency situations to remove excessive accumulations of **blood** or fluid from the pericardial sac, such as with cardiac

KEY TERMS

Cardiac tamponade—Compression and restriction of the heart that occurs when the pericardium fills with blood or fluid. This increase in pressure outside the heart interferes with heart function and can result in shock and/or death.

Catheter—A long, thin, flexible tube used to drain or administer fluids.

Echocardiogram—An imaging test using high-frequency sound waves to obtain pictures of the heart and surrounding tissues.

Electrocardiogram—A cardiac test that measures the electrical activity of the heart.

Myocardium—The middle layer of the heart wall.

Pericardium—A double membranous sac that envelops and protects the heart.

tamponade. When fluid builds up too rapidly or excessively in the pericardial cavity, the resulting compression on the heart impairs the pumping action of the vascular system. Cardiac tamponade is a life-threatening condition that requires immediate treatment.

Precautions

Whenever possible, an echocardiogram (ultrasound test) should be performed to confirm the presence of the pericardial effusion and to guide the pericardiocentesis needle during the procedure. Because of the risk of accidental puncture to major arteries or organs in pericardiocentesis, surgical drainage may be a preferred treatment option for pericardial effusion in non-emergency situations.

Description

The patient's **vital signs** are monitored throughout the procedure, and an ECG tracing is continuously run. If time allows, sedation is administered, the puncture site is cleaned with an antiseptic iodine solution, and a local anesthetic is injected into the skin to numb the area. The patient is instructed to remain still. The physician performing pericardiocentesis will insert a syringe with an attached cardiac needle slowly into the chest wall until the needle tip reaches the pericardial sac. The patient may experience a sensation of pressure as the needle enters the membrane. When the needle is in the correct position, the physician will aspirate, or withdraw, fluid from the pericardial sac.

When the procedure is performed for diagnostic purposes, the fluid will be collected into specimen tubes for laboratory analysis. If the pericardiocentesis is performed to treat a cardiac tamponade or other significant fluid build-up, a pericardial catheter may be attached to the needle to allow for continuous drainage.

After the cardiac needle is removed, pressure is applied to the puncture site for approximately five minutes, and the site is then bandaged.

Preparation

Prior to pericardiocentesis, the test procedure is explained to the patient, along with the risks and possible complications involved, and the patient is asked to sign an **informed consent** form. If the patient is incapacitated, the same steps are followed with a family member.

No special diet or fasting is required for the test. After the patient changes into a hospital gown, an intravenous line is inserted into a vein in the arm. The IV will be used to administer sedation, and any required medications or blood products. Leads for an electrocardiogram (ECG) tracing are attached to the patient's right and left arms and legs, and the fifth lead is attached to the cardiac needle used for the procedure. The patient is instructed to lie flat on the table, with the upper body elevated to a 60-degree angle.

Aftercare

The site of the puncture and any drainage catheter should be checked regularly for signs of infection such as redness and swelling. **Blood pressure** and pulse are also monitored following the procedure. Patients who experience continued bleeding or abnormal swelling of the puncture site, sudden **dizziness**, difficulty breathing, or chest pains in the days following a pericardiocentesis procedure should seek immediate medical attention.

Risks

Pericardiocentesis is an invasive procedure, and infection of the puncture site or pericardium is always a risk. Possible complications include perforation of a major artery, lung, or **liver**. The myocardium, the outer muscle layer of the heart, could also be damaged if the cardiac needle is inserted too deeply.

Normal results

Normal pericardial fluid is clear to straw-colored in appearance with no **bacteria**, blood, **cancer** cells or pathogens. There is typically a minimal amount of the fluid (10–50 mL) in the pericardial cavity.

Abnormal results

A large volume of pericardial fluid (over 50 mL) indicates the presence of pericardial effusion. Laboratory analysis of the fluid can aid in the diagnosis of the cause of pericarditis. The presence of an infectious organism such as *staphylococcus aureus* is a sign of bacterial pericarditis. Excessive protein is present in cases of systemic lupus erythematosus or myocardial infarction (heart attack). An elevated white blood count may point to a fungal infection. If the patient has a hemorrhage, a cardiac rupture, or cancer, there may be blood in the pericardial fluid.

Resources

BOOK

Maisch, Bernhard, et al. *Interventional Pericardiology: Pericardiocentesis, Pericardioscopy, Pericardial Biopsy, Balloon Pericardiotomy, and Intrapericardial Therapy.* New York: Springer, 2010.

ORGANIZATION

American Heart Association National Center, 7272 Greenville Avenue, Dallas, TX 75231, ((800)) 242-8721, Review. personal.info@heart.org

Paula Anne Ford-Martin

Pericarditis

Definition

Pericarditis is an inflammation of the two layers of the thin, sac-like membrane that surrounds the **heart**. This membrane is called the pericardium, so the term pericarditis means inflammation of the pericardium.

Description

Pericarditis is fairly common. It affects approximately one in 1,000 people. The most common form is caused by **infection** with a virus. People in their 20s and 30s who have had a recent upper respiratory infection are most likely to be affected, along with men aged 20–50. One out of every four people who have had pericarditis will get it again, but after two years these relapses are less likely.

Causes and symptoms

The **viruses** that cause pericarditis include those that cause **influenza**, polio, and rubella (German measles). In children, the most common viruses that cause pericarditis are the adenovirus and the cocksackievirus (which is most likely to affect children during warmer weather).

Although pericarditis is usually caused by a virus, it also can be caused by an injury to the heart or it can follow a heart attack. It may also be caused by certain inflammatory diseases such as **rheumatoid arthritis** or systemic lupus erythematosus. **Bacteria, fungi, parasites, tuberculosis, cancer** or kidney failure may also affect the pericardium. Sometimes the cause is unknown.

There are several forms of pericarditis, depending on the cause.

Acute pericarditis

This is caused by infection with a virus, bacteria, or fungus—usually in the **lungs** and upper respiratory tract. This form of the disease causes a sharp, severe **pain** that starts in the region of the breastbone. If the pericarditis is caused by a bacteria, it is called bacterial or purulent pericarditis.

Cardiac tamponade

Sometimes fluid collects between the heart and the pericardium. This is called **pericardial effusion**, and may lead to a condition called cardiac tamponade. When the fluid accumulates, it can squeeze the heart and prevent it from filling with **blood**. This keeps the rest of the body from getting the necessary supply of oxygen and can cause dangerously low **blood pressure**. A cardiac tamponade can happen when the chest is injured during surgery, radiation therapy, or an accident. Cardiac tamponade is a serious medical emergency and must be treated immediately.

Constrictive pericarditis

When the pericardium is scarred or thickened, the heart has difficulty contracting. This is because the pericardium has shrunken or tightened around the heart, constricting the muscle's heart movement. This usually occurs as a result of tuberculosis, which now is rarely found in the United States, except in immigrant, **AIDS**, and prison populations.

Computed tomography (CT) scan—A CT scan uses x rays to scan the body from many angles. A computer compiles the x rays into a picture of the area being studied. The images are viewed on a monitor and printed-out.

Echocardiogram—An echocardiogram bounces sound waves off the heart to create a picture of its chambers and valves.

Electrocardiogram (ECG)—An ECG is a test to measure electrical activity in the heart.

Heart catheterization—A heart catheterization is used to view the heart's chamber and valves. A tube (catheter) is inserted into an artery, usually in the groin. A dye is then put into the artery through the tube. The dye makes its way to the heart to create an image of the heart on x-ray film. The image is photographed and stored for further examination.

Pericardiocentesis—Pericardiocentesis is a procedure used to test for viruses, bacteria, and fungus. The physician puts a small tube through the skin, directly into the pericardial sac, and withdraws fluid. The fluid then is tested for viruses, bacteria, and fungus.

Pericardium—The pericardium is the thin, sac-like membrane that surrounds the heart. It has two layers: the serous pericardium and the fibrous pericardium.

Symptoms of pericarditis

Symptoms likely to be associated with pericarditis include:

- rapid breathing
- breathlessness
- dry cough
- fever and chills
- weakness
- broken blood vessels (hemorrhages) in the mucus membrane of the eyes, the back, the chest, fingers, and toes
- feelings of anxiety
- A sharp or dull pain that starts in the front of the chest under the breastbone and radiates to the left side of the neck, upper abdomen, and left shoulder the pain is less intense when the patient sits up or leans forward and worsens when lying down; it may worsen with a deep breath, like pleurisy, which may accompany pericarditis

In cardiac tamponade, neck veins may be swollen and blood pressure may be very low.

Diagnosis

The heart of a person with pericarditis is likely to produce a grating sound (friction rub) when heard through a **stethoscope**. This sound occurs because the roughened pericardium surfaces are rubbing against each other.

The following tests will also help diagnose pericarditis and what is causing it:

- electrocardiograph (ECG) and echocardiogram to distinguish between pericarditis and a heart attack.
- x ray to show the traditional "water bottle" shadow around the heart that is often seen in pericarditis where there is a sufficient fluid build up.
- computed tomography scan (CT scan) of the chest.
- heart catheterization to view the heart's chambers and valves.
- pericardiocentesis to test for viruses, bacteria, fungus, cancer, and tuberculosis.
- blood tests such as LDH and CPK to measure cardiac enzymes and distinguish between a heart attack and pericarditis, as well as a complete blood count (CBC) to look for infection.

Treatment

Since most pericarditis is caused by a virus and will heal naturally, there is no specific, curative treatment. Ordinary **antibiotics** do not work against viruses. Pericarditis that comes from a virus usually clears up in two weeks to three months. Medications may be used to reduce inflammation, however. They include **nonsteroidal anti-inflammatory drugs** (NSAIDs), such as ibuprofen and aspirin. **Corticosteroids** are helpful if the pericarditis was caused by a heart attack or systemic lupus erythematosus. **Analgesics** (painkillers such as aspirin or acetaminophen) also may be given.

If the pericarditis recurs, removal of all or part of the pericardium (pericardiectomy) may be necessary. In the case of constrictive pericarditis, the pericardiectomy may be necessary to remove the stiffened parts of the pericardium that are preventing the heart from beating correctly.

If a cardiac tamponade is present, it may be necessary to drain excess fluid from the pericardium. **Pericardiocentesis**, the same procedure used for testing, will be used to withdraw the fluid.

For most people, **home care** with rest and medications to relieve pain are sufficient. A warm heating pad or compress also may help relieve pain. Sitting in an upright position and bending forward helps relieve discomfort. A person with pericarditis may also be kept in bed, with the head of the bed elevated to reduce the heart's need to work hard as it pumps blood. Along with painkillers and antibiotics, diuretic drugs ("water pills") to reduce fluids may also be used judiciously.

Prognosis

Prognosis is good. Most people recover within three weeks to several months and do not need any additional treatment.

Prevention

There is no way to prevent pericarditis, but a healthy lifestyle with proper **nutrition** and **exercise** will help keep the body's **immune system** strong and more likely to fight off invading microorganisms.

ORGANIZATIONS

American Heart Association National Center, 7272 Greenville Avenue, Dallas, TX 75231, ((800)) 242-8721, Review. personal.info@heart.org

National Heart Lung and Blood Institute Health Information Center, P.O. Box 30105, Bethesda, MD 20824-0105, ((301)) 592-8573, Fax: ((240)) 629-3246, http://www.nhlbi.nih.gov

Christine Kuehn Kelly

Perinatal infection

Definition

Perinatal infections are those infections affecting the mother during a **pregnancy**, and may be transmitted to the fetus during pregnancy, during delivery through the birth canal, or after delivery through the breast milk.

Description

Perinatal infections may be bacterial, fungal, or viral in nature. The degree to which the mother is affected by the **infection** is not an indication of its impact on the fetus. The mother may have slight or no symptoms, and yet the fetus may be significantly affected by the infection. The woman's sexual partner (s) may also be affected by these infections and should seek medical treatment. The more common perinatal infections significantly affecting the fetus are discussed below.

Causes and symptoms

Chlamydia

According to the Centers for Disease Control (CDC), chlamydia trachomatis is the most frequently reported bacterial **sexually transmitted disease** in the United States, with about 834,555 cases reported in 2002 and 1,244,180 cases reported in 2009. It is often referred to as a silent disease, because so many infected individuals are asymptomatic. While about 75% of women are unaware of their infection, symptoms include purulent endocervical discharge, inflammation, **edema**, and bleeding. Chlamydial infection can permanently damage the reproductive tract. While asymptomatic, women can experience inflammation of the fallopian tubes, chronic pelvic **pain**, pelvis inflammatory disease, an increased risk for ectopic pregnancy, and **infertility**. For pregnant woman, chlamydial infection increases the risk for premature rupture of membranes, preterm delivery, and neonatal conjunctival or pneumonic infection. About 65% of infected neonates acquired the disease during a vaginal delivery.

Cytomegalovirus (CMV)

CMV is a common congenital viral infection, belonging to the herpes virus group of infections. Maternal infection usually occurs through sexual intercourse, including kissing, with an infected individual. Maternal infection may be asymptomatic, or the mother may present with mononucleosis-like symptoms, fatigue, lymphadenopathy, or **fever**. Transmission to the fetus can occur if the mother becomes infected during pregnancy, or if she has a flaring of a pre-exisisting CMV infection. Some immunity is transferred to the fetus if the mother has had a prior CMV infection. Infants infected in utero with CMV may be asymptomatic, or may have a delayed reaction, manifesting as mental retardation or deafness. About 10% of newborns with congenital CMV have evidence of disease at birth. CMV can also be acquired by the newborn through cervical secretions, saliva, urine, or breast milk. It can also be acquired in the newborn nursery by contact with infected individuals. Individuals with a compromised **immune system**, organ recipients, and those with HIV/AIDS are more likely to suffer severe consequences.

Genital herpes

Genital herpes is a sexually transmitted disease (STD) caused by the herpes simplex virus (HSV), and is considered a life-long infection. It may be contracted in two types, HSV-1 and HSV-2. According to a June 2001 report by the CDC, about 45 million Americans aged 12 and older have contracted HSV-2. The most recent data (2010) from the CDC, reports that nationwide, about one out of six, people 14 to 49 years of age have the genital HSV-2 infection.

The infections may exist subclinically, and later erupt in lesions. The risk of contracting the disease increases with the number of sexual partners. If genital herpes occurs for the first time during pregnancy, first trimester **miscarriage** and third trimester preterm birth may be the result. The greatest risk for the fetus occurs when genital herpes is contracted near term. Intrauterine transmission does occur, although it is more rare, and can take place across the placenta. After birth, neonates can also contract the disease from an infected newborn in the nursery.

Hepatitis B virus (HBV)

HBV is contracted through direct contact with the **blood** or other body fluids of an infected individual. It is sexually transmitted, through infected blood or blood products, and to the infant during a vaginal birth. In infants with HBV, 90% contract it at birth. The disease may present in very mild form, with no symptoms and only detected through **liver function tests**, or may be severe, even fatal, if it has advanced to **liver** necrosis. Symptoms of HBV infection include:

- jaundice
- fatigue
- rash
- fever that is usually either not present, or very mild
- vague abdominal discomfort
- abdominal pain
- loss of appetite
- nausea
- vomiting
- joint pain

Human immunodeficiency virus (HIV)

HIV is transmitted through direct contact with an infected individual's blood and body fluids (such as semen, amniotic fluid, breast milk, and vaginal and cervical secretions), and leads to the development of acquired **immunodeficiency** syndrome (**AIDS**). The majority of pediatric AIDS cases are due to vertical transmission from the mother to the fetus, and is a leading cause of death in children aged one to four years old. Transmission from the mother to the fetus occurs during pregnancy through the placenta, during a vaginal delivery or with premature rupture of membranes, or through the breast milk. Symptoms of an impaired immune system suspicious of HIV infection include:

- fever
- weight loss
- malaise
- oral candidiasis
- central nervous system dysfunction

Human papillomavirus (HPV)

HPV is a STD than can cause genital warts. However, many infected individuals are asymptomatic. This variability is due to the fact that there are about 40 types of HPV. The CDC estimates about 6 million new cases of HPV a year, with about 20 million people infected to date. About 28–46% of women under the age of 25 have HPV. Individuals who are immunocompromised, such as those with HIV, are at higher risk of contracting the disease. This is also true of those who are pregnant. Genital warts appear to grow more quickly during pregnancy, and can be large enough to obstruct the cervix for a vaginal delivery. Disruption to the warts of the genital tract during pregnancy or delivery can lead to significant maternal blood loss.

Rubella

Rubella is a contagious disease, and is spread through the respiratory tract. Because of effective **vaccination**, it is rare in pregnancy. However, it can be passed to the fetus through the placenta if the mother becomes infected during pregnancy. Maternal symptoms include:

- low-grade fever
- swollen glands
- rash starting at the face and moving down toward the extremities
- joint pain
- conjunctivitis

Streptococcus

Group B streptococcus (GBS) is a contagious, bacterial infection that is particularly harmful to pregnant women, newborns, the elderly, and those who are immunocompromised by other illnesses. According to the CDC, it is the most common cause of life-threatening illness in neonates. In pregnant women it can cause bladder infections, amnionitis, endometritis, and still-birth. Newborns may develop early-onset disease, from day one to day seven, or late-onset disease, from day seven to several months postpartum. In early-onset disease, infants may present with **sepsis**, respiratory distress, apnea, **pneumonia**, **shock**, or **meningitis**. Late-onset disease may present as sepsis or meningitis. Individuals may harbor GBS without symptoms, but be able to transmit it to another individual. **Premature infants** are particularly vulnerable.

Syphilis

Syphilis is a sexually-transmitted disease caused by the bacterium *Treponema pallidum*. It progresses in three stages. In the primary stage, shortly after infection, a small, round, firm chancre sore develops at the site of transmission. Multiple sores may also exist, usually in the vagina, anus, rectum, lips, or mouth. It heals on its own, and may go unnoticed. Untreated, the disease progresses to the secondary stage. In this stage multiple locations break out in a **rash** of red or brown spots that do not itch. It may be accompanied by fever, weight loss, fatigue, or muscle pain. If untreated, the disease can progress to late-stage syphilis. In this stage, damage to internal organs, the **central nervous system**, and body systems develops. This stage can lead to **paralysis**, numbness, blindness, **dementia**, and death. A mother can pass the disease on to her fetus, who may be stillborn or die shortly after birth.

Toxoplasmosis

A pregnant woman can become infected with toxoplasmosis either by handling infected cat feces, or by ingesting raw or undercooked infected meat. The risk of maternal to fetal transmission is greater when the mother is suffering from an acute, rather than a chronic, infection of toxoplasmosis.

Diagnosis

Chlamydia

In women, chlamydia is diagnosed by evaluating a sample taken of the cervical secretions. A urine test is also available. The Pap smear does not test for chlamydia. To properly diagnose the disease, the endocervical sample needs to be adequate in amount and contain columnar epithelial cells.

Cytomegalovirus

A blood sample can be evaluated for the presence of a CMV-specific antibody, but about 20% of women will show no antibody presence. Prevalence of CMV among the adult general population is high, in some regions occurring in 40–100% of the population. About 33–66% of pregnant women test positive to the CMV IgG antibody. Ultrasound can detect fetal infection, presenting as intrauterine growth retardation, polyhydramnios, and central nervous system abnormalities.

Genital herpes

When lesions are present, tissue sample scrapings or a biopsy can be taken and cultured to confirm the diagnosis. When the condition is latent, diagnosis is more difficult. Blood tests are available, but accuracy of results is not guaranteed. At the first prenatal visit, mothers should be questioned about a prior history of lesions.

Hepatitis B

Diagnosis for HBV is through evaluation of a blood sample for the presence of antigens or **antibodies**.

Human immunodeficiency virus (HIV)

The HIV infection affects the immune system, causing progressive deterioration during which the individual becomes susceptible to infections and neoplasms rarely seen in those with an intact immune system, such as wasting syndrome, Pneumocystis carini, and Karposi's sarcoma. The diagnosis of these conditions promotes further evaluation for the presence of HIV/AIDS. The average latency between HIV infection and the development of AIDS is about 11 years. A blood sample is used to detect the presence of HIV infection.

Human papillomavirus

Genital warts are diagnosed during a clinical exam.

Rubella

Because rashes can mimic several diseases, the best diagnostic evaluation for rubella is a blood test for the presence of a rubella-specific IgM antibody. The test can also be performed by evaluating samples of nasal or throat secretions, as well as cerebrospinal fluid.

Streptococcus

Diagnosis is done through cultures of rectal or vaginal secretions taken during the third trimester. In the neonate, blood samples can be taken.

Syphilis

Syphilis diagnoses are often missed because the signs can mimic other conditions or be so mild in appearance as to go unnoticed. Samples from chancre sores can be evaluated for the presence of syphilis, or a blood test can be run. While antibodies do develop, they diminish as time passes, and the individual may become reinfected.

Toxoplasmosis

Maternal infection with toxoplasmosis may be asymptomatic. About 10–20% of infected women may present with lymphadenopathy. Fatigue and mononucleosis-like symptoms may also be present. A blood sample can be evaluated for the maternal presence of a toxoplasmosis-specific IgM antibody. Amniotic sampling can detect fetal infection. Infected neonates may present with liver or spleen enlargement, **jaundice**, fever, **hydrocephalus**, or microcephalus.

Treatment

Chlamydia

The drugs azithromycin, doxycycline, and oflaxacin are the first-choice treatment for chlamydia, but are contraindicated in pregnancy. Erythromycin and amoxicillin are used during pregnancy. Repeat testing is recommended three weeks after the conclusion of treatment.

Cytomegalovirus

Since no fetal treatment exists for CMV, maternal testing is usually not recommended. In affected infants, acyclovir (Zovirax) and ganciclovir have been used to suppress the infection. However, the infection reappears once the medication is discontinued.

Genital herpes

Antiviral medical treatment does not cure herpes, but rather shortens the course of the disease. For severe maternal complications, intravenous acyclovir may be used. Acyclovir should be given to all neonates with the disease. Treatment can prevent disease progression to serious consequences. Even with antiviral treatment, if the HSV has spread throughout the infant, mortality may be as high as 50%.

Hepatitis B

Because HBV affects the liver, alcohol should be avoided. HBV-infected individuals should have their liver evaluated for signs of disease. The CDC reports that the use of alpha interferon and lamivudine are effective for about 40% of patients. The use of these medications in pregnancy is contraindicated.

Human immunodeficiency virus (HIV)

Careful monitoring of the mother's immune status is an essential component of HIV management. For pregnant HIV-positive women, the medical focus is to maximize benefit for the mother herself, while avoiding vertical transmission, if at all possible. The use of zidovudine (ZDV) reduces the incidence of maternal transmission to the fetus. The pregnant state also balances the side effects of treatment on the mother. The use of ritonavir and nelfinavir (Virocept) are first-line protease inhibitor choices for the pregnant woman. The treatment plan of the HIV-infected individual is determined by the amount of virus present in the body, referred to as *viral load*. The greater the viral load, the greater the degree to which the maternal immune system is compromised, and the higher the risk of transmission to the fetus. During the first trimester of pregnancy, the teratogenic effects of the antiviral agents given to the mother are the greatest for the fetus.

Human papillomavirus

Direct treatment of the warts is done to provide symptomatic relief. However, the nearby normal-looking tissue can also harbor the HPV. The drugs podophyllin, podofilox, and imiquimod are not used during pregnancy. Instead, laser therapy, surgical excision, cryosurgery, or trichloroacetic acid may be used. To avoid transmission of the disease during vaginal delivery, cesarean birth may be performed. Despite the treatment used, the likelihood of recurrence is high.

Rubella

There is no antiviral treatment for rubella. Prevention through vaccination is the best means of avoiding contracting the disease.

Streptococcus

Penicillin or ampicillin are the drugs of choice, but penicillin-resistant strains exist. Severe infection may warrant the use of an aminoglycoside in addition to the penicillin.

Syphilis

If the infection is within a year, a single dose of penicillin can cure the disease, according to the CDC. A greater dose will be needed if the infection has been present for more than a year. The antibiotic will cure the disease, but not any damage that has already occurred. Mothers with syphilis can be treated while pregnant. The infant may require antibiotic treatment as well after birth.

Toxoplasmosis

Pregnant women infected with toxoplasmosis may be treated with pyrimethamine, folinic acid, spiramycin, and sulfonamide. Maternal treatment may prevent transmission to the fetus. Pyrimethamine can be teratogenic if given in the first trimester.

Prognosis

Chlamydia

Chlamydia infection can have serious consequences for the fetus and neonate. These include:

- spontaneous abortion
- premature rupture of membranes
- preterm delivery
- stillbirth
- neonatal death
- pneumonia

The prognosis for the mother depends on the degree of damage to the reproductive tract prior to treatment. Chlamydia responds well to antibiotic treatment.

Cytomegalovirus

Prognosis overall is good, as many infected individuals are asymptomatic. However, fetal death may occur, and infected infants born with mental retardation, chronic liver disease, motor disabilities, or deafness have life-long consequences.

Genital herpes

About 30–50% of infants exposed to genital herpes near term will contract the disease. This is in comparison to the 3–5% rate of infection for infants exposed to recurrent genital herpes during pregnancy. Infants exposed to the virus during a vaginal birth have higher rates of the disease than those born via cesarean delivery. Infants with HSV localized to the eyes, skin, or mouth have the best outcome. HSV in infants can lead to death through disseminated intravascular coagulation, pneumonitis, or **encephalitis**.

Hepatitis B

According to the CDC, the number of new infections has declined from 450,000 in the 1980s to 80,000 in 1999. The area of highest growth is in those aged 20 to 49. Because of vaccinations of younger children, those numbers are declining.

Human immunodeficiency virus (HIV)

While long-term prognosis remains poor, short-term prognosis has been improving. Most studies have been done on men, with research focused on women trailing behind. Pregnancy does not appear to alter the course of the disease.

Human papillomavirus

HPV puts women at increased risk for cervical and anal **cancer**. Infants born via vaginal delivery may also develop papillomas in the larynx or conjunctiva.

Rubella

Rubella is most commonly seen in non-vaccinated children. In children, the disease course is milder than in adults. Fetal contraction of the disease can lead to fetal death, preterm delivery, and congenital defects such as **heart** anomalies, mental retardation, blindness, and deafness. The stage of gestation is a critical factor in the degree of impairment to the fetus. All fetal body organs and systems can be affected.

Streptococcus

GBS responds well to antibiotic treatment. Unrecognized or untreated, the effect on the neonate can be severe, including sepsis, pneumonia, or meningitis.

Syphilis

Prognosis depends on the stage to which the disease has progressed. Untreated infants may be asymptomatic, and if untreated may have seizures and die soon after birth.

Toxoplasmosis

The later in the pregnancy the infection is contracted, the better the chance of recovery. A chronic infection in which the mother is infected prior to pregnancy is less likely to be transmitted to the fetus. Fetal death may occur in about 10% of cases occurring in the first trimester of pregnancy. Fetal death is rare when the infection occurs in the third trimester. An acute infection is associated with premature birth and stillbirth. Spontaneous **abortion** is rare.

Prevention

Chlamydia

When a woman has multiple partners, the use of condoms every time a woman has sexual intercourse can decrease the risk of becoming infected. Limiting the number of sexual partners also decreases the risk of chlamydial infection.

Cytomegalovirus

CMV can be shed in body fluids, so care must be taken when handling these substances. This includes the handling of diapers, especially in day care environments. Those working in a hospital environment should always observe **universal precautions** when handling any body fluid or secretion. Careful hand washing can decrease the risk of transmission. Since CMV is shed in cervical secretions, cesarean birth may decrease the risk of transmission, although infection during the first two trimesters of pregnancy carries the greatest fetal risk. Research is investigating the usefulness of a preconception vaccine.

Genital herpes

Cesarean delivery can substantially reduce **disease transmission** to the neonate. For mothers with genital herpes, delivery following premature rupture of membranes (PROM) should be considered, as the risk of disease transmission increases by six hours after PROM. If maternal HSV is suspected, a fetal scalp monitor should be avoided, as this creates a direct portal of entry for the infection.

Hepatitis B

The HBV vaccine is considered the best prevention. It is a series of three injections over seven months. It is not contraindicated in pregnancy. Use of latex condoms will help reduce the risk of transmission. Avoiding high-risk contact, such as contact with blood and other body fluids, will also lessen the risk of HBV. The CDC recommends that newborns born to HBV-infected mothers receive hepatitis B immune globulin after birth as well as the first dose of the vaccine within 12 hours postpartum.

Human immunodeficiency virus (HIV)

In the early 1990s, studies of ZDV used during pregnancy and given to the neonate for six weeks postpartum resulted in a 70% decrease in maternal HIV transmission to the infant. Cesarean birth also reduces transmission, as compared with vaginal birth. Knowledge of the mother's HIV status during pregnancy is therefore important in reducing the transmission risk. Testing for HIV status should be offered to all pregnant women. Avoidance of breast-feeding can also decrease the risk of transmission. If untreated, about 20–30% of infants born to HIV-positive women will be infected. Treatment with ZDV and avoidance of breast-feeding has been reported to lower transmission to about 2–3%. In 1999, a Ugandan study reported that a single dose of nevirapine given to infected mothers during labor in addition to a single dose given to the neonate within three days of birth cut the transmission rate in half, as compared with those treated with AZT throughout pregnancy and during the first six weeks of life.

Human papillomavirus

Use of a condom and limiting the number of sexual partners decreases the risk of contracting the disease.

Rubella

Women in childbearing age should have a titer draw to test for immune status. If they have not been exposed to rubella, they can be vaccinated against the disease, but should not become pregnant for three months following

QUESTIONS TO ASK YOUR DOCTOR

- What are the indications that I may have a perinatal infection?
- What diagnostic tests are needed for a thorough assessment?
- What treatment options do you recommend for me?
- What are the side effects associated with the medications you have prescribed for me?
- What tests or evaluation techniques will you perform to see if treatment has been beneficial for me?
- Does having a perinatal infection put me at risk for other health conditions?
- Does having a perinatal infection put my baby at risk for health problems?
- What infection–related concerns should I be aware of during my pregnancy?
- What measures can be taken to prevent a perinatal infection?
- What symptoms are important enough that I should seek immediate treatment?
- Can you recommend an organization that will provide me with additional information and specifics about my perinatal infection?

the vaccination, due to potential devastating effects on the fetus.

Streptococcus

Prevention of transmission of GBS from the mother to the infant can be enhanced by careful monitoring of the mother during labor for potential signs of infection such as fever, urinary tract infection, or PROM before 37 weeks or 18 hours or more before delivery. Treating the mother with IV **antibiotics** during labor limits the risk of transmission.

Syphilis

Use of a latex condom can reduce the risk of contracting the disease. However, the condom may not cover the area of infection. A blood test is the best way of finding out if one has syphilis, as the sores may be in hidden areas.

Toxoplasmosis

Infection through cat feces is best prevented by having someone other than the mother clean the cat litter, and to avoid inhalation of airborne oocytes. If this is not possible, cat litter should be changed daily, as spores develop in one to five days in the litter. Cats become infected by eating contaminated wildlife, so keeping the cat completely indoors significantly reduces the risk of contagion. Infection through meat can be avoided by avoiding raw meat and by cooking meat to at least 159 °F (71 °C). Garden soil can be contaminated, so the use of gloves when gardening with thorough hand washing afterward, can decrease infection. Outdoor sandboxes should be covered to avoid contamination by stray cats.

Health care team roles

Laboratory technicians and phlebotomists need to observe standard universal precautions in drawing and handling blood and other body fluids, as the complete infection status of a patient will not be known. This includes the use of gloves, eye protection such as a facemask or goggles, and personal protective clothing. **Radiology** technicians will be involved in ultrasound scanning to detect fetal compromise as a result of infection. Ultrasound-guided sampling of amniotic fluid or fetal tissue may be used to diagnose fetal infection. Through individual discussion, waiting room videos, and pamphlets, nurses can educate pregnant mothers during routine visits about ways to prevent infection by these agents. Nurses can play a significant role in emphasizing the need for retesting after treatment (when required) and discussing the importance of having the woman's sexual partner tested and treated to avoid reinfection.

Resources

BOOKS

Gross, Gerd., and Stephen K. Tyring, eds. *Sexually Transmitted Infections and Sexually Transmitted Diseases.* New York, NY: Springer, 2012.

Marr, Lisa, MD. *Sexually Transmitted Diseases: A Physician Tells You What You Need to Know,* 2nd ed. Baltimore, MD: The Johns Hopkins University Press, 2007.

Wilson, Michael R., MD. *Pelvic Inflammatory Disease.* New York, NY: Rosen Publishing Group, 2009.

OTHER

Cytomegalovirus (CMV) Infection. National Center for Infectious Diseases, CDC. May 22, 2009 [cited May 6, 2012]. http://www.cdc.gov/cmv/index.html.

"Genital Herpes." National Institute of Allergy and Infectious Disease. April 8, 2009 [cited May 6, 2012]. http://www. niaid.nih.gov/topics/genitalHerpes/Pages/default.aspx.

"Gonorrhea." National Institute of Allergy and Infectious Disease. March 27, 2009 [cited May 6, 2012]. http://www.niaid.nih.gov/topics/gonorrhea/Pages/default.aspx.

"Group B Streptococcal Disease (GBS)." Disease Information. Division of Bacterial and Mycotic Diseases, CDC. October 11, 2005 [cited May 6, 2012]. http://www.cdc.gov/groupbstrep/index.html.

"HIV/AIDS:Prevention of Mother–To–Infant Transmission." National Institute of Allergy and Infectious Disease. HIV Prevention Site, Division of AIDS, NIAID. November 11, 2009 [cited May 6, 2012]. http://www.niaid.nih.gov/topics/HIVAIDS/Research/prevention/Pages/mtct.aspx.

"HIV and Pregnancy." AIDSinfo. Health Information for Patients, U.S. Department of Health and Human Services. October 2007 [cited May 6, 2012]. http://www.aidsinfo.nih.gov/contentfiles/HIVandPregnancy_FS_en.pdf.

"Human Papillomavirus and Genital Warts." National Institute of Allergy and Infectious Disease. May 12, 2010 [cited May 6, 2012]. http://www.niaid.nih.gov/topics/genital-warts/pages/default.aspx.

Pregnant Women and Hepatitis B. Hepatitis B Foundation. February 2007. [Cited May 6, 2012]. http://www.hepb.org/pdf/pregnancy.pdf.

"STDs & Pregnancy." STD Prevention. National Center for HIV, SID and TB Prevention, CDC. January 4, 2008. [Cited May 6, 2012]. http://www.cdc.gov/std/pregnancy/STDFact-Pregnancy.htm.

ORGANIZATIONS

American Congress of Obstetricians and Gynecologists. PO Box 70620, Washington, DC. 20024-9998. 202-638-5577. http://www.acog.org.

American Social Health Association. PO Box 13827, Research Triangle Park, NC 27709-3827. 919-361-8400. http://www.ashastd.org.

American Society for Reproductive Medicine. 1209 Montgomery Highway,, Birmingham, AL 35216-2809. (205) 978-5000. http://www.asrm.com

Association of Women's Health, Obstetric and Neonatal Nurses. 2000 L Street NW, Suite 740, Washington, DC. 20036. 800-673-8499. 202-261-2400. http://www.awhonn.org.

Centers for Disease Control and Prevention. 1600 Clifton Road, Atlanta, GA 30333. 888-232-3228. http://www.cdc.gov.

Hepatitis B Foundation. 3805 Old Easton Road, Doylestown, PA 18902. 215-489-4900. http://www.hepb.org.

National Institutes of Health (NIH), 9000 Rockville Pike, Bethesda, MD 20892, (301) 496-4000, http://www.nih.gov/index.html

National Women's Health Network. 514 10th Street NW, Suite 400,, Washington, DC 20004. (202) 628-7814. http://www.nwhn.org

RESOLVE, 8405 Greensboro Drive, Suite 800,, McLean,, VA 22102-5120. (703) 556-7172. http://www.resolve.org

U.S. National Library of Medicine, 8600 Rockville Pike, Bethesda, MD 20894, http://www.nlm.nih.gov/medlineplus/medlineplus.html.

Esther Csapo Rastegari, R.N., B.S.N., Ed.M.
Laura Jean Cataldo, RN, Ed.D.

Periodontal abscess *see* **Dental abscess**

Periodontal charting *see* **Dental and periodontal charting**

Periodontal disease *see* **Periodontitis**

Periodontal index *see* **Dental indices**

Periodontics *see* **Dental specialties**

Periodontitis

Definition

Periodontitis is a form of periodontal disease resulting in inflammation within the supporting structures of the teeth, progressive attachment, and **bone** loss. If left untreated, periodontitis can lead to tooth loss.

Description

Periodontal diseases involve the gum, and include **gingivitis** and periodontitis. These are both serious infections that begin when **bacteria** in plaque (a sticky, colorless film that constantly forms on the teeth) cause inflammation of the gums. Undiagnosed or ignored gingivitis—in either case, untreated—can result in periodontitis. When this occurs, plaque may spread and invade below the gum line. When toxins made by the bacteria in the plaque irritate the gums, an inflammatory response is elicited. This response becomes chronic; the body turns on itself and the disease advances. Tissues and bones that support the teeth break down. Pockets, or spaces between the teeth and gums, form—the result of severe **infection** of the periodontal tissue and gums (the gingiva, periodontal ligament, cementum, and alveolar bone). With progression of periodontitis, the pockets deepen. Destruction of the gum tissue and bone worsens. Despite the frequent presentation of very mild symptoms, teeth that have become loose because of these changes may have to be removed.

Plaque and tartar (calculus) accumulate at the base of the teeth. Inflammation causes a pocket to develop between the gums and the teeth, which fills with plaque and tartar. Soft tissue swelling traps this plaque in the pocket, and the bacteria from the plaque begin to develop and grow. Continued inflammation and bacteria growth eventually causes destruction of the tissue surrounding the tooth. An **abscess** may also develop, which increases the rate of bone destruction. Several bacterial products that diffuse through tissue are thought to play a role in disease formation.

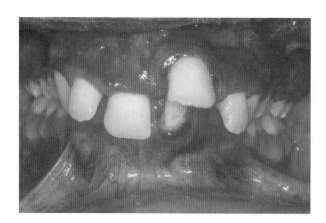

(Juvenile periodontal disease (red gums, crooked teeth), photograph by Edward H. Gill. Custom Medical Stock Photo. Reproduced by permission.)

Bacterial endotoxin is a toxin produced by some bacteria that can kill cells. The amount of endotoxin present correlates with the severity of the periodontitis. Other bacterial products include proteolytic enzymes (molecules that digest protein found in cells), thereby causing cell destruction. The **immune response** has also been implicated in tissue destruction. As part of the normal immune response, WBCs enter regions of inflammation to destroy bacteria. In the process of destroying bacteria, periodontal tissue is also destroyed.

Onset of periodontitus at an early age and an infection characterized by necrosis of the gingival tissue, periodontal ligament, and alveolar bone, have most commonly been observed with individuals with medical conditions including **Down syndrome**, **Crohn's disease**, **AIDS**, and any disease that reduces the number of white **blood** cells (WBCs) in the body for extended periods of time. Reduction of the number of WBCs makes it difficult for the body to fight off infection.

Distinct types of periodontitis

Although there are many kinds of periodontitis, the following are the ones most often presented at the dentist's office:

• Gingivitis. The mildest type of periodontal disease, gingivitis is the reason that gums redden, swell, and bleed easily. Reversible with professional management and good home care, gingivitis is usually relatively painless or pain free.

• Aggressive periodontitis. This occurs in patients with relative good health, clinically. Aggressive periodontitis includes rapid ligament attachment loss and bone destruction.

• Chronic periodontitis. Patients with inflammation within the supporting tissues of the teeth and progressive attachment of the ligament and bone structure, characterized by pocket formation and/or recession of the gum tissue, are known to have chronic periodontitis. Although it occurs most frequently in adults, it can affect anyone, of any age. This progressive periodontitis affects gums and bones slowly, but can has also been known to advance quickly.

• Periodontitis as a manifestation of systemic disease. In this case, the onset is often at a young age. It is generally associated with one of several physiogenic diseases, such as diabetes.

• Necrotizing periodontal disease. This type of periodontal disease is characterized by necrosis (cell death) of gingival tissues, periodontal ligament, and alveolar bone. People with systemic conditions usually present with these symptoms; they may be malnourished, immunosuppressed, or have the human immunodeficiency virus (HIV).

Causes and symptoms

The initial symptoms of periodontitis are bleeding, inflamed gums, and bad breath. Periodontitis follows cases of gingivitis, which may not be severe enough to cause a patient to seek dental help. Although the symptoms of periodontitis are also seen in other forms of periodontal diseases, the key characteristic in periodontitis is a large pocket that forms between the teeth and gums. Another characteristic of periodontitis is that **pain** usually does not develop until late in the disease, when a tooth loosens or an abscess forms.

Several risk factors play a role in the development of periodontal disease. The most important are age and **oral hygiene**. The number and type of bacteria present on the gingival tissues also play a role in the development of periodontitis. The presence of certain species of bacteria in large enough numbers in the gingival pocket and related areas correlates with the development of this disease.

There are a number of other factors that can affect gum health. These include **smoking** and using tobacco, genetics, **pregnancy**, **puberty**, **stress**, medications, clenching or grinding one's teeth, diabetes, poor **nutrition**, and other systemic diseases. For example, poor nutrition can contribute to compromising the body's **immune system**. This will make it more difficult for it to fight infection. There are also some drugs—such as a few **heart** medicines, antidepressants, and oral contraceptives—that can affect one's health. Smoking can cause bone loss and gum recession; they are much more likely

Periodontal case types

Case Type 1— gingival disease	Inflammation of the gingiva characterized by changes in color, gingival form, position, surface appearance, and presence of bleeding and/or exudate.
Case Type II— early or slight periodontitis	Progression of the gingival inflammation into the deeper periodontal structures and alveolar bone crest, with slight bone loss. There is usually a slight loss of connective tissue attachment and alveolar bone.
Case Type III— moderate periodontitis	A more advanced stage of the preceding condition, with increased destruction of the periodontal structures and noticeable loss of bone support, possibly accompanied by an increase in tooth mobility. There may be furcation involvement in multirooted teeth.
Case Type IV— advanced periodontitis	Further progression of periodontitis with major loss of alveolar bone support usually accompanied by increased tooth mobility. Furcation involvement in multirooted teeth is likely.
Case Type V— refractory progressive periodontitis	Includes patients with multiple disease sites that continue to demonstrate attachment loss after appropriate therapy. These sites presumably continue to be infected by periodontal pathogens no matter how thorough or frequent the treatment provided. Also includes patients with recurrent disease at single or multiple sites.

SOURCE: American Academy of Periodontology, 1991.

than nonsmokers to have calculus form on their teeth, even when no periodontal disease is indicated. Smoking exacerbates inflammation by an overactive response of the immune system. It contributes to the early onset of periodontal disease. Serious diseases, such as heart disease, respiratory disease, or diabetes, may put one at higher risk for the development of infection of the gums. Individuals with diabetes may have more difficulty controlling infections.

Contrary to general opinion, age may not be a risk factor in the development of periodontal disease. There are risk factors that may make older people more prone to health problems, such as decreased immune status, taking medications, diminished saliva flow, depression, and general poor health. However, **aging**, in and of itself, does not constitute a serious risk factor for periodontal disease.

Symptoms of periodontitis are:

- gum tissue that is red, swollen, or tender
- gum tissue that bleeds easily; for example, during brushing or flossing
- gums that seem to have pulled away from the teeth
- a bad taste in the mouth; persistent bad breath due to the collection of debris and bacteria in the mouth
- pus between the gums and teeth
- loose or separating teeth
- changes in the way the teeth meet when the mouth closes

Early signs of periodontitis may be mistaken for gingivitis, but warning signs should be heeded and professional dental care attention should be sought promptly.

Diagnosis

Diagnosis is made by clinical and radiologic evaluation of infected gums and bones. A medical history will be taken by the health care provider to assess the patient's overall systemic health. The patient may have a condition that is contributing to the presenting infection. A general dentist is usually the first person to diagnose and characterize the various stages of periodontitis.

Diagnosis of periodontitis includes measuring the size of the pockets formed between the gums and teeth. Normal gingival pockets are shallow. If periodontal disease is severe, bone loss will be detected in x-ray images of the teeth. If too much bone is lost, the teeth become loose and can change position. This will also be seen in x-ray images.

Treatment

The goal of treating periodontitis is to reduce inflammation and rid the mouth of the causes of the disease. Treatment requires professional dental care, commonly accomplished in the dental office by a registered **dental hygienist** (RDH). The pockets around the teeth must be cleaned, and all tartar and plaque removed. In periodontitis, tartar and plaque can extend far down the tooth root. Normal dental hygiene—brushing and flossing—cannot reach deep enough to be effective in treating periodontitis. In cases where pockets are very deep (more than 0.25 in, or 0.6 cm), surgery is required to clean the pocket. Over-the-counter (OTC) pain medications can be useful if the treatment is uncomfortable. These include Tylenol (acetaminophen), Advil (ibuprofen), and Motrin (ibuprofen).

A periodontist performs surgery in a dental office as an out patient procedure. Sections of gum that are not likely to reattach to the teeth may be removed to promote healing by healthy sections of gum. Abscesses are treated with a combination of **antibiotics** and surgery. The antibiotics may be delivered directly to the infected gum and bone tissues to ensure that high concentrations of the antibiotic reach the infected area such as Periostat. Abscess infections, especially of bone, are difficult to treat and require long-term antibiotic treatments to prevent a recurrence of infection, such as augmentin or tetracycline.

Prognosis

Periodontitis can be treated. Prognosis will be good if bone loss has not been too extreme. Removal of the plaque and tartar may be uncomfortable, but any discomfort will subside as the healing process begins. Bleeding and tenderness of the gum tissue will diminish within one or two weeks after treatment. The gums usually heal and resume their normal shape and function. After successful treatment for periodontitis, pathologic pockets are less deep, and reattachment of the ligament will have occurred in most areas.

Health care team roles

A general dentist is commonly the first person seen in the dental field by a patient presenting periodontitis. The dentist evaluates the case and may recommend that the patient see a periodontist for further treatment. The periodontist will then re-evaluate the case and refer for deep pocket scaling and cleanings by the RDH or suggest surgery. The registered dental assistant (RDA) may assist the general dentist or periodontist in treatment and aiding in **patient education**. All staff members are part of the team effort to treat a patient with periodontitis. Patient care and understanding will aid in the reduction of this disease and the reduction of the time spent in the office. Patient education is vital in this treatment.

Prevention

Periodontitis can be prevented with good oral hygiene, including thorough toothbrushing and flossing. Regular professional dental cleanings and dental check ups are the best measures of prevention. Daily use of a toothbrush and flossing is sufficient to prevent most cases of periodontitis. Tartar control toothpastes help prevent tartar formation, but do not remove tartar once it has formed. Patient education is also important in teaching what environmental products aid in the development of periodontitis and what to avoid.

Resources

PERIODICAL

Mullally, Brian H., Blanaid Breen, and Gerard J. Linden. "Smoking and Patterns of Bone Loss in Early-Onset Periodontitis." *Journal of Periodontology* (April 1999).

ORGANIZATIONS

Adam.com Health and Medical Association Online. Atlanta Corporate Office 1600 River Edge Parkway, Suite 800 Atlanta, Georgia 30328 (770) 980-0888. http://www.adam.com/home.htm.

American Academy of Periodontology, 4157 Mountain Road, PBN 249 Pasadena, MD 21122. (410) 437-3749. http://www.perio.org.

American Dental Association, 211 East Chicago Avenue, Chicago, IL 60611. (312) 440-2500. http://www.ada.org.

OTHER

"Periodontitis Overview." Adam.com Health Issues. http://merckmedco.adam.com/ency/article/001059.htm..

"Periondontal Disease." WebMDHealth. http://www.my.webmd.com/content/dmk/dmk_article_40068.htm.

Cindy F. Ovard, RDA

Peripheral nervous system *see* **Nervous system, somatic**

Peripheral neuropathy

Definition

The term peripheral neuropathy encompasses a wide range of disorders in which the nerves outside of the **brain** and spinal cord—peripheral nerves—have been damaged. Peripheral neuropathy may also be referred to as peripheral neuritis, or if many nerves are involved, the terms polyneuropathy or polyneuritis may be used.

Demographics

Leprosy is extremely rare in the United States, where diabetes is the most commonly known cause of peripheral neuropathy. It has been estimated that upwards of 20 million Americans suffer from peripheral neuropathy and more than 17 million people in the United States and Europe have diabetes-related polyneuropathy. Many neuropathies are idiopathic, meaning that no known cause can be found. The most common of the inherited peripheral neuropathies in the United States is Charcot-Marie-Tooth disease, which affects approximately 125,000 persons.

Description

Peripheral neuropathy is a widespread disorder, and there are many underlying causes. Some of these causes are common, such as diabetes, and others are extremely rare, such as acrylamide **poisoning** and certain inherited disorders. The most common worldwide cause of peripheral neuropathy is leprosy. Leprosy is caused by the bacterium *Mycobacterium leprae*, which attacks the peripheral nerves of affected people. According to statistics gathered by the World Health Organization, an estimated 1.15 million people have leprosy worldwide.

Another of the better known peripheral neuropathies is Guillain-Barré syndrome, which arises from complications associated with viral illnesses, such as cytomegalovirus, Epstein-Barr virus, and human **immunodeficiency** virus (HIV), or bacterial **infection**, including *Campylobacter jejuni* and Lyme disease. The worldwide incidence rate is approximately 1.7 cases per 100,000 people annually. Other well-known causes of peripheral neuropathies include chronic **alcoholism**, infection of the varicella-zoster virus, botulism, and poliomyelitis. Peripheral neuropathy may develop as a primary symptom, or it may be due to another disease. For example, peripheral neuropathy is only one symptom of diseases such as amyloid neuropathy, certain cancers, or inherited neurologic disorders. Such diseases may affect the peripheral nervous system (PNS) and the **central nervous system** (CNS), as well as other body tissues.

To understand peripheral neuropathy and its underlying causes, it may be helpful to review the structures and arrangement of the PNS.

Nerve cells and nerves

Nerve cells are the basic building block of the nervous system. In the PNS, nerve cells can be threadlike (i.e., their width is microscopic, but their length can be measured in feet). The long, spidery extensions of nerve cells are called axons. When a nerve cell is stimulated, by touch or **pain**, for example, the message is carried along the axon, and neurotransmitters are released within the cell. Neurotransmitters are chemicals within the nervous system that direct nerve cell communication.

Certain nerve cell axons, such as the ones in the PNS, are covered with a substance called myelin. The myelin sheath may be compared to the plastic coating on electrical wires—it is there both to protect the cells and to prevent interference with the signals being transmitted. Protection is also given by Schwann cells, special cells within the nervous system that wrap around both myelinated and unmyelinated axons. The effect is similar to beads threaded on a necklace.

Nerve cell axons leading to the same areas of the body may be bundled together into nerves. Continuing the comparison to electrical wires, nerves may be compared to an electrical cord—the individual components are coated in their own sheaths and then encased together inside a larger protective covering.

Peripheral nervous system

The nervous system is classified into two parts: the CNS and the PNS. The CNS is made up of the brain and the **spinal cord**, and the PNS is composed of the nerves that lead to or branch off from the CNS.

The peripheral nerves handle a diverse array of functions in the body. This diversity is reflected in the major divisions of the PNS: the afferent and the efferent divisions. The afferent division is in charge of sending sensory information from the body to the CNS. When afferent nerve cell endings, called receptors, are stimulated, they release neurotransmitters. These neurotransmitters relay a signal to the brain, which interprets it and reacts by releasing other neurotransmitters.

Some of the neurotransmitters released by the brain are directed at the efferent division of the PNS. The efferent nerves control voluntary movements, such as moving the arms and legs, and involuntary movements, such as making the **heart** pump **blood**. The nerves controlling voluntary movements are called motor nerves, and the nerves controlling involuntary actions are referred to as autonomic nerves. The afferent and efferent divisions continually interact with each other. For example, if a person were to touch a hot stove, the receptors in the skin would transmit a message of heat and pain through the sensory nerves to the brain. The message would be processed in the brain and a reaction, such as pulling back the hand, would be transmitted via a motor nerve.

Neuropathy

NERVE DAMAGE. When an individual has a peripheral neuropathy, nerves of the PNS have been damaged. Nerve damage can arise from a number of causes, including disease, physical injury, poisoning, or malnutrition. These agents may affect either afferent or efferent nerves. Depending on the cause of damage, the nerve cell axon, its protective myelin sheath, or both may be injured or destroyed.

CLASSIFICATION. There are hundreds of peripheral neuropathies. Reflecting the scope of PNS activity, symptoms may involve sensory, motor, or autonomic functions. To aid in diagnosis and treatment, the symptoms are classified into principal neuropathic syndromes based on the type of affected nerves and how long symptoms have been developing. Acute development refers to symptoms that have appeared within days, and subacute refers to those that have evolved over a number of weeks. Early chronic symptoms are those that take months to a few years to develop, and late chronic symptoms have been present for several years.

The classification system is composed of six principal neuropathic syndromes, which are subdivided into more specific categories. By narrowing down the possible diagnoses in this way, specific medical tests can be used more efficiently and effectively. The six syndromes and a few associated causes are listed below:

• Acute motor paralysis, accompanied by variable problems with sensory and autonomic functions. Neuropathies associated with this syndrome are mainly accompanied by motor nerve problems, but the sensory and autonomic nerves may also be involved. Associated disorders include Guillain-Barré syndrome, diphtheritic polyneuropathy, and porphyritic neuropathy.

• Subacute sensorimotor paralysis. The term sensorimotor refers to neuropathies that are mainly characterized by sensory symptoms but also have a minor component of motor nerve problems. Poisoning with heavy metals (e.g., lead, mercury, and arsenic), chemicals, or drugs are linked to this syndrome. Diabetes, Lyme disease, and malnutrition are also possible causes.

• Chronic sensorimotor paralysis. Physical symptoms may resemble those in the above syndrome, but the time scale of symptom development is extended. This syndrome encompasses neuropathies arising from cancers, diabetes, leprosy, inherited neurologic and metabolic disorders, and hypothyroidism.

• Neuropathy associated with mitochondrial diseases. Mitochondria are organelles—structures within cells—responsible for handling a cell's energy requirements. If the mitochondria are damaged or destroyed, the cell's energy requirements are not met and the cell can die.

• Recurrent or relapsing polyneuropathy. This syndrome covers neuropathies that affect several nerves and may come and go, such as Guillain-Barré syndrome, porphyria, and chronic inflammatory demyelinating polyneuropathy.

• Mononeuropathy or plexopathy. Nerve damage associated with this syndrome is limited to a single nerve or a few closely associated nerves. Neuropathies related to physical injury to the nerve, such as carpal tunnel syndrome and sciatica, are included in this syndrome.

Causes and symptoms

Typical symptoms of neuropathy are related to the type of affected nerve. If a sensory nerve is damaged, common symptoms include numbness, tingling in the area, a prickling sensation, or pain. Pain associated with neuropathy can be quite intense and may be described as cutting, stabbing, crushing, or burning. In some cases, a nonpainful stimulus may be perceived as excruciating or pain may be felt even in the absence of a stimulus. Damage to a motor nerve is usually indicated by **weakness** in the affected area. If the problem with the motor nerve has continued over a length of time, muscle shrinkage (atrophy) or lack of muscle tone may be noticeable. Autonomic nerve damage is most noticeable when an individual stands upright and experiences problems such as light-headedness or changes in **blood pressure**. Other indicators of autonomic nerve damage are lack of sweat, tears, and saliva; constipation; urinary retention; and impotence. In some cases, heart beat irregularities and respiratory problems can develop.

Symptoms may appear over days, weeks, months, or years. Duration of symptoms and the ultimate outcome of the neuropathy are linked to the cause of the nerve damage. Potential causes include diseases, physical injuries, poisoning, malnutrition, or alcohol abuse. In some cases, neuropathy is not the primary disorder, but a symptom of an underlying disease.

Disease

Diseases that cause peripheral neuropathies may either be acquired or inherited; in some cases, it is difficult to make that distinction. The diabetes-peripheral neuropathy link has been well established. A typical pattern of diabetes-associated neuropathic symptoms includes sensory effects that first begin in the feet. The associated pain or pins-and-needles, burning, crawling, or prickling sensations form a typical "stocking" distribution in the feet and lower legs. Other diabetic neuropathies affect the autonomic nerves and have potentially fatal cardiovascular complications.

Several other metabolic diseases have a strong association with peripheral neuropathy. Uremia, or **chronic kidney failure**, carries a 10–90% risk of eventually developing neuropathy, and there may be an association between **liver** failure and peripheral neuropathy. Accumulation of **lipids** inside **blood vessels** (**atherosclerosis**) can choke-off blood supply to certain peripheral nerves. Without oxygen and nutrients, the nerves slowly die. Mild polyneuropathy may develop in persons with low thyroid hormone levels. Individuals with abnormally enlarged skeletal extremities (acromegaly), caused by an overabundance of growth hormone, may also develop mild polyneuropathy.

Neuropathy can also result from severe vasculitides, a group of disorders in which blood vessels are inflamed. When the blood vessels are inflamed or damaged, blood supply to the nerve can be affected, injuring the nerve.

Both viral and bacterial infections have been implicated in peripheral neuropathy. Leprosy is caused by the **bacteria** *M. leprae*, which directly attack sensory nerves. Other bacterial illness may set the stage for an immune-mediated attack on the nerves. For example, one theory about Guillain-Barré syndrome involves complications following infection with *Campylobacter jejuni*, a bacterium commonly associated with food poisoning. This bacterium carries a protein that closely resembles components of myelin. The **immune system** launches an attack against the bacteria, but, according to the theory, the immune system confuses the myelin with the bacteria in some cases and attacks the myelin sheath as well. The underlying cause of neuropathy associated with Lyme disease is unknown; the bacteria may either promote an immune-mediated attack on the nerve or inflict damage directly.

Infection with certain **viruses** is associated with extremely painful sensory neuropathies. A primary example of such a neuropathy is caused by **shingles**. After a case of chickenpox, the causative virus, varicella-zoster virus, becomes inactive in sensory nerves. Years later, the virus may be reactivated. Once reactivated, it attacks and destroys axons. Infection with HIV is also associated with peripheral neuropathy, but the type of neuropathy that develops can vary. Some HIV-linked neuropathies are noted for myelin destruction rather than axonal degradation. Also, HIV infection is frequently accompanied by other infections, both bacterial and viral, that are associated with neuropathy.

Several types of peripheral neuropathies are associated with inherited disorders. These inherited disorders may primarily involve the nervous system, or the effects on the nervous system may be secondary to an inherited metabolic disorder. Inherited neuropathies can fall into several of the principal syndromes, because symptoms may be sensory, motor, or autonomic. The inheritance patterns also vary, depending on the specific disorder. The development of inherited disorders is typically drawn out over several years and may herald a degenerative condition, a condition that becomes progressively worse over time. Even among specific disorders there may be a degree of variability in inheritance patterns and symptoms. For example, Charcot-Marie-Tooth disease is usually inherited as an autosomal dominant disorder, but it can be autosomal recessive or, in rare cases, linked to the X chromosome. Its estimated frequency is approximately one in 2,500 people. Age of onset and sensory nerve involvement can vary. The main symptom is a degeneration of the motor nerves in legs and arms, and resultant muscle atrophy. Other inherited neuropathies have a distinctly metabolic component. For example, in familial amyloid **polyneuropathies**, protein components that make up the myelin are constructed and deposited incorrectly.

Physical injury

Accidental **falls** and mishaps during sports and recreational activities are common causes of physical injuries that can result in peripheral neuropathy. The common types of injuries in these situations occur from placing too much pressure on the nerve, exceeding the nerve's capacity to stretch, blocking adequate blood supply of oxygen and nutrients to the nerve, and tearing the nerve. Pain may not always be immediately noticeable, and obvious signs of damage may take a while to develop.

These injuries usually affect one nerve or a group of closely associated nerves. For example, a common injury encountered in contact sports such as football is the "burner," or "stinger," syndrome. Typically, a stinger is caused by overstretching the main nerves that span from the neck into the arm. Immediate symptoms are numbness, tingling, and pain that travels down the arm, lasting only a minute or two. A single incident of a stinger is not dangerous, but recurrences can eventually cause permanent motor and sensory loss.

Poisoning

The poisons, or toxins, that cause peripheral neuropathy include drugs, industrial chemicals, and environmental toxins. Neuropathy that is caused by drugs usually involves sensory nerves on both sides of the body, particularly in the hands and feet, and pain is a common symptom. Neuropathy is an unusual side effect of medications; therefore, most people can use these drugs safely. Drugs that have been linked with peripheral neuropathy include metronidazole, an antibiotic; phenytoin, an anticonvulsant; and simvastatin, a cholesterol-lowering medication.

Certain industrial chemicals have been shown to be poisonous to nerves (neurotoxic) following work-related exposures. Chemicals such as acrylamide, allyl chloride, and carbon disulfide have all been strongly linked to development of peripheral neuropathy. Organic compounds, such as N-hexane and toluene, are also encountered in work-related settings, as well as in glue-sniffing and solvent abuse. Either route of exposure can produce severe sensorimotor neuropathy that develops rapidly.

Heavy metals are the third group of toxins that cause peripheral neuropathy. Lead, arsenic, thallium, and mercury usually are not toxic in their elemental form but rather as components in organic or inorganic compounds. The types of metal-induced neuropathies vary widely. Arsenic poisoning may mimic Guillain-Barré syndrome; lead affects motor nerves more than sensory nerves; thallium produces painful sensorimotor neuropathy; and the effects of mercury are seen in both the CNS and PNS.

Malnutrition and alcohol abuse

Burning, stabbing pains, and numbness in the feet and sometimes in the hands are distinguishing features of alcoholic neuropathy. The level of alcohol consumption associated with this variety of peripheral neuropathy has been estimated as approximately 3 L of beer or 300 mL of liquor daily for three years. It is unclear whether alcohol alone is responsible for the neuropathic symptoms because chronic alcoholism is strongly associated with malnutrition.

Malnutrition refers to an extreme lack of nutrients in the diet. It is unknown precisely which nutrient deficiencies cause peripheral neuropathies in alcoholics and famine and starvation patients, but it is suspected that the B **vitamins** have a significant role. For example, **thiamine** (vitamin B_1) deficiency is the cause of beriberi, a neuropathic disease characterized by **heart failure** and painful polyneuropathy of sensory nerves. **Vitamin E** deficiency seems to have a role in both CNS and PNS neuropathy.

Diagnosis

Clinical symptoms can indicate peripheral neuropathy, but an exact diagnosis requires a combination of medical history, medical tests, and possibly a process of exclusion. Certain symptoms can suggest a diagnosis, but more information is commonly needed. For example, painful, burning feet may be a symptom of alcohol abuse, diabetes, HIV infection, or an underlying malignant tumor, among other causes. Without further details, effective treatment would be difficult.

During a **physical examination**, an individual is asked to describe the symptoms very carefully. Detailed information about the location, nature, and duration of symptoms can help exclude some causes or even pinpoint the actual problem. The person's medical history may also provide clues as to the cause, because certain diseases and medications are linked to specific peripheral neuropathies. A medical history should also include information about diseases that run in the family, because some peripheral neuropathies are genetically linked. Information about hobbies, recreational activities, alcohol consumption, and workplace activities can uncover possible injuries or exposures to poisonous substances.

The physical examination also includes blood tests, such as those that check levels of glucose and creatinine to detect diabetes and kidney problems, respectively. A blood count is also done to determine levels of different blood cell types. **Iron**, **vitamin B_{12}**, and other factors may be measured as well, to rule out malnutrition. More specific tests, such as an assay for heavy metals or poisonous substances, or tests to detect vasculitis, are not typically done unless there is reason to suspect a particular cause.

An individual with neuropathy may be sent to a doctor who specializes in nervous system disorders (neurologist). By considering the results of the physical examination and observations of the referring doctor, the neurologist may be able to narrow down the possible diagnoses. Additional tests, such as nerve conduction studies and **electromyography**, which tests muscle reactions, can confirm that nerve damage has occurred and may also be able to indicate the nature of the damage. For example, some neuropathies are characterized by destruction of the myelin. This type of damage is shown by slowed nerve conduction. If the axon itself has suffered damage, the nerve conduction may be slowed, but it will also be diminished in strength. Electromyography adds further information by measuring nerve conduction and muscle response, which determines whether the symptoms are due to a neuropathy or to a muscle disorder.

In approximately 10% of peripheral neuropathy cases, a nerve biopsy may be helpful. In this test, a small part of the nerve is surgically removed and examined under a **microscope**. This procedure is usually the most helpful in confirming a suspected diagnosis, rather than as a diagnostic procedure by itself.

Treatment

Treat the cause

Attacking the underlying cause of the neuropathy can prevent further nerve damage and may allow for a better recovery. For example, in cases of bacterial infection such as leprosy or Lyme disease, **antibiotics** may be given to destroy the infectious bacteria. Viral infections are more difficult to treat, because antibiotics are not effective against them. Neuropathies associated with drugs, chemicals, and toxins are treated in part by stopping exposure to the damaging agent. Chemicals such as ethylenediaminetetraacetic acid (EDTA) are used to help the body concentrate and excrete some toxins. Diabetic neuropathies may be treated by gaining better control of blood sugar levels, but chronic kidney failure may require dialysis or even kidney transplant to prevent or reduce nerve damage. In some cases, such as compression injury or tumors, surgery may be considered to relieve pressure on a nerve.

In a crisis situation, as in the onset of Guillain-Barré syndrome, plasma exchange, intravenous immunoglobulin, and steroids may be given. Intubation, in which a tube is inserted into the trachea to maintain an open airway, and ventilation may be required to support the **respiratory system**. Treatment may focus more on symptom management than on combating the underlying cause, at least until a definitive diagnosis has been made.

Pain management

Because pain is associated with many of the neuropathies, a **pain management** plan may need to be mapped out, especially if the pain becomes chronic. Mild symptoms may be relieved by over-the-counter pain medications and as in any chronic disease, narcotics are best avoided due to the potential for dependence and side effects such as sedation.

The choice of proven drug therapies has broadened during the past decade. Four main classes of drugs are available for nerve pain management, alone or in combination. These include:

- anticonvulsants such as gabapentin (Neurontin), topiramate (Topamax), pregabalin (Lyrica), carbamazepine (Tegretol), and phenytoin (Dilantin)

- antidepressants such as duloxetine hydrochloride (Cymbalta), and Tricyclic antidepressants such as amitriptyline (Elavil), nortriptyline (Pamelor), and imipramine (Tofranil)

- narcotic analgesics such as codeine and morphine

- antiarrhythmics

In addition, topical medications administered via a skin patch (transdermal patch), may be effective for pain relief. The topical anesthetic, Lidocaine, may be administered via patch to the affected area. Capsaicin cream rubbed over the area may be beneficial, as well.

Supportive care and long-term therapy

Some peripheral neuropathies cannot be resolved or require time for resolution. In these cases, long-term monitoring and supportive care is necessary. Medical tests may be repeated to chart the progress of the neuropathy. If autonomic nerve involvement is a concern, regular monitoring of the **cardiovascular system** may be carried out.

Transcutaneous electrical nerve stimulation (TENS) may be administered via a TENS unit. This therapy utilizes electrodes that adhere to the skin and deliver varying frequencies of electric current. Some patients find minimal to moderate pain relief when this therapy is done on a frequent and ongoing basis.

Physical therapy and physician-directed exercises can help maintain or improve function. In cases in which motor nerves are affected, braces and other supportive equipment can aid an individual's ability to move about.

Prognosis

The outcome for peripheral neuropathy depends heavily on the cause. Peripheral neuropathy ranges from a reversible problem to a potentially fatal complication. In the best cases, a damaged nerve regenerates. Nerve cells cannot be replaced if they are killed, but they are capable of recovering from damage. The extent of recovery is tied to the extent of the damage and a person's age and general health status. Recovery can take weeks to years, because **neurons** grow very slowly. Full recovery may not be possible and it may also not be possible to determine the prognosis at the outset.

If the neuropathy is a degenerative condition, such as Charcot-Marie-Tooth disease, an individual's condition will become worse. There may be periods of time when the disease seems to reach a plateau, but cures have not yet been discovered for many of these degenerative diseases. Therefore, continued symptoms, potentially worsening to disabilities are to be expected.

A few peripheral neuropathies are eventually fatal. Fatalities have been associated with some cases of diphtheria, botulism, and others. Some diseases associated with neuropathy may also be fatal, but the ultimate cause of death is not necessarily related to the neuropathy, such as with **cancer**.

Prevention

Peripheral neuropathies are preventable only to the extent that the underlying causes are preventable. Steps that a person can take to prevent potential problems include vaccines against diseases that cause neuropathy, such as polio and diphtheria. Treatment for physical injuries in a timely manner can help prevent permanent or worsening damage to nerves. Precautions when using certain chemicals and drugs are well advised in order to prevent exposure to neurotoxic agents. Control of chronic diseases such as diabetes may also reduce the chances of developing peripheral neuropathy.

Although not a preventive measure, genetic screening can serve as an early warning for potential problems. Genetic screening is available for some inherited conditions, but not all. In some cases, presence of a particular gene may not mean that a person will necessarily develop the disease, because there may be environmental and other components involved.

Resources

BOOKS

Ali, Naheed. *Diabetes and You: A Comprehensive, Holistic Approach.* Lanham, MD: Rowman & Littlefield, 2011.

Aminoff, Michael J. *Neurology and General Medicine,* 4th ed. London: Churchill Livingstone, 2007.

Birch, Rolfe. *Surgical Disorders of the Peripheral Nerves.* 2nd ed. New York: Springer, 2011.

Tesfaye, Solomin, and Andrew Boulton. *Diabetic Neuropathy.* New York: Oxford University Press, 2009.

ORGANIZATIONS

American Academy of Neurology (AAN), 1080 Montreal Avenue, Saint Paul, MN 55116, (651) 695-2717, (800) 879-1960, Fax: (651) 695-2791, memberservices@aan.com, http://www.aan.com

American Academy of Physical Medicine and Rehabilitation, 9700 West Bryn Mawr Avenue, Suite 200, Rosemont, IL 60018-5701, (847) 737-6000, Fax: (847) 737-6001, info@aapmr.org, http://www.aapmr.org

American Diabetes Association, 1701 North Beauregard Street, Alexandria, VA 22311, (800) DIABETES, askADA@diabetes.org, http://www.diabetes.org

American Neurological Association, 5841 Cedar Lake Road, Suite 204, Minneapolis, MN 55416, (952) 545-6284, http://www.aneuroa.org

Juvenile Diabetes Foundation, 26 Broadway, 14th Floor, New York, NY 10004, (800) 533-CURE, info@jdrf.org, http://www.jdf.org

Myelin Project Headquarters, P.O. Box 39, Pacific Palisades, CA 90272-0039, (310) 459-1071, (800) 8-MYELIN, Fax: (310) 230-4298, http://www.myelin.org

National Institute of Neurological Disorders and Stroke (NINDS), P.O. Box 5801, Bethesda, MD 20824, (301) 496-5751, (800) 352-9424, http://www.ninds.nih.gov

National Institutes of Health (NIH), 9000 Rockville Pike, Bethesda, MD 20892, (301) 496-4000, NIHinfo@od.nih.gov, http://www.nih.gov/index.html

Neuropathy Association, 60 East 42nd Street, Suite 942, New York, NY 10165, (212) 692-0662, Fax: (212) 692-0668, info@neuropathy.org, http://www.neuropathy.org

U.S. National Library of Medicine, 8600 Rockville Pike, Bethesda, MD 20894, (301) 594-5983, (888) 346-3656, Fax: (301) 402-1384, custserv@nlm.nih.gov, http://www.nlm.nih.gov.

Julia Barrett
Laura Jean Cataldo, RN, EdD

Peripheral neuropathy *see* **Polyneuropathies**

Peripheral vascular disease

Definition

Peripheral vascular disease is a narrowing of **blood vessels** that restricts **blood** flow. It mostly occurs in the legs, but is sometimes seen in the arms.

Description

Peripheral vascular disease includes a group of diseases in which blood vessels become restricted or blocked. Typically, the patient has peripheral vascular disease from **atherosclerosis**. Atherosclerosis is a disease in which fatty plaques form in the inside walls of blood vessels. Other processes, such as blood clots, further restrict blood flow in the blood vessels. Both veins and arteries may be affected, but the disease is usually arterial. All the symptoms and consequences of peripheral vascular disease are related to restricted blood flow. Peripheral vascular disease is a progressive disease that can lead to **gangrene** of the affected area. Peripheral vascular disease may also occur suddenly if an **embolism** occurs or when a blot clot rapidly develops in a blood vessel already restricted by an atherosclerotic plaque, and the blood flow is quickly cut off.

Causes and symptoms

There are many causes of peripheral vascular disease. One major risk factor is **smoking** cigarettes. Other diseases predispose patients to develop peripheral vascular disease. These include diabetes, Buerger's disease, **hypertension**, and Raynaud's disease. The main symptom is **pain** in the affected area. Early symptoms include an achy, tired sensation in the affected muscles. Since this disease is seen mainly in the legs, these sensations usually occur when walking. The symptoms may disappear when resting. As the disease becomes worse, symptoms occur even during light exertion and, eventually, occur all the time, even at rest. In the severe stages of the disease the leg and foot may be cold to the touch and will feel numb. The skin may become dry and scaly. If the leg is even slightly injured, ulcers may form because, without a good blood supply, proper healing cannot take place. At the most severe stage of the disease, when the blood flow is greatly restricted, gangrene can develop in those areas lacking blood supply. In some cases, peripheral vascular disease occurs suddenly. This happens when an embolism rapidly blocks blood flow to a blood vessel. The patient will experience a sharp pain. followed by a loss of sensation in the affected area. The limb will become cold and numb, and loose color or turn bluish.

Diagnosis

Peripheral vascular disease can be diagnosed by comparing blood pressures taken above and below the point of pain. The area below the pain (downstream from the obstruction) will have a much lower or undetectable **blood pressure** reading. **Doppler ultrasonography** and **angiography** can also be used to diagnose and define this disease.

Treatment

If the person is a smoker, they should stop smoking immediately. **Exercise** is essential to treating this disease. The patient should walk until pain appears, rest until the pain disappears, and then resume walking. The amount of walking a patient can do should increase gradually as the symptoms improve. Ideally, the patient should walk 30–60 minutes per day. Infections in the affected area should be treated promptly. Surgery may be required to attempt to treat clogged blood vessels. Limbs with gangrene must be amputated to prevent the death of the patient.

Prognosis

The prognosis depends on the underlying disease and the stage at which peripheral vascular disease is discovered. Removal of risk factors, such as smoking, should be done immediately. In many cases, peripheral vascular disease can be treated successfully but co-existing cardiovascular problems may ultimately prove to be fatal.

Resources

BOOKS

Miller, Max. *The Quit Smoking Companion: the daily guide to freedom from cigarettes.* Charleston, SC: BookSurge Publishing, 2009.

Mohler, Emile R. III, and Alan T. Hirsch.*100 Questions & Answers About Peripheral Artery Disease.* Sudbury, MA: Jones and Bartlett Publishers, 2009.

Rokavec, Kathleen A., MD. *The Hospital Book.* Raleigh, NC: lulu.com., 2009.

Wallach, Jacques. *Interpretation of Diagnostic Tests,* 8th ed. Philadelphia, PA: Lippincott Williams & Wilkins, 2006.

Zimring, Michael P., MD. *Healthy Travel: Don't Travel Without It!* Laguna Beach, CA: Basic Health Publications, Inc., 2009.

OTHER

Avoid Deep Vein Thrombosis: Keep the Blood Flowing. MedicineNet Website, 2010. www.medicinenet.com/script/main/art.asp?articlekey=40582 .

ORGANIZATIONS

American Heart Association, 7272 Greenville Ave., Dallas, TX 75231, (301) 223-2307, (800) 242-8721, http://www.americanheart.org

Centers for Disease Control (CDC). Division for Heart Disease and Stroke Prevention, 4770 Buford Hwy NE, Atlanta, GA 30341-3717, 770-488-2424, www.cdc.gov/cholesterol/faqs.htm

National Heart, Lung, and Blood Institute, P.O. Box 30105, Bethesda, MD 20824-0105, (301) 592-8573, Fax: (204) 629-3246, nhlbiinfo@nhlbi.nih.gov, http://www.nhlbi.nih.gov

Society of Interventional Radiology, 10201 Lee Highway, Suite 500, Fairfax, VA 22030, 703-691-1805, http://www.sirweb.org.

John T. Lohr, Ph.D.
Laura Jean Cataldo, RN, Ed.D.

Peripherally inserted central cather maintenance *see* **Central catheter maintenance**

Peritoneal dialysis

Definition

Dialysis is the medical process of removing fluid and waste products from the body, a function usually performed by the **kidneys**. There are two types of dialysis: hemodialysis and peritoneal dialysis. Peritoneal dialysis accomplishes the removal of waste and excess fluid by using the abdominal lining, called the peritoneal membrane, as a filter.

Purpose

The purpose of peritoneal dialysis is to replace the function of the kidneys in patients who have kidney disease. Because peritoneal dialysis can be done continuously, it more closely imitates the function of the kidneys than hemodialysis does. Peritoneal dialysis is also easy to do when away from home, which makes it an appealing choice for patients who do not wish to be tied down to a dialysis infusion site's location or schedule.

Peritoneal dialysis is a relatively slow process compared to hemodialysis. This is especially useful for patients with cardiovascular disease because rapid changes in **blood** urea (a waste product), glucose, electrolytes, or fluid volume can exacerbate cardiovascular disease. Peritoneal dialysis is a commonly prescribed method of dialysis for diabetic patients because insulin can be added to the dialysate. It also reduces the risk of retinal hemorrhage since, unlike with hemodialysis, heparin (an anticoagulant) is not used. Peritoneal dialysis is the treatment of choice for children as it does not interfere with growth.

Precautions

Peritoneal dialysis is contraindicated in patients with hypercatabolism because adequate clearance of uremic toxins cannot be achieved with this method of dialysis. Peritoneal adhesions and scarring are also contraindications. Caution should be used when prescribing peritoneal dialysis for patients with a history of ruptured diverticuli, respiratory disease, recurrent peritonitis (**infection** of the peritoneum), abdominal malignancies, severe vascular disease, back problems, and those who are obese.

Description

Before peritoneal dialysis begins, patients have a catheter surgically inserted into their peritoneal cavity. The catheter is usually placed 1.2–2 in (3–5 cm) below the umbilicus. When dialysis is ready to begin, a bag of fluid (dialysate) containing sterile water, normal plasma, electrolytes, and glucose is infused into the abdominal cavity. The volume of dialysate used can range from 1.5–3 qts (1.5–3 l), and the concentration of electrolytes and glucose is altered according to what the physician prescribes. The dialysate is left in the abdominal cavity for anywhere from one hour to 10 hours, depending on the type of dialysis. The period of time that the dialysate is left in the abdominal cavity is called the dwell time. At the end of the prescribed dwell time, the dialysate is drained out of the abdominal cavity through the catheter. The drained dialysate takes waste products with it. This process of instilling a bag of dialysate, dwell time, and emptying the dialysate is called an exchange. The amount and timing of exchanges performed by patients depends on the type of dialysis, the recommendation of the physician, and the lifestyle of the patient.

Peritoneal dialysis works based on the principles of osmotic pressure and diffusion. Osmotic pressure is the moving of fluid toward the solution with a higher solute concentration. Diffusion is the passing of particles from an area of high concentration to an area of lower concentration. The dialysate infused into the abdominal cavity is prepared with specific concentrations of electrolytes and glucose that will draw the waste products and excess fluid across the peritoneal membrane using diffusion and osmotic pressure. The pores in the peritoneal membrane are large enough to allow the waste to pass through into the abdominal cavity, but small enough that blood cells and other protein molecules are unable to pass through.

There are two types of peritoneal dialysis: continuous ambulatory peritoneal dialysis (CAPD) and automated peritoneal dialysis (APD). Within APD, there are three different scheduling methods, including continuous cyclic peritoneal dialysis (CCPD), intermittent peritoneal dialysis (IPD), and nightly peritoneal dialysis (NPD).

With CAPD, dialysate is instilled into and drawn out of the abdominal cavity by gravity alone. No machine is needed. The dwell time for CAPD ranges from four to 10 hours. The CAPD patient usually performs four exchanges per day, including an eight-hour overnight dwell. This continuous exchange most closely resembles normal renal function, and it is also convenient because the exchanges can be performed anywhere since no equipment is required.

The automated dialysis methods require a peritoneal cycling machine. Patients using CCPD set their cyclers to do three exchanges at night and one eight-hour daytime dwell, which frees up the patient during the day. NPD performs several exchanges at night over an eight- to 12-hour period, and does not require a daytime dwell. This is preferred by many patients who are self-conscious about the way they look with the extra fluid in their abdominal cavity. IPD is performed for 10 to 14 hours three to four times a week. This type of treatment is usually performed in the hospital.

Preparation

Strict sterile technique should be used when preparing to do an exchange to prevent infection.

KEY TERMS

Automated peritoneal dialysis (APD)—A type of peritoneal dialysis that requires a cyclic machine to complete exchanges.

Continuous ambulatory peritoneal dialysis (CAPD)—A type of peritoneal dialysis that uses gravity to infuse and empty dialysate instead of a machine.

Dialysate—The solution that is used during peritoneal dialysis.

Dialysis—The process of removing fluid and waste products from the body through artificial means.

Dwell time—Stage of a dialysis exchange when the dialysate is inside the abdominal cavity, which is when the filtration takes place.

Exchange—A complete dialysis cycle, starting with infusing the dialysate and ending with the emptying out of the used dialysate solution.

Hypercatabolism—A state in which the body is metabolizing proteins at an exaggerated rate.

Peritoneal dialysis—A removal system for waste products and excess fluid in patients whose kidneys are failing. This system uses the abdominal lining or peritoneal membrane as a filter.

Peritonitis—An infection of the peritoneum.

Uremic toxins—Waste products carried in the blood stream that are usually excreted by the kidneys.

Dialysate should be warmed to 98.6 °F (37 °C) to provide comfort to the patient; this also is the optimal temperature for clearance of uremic metabolites. The catheter tubing should be flushed so that air does not enter the abdominal cavity.

Aftercare

When not in use, the dialysis catheter can be clamped and tucked under clothing for concealment. If a method of peritoneal dialysis is chosen with dwell times during the day, the patient may have to wear larger, loose-fitting clothes to account for the additional fluid in the abdominal cavity.

Complications

The major complication that can be encountered by peritoneal dialysis patients is peritonitis, an infection of

the peritoneum. Symptoms of peritonitis include **fever**, rebound tenderness, nausea, malaise, and cloudy dialysate output. Peritonitis is treated with **antibiotics** placed in the dialysate or taken orally. To avoid peritonitis, patients must be taught to handle the catheter and other dialysis equipment with sterile technique.

Other complications associated with peritoneal dialysis are problems with the catheter such as obstruction, as well as bowel and bladder perforations caused by the insertion of the catheter. Dialysis-related complications include fluid and electrolyte imbalances, **hypotension**, **pain**, hyperglycemia (high blood glucose levels), and respiratory difficulties due to the presence of the dialysate fluid and the pressure it puts on the diaphragm.

Results

When the proper type of peritoneal dialysis is prescribed, and the patient complies with the regimen, peritoneal dialysis can be very successful in maintaining the fluid and **electrolyte balance** and removing waste when the kidneys are unable to perform these tasks. Peritoneal dialysis allows patients to live full and productive lives by providing flexibility of time and place in dialysis treatment.

Health care team roles

Peritoneal dialysis is primarily performed at home by patients and their family members. It is the responsibility of health care providers to educate patients in the proper use of peritoneal dialysis so that the patient complies with the regimen and avoids complications. **Patient education** must include instruction on aseptic measures to prevent infection, timing and number of exchanges to be performed, appropriate dwell times, use of the cycler if automated dialysis is chosen, obtaining the proper dialysate solutions, and storage of solutions and equipment.

Resources

BOOK

Black, Joyce M., and Esther Matassarin-Jacobs. *Medical-Surgical Nursing Clinical Management For Continuity of Care, 5th Edition*. Philadelphia: W.B. Saunders Company, 1997.

ORGANIZATION

National Diabetes Information Clearinghouse. 1 Information Way, Bethesda, MD 20892-3560. http://www.niddk.nih.gov/health/diabetes/pubs/esrd/esrd.htm.

Jennifer Lee Losey, R.N.

Peritoneal fluid analysis *see* **Paracentesis**

Permanent tooth development *see* **Tooth development, permanent**

Personal hygiene for cognitive impairment

Definition

Personal hygiene refers to maintaining cleanliness of one's body and clothing to preserve overall health and well-being. It includes a number of different activities related to the following general areas of self-care: washing or bathing, **oral hygiene**, grooming and dressing, keeping one's clothes clean, and toileting. These are sometimes described (along with such other daily tasks as preparing meals or managing finances) as activities of daily living or ADLs. Cognitive impairment may affect a person's ability to maintain personal hygiene in all these areas.

Cognitive impairments refer to limitations on a person's ability to think, pay attention, perceive, and remember. They may be associated with a variety of diseases and disorders, including:

- developmental disorders of childhood including autism, Asperger's syndrome, pervasive developmental disorder (PDD), and others that are sometimes grouped together as autistic spectrum disorders

- mental retardation

- psychotic disorders, including schizophrenia, which is a mental disorder characterized by delusions, hallucinations, and other deficits in reality testing

- mood disorders, particularly depression and bipolar disorder

- substance abuse disorders

- multiple sclerosis (MS), which often affects the patient's visual perception as well as memory and abstract reasoning

- stroke

- dementing illnesses, including Alzheimer's disease and AIDS-related dementia

- mild cognitive impairment (MCI). MCI is a condition found in older adults in which the person has some memory loss but is able to carry out ordinary activities of daily life with the help of notes, calendars, or other written reminders

Purpose

Personal hygiene is a preventive health measure that serves emotional and social as well as physical well-being. Personal hygiene:

- protects against the spread of disease from external parasites (such as body or head lice) or from contact with contaminated feces or other body fluids

- protects the skin against rashes and sores from contact with urine

- protects against malnutrition or swallowing difficulties caused by lack of oral care

- minimizes the chances of social embarrassment, job loss or educational failure, and eventual isolation from others

- keeps up morale and helps avoid depression

Precautions

Inattention to personal cleanliness or grooming in adults or adolescents may be one of the earliest signs of depression, dementing illnesses, **substance abuse** disorders, and psychotic disorders. Therefore, accurate diagnosis of the cause or causes of the person's cognitive impairment is critical. It is also important to remember that depression may coexist with other disorders, and may require separate treatment. In the case of children with mental retardation or developmental disorders, an evaluation of the child's capacity to learn self-care is necessary. Children with mild cognitive impairments can often learn to perform ADLs related to personal hygiene with appropriate instruction, repetition, and coaching.

Description

Inability or unwillingness to carry out bathing, grooming, or other activities related to personal hygiene is often an early sign of cognitive impairment, particularly in older adults or in adolescents diagnosed with **schizophrenia**. For this reason, geriatric and other medical assessment checklists include personal hygiene as one of the items to be evaluated in determining whether the impaired person is still capable of living independently.

The onset of a patient's difficulties with personal cleanliness may be either gradual or sudden. In patients with schizophrenia, neglect of self-care often indicates that the patient is relapsing.

Complications

Some types of cognitive impairment present specific difficulties with regard to maintaining the patient's personal cleanliness and grooming.

KEY TERMS

Activities of daily living (ADLs)—A shorthand term for the everyday tasks that must be carried out to maintain basic cleanliness, nutrition, contact with others, etc.

Catastrophic reaction—An emotional outburst or overreaction to a situation or event. Catastrophic reactions are common in patients with dementing illnesses.

Cognitive—Pertaining to such mental activities as perceiving, thinking, and remembering.

Cognitive therapy—An approach to psychotherapy that focuses on interrupting and correcting the patient's present faulty thinking patterns rather than on exploring emotions or childhood memories. It appears to be particularly helpful in treating depression.

Dementia—A decline in a person's level of intellectual functioning. Dementia includes memory loss as well as difficulties with language, simple calculations, planning or decision-making, and motor (muscular movement) skills.

Incontinence—Inability to control one's bowel or bladder functions.

Mild cognitive impairment (MCI)—A transitional phase of memory loss in older people that may eventually progress to dementia or Alzheimer's disease.

Psychosis—A type of mental disorder in which the patient's contact with reality is severely impaired. It is characterized by delusions, hallucinations, incoherent speech, and disorganized behavior. Schizophrenia is one type of psychosis.

• dementia. Patients with a dementing illness often lose their ability to control their emotions as well as their thought processes. It is not unusual for these patients to have what is called a catastrophic reaction when they are asked to take a bath or shower. A catastrophic reaction is an emotional outburst or overreaction to a situation or event. Patients with dementia may become upset about bathing because they are embarrassed by having to disrobe in front of someone else, they are disoriented, they feel rushed, panicked or cold, or because they cannot remember all the steps involved in taking a bath. Many caregivers recommend coaching the patient through one step at a time and allowing him or her to have as much control as possible over the time of day for bathing and the choice of a bath or shower.

• schizophrenia. Smoking is a common behavior in schizophrenic patients that complicates personal hygiene, particularly oral care and keeping clothes clean. About 80% of patients with schizophrenia—three times the rate in the general population—are addicted to nicotine. Stopping smoking is particularly difficult for these patients because nicotine withdrawal often causes their psychotic symptoms to worsen. It is not yet known whether there is a biological basis for the high level of nicotine craving in many persons with schizophrenia.

• children and adolescents with learning or developmental disorders living in troubled homes. Some young people with these disorders react to abuse or other problems in their families by neglecting personal hygiene or refusing to bathe and otherwise care for themselves. A social worker's evaluation of the home situation is usually necessary.

Results

Results depend on the reason(s) for and degree of the patient's cognitive impairment, and whether or not he or she is also physically impaired. A physically healthy young person with mild mental retardation may be able to live independently and maintain a reasonable level of personal hygiene and grooming with occasional instruction or reminders from others, whereas an elderly patient with late-stage **Alzheimer's disease** will be completely bedridden, incontinent and unable to think clearly or even speak.

Health care team roles

Depending on the age of a patient with cognitive impairment and the cause(s) of it, most or all of the following health professionals will be involved:

• primary care physician.

• dentist and dental hygienist. These professionals may be able to give instruction in care of the mouth and gums as well as perform examinations and routine cleaning of the teeth.

• psychiatrist, neurologist, gerontologist, or clinical psychologist. These specialists may help to diagnose the cause or causes of the cognitive impairments. A psychiatrist usually prescribes and monitors medications for psychotic and mood disorders. A neurologist may be needed to evaluate the patient for evidence of a stroke or other organic brain damage, while a clinical psychologist may administer tests to determine the type and severity of learning or developmental disorders. Gerontologists specialize in the care of the elderly.

• psychotherapist. Patients recovering from depression or substance abuse disorders are often helped by individual or group psychotherapy. Cognitive therapy appears to be useful in treating depressed patients by interrupting and correcting the distorted thought patterns that underlie and maintain depression.

• case manager, social worker, occupational therapist, and/or personal support worker or "coach." Many patients with schizophrenia or mental retardation are capable of living in the community and holding jobs with the help of these professionals.

• physical therapist. May design physical exercises for stroke patients to speed recovery, minimize loss of cognitive function, and minimize the risk of depression.

• home care aide. May be needed to help moderately cognitively impaired patients with ADLs related to personal care.

• twelve-step or similar support group. Important in helping persons recovering from substance abuse to maintain self-care as well as other aspects of recovery.

Resources

BOOKS

Beck, Aaron T., A. John Rush, Brian F. Shaw, and Gary Emery. *Cognitive Therapy of Depression.* New York: The Guilford Press, 1987.

Crissey, Pat. *Personal Hygiene? What's That Got to Do with Me?* Philadelphia: Jessica Kingsley, 2005.

Diagnostic and Statistical Manual of Mental Disorders Revised IV. Washington, DC: American Psychiatric Press, 2000.

Mace, Nancy L., and Peter V. Rabins. *The 36-Hour Day,* revised and updated edition. New York: Warner Books, Inc., 2001; by arrangement with The Johns Hopkins University Press.

Marcantonio, Edward, MD. "Dementia." *The Merck Manual of Geriatrics, Mark H. Beers, and Robert Berkow, eds.* Whitehouse Station, NJ: Merck Research Laboratories, 2004.

Morris, Virginia. *How to Care for Aging Parents,* revised edition. New York: Workman Publishing, 2004.

Schizophrenia and Related Disorders. Section 15, Chapter 193 in *The Merck Manual of Diagnosis and Therapy*, Mark H. Beers, and Robert Berkow, eds. Whitehouse Station, NJ: Merck Research Laboratories, 2004.

Ziefert, Penelope, Mark Leary, and Alicia A. Boccellari. *AIDS and the Impact of Cognitive Impairment.* San Francisco: University of California at San Francisco AIDS Health Project, 1995.

PERIODICALS

Dunn, Joshua C., Brenda Thiru-Chelvam, and Charles H. M. Beck. "Bathing: Pleasure or Pain?" *Journal of Gerontological Nursing* 28 (November 2002): 6–13.

Rao, Stephen M. "Cognitive Function in Patients with Multiple Sclerosis: Impairment and Treatment." *International Journal of MS Care* 1 (2004): 9–22.

Shankle, William R., A. Kimball Romney, Junko Hara, et al. "Methods to Improve the Detection of Mild Cognitive Impairment." *Proceedings of the National Academy of Sciences* 102 (March 29, 2005): 4919–4924.

ORGANIZATIONS

Alzheimer's Association. 225 North Michigan Avenue, Floor 17, Chicago, IL 60601. (800) 272-3900. http://www.alz.org.

American Academy of Child and Adolescent Psychiatry. 3615 Wisconsin Avenue, NW, Washington, DC 20016-3007. (202) 966-7300. Fax: (202) 966-2891. www.aacap.org.

American Association on Mental Retardation (AAMR). 444 North Capitol Street, Washington, DC 20001-1512. (202) 387-1968. Fax: (202) 387-2193. http://www.aamr.org.

American Physical Therapy Association (APTA). 1111 North Fairfax Street, Alexandria, VA 22314-1488. (703) 684-APTA. Fax: (703) 684-7343. http://www.apta.org.

National Alliance on Mental Illness (NAMI). Colonial Place Three, 2107 Wilson Blvd., Suite 300, Arlington, VA 22201-3042. (800) 950-NAMI or (703) 524-7600. Fax: (703) 524-9094. www.nami.org.

National Institute of Mental Health (NIMH). 6001 Executive Boulevard, Room 8184, MSC 9663, Bethesda, MD 20892-9663. (301) 443-4513 or (866) 615-NIMH. Fax: (301) 443-4279. www.nimh.nih.gov.

Rebecca J. Frey, PhD

Personal hygiene for physical impairment

Definition

Personal hygiene refers to maintaining cleanliness of one's body and clothing to preserve overall health and well-being. It includes a number of different activities related to the following general areas of self-care: washing or bathing, **oral hygiene**, grooming and dressing, keeping one's clothes clean, and toileting. These are sometimes described (along with such other daily tasks as preparing meals or managing finances) as activities of daily living or ADLs. Physical impairments may affect a person's ability to maintain personal hygiene in all these areas or in only one or two.

Purpose

Personal hygiene is a preventive health measure that serves emotional and social as well as physical well-being. Personal hygiene:

- protects against the spread of disease from external parasites (such as body or head lice) or from contact with contaminated feces or other body fluids
- protects the skin against rashes and sores from contact with urine
- protects against malnutrition or swallowing difficulties caused by lack of oral care
- minimizes the chances of social embarrassment, job loss or educational failure, and eventual isolation from others
- keeps up morale and helps avoid depression

Precautions

Maintaining personal hygiene in someone with physical impairments requires a thorough assessment of the patient's living circumstances, as well as the nature and severity of the impairment itself. Factors that should be evaluated include the following:

- duration of the impairment; that is, whether it is temporary or permanent. A person recovering from joint replacement surgery has only temporary limitations on their mobility compared to someone permanently paralyzed below the waist.
- organs or organ systems affected. Limited mobility leads to a different pattern of problems for maintaining personal cleanliness than impaired hands or wrists (the most common single impairment in patients with osteoarthritis), an ostomy, or impaired vision or hearing.
- severity of the impairment. Some patients may be able to take care of personal cleanliness and grooming with the help of personal assistive devices (canes, walkers, etc.), special tools or devices designed for arthritic hands, or environmental changes (furniture rearrangement, installation of grab bars, a seat and hose attachment in the shower, a raised toilet, etc.), while those who are completely bedridden may need help with nearly all aspects of personal hygiene.
- coexisting cognitive or emotional impairments. These can complicate maintaining personal hygiene in persons with physical impairments.

In the specific case of incontinence (inability to control the passage of urine or bowel movements), a doctor should examine the patient to determine the cause. There are several different physical causes that may contribute to incontinence: structural abnormalities or weak muscles in the area of the bladder or anus; diseases that affect the nerves leading to and from the colon or bladder; medications that interfere with normal patterns of elimination; or difficulty reaching the bathroom quickly because of mobility impairments. **Urinary incontinence** is a particularly important hygienic problem because it is the single most common reason for institutionalizing physically impaired elderly patients.

Relatives or health care professionals who may provide short- or long-term assistance with personal care should be sensitive to the psychological impact of needing help with such activities as bathing, toileting, or dressing. These are basic markers of independence in children as well as adults, and are also usually carried out in private. To have someone else look at or touch one's body in order to maintain basic cleanliness is uncomfortable for most people. In general, it is best to let the patient do as much of the washing or toileting as he or she is able to perform.

Description

It is difficult to describe a typical routine for maintaining personal for a patient with physical impairments because of the variety of types of impairment, as well as the wide range of severity associated with physical impairments. In the case of a patient who needs assistance with all aspects of personal cleanliness, the following is a summary description:

- bathing or washing. The caregiver must be careful to support the person (if a stool or bath seat is not used) at all times. They should *never* leave the patient alone in the tub or shower, as falls or other accidents can easily occur. It is also important to check the temperature of the water to make sure it is not too hot. The patient may be able to wash him- or herself once seated; if not, the caregiver must be careful to wash the genital areas and all body folds (including the area under the breasts in women). Bubble bath and bath oils should be avoided, as they can make the tub or shower slippery. Soap should be thoroughly rinsed off to avoid irritating the skin. The patient should be dried off completely with a towel. During the bath or shower, the caregiver should check for skin rashes, pressure sores, or similar problems and report them to the doctor. If the patient is completely bedridden, a sponge bath can be given, using a bowl of warm water with a small amount of soap and a soft washcloth.
- dressing and grooming. Looking one's best is important to self-esteem. It is helpful, however, to simplify

KEY TERMS

Activities of daily living (ADLs)—A shorthand term for the everyday tasks that must be carried out to maintain basic cleanliness, nutrition, contact with others, etc.

Incontinence—Inability to control one's bowel or bladder functions.

Ostomy—A general term for a surgical procedure in which an artificial opening is made for the drainage of body wastes.

dressing and grooming for a physically impaired person by choosing clothes and shoes with pull-on styling or Velcro fasteners and to arrange the hair in a simple style that is easy to wash and does not need setting. The caregiver may also need to do the patient's laundry or periodically trim fingernails and toenails if the patient cannot do these things.

- oral hygiene. The caregiver may need to brush the patient's teeth or clean their dentures, which must be done on a daily basis. Some dentists recommend foam applicators instead of brushes for cleaning the teeth of persons with physical impairments. If a brush is used, an electric model may be more efficient than a standard toothbrush. The caregiver should also check the person's mouth and gums for ulcers or irritated areas.

- toileting. Many persons with physical impairments find it easier to use a toilet with an elevated seat There should be supports or grab bars on each side of the toilet to minimize the risk of falls. It is important to remove soiled or wet clothing and cleanse the patient's body as quickly as possible if they cannot get to the toilet in time or are chronically incontinent. The area around the urethra or anus should be washed and carefully dried to prevent skin irritation. Baby powder or corn starch may be used to help keep the skin dry.

Preparation

Preparation for maintaining personal hygiene in a physically impaired person should include the following considerations:

- a safety evaluation of the person's apartment or room for such features as adequate lighting, non-slip flooring, hand rails or grab bars, properly secured electrical cords and household chemicals, and similar considerations. The temperature setting of the hot water supply should be checked to prevent accidental scalding.

- assessment of the type and frequency of assistance needed, if any, and the qualifications of the caregiver, if one is required.

- storing clothing, personal care supplies, assistive devices, etc. close to where they are used.

Health care team roles

A person with physical impairments may require the assistance of one or more of the following health care professionals, depending on the extent and complexity of their impairment:

- occupational therapist. Some patients may be able to manage bathing, dressing, and oral care with instruction or rehabilitation techniques.

- physical therapist. Patients whose impairments are temporary may benefit from exercises designed by the therapist to help them with ADLs as well as regain general mobility and functioning.

- homemaker. Some patients may require assistance with laundry, changing bed linens, or shopping for food, personal care items and clothing. Homemakers do not usually provide direct assistance with personal care, however.

- home health aide. Home health aides are trained to assist patients who require help with bathing, toileting, oral care, and other ADLs. They may also give advice or instruction about personal cleanliness and self-care.

- social worker or registered nurse. These professionals typically supervise aides employed by home healthcare agencies; they may or may not have direct contact with the patient.

Resources

BOOKS

Beers, Mark H. and Thomas V. Jones. Section 1, "Basics of Geriatric Care," in *The Merck Manual of Geriatrics*, 3rd ed. Whitehouse Station, NJ: Merck, 2005.

Mace, Nancy L. and Peter V. Rabins. *The 36-Hour Day*, revised and updated edition. New York: Warner Books, Inc., 2001; by arrangement with The Johns Hopkins University Press

Morris, Virginia. *How to Care for Aging Parents*, revised edition. New York: Workman Publishing, 2004.

Silber, Irwin. *A Patient's Guide to Knee and Hip Replacement*. New York: Simon & Schuster, 1999.

PERIODICALS

Dunn, Joshua C., Brenda Thiru-Chelvam, and Charles H. M. Beck. "Bathing: Pleasure or Pain?" *Journal of Gerontological Nursing* 28 (November 2002): 6–13.

Quinn, M. E., M. A. Johnson, E. L. Andress, et al. "Health Characteristics of Elderly Personal Care Home Residents." *Journal of Advanced Care Nursing* 30 (August 1999): 410–417.

Westhoff, G., J. Listing, and A. Zink. "Loss of Physical Independence in Rheumatoid Arthritis: Interview Data from a Representative Sample of Patients in Rheumatologic Care." *Arthritis Care and Research* 13 (February 2000): 11–22.

ORGANIZATIONS

American Physical Therapy Association (APTA). 1111 North Fairfax Street, Alexandria, VA 22314-1488. (703) 684-APTA. Fax: (703) 684-7343. http://www.apta.org.

National Association for Home Care and Hospice (NAHC). 228 Seventh Street, SE, Washington, DC 20003. (202) 547-7424. Fax: (202) 547-3540. http://www.nahc.org.

National Association of Certified Caregivers/Personal Support Workers (NACPSW). P.O. Box 175, Owen Sound, ON, Canada N4K 5P2. (519) 376-7396. Fax: (519) 376-6772. http://www.nacpsw.org.

Rebecca J. Frey, PhD

Personal oral hygiene *see* **Oral hygiene**

Personality disorders

Definition

Personality disorders are a group of personality flaws defined by the fourth (2000) edition of the *Diagnostic and Statistical Manual of Mental Disorders (Text Revision) (DSM-IV-TR)* as "enduring pattern[s] of inner experience and behavior" that are sufficiently rigid and deep-seated to bring a person into repeated conflicts with his or her social and occupational environment. *DSM-IV-TR* specifies that these dysfunctional patterns must be regarded as non-conforming or deviant by the person's culture, and cause significant emotional **pain** and/or difficulties in relationships and occupational performance. In addition, the patient usually sees the disorder as being consistent with his or her self-image (ego-syntonic) and may blame others.

Description

To meet the diagnosis of personality disorder, which is sometimes called character disorder, the patient's problematic behaviors must appear in two or more of the following areas:

- perception and interpretation of the self and other people

- intensity and duration of feelings and their appropriateness to situations

- relationships with others

- ability to control impulses

Personality disorders have their onset in late adolescence or early adulthood. Doctors rarely give a diagnosis of personality disorder to children on the grounds that children's personalities are still in the process of formation and may change considerably by the time they are in their late teens. But, in retrospect, many individuals with personality disorders could be judged to have shown evidence of the problems in childhood.

It is difficult to accurately estimate the percentage of the population that suffer from personality disorders. Patients with certain personality disorders, including antisocial and borderline disorders, are more likely to get into trouble with the law or otherwise attract attention than are patients whose disorders chiefly affect their capacity for intimacy. On the other hand, some patients, such as those with narcissistic or obsessive-compulsive personality disorders, may be outwardly successful because their symptoms are useful within their particular occupations. It has, however, been estimated that about 15% of the general population of the United States suffers from personality disorders, with higher rates in poor or troubled neighborhoods. The rate of personality disorders among patients in psychiatric treatment is between 30% and 50%. It is possible for patients to have a so-called dual diagnosis; for example, they may have more than one personality disorder, or a personality disorder together with a substance-abuse problem.

DSM-IV-TR classifies personality disorders into three clusters based on symptom similarities:

- Cluster A (paranoid, schizoid, schizotypal): Patients appear odd or eccentric to others.

- Cluster B (antisocial, borderline, histrionic, narcissistic): Patients appear overly emotional, unstable, or self-dramatizing to others.

- Cluster C (avoidant, dependent, obsessive-compulsive): Patients appear tense and anxiety-ridden to others.

The *DSM-IV-TR* clustering system does not mean that all patients can be fitted neatly into one of the three clusters. It is possible for patients to have symptoms of more than one personality disorder or to have symptoms from different clusters.

Since the criteria for personality disorders include friction or conflict between the patient and his or her social environment, these syndromes are open to redefinition as societies change. Successive editions of *DSM* have tried to be sensitive to cultural differences, including changes over time, when defining personality disorders. One category that had been proposed for *DSM-III-R,* self-defeating personality disorder, was excluded from *DSM-IV-TR* on the grounds that its definition reflected prejudice against women. *DSM-IV-TR* recommends that doctors take a patient's background, especially recent immigration, into account before deciding that he or she has a personality disorder. One criticism that has been made of the general category of personality disorder is that it is based on Western notions of individual uniqueness. Its applicability to people from other cultures is thus open to question. Furthermore, even within a culture, it can be difficult to define the limits of "normalcy."

The personality disorders defined by *DSM-IV-TR* are described below. Certain personality disorders, such as paranoid, schizoid, and schizotypal, should not be confused with psychotic disorders with the same or similar names. Psychotic disorders are characterized by more seriously disordered thinking, frequently involving hallucinations (seeing things that aren't present or **hearing** voices) and delusions (having unrealistic beliefs, such as thinking one has god-like powers), with an inability to distinguish reality from fantasy.

Paranoid

Patients with paranoid personality disorder are characterized by suspiciousness and a belief that others are out to harm or cheat them. They have problems with intimacy and may join cults or groups with paranoid belief systems. Some are litigious, bringing lawsuits against those they believe have wronged them. Although not ordinarily delusional, these patients may develop psychotic symptoms under severe **stress**. It is estimated that 0.5–2.5% of the general population meet the criteria for paranoid personality disorder.

Schizoid

Schizoid patients are perceived by others as "loners" without close family relationships or social contacts. Indeed, they are aloof and really do prefer to be alone. They may appear cold to others because they rarely display strong emotions. They may, however, be successful in occupations that do not require personal interaction. About 2% of the general population has this disorder. It is slightly more common in men than in women.

Schizotypal

Patients diagnosed as schizotypal are often considered odd or eccentric because they pay little attention to their clothing and sometimes have peculiar speech mannerisms. They are socially isolated and uncomfortable in parties or other social gatherings. In addition, people with schizotypal personality disorder often have oddities of thought, including "magical" beliefs or peculiar ideas (for example, a belief in telepathy) that are outside of their cultural norms. It is thought that 3% of the general population has schizotypal personality disorder. It is slightly more common in males. There is some evidence that schizotypal personality disorder and the psychotic disorder, **schizophrenia**, are genetically related.

Antisocial

Patients with antisocial personality disorder are sometimes referred to as sociopaths or psychopaths. They are characterized by lying, manipulativeness, and a selfish disregard for the rights of others; some may act impulsively. People with antisocial personality disorder are frequently chemically dependent and sexually promiscuous. It is estimated that 3% of males in the general population and 1% of females have antisocial personality disorder.

Borderline

Patients with borderline personality disorder (BPD) are highly unstable, with wide mood swings, a history of intense but stormy relationships, impulsive behavior, and confusion about career goals, personal values, or sexual orientation. These often highly conflicting ideas may correspond to an even deeper confusion about their sense of self (identity). People with BPD frequently cut or burn themselves, or threaten or attempt suicide. Many of these patients have histories of severe childhood abuse or **neglect**. About 2% of the general population have BPD; 75% of these patients are female.

Histrionic

Patients diagnosed with this disorder impress others as overly emotional, overly dramatic, and hungry for attention. They may be flirtatious or seductive as a way of drawing attention to themselves, yet they are emotionally shallow. Histrionic patients often live in a romantic fantasy world and are easily bored with routine. About 2–3% of the population is thought to have this disorder. Although historically, in clinical settings, the disorder has been more associated with women, there may be bias toward diagnosing women with this personality disorder.

Narcissistic

Narcissistic patients are characterized by a sense of self-importance, a craving for admiration, and exploitative attitudes toward others. They have unrealistically inflated views of their talents and accomplishments, and may become extremely angry if they are criticized or outshone by others. Narcissists may be professionally successful but rarely have long-lasting intimate relationships. Fewer than 1% of the population has this disorder; about 75% of those diagnosed with it are male.

Avoidant

Patients with avoidant personality disorder are fearful of rejection and shy away from situations or occupations that might expose their supposed inadequacy. They may reject opportunities to develop close relationships because of their fears of criticism or humiliation. Patients with this personality disorder are often diagnosed with dependent personality disorder as well. Many also fit the criteria for social phobia. Between 0.5–1.0% of the population have avoidant personality disorder.

Dependent

Dependent patients are afraid of being on their own and typically develop submissive or compliant behaviors in order to avoid displeasing people. They are afraid to question authority and often ask others for guidance or direction. Dependent personality disorder is diagnosed more often in women, but it has been suggested that this finding reflects social pressures on women to conform to gender stereotyping or bias on the part of clinicians.

Obsessive-compulsive

Patients diagnosed with this disorder are preoccupied with keeping order, attaining perfection, and maintaining mental and interpersonal control. They may spend a great deal of time adhering to plans, schedules, or rules from which they will not deviate, even at the expense of openness, flexibility, and efficiency. These patients are often unable to relax and may become "workaholics." They may have problems in employment as well as in intimate relationships because they are very "stiff" and formal, and insist on doing everything their way. About 1% of the population has obsessive-compulsive personality disorder; the male/female ratio is about 2:1.

Causes and symptoms

Personality disorders are thought to be a disparity between a child's temperament or character and his or her family or social relationships. Temperament can be defined as a person's innate or biologically shaped basic disposition. Human infants vary in their sensitivity to light or noise, their level of physical activity, their adaptability to schedules, and other aspects. Even traits such as "shyness" and "novelty-seeking" may be, at least in part, determined by the biology of the **brain** and the genes one inherits.

Character is defined as the set of attitudes and behavior patterns that the individual acquires or learns over time. It includes such personal qualities as work and study habits, moral convictions, neatness or cleanliness, and consideration of others. Since children must learn to adapt to their specific families, they may develop personality disorders in the course of struggling to survive psychologically in disturbed or stressful families. For example, nervous or high-strung parents might be unhappy with a baby who is very active and try to restrain him or her at every opportunity. The child might then develop an avoidant personality disorder as the outcome of coping with constant frustration and parental disapproval. As another example, **child abuse** is believed to play a role in shaping borderline personality disorder. One reason that some therapists use the term developmental damage instead of personality disorder is that it takes the presumed source of the person's problems into account.

Some patients with personality disorders come from families that appear to be stable and healthy. It has been suggested that these patients are biologically hypersensitive to normal family stress levels. Levels of the brain chemical (neurotransmitter) dopamine may influence a person's level of novelty-seeking, and serotonin levels may influence aggression.

Diagnosis

Diagnosis of personality disorders is complicated by the fact that persons suffering from them rarely seek help until they are in serious trouble or until their families (or the law) pressure them to get treatment. The reason for this slowness is that the problematic traits are so deeply entrenched that they seem normal (ego-syntonic) to the patient. Diagnosis of a personality disorder depends in part on the patient's age. Although personality disorders originate during the childhood years, they are considered to be adult disorders. Some patients, in fact, are not diagnosed until late in life because their symptoms had been modified by the demands of their job or by marriage. After retirement or the spouse's death, however, these patients' personality disorders become fully apparent. In general, however, if the onset of the patient's problem is in mid- or late-life, the doctor will rule out **substance abuse** or personality change caused by medical or neurological problems before considering the diagnosis of a personality disorder. It is unusual for people to develop personality disorders "out of the blue" in mid-life.

There are no tests that can provide a definitive diagnosis of personality disorder. Most doctors will evaluate a patient on the basis of several sources of information collected over a period of time in order to determine how long the patient has been having difficulties, how many areas of life are affected, and how severe the dysfunction is. These sources of information may include:

Interviews

The doctor may schedule two or three interviews with the patient, spaced over several weeks or months, in order to rule out an adjustment disorder caused by job loss, bereavement, or a similar problem. An office interview allows the doctor to form an impression of the patient's overall personality as well as obtain information about his or her occupation and family. During the interview, the doctor will note the patient's appearance, tone of voice, body language, eye contact, and other important non-verbal signals, as well as the content of the conversation. In some cases, the doctor may contact other people (family members, employers, close friends) who know the patient well in order to assess the accuracy of the patient's perception of his or her difficulties. It is quite common for people with personality disorders to have distorted views of their situations, or to be unaware of the impact of their behavior on others.

Psychological testing

Doctors use psychological testing to help in the diagnosis of a personality disorder. Most of these tests require interpretation by a professional with specialized training. Doctors usually refer patients to a clinical psychologist for this type of test.

PERSONALITY INVENTORIES. Personality inventories are tests with true/false or yes/no answers that can be used to compare the patient's scores with those of people with known personality distortions. The single most commonly used test of this type is the Minnesota Multiphasic Personality Inventory, or MMPI. Another test that is often used is the Millon Clinical Multiaxial Inventory, or MCMI.

PROJECTIVE TESTS. Projective tests are unstructured, meaning that instead of giving one-word answers to questions, the patient is asked to talk at some length about a picture that the psychologist presents, or to supply an ending for the beginning of a story. Projective tests allow the clinician to assess the patient's patterns of thinking, fantasies, worries or anxieties, moral concerns, values, and habits. Common projective tests include the Rorschach, in which the patient responds to a set of 10 inkblots; and the Thematic Apperception Test (TAT), in which the patient is shown drawings of people in different situations and then tells a story about the picture.

Prognosis

At one time psychiatrists thought that personality disorders did not respond very well to treatment. This opinion was derived from the notion that human personality is fixed for life once it has been molded in childhood, and from the belief among people with personality disorders that their own views and behaviors are correct, and that others are the ones at fault. More recently, however, doctors have recognized that humans can continue to grow and change throughout life. Most patients with personality disorders are now considered to be treatable, although the degree of improvement may vary. The type of treatment recommended depends on the personality characteristics associated with the specific disorder.

Treatment

A number of treatments are available for patients with personality disorders. One of the newer treatments is the use of certain antidepressant medications such as the SSRI (selective serotonin reuptake inhibitors) antidepressants.

Hospitalization

Inpatient treatment is rarely required for patients with personality disorders, with two major exceptions: borderline patients who are threatening suicide or suffering from drug or alcohol withdrawal; and patients with paranoid personality disorder who are having psychotic symptoms.

Psychotherapy

Psychoanalytic **psychotherapy** is suggested for patients who can benefit from insight-oriented treatment. These patients typically include those with dependent, obsessive-compulsive, and avoidant personality disorders. Doctors usually recommend individual psychotherapy for narcissistic and borderline patients, but often refer these patients to therapists with specialized training in these disorders. Psychotherapeutic treatment for personality disorders may take as long as three to five years.

Insight-oriented approaches are not recommended for patients with paranoid or antisocial personality disorders. These patients are likely to resent the therapist and see him or her as trying to control or dominate them.

Supportive therapy is regarded as the most helpful form of psychotherapy for patients with schizoid personality disorder.

Cognitive-behavioral therapy

Cognitive-behavioral approaches are often recommended for patients with avoidant or dependent personality disorders. Patients in these groups typically have mistaken beliefs about their competence or likableness. These assumptions can be successfully challenged by cognitive-behavioral methods.

Group therapy

Group therapy is frequently useful for patients with schizoid or avoidant personality disorders because it helps them to break out of their social isolation. It has also been recommended for patients with histrionic and antisocial personality disorders. These patients tend to act out, and pressure from peers in group treatment can motivate them to change. Because patients with antisocial personality disorder can destabilize groups that include people with other disorders, it is usually best if these people meet exclusively with others with the same disorder (in "homogeneous" groups).

Family therapy

Family therapy may be suggested for patients whose personality disorders cause serious problems for members of their families. It is also sometimes recommended for borderline patients from overinvolved or possessive families.

Medications

Medications may be prescribed for patients with specific personality disorders. The type of medication depends on the disorder.

ANTIPSYCHOTIC DRUGS. **Antipsychotic drugs**, such as haloperidol (Haldol), may be given to patients with paranoid personality disorder if they are having brief psychotic episodes. Patients with borderline or schizotypal personality disorder are sometimes given

antipsychotic drugs in low doses; however, the efficacy of these drugs in treating personality disorder is less clear than in schizophrenia.

MOOD STABILIZERS. Carbamazepine (Tegretol) is a drug that is commonly used to treat seizures, but is also helpful for borderline patients with rage outbursts and similar behavioral problems. Lithium and valproate may also be used as mood stabilizers, especially among people with borderline personality disorder.

ANTIDEPRESSANTS AND ANTI-ANXIETY MEDICATIONS. Medications in these categories are sometimes prescribed for patients with schizoid personality disorder to help them manage **anxiety** symptoms while they are in psychotherapy. Antidepressants are also commonly used to treat people with borderline personality disorder.

Treatment with medications is not recommended for patients with avoidant, histrionic, dependent, or narcissistic personality disorders. The use of potentially addictive medications should be avoided in people with borderline or antisocial personality disorders. However, some avoidant patients who also have social phobia may benefit from monoamine oxidase inhibitors (MAO inhibitors), a particular class of antidepressant.

Prognosis

The prognosis for recovery depends in part on the specific disorder and the existence of a mood disorder or coexisting psychiatric diagnosis. Although some patients improve as they grow older and have positive experiences in life, personality disorders are generally life-long disturbances with periods of worsening (exacerbations) and periods of improvement (remissions). Others, particularly schizoid patients, have better prognoses if they are given appropriate treatment. Patients with paranoid personality disorder are at some risk for developing delusional disorders or schizophrenia. The personality disorders with the poorest prognoses are the antisocial and the borderline. Borderline patients are at high risk for developing substance abuse disorders or bulimia. About 80% of hospitalized borderline patients attempt suicide at some point during treatment, and about 5% succeed in committing suicide.

Health care team roles

Nursing staff and allied health professionals can assist in the treatment of personality disorders by being aware of the symptoms of each cluster. Since personality disorders often present as relationship difficulties, nursing staff and allied health professionals may recognize personality disorders in particularly problematic patients.

During the treatment phase, nursing staff and allied health professionals can help patients by providing them with appropriate educational materials and referrals for ongoing psychotherapy or group therapy, if applicable.

Prevention

The most effective preventive strategy for personality disorders is early identification and treatment of children and adults who are at risk. High-risk groups

---

QUESTIONS TO ASK YOUR DOCTOR

- Are there "clues" that I can watch for that warn of possible personality disorders in my aging parents?

- If personality disorders have their origin in childhood, are there specific behaviors I can employ or avoid to prevent my children from developing such behaviors?

- What medical professionals are available locally to provide me with additional information about possible personality disorders I suspect in my family?

- What kinds of tests are available for diagnosing personality disorders, and what information do they provide you about a person's problems?

- How valid do you think projective tests like the Rorschach are for diagnosing personality disorders?

- How are personality disorders different from psychoses?

---

include abused children, children from troubled families, children with close relatives diagnosed with personality disorders, children of substance abusers, and children who grow up in cults or political extremist groups.

Resources

BOOKS

American Psychiatric Association. *Diagnostic and Statistical Manual of Mental Disorders: DSM-IV-TR.* Arlington, TX: American Psychiatric Association, 2000.

Townsend, Mary C. *Essentials of Psychiatric Mental Health Nursing: Concepts of Care in Evidence-based Practice.* Philadelphia: F.A. Davis, 2011.

OTHER

Bienenfeld, David. *Personality Disorders.* http://emedicine. medscape.com/article/294307-overview (accessed May 9, 2012).

Mayo Clinic Staff. *Personality Disorders.* http://www. mayoclinic.com/health/personality-disorders/DS00562 (accessed May 9, 2012).

Personality Disorders. Mental Health Net. http://www.mental-help.net/poc/center_index.php?id=8 (accessed May 9, 2012).

Personality Disorders. Medline Plus. http://www.nlm.nih.gov/ medlineplus/personalitydisorders.html (accessed May 9, 2012).

Bethanne Black

PET scan *see* **Positron emission tomography (PET)**

PET unit *see* **Positron emission tomography (PET) unit**

Phantom limb

Definition

Phantom limb is the term for abnormal sensations perceived from a previously amputated limb. The abnormal sensations may be painful or nonpainful. It is presumed to be due to central and peripheral nervous system reorganization as a response to injury. Phantom limb **pain** is often considered to be a form of neuropathic pain, a group of pain syndromes associated with damage to nerves.

Demographics

The incidence of phantom limb pain is estimated in 50–80% of all amputees. It is more prevalent in upper limb amputees (82%) than lower limb amputees (54%). There is no known association with age, gender, or which limb is amputated. Studies have shown a decreased incidence of phantom limb syndrome in those born without limbs versus actual amputees.

Description

Silas Weir Mitchell, an American neurologist, coined the term "phantom limb" in 1871. Phantom limb syndrome was first described by Ambroise Paré in 1552. Paré, a French surgeon, noticed this phenomenon in soldiers who felt pain in their amputated limbs. Phantom limb syndrome can be subdivided into phantom limb sensation and phantom limb pain. Stump or residual limb pain refers to pain that may persist at the residual site of amputation and may be grouped under phantom limb syndrome as well.

The onset of pain after amputation usually occurs within days to weeks, although it may be delayed months or years. Pain may last for years and tends to be intermittent rather than constant. Pain may last up to 10–14 hours a day and can vary in severity from mild to debilitating. The abnormal "phantom" sensations and pain are usually located in the distal parts of the missing limb. Pain and tingling may be felt in the fingers and hand and in the lower limbs, in the toes and the feet.

Causes and symptoms

Causes

The exact etiology of phantom limb pain is unknown. Phantom limb is thought to be secondary to the **brain** plasticity and reorganization. The human brain has an enormous capacity to alter its connections and function in response to everyday learning or to the setting of injury. These processes of reorganization may occur in retained nerves in the amputated limbs, the **spinal cord**, or various parts of the brain, including the thalamus and the cerebral cortex.

Although phantom pain is presumably a result of a response to amputation injury, phantom limb pain may occur in non-amputees with spinal cord damage causing loss of sensation. This suggests that the phantom limb phenomenon may be a result of damage to pathways responsible for painful sensation in general. Research studies in primates and patients with limb amputation have shown that after amputation, the area of the brain that is responsible for processing the sensations from the missing limb are taken over by areas neighboring the missing limb.

Symptoms

Patients may feel a variety of sensations emanating from the absent limb. The limb may feel completely intact despite its absence. Nonpainful sensations may include changes in temperature, **itching**, tingling, shock-like sensations, or perceived motion of the phantom limb. The limb may feel as if it is retracting into the stump, a phenomenon called telescoping. Painful sensations include burning, throbbing, or stabbing in nature. Touching the remaining stump may elicit sensations from the phantom. The quality of the pain may change over time and may not remain constant. Patients may also feel pain from the retained stump itself. Stump pain is often associated with phantom limb sensations and may be related in etiology.

Diagnosis

The diagnosis of phantom limb is a clinical one. A history of previous limb amputation and the subsequent symptoms of abnormal sensations from the missing limb are key to the diagnosis. Spinal cord damage affecting pathways mediating sensation may also be associated with phantom limb. There are no imaging or clinical tests useful in diagnosing phantom limb.

Treatment team

The treatment team for phantom limb pain may involve the participation of neurologists, pain specialists, physical therapists, neurosurgeons, or **reha-bilitation** specialists. Neurologists and pain specialists may help in prescribing medications to treat the phantom limb pain. Physical therapists may help to facilitate and maintain mobility. Neurosurgeons may perform surgery to place electrical nerve stimulators in the spinal cord or lesion procedures to help treat the pain.

Treatment

There are few controlled clinical studies on phantom limb treatment, and therefore no consensus on the best treatment. Treatment is directed toward the management of painful symptoms. Nonpainful symptoms rarely require treatment. Treatment for phantom limb pain involves the use of medications, as well as non-medical, electrical, and surgical therapy.

Medical treatment of phantom limb pain involves agents typically used for neuropathic pain. Medications such as anticonvulsants, **muscle relaxants**, and antidepressants may be tried. Opiate medications have also been used. Ketamine, an anesthetic agent, or calcitonin has been shown to be effective in some clinical studies.

Various electrical and nonmedical treatments may be tried. Transcutaneous electrical nerve stimulation (TENS), vibration therapy, and biofeedback may be used. Massage, ultrasound, hypnosis, and **acupuncture** modalities may be tried as well. Training patients to discriminate sensory signals in the stump appears to be helpful in reducing pain. In research studies, allowing individuals to see a reflection of the normal, intact limb moving in the position of the amputated limb helped alleviate symptoms of phantom limb pain.

Mirror box therapy is another treatment modality for phantom limb pain. This therapy, developed in 1995 by Vilayanur Ramachandran, involves artificial visual feedback using two mirrors to train individuals to sense movement and guiding of the phantom limb into a position of comfort. Repeated training is necessary and has led to improvement of pain for some individuals.

Immersive virtual reality is a relatively new treatment modality being developed by a team of researchers at the University of Manchester in England. After attaching their real limb to a specially designed interface, computer simulation allows the individual to view two limbs moving, creating an illusion to "trick" sensory areas in the brain to help decrease discomfort in the phantom limb. Research is ongoing to further develop this therapy.

Surgical treatments for phantom limb pain are limited in benefit. Lesions of various pain centers in the spinal cord and brain can be performed and may provide short-term relief on most occasions.

Recovery and rehabilitation

Prospective studies of phantom pain show that, in two years, many amputees will experience a reduction of symptoms. Physical and occupational therapists may help in the treatment of phantom limb pain by maintaining range of motion and mobility.

Clinical trials

There are ongoing clinical trials conducted by the National Institute of Neurological Disorders and **Stroke** (NINDS) studying touch perception in patients with upper limb amputation. Individuals who wish to participate can find a list of clinical trials currently enrolling volunteers at http://clinicaltrials.gov. There is no cost to the patient to participate in a clinical trial.

Prognosis

The prognosis for phantom limb varies from individual to individual. Medical treatment shows the most benefit in treating symptoms. Some studies show that in a two-year period, many amputees will experience a reduction or disappearance of their phantom limb pain. The results of the studies are somewhat limited due to the heterogeneity of the populations studied.

Special concerns

Social needs

Phantom limb may have a chronic course and may lead to feelings of depression or **anxiety**. These feelings may require treatment by a psychiatrist. Patients with phantom limb should continue to be active and participate in community and social activities. There are various support groups for amputees.

Resources

BOOKS

Aminoff, Michael J. *Neurology and General Medicine,* 4th ed. London: Churchill Livingstone, 2007.

Gallagher, Pamela, Deirdre Desmond, and Malcolm Macla-chlan, eds. *Psychoprosthetics.* New York: Springer, 2010.

Moore, Rhonda J., ed. *Biobehavioral Approaches to Pain.* New York: Springer, 2009.

Rosenquist, Richard W. *A Practical Approach to Pain Management.* New York: Lippincott Williams & Wilkins, 2012.

Schaefer, Michael. *Body in Mind: A New Look at the Somatosensory Cortices.* New York: Nova Science, 2010.

Sherman, Richard A. *Phantom Pain.* New York: Springer, 2010.

PERIODICALS

Chapman, Suzanne. "Pain management in patients following limb amputation." *Nursing Standard* 25.19 (2011): 35.

Chernev, Ivan, Delia G. Wilcher, and Kun Yan. "Combined mirror visual and auditory feedback therapy for upper limb phantom pain: a case report." *Journal of Medical Case Reports* 5 (2011): 41.

Jacobs, Michael Bradley, and Richard C. Niemtzow. "Treatment of phantom limb pain with laser and needle auricular acupuncture: a case report." *Medical Acupuncture* 23.1 (2011): 57.

Murray, Craig D. "A review of the use of virtual reality in the treatment of phantom limb pain." *Journal of CyberTherapy and Rehabilitation* 2.2 (2009): 105.

ORGANIZATIONS

American Academy of Neurology (AAN), 1080 Montreal Avenue, Saint Paul, MN 55116, (651) 695-2717, (800) 879-1960, Fax: (651) 695-2791, memberservices@aan.com, http://www.aan.com

American Academy of Physical Medicine and Rehabilitation, 9700 West Bryn Mawr Avenue, Suite 200, Rosemont, IL 60018-5701, (847) 737-6000, Fax: (847) 737-6001, info@aapmr.org, http://www.aapmr.org

American Chronic Pain Association (ACPA), P.O. Box 850, Rocklin, CA 95677, (916) 632-0922, (800) 533-3231, Fax: (916) 632-3208, ACPA@pacbell.net, http://www.theacpa.org

American Neurological Association, 5841 Cedar Lake Road, Suite 204, Minneapolis, MN 55416, (952) 545-6284, http://www.aneuroa.org

American Pain Foundation, 201 North Charles Street, Suite 710, Baltimore, MD 21201, (888) 615-PAIN, info@painfoundation.org, http://www.painfoundation.org

National Institute of Neurological Disorders and Stroke (NINDS), P.O. Box 5801, Bethesda, MD 20824, (301) 496-5751, (800) 352-9424, http://www.ninds.nih.gov

National Institutes of Health (NIH), 9000 Rockville Pike, Bethesda, MD 20892, (301) 496-4000, NIHinfo@od.nih.gov, http://www.nih.gov/index.html

The Pain Relief Foundation, Clinical Sciences CentreUniversity Hospital AintreeLower Lane, Liverpool, United Kingdom L9 7AL, (0151) 529-5820, Fax: (0151) 529-5821, secretary@painrelieffoundation.org.uk, http://www.painrelieffoundation.org.uk

U.S. National Library of Medicine, 8600 Rockville Pike, Bethesda, MD 20894, (301) 594-5983, (888) 346-3656, Fax: (301) 402-1384, custserv@nlm.nih.gov, http://www.nlm.nih.gov.

Peter T. Lin, MD
Laura Jean Cataldo, RN, EdD

Pharmacology

Definition

Pharmacology is the branch of medicine that deals with the study of drug actions in living organisms. The English word is derived from two Greek words that mean "drug" and "study of."

Description

Pharmacology is the science of understanding how drugs act on the body and conversely, how the body acts on drugs. Pharmacology is not to be confused with pharmacy, which deals with the preparation and dispensing of drugs. Drugs can be defined as chemical compounds with a specific therapeutic function, such as **fever** reduction or **pain** relief. Pharmacology focuses on how a drug enters the body, where the drug acts within the body, and how the body clears (gets rid of) a drug. In addition, a pharmacologist will also study the therapeutic potential of a drug, the interaction of a drug with other drugs, and analyze adverse drug reactions, otherwise known as toxicities. There are several subdivisions and subdisciplines of pharmacology that apply the basic principles of pharmacology in different ways.

Pharmacology can be divided into subdivisions based on the body organ being studied. These include, but are not limited to, neuropharmacology, cardiovascular pharmacology, endocrine pharmacology, and **chemotherapy**. Neuropharmacology deals with the effect of drugs on the nervous system, which includes the **brain**, **spinal cord**, and nerves. Neuropharmacology includes the study of drugs of abuse such as heroin and also drugs used to treat nervous system disorders such as L-dopa, which is given to **Parkinson's disease** patients. Cardiovascular pharmacology focuses on drugs that modify the **heart** and vascular system. **Blood pressure** medications would be studied under this category. Endocrine pharmacology focuses on the interaction of drugs with various hormones or hormonal systems. Birth control pills would fall under the division of endocrine pharmacology. Lastly, the division of chemotherapy studies the pharmacology of drugs used to treat **cancer** such as tamoxifen used in **breast cancer**.

In addition to dividing the field of pharmacology on the basis of the targeted organ system, pharmacology can also be divided into subdisciplines. These subdisciplines include but are not limited to molecular pharmacology, behavioral pharmacology, and clinical pharmacology. Molecular pharmacology studies the interaction of drugs at the cellular level. This includes studies on the interaction of drugs with protein receptors expressed on the surface of the cell. For example, the **asthma** drug, albuterol, interacts with beta receptors in the lung to increase airflow. The effect of drugs on behavior is the basis for the behavioral pharmacology discipline. Behavioral pharmacology includes addiction research. which tries to understand why people become addicted to drugs like alcohol. The field of clinical pharmacology focuses more on the therapeutic use of drugs, the interactions of drugs with one another in the body, and the nature of adverse drug reactions.

Other subdisciplines include:

• Pharmacognosy: the study of drugs derived from plants and other natural sources. Although most researchers in this field investigate botanicals, others study drugs derived from marine organisms and microbes.

• Pharmacogenomics: the application of genomic technologies to the discovery of new drugs and better understanding of older drugs.

• Psychopharmacology: the study of the effects of drugs on the brain and central nervous system, including their effects on mood, cognition, sensation, and behavior.

• Pharmacoepidemiology: the study of the effects of medications in large populations.

• Toxicology: the study of the harmful or poisonous effects of drugs.

• Veterinary pharmacology: the study of how drugs work in animals, safe dosages, the discovery of new drugs, etc. It is more complicated than human pharmacology because researchers must study the effects of medications across a number of species, not in only one.

The various subdivisions and disciplines of pharmacology pursue the discovery and understanding of drugs for the purpose of treating a disease or condition, such as high **blood** pressure.

The basic principles of pharmacokinetics, pharmacodynamics, and efficacy are universal across the various areas of pharmacology. A significant amount of pharmacology research is spent on identifying new drugs to treat disease. In addition, it is important to predict drug toxicities or adverse reactions. This prediction is accomplished by studying the pharmacokinetics of a drug. Pharmacokinetics is basically a determination of the ways in which drugs are introduced into the body, how they are used within the body, and how they are cleared (excreted). It describes the relationships between drug dosage and drug blood levels, which can be influenced by individual differences in drug absorption, distribution, **metabolism**, and elimination. This is important because if a drug is eliminated by the **kidneys** and a patient has damaged kidneys, then the drug could accumulate in the patient to fatal levels. Pharmacokinetic

KEY TERMS

Clearance—Measurement of the kidneys' ability to excrete (clear) the metabolites of a drug.

Efficacy—The effectiveness of a drug in treating a disease or condition.

Pharmacodynamics—The ways in which a drug acts on tissues and cells in the body.

Pharmacokinetics—The route and rate at which a drug enters and leaves the body.

calculations can be used to determine the dose needed to give safe and effective blood levels in this situation.

A significant amount of pharmacology research is also spent on understanding how drugs act on the body. This is important to understanding adverse reactions, **drug interactions**, and also for the design of better drugs. This area is known more specifically as pharmacodynamics. Pharmacodynamics basically refers to the ways in which drugs interact with the body. Many drugs bind to protein receptors on the surface of a cell. Pharmacodynamics strives to understand how tightly a drug binds to its receptor, what happens inside the cell upon drug binding, and whether the drug has desired or toxic effects on the body.

Lastly, the overall outcome of drugs on the human or animal condition is studied and this is known as efficacy. Efficacy deals with analyzing how well a drug may correct a condition such as arthritis. All three principles, pharmacodynamics, pharmacokinetics, and efficacy, play a pivotal role in pharmacology research.

Work settings

Many pharmacologists work in a laboratory research setting conducting experiments with various drugs. These experiments may be done in animal models of disease or at the biochemical level. Pharmacologists are employed by universities, commercial companies such as a pharmaceutical company, or by the government. University settings are often associated with medical centers and pharmacology research projects are largely funded by grants from outside resources. Many pharmacologists in academic settings study tightly focused areas in which they are interested. Academic labs are headed by a Ph.D. scientist who will lead a team of technicians and students. Academic pharmacology projects tend to focus on how different drugs work and why. Veterinary pharmacologists in university settings are usually found only at institutions that have schools of veterinary medicine.

Pharmaceutical company settings usually have a basic pharmacology research division, a clinical trials division, a production area, and a quality assurance team. A pharmaceutical company may hire a pharmacologist to discover new drugs or to study existing ones for adverse reactions. Pharmaceutical companies conduct very detailed clinical trials in order to have drugs approved by the FDA (U.S. Department of Health and Human Services Food and Drug Administration). Pharmaceutical companies spend a significant amount of money and employ many scientists in order to prove that a drug is safe and useful in treating a particular disease or condition. A pharmacologist may also be hired by a government agency such as the FDA to conduct research on drugs or to review drug approval applications. The FDA is also responsible for monitoring the safety of already approved drugs and therefore hires pharmacologists to monitor approved drugs as well as establish guidelines. All three settings, academic, commercial, and government, provide viable and exciting opportunities for a pharmacologist.

A typical workday for a pharmacologist depends on the subdiscipline the pharmacologist works in. A molecular pharmacologist may spend a significant portion of the day at the lab bench conducting experiments in test tubes. A behavioral pharmacologist may spend the day observing animals treated with certain drugs. A clinical pharmacologist is more likely to spend time evaluating data from patients taking certain medications. These workdays are typical of traditional research pharmacologists. Pharmacologists in less traditional careers may be involved in the business or legal side of science. In other words, pharmacologists are not limited to just experimental research in a laboratory setting.

Education and training

A college degree is required to become a pharmacologist. High school students should take biology, chemistry, and math classes. Several undergraduate institutions now offer a bachelor of science degree in pharmacology. College-level courses in biology, **biochemistry**, **anatomy**, and **physiology** are required. The field of pharmacology also requires knowledge of statistics and laboratory mathematics, and students should complete a statistics course. Undergraduate pharmacology majors should also take chemistry courses, including basic chemistry and organic chemistry. The undergraduate science courses should have a practical laboratory component to prepare students for careers in a laboratory research setting. Students should also pursue undergraduate research projects and look for internship opportunities at pharmaceutical or biotechnology

companies. Research associate positions in industry are available for pharmacology college majors, but experience in a laboratory research setting is a must for many of these job opportunities. Universities also hire lab technicians with a college-level pharmacology background.

Advanced education and training

Most pharmacologists have advanced degrees at the master's or doctoral level. Over 120 American and 10 Canadian universities offer graduate degree programs in pharmacology or **toxicology** as of 2012. Students pursuing a graduate degree should have a baccalaureate degree in biology, chemistry, or a related field. Ph.D. students take in depth courses in physiology and pharmacology. In addition, a major requirement for a Ph.D. is a dissertation research project that is conducted over several years. The Ph.D. student is required to publish novel findings in peer-reviewed scientific journals. After completing a Ph.D. in pharmacology, many graduates go on to postdoctoral research training. Postdoctoral training may take place in an academic or commercial setting. This training period has an indefinite time length. Many pharmacologists will then go on to become professors at universities or enter the commercial workforce as research scientists.

Future outlook

The field of pharmacology is experiencing rapid growth and prospects for pharmacologists continue to look good in 2012, according to *U.S. News*. The average salary for a pharmacologist is $81,000 as of 2012. The mapping of the human genome will provide new insights into designing better drugs and will create a need for more pharmacologists to make use of this new information. Many pharmaceutical companies are hiring pharmacologists for their drug discovery research projects.

According to the U.S. Department of Labor, the number of jobs for all medical scientists (which includes pharmacologists) is expected to increase by 36% between 2010 and 2020—a higher than average rate of job increase.

Resources

BOOKS

Acosta, W. Renée. *Pharmacology for Health Professionals*, 2nd ed. Philadelphia: Wolters Kluwer/Lippincott Williams and Wilkins Health, 2013.

Edmunds, Marilyn Winterton. *Introduction to Clinical Pharmacology*, 7th ed. St. Louis, MO: Elsevier/Mosby, 2013.

Moini, Jahangir. *Focus on Pharmacology: Essentials for Health Professionals*, 2nd ed. Boston, MA: Pearson Education, 2013.

PERIODICALS

Aronson, J.K. "What Do Clinical Pharmacologists Do? A Questionnaire Survey of Senior UK Clinical Pharmacologists." *British Journal of Clinical Pharmacology* 73 (February 2012): 161–169.

Carpenter, D., and D.A. Tobbell. "Bioequivalence: The Regulatory Career of a Pharmaceutical Concept." *Bulletin of the History of Medicine* 85 (Spring 2011): 93–131.

Doggrell, S.A. "Found in Translation: Integrated Approaches to Drug Development."

Mancuso, C., et al. "Pharmacologists and Alzheimer Disease Therapy: To Boldly Go Where No Scientist Has Gone Before." *Expert Opinion on Investigational Drugs* 20 (September 2011): 1243–1261.

Zhang, L., et al. "Fostering Culture and Optimizing Organizational Structure for Implementing Model-based Drug Development." *Journal of Clinical Pharmacology* 50 (September 2010): Suppl. 9: 146S–150S.

WEBSITES

American College of Clinical Pharmacology (ACCP). "Student Outreach." This is the ACCP's program for assisting the development of graduate and postdoctoral students. http://www.accp1.org/student_outreach.shtml (accessed May 16, 2012).

American Society for Pharmacology and Experimental Therapeutics (ASPET) Career Center. http://careers.aspet.org/ (accessed May 16, 2012).

U.S. Department of Labor (DOL) Occupational Outlook Handbook. "Medical Scientists." http://www.bls.gov/ooh/life-physical-and-social-science/medical-scientists.htm (accessed May 16, 2012).

U.S. News University Directory. "Pharmacology Majors See Growing Number of Job Opportunities." http://www.usnewsuniversitydirectory.com/articles/pharmacology-majors-see-growing-number-of-job-oppo_12190.aspx (posted February 15, 2012; accessed May 16, 2012).

ORGANIZATIONS

American College of Clinical Pharmacology (ACCP), 416 Hungerford Dr., Suite 300, Rockville, MD United States 20850, (240) 399-9070, Fax: (240) 399-9071, http://www.accp1.org/

American Society for Pharmacology and Experimental Therapeutics (ASPET), 9650 Rockville Pike, Bethesda, MD United States 20814-3995, (301) 634-7060, Fax: (301) 634-7061, http://www.aspet.org/

Food and Drug Administration (FDA), 10903 New Hampshire Avenue, Silver Spring, MD United States 20993, (888) INFO-FDA (463-6332), http://www.fda.gov/default.htm

Susan M. Mockus, Ph.D.
Rebecca J. Frey, Ph.D.

Pharmacy technician

Definition

Pharmacy technicians assist licensed pharmacists in preparing medications for patients.

Description

Pharmacy technicians, who may also be called pharmacy assistants or pharmacy aides, assist licensed pharmacists in preparing medication for patients. Depending on the work setting and the laws of the individual state, this may involve a number of different tasks.

The primary responsibility of most technicians is to fill orders or prescriptions under the direction and supervision of a pharmacist. The extent of this involvement is often subject to state law, which limits certain activities to performance by a licensed pharmacist. The following discussion will vary with the specific location.

When a medication order or prescription is received, it is reviewed by the pharmacist. This review assures that the order is properly written, and is for a safe and effective dose considering the patient's medical condition and the other drugs being taken. Once the order has been reviewed, the technician locates the medication, counts the required number of doses, prepares a label, and performs other required tasks such as pricing the prescription. This work is subject to review by the pharmacist, who is also responsible for giving the medication to the patient and for providing information about the proper way in which the medication should be taken.

Preparing medication for dispensing may take varying forms, depending on the work setting. In some hospitals, technicians, following written protocols, prepare injections. This requires familiarity with **infection control** procedures and specialized machinery. Extreme care in measuring and technical proficiency in the use of equipment are also required. Technicians may also prepare ointments, solutions, or fill capsules.

Technicians may be expected to do stock work. This may require taking inventories of drugs, checking inventories for expiration dates, preparing orders, and checking in deliveries.

Technicians may be responsible for maintaining patient medication profiles. These are records of a patient's prescriptions or drug orders, and are used by the pharmacist to review all the drugs a patient is taking. After the order has been reviewed, the technician may transcribe the information onto the profile, either by hand or using a computer. This task requires familiarity with drugs names and doses, as well as knowledge of common medical abbreviations and terminology. The technician must be extremely diligent and precise.

Technicians commonly prepare insurance claim forms. This requires the same familiarity with terminology as preparing medication profiles, plus familiarity with insurance claims procedures.

Technicians routinely clean and maintain equipment, including computers and dispensing machinery. Because the cleaning process prevents medication from becoming contaminated by other drugs, this task requires extreme thoroughness.

In some work locations, the technician may be expected to serve as a cashier. This requires knowledge of cash register operation and additional diligence.

Work settings

Pharmacy technicians work in a pharmacy. Seventy percent work in retail pharmacies, either independent stores or those that are part of chains. The stores may be drug stores or supermarkets that contain a pharmacy. Most other pharmacy technicians work in hospitals, although a small percentage may find employment with wholesale pharmacies, clinics, or in other settings.

Pharmacy technicians normally work as part of a team, under the direction of one licensed pharmacist, with another technician or other unlicensed person. Most states limit the ratio of technicians or other unlicensed personnel who can be supervised by a single pharmacist. The most common ratio is two unlicensed people to one pharmacist, but this may vary. Other possible team members include cashiers, pharmacy interns, graduates of a college of pharmacy who have not yet been licensed, and pharmacy aides, who may do some of the stock and inventory work but do not prepare medication orders.

Hours are variable, and may include evenings, nights, weekends, and holidays.

The physical work-load depends on circumstances, and may be very light, or may require heavy lifting.

Education and training

Training varies by state, with many states having no requirements for pharmacy technician training. California requires a formal 240-hour training program with at least 120 hours devoted to lecture, rather than on-the-job training, and a letter certifying completion of the program. Louisiana requires that all pharmacy technicians pass an examination given by the State, but does not specify how training is to be provided.

Some technical and community colleges offer courses leading to a career as a pharmacy technician, and in other places, labor unions have developed educational programs for their members. A typical program, such as the one described by the Indiana State Board of Pharmacy "includes **medical terminology** specific to the pharmacy, reading and interpreting prescriptions and defining drugs by brand name. Students receive a **pharmacology** overview and learn dosage calculations, I.V. flow rates, drug compounding and dose conversions. Dispensing of prescriptions, inventory control, billing and reimbursement also are covered."

A number of on-line programs and books are also available for technician training.

Although there are no formal education requirements, the Pharmacy Technician Certification Board (PTCB) administers a national certification examination. Admission to the certification examination requires a high school diploma or equivalent. Certification is not required for employment, but many employers prefer to hire certified technicians, and some states may require certification for employment in the future. Maintenance of certification requires participation in 10 hours each year of continuing education, at least one hour of which must be in the area of pharmacy law.

Advanced education and training

Pharmacy technicians may continue their studies and eventually become pharmacists.

Future outlook

There are currently an estimated 170,000 to 200,000 pharmacy technicians in the United States, of which about 50,000 are certified. Although it has been estimated that the growth of this occupation will be no greater than average for all occupations, the current and projected shortage of licensed pharmacists may lead to increased job opportunities for trained technicians. This shortage, combined with an **aging** population and increased used of drug therapy, has led to recommendations that the ratio of technicians to pharmacists be increased.

Resources

BOOKS

Occupational Outlook Handbook, 2011-2012 Ed. Washington, DC: Department of Labor, 2011.

The Pharmacy Technician. 4th ed. Morton Publishing Company, 2010.

ORGANIZATION

American Association of Pharmacy Technicians, P.O. Box 1447 Greensboro, NC 27402.

Samuel D. Uretsky, PharmD

Pharyngitis *see* **Sore throat**

Phenylketonuria testing *see* **Amino acid disorders screening**

Phimosis

Definition

A tightening of the foreskin of the penis that may close the opening of the penis.

Description

The foreskin of a newborn boy is always closely contracted around the penis head (glans). Only a small passage allows the urine to pass through. In the first months the foreskin is stuck to the glans and cannot be pulled back and one should not attempt to do so. During the first couple of years, the foreskin will become gradually looser and in many boys it can in time be pulled back without trouble. Half of all three-year-olds can pull back their foreskin. It is not advisable to try pulling the foreskin back using force, since this may cause small cuts in the foreskin with scars which could finally cause a regular foreskin contraction.

Foreskin contraction, called phimosis, can last throughout life and not cause any trouble at all. It is a voluntary decision whether to have a **circumcision** operation or not. If any problems do arise, they happen after **puberty**. The contraction may occur for the first time as an adult and usually requires circumcision, the surgical removal of the foreskin.

Causes & symptoms

Phimosis is caused by the inability of the foreskin to retract from around the opening of the penis. In adults, phimosis can lead to chronic inflammation and **cancer**.

Diagnosis

A physician usually diagnoses phimosis when there are persistent problems urinating, when there are recurrent infections under the foreskin, or when the opening to the penis is completely blocked by the foreskin. Phimosis is a tight ring of foreskin often made of scar tissue preventing retraction of the foreskin. It may be primary, or secondary to recurrent **infection**. It may produce urinary obstruction with ballooning of the foreskin. Phimosis is different than having a non-retractable foreskin, which is normal in many boys.

Treatment

If the foreskin cannot be pulled back into place treatment should be sought. If the **blood** flow to the penis is restricted then emergency treatment is required and if the foreskin cannot be pulled back a surgical cut to the trapped foreskin may be required. Failure to seek treatment can result in permanent damage to the penis. Once phimosis is diagnosed, the available treatments include topical **corticosteroids**, manual stretching, foreskin surgical repair or **plastic surgery**, and circumcision. Conservative treatments should be tried in the first instance and surgery used as the treatment of last resort.

KEY TERMS

Balanitis xerotica obliterans (BXO)—A chronic, progressive, hardening skin inflammation of the penis.

Buck's fascia—The deep connective tissue of the penis.

Circumcision—The removal of all or part of the foreskin from the penis.

Corticosteroids—A synthetic drug similar or identical to a natural corticosteroid, used to reduce inflammation.

Glans—The head of the penis.

Paraphimosis—The entrapment of a retracted foreskin behind the coronal sulcus, a groove that separates the shaft and head of the penis.

A number of studies show that phimosis can be safely and effectively treated by the application of topical steroids in 80–90% of cases. Betamethasone cream 0.05% should be applied to the exterior and interior of the tip of the foreskin two or three times a day. The treatment should be discontinued as ineffective after three months if the foreskin has not become retractile during this time.

A number of corrections are available for the adult or adolescent non-retractable foreskin. These include surgery to repair the foreskin, in which an incision is made through the constrictive band of the foreskin. The underlying tissue is spread with forceps to expose the Buck's fascia (the deep, connective tissue of the penis) and the incision is closed with absorbable sutures. This procedure has less risk of disease and infection than circumcision, and allows the foreskin to be retained.

Circumcision is very traumatic to a child. It is essentially irreversible and should be the treatment of last resort. Phimosis due to *balanitis xerotica obliterans* (BXO), a chronic, progressive, hardening skin inflammation of the penis, has been considered the one common absolute indication for circumcision.

Alternative treatment

There are no **alternative medicine** treatments for phimosis.

Prognosis

In most men, phimosis is not a serious problem and will not require treatment. However, it is not expected to improve on its own. With treatment, phimosis in most males can be managed or corrected.

Prevention

Proper hygiene is the most important preventative measure. The American Academy of **Pediatrics** recommends that the immature foreskin of boys not be forced back for cleaning. The only person who should clean and retract the foreskin is the boy himself. Bubble bath products and other chemical irritants can cause the foreskin to tighten and it is recommended they should be avoided by males with foreskins.

Resources

PERIODICALS

Berk, David R. "Paraphimosis in a Middle-Aged Adult After Intercourse."*American Family Physician*(February 15, 2004): 807.

GP Registrar: Pictorial-Case Study (Diagnosis of Phimosis). *GP* (February 11, 2005): 66.

OTHER

Circumcision Information and Resource Pages. Conservative Treatment of Phimosis: Alternatives to Radical Circumcision. http://www.cirp.org/library/treatment/ phimosis/.

ORGANIZATION

American Urological Association Foundation, 1000 Corporate Blvd., Linthicum, MD 21090, ((410)) 689-3700 Fax: ((410)) 689-3800, ((866)) 746-4282, auafoundation@auafoundation. org, http://www .urologyhealth.org/

Ken R. Wells

Phlebography

Definition

Phlebography is an x-ray test that provides an image of the leg veins after a contrast dye is injected into a vein in the patient's foot.

Purpose

Phlebography is primarily performed to diagnose deep vein thrombosis—a condition in which clots form in the veins of the leg that can lead to **pulmonary**

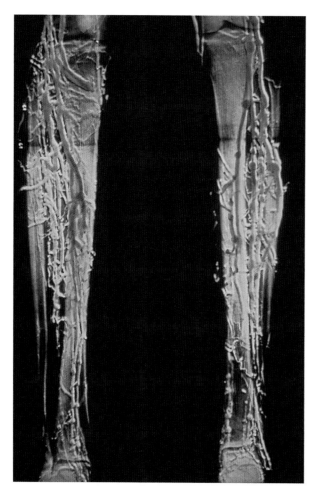

(Venography (varicose veins), photograph. © 1992 Science Photo Library/Custom Medical Stock Photo. Reproduced by permission.)

embolism in which those clots break off, travel to the **lungs** and pulmonary artery. Phlebography can also be used to distinguish **blood** clots from obstructions in the veins, to evaluate congenital vein problems, to assess the function of the deep leg vein valves, and to identify a vein for arterial bypass grafting. Ultrasound has replaced phlebography in many cases; but phlebography is the "gold standard" or the best test by which others are judged, but not used as a standard practice.

Precautions

Phlebography is usually not performed in patients with kidney (renal) problems.

Description

Phlebography, also called venography, ascending contrast phlebography, or contrast phlebography, is an invasive diagnostic test that provides a constant image of leg veins on a **fluoroscope** screen. Phlebography identifies the location, extent, and degree of attachment of blood clots, and enables the condition of the deep leg veins to be assessed. It is especially useful when there is a strong suspicion of **deep vein thrombosis**, after noninvasive tests have failed to identify the disease.

Phlebography is the most accurate test for detecting deep vein thrombosis. It is nearly 100% sensitive and specific in making this diagnosis (pulmonary **embolism** is diagnosed in other ways). Accuracy is crucial since deep vein thrombosis can lead to pulmonary embolism, a condition that can be fatal.

Phlebography is not used often, however, because it is painful, expensive, exposes the patient to a fairly high dose of radiation, and can cause complications. In about 5% of cases, there are technical problems in conducting the test. In addition, the test is less accurate in diagnosing problems below the knee.

Phlebography takes between 30 to 45 minutes and can be done in a physician's office, a laboratory, or a hospital. During the procedure, the patient lies on a tilting x-ray table. The area where the catheter will be inserted is sometimes shaved, if necessary, and cleaned. Sometimes a local anesthetic is injected to numb the skin at the site of the insertion. A small incision may be required to make a point for insertion. The catheter is inserted and the contrast solution (or dye) is slowly injected. Injection of the dye causes a warm, flushing feeling in the leg that may spread through the body. The contrast solution may also cause slight nausea. About 18% of patients experience discomfort from the contrast solution.

In order to fill the deep venous system with dye, a tight band (tourniquet) may be tied around the ankle or below the knee of the side into which the dye is injected, or the lower extremities may be tilted. The patient is asked to keep the leg still. The doctor also observes the movement of the solution through the vein with a fluoroscope. At the same time, a series of x rays is taken. When the test is finished, fluid is injected to clear the dye from the veins, the catheter is removed, and a bandage is applied over the site of the injection.

Preparation

Fasting or drinking only clear liquids is necessary for four hours before the test, although the test may be done in an emergency even if the patient has eaten. The contrast solution contains iodine, to which some people are allergic. Patients who have **allergies** or hay **fever**, or

KEY TERMS

Contrast solution—A liquid dye injected into the body that allows veins to be seen by x rays. Without the dye, the veins could not be seen on x rays.

Deep vein thrombosis—The development or presence of a blood clot in a vein deep within the leg. Deep vein thrombosis can lead to pulmonary embolism.

Invasive—A diagnostic test that invades healthy tissue; in the case of phlebography, through an incision in a healthy vein.

Pulmonary embolism—An obstruction of a blood vessel in the lungs, usually due to a blood clot that blocks a pulmonary artery. A pulmonary embolism can be very serious and in some cases is fatal.

have had a bad reaction to a contrast solution, should tell their doctor.

Aftercare

Patients should drink large amounts of fluids to flush the remaining contrast solution from their bodies. The area around the incision will be sore for a few days. If there is swelling, redness, **pain**, or fever, the doctor should be notified. Pain medication may be needed. In most cases, the patient can resume normal activities the next day.

Complications

Phlebography can cause complications such as phlebitis, tissue damage, and the formation of deep vein thrombosis in a healthy leg. A rare side effect in up to 8% of cases is a severe allergic reaction to the dye. This usually happens within 30 minutes after injection of the dye and requires medical attention.

Results

Normal phlebography results show proper blood flow through the leg veins.

Abnormal phlebography results show well-defined filling defects in veins. Findings include:

• blood clots

• consistent filling defects

• an abrupt end of a test dye column

• major deep veins that are unfilled

• dye flow that is diverted (These results confirm a diagnosis of deep vein thrombosis.)

Health care team roles

A phelbography is generally performed in a hospital, or in an outpatient or freestanding facility. A qualified x-ray lab technician, nurse, or doctor might perform the test, with a radiologist reading or interpreting the results that are presented to the patient either directly, or through the primary care physician. Because the patient will be asked to lie on the x-ray table and a vein is punctured in order for the test to be taken, an attending nurse or other medical assistant in addition to the person performing the test should be present to assist when necessary. A professional will be prepared to handle any possible complication, especially if a patient experiences an allergic reaction to the test medium.

Resources

BOOKS

DeBakey, Michael E., and Antonio M. Gotto, Jr. "Invasive Diagnostic Procedures." In *The New Living Heart.* Holbrook, MA: Adams Media Corporation, 1997, 78.

Phlebography. In *Mayo Clinic Practice of Cardiology,* 3rd ed. St. Louis, MO: Mosby, 1996, 1840-1841.

Texas Heart Institute. "Diseases of the Peripheral Arteries and Veins." In *Texas Heart Institute Heart Owner's Handbook.* New York: Wiley & Sons, 1996.

Venous Imaging. In *Diagnostic Nuclear Medicine,* 3rd ed., Vol. 1. Baltimore, MD: Williams & Wilkins, 1996, 586-587.

Lori De Milto
Stéphanie Islane Dionne

Phlebotomy

Definition

Phlebotomy is the act of drawing or removing **blood** from the circulatory system through a cut (incision) or puncture in order to obtain a sample for analysis and diagnosis. Phlebotomy is also done as part of the patient's treatment for certain blood disorders.

Purpose

Treatment

Phlebotomy that is part of treatment (therapeutic phlebotomy) is performed to treat polycythemia vera, a condition that causes an elevated red blood cell volume (**hematocrit**). Phlebotomy is also prescribed for patients with disorders that increase the amount of **iron** in their blood to dangerous levels, such as hemochromatosis, hepatitis B, and hepatitis C. Patients with pulmonary **edema** may undergo phlebotomy procedures to decrease their total blood volume.

Diagnosis

Phlebotomy is also used to remove blood from the body during blood donation and for analysis of the substances contained within it.

Precautions

Patients who are anemic or have a history of cardiovascular disease may not be good candidates for phlebotomy.

Description

Phlebotomy, which is also known as venesection, is performed by a nurse or a technician known as a phlebotomist. Blood is usually taken from a vein on the back of the hand or inside of the elbow. Some blood tests, however, may require blood from an artery. The skin over the area is wiped with an antiseptic, and an elastic band is tied around the arm. The band acts as a tourniquet, slowing the blood flow in the arm and making the veins more visible. The patient is asked to make a fist, and the technician feels the veins in order to select an appropriate one. When a vein is selected, the technician inserts a needle into the vein and releases the elastic band. The appropriate amount of blood is drawn and the needle is withdrawn from the vein. The patient's pulse and **blood pressure** may be monitored during the procedure.

For some tests requiring very small amounts of blood for analysis, the technician uses a finger stick. A lance, or small needle, makes a small cut in the surface of the fingertip, and a small amount of blood is collected in a narrow glass tube. The fingertip may be squeezed to get additional blood to surface.

The amount of blood drawn depends on the purpose of the phlebotomy. Blood donors usually contribute a unit of blood (500 mL) in a session. The volume of blood needed for laboratory analysis varies widely with the type of test being conducted.

Therapeutic phlebotomy removes a larger amount of blood than donation and blood analysis require. Phlebotomy for treatment of hemochromatosis typically involves removing a unit of blood–or 250 mg of iron– once a week. Phlebotomy sessions are required until iron levels return to a consistently normal level, which may take several months to several years. Phlebotomy for polycythemia vera removes enough blood to keep the patient's hematocrit below 45%. The frequency and duration of sessions depends on the patient's individual needs.

Preparation

Patients having their blood drawn for analysis may be asked to discontinue medications or to avoid food (to fast) for a period of time before the blood test. Patients donating blood will be asked for a brief medical history, have their blood pressure taken, and have their hematocrit checked with a finger stick test prior to donation.

Aftercare

After blood is drawn and the needle is removed, pressure is placed on the puncture site with a cotton ball to stop bleeding, and a bandage is applied. It is not uncommon for a patient to feel dizzy or nauseated during or after phlebotomy. The patient may be encouraged to rest for a short period once the procedure is completed. Patients are also instructed to drink plenty of fluids and eat regularly over the next 24 hours to replace lost blood volume. Patients who experience swelling of the puncture site or continued bleeding after phlebotomy should get medical help at once.

Risks

Most patients will have a small bruise or mild soreness at the puncture site for several days. Therapeutic phlebotomy may cause thrombocytosis and chronic iron deficiency (anemia) in some patients. As with any invasive procedure, **infection** is also a risk. This risk can be minimized by the use of prepackaged sterilized equipment and careful attention to proper technique.

Normal results

Normal results include obtaining the needed amount of blood with the minimum of discomfort to the patient.

Resources

BOOKS

McCall, Ruth E., and Cathee M. Tankersley. *Phlebotomy Essentials,* 5th edition. Lippincott Williams & Wilkins, 2011.
Strasinger, Susan, and Marjorie Di Lorenzo. *The Phlebotomy Textbook,* 3rd edition. F.A. Davis Company, 2011.

PERIODICALS

Kosiborod, Mikhail, and Adam C Salisbury. "Diagnostic blood sampling: how much is too much?" *Expert Review of Hematology* 5.1 (2012): 5.
Lipley, Nick. "Staff require training in phlebotomy to ensure accurate blood test results: researchers find that doctors use outdated equipment and follow the wrong procedures when taking samples." *Emergency Nurse* (November 2011): 9.
"Phlebotomy or bloodletting: from tradition to evidence-based medicine." *Transfusion* 52.3 (2012): 460.

Paula Anne Ford-Martin

Phonophoresis

Definition

Phonophoresis is a procedure that delivers drugs through the skin (transdermally) through the use of ultrasound. Phonophoresis is sometimes called sonophoresis.

Purpose

Ultrasound has been used to as a treatment for musculoskeletal disorders for almost 40 years. The application of low-frequency sound waves (ultrasound) to the skin increases the permeability of the skin and raises the temperature 7–9 °F(4–5 °C) up to 3 in (8 cm) below the skin surface within a localized area. In phonophoresis, drugs are applied to the skin before ultrasound treatment. The idea is that the ultrasound waves disrupt the lipid (fat) layer in the cell membrane of the skin cells on the surface of the body. These cells create the strongest barrier to drug penetration.

The theory behind phonophoresis is that ultrasound creates a channel in the cell membrane and drives the drug through the barrier and deeper into the tissue. Phonophoresis is used to treat **pain** caused by musculoskeletal disorders, mainly arthritis and **sports injuries**. Some insurance companies consider phonophoresis an investigational or alternative treatment and do not cover its cost.

Precautions

Phonophoresis is non-invasive and involves minimal risks. It should not be performed over areas where the skin is broken or over a fracture. Allergic reactions can also occur to drugs used during phonophoresis.

Description

The skin is cleaned and the medication is applied. The medication is usually in the form of a cream. Drugs used during phonophoresis are usually **nonsteroidal anti-inflammatory drugs** such as ibuprofen, steroid drugs, or local anesthetics.

The area to be treated is then exposed to either pulsed or continuous ultrasound. Pulsed treatments tend to be preferred for acute injuries and continuous treatment for chronic conditions. Treatment continues for five to eight minutes, after which the skin is cleaned again.

Preparation

No special preparation is needed before phonophoresis.

Aftercare

After washing the skin, no special aftercare is needed, No disability or delayed recovery is expected from this treatment.

Complications

No complications are expected with this procedure.

Results

Few large, well-designed, controlled studies of phonophoresis exist. The ones that do use a variety of different drugs and show mixed results. Some steroid drugs appear to penetrate the skin and move into deep tissue layers. However a controlled study of the nonsteroidal anti-inflammatory drug ibuprofen showed no greater improvement among individuals who received plain ultrasound and those who received phonophoresis (ultrasound plus the drug). The authors concluded that any improvement seen by patients in either treatment group was from the heating effects of the ultrasound rather than from penetration of the drug. Because there is no clear-cut benefit of phonophoresis over ultrasound treatment alone, many insurers will not pay for the procedure.

Health care team roles

Phonophoresis is almost always performed by a physical therapist or sports medicine technician in an outpatient setting.

Resources

PERIODICALS

Cagnie, Barbara et al. "Phonophoresis versus Topical Application of Ketoprofen: Comparison Between Tissue and Plasma Levels." *Physical Therapy.* 83 (August 2003): 707-713.

Koznoglu, Erkan, et al. "Short Term Efficacy of Ibuprofen Phonophoresis Versus Continuous Ultrasound Therapy in Knee Osteoarthritis." *Swiss Medical Weekly.* 2003:133:333-338.

Meidan, V.M. and B.B. Michniak. "Emerging Technologies in Transdermal Theraputics" *American Journal of Therapy.* 4 (July-August 2004): 312-316.

OTHER

"Phonophoresis of Topical Medications." Leigh University Department of Athletics. 2003. http://www.lehighsports.com/uploads/files/Phonophoresis.PDF

Tish Davidson, A.M.

Phosphorus

Description

Phosphorus (chemical symbol P) is a mineral discovered by the German alchemist Henig Brand in 1699. It plays an essential part in multiple biochemical reactions for both plants and animals and is essential to all life. Phosphorus is found in living things, in soil and rock, mostly as chemical compounds known as phosphates. Rock and soil phosphorus are mined extensively throughout the world, but especially in the Peoples' Republic of China and the United States.

Phosphorus extracted from rock is classified as either white, red, or black. White (also called yellow or common) phosphorus is a wax-like substance created by heating phosphate rock until it vaporizes and the condensation solidifies. One of this form's characteristics has given the English language the adjective phosphorescent, from white phosphorus's capacity to glow in the dark when exposed to air.

White phosphorus is highly toxic, causes **burns** if it comes in contact with skin, and is so combustible that it has to be stored underwater for safety. Red phosphorus is a rust-colored powder created by heating white phosphorus and exposing it to sunlight. It is not as combustible as the white form. Black phosphorus is made by heating white phosphorus under extremely high pressure until it resembles graphite.

In plants, phosphorus is necessary for photosynthesis to take place. In the human body, phosphorus works in tandem with another element, **calcium**, in much the same way that two other electrolyte components, sodium and potassium, do. Though phosphorus is found in every cell of the human body and accounts for 1% of the body's total weight, its primary function is working in conjunction with calcium to form teeth and bones.

Eighty-five percent of the phosphorus found in the body is located in these structures. In a delicately balanced chemical reaction, substances known as PTH (parathyroid hormone), calcitonin, and 25-dihydroxy **vitamin D** regulate the absorption of both calcium and phosphorus from the intestinal tract, thus making it available for the production of bones and teeth. If an excessive amount of phosphorus is absorbed, this will result in the phosphorus combining with all available calcium and preventing the calcium's efficient use in making and maintaining bones and teeth.

PTH balances the proportions of calcium and phosphorus in the body by increasing the release of calcium and phosphate from **bone** and the loss of phosphorus via the **kidneys** while limiting the excretion of calcium. PTH also increases the activity of the 25-dihydroxy vitamin D, which, in contrast, increases the absorption of both phosphorus and calcium from the intestinal tract.

General use

White phosphorus is a component of fertilizers, detergents and water softeners. It is also used in the manufacture of steel, plastics, insecticides, medical drugs, and animal feeds. Both white and red phosphorus are used in the making of safety matches and pesticides, including rat poison.

But the 15% of this element found in the **blood** stream and in other soft tissue also has a highly significant part to play in a variety of other body functions. Working with vitamin B, phosphorus is

KEY TERMS

Anorexia nervosa—A serious and sometimes fatal eating disorder characterized by intense fear of being fat and severe weight loss. It primarily affects teenage and young adult females. Sufferers have a distorted body image wherein they see themselves as being fat even when they are at normal weight or even emaciated.

Bulimia—An eating disorder characterized by bouts of gross overeating usually followed by self-induced vomiting.

Calcitonin—A hormone produced by the thyroid gland that controls the calcium level in the blood. It does this by slowing the rate that calcium is lost from bone.

Deciliter—A fluid measurement that is equal to one-tenth of a liter, or 100 cubic centimeters (27 fluid drams or teaspoonfuls).

Diabetic ketoacidosis—A potentially serious condition in which ketones become present in the blood stream because of the metabolism of fats burned in lieu of carbohydrates that would normally be used. This occurs because there is insufficient insulin available to cause carbohydrates to be used as fuel.

Electrolyte—Substances that split into ions, or electrically-charged particles, within the body to regulate many important bodily processes. Examples of electrolytes would be sodium, potassium, hydrogen, magnesium, calcium, bicarbonate, phosphates, and chlorides.

Multiple endocrine neoplasia—Tumor formation characterized by a progressive, abnormal multiplication of cells that are not necessarily malignant in any of the glands that secrete chemicals directly into the blood stream, such as the thyroid gland, adrenal glands, or ovaries.

Osteomalacia—Softening, weakening, and removal of the minerals from bone in adults caused by vitamin D deficiency.

Osteoporosis—Loss of formative protein tissue from bone, causing it to become brittle and easily fractured. It is considered to be a normal part of aging, but does have hormonal causes that make it much more common in women than men.

Sarcoidosis—A rare disease of currently unknown cause that occurs mostly in young adults. Inflammation occurs in the lymph nodes and other tissues throughout the body, usually including the lungs, liver, skin, and eyes.

involved in the **metabolism** of fats and **carbohydrates**, in both the repair of damaged cells and tissues and the routine maintenance of healthy ones. Phosphorus is necessary for the regularity of the heartbeat, and aids in the contraction of all other muscles throughout the body. Phosphorus is needed for the functioning of the kidneys and plays a part in the conduction of impulses along the network that makes up the nervous system.

Preparations

According to the American Dietetic Association, phosphorus intake in the United States is generally above what is needed, and in recent years has actually increased. Therefore, under normal circumstances with normal food intake, there is seldom if ever a need to supplement intake of phosphorus. Persons suffering from eating disorders such as anorexia and bulimia can be deficient in phosphorus intake, as well as other nutrients. As the best source of phosphorus is in protein foods such as meat, eggs, and milk products, some vegetarians may also need to evaluate their intake of this element. Excess

consumption of processed foods, and inadequate intake of whole foods, plus fertilizers and pesticides are some of the causes for excess phosphorus.

Beside high-protein foods, phosphorus is also found in decreasing quantities in whole grain breads and cereals, especially unprocessed ones, and in minute amounts in fruits and vegetables. The phosphorus present in whole grain breads and cereals, however, exists as a substance called phytin. Phytin combines with calcium to create a salt that the human body is incapable of absorbing, thus making unprocessed, unenriched grains a negligible source of phosphorus. But both commercially prepared cereals and breads may provide this element as they are frequently enriched with it. Phosphates can also be taken by mouth as a tablet.

Precautions

White phosphorus is poisonous. Red phosphorus is not. As noted, white phosphorus is a highly toxic, flammable substance capable of burning the skin if it makes contact, and of igniting at room temperature. It should be handled with extreme care. Accidental phosphorus **poisoning** can happen from both fertilizers and pesticides. Phosphates sometimes are leached into water systems through sewage and can drastically alter the chemical makeup of lakes and rivers. In sufficient quantities, they can lead to the death of nearly all forms of aquatic life.

A normal blood serum level of phosphorus is 2.4–4.1 mg per deciliter of blood. An abnormal serum phosphorus level should be evaluated by a physician.

Phosphorus levels higher than normal can indicate a diet that includes an excessive phosphorus intake, inadequate intake of calcium, or lack of PTH (parathyroid hormone) in the system. It can be related to bone metastasis associated with **cancer**, **liver** or kidney disease, or sarcoidosis.

Serum phosphorus levels that are below normal can be related to insufficient phosphorus or vitamin D in one's diet leading to rickets in children and osteomalacia in adults. Disorders of the parathyroid gland, causing it to secrete excessive quantities of PTH, or of the **pancreas**, causing it to secrete too much insulin, also affect blood levels of phosphorus. Diabetic ketoacidosis or too much calcium are other possible causes. Multiple endocrine neoplasia (MEN) is yet another condition that often is associated with lower than normal levels of phosphorus.

Side effects

Phosphorus preparations taken to supplement low phosphorus levels in the body can cause **diarrhea**.

Interactions

Antacids can decrease the absorption of phosphorus. **Laxatives** and enemas that contain the chemical compound sodium phosphate and excessive intake of vitamin D can increase phosphorus levels in the body. Administration of intravenous glucose solutions will cause phosphorus to combine with the glucose that is being absorbed by the cells.

Resources

BOOKS

Busch, Marianna A., Ph.D. *Phosphorus, World Book.* Chicago, IL: World Book, Inc., 1999.
Clayman, Charles B., M.D. *The American Medical Association Home Medical Encyclopedia.* New York: Random House, 1989.

OTHER

"Phosphorus in the Diet." http://www.Healthcentral.com. (June 2000).
"Serum Phosphorus." http://www.Healthcentral.com. (June 2000).

"Vitamin D." http://www.Healthcentral.com. (June 2000).

Joan Schonbeck

Photorefractive keratectomy *see* **Refractive eye surgeries**

Phototherapy
Definition

Phototherapy, or light therapy, is the administration of doses of bright light in order to treat a variety of disorders. It is most commonly used to re-regulate the body's internal clock and/or relieve depression.

Origins

Light, both natural and artificial, has been prescribed throughout the ages for healing purposes. Sunlight has been used medicinally since the time of the ancient Greeks; Hippocrates, the father of modern medicine, prescribed exposure to sunlight for a number of illnesses. In the late nineteenth and early twentieth centuries, bright light and fresh air were frequently prescribed for a number of mood and **stress** related disorders. In fact, prior to World War II, hospitals were regularly built with solariums, or sun rooms, in which patients could spend time recuperating in the sunlight.

In the 1980s, phototherapy began to make an appearance in the medical literature as a treatment for seasonal affective disorder, or SAD. Today, it is widely recognized as a front-line treatment for the disorder.

Benefits

Phototherapy is most often prescribed to treat seasonal affective disorder, a form of depression most often associated with shortened daylight hours in northern latitudes from the late fall to the early spring. It is also occasionally employed to treat sleep-related disorders such as insomnia and jet lag.

When used for SAD treatment, phototherapy has several advantages over prescription antidepressants. Phototherapy tends to work faster than medications, alleviating depressive symptoms within two to 14 days after beginning phototherapy as opposed to an average of four to six weeks with medication. And unlike antidepressants, which can cause a variety of side effects from nausea to concentration problems, phototherapy is extremely well tolerated. Some side effects are possible with light but are generally not serious enough to cause discontinuation of the therapy.

Description

Phototherapy is generally administered at home. The most commonly used phototherapy equipment is a portable lighting device known as a light box. The light box may be a full spectrum box, in which the lighting element contains all wavelengths of light found in natural light (including UV rays), or it may be a bright light box, in which the lighting element emits non-UV white light. The box may be mounted upright to a wall, or slanted downwards towards a table.

The patient sits in front of the box for a prescribed period of time (anywhere from 15 minutes to several hours). For patients just starting on the therapy, initial sessions are usually only 10–15 minutes in length. Some patients with SAD undergo phototherapy session two or three times a day, others only once. The time of day and number of times treatment is administered depends on the physical needs and lifestyle of the individual patient. If phototherapy has been prescribed for the treatment of SAD, it typically begins in the fall months as the days begin to shorten, and continues throughout the winter and possibly the early spring. Patients with a long-standing history of SAD are usually able to establish a time-table or pattern to their depressive symptoms, and can initiate treatment accordingly before symptoms begin.

The light from a slanted light box is designed to focus on the table it sits upon, so patients may look down to read or do other sedentary activities during therapy. Patients using an upright light box must face the light source, and should glance toward the light source occasionally without staring directly into the light. The light sources in these light boxes typically range from 2,500–10,000 lux (in contrast, average indoor lighting is 300–500 lux; a sunny summer day is about 100,000 lux).

Light boxes can be purchased for between $200 and $500. Some health care providers and health care supply companies also rent the fixtures. This gives a patient the opportunity to have a trial run of the therapy before making the investment in a light box. Recently, several new light box products have become available. Dawn simulators are lighting devices or fixtures that are programmed to gradually turn on, from dim to bright light, to simulate the sunrise. They are sometimes prescribed for individuals who have difficulty getting up in the morning due to SAD symptoms. Another device, known as a light visor, was designed to give an individual more mobility during treatment. The visor is a lighting apparatus that is worn like a sun visor around the crown of the head. Patients with any history of eye problems should consult their health care professional before attempting to use a light visor.

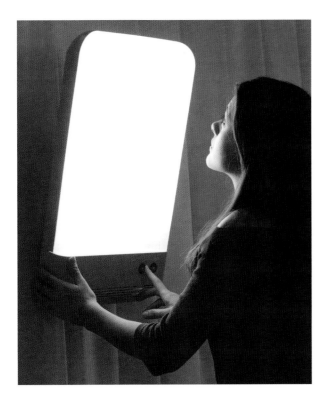

(Science & Society Picture Library/Getty Images)

There are several other different applications for phototherapy, including:

- Full-spectrum/UV phototherapy for disorders of the skin. A subtype of phototherapy that is often prescribed to treat skin diseases, rashes, and jaundice.

- Cold laser therapy. The treatment involves focusing very low-intensity beams of laser light on the skin, and is used in laser acupuncture to treat a myriad of symptoms and illnesses, including pain, stress, and tendinitis.

- Colored phototherapy. In colored phototherapy, different colored filters are applied over a light source to achieve specific therapeutic effects. The colored light is then focused on the patient, either with a floodlight which covers the patient with the colored light, or with a beam of light that is focused on the area of the illness.

- Back of knee phototherapy. A 1998 report published in the journal *Science* reported that the area behind the human knee known as the popliteal region contains photoreceptors which can help adjust the body's circadian rhythms. The authors of the study found that they could manipulate circadian rhythms by focusing a bright light on the popliteal region. Further studies are needed to determine the efficacy of this treatment on disorders such as SAD and jet lag.

KEY TERMS

Neurotransmitter—A chemical in the brain that transmits messages between neurons, or nerve cells.

Seasonal affective disorder—SAD is a mood disorder characterized by depression during the winter months. An estimated 4–6% of the U.S. population suffers from SAD.

Preparations

Full-spectrum light boxes do emit UV rays, so patients with sun-sensitive skin should apply a sun screen before sitting in front of the box for an extended period of time.

Precautions

Patients with eye problems should see an opthamologist regularly both before and during phototherapy. Because UV rays are emitted by the light box, patients taking photosensitizing medications should consult with their health care provider before beginning treatment. In addition, patients with medical conditions that make them sensitive to UV rays should also be seen by a health care professional before starting phototherapy.

Patients beginning phototherapy for SAD may need to adjust the length, frequency, and timing of their phototherapy sessions in order to achieve the maximum benefits. Patients should keep their health care provider informed of their progress and the status of their depressive symptoms. Occasionally, additional treatment measures for depression (i.e., antidepressants, herbal remedies, **psychotherapy**) may be recommended as an adjunct, or companion treatment, to phototherapy.

Side effects

Some patients undergoing phototherapy treatments report side effects of eyestrain, headaches, insomnia, fatigue, sunburn, and dry eyes and nose. Most of these effects can be managed by adjusting the timing and duration of the phototherapy sessions. A strong sun block and eye and nose drops can alleviate the others. Long-term studies have shown no negative effects to eye function of individuals undergoing phototherapy treatment.

A small percentage of phototherapy patients may experience hypomania, a feeling of exaggerated, hyper-elevated mood. Again, adjusting the length and frequency of treatment sessions can usually manage this side effect.

Research and general acceptance

Phototherapy is widely accepted by both traditional and **complementary medicine** as an effective treatment for SAD. The exact mechanisms by which the treatment works are not known, but the bright light employed in phototherapy may act to readjust the body's circadian rhythms, or internal clock. Other popular theories are that light triggers the production of serotonin, a neurotransmitter believed to be related to **depressive disorders**, or that it influences the body's production of melatonin, a hormone that may be related to circadian rhythms.

Wide spectrum UV light treatment for skin disorders such as **psoriasis** is also considered a standard treatment option in clinical practice. However, other light-related treatments such as cold laser therapy and colored phototherapy are not generally accepted, since few or no scientific studies exist on the techniques.

Training and certification

Psychiatrists, psychologists, and other mental health care professional prescribe phototherapy treatment for SAD. Holistic health care professionals and light therapists who specialize in this treatment are also available; in some states, these professionals require a license, so individuals should check with their state board of health to ensure their practitioner has the proper credentials. Phototherapy for skin disorders should be prescribed by a dermatologist or other health care professional with expertise in skin diseases and phototherapy treatment.

Resources

BOOKS

Diagnostic and Statistical Manual of Mental Disorders Revised IV. Washington, DC: American Psychiatric Press, 2000.

Lam, Raymond, ed. *Seasonal Affective Disorder and Beyond: Light Treatment for SAD and non-SAD conditions.* Washington, DC: American Psychiatric Press, 1998.

Rosenthal, Norman. *Winter Blues: Seasonal Affective Disorder—What it is and how to overcome it.* New York: Guilford Press, 1998.

PERIODICAL

Jepson, Tracy, et al. "Current Perspectives on the Management of Seasonal Affective Disorder." *Journal of the American Pharmaceutical Association* 39, no. 6 (1999): 822–829.

ORGANIZATIONS

National Depressive and Manic Depressive Association. 730 Franklin Street, Suite 501, Chicago, IL 60610. (800) 826–3632. http://www.ndmda.org.

Society for Light Treatment and Biological Rhythms. 824 Howard Ave., New Haven, CT 06519. Fax (203) 764–4324. http://www.sltbr.org. sltbr@yale.edu.

Paula Ford-Martin

Physical development in children *see*
Human growth and development

Physical examination

Definition

A physical examination is the evaluation of a body to determine its state of health. The techniques of inspection, palpation (feeling with the hands), percussion (tapping with the fingers), auscultation (listening), and **smell** are used. A complete health assessment also includes gathering information about a person's medical history and lifestyle, conducting laboratory tests, and screening for disease. These elements constitute the data on which a diagnosis is made and a plan of treatment is developed.

Purpose

The term annual physical examination has been replaced in most health care circles by periodic health examination. The frequency with which it is conducted depends on factors such as the age, gender, and the presence of risk factors for disease in the person being examined. Health care professionals often use guidelines that have been developed by organizations such as the United States Preventative Services Task Force. Organizations such as the American Cancer Society or American **Heart** Association, which promote detection and prevention of specific diseases, generally recommend more intensive or frequent examinations or that examinations be focused on particular organ systems of the body.

Comprehensive physical examinations provide opportunities for health care professionals to obtain baseline information about individuals that may be useful in the future. They also allow health care providers to establish relationships before problems occur. Physical examinations are appropriate times to answer questions and teach good health practices. Detecting and addressing problems in their early stages can have beneficial long-term results.

Precautions

The individual being examined should be comfortable and treated with respect throughout the examination. As the examination continues, the examiner should explain what they are doing and share any relevant findings. Using language appropriate to the person being examined improves the effectiveness of communications and ultimately fosters better relations between examiners and examinees.

Description

A complete physical examination usually starts at the head and proceeds all the way to the toes. However,

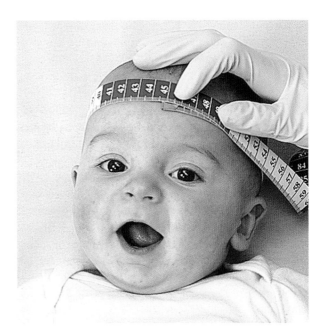

(Gloved hand measuring infant's head circumference, baby looking directly at camera, close-up, photograph. From Delmar's Nursing Image Library 1st Edition by DELMAR. © 2001. Reprinted with permission of Delmar Learning, a division of Thomson Learning: wwww.thomsonrights.com. Fax 800-730-2215.)

the exact procedure will vary according to the needs of the person being examined and the preferences of the examiner. An average examination takes about 30 minutes. The cost of an examination will depend on the charge for the professional's time and any tests that are included. Most health plans cover routine physical examinations including some tests.

The examination

Before examiners even speak, they will observe a person's overall appearance, general health, and behavior. Measurements of height and weight are made. **Vital signs** such as pulse, breathing rate, body temperature, and **blood pressure** are recorded.

With the person being examined in a sitting position, the following systems are reviewed:

- Skin. The exposed areas of the skin are observed. The size and shape of any lesions are noted.

- Head. The hair, scalp, skull, and face are examined.

- Eyes. The external structures are observed. The internal structures can be observed using an ophthalmoscope (a lighted instrument) in a darkened room.

- Ears. The external structures are inspected. A lighted instrument called an otoscope may be used to inspect internal structures.

- Nose and sinuses. The external nose is examined. The nasal mucosa and internal structures can be observed with the use of a penlight and a nasal speculum.
- Mouth and pharynx. The lips, gums, teeth, roof of the mouth, tongue, and pharynx are inspected.
- Neck. The lymph nodes on both sides of the neck and the thyroid gland are palpated (examined by feeling with the fingers).
- >Back. The spine and muscles of the back are palpated and checked for tenderness. The upper back, where the lungs are located, is palpated on the right and left sides and a stethoscope is used to listen for breath sounds.
- Breasts and armpits. A woman's breasts are inspected with the arms relaxed and then raised. In both men and women, the lymph nodes in the armpits are felt with the examiner's hands. While the person is still sitting, movement of the joints in the hands, arms, shoulders, neck, and jaw can be checked.

While the person is lying down on the examining table, the examination includes:

- Breasts. The breasts are palpated and inspected for masses.
- Front of chest and lungs. The area is inspected with the fingers, using palpation and percussion. A stethoscope is used to listen to internal breath sounds.

The head should be slightly raised for:

- Heart. A stethoscope is used to listen to the heart's rate and rhythm. The blood vessels in the neck are observed and palpated.

The person being examined should lie flat for:

- Abdomen. Light and deep palpation is used on the abdomen to feel the outlines of internal organs including the liver, spleen, kidneys, and aorta, a large blood vessel.
- Rectum and anus. With the person lying on the left side, the outside areas are observed. An internal digital examination (using a gloved finger), is usually done for persons over 40 years old. In men, the prostate gland is also palpated.
- Reproductive organs. The external sex organs are inspected and the area is examined for hernias. In men, the scrotum and testicles are palpated. In women, a pelvic examination is completed using a speculum and a Papanicolaou test (Pap test) may be taken.
- Legs. While lying flat, the legs are inspected for swelling, and pulses in the knee, thigh, and foot area are found. The groin area is palpated for the presence of lymph nodes. The joints and muscles are observed.
- Musculoskeletal system. With the person standing, the straightness of the spine and the alignment of the legs and feet is noted.

- Blood vessels. The presence of any abnormally enlarged veins (varicose), usually in the legs, is noted.

In addition to evaluating a person's alertness and mental ability during the initial conversation, additional inspection of the nervous system may be conducted:

- Neurologic screen. The person's ability to take a few steps, hop, and do deep knee bends is observed. The strength of the hand grip is felt. While sitting in an upright position, the reflexes in the knees and feet can be tested with a small hammer. The sense of touch in the hands and feet can be evaluated by testing reaction to pain and vibration.
- Sometimes additional time is spent examining the 12 nerves in the head (cranial) that are connected directly to the brain. They control the senses of smell and taste, strength of muscles in the head, reflexes in the eye, facial movements, gag reflex, vision, hearing, and muscles in the jaw. General muscle tone and coordination, and the reaction of the abdominal area to stimulants like pain, temperature, and touch may also be evaluated.

Preparation

Before visiting a health care professional, individuals should write down important facts and dates about their own medical history, as well as those of family members. There should be a complete listing of all medications and their dosages. This list should include over-the-counter preparations, **vitamins**, and herbal supplements. Some people bring their bottles of medications with them. Any questions or concerns about medications should be written down.

Before the physical examination begins, the bladder should be emptied. A urine specimen is usually collected in a small container at this time. The urine is tested for the presence of glucose (sugar), protein, and **blood** cells. For some blood tests, individuals may be told ahead of time not to eat or drink after midnight.

Individuals being examined usually remove all clothing and put on a loose-fitting hospital gown. An additional sheet is provided to keep persons covered and comfortable during the examination.

Aftercare

Once a physical examination has been completed, the person being examined and the examiner should review what laboratory tests have been ordered, why they have been selected, and how the results will be shared with the patient. A health professional should discuss any recommendations for treatment and follow-up visits. Special instructions should be put in writing. This is also an opportunity for persons to ask any remaining questions about their own health concerns.

KEY TERMS

Auscultation—The process of listening to sounds that are produced in the body. Direct auscultation uses the ear alone, such as when listening to the grating of a moving joint. Indirect auscultation involves the use of a stethoscope to amplify sounds from within the body, such as those coming from the heart or intestines.

Hernia—The bulging of an organ, or part of an organ, through the tissues normally containing it; also called a rupture.

Inspection—The visual examination of the body using the eyes and a lighted instrument if needed. The sense of smell may also be used.

Ophthalmoscope—Lighted device for studying the interior of the eyeball.

Otoscope—An instrument with a light for examining the internal ear.

Palpation—The examination of the body using the sense of touch. There are two types: light and deep.

Percussion—An assessment method in which the surface of the body is struck with the fingertips to obtain sounds that can be heard or vibrations that can be felt. It can determine the position, size, and consistency of an internal organ. It is performed over the chest to determine the presence of normal air content in the lungs, and over the abdomen to evaluate air in the loops of the intestine.

Reflex—An automatic response to a stimulus.

Speculum—An instrument for enlarging the opening of any canal or cavity in order to facilitate inspection of its interior.

Stethoscope—A Y-shaped instrument that amplifies body sounds such as heartbeat, breathing, and air in the intestine. Used in auscultation.

Varicose veins—The permanent enlargement and twisting of veins, usually in the legs. They are most often seen in people working in occupations requiring long periods of standing, and in pregnant women.

Complications

Complications with the process of a physical examination are unusual. Occasionally, a useful piece of information or data may be overlooked. More commonly, results of associated laboratory tests compel physicians to recheck an individual of to re-examine portions of the body already reviewed. In a sense, complications may arise from the findings of a physical examination. These usually trigger further investigations or initiate treatment. They are really more beneficial than negative as they often begin a process of treatment and recovery.

Results

Normal results of a physical examination correspond to the healthy appearance and normal functioning of the body. For example, appropriate **reflexes** will be present, no suspicious lumps or lesions will be found, and vital signs will be normal.

Abnormal results of a physical examination include any findings that indicate the presence of a disorder, disease, or underlying condition. For example, the presence of lumps or lesions, **fever**, muscle **weakness** or lack of tone, poor reflex response, heart arhythmia, or swelling of lymph nodes will indicate possible health problems.

Health care team roles

When considering a physical examination, the leader of a health care team is usually an examining physician, although **advanced practice nurses** and physician assistants also perform the procedures. This individual has the responsibility for coordinating and interpreting the results of any needed laboratory tests and managing any post-examination activities or treatment. A physician assistant may perform some components of a routine physical examination. A nurse may assist in aspects of many examinations. Laboratory technicians collect and analyze bodily samples such as blood, urine, sputum, and tissue. They supply data to an examining physician for analysis and interpretation.

Resources

BOOKS

Bickley, Lynn S., Robert A. Hoekelman, and Barbara Bates. *Bates' Guide to Physical Examination and History Taking.* Philadelphia, PA: Lippincott, 1999.

DeGowin, Robert L., and Donald D. DeGowin. *DeGowin's Diagnostic Examination, 7th ed.* New York, NY, McGraw Hill, 1999.

Seidel, Henry M. *Mosby's Guide to Physical Examination, 4th ed.* St. Louis, MO. Mosby-Year Book, 1999.

Shwartz, Mark A., and William Schmitt. *Textbook of Physical Diagnosis: History and Examination, 3rd ed.* Philadelphia, PA. Saunders, 1998.

OTHER

Karolinska Institute. http://isp.his.ki.se/text/physical.htm.

Loyola University Chicago Stritch School of Medicine. http://www.meddean.luc.edu/lumen/MedEd/MEDICINE/PULMONAR/PD/Pdmenu.htm.

University of Maryland Medical System. http://umm.drkoop.com/conditions/ency/article/002274.htm.

L. Fleming Fallon, Jr., MD, PhD, DrPH

Physical restraint use *see* **Restraint use**

Physical therapy

Definition

Physical therapists provide services to restore function, improve mobility, relieve **pain**, and prevent or limit permanent physical disabilities among those suffering from injuries, disabilities, or disease.

Description

Organized physical therapy began during World War I with 800 reconstruction aides. Today there are more than 80,000 licensed physical therapists in the United States.

Physical therapists treat patients with a variety of health conditions and diseases including accident victims and individuals with disabling conditions such as low **back pain**, arthritis, **heart** disease, **fractures**, head injuries, and **cerebral palsy**.

In an effort to restore, maintain, and promote overall fitness and health, physical therapists examine patients' medical histories, as well as test and measure patients' strength, range of motion, balance, coordination, posture, muscle performance, respiration, and motor function. Physical therapists determine patients' ability to be independent and reintegrate into the community or workplace. Based on a patient's medical history and test results, physical therapists develop treatment plans that describe treatment strategy, purpose, and anticipated outcome.

A physical therapist's treatment often includes **exercise** for patients who have been immobilized or who lack flexibility, strength, or endurance. As part of the treatment, physical therapists encourage patients to improve flexibility, range of motion, strength, balance, coordination, and endurance. The goal is to improve an individual's function at work and home.

Physical therapists may use electrical stimulation, hot packs, cold compresses, or ultrasound to relieve pain and reduce swelling. They may use traction or deep-tissue massage to relieve pain. Therapists also teach patients to use assistive and adaptive devices including **crutches**, prostheses, and wheelchairs. They may also show patients how to perform exercises to do at home.

During treatment, physical therapists document the patient's progress, conduct periodic examinations, and modify treatments when necessary. Physical therapists rely on this documentation to track the patient's progress and identify areas requiring more or less attention.

Physical therapists often consult and practice with physicians, dentists, nurses, educators, social workers, occupational therapists, speech-language pathologists, and audiologists.

Some physical therapists treat a wide range of ailments while others specialize in areas such as **pediatrics**, geriatrics, **orthopedics**, sports medicine, **neurology**, and cardiopulmonary physical therapy.

Physical therapist assistants and aides

Physical therapist assistants, under the direction and supervision of a physical therapist, may be involved in implementing patient treatment plans. For example, physical therapist assistants perform treatment procedures including exercises, massages, electrical stimulation, paraffin baths, hot and cold packs, traction, and ultrasound. Physical therapist assistants record patients' treatment responses and report these responses to the physical therapist.

Physical therapist aides work under the direct supervision of a physical therapist or a physical therapist assistant. Aides help make therapy sessions productive and are often responsible for keeping the treatment area clean and organized, preparing for each patient's therapy, and assisting patients who need help in moving to or from a treatment area. Because they are not licensed, aides are only able to perform a limited range of tasks.

Physical therapist aides' duties include clerical tasks such as ordering supplies, answering the phone, filling out insurance forms, and other paperwork. The extent of an assistant's or an aide's clerical responsibilities depend on the size and location of the facility.

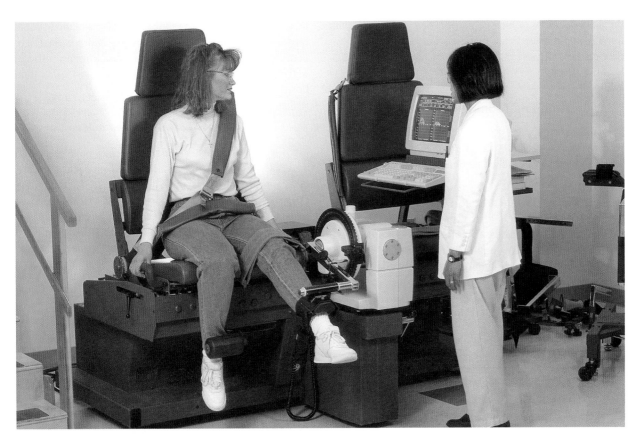

(Patient on physical therapy machine, photograph. UPI/Corbis Bettmann. Reproduced by permission.)

Work settings

Physical therapists practice in hospitals, clinics, and private offices. They may also treat patients in the patient's home or at school.

Most physical therapists work a 40-hour week, which may include some evenings and weekends depending on their patients' schedules. The job can be physically demanding, because therapists often have to stoop, kneel, crouch, lift, or stand for long periods of time. In addition, physical therapists move heavy equipment, lift patients, or help them turn, stand, or walk.

In 1998, approximately 75% of the physical therapists employed in approximately 120,000 jobs worked full time. Approximately 10% of physical therapists held more than one job.

Over two-thirds of physical therapists are employed in either hospitals or physical therapists' offices. Other work settings include home health agencies, outpatient **rehabilitation** centers, physicians' offices and clinics, and **nursing homes**. Some physical therapists maintain a private practice and provide services to individual patients or contract to provide services in hospitals, rehabilitation centers, nursing homes, home health agencies, adult daycare programs, or schools. They may be engaged in individual practice or be part of a consulting group. Some physical therapists teach in academic institutions and conduct research.

Physical therapist assistants and aides

Physical therapist assistants and aides work varying schedules, depending on the facility and whether they are full or part-time employees. To accommodate patients' schedules, many outpatient physical therapy offices and clinics remain open during evenings and weekends.

Physical therapist assistants and aides are required to have a moderate degree of strength due to the physical exertion needed in assisting patients with their treatment. In some cases, for example, assistants and aides help lift patients. In addition, these jobs typically require a good deal of kneeling, stooping, and standing for long periods.

Physical therapist assistants and aides held 82,000 jobs in 1998. Although they work alongside physical therapists in a variety of settings, over two-thirds of all assistants and aides work in hospitals or physical therapists' offices. Other assistants and aides work in nursing and personal care facilities, outpatient rehabilitation centers, physicians' offices and clinics, and home health agencies.

Education and training

Before they can practice, physical therapists are required to pass a licensure exam after graduating from an accredited physical therapist educational program.

According to the American Physical Therapy Association, in 1999 there were 189 accredited physical therapist programs. Of the accredited programs, 24 offered bachelor's degrees, 157 offered master's degrees, and eight offered doctoral degrees. By 2002, the Commission on Accreditation in Physical Therapy Education will require all physical therapist programs seeking accreditation to offer degrees at the post-baccalaureate level.

Physical therapist programs start with basic science courses such as biology, chemistry, and physics, followed by specialized courses such as **biomechanics**, neuroanatomy, **human growth and development**, manifestations of disease, examination techniques, and therapeutic procedures. Besides classroom and laboratory instruction, students receive supervised clinical experience.

Admission to physical therapist education programs is very competitive. Interested students may improve their admission potential by attaining superior grades, especially in science courses. Interested students should take courses such as **anatomy**, biology, chemistry, social science, mathematics, and physics. Before granting admission, many programs require that the student at least have experience as a volunteer in a hospital or clinic physical therapy department.

Physical therapists need strong interpersonal skills to successfully educate patients about their physical therapy treatments and to interact with the patient's family. Therapists should also be compassionate and posses a desire to help patients.

Physical therapists are expected to remain current in their professional development by participating in continuing education courses and workshops. A number of states require continuing education to maintain licensure.

In 1998, physical therapists earned a median annual income of $56,600. The lowest 10% earned less than $35,700 while the highest 10% earned in excess of $90,870 a year. Those in the middle 50% earned between $44,460 and $77,810 a year. In 1997, physical therapists' median annual earnings in the industries employing the largest number of physical therapists included home health care services, $65,600; nursing and personal care facilities, $60,400; health care practitioner offices, $56,600; physicians' offices and clinics, $55,100; and hospitals, $50,100.

Physical therapist assistants and aides

Physical therapist assistants typically have earned an associate's degree from an accredited physical therapist assistant program. As of January 1997, 44 states and Puerto Rico regulated assistants. Physical therapist assistants are also required to have certifications in **CPR** and other **first aid**, along with a specified minimum number of hours of clinical experience. Physical therapist aides are also trained on the job.

In 1999, according to the American Physical Therapy Association, there were 274 accredited physical therapist assistant programs in the United States. Accredited physical therapist assistant programs are designed to last two years or four semesters. Those who successfully complete the program are awarded an associate's degree. Admission into physical therapist assistant programs is competitive. Programs are divided into academic study and hands-on clinical experience. Academic coursework includes algebra, anatomy, **physiology**, biology, chemistry, and psychology. Before students begin their clinical field experience, many programs require that they complete a semester of anatomy and physiology and have certifications in CPR and other first aid. Employers and educators view clinical experience as essential to ensuring that students understand the responsibilities of a physical therapist assistant.

Employers typically require physical therapist aides to have a high school diploma, strong interpersonal skills, and a desire to assist people in need. Most employers provide clinical on-the-job training.

Future outlook

Employment for physical therapists is expected to grow by 21–35% through 2008. For a variety of reasons, the demand for physical therapists should continue to rise. As the baby boom generation ages, the number of individuals with disabilities requiring therapy services should increase, as well as patients who will require cardiac and physical rehabilitation after a heart attack or **stroke**. In addition, the need for physical therapy will be increased as technological advances save the lives of a larger number of newborns with severe **birth defects**.

Future medical developments will also increase trauma victims' survival rate, thereby creating additional demand for rehabilitative care. Growth may also result from advances in medical technology which permit treatment of more disabling conditions.

Widespread interest in health promotion may also increase demand for physical therapy services. A growing number of employers are seeking the services of physical therapists to evaluate worksites, develop exercise programs, and teach safe work habits to employees in the hope of reducing injuries.

Physical therapist assistants and aides

Employment for physical therapist assistants and aides is expected to increase by at least 36% through the year 2008. As with the future outlook for physical therapists, the demand for physical therapist assistants and aides will continue to rise to keep pace with the increase in the number of individuals with disabilities and the rapidly growing elderly population, many of whom are particularly vulnerable to chronic and debilitating conditions that require therapeutic services. These patients often need additional assistance in their treatment, making the roles of assistants and aides vital. As the large baby-boom generation reaches the prime age for heart attacks and strokes, the demand for cardiac and physical rehabilitation will also increase. In addition, future medical developments should permit an increased percentage of trauma victims to survive, creating an additional demand for therapy services.

In 1998, physical therapist assistants and aides earned a median annual income of $21,870. The lowest 10% earned less than $13,760 while the highest 10% earned more than $39,730 a year. The middle 50% earned between $16,700 and $31,260 a year. In 1997, the median annual income earned by physical therapist assistants and aides working in the industries employing the largest number of physical therapist assistants and aides included hospitals, $21,200; health care practitioners offices, $20,700; and nursing and personal care facilities, $19,200.

Resources

BOOKS

American Physical Therapy Association. *Guide to Physical Therapist Practice, 2nd Edition.* American Physical Therapy Association, 2001.

Carr, Janet and Shepherd, Roberta. *Movement Science: Foundations for Physical Therapy in Rehabilitation, 2nd Edition.* Aspen Publishers, Inc., 2000.

Krumshansl, Bernice. *Opportunities in Physical Therapy Careers.* VGM Career Horizons, 1999.

U.S. Department of Labor. *Occupational Outlook Handbook 2000-2001 Edition.* Bureau of Labor Statistics.

ORGANIZATION

The American Physical Therapy Association, 1111 North Fairfax Street, Alexandria, VA 22314-1488. http://www.apta.org.

Bill Asenjo, MS, CRC

Physical therapy assisting

Definition

Physical therapy assistants are skilled health care providers who work under the direction or supervision of one or more physical therapists. Their role is to facilitate care and treatment of patients with injuries, diseases, or disabilities that involve mobility or other basic physical functioning. Duties include patient instruction and monitoring, reporting progress and problems to the therapist, and providing or assisting in various forms of treatment.

Description

Physical therapy assisting is an adjunct to the profession of physical therapy and comprises workers with at least a two-year education and clinical experience. Physical therapist assistants (PTAs) are in the role of supporting the physical therapist by providing different types of patient treatment and education, and tracking patient progress. Some kinds of treatment PTAs can provide or assist with include massage, heat and cold therapy, traction, ultrasound, electrical stimulation, and helping patients learn and perform various therapeutic exercises. PTAs may also work with patients who need to learn to use corrective equipment, such as braces or prostheses, wheelchairs or **crutches**, or other supportive devices. Other PTA responsibilities include organization and maintenance of treatment areas and equipment, and occasional performance of clerical tasks.

Patients with whom PTAs work may include children, the elderly, athletes, accident victims, and those with diseases like low **back pain**, arthritis, **cerebral palsy**, as well as people who have sustained **fractures** and head injuries. PTAs also assist people who need help managing **pain** and restoring, acquiring, or maintaining mobility and other functions. Coworkers may include physical therapists, other health care and **rehabilitation** professionals. Physical therapy aides also work with PTAs; aides perform a more limited range of functions, albeit similar, along with clerical, maintenance, and

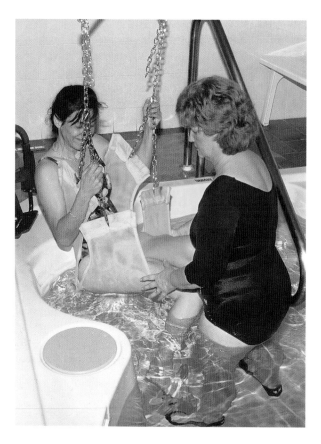

(Paraplegic patient, being assisted by physical therapist into pool, photograph. Custom Medical Stock Photo, Inc. Reproduced by permission.)

Advanced education and training

Some PTAs may choose to complement their education by obtaining a baccalaureate degree in a related health field (APTA). The PTA curriculum does not meet the prerequisites for a physical therapy degree. PTAs, therefore, cannot directly advance to the status of physical therapist through supplementary education. There are programs, however, that help PTAs earn a master's degree in physical therapy while remaining employed as PTAs. PTAs who would like to participate in the clinical education of PTA students can also earn a Clinical Instructor Credentialing Certificate from the APTA.

Future outlook

According to the *Occupational Outlook Handbook (OOH)*, employment opportunities for PTAs (and physical therapy aides) are expected to grow faster than average through 2008, with the majority of the growth in the latter part of the period. Some of the reasons for expected growth are an increasing elderly population, the **aging** of the baby boom generation, and increased survival potential of trauma victims. In California, for example, physical therapy assistants and aides are in the Top Fifty Fastest Growth Occupations, as noted by California's Employment Development Department.

Resources

BOOK

U.S. Department of Labor. "Physical Therapist Assistants and Aides." In *Occupational Outlook Handbook (OOH).* Washington, D.C.

ORGANIZATIONS

American Physical Therapy Association (APTA). 1111 North Fairfax Street. Alexandria, VA 22314. (703) 684-2782. (800) 999-2782. www.apta.org.

State of California, Employment Development Department. Labor Market Information Division. Information Services Group. (916) 262-2162.

Diane Fanucchi, B.A., C.M.T.

other supportive duties. Aides usually receive their training on the job.

Work settings

Physical therapy assistants may work in hospitals, private physical therapy offices, **nursing homes**, rehabilitation centers, sports facilities, schools, and other institutions. Some degree of bodily strength and endurance is necessary because of the physical handling of patients with limited mobility.

Education and training

A two-year associate's degree, usually from a community or junior college, is generally required. More than half of the states in the United States require licensure, registration, or an American Physical Therapy Association (APTA) certification. **Cardiopulmonary resuscitation** and **first aid** certification, as well as clinical experience hours are also required, although the amount of hours varies by state.

Physiology

Definition

Physiology is the branch of biology that studies how living things function, including growth, development, nutrient use, and the physical and biological functioning of various organ systems.

Description

The study of human physiology is a core competency necessary for anyone from a personal trainer to a physician who wishes to enter a career in the health sciences. Physiology examines how the major organ systems of the body—circulatory, nervous, musculoskeletal, respiratory, gastrointestinal, integumentary, urinary, reproductive, endocrine, and immune systems—work together. Although everyone who works in an allied health field needs a background in physiology, only a few people, mostly research scientists, consider themselves physiologists. Most research physiologists have a doctor of philosophy (PhD) degree in biology or physiology. These researchers rarely work with human subjects. However, some physiologists have a PhD degree and are medical doctors (MDs) or doctors of **osteopathy** (DOs). These physiologists may work in clinical settings with human subjects.

Exercise physiology is a subspecialty of kinesiology. Exercise physiologists study the short-term response to exercise and adaption of the body to regular exercise. Exercise physiologists often work with athletes as trainers or conditioning experts. They also work under medical supervision with individuals who have chronic diseases such as chronic **heart** and lung diseases.

Origins

The study of physiology is as old as the study of the human body. As far back as 420 BC, Hippocrates, considered the father of medicine, believed that it essential to understand the relationship between structure and function of various organs in the body. However, because of religious and legal prohibitions about dissecting human cadavers, much of the understanding of how the human body worked was extrapolated from the dissection of pigs, monkeys, dogs and other animals.

Although illegal and semi-legal dissections were quietly carried out, it was not until 1752 that England allowed the legal dissection of criminals hanged for murder. The supply of bodies available for dissection

> **Kinesiology**—The study of how physical activity affects human mental and physical health.

remained quite limited until the mid-1800s. After that, knowledge of the way the body functioned increased rapidly as did technical innovations that allowed scientists to study the body in new ways. Most of the early work in physiology was carried out by medical doctors. Today academic researchers do much basic research in the laboratory. Medical and allied health professionals then apply their research findings in clinical settings.

Purpose

The purpose of human physiology is to understand how the body functions in order to prevent and cure disease and maximize performance.

Training and certification

Research physiologists uaually have a PhD degree and may also have a medical degree. A PhD requires a four-year undergraduate degree in biology or a related science and four to five years of graduate study and original research. Medical degrees require four years of undergraduate study and an additional four years of medical school followed by three to four years of internship and residency. Combined MD/PhD programs can reduce the time it takes to acquire a joint degree.

The education and training requirements for allied health professionals vary greatly depending on the position and state licensing laws. Generally, exercise physiologists who work with chronically ill individuals under medical supervision are required to have a four-year college degree in kinesiology or exercise physiology and a hands-on internship. Many have master's degrees. The American Society of Exercise Physiologists, founded in 1997, has developed a board certification program for exercise physiologists.

The American College of Sports Medicine offers a variety of health and fitness, clinical, and specialty certifications. In some states and in some positions (e.g., personal trainer), certification is optional while in others it is required. Other organizations for allied health professionals have their own standards for certification, many of which are legally required, and all of which demand a basic understanding of physiology.

Resources

BOOKS

Boron, Walter F., and Emile L. Boulpaep. *Medical Physiology*, 2nd edition. Saunders, 2011.

Hall, John E. *Guyton and Hall Textbook of Medical Physiology*, 12th edition. Saunders, 2010.

OTHER

Davis, Paul. Careers in Exercise Physiology. American Kinesiology Association. Undated [accessed August 27, 2012].

National Health Service (United Kingdom). Careers In Physiological Sciences. Undated. [accessed August 26, 2012]. http://www.nhscareers.nhs.uk/explore-by-career/healthcare-science/careers-in-healthcare-science/careers-in-physiological-sciences/

ORGANIZATIONS

American College of Sports Medicine, 401 West Michigan Street, Indianapolis, IN 46206-3233, (317) 637-9200, Fax: (317) 634-7817, http://www.acsm.org

American Kinesiology Association, P.O. Box 5076, Champaign, IL 61825-5076, Fax: (217) 351-154, http://www.americankinesiology.org

American Physiological Association, 9650 Rockville Pike, Bethesda, MD 20814-3991.http://www.the-aps.org

American Society of Exercise Physiologists, 1200 Kenwood Avenue, Duluth, MN 55811, (218) 723-6297, Fax: (218) 723-6472, http://www.asep.org

Tish Davidson, AM

PIH *see* **Preeclampsia and eclampsia**

Pitocin *see* **Uterine stimulants**

Pituitary gland

Definition

The pituitary gland is located at the base of the **brain** and is part of the **endocrine system**. It is sometimes called the *hypophysis*, from two Greek words that mean "to grow beneath." The pituitary is responsible for the hormonal regulation of several body processes, including water retention, breast milk synthesis and release, human growth, and **thyroid gland** secretions.

Description

The pituitary is one of the most extensively researched glands in the endocrine system. In humans, it is located at the base of the brain just beneath the hypothalamus. There are three separate lobes (or sections) of the pituitary: the anterior lobe, the posterior lobe and the intermediate lobe. Therefore, it is sometimes considered as three different glands. In addition, there is a small stem called the pituitary stalk that connects the pituitary to the hypothalamus.

The pituitary gland is formed during early **fetal development**. An understanding of its formation explains its position in the endocrine system as well as its neurological importance. Early in the development of the fetus, a small sac of cells forms at the top of the oral cavity and moves upward. These cells are known as Rathke's pouch. At the same time, a small fold of neural tissue extends downward from the hypothalamus. During fetal development, the two structures continue to move toward each other; they meet and fuse to form the anterior (originally Rathke's pouch) and posterior (from the hypothalamus) lobes of the pituitary.

The hypothalamus, which is located just above the pituitary gland, is a region in the forebrain that is responsible for regulating all lobes of the pituitary. The pituitary releases, but does not necessarily synthesize, nine different hormones. Neurohormones are synthesized by the hypothalamus and transported to the posterior pituitary. The release of hormones from each lobe of the pituitary is regulated differently.

Anterior pituitary

The anterior pituitary is sometimes called the adenohypophysis. It constitutes about 80% of the pituitary by weight. The cells of the anterior pituitary act like true endocrine cells. Instead of containing **neurons**, the anterior pituitary receives chemical signals through the **blood** and releases hormones in response. It has a direct connection with the hypothalamus through **blood vessels**. Various cells in the anterior pituitary release the following hormones:

- Gonadotrophs release luteinizing hormone (LH) and follicle-stimulating hormone (FSH).
- Lactotrophs release prolactin (PRL).
- Corticotrophs release adrenocorticotropic hormone (ACTH).
- Somatotrophs release growth hormone (GH).
- Thyrotrophs release thyroid-stimulating hormone (TSH).

Posterior pituitary

The posterior pituitary is sometimes referred to as the neurohypophysis because it acts like an extension of the nervous system. As opposed to the anterior pituitary, which is connected to the hypothalamus via the circulatory system, the posterior pituitary receives nerve impulses from the same nerve cells that innervate the hypothalamus. The posterior pituitary releases oxytocin and antidiuretic hormone (ADH, or vasopressin).

Intermediate pituitary

The intermediate lobe is not a complete "lobe" in humans. Instead it is a simple structure comprised of just a few cells. The intermediate pituitary is an important structure in many lower vertebrates, but it has very little significance in humans. In lower vertebrates, the intermediate pituitary releases melanocyto-stimulating hormone. This hormone stimulates the growth of melanocytes, which are cells that produce a dark pigment called melanin.

Function

The pituitary gland is an organ that is part of the endocrine system, along with many other glands and organs. It is regulated by the hypothalamus, and it in turn regulates the secretion of many different hormones that are essential to human health.

Role in human health

Hormones released from the anterior and posterior pituitary have far-reaching effects on many different organ systems and physiological processes.

Hormones of the anterior pituitary

Luteinizing hormone and follicle stimulating hormone are called gonadotropins. As the name suggests, the target tissues of these hormones are the gonads (ovaries and testes). They have two main functions. The first is to promote the development and maturation of sperm and eggs. Second, they stimulate the production and release of such sex steroid hormones as estradiol and testosterone in women and men respectively.

Prolactin is responsible for stimulating cells in the female breast to produce milk. Therefore, lactotrophs located in the anterior pituitary of women that are breastfeeding are large and numerous, indicating an increased amount of prolactin production. These lactotrophs comprise about 30% of the cells in the anterior pituitary. The pituitary in women doubles in size during **pregnancy** because of the increase in size and number of lactotrophs.

The target tissue of adrenocorticotropic hormone is the adrenal cortex (part of the adrenal gland that is located above the kidney). ACTH stimulates the production of cortisol and also causes the cells of the adrenal gland to grow. Cortisol has many effects on **metabolism** in various tissues.

Growth hormones have many different target tissues and promote the growth of each of them. For this reason human growth hormone (GH) is considered an anabolic hormone, indicating that it is responsible for building tissue **proteins**. For example, GH directly increases protein synthesis in muscles and the **liver**; and it decreases the size of adipose tissue. It also has an indirect effect by stimulating other hormones. Growth hormones indirectly affect the bones by increasing protein synthesis, collagen synthesis and cell proliferation. In many other tissues, the indirect effects of growth hormone are responsible for protein, RNA and DNA synthesis. The overall effect of growth hormone is to promote skeletal growth and a lean body mass.

As its name implies, thyroid-stimulating hormone (TSH) promotes cell growth in the thyroid gland. TSH also triggers the secretion of thyroid hormones that affect many metabolic processes in the body.

Hormones of the posterior pituitary

Both oxytocin and antidiuretic hormone (ADH) are peptide hormones that are synthesized in the cell bodies of the nerves originating in the hypothalamus and then delivered through the axons to the posterior pituitary. Thus, they are good examples of neuroendocrine hormones.

The primary target organ of ADH is the kidney. ADH is responsible for increasing water retention by the kidney, resulting in an increase in extracellular fluid and a decrease in urine volume. Receptors in the hypothalamus called osmoreceptors can sense the concentration of water in the extracellular fluid through changes in extracellular fluid osmolarity. The osmoreceptors in turn determine the release of ADH by the posterior pituitary. The consumption of alcohol decreases the amount of ADH released. As a result, more fluid is lost through urination, resulting in excessive water loss and thirst.

The primary site of action of oxytocin is female breast tissue. Oxytocin stimulates the contraction of smooth muscle cells in the breast, transferring milk from the place of synthesis to the larger ducts of the breast. Oxytocin is secreted by the stimulation of touch sensors when an infant is suckling. Other psychological factors, such as the sound of a baby crying, can stimulate the release and action of oxytocin. The role of oxytocin in the onset of labor contractions is not fully clear. There is no known stimulus for the secretion of oxytocin in the human male.

Common diseases and disorders

Hypopituitarism

Disorders of the pituitary gland can have severe effects on normal growth and sexual maturation. A general condition known as **hypopituitarism**, also

KEY TERMS

Acromegaly—Abnormal enlargement of such parts of the body as the hands, face, head, and feet.

Adenohypophysis—Another name for the anterior lobe of the pituitary.

Antidiuretic hormone (ADH)—A hormone released by the posterior lobe of the pituitary gland that increases the absorption of water by the kidneys. It is also known as vasopressin.

Diabetes insipidus—A disorder characterized by increased urine production resulting from inadequate levels of ADH.

Gonadotropins—Hormones that affect the development or activity of the ovaries or testes.

Hypophysis—Another name for the pituitary gland.

Hypopituitarism—A condition produced by deficient activity of the anterior lobe of the pituitary gland. It is characterized by obesity, incomplete sexual maturation, and in extreme cases, dwarfism.

Hypothalamus—A region in the forebrain that regulates the functions of the autonomic nervous system by vascular communication. The hypothalamus governs the functions of both lobes of the pituitary gland.

Neurohypophysis—Another name for the posterior lobe of the pituitary.

Oxytocin—A hormone produced by the posterior pituitary that stimulates the movement of breast milk from the sacs in which the milk is produced to the larger ducts from which the milk is ejected.

Peptide—A compound containing two or more amino acids, in which the carboxyl group of one acid is linked to the amino group of the other.

Vasopressin—Another name for ADH.

known as pituitary dwarfism, is characterized by a decrease in one or more of the hormones produced by the anterior pituitary. Sexual immaturity and metabolic dysfunction leading to **obesity** are symptoms of this syndrome. When hypopituitarism occurs in childhood, growth is slowed. Tumors are often the cause of hypopituitarism; however, sometimes there is no identifiable cause. If there is a decrease in the levels of hormones released from the hypothalamus, then hypopituitarism results. The symptoms vary according to the number and amount of hormones that are deficient. The most effective treatment is the administration of replacement hormones.

Hyperpituitarism

The overproduction of growth hormone during childhood produces a condition known as gigantism or acromegaly. Excessive secretion of anterior pituitary hormones is known as hyperpituitarism. Growth hormone influences the overgrowth of the skeleton and all other tissues. A person may grow to 8 ft (2.4 m) or more in height. It is still unclear, but researchers think that overproduction of growth hormone may be caused by an adenoma (tumor) on the anterior pituitary. Sometimes, this condition occurs in more than one member of the family, suggesting that there is a genetic component. Gigantism is treated by removing the tumor and administering medications (bromocriptine and octreotide) that inhibit the production of growth hormone.

Diabetes insipidus

A disorder related to both the hypothalamus and the posterior lobe of the pituitary is **diabetes insipidus**, not to be confused with **diabetes mellitus**. Diabetes insipidus, or DI, is caused by a deficiency of antidiuretic hormone (ADH). As a result, water is rapidly released from the body through large volumes of urine (3–30 quarts per day). DI may result from an inherited trait; from damage to the hypothalamus, which synthesizes ADH; or from damage to the posterior pituitary, which stores the ADH. Diabetes insipidus occurs more frequently in men than in women. In mild cases, no treatment is necessary other than water replacement. In extreme cases, the patient can be treated by hormone replacement therapy.

Resources

BOOKS

Cahill, Matthew, ed. *Professional Guide to Diseases*, 6th ed. Springhouse, PA: Springhouse Corporation, 1998.

Greenspan, Francis S., and David G. Gardner. *Basic and Clinical Endocrinology*, 6th ed. New York: Lange Medical Books/McGraw-Hill, 2001.

Hypothalamic-Pituitary Relationships. Chapter 6 in *The Merck Manual of Diagnosis and Therapy*, edited by Mark H. Beers, MD, and Robert Berkow, MD. Whitehouse Station, NJ: Merck Research Laboratories, 1999.

Martin, John H., PhD. *Neuroanatomy: Text and Atlas*, 2nd ed. Norwalk, CT: Appleton & Lange, 1996.

Pituitary Disorders. in *The Merck Manual of Diagnosis and Therapy*, edited by Mark H. Beers, MD, and Robert Berkow, MD. Whitehouse Station, NJ: Merck Research Laboratories, 2004.

Vander, Arthur, et al, eds. *Human Physiology: The Mechanisms of Body Function,* 7th ed. Boston, MA: WBC/McGraw-Hill, 1998.

Sally C. McFarlane-Parrott

Pituitary hormone tests

Definition

Pituitary hormones include growth hormone, adrenocorticotropic hormone, thyroid stimulating hormone, follicle stimulating hormone, luteinizing hormone, prolactin, antidiuretic hormone, and oxytocin. This cluster of hormones has a vast and complex impact on the growth, fertility, and function of the human body via the effect of the hormones on their target organs. Tests measure hormone levels to test for various diseases and conditions.

Purpose

Measurement of several pituitary hormones may be requested to investigate pituitary dysfunction in general. The entire gland may cease to function normally due to a hypothalamic disease, surgery, pituitary tumor, or trauma (e.g., Sheehan's syndrome, pituitary failure caused by hemorrhage into the gland after obstetric delivery). Alternatively, one or more specific hormones may be measured to investigate dysfunction of a target organ. For example, LH, FSH, and prolactin are commonly measured along with estrogen (estradiol) and progesterone to investigate ovarian failure. ACTH is needed to investigate the cause of adrenocortical excess or insufficiency. TSH is specifically used to diagnose thyroid under- or overactivity. Growth hormone is used to test for growth impairment or acromegaly. ADH testing is used to investigate disturbances in electrolytes (sodium and potassium) that will be abnormal when either too much or too little water is reabsorbed by the **kidneys**. Oxytocin is rarely measured, but may be used to identify ectopic production by tumor cells (e.g., lung carcinoma) that secrete the hormone.

Precautions

Each of these hormones is involved in intricate relationships with other organ systems. Levels may vary markedly depending on time of sampling (hGH, ACTH, prolactin), phase of the menstrual or reproductive cycle (FSH, LH), age, sex, physical activity, and a variety of psychological and nutritional factors. A thorough history of the patient's physical activities and medications is very helpful in interpreting **blood** test results. Pituitary hormones may be measured on plasma or urine. The nurse or phlebotomist collecting the sample should observe **universal precautions** for the prevention of transmission of bloodborne pathogens.

Many drugs are known to affect the level of pituitary hormones. For example, TSH test results may be influenced by medications such as lithium, potassium iodide, aspirin, dopamine, heparin, and **corticosteroids**. In addition, small fibrin clots and heterophile **antibodies** (HAMA) have been known to cause erroneous results with some immunoassays.

Description

Growth hormone (hGH), or somatotropin, is responsible for normal body growth and development, and regulates carbohydrate and **protein metabolism**. Adrenocorticotropic hormone (ACTH) regulates cortisol release from the **adrenal glands**. Thyroid stimulating hormone (TSH) regulates the synthesis and release of thyroid hormones. Follicle stimulating hormone (FSH) controls the maturation of the ovarian follicle in females and the development of the seminiferous tubules and sperm production in males. In females, luteinizing hormone (LH) causes release of the ovum from the ovary and supports the corpus luteum after ovulation. In males, LH supports testosterone production. Both FSH and LH are found at highest concentrations in plasma immediately before a woman ovulates. Prolactin promotes **lactation**, or milk production, after **childbirth**. Antidiuretic hormone (ADH), also called vasopressin, acts on the kidneys (collecting tubules) to increase the reabsorption of water. Oxytocin is released during labor and breastfeeding. It causes smooth muscle contractions needed for delivery and promotes the release of breast milk.

Growth hormone

Human growth hormone (hGH), or somatotropin, is a protein made up of 191 amino acids. It is secreted by the anterior **pituitary gland** and coordinates normal growth and development. Human growth is characterized by two spurts, one at birth and the other at **puberty**. hGH plays an important role at both of these times. Receptors that respond to hGH exist on cells and tissues throughout the body. The most pronounced effect of hGH is on linear skeletal development, but hGH also greatly increases lean muscle mass. Humans have two forms of hGH, and the functional difference between the two is unclear. hGH is produced in the anterior portion of the pituitary gland by somatotrophs under the control of hormonal peptides from the hypothalamus. The primary hypothalamic hormone regulating hGH is growth hormone-releasing hormone (GHRH). When blood glucose levels fall, GHRH triggers the secretion of stored hGH. As blood glucose levels rise, GHRH release is turned off. Increases in blood protein levels trigger a similar response. GHRH is opposed by growth hormone-inhibiting hormone (GHIH), which is a neuropeptide causing decreased release of hGH and TSH and which inhibits gastrin, secretin, and insulin. As a result of this hypothalamic feedback loop, hGH levels fluctuate throughout the day.

Because of its critical role in producing hGH and other hormones, an aberrant pituitary gland will often yield altered growth. Dwarfism (very small stature) can be caused by underproduction of hGH or insulin-like growth factor I (IGF-I), or by a flaw in the target tissue response to either of these. Overproduction of hGH or IGF-I, or an exaggerated response to these hormones, can lead to gigantism or acromegaly, both of which are characterized by a very large stature. Gigantism is the result of hGH overproduction in early childhood leading to a skeletal height up to 8 feet (2.4 m) or more. In this condition, the epiphyseal plates of the long bones do not close, and they remain responsive to hGH. Acromegaly results when hGH is overproduced after the onset of puberty. This disorder is characterized by an enlarged **skull**, hands and feet, nose, neck, and tongue owing to proliferation of connective tissue. Use of hGH supplementation by athletes to "cheat" during competition is a concern among agencies that oversee athletic competitions. As of summer 2004, there was no screening test for hGH doping.

Growth hormone in plasma or urine is usually measured by radioimmunoassay (RIA). Some fluorescent and chemiluminescent enzyme immunoassays are available as well. In children, hGH in plasma is often too low to detect or permit differentiation of normal and deficient levels. A child below average in height who has normal pituitary function may have a low level of growth hormone as a result of normal physiological variation. Diagnosis is made either by a provocative test or measurement of IGF-I. A deficiency of IGF-I occurs in both hGH deficiency and protein malnutrition. Provocative testing for hGH deficiency involves administration of a drug known to stimulate release of growth hormone, or vigorous **exercise**, which does the same. Drugs used include arginine, insulin, glucagon, and propranolol. In the exercise test, a blood sample is measured for hGH immediately following exercise performed vigorously for 20 minutes. A level greater than 6 nanograms per mL rules out growth hormone deficiency. A lower response is suggestive and is followed by a drug stimulation test. Growth hormone is increased in approximately 90% of

persons with acromegaly. Acromegaly is caused by an adenoma in the pituitary that produces hGH. For suspected cases that do not demonstrate an elevated plasma level, a glucose suppression test is needed for diagnosis. The test is performed by giving 100 grams of glucose orally, and collecting a blood sample one hour later. The gluocse should suppress hGH to below 1 ng/mL. Failure to do so is evidence of acromegaly.

Adrenocorticotropic hormone

ACTH production is controlled by the production of corticotropin-releasing hormone (CRH) by the hypothalamus. The release of this neuropeptide is inhibited by plasma cortisol via negative feedback. When plasma cortisol is elevated, CRH is inhibited, and less ACTH is produced. As a result the adrenal cortex produces less cortisol, and ACTH levels return to normal. Conversely, if cortisol levels fall, CRH is released, causing increased secretion of ACTH by the pituitary. ACTH levels rise in response to **stress**, emotions, injury, **infection**, **burns**, surgery, and decreased **blood pressure**.

Cushing's disease is caused by an abnormally high level of circulating cortisol (hydrocortisone). The high level may be the result of an adrenal gland tumor; enlargement of both adrenal glands due to a pituitary tumor; production of ACTH by a tumor outside the pituitary gland (ectopic production); or excessive administration of corticosteroid drugs. Corticosteroid drugs are widely used for reducing inflammation in disorders such as **rheumatoid arthritis**, inflammatory bowel disease, and **asthma**.

Addison's disease is a rare disorder in which symptoms are caused by a deficiency of cortisol and aldosterone. The most common cause of this disease is an autoimmune disorder. Addison's disease generally progresses slowly, with symptoms developing gradually over months or years. However, acute episodes, called Addisonian crises, are brought on by infection, injury, or other stresses.

ACTH is measured by RIA or fluorescent and chemiluminescent enzyme immunoassay. ACTH in plasma is measured in order to help differentiate the cause of Cushing's disease. Approximately half of persons with Cushing's disease (pituitary Cushing's) have a normal ACTH level and half will have an elevated level. Most persons with adrenal tumors will have low (less than 10 picograms/L) or undetectable ACTH in the plasma owing to suppression by cortisol. Most persons with ectopic ACTH secreting tumors will have elevated levels in excess of 200 pg/L. Persons with primary Addison's disease will usually have high ACTH levels (greater than 150 picrograms/L) caused by negative feedback (low cortisol) while those with secondary

Addison's disease will have low or normal ACTH levels owing to pituitary failure or hypothalmic suppression.

Thyroid stimulating hormone

Thyroid stimulating hormone is released by the anterior pituitary in response to thyroid releasing hormone (TRH) from the hypothalamus. It results in synthesis, storage, and release of T3 and T4, the thyroid hormones. Elevated levels of free T3 and T4 exert negative feedback on the hypothalamus inhibiting the release of TRH, which reduces TSH. Thyroid hormones have pronounced effects on the body's rate of **metabolism**. Decreased levels are responsible for myxedema, which produces a constellation of symptoms such as **edema**, low **heart** rate, intolerance to cold, hyperlipidemia, and anemia. The most common cause of myxedema is Hashimoto's disease, an autoimmune condition causing chronic hypothyroidism. Increased levels of the thyroid hormones (hyperthyroidism) causes a condition called thyrotoxicosis. It is characterized by exophthalmia (protruding eyeballs), tachycardia, insomnia, and weight loss. The most common cause of hyperthyroidism is Graves' disease.

TSH is commonly measured by enzyme immunoassay, and is the best screening test for diagnosis of both hypothyroidism and hyperthyroidism. It also is used as part of the diagnosis of congenital hypothyroidism in newborns. In primary hypothyroidism, the plasma level of free T4 will be low and TSH will be elevated. In primary hyperthyroidism, the plasma level of free T3 will be high and TSH will be low. In thyroid disease caused by pituitary failure, the TSH and thyroid hormones will move in the same direction. For example, in secondary hypothyroidism, both free T4 and TSH will be low. Researchers have developed a new TSH immunoassay that allows observation of reaction kinetics in real-time.

Follicle-stimulating hormone and luteinizing hormone

Both FSH and LH are regulated by the hypothalamic release of gonadotropin-releasing hormone. In males, both hormones are inhibited via negative feedback by testosterone. In females, both hormones are inhibited via negative feedback by estrogen and progesterone. Levels of these hormones show pulse variation; this is especially true of LH and for this reason, 24-hour urine levels are preferred by some clinicans over plasma measurements. FSH and LH are performed when a person exhibits abnormal reproductive function. In women conditions such as precocious puberty, polycystic ovaries, failure to ovulate, dysmenorrhea, and the onset of **menopause** are the primary reasons for measuring these hormones. In males, these hormones are measured along with testosterone to diagnose and differentiate the cause of gonadal failure.

Levels of FSH and LH are somewhat constant prior to puberty. At puberty, both hormone levels increase significantly. In women the levels of both hormones vary with the phase of the menstrual cycle. Both FSH and LH peak in the midcycle just prior to ovulation. Prior to this peak, levels are somewhat higher than they are after ovulation. The midcycle peak has been used to identify the best opportunity to conceive. A urine LH detection kit is available for use at home. This test is sometimes called an "ovulation test" and is similar to a home **pregnancy test**. A sample of the woman's first morning urine is tested with the materials provided in the kit. These home tests may be used by women who want to become pregnant. By monitoring levels of LH and watching for the surge signaling ovulation, a couple can time sexual intercourse to increase the chance that the egg will be fertilized.

LH and FSH are measured mainly by enzyme or chemiluminescent immunoassays. In males, testosterone RIA is used along with FSH and LH to differentiate the cause of gonadal failure. A low testosterone with low LH or FSH points to a hypothalmic-pituitary cause. A low testosterone with an increased LH and/or FSH indicates primary testicular failure. In females, LH and FSH are measured along with estrogen, progesterone, and prolactin to investigate the cause of abnormal gonadal function. In menopause, the midcycle peaks for both LH and FSH are usually higher than in normal menstruating females. Prior to menopause, the LH peak is greater in magnitude than FSH. However, in menopause, this pattern reverses. In females, low plasma estrogen and progesterone seen with elevated serum or urinary levels of LH and FSH signal primary ovarian failure. Conversely, low estrogen and progesterone in association with low levels of LH and FSH indicate pituitary (secondary) hypogonadism. Home kits also have been developed for testing FSH levels to indicate menopause, but in 2005, the Canadian Society of Obstetricians and Gynecologists warned against use of these kits. The society also did not recommend FSH testing for menopause by health care providers. Prolactin levels should also be performed when evaluating hypogonadism in females. High plasma prolactin caused by pituitary adenoma causes inhibition of LH and FSH by negative feedback. Therefore, prolactinoma may be responsible for ovarian failure.

Prolactin

Prolactin is also known as the lactogenic hormone or lactogen. It is essential for enlargement of the mammary glands during **pregnancy**, and for stimulating and maintaining lactation after childbirth. Like hGH, prolactin acts directly on tissues, and levels rise in response to sleep and to physical or emotional stress. During sleep, prolactin levels in nonpregnant females can reach as high as those seen in pregnant women (as high as ten to twenty times the normal level). Prolactin secretion is controlled by prolactin-releasing and prolactin-inhibiting factors secreted by the hypothalamus. In addition, TRH can also stimulate prolactin secretion.

Prolactin deficiency is rare, and like hGH it cannot be diagnosed without a provocative test because low and normal levels overlap. As with hGH, a normal or elevated level will rule out a deficiency. Documentation of prolactin deficiency requires the use of the TRH stimulation test and demonstration of a subnormal response. Elevated prolactin is the most common pituitary abnormality. Microadenomas of the pituitary that produce prolactin are the most common pituitary tumors. Depending on the type of cell involved, these tumors are also called prolactin-secreting pituitary acidophilic or chromophobic adenomas. However, there are several other conditions that increase plasma prolactin including pregnancy, drugs, hypothyroidism, and renal failure. Prolactinoma is typically associated with a plasma prolactin level greater than 200 nanograms per mL. Because about half of microadenomas are too small to see by imaging tests such as **CT scans**, plasma prolactin levels above 200 ng/mL, together with the absence of other known causes, are used to diagnose prolactinoma.

Pituitary neoplasia

Pituitary tumors are often responsible for increases in one or more pituitary hormones. About 30% of pituitary adenomas produce prolactin and about 20% produce FSH. Ectopic hormones may also be produced, for example, ACTH by squamous cell carcinoma of the lung. In addition, the pituitary gland is often involved in multiple endocrine neoplasia type 1 (MEN-1). This condition is inherited as an autosomal dominant disorder. It involves enlargement of at least two endocrine glands, which may be the result of hyperplasia, adenoma, or adenocarcinoma. One or more pituitary hormones will be secreted when the gland is involved. Therefore, plasma levels of pituitary hormones are sometimes measured to diagnose and monitor various malignant diseases.

Posterior pituitary hormones

The purpose of ADH is to control the amount of water reabsorbed by the kidneys. Water is continually being taken into the body in food and drink, as well as being produced by chemical reactions in cells. Water is also continually lost in urine, sweat, feces, and in the breath as water vapor. ADH acts to keep blood and extracellular fluid volumes constant under conditions of changing water and solute intake. Under normal conditions, the blood volume expands when excess water is absorbed. This reduces the plasma osmolality, which inhibits the release of ADH causing water to be lost in the urine. Under conditions of water deprivation, plasma osmolality increases. This stimulates the osmoreceptors in the carotid sinus and ADH is released. The distal collecting tubule of the kidney reabsorbs more water, causing the osmolality to fall until blood volume is restored. Various factors can affect ADH production, thereby disturbing the body's water balance. Physical stress, surgery, and high levels of **anxiety** can stimulate ADH release. Alcohol consumption reduces ADH production by direct action on the **brain**, resulting in a temporarily increased production of urine. Abnormal water balance occurs in **diabetes insipidus**, when the pituitary gland produces insufficient ADH; and in chronic renal disease, when the kidneys fail to respond to ADH. The reverse effect, water retention, can result from temporarily increased ADH production after a major operation or accident. Water retention may also be caused by the secretion of ADH by some tumors, especially of the brain and lung. Any condition other than the thirst response that causes increased release of ADH is referred to as the syndrome of inappropriate ADH release (SIADH). Ectopic ADH production by tumors is the most common cause.

Antidiuretic hormone is measured by RIA. It is used in conjunction with serum and urine osmolality or sodium measurements to differentiate SIADH from psychogenic polydipsia and other causes of low electrolytes and to differentiate neurogenic (pituitary) diabetes insipidus from nephrogenic (renal) diabetes insipidus.

Oxytocin is released by the posterior pituitary to cause strong uterine contractions in labor and delivery, and it also acts on muscle cells in lactating breast tissue to aid in the release of milk. Oxytocin levels are rarely measured, but oxytocin is often used in the hospital setting to induce or reinforce uterine contractions in labor. It is also useful in its natural or commercial form for helping the uterus to stay small and contracted after delivery, minimizing blood loss. Oxytocin is produced by males as well, and its function is thought to be related to sperm transportation.

Preparation

Pituitary hormones demonstrate both diurnal and pulse variation, and it is important to note the time of day that the sample is collected. Samples for both ACTH and ADH should be drawn in the fasting state. Blood for ACTH is usually drawn early in the morning, when ACTH is anticipated to be at its peak, and is also assessed in the evening when it is expected to be at its lowest level. ACTH fluctuates and should be collected in EDTA using plastic tubes. The blood should be centrifuged immediately (preferably in the cold) and the plasma removed and frozen until the time of assay. FSH and LH vary greatly depending upon the time of collection. For this reason, results should be evaluated with regard to the time of sampling. Since levels vary greatly during the menstrual cycle, the levels must be evaluated with regard to the menstrual phase. Some clinicians prefer to pool plasma specimens collected across the menstrual cycle for a single measurement, or to use 24-hour urine samples for measurement. Growth hormone specimens should be collected using heparin or EDTA from a fasting patient. The various tests used to investigate human growth hormone are highly influenced by the fasting or non-fasting state, as well as the presence or absence of recent exercise. Prolactin levels should be drawn in the morning at least two hours after the patient wakes. (Samples drawn earlier may show sleep-induced peak levels.) No specific preparation is necessary for drawing TSH levels, but illness and stress can affect results significantly.

Aftercare

No special care is necessary after collection of blood or urine for pituitary hormone assessment. Patients should return to normal eating and exercise, and resume routine medications. Following venipuncture for blood plasma hormone tests, the laboratory technologist, nurse, or phlebotomist drawing the sample should inspect the venipuncture site to make sure that the wound has closed and no bleeding is present. The site should be covered with an adhesive bandage. There is no notable aftercare for patients undergoing 24-hour urine hormone tests. Patients should be reminded to resume foods and medications that were restricted prior to testing.

Complications

Complications from drawing blood are minimal and may include slight bleeding from the venipuncture site, fainting, or lightheadedness after the blood sample is drawn. Blood may accumulate under the puncture site (hematoma) if pressure is not applied to the site immediately after drawing blood. There are no complications for the urine test. Some of the test protocols for growth hormone assessment involve administering drugs, such that nausea, sleepiness, sweating and/or

nervousness may occur. Severe **hypoglycemia** could theoretically occur with insulin, but this is unlikely if the patient is closely monitored and treated appropriately.

Results

The normal ranges for pituitary hormone tests are highly method-dependent, resulting in significant laboratory variation. Also, age, sex, and sampling time must be taken into consideration when interpreting results.

Generally, hGH ranges from undetectable to 5ng/mL for adult men, up to 10 ng/mL for adult women, and as high as 16 ng/mL in children over six years. Arginine (an amino acid), insulin, and other substances are sometimes used to try to elicit higher levels of hGH to investigate a possible deficiency. Decreased levels are seen in hGH deficiency, dwarfism, hyperglycemia, failure to thrive, and delayed sexual maturity. Excess hGH is responsible for the syndromes of gigantism and acromegaly. Excess secretion is stimulated by **anorexia nervosa**, stress, hypoglycemia, and exercise.

Representative normal values for ACTH range from 8–100 pg/mL between 4 and 8 AM, and less than 50 pg/mL between 8 and 10 PM. High levels of ACTH may be caused by ACTH-producing tumors. These tumors may be either in the pituitary or in another area (such as tumors from **lung cancer** or ovarian **cancer**). In Addison's disease, the adrenal glands fail, and the pituitary gland secretes very high levels of ACTH in an attempt to restore normal adrenal hormone. Low levels of ACTH may occur because of decreased pituitary function. Low ACTH levels may result from adrenal adenoma which causes high levels of cortisol. The cortisol causes negative feedback to the pituitary.

Representative adult normal values for TSH are 0.2–4.7 microunits per mL (uU/mL). Higher values may by caused by congenital hypothyroidism (cretinism) or primary hypothyroidism (**thyroid gland** failure). Low values may be due to hyperthyroidism such as in Graves' disease or thyroiditis, or secondary hypothyroidism (hypothalamic or pituitary failure).

FSH test results vary according to age and sexual maturity. The phase of a woman's menstrual cycle or use of birth-control pills also affects test results. For an adult male, normal results range from 4–25 U/L. For a premenopausal woman, normal values range from 4–30 U/L. In a pregnant woman, FSH levels are too low to measure. After menopause, normal values range from 40–250 U/L. FSH levels fluctuate during premenopause. FSH is not a good marker for menopause, according to many obstetrics physicians. Anorexia nervosa and disorders of the hypothalamus or pituitary gland can result in abnormally low FSH levels. Abnormal

KEY TERMS

Adrenal glands—A pair of endocrine glands that lie on top of the kidneys, which produce natural steroid-based hormones.

Anovulatory bleeding—Bleeding without release of an egg from an ovary.

Klinefelter's syndrome—Inheritance of an extra X chromosome that results in small testes and male infertility.

Polycystic ovarian syndrome—A condition in which a woman has little or no menstruation, is infertile, has excessive body hair, and is usually obese. The ovaries may contain several cysts.

levels can also indicate precocious puberty, **hypopituitarism** (diffuse failure of the pituitary to make hormones), Klinefelter's syndrome (in men), Turner syndrome, testicular failure, and polycystic ovarian syndrome.

The normal range for LH in males is 1–8 mU/mL and in children is 1–5 mU/mL. Levels in females vary dramatically based upon the phase of the menstrual cycle. In the follicular phase, levels are normally in the range of 1.7–15 mU/mL; in the midcycle peak they are normally between 16–104 mU/mL; and in the luteal phase they normally range from 0.6–16 mU/mL. LH in postmenopausal women is normally in the range of 16–66 mU/mL. Abnormally high levels may be found in primary gonadal dysfunction, polycystic ovarian syndrome, and pituitary adenoma. Abnormally low levels can be seen with delayed puberty, congenital adrenal hyperplasia, stress, malnutrition and diffuse pituitary or hypothalamic problems.

Reference ranges for prolactin vary from laboratory to laboratory, but are generally between 3–15 ng/mL for adult males and 3.8–23 ng/mL for nonpregnant adult females. Prolactin levels in pregnancy vary greatly with the time of gestation. Normal values in the third trimester are 95–475 ng/mL. Increased prolactin levels are found in galactorrhea, amenorrhea, hypothyroidism, prolactin-secreting pituitary tumors, infiltrative diseases of the hypothalamus, and metastatic cancer of the pituitary gland. Higher levels than normal are also seen in stress, which may be produced by anorexia nervosa, surgery, strenuous exercise, trauma, and in renal (kidney) failure. Decreased prolactin levels are seen in pituitary failure.

ADH normal ranges are also laboratory-specific but can range from 1–5 pg/mL or 1–5 ng/L (SI units). Patients who are dehydrated, who have a decreased amount of blood in the body (hypovolemia), or who are undergoing severe physical stress (e.g., trauma, **pain** or prolonged **mechanical ventilation**) may exhibit increased ADH levels as a normal response to the needs of the body. Similarly, patients who are overly hydrated may have decreased ADH levels. Abnormal conditions that cause increased levels (SIADH) include **central nervous system** tumors, ectopic tumors, and infection. ADH deficiency is called diabetes insipidus, and results in severe water losses from the body. It is easily treated with nasally administered vasopressin.

Health care team roles

A physician will order pituitary tests and will interpret the results, often with the aid of an endocrinologist. A nurse or phlebotomist will draw blood samples and give instructions for 24-hour urine collection if needed. Nurses are also responsible for accurate history-taking in order to document medications, stressors, or exercise that may influence test results. Clinical laboratory scientists/medical technologists perform the various hormone assays. Tests for hGH, ACTH, and ADH are usually performed by reference laboratories.

Resources

BOOKS

Malarkey, Louise M., and Mary Ellen McMorrow. *Nurse's Manual of Laboratory Tests and Diagnostic Procedures,* 2nd ed. W.B. Saunders Company, 2000:580–584, 552–555, 683–696.

Pagana, Kathleen Deska, and Timothy James Pagana. *Mosby's Diagnostic and Laboratory Test Reference,* 4th ed. Mosby, 1998:23–28.

Tierney, Lawrence M., Stephen J. McPhee and Maxine A. Papadakis. *Current Medical Diagnosis and Treatment 2001.* Lange Medical Books/McGraw-Hill, 2001:1092-1102.

PERIODICALS

Lanting, Caren I., et al. "Clinical Effectiveness and Cost-effectiveness of the Use of the Thyroxine/Thyroxine-binding Globulin Ratio to Detect Congenital Hypothyroidism of Thyroidal and Central Origin in a Neonatal Screening Program." *Pediatrics* (July 2005): 168–174.

Unnecessary to Test for FSH. *A Friend Indeed* (March-April 2005): 8.

OTHER

National Library of Medicine. Medline. http://www.nlm.nih.gov/medlineplus/ency/article/000343.htm.

National Library of Medicine. Medline. http://www.nlm.nih.gov/medlineplus/ency/article/003684.htm.

University of Toledo. http://www.neurosci.pharm.utoledo.edu/MBC3320/vasopressin.htm.

Erika J. Norris
Teresa G. Odle

Pivot joint

Definition

A pivot joint is a synovial joint in which the ends of two bones meet—one end being a central bony cylinder, the other end being a ring (or ring-like structure) made of **bone** and ligament. In some joints, the cylinder rotates inside the ring. In other joints, the ring rotates around the cylinder. The rotation of the **skull** is made possible by a pivot joint. (A synovial joint is the living material that holds two or more bones together, but also permits these bones to move relative to each other.)

A more precise rendering of the international Latin anatomical term for pivot joint would be "wheel joint." A wheel rotates around an axis or pivot (for example, the axle around which automobile tires rotate). The Latin term (itself borrowed from Greek) refers directly to the ring made of bone and ligament. The English term refers directly to the cylindrical end of the bone.

Description

Pivot joints hold the two bones of the forearm together. That is, a pivot joint, located near the elbow, joins the bones of the forearm (called the ulna and the radius) to each other. These two bones are also joined to each other near the wrist by another pivot joint. A different pivot joint, located at the base of the skull, joins the first vertebra of the spine to the second vertebra and thus permits the head to rotate (since the first vertebra is joined to the skull).

If the bony surfaces of two bones that meet at a joint actually touched each other, then motion would cause friction, which would soon produce wear and tear on the touching ends of the bones. An engineer designing a mechanical counterpart would arrange for lubricating oil to prevent such wear and tear and facilitate smooth movement between the two metal "bones." A joint thus holds bones together (it is called a "joint" because it "joins" them) but also keeps them slightly separated to prevent their damaging each other in motion.

A kind of cartilage special to joints covers the ends of the bones being joined. A membrane hermetically seals two (or more) bone-ends with their cartilage, enclosing them in a kind of living capsule. For the sake of simplicity, the following example discusses a joint with only two bones. Inside this membrane capsule, there is a short distance between the cartilage of one bone and the cartilage of the other, because even cartilage rubbing directly against cartilage would produce wear and tear. But the gap between the cartilage surfaces is not a vacuum and is not filled with air. It is filled with synovial fluid. This fluid is in a sense the equivalent of the motor oil that lubricates moving parts of an automobile engine.

The interior of a synovial joint has negative pressure in relation to air pressure. For this reason, air pressure pushes the bones together tightly into the membrane capsule while the fluid keeps them from actually touching. The hermetically sealed membrane capsule in this paradoxical fashion aids the tight joining while it ensures the slight separation.

This negative pressure in the joint continues to work even after death. Of course, the two bones are kept together in a living body not only by the membrane capsule and the synovial fluid, but also by the tissues around the bones. If, while dissecting a corpse, one removes the tissues leaving only the membrane capsule, the pair of bones will remain tightly joined. But if one pierces the capsule and allows air to rush inside, one then has normal atmospheric pressure inside the capsule instead of the negative pressure of the interior of the living joint when it is hermetically sealed by the capsule, and now the bones come easily apart.

Synovial fluid has another important quality. Most bodily tissues are nourished by **blood vessels**, but the cartilage on bone-ends in joints does not have **blood** vessels. Synovial fluid provides the **nutrition** for the cartilage that keeps it alive, strong, and healthy. The wall of the membrane capsule has two layers. The outer layer is fibrous. The inner layer produces the synovial fluid, and hence is called the synovial layer.

Function

A pivot joint allows movement in one plane, such as rotation about an axis. Pivot joints, for example, permit one, after bending the elbow, to turn the palm of one's hand upward or downward by rotating the forearm. The two bones of the forearm (the ulna and the radius) twist around each other using a pivot joint.

Role in human health

The role of pivot joints in human health (the same as that played by the other types of synovial joints) is to allow freedom of movement and thus provide flexibility to the skeleton.

Common diseases and disorders

The pivot joints (and the other joints) can be affected by such conditions as the following:

• Ankylosis: The fusion of bones across a joint. It is often a complication of arthritis.

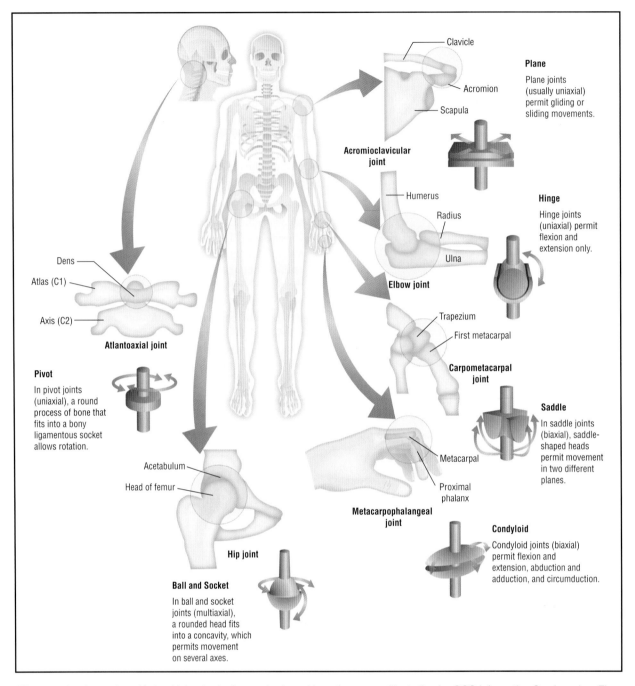

(Diagram showing various kinds of joints in the human body and how they move. Illustration by GGS Information Services, Inc. The Gale Group.)

- Ankylosing spondylitis: A type of inflammatory arthritis that progresses to ankylosis. It occurs chiefly in young men.

- Capsulitis: Inflammation of the membrane capsule that produces and encloses the synovial fluid.

- Dislocation: The displacing of a bone from its normal position, causing tendons to stretch and strain.

- Neoplasms: Abnormal growths (neoplasms) involving the pivot joints are rare. Such growths as do occur usually involve non-cancerous (benign) growths of cartilage or of tendons and their sheaths. Synovial sarcoma is a cancerous (malignant) growth of cells resembling those of the synovial layer of the membrane capsule. It is found at the contact surfaces of bones in a joint, usually in the larger joints of young adults.

KEY TERMS

Articulation—A synonym of "joint."

Carpals—The eight small bones that form the wrist and are joined to the metacarpals of the hand and to the bones of the forearm.

Humerus—The bone of the upper part of the arm.

Neoplasm—New and abnormal growth of tissue, which may be non-cancerous (benign) or cancerous (malignant).

Pronation—Motion of the forearm and hand by which, after one bends the elbow, the palm is turned downward.

Radius—One of the two bones of the forearm. A pivot joint joins it with the ulna near the elbow. A second pivot joint joins the other end of the radius to the other end of the ulna near the wrist.

Supination—Motion by which, after one bends one's elbow, a palm is turned upward.

Synovial fluid—A transparent, sticky fluid that lubricates joints and nourishes the cartilage in a joint. (It is also found in tendons, sheaths, and bursae.)

Ulna—One of the two bones of the forearm. Two pivot joints join it to the radius, one near the elbow, one near the wrist.

- Rheumatoid arthritis: A common form of chronic inflammation of the joints. It causes swelling, pain, stiffness, elevated temperature, and redness of the joints. It is a disease of connective tissue and leads to the destruction of bone, cartilage, and ligaments in the joints.

Resources

BOOKS

Dimon, Theodore and Megan Day. *Anatomy of the Moving Body: A Basic Course in Bones, Muscles, and Joints.* Berkeley, CA: North Atlantic Books, 2001.

Hoffmann, David. *Healthy Bones and Joints: A Natural Approach to Treating Arthritis, Osteoporosis, Tendinitis, Myalgia, Bursitis.* Pownal, VT: Storey Books, 2000 (A Storey Medicinal Herb Guide).

OTHER

LaStayo, Paul C., Ph.D., P.T., C.H.T., Northern Arizona University, Physical Therapy Program. "Differentiating Joint and Muscle Disorders." http://jan.ucc.nau.edu/~pcl/diagnosispt680/jmd.htm (2.5 KB, 29 January 2001).

Monique Laberge, Ph.D.

Placenta previa

Definition

Placenta previa is an abnormal condition of **pregnancy** in which the placenta is attached to the lower section of the uterus, partially or completely covering the cervix. It occurs in about 0.5% of pregnancies.

Description

The placenta is a hormone-producing fetal organ, rich in **blood vessels**, that connects the baby to the mother via the umbilical cord. It begins to develop along with the embryo right after conception. The placenta normally implants high on the uterine wall and securely attaches into the wall through finger-like projections. The umbilical cord is created by the interweaving of two arteries and one vein that connect the placenta to the fetus. The nutrients and oxygen from the mother pass through the placenta and into the fetus. Carbon dioxide and waste products excreted by the fetus pass through the placenta and into the mother's circulation for removal. The placenta functions as a lifeline for the fetus.

In placenta previa, the placenta has attached itself towards the bottom of the uterus, near or on the cervix. Its usual implantation site is high up on the uterine wall. During a vaginal birth the cervix thins and opens sufficiently for the fetus to pass through the cervix, into the birth canal, and out the mother's vagina. As the cervix begins to dilate during labor, the force on the low-lying placenta causes tearing and subsequent bleeding. Excessive bleeding, or hemorrhage, can be dangerous for both the mother and fetus. If the placenta tears, the fetus is deprived of nutrients and oxygen and can suffer **brain** damage or even death.

In some pregnancies, the low placement may not provide a sufficiently large area for good exchange of nutrients and gases. This may impede fetal growth. In most cases of placenta previa, the condition becomes a concern towards the end of the pregnancy, often around 30 weeks gestation. At this point the uterus starts to undergo changes in preparation for labor and delivery. It is when these changes occur that the placenta may begin to tear and bleed. Infants born to mothers with placenta previa also have a greater risk of **respiratory distress syndrome**. In a study published in October of 2000, researchers found that mothers carrying a male fetus are at greater risk of placenta previa than those carrying a female fetus.

There are four degrees of placenta previa:

- Low-lying implantation. The placenta lies abnormally low on the uterine wall, but is not yet approximating the cervix.

- Marginal implantation. The placenta is within 2 centimeters of the internal cervical os.
- Partial previa. The placenta covers part of the cervix. The distinction between partial and complete previa is somewhat unclear while the cervix is still closed.
- Total previa. The placenta completely covers the cervical os.

Causes and symptoms

The exact cause of placenta previa is unknown. However, contributing factors include:

- Uterine shape abnormality.
- Increased parity, i.e. the mother has been pregnant before.
- Previous cesarean births.
- Older maternal age. Women over the age of 35 have an increased risk of placenta previa by 4.7 times. When the mother is over 40, the risk rises to 9 times.
- Previous dilation and curettage of the uterus.
- Multiple gestation (twins, triplets, etc.).
- Previous placenta previa.
- Cigarette smoking.

Placenta previa is characterized by painless vaginal bleeding that often starts abruptly. The bleeding may continue, or it may stop as abruptly as it started. By the time the woman is seen by her obstetrical provider, there may be some spotting, or perhaps no bleeding at all. Even if the bleeding has stopped, placenta previa is an emergency situation and the mother needs to be seen right away. Bleeding indicates that the placenta has begun to tear. The mother is now at risk of hemorrhage if no intervention is made. The fetus may be compromised as the level of oxygen available to it has changed.

Diagnosis

Most pregnant women undergo at least one routine ultrasound during their pregnancy. During the ultrasound the placement and position of the placenta is identified. When a low-lying placenta is detected, the degree to which the placenta covers the cervical os is described in percentages. For example, a complete placenta previa is 100%. Once placenta previa has been diagnosed, the pregnancy is considered high risk. However, the position of the placenta can change as the uterus grows, and so periodic ultrasounds may be ordered. A transvaginal ultrasound may be ordered following an **abdominal ultrasound** to more accurately assess how low the placenta is lying. There is a false-negative and false-positive risk of 7% with abdominal ultrasound. For this condition, transvaginal ultrasound appears to be far more reliable. In addition, the placenta is able to creep upwards over time.

If a woman experiences sudden, painless, bright red bleeding at any point in the pregnancy, she should be seen right away, even if the bleeding has stopped. An ultrasound will usually be done in order to reassess the position of the placenta, and to evaluate the fetus. A manual examination of the cervix is not done, as this could disturb the placenta.

Treatment

The treatment plan will depend on the gestational age, the severity of the bleeding, and the risks to mother and fetus. If the fetus is sufficiently mature and the pregnancy is near term, immediate cesarean birth may be suggested. If it is too early for the fetus to survive outside the womb, and the mother's condition is stable, the mother may be placed on bed rest in the hospital with medications to prevent uterine contractions. Close monitoring of the fetus and mother will continue. If there has been no bleeding for a few days, the mother may be sent home, and may be prescribed medication to improve the fetus' lung maturity so that if a preterm birth is necessary, the fetus has a better chance for healthy survival. The position of the placenta will determine if a vaginal birth is possible, or if the safest delivery will be by **cesarean section**.

Prognosis

Prognosis for mother and fetus have significantly improved with accurate imaging technology that identifies the condition in advance and allows for proper high-risk management of the pregnancy. A planned cesarean birth rather than unexpected, profuse bleeding at the time of labor is a part of placenta previa management. The prognosis for the fetus depends on how well developed it is at the time of delivery, and whether the bleeding caused any significant oxygen deprivation. The mother has an excellent prognosis unless hemorrhage occurs and is not well managed.

Health care team roles

The radiologic technologist usually performs the ultrasound, but the obstetrical provider may choose to do it if bleeding has begun. Any reassuring signs should be mentioned to the mother. Bleeding during pregnancy is frightening, and speaking in a calm voice and providing a comfortable environment can allow the mother the opportunity to relax somewhat. The nurse places the woman on her side to ensure better **blood**

Cervix—The cervix, or cervical os, is the opening between the vagina and the uterus. During labor the cervix thins and dilates, allowing the fetus to pass through, entering the birth canal and leaving through the vagina.

Cesarean birth—The terms cesarean section, birth, or delivery may be used interchangeably. This procedure to deliver a baby involves an abdominal incision made through the abdominal wall and into the uterus to extract the baby.

Hemorrhage—Hemorrhage refers to an excessive amount of blood lost within a very short time period. With massive blood loss the mother may have a rapid, weak pulse, drop in blood pressure, dizziness, pallor, clammy skin and appear disoriented. Hemorrhage is an emergency situation.

Placental abruption—This condition of pregnancy, also called abruptio placentae, is characterized by sharp pain, a hard, rigid abdomen and vaginal bleeding due to the detachment of the placenta from the uterine wall, placing the mother and fetus at great risk.

flow once she arrives at the health care facility, and obtains baseline **vital signs**, particularly **blood pressure** and pulse rate. Questions to ask the mother include:

- How far along is the pregnancy?

- When did the bleeding begin?

- What color was the bleeding? Bright red indicates fresh, or ongoing bleeding.

- Was there pain with the bleeding?

- How many sanitary pads have you used since the bleeding started? This is to estimate amount of blood loss.

- Did you use anything to stop the blood flow, such as a tampon? Tampons will absorb the blood, and the true amount of bleeding may be masked.

- Is this the first episode of bleeding in this pregnancy? If not, obtain details about previous episodes.

The woman should be closely monitored for any signs of hemorrhage. The health of the fetus is monitored externally. Once bleeding has stopped and the mother must wait for the delivery, she can be at risk of perceiving the pregnancy as failed. This could result in her taking less care of herself, and thereby

putting the fetus at risk. Continued reassurance for the mother helps prevent this from happening.

Prevention

Placenta previa is not preventable, as it is not possible to affect where the placenta will implant. However, once diagnosed, the mother may be instructed to avoid intercourse, get enough rest, and telephone the provider if any bleeding occurs.

Resources

BOOKS

Creasy, Robert K. and Robert Resnik. *Maternal-Fetal Medicine.* Philadelphia: W.B. Saunders Company, 1999.

Feinbloom, Richard I. *Pregnancy, Birth, and the Early Months.* Cambridge, MA: Perseus Publishing, 2000.

Pillitteri, Adele. *Maternal & Child Health Nursing.* 3rd ed. Philadelphia: Lippincott, 1999.

ORGANIZATION

American College of Obstetricians and Gynecologists. 409 12th St., S.W., PO Box 96920 Washington, D.C. 20090-6920. http://www.acog.org.

Esther Csapo Rastegari, R.N., B.S.N., Ed.M.

Placental abruption

Definition

Placental abruption is a condition in **pregnancy** in which the placenta prematurely separates from the uterine wall while the fetus is still *in utero*. While it is seen most often during the third trimester of pregnancy, especially during the labor process, the term can be applied from 20 weeks gestation through term. Severe bleeding, even hemorrhage, can result, putting both the mother and fetus at significant risk. It is also known as placenta abruptio and abruptio placentae.

Description

In most cases placental abruption occurs in a normally implanted placenta, one that is located high on the uterine wall. However, it can occur in tandem with **placenta previa**. In a normal vaginal delivery, the delivery of the placenta follows that of the neonate within about 30 minutes. Because the neonate has been born and is now breathing on his or her own, the separation of the

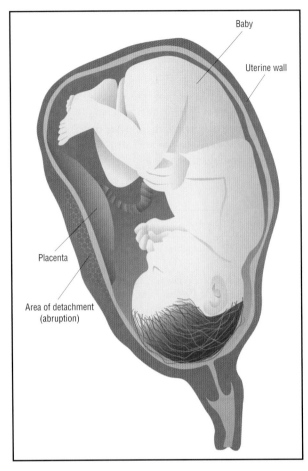

(Diagram showing a baby in the womb and a detached placenta. Illustration by GGS Information Services, Inc. The Gale Group.)

placenta from the uterine wall causes no distress. In placental abruption, however, the premature separation of the placenta deprives the fetus of the oxygen, nutrients, and **gas exchange** taking place at the site of the separation. The cost to the fetus depends on the degree and size of the separation. The risk to the mother depends on the amount of **blood** lost, the subsequent change in circulating blood volume, and its accompanying decrease in tissue perfusion.

Placental abruption occurs in about one in 120 deliveries. Severe abruption leading to fetal death occurs in about one in 420 deliveries. **Cocaine** use increases the risk of abruption by increasing vasoconstriction, and about 10% of mothers using cocaine in the third trimester succumb to placental abruption.

Causes and symptoms

The causes of abruption are not fully understood, but it appears that it may be the end result of a series of fetal-maternal vascular abnormalities. Impaired blood vessel

integrity and suppressed immune function may lie at the core of the development of abruption. Some of the factors leading to placental abruption include:

• Trauma. An abdominal blow, such as that incurred during an automobile accident may cause abruption. Mothers experiencing a severe blow to the abdomen, with subsequent uterine contractions, should be monitored for about 24 hours, even in the absence of vaginal bleeding. This is because there could be a delay in symptoms. Observation of the mother should also include fetal monitoring to assure fetal well-being.

• Maternal hypertension. Mothers who have either chronic high blood pressure or hypertension induced by pregnancy are at increased risk of abruption.

• Maternal age. Placental abruption is seen more often in older women. However, it is unclear whether the advanced age or the increased likelihood of previous gestations is the primary factor.

• Uterine and umbilical cord abnormalities, such as a short cord or a uterine myoma at the placental implantation site.

• Placental abnormalities resulting in poor implantation.

• Cigarette smoking. As the number of cigarettes per day increases, so does the risk of abruption. This may be because of the harmful effect of nicotine on blood vessel integrity.

• Previous placental abruption. The risk of recurrence may be almost 17%.

The classic symptoms of abruption include sharp **abdominal pain**, rigid **abdomen**, vaginal bleeding, uterine contractions, and uterine tenderness. However, these signs are not always present. About 10% of women may have no vaginal bleeding. This is because the blood is pooling behind the placenta that has detached in the center. If the abruption occurred in tandem with labor contraction, and if the abruption is mild or moderate, the **pain** of labor contractions may mask the underlying abdominal pain and uterine tenderness of the abruption. This variability of symptoms emphasizes the need for careful diagnosis.

Diagnosis

Diagnosis of placental abruption, especially when mild or moderate, can be elusive. A thorough maternal history can play a significant role in identifying mothers at increased risk. Severity of abruption cannot be determined only from the volume of visible blood lost, as concealed hemorrhage may be taking place. Pain may be primarily in the back instead of abdominal. It may be sharp and severe, or dull and intermittent. It may be accompanied by nausea and **vomiting**. The uterine

KEY TERMS

Disseminated intravascular coagulation—DIC is a serious medical complication in which the mother's blood no longer clots in the usual manner because of extreme loss of blood. Bruising is visible on the skin, and blood can seep from sites of IV insertion. This is a medical emergency, as it can quickly lead to massive hemorrhage.

Gestation—The age of the fetus in weeks since conception.

Myoma—A benign fibroid tumor of the uterine muscle.

Placenta previa—Placenta previa is a condition of pregnancy in which the placenta, which normally is implanted high on the uterine wall, is instead implanted near the cervical opening. As the uterus begins to change in preparation for labor and delivery, the force exerted on the placenta can cause it to tear, depriving the fetus of nutrition and oxygen, and putting the mother at risk of hemorrhage.

contraction pattern tends to be low in amplitude but high in frequency. If the uterus and abdomen are rigid, external monitoring or contractions may be inaccurate. Uterine tenderness may be localized to the site of detachment, but may also present as generalized. Unfortunately, ultrasound is not very reliable in establishing the presence of placental abruption. Blood work may be done to check on the presence of an abnormal clotting process. Diagnosis may become the piecing together of a puzzle of symptoms, with the experienced practitioner being more likely to solve the puzzle.

Placental abruption is categorized into four degrees of separation. These are:

• Grade 0. Abruption was diagnosed after delivery, upon inspection of the placenta. The placenta will show a small area of clotting on the side of maternal attachment. No other visible maternal or fetal signs of abruption were present.

• Grade 1. Some separation occurred with some vaginal bleeding and changes in maternal vital signs. No fetal distress was noted.

• Grade 2. Moderate separation, fetal distress, uterus is tender to touch.

• Grade 3. Extreme separation; without emergency intervention mother and fetus are at risk of shock, hemorrhage, or death.

Separation may be partial, with vaginal bleeding; partial without vaginal bleeding (known as concealed hemorrhage); complete separation, with vaginal bleeding (likely hemorrhage); or complete separation with concealed hemorrhage. Concealed bleeding is very dangerous because the lack of vaginal bleeding masks the true severity of the condition. Then, if the mother goes into **shock**, it may be unexpected and result in a poor outcome. If the placenta detached in the center, concealed bleeding is more likely to occur. Blood may seep into the uterine wall and result in a condition called *couvelaire uterus*, which is characterized by a hard uterus, no bleeding, and no signs of impending maternal shock. Shock results from the blood loss into the uterine tissue.

Treatment

A mother with suspected placental abruption needs to be admitted to the hospital. As complete a history as possible should be taken. If the mother is in crisis, family or friends may be able to assist with the history. Blood work to check for clotting disorders is done, as placental abruption may be accompanied by disseminated intravascular coagulation (DIC) which can lead to massive hemorrhage. Intravenous (IV) fluids and blood transfusions may be necessary to replace blood lost. Oxygen may be administered. Continuous fetal monitoring is done to assess for signs of fetal distress. Decreased maternal urine output indicates a compromised blood volume with poor tissue perfusion. The severity of the abruption determines the course of treatment. If a small separation has occurred, the pregnancy may be maintained as long as the mother is stable and the fetus does not show signs of distress. If the separation is a grade 0 or 1, and the fetus is near term, a vaginal delivery may be attempted. A separation of grade 3 or 4 necessitates delivery even if the fetus is not sufficiently mature, as the separation has compromised adequate nutrients and oxygen from reaching the fetus, and the accompanying blood lost has put the mother's well-being at risk. If DIC has begun, prompt evacuation of the uterus of the fetus and the placenta can allow for a positive prognosis for the mother. However, surgery poses great risk to the mother because of her compromised ability to clot. Severe hemorrhage, organ failure, and death could occur.

Prognosis

Prognosis is dependent on many factors such as the frequent monitoring of **vital signs**, the degree of separation, amount of blood lost, preexisting fetal complications such as growth retardation and congenital abnormalities, gestational age of the fetus, any permanent organ damage to the mother, and degree of oxygen deprivation. Prompt diagnosis enhances chances for a successful outcome.

Health care team roles

Nurses play a significant role in obtaining a full and accurate patient history. Questions should include maternal symptoms, time elapsed since symptoms began, presence and quality of pain (sharp, dull, constant, intermittent), bleeding (amount and color), and any actions taken, such as medication for pain or use of tampons.

Prevention

While most factors contributing to abruption are not preventable, cigarette **smoking**, cocaine use, and seat belt use with proper placement are important areas on which to focus during **prenatal care**. Identifying a mother at high risk and having a management plan in place can expedite diagnosis, especially if the mother arrives through the emergency department in crisis, and result in a more successful outcome for both mother and baby.

Resources

BOOKS

Creasy, Robert K., and Robert Resnik. *Maternal-Fetal Medicine.* Philadelphia: W.B. Saunders Company, 1999.

Feinbloom, Richard I. *Pregnancy, Birth, and the Early Months.* Cambridge, MA: Perseus Publishing, 2000.

Pillitteri, Adele. *Maternal & Child Health Nursing.* 3rd ed. Philadelphia: Lippincott, 1999.

ORGANIZATION

American College of Obstetricians and Gynecologists. 409 12th St., S.W., PO Box 96920, Washington, D.C. 20090-6920. http://www.acog.com.

Esther Csapo Rastegari, R.N., B.S.N., Ed.M.

Plasma protein tests

Definition

Plasma protein tests are laboratory tests used to evaluate the levels of specific **proteins** in the **blood**. A decrease or increase in the concentration of the protein is associated with one or more clinical conditions. Prior to measuring a specific protein, a comprehensive metabolic profile is usually performed. This profile includes tests for the total protein and albumin. If either of these tests is abnormal, serum protein electrophoresis may be performed in order to determine the cause. Abnormalities seen on the **protein electrophoresis test** as well as other clinical information are used to determine the necessity for specific protein tests. The most frequently measured plasma proteins include alpha-1 antitrypsin (AAT), ceruloplasmin (CER), C3 and C4 (complement proteins), C-reactive protein (CRP), haptoglobin (Hp, HAP), immunoglobulins (IgG, IgA, IgM),transferrin (TRF),and transthyretin (TTR).

Purpose

Plasma protein tests are used to determine whether a specific protein or proteins have increased or decreased in concentration. An abnormal level of total protein or of a specific protein indicates particular diseases or conditions associated with the respective change. Some protein tests are useful for establishing a diagnosis, while others are useful in determining the extent of a condition such as **dehydration** or inflammation.

Precautions

A nurse or phlebotomist who collects the sample for a plasma protein test should follow standard precautions for the prevention of transmission of bloodborne pathogens. Total protein and albumin concentrations are approximately 10% higher in ambulatory persons. Plasma total protein is approximately 0.2–0.4 g/dL higher than serum. Some drugs, especially estrogens and **corticosteroids**, may increase the concentration of specific proteins.

Description

Proteins are vital to the proper functioning of the body. There are more than 3,000 proteins found in a single human cell. Some proteins, such as enzymes, hormones, coagulation factors, lipoproteins, and hemoglobin, are measured routinely and are described in other topics. The proteins considered here are those which are sufficient in concentration to affect results of the total protein or protein electrophoresis tests or are measured by immunonephelometry. Each of the proteins described below, with the exception of total protein and albumin, are measured by this method. In immunonephelometry, plasma or serum is added to a buffer containing an excess of a specific antibody (e.g., anti-haptoglobin). The **antibodies** will bind to the haptoglobin molecules (antigen), forming small soluble immune complexes. Monochromatic light (usually 450-550 nm) passing through the reaction tube will be scattered by the immune complexes as they form. Forward-angle light scatter is measured by a light detector (photomultiplier tube) placed at an angle (usually 70 degrees) to the incident light. The combination of antibody and antigen molecules occurs rapidly, and the photodector current increases with time until a peak signal is reached. This peak is proportional to antigen concentration. To insure that the antibody molecules are in excess, an addition of reagent antigen is injected into the reaction mixture after the peak rate is obtained. This will produce an increase in light scattering provided that sufficient antibody remains. The clinical significance of each protein test is described below.

Total protein: The total protein of plasma or serum is measured by a colorimetric reaction called the biuret method. The sample is added to an alkaline solution of **copper** II sulfate. The copper ions form coordinate bonds with the carbonyl and imine groups of the protein. This causes the reagent to change from a sky blue to a purple color. The absorbance of the solution at 540 nm is proportional to protein concentration.

Total protein is increased in conditions causing dehydration. They include **vomiting**, **diarrhea**, **diabetes insipidus**, **diabetes mellitus**, and Addison's disease. Total protein is increased in conditions that cause inflammation. These include **cancer**, autoimmune diseases, and chronic or severe infections. Total protein is also increased by monoclonal immunoglobulin production caused by benign or malignant proliferation of antibody-secreting cells (plasma cells) such as **multiple myeloma**. Low total protein can result from protein loss, as occurs in hemorrhage, glomerulonephritis, nephrosis, protein-losing gastroenteropathy, and **burns**; excessive hydration as occurs in salt retention syndromes and the syndrome of inappropriate antidiuretic hormone (SIADH); or decreased synthesis resulting from starvation and chronic **liver** disease.

Albumin: The albumin in plasma comprises 50-65% of the total protein. In addition to holding water in the vascular bed (maintenance of oncotic pressure) albumin is primarily a transport protein and is responsible for the protein binding of most drugs. It is measured by a dye binding method using either bromcresol green (BCG) or bromcresol purple (BCP). These dyes selectively bind to albumin, forming a colored complex. The color formed is proportional to albumin concentration. Plasma albumin is increased by dehydration or intravenous infusion of albumin as a blood volume expander. It is decreased in hemorrhage, renal disease, salt retention, SIADH, liver disease, starvation, inflammation, malignancy, and **infection**.

Alpha-1 antitrypsin: ATT is a glycoprotein (molecular weight 52,000) made by the liver. ATT is an inhibitor of the enzyme trypsin as well as of other proteolytic enzymes (serine proteases) that are released from phagocytic white blood cells during inflammation. ATT reduces the damage to tissues caused by the **immune response**, and plasma levels increase up to two-fold in acute and chronic inflammatory conditions. Proteins such as ATT that are increased in response to inflammation are called acute phase proteins. They are sensitive markers for tissue injury, **myocardial infarction**, infection, malignancy, and autoimmune diseases.

A deficiency of AAT results in excessive inflammation in tissues that are exposed to **bacteria** and other foreign cells, commonly the **lungs** and gastrointestinal organs. AAT deficiency is usually inherited. Expression of the genes for AAT is codominant. The most common normal phenotype is MM. The phenotype ZZ (homozygous for the Z variant) produces only about 10% of normal activity and is most commonly associated with immunological damage. The most frequent complications involve the lungs (**emphysema**) and the hepatobiliary tract (hepatitis and **cirrhosis**). A deficiency of AAT is suspected when the alpha-1 band of serum protein electrophoresis is absent or below 1% of the total protein. The AAT concentration is measured by immunonephelometry and the variant proteins can be identified by high-resolution gel electrophoresis.

Ceruloplasmin: CER is a protein (molecular weight 120,000) produced by the liver. It is an acute phase protein, and increased CER may contribute slightly to the size of the alpha-2 band on electrophoresis. Ceruloplasmin is measured as an aid to the diagnosis of Wilson's disease. This is an autosomal recessive disease in which the binding of copper by CER and the excretion of copper into the bile are impaired. Copper accumulates in the tissues, principally the liver, **central nervous system**, and eyes. Deposition in the eyes produces Kayser-Fleischer rings (green to brown rings around the edge of the cornea), a classic sign on physical exam. Copper deposition damages tissues, causing cirrhosis of the liver and damage to the lenticular area of the **brain** (hepatolenticular degeneration). It may also cause **osteoporosis**, renal, joint, cardiac, and other damage. Plasma levels below half the lower limit of normal and low plasma copper are suggestive but are not conclusive in the absence of clinical signs. CER is measured by immunonephelometry.

C3 and C4: C3 and C4 are glycoproteins that act along with other complement proteins to facilitate lysis of antibody-coated cells. The complement system consists of nine proteins in the classical pathway and an additional five that act in the alternative pathway. Deficiencies of 10 complement proteins have been described. A deficiency of C3 or C4 is associated with systemic lupus erythematosus (SLE) and other autoimmune diseases. The deficiency of either complement component may be responsible in part for the development of the disease by preventing the effective removal of immune complexes. C3 and C4 deficiency are also associated with severe recurrent infections. In active SLE, glomerulonephritis, cirrhosis, and **sepsis**, C3, C4, and complement activity may be reduced due to consumption by immune complex formation. In **rheumatoid arthritis**, **rheumatic fever**, and some chronic dermatologic diseases, C3 and C4 levels are elevated owing to increased complement activation.

C-reactive protein (CRP): C-reactive protein is a protein consisting of five subunits (molecular weight 120,000) produced mainly in the liver. Its name is derived from the fact that it binds to the C-polysaccharide of the capsule of *Streptococcus pneumoniae*. Increased levels are seen in patients with pneumococcal **pneumonia** as well as other acute infections and inflammatory conditions. In the absence of inflammation, CRP levels in plasma are very low (<4 mg/L). Levels in inflammation can reach several hundred-fold above normal, causing a small but distinct band in the gamma zone on electrophoresis. Recent studies have shown that a CRP near the upper limit of normal (5-10 mg/L) in persons with a history of chronic inflammation is a risk factor for **coronary artery disease**. A new test, called high-sensitivity CRP, can measure CRP levels below 1 mg/L and is being used by some cardiologists to predict the risk of coronary artery disease in persons with normal total **cholesterol** who have no history of **angina** or **heart** disease. CRP is measured by immunonephelometry or enzyme immunoassay.

Haptoglobin: Hp is a glycoprotein (molecular weight 85,000-100,000) made by the liver. Hp binds to free plasma hemoglobin, transporting it to the liver, where the complex is removed by the reticuloendothelial cells. Low levels are seen in persons with intravascular hemolysis (e.g., following an intravascular transfusion reaction). Haptoglobin is also an acute phase protein. Hp and alpha-2 macroglobulin are responsible for the increased density of the alpha-2 band on electrophoresis seen in acute and chronic inflammatory states. Hp is measured by immunonephelometry.

Immunoglobulins G, A and M (IgG, IgA, and IgM): Immunoglobulins are antibodies produced by B lymphocytes and secreted by plasma cells. They will be increased in response to infections, malignancy, and autoimmune diseases—all of which produce a polyclonal response (i.e., a general increase in all three immunoglobulin classes). This response causes a diffuse increase in the density of the gamma zone on electrophoresis. In malignant or benign plasma cell disorders, proliferation of a single clone of plasma cells results in the accumulation of identical antibody molecules called a

KEY TERMS

Edematous—The state of having swelling (edema) caused by the collection of excess fluid within tissues.

Hematoma—Swelling and subsequent bruising when blood leaks from a vein into local tissues; can be caused by improper venipuncture when the needle has gone through a vein or when the needle has been inserted incorrectly.

Hemolytic—Destructive to red blood cells.

Venipuncture—Puncture of a vein with a needle for the purpose of withdrawing a blood sample for analysis.

Wilson's disease—A genetic disorder that creates excessive amounts of copper in the body. Patients often have damaging deposits of copper in the brain, liver, and other organs, and a green discoloration from copper around the iris of the eyes. This disease is also called hepatolenticular degeneration.

monoclonal gammopathy. This may be recognized on electrophoresis as an area of restricted mobility in the gamma zone. Decreased plasma concentration of one or more immunoglobulin classes may be associated with immunologic impairment and result in both recurrent and opportunistic infections. Both increases and decreases of each immunoglobulin class can be detected by immunonephelometry, using antibodies specific for each. For example, rabbit anti-human IgG can be used to measure the plasma concentration of IgG.

Transferrin: TRF is a glycoprotein (molecular weight 77,000) made by the liver. It is responsible for transport of **iron** from the gut to the **bone** marrow. The concentration of transferrin in the plasma is directly related to the total iron binding capacity (TIBC). In iron deficiency, the transferrin level is increased, causing an increase in the density of the beta globulin band on electrophoresis. Transferrin levels are decreased in nephrosis, liver disease, starvation, and chronic illness. Like albumin, transferrin is reduced in acute and chronic inflammation and is referred to as a negative acute phase protein.

Transthyretin: Transthyretin or prealbumin is a glycoprotein (molecular weight 54,000) made in the liver. TTR has a very short half-life making it a useful marker for protein calorie malnutrition. In persons with deficient protein intake, the plasma level of TTR decreases before those of most other proteins. The level of TTR can be monitored to assess the efficacy of dietary intervention in malnourished persons. TTR is measured by immunonephelometry.

Preparation

Prior to performing the venipuncture, the nurse or other health care professional should document any medications the patient is currently taking, and any medical conditions that could influence the protein tests. For example, oral contraceptives, estrogen-containing drugs, or **pregnancy** can increase the level of ceruloplasmin.

Aftercare

The patient may feel discomfort when blood is drawn from a vein. Bruising may occur at the puncture site, or the person may feel dizzy or faint. Pressure should be applied to the puncture site until the bleeding stops, to reduce bruising. Warm packs can also be placed over the puncture site to relieve discomfort.

Complications

In normal circumstances, a blood draw for protein tests takes only a few minutes, and the patient experiences only minor discomfort from the puncture.

Results

The physician will carefully consider the results from the specific protein test within the context of the patient's current health status to make decisions on further testing, diagnosis, and treatment. The protein test results must be interpreted by comparison with standard reference ranges provided by the laboratory that has performed the test. The normal ranges shown below are frequently cited for the methods described previously.

- total protein: 6.0–8.0 g/dL nonambulatory; 6.5–8.5 g/dL ambulatory
- albumin: 3.0–5.0 g/dL nonambulatory; 3.5–5.5 g/dL ambulatory
- alpha-1 antitrypsin: 90–200 mg/dL
- ceruloplasmin: 20–60 mg/dL
- C-reactive protein: 0.7–8.2 mg/L
- Hs-CPR: 0.08–3.1 mg/L
- C3: 90–180 mg/dL
- C4: 10–40 mg/dL
- haptoglobin: 30–200 mg/dL
- immunoglobulins: IgG: 700–1600 mg/dL; IgA: 70–400 mg/dL; IgM: 40–230 mg/dL
- transferrin: 200–360 mg/dL
- transthyretin: 20–40 mg/dL

Health care team roles

In accordance with the physician's orders, the nurse, phlebotomist, or laboratory professional usually prepares the patient, performs the blood draw, and readies the specimen for transport to the laboratory for analysis. A clinical laboratory scientist, CLS(NCA)/medical technologist, MT(ASCP) or clinical laboratory technician CLT(NCA)/medical laboratory technician MLT(ASCP) performs the testing. Results are interpreted by a physician.

Resources

BOOKS

Fischbach, Frances. "Diagnostic Testing." In *A Manual of Laboratory & Diagnostic Tests,* 6th ed. Philadelphia: Lippincott Williams & Wilkins, 2000, pp. 1-25.

Johnson, A. Myron, Elizabeth M. Rohlfs, and Lawrence M. Silverman. "Proteins." In *Tietz Textbook of Clinical Chemistry,* 3rd ed., edited by Carl A. Burtis and Edward R. Ashwood. Philadelphia: W. B. Saunders Company, 1999, pp. 478-523.

Kee, Joyce LeFever. *Laboratory & Diagnostic Tests with Nursing Implications.* 5th ed. Stamford, CT: Appleton & Lange, 1999, pp. xv-xix, 27-29, 111-112, 214-215, 269-271, 362-364.

Sacher, Ronald A., Richard A. McPherson, with Joseph M. Campos. "Special Tests in Evaluation of Liver Disease." In *Widmann's Clinical Interpretation of Laboratory Tests,* 11th ed. Philadelphia: F. A. Davis Company, 2000, pp. 586-593.

ORGANIZATIONS

The American Society for Clinical Laboratory Science. 7910 Woodmont Ave., Suite 523, Bethesda, MD 20814. (301) 657-2768. http://www.ascls.org.

Wilson's Disease Association. 4 Navaho Dr., Brookfield, CT 06804. (800) 399-0266. http://www.wilsonsdisease.org.

Linda D. Jones, B.A., PBT (ASCP)

Plasma renin activity

Definition

Renin is an enzyme released by the **kidneys** to help control the body's sodium-potassium balance, fluid volume, and **blood pressure**. Renin splits angiotensinogen in plasma-forming angiotensin I. This compound is acted upon by plasma converting enzymes produced in the **lungs** to form angiotensin II or III. These powerful vasoconstrictors increase **blood** pressure and stimulate aldosterone release by the adrenal cortex.

Purpose

Plasma renin activity (PRA), also called plasma renin assay, is used to investigate the cause of **hypertension**. PRA is increased in persons with hypertension of renal origin. It is used to classify persons with essential hypertension. A PRA test, along with a measurement of the plasma aldosterone level, is used for the differential diagnosis of primary and secondary aldosteronism. The latter condition is caused by increased renin release by the kidney(s), and therefore, elevated PRA. Patients with primary hyperaldosteronism (caused by an adrenal tumor that overproduces aldosterone) will have an increased aldosterone level with decreased renin activity.

Precautions

Patients taking diuretics, antihypertensives, vasodilators, oral contraceptives, and licorice should discontinue use of these substances for two to four weeks before the test. It should be noted that renin activity is increased in **pregnancy** and in diets with reduced salt intake. Also, since renin is affected by body position, as well as by diurnal variation, blood samples should be drawn in the morning, and the position of the patient (sitting or lying down) should be noted.

The nurse or plebotomist performing the venipuncture should follow **universal precautions** for the prevention of transmission of bloodborne pathogens. Blood should be collected in EDTA in a chilled syringe, and the sample immediately placed on ice. The plasma should be separated from the cells immediately and then frozen until assay.

Description

The kidneys normally release renin in response to decreased blood volume, low plasma sodium, and high plasma potassium levels. The release of renin is the first step in the renin-angiotensin-aldosterone cycle. Renin is produced and secreted by specialized cells called juxtaglomerular cells, located at the junction where the distal tubule meets the afferent and efferent arterioles. These cells secrete renin in response to a decreased flow of blood through the afferent arteriole. Renin is a proteolytic enzyme; it splits angiotensinogen in the plasma forming angiotensin I, which in turn is converted to angiotensin II or III by a converting enzyme produced by the lungs. Angiotensins II and III are powerful blood

vessel constrictors. In addition, they stimulate the release of aldosterone from the cortex of the **adrenal glands**. Aldosterone causes increased sodium reabsorption by the kidneys. As sodium is reabsorbed, the osmotic pressure (osmolality) of the plasma rises, and this stimulates osmoreceptors in the **central nervous system**. These cause secretion of antidiuretic hormone (vasopressin) from the posterior **pituitary gland**. Vasopressin causes more water to be reabsorbed by the kidney. This increases blood volume and restores the blood pressure in the afferent arterioles reducing renin release. Together, angiotensin and aldosterone increase the blood volume, the blood pressure, and the blood sodium to re-establish the body's sodium-potassium and fluid volume balance.

High blood pressure affects about 20 million people in the United States and is a major risk factor for cardiovascular disease and **stroke**. More than 90% of hypertension is due to essential (primary) hypertension. This form of high blood pressure is genetic and its causes are unknown. Essential hypertension is aggravated by excess sodium intake, and affected individuals vary in their response to treatment. Plasma renin activity can be used to classify persons with essential hypertension into groups (high, normal, or low PRA) that respond differently to treatment. For instance, low PRA-type essential hypertension results from excessive aldosterone secretion (primary aldosteronism), and is effectively treated by diuretic therapy.

Measurement

Renin itself is not actually measured in the PRA test. There are two forms of this test. The classic test is called the plasma renin activity (PRA) test, and the newer form is called the plasma renin concentration (PRC) test. Both tests measure the conversion of angiotensinogen to angiotensin I by renin. The difference between the two is that the former uses endogenous (i.e., the patient's own) plasma angiotensinogen as the substrate, while the latter uses excess angiotensinogen from an exogenous source such as sheep plasma. To perform the activity test, the plasma is thawed and a small measured amount is added to a buffered solution at pH 6 that contains phenylmethyl sulfonyl fluoride to inhibit plasma angiotensinases that also split angiotensinogen. The mixture is incubated for one hour at 98.6°F(37°C) and then refrigerated to stop the enzyme activity. Following this, the angiotensin I produced is measured by radioimmunoassay (RIA). To correct for the endogenous angiotensin I present beforehand, an equal amount of the thawed sample is kept at 4°C and then measured for angiotensin I activity by RIA. This value is subtracted from the test result obtained from the 98.6°F(37°C) incubation. The plasma renin concentration test is performed as described above, except that the test plasma is first treated with an acid buffer to destroy the endogenous angiotensinogen. A measured volume of the treated plasma is added to a buffered solution containing an excess amount of exogenous angiotensinogen. The amount of angiotensin I produced following the incubation is equivalent to the maximum rate of enzyme activity, and is a more accurate reflection of renin concentration because it is independent of the plasma angiotensinogen

Both the PRA and the PRC are extremely difficult to perform. Not only is renin itself unstable, but the patient's body position and the time the specimen is collected affect the results. Also, the sample must be collected properly: drawn into a chilled syringe and collection tube, placed on ice, and sent to the laboratory immediately. Even when all these procedures are followed, results can vary significantly. An alternative method is the measurement of plasma renin mass by double antibody sandwich immunoassay. This assay uses two **monoclonal antibodies**, one that binds to the prorenin molecule and a second that binds to renin. This assay detects only active renin because the inactive enzyme is not bound by the second antibody. The mass unit assay is independent of angiotensinogen and therefore not as subject to procedural errors related to temperature inactivation of the enzyme.

Renin stimulation tests

A renin stimulation test is performed to help diagnose and distinguish primary from secondary aldosteronism. The test protocol involves either stimulating salt loss by administration of furosemide, a diuretic; or restricting the patient's salt intake for three to five days. A low sodium level and standing posture stimulate renin release in normal persons, resulting in a two to three fold increase in PRA. Persons with secondary aldosteronism (renin-mediated aldosteronism) typically show a five-fold increase in PRA. Persons with primary aldosteronism show no increase in PRA over the baseline.

One example of a stimulation test is performed as follows. With the patient having been on a low-salt diet and lying down for the test, a blood sample for PRA is obtained. The PRA is repeated with the patient still on the low-salt diet, but now standing upright for two or more hours. In cases of primary hyperaldosteronism, the blood volume is greatly expanded, and a change in position or reduced salt intake does not result in decreased renal blood flow or decreased blood sodium. As a result, renin levels do not increase. However, in secondary hyperaldosteronism, blood sodium levels decrease with a lowered salt intake, and when the patient is standing upright, the renal blood flow decreases as well. Consequently, renin levels will increase.

Captopril suppression test

The captopril test is a screening test for renovascular hypertension. This is a common form of secondary aldosteronism. For this test, a baseline PRA test is measured; then the patient receives an oral dose of captopril, an angiotensin-converting enzyme (ACE) inhibitor. Blood pressure measurements are taken at this time and again at 60 minutes, when another PRA test is done. Patients with kidney-based hypertension demonstrate greater falls in blood pressure and increases in PRA after captopril administration than do those with essential hypertension. Consequently, the captopril test is an excellent screening procedure to determine the need for a more invasive radiographic evaluation such as renal arteriography.

Preparation

This test requires a blood sample. For the PRA, the patient should maintain a normal diet with a normal amount of sodium (approximately 3 g per day) for three days before the test, unless specified otherwise as for a stimulation test. It is recommended that the patient be fasting (nothing to eat or drink) from midnight on the day of the test.

Aftercare

Discomfort or bruising may occur at the puncture site. Applying pressure to the puncture site until the bleeding stops helps to reduce bruising; warm packs relieve discomfort. Some people feel dizzy or faint after blood has been drawn and should be treated accordingly.

Complications

Other than potential bruising at the puncture site, and/or **dizziness**, there are no complications associated with this test.

Results

Reference values for the PRA test are laboratory-specific and depend upon the patient's diet (sodium restricted or normal), the age of the patient, and the patient's posture at the time of the test. Values are also affected if renin has been stimulated or if the patient has received an ACE inhibitor like captopril. A representative normal range for the PRA test in adults on a normal diet is 0.2-3.3 nanograms angiotensin I per mL per hour. For the monoclonal double antibody sandwich assay (direct

KEY TERMS

Aldosteronism—A disorder caused by excessive production of the hormone aldosterone, which is produced by a part of the adrenal glands called the adrenal cortex. Causes include a tumor of the adrenal gland (Conn's syndrome), or a disorder reducing the blood flow through the kidney. This leads to overproduction of renin and angiotensin, and in turn causes excessive aldosterone production. Symptoms include hypertension, impaired kidney function, thirst, and muscle weakness.

Conn's syndrome—A disorder caused by excessive aldosterone secretion by a benign tumor of one of the adrenal glands. This results in malfunction of the body's salt and water balance and subsequently causes hypertension. Symptoms include thirst, muscle weakness, and excessive urination.

renin assay), the normal range is 7-76 U/mL for persons not lying down.

Increased PRA levels are seen in up to 15% of persons with essential hypertension (associated with renal injury or vascular disease), malignant hypertension, and kidney-based (renovascular) hypertension. Renin-producing renal and other tumors, while rare, can also cause elevated levels, as can cirrhosis, low blood volume due to hemorrhage, and diminished adrenal function (Addison's disease). Decreased renin levels may indicate increased blood volume due to a high-sodium diet, salt-retaining steroids, primary aldosteronism, or licorice ingestion syndrome. About 25% of persons with essential hypertension will have low renin levels.

Health care team roles

Physicians order PRA tests and interpret the results. A nurse or phlebotomist usually collects the blood and is responsible for icing the sample and transporting to the laboratory. Clinical laboratory scientists/medical technologists perform the renin (and angiotensin I) tests.

Resources

BOOKS

Jacobs, David S. *Laboratory Test Handbook,* 4th ed. Hudson, OH: Lexi-Comp Inc., 1996.

Pagana, Kathleen Deska. *Mosby's Manual of Diagnostic and Laboratory Tests.* St. Louis, MO: Mosby, Inc., 1998.

Victoria E. DeMoranville

Plasmapheresis

Definition

Plasmapheresis is a **blood** purification procedure used to treat several autoimmune diseases. It is also known as therapeutic plasma exchange.

Purpose

In an autoimmune disease, the **immune system** attacks the body's own tissues. In many autoimmune diseases, the chief weapons of attack are **antibodies**, **proteins** that circulate in the bloodstream until they meet and bind with the target tissue. Once bound, they impair the functions of the target, and signal other immune components to respond as well.

Plasmapheresis is used to remove antibodies from the bloodstream, thereby preventing them from attacking their targets. It does not directly affect the immune system's ability to make more antibodies, and therefore may only offer temporary benefit. This procedure is most useful in acute, self-limited disorders such as Guillain-Barré syndrome, or when chronic disorders, such as myasthenia gravis, become more severe in symptoms. In these instances, a rapid improvement could save the patient's life. Neurologic diseases comprise 90% of the diseases that could profit from plasmapheresis.

Precautions

Patients with clotting disorders may not be suitable candidates for plasmapheresis.

Description

The basic procedure consists of removal of blood, separation of blood cells from plasma, and return of these blood cells to the body's circulation, diluted with fresh plasma or a substitute. Because of concerns over viral **infection** and allergic reaction, fresh plasma is not routinely used. Instead, the most common substitute is saline solution with sterilized human albumin protein. During the course of a single session, two to three liters of plasma is removed and replaced.

Plasmapheresis requires insertion of a venous catheter, either in a limb or central vein. Central veins allow higher flow rates and are more convenient for repeat procedures, but are more often the site of complications, especially bacterial infection.

When blood is outside the body, it must be treated to prevent it from clotting. While most of the anticlotting agent is removed from the blood during treatment, some is returned to the patient.

KEY TERMS

Anaphylaxis—Also called anaphylactic shock, it is a severe allergic reaction to a foreign substance that the patient has had contact with. Penicillin is an example of a substance that causes severe allergic reactions for some people.

Antibody—Chemicals produced by the body to defend it against bacteria, viruses, or other cells foreign to the body (antigens). Each specific antibody reacts against a specific foreign body. Antibodies are also termed immunoglobulins.

Autoimmune—Autoimmune refers to the body's development of intolerance of the antigens on its own cells.

Hemodialysis—A method to take out unwanted parts of the blood. The patient's blood is run through a catheter and tubing into a machine called a dialyzer, which filters out the unwanted blood component.

Plasma—Plasma makes up 50% of human blood. It is a watery fluid that carries red cells, white cells, and platelets throughout the body.

Three procedures are available:

- "Discontinuous flow centrifugation." Only one venous catheter line is required. Approximately 300 mL of blood is removed at a time and centrifuged to separate plasma from blood cells.

- "Continuous flow centrifugation." Two venous lines are used. This method requires slightly less blood volume to be out of the body at any one time.

- "Plasma filtration." Two venous lines are used. The pasma is filtered using standard hemodialysis equipment. It requires less than 100 mL of blood to be outside the body at one time.

A single plasmapheresis session may be effective, although it is more common to have several sessions per week over the course of two weeks or more.

Preparation

Good **nutrition** and plenty of rest make the procedure less stressful. The treating physician determines which of the patient's medications should be discontinued before the plasmapheresis session.

Aftercare

The patient may experience **dizziness**, nausea, numbness, tingling, or lightheadedness during or after the procedure. These effects usually pass quickly, allowing the patient to return to normal activities the same day.

Risks

Reinfusion (replacement) with human plasma may cause **anaphylaxis**, a life threatening allergic reaction. All procedures may cause a mild allergic reaction, leading to

fever, chills, and **rash**. Bacterial infection is a risk, especially when a central venous catheter is used. Reaction to the citrate anticoagulant used may cause cramps and numbness, though these usually resolve on their own. Patients with impaired kidney function may require drug treatment for the effects of citrate **metabolism**.

Plasma contains clotting agents, chemicals that allow the blood to coagulate into a solid clot. Plasma exchange removes these. Bleeding complications are rare following plasmapheresis, but may require replacement of clotting factors.

Normal results

Plasmapheresis is an effective temporary treatment for:

- Guillain-Barré syndrome (an acute neurological disorder following a viral infection that produces progressive muscle weakness and paralysis)

- Myasthenia gravis (an autoimmune disease that causes muscle weakness)

- chronic inflammatory demyelinating polyneuropathy (a chronic neurological disorder caused by destruction of the myelin sheath of peripheral nerves, which produces symptoms similar to Guillain-Barré syndrome)

- thrombotic thrombocytopenic purpura (a rare blood disorder)

- Paraproteinemic peripheral neuropathies (a neurological disorder affecting the peripheral nerves)

- blood that is too thick (hyperviscosity)

Other conditions may respond to plasmapheresis as well. Beneficial effects are usually seen within several days. Effects commonly last up to several months, although longer-lasting changes are possible, presumably by inducing shifts in **immune response**.

Resources

BOOKS

Brenner, Barry M., and Floyd C. Rector. *Brenner & Rector's the Kidney*. Philadelphia: Saunders Elsevier, 2008.

Richard Robinson

Plasmodium infection *see* **Malaria**

Plastic, reconstructive, and cosmetic surgery

Definition

Plastic, reconstructive, and cosmetic surgery procedures are a variety of operations performed in order to repair or restore body parts to look normal, or to change a body part to look better. These types of surgery are highly specialized. They are characterized by careful preparation of a person's skin and tissues, by precise cutting and suturing techniques, and by care taken to minimize scarring. Recent advances in the development of miniaturized instruments, new materials for artificial limbs and body parts, and improved surgical techniques have expanded the range of plastic surgery procedures that can be performed.

Purpose

Although these three types of surgery share some common techniques and approaches, they have somewhat different emphases. Plastic surgery is usually performed to treat **birth defects** and to remove skin blemishes such as warts, acne scars, or birthmarks. Cosmetic surgery procedures are performed to make persons look younger or enhance their appearance in other ways. Reconstructive surgery is used to reattach body parts severed in combat or accidents, to perform skin grafts after severe **burns**, or to reconstruct parts of person's body that were missing at birth or removed by surgery. Reconstructive surgery is the oldest form of plastic surgery, having developed out of the need to treat wounded soldiers in wartime.

Demographics

The top 10 most commonly performed elective cosmetic surgeries in the United States include the following:

- liposuction
- breast augmentation
- eyelid surgery
- face lift
- tummy tuck
- collagen injections
- chemical peel
- laser skin resurfacing
- rhinoplasty
- forehead lift

There were approximately 31 million surgical procedures performed in the United States in 2006. Because many plastic and reconstructive surgical procedures are performed in private professional offices or as outpatient procedures, accurate statistics concerning the number of procedures performed are not available.

Description

Plastic surgery

Plastic surgery includes a number of different procedures that usually involve skin. Operations to remove excess fat from the **abdomen** ("tummy tucks"), dermabrasion to remove acne scars or tattoos, and reshaping the cartilage in children's ears (otoplasty) are common applications of plastic surgery.

Cosmetic surgery

Most cosmetic surgery is done on the face. It is intended either to correct disfigurement or to enhance a person's features. The most common cosmetic procedure for children is correction of a cleft lip or palate. In adults, the most common procedures are remodeling of the nose (rhinoplasty), removal of baggy skin around the eyelids (blepharoplasty), face lifts (rhytidectomy), or changing the size or shape of the breasts (mammoplasty). Although many people still think of cosmetic surgery as only for women, growing numbers of men are choosing to have face lifts and eyelid surgery, as well as hair transplants and "tummy tucks."

Reconstructive surgery

Reconstructive surgery is often performed on burn and accident victims. It may involve the rebuilding of severely fractured bones, as well as skin grafting. Reconstructive surgery includes such procedures as the reattachment of an amputated finger or toe, or implanting a prosthesis. Prostheses are artificial structures and materials that are used to replace missing limbs or teeth, or arthritic hip and knee joints.

KEY TERMS

Blepharoplasty—Surgical reshaping of the eyelid.

Dermabrasion—A technique for removing the upper layers of skin with planing wheels powered by compressed air.

Face lift—Plastic surgery performed to remove sagging skin and wrinkles from an individual's face.

Liposuction—A surgical technique for removing fat from under the skin by vacuum suctioning.

Mammoplasty—Surgery performed to change the size or shape of breasts.

Rhinoplasty—Surgery performed to change the shape of the nose.

Diagnosis/Preparation

General preparation

Preparation for nonemergency plastic or reconstructive surgery includes individual education, as well as medical considerations. Some operations, such as nose reshaping or the removal of warts, small birthmarks, and tattoos can be done as outpatient procedures under **local anesthesia**. Most plastic and reconstructive surgery, however, involves a stay in the hospital and **general anesthesia**.

Medical preparation

Preparation for plastic surgery includes the surgeon's detailed assessment of the parts of an individual's body that will be involved. Skin grafts require evaluating suitable areas of skin for the right color and texture to match the skin at the graft site. Face lifts and cosmetic surgery in the eye area require very close attention to the texture of the skin and the placement of surgical cuts (incisions).

Persons scheduled for plastic surgery under general anesthesia will be given a **physical examination**, **blood** and urine tests, and other tests to make sure that they do not have any previously undetected health problems or blood clotting disorders. The surgeon will check the list of prescription medications that the prospective patient may be taking to make sure that none of them will interfere with normal blood clotting or interact with the anesthetic.

Individuals are asked to avoid using aspirin or medications containing aspirin for a week to two weeks before surgery, because these drugs lengthen the time of blood clotting. Smokers are asked to stop **smoking** two weeks before surgery because smoking interferes with the healing process. For some types of plastic surgery, individuals may be asked to donate several units of their own blood before the procedure, in case a transfusion is needed during the operation. The prospective patient will be asked to sign a consent form before the operation.

Personal education

The surgeon will meet with the prospective patient before the operation is scheduled, in order to explain the procedure and to be sure that the individual is realistic about the expected results. This consideration is particularly important for people undergoing cosmetic surgery.

Medical considerations

Some people should not have plastic surgery because of certain medical risks. These groups include:

- persons recovering from a heart attack, severe infection (for example, pneumonia), or other serious illnesses
- people with infectious hepatitis or HIV infections
- individuals with cancer whose cancer might spread (metastasize)
- people who are extremely overweight (Individuals who are more than 30% overweight should not have liposuction.)
- persons with blood clotting disorders

Psychological

Plastic, cosmetic, and reconstructive surgeries have an important psychological dimension because of the high value placed on outward appearance in Western society. Many people who are born with visible deformities or disfigured by accidents later in life develop emotional problems related to social rejection. Other people work in fields such as acting, modeling, media journalism, and even politics, where their employment depends on how they look. Some people have unrealistic expectations of cosmetic surgery and think that it will solve all their life problems. It is important for anyone considering non-emergency plastic or cosmetic surgery to be realistic about its results. One type of psychiatric disorder, called body dysmorphic disorder, is characterized by an excessive preoccupation with imaginary or minor flaws in appearance. Persons with this disorder frequently seek unnecessary plastic surgery.

Aftercare

Medical

Medical aftercare following plastic surgery under general anesthesia includes bringing patients to a recovery room, monitoring their **vital signs**, and giving medications to relieve **pain** as necessary. Persons who have had fat removed from the abdomen may be kept in bed for as long as two weeks. Individuals who have had mammoplasties, breast reconstruction, and some types of facial surgery typically remain in the hospital for a week after the operation. Those who have had liposuction or eyelid surgery are usually sent home in a day or two.

People who have had outpatient procedures are usually given **antibiotics** to prevent **infection** and are sent home as soon as their vital signs are normal.

Psychological

Some individuals may need follow-up **psychotherapy** or counseling after plastic or reconstructive surgery. These people typically include children whose schooling and social relationships have been affected by birth defects, as well as persons of any age whose deformities or disfigurements were caused by trauma from accidents, war injuries, or violent crimes.

Risks

The risks associated with plastic, cosmetic, and reconstructive surgery include the postoperative complications that can occur with any surgical operation under anesthesia. These complications include wound infection, internal bleeding, **pneumonia**, and reactions to the anesthesia.

In addition to these general risks, some plastic, cosmetic, and reconstructive surgical procedures carry specific risks:

- formation of undesirable scar tissue

- development of persistent pain, redness, or swelling in the area of the surgery

- infection inside the body related to inserting a prosthesis (These infections can result from contamination at the time of surgery or from bacteria migrating into the area around the prosthesis at a later time.)

- anemia or fat embolisms from liposuction

- rejection of skin grafts or tissue transplants

- loss of normal feeling or function in the area of the operation (For example, it is not unusual for women who have had mammoplasties to lose sensation in their nipples.)

- complications resulting from unforeseen technological problems (The best-known example of this problem was the discovery in the mid-1990s that breast implants made with silicone gel could leak into the recipient's body.)

Normal results

Normal results include an individual's recovery from the surgery with satisfactory results and without complications.

Morbidity and mortality rates

Morbidity and mortality rates vary with the complexity and severity of different procedures. Mortality is similar to that associated with all surgical procedures. Morbidity is influenced by personal expectations. From a surgical perspective, most morbidity is due to errors associated with anesthesia, procedure, pain medications, and after care. From an individual's perspective, morbidity involves the degree to which actual results compared to expected outcomes. The latter distinction is very subjective.

Alternatives

Alternatives to plastic, reconstructive, and cosmetic surgical procedures include using various products that may be affixed to articles of clothing or the surface of the body.

Resources

BOOKS

Loftus, J. M. *The Smart Woman's Guide to Plastic Surgery.* 2nd ed. New York: McGraw-Hill, 2007.

Mendelson, R. *The Chase for Beauty.* Garden City, NY: Morgan James, 2008.

Papel, I. D. *Facial Plastic and Reconstructive Surgery.* 3rd ed. New York: Thieme Medical, 2008.

Shiffman, M. A., S. J. Mirrafati, S. M. Lam, and C. G. Cueteeaux. *Simplified Facial Rejuvenation.* New York: Springer, 2007.

Thorne, C. H., S. P. Bartlett, R. W. Beasley, S. J. Aston, and G. C. Gurtner. *Grabb and Smith's Plastic Surgery.* 6th ed. Philadelphia: Lippincott Williams and Wilkins, 2006.

PERIODICALS

Davison, S. P. "Essentials of plastic surgery." *Plastic and Reconstructive Surgery* 120, no. 7 (2007): 2112–2125.

Doer, T. D. "Lipoplasty of the face and neck." *Current Opinions in Otolaryngology, Head and Neck Surgery* 15, no. 4 (2007): 228–232.

Jose, R. M. "Plastic surgery: discipline defined by techniques." *Plastic and Reconstructive Surgery* 120, no. 2 (2007): 576–577.

Wallace, D. L., S, M. Jones, C. Milroy, and M. A. Pickford. "Telemedicine for acute plastic surgical trauma and burns." *Journal of Plastic, Reconstructive and Aesthetic Surgery* 61, no. 1 (2008): 31–36.

Whitaker, I. S., R. O. Karoo, G. Spyrou, and O. M. Fenton. "The birth of plastic surgery: the story of nasal reconstruction from the Edwin Smith Papyrus to the twenty-first century." *Plastic and Reconstructive Surgery* 120, no. 1 (2007): 327–336.

OTHER

American Academy of Cosmetic Surgery. Information about Plastic and Reconstructive Surgery. 2007 (accessed December 30, 2007). http://www.cosmeticsurgery.org/Surgeons/education.asp.

American Board of Facial Plastic and Reconstructive Surgery. Information about Plastic and Reconstructive Surgery. 2007 (accessed December 30, 2007). http://www.abfprs.org.

Canadian Society of Plastic Surgery. Information about Plastic and Reconstructive Surgery. 2007 (accessed December 30, 2007). http://www.plasticsurgery.ca.

Mayo Clinic. Information about Plastic and Reconstructive Surgery. 2007 (accessed December 30, 2007). http://www.mayoclinic.org/plasticsurgery-rst.

National Library of Medicine. Information about Plastic and Reconstructive Surgery. 2007 (accessed December 30, 2007). http://www.nlm.nih.gov/medlineplus/plasticandcosmeticsurgery.html.

ORGANIZATIONS

American Academy of Facial Plastic and Reconstructive Surgery, 310 S. Henry Street, Alexandria, VA 22314, (703) 299-9291, http://www.aafprs.org

American Board of Plastic Surgery, Seven Penn Center, Suite 400, 1635 Market Street, Philadelphia, PA 19103-2204, (215) 587-9322, http://www.abplsurg.org

American Society for Aesthetic Plastic Surgery, 11081 Winners Circle, Los Alamitos, CA 90720, (888) 272-7711, http://www.surgery.org

American Society of Plastic Surgeons, 444 E. Algonquin Road, Arlington Heights, IL 60005, (847) 228-9900, http://www.plasticsurgery.org.

L. Fleming Fallon, Jr., MD, DrPH
Brenda W. Lerner

Platelet aggregation test

Definition

Platelets (thrombocytes) are small anucleate (i.e. without a nucleus) disk-shaped **blood** cells that play a major role in the blood-clotting process. When a blood vessel wall is cut or injured, platelets adhere to the

damaged site and aggregate (clump) together to form a barrier to the escape of blood. The platelet aggregation test is a measure of the platelet clumping function.

Purpose

The platelet aggregation test aids in the evaluation of **bleeding disorders** by measuring the rate and degree to which platelets aggregate after the addition of a chemical, an agonist, that stimulates platelet clumping. The test can be used to differentiate between several inherited and acquired disorders of platelet function.

Precautions

There are many medications that can affect the results of the platelet aggregation test. The patient should discontinue as many of these as possible beforehand. Some of the drugs that can decrease platelet aggregation include aspirin, some **antibiotics**, beta-blockers, dextran (Macrodex), alcohol, heparin (Lipo-Hepin), **nonsteroidal anti-inflammatory drugs** (NSAIDs), tricyclic antidepressants, and warfarin (Coumadin).

Description

There are many factors involved in blood clotting (coagulation). One of the first steps in the process involves small cells in the bloodstream called platelets, which are produced in the **bone** marrow. Platelets gather at the site of an injury, adhere to the damaged vessel wall, and aggregate together forming a plug that helps to limit the loss of blood and promote healing. Normal aggregation depends upon the release of platelet granules, normal membrane receptors on the platelets, and a normal level of plasma fibrinogen.

A defect in platelet aggregation will result in a prolonged bleeding time. Abnormal platelet aggregation may be caused by an inherited bleeding disorder (e.g., von Willebrand's disease); certain acquired bleeding disorders that occur as a consequence of another disease or condition (e.g. connective tissue or collagen disorders, kidney or **liver** failure, leukemia, myeloma); or by certain medications (e.g., aspirin, heparin, and NSAIDs).

The platelet aggregation test uses an instrument called an aggregometer to measure the optical density (turbidity) of platelet-rich plasma. The plasma should stand at room temperature for 30 minutes prior to the assay, but the tests should be performed within three hours of sample collection. Several different substances called agonists are used in the test. These agonists include adenosine diphosphate (ADP), epinephrine, thrombin, collagen, arachidonic acid, and ristocetin. The addition of an agonist to a plasma sample causes the platelets to aggregate, making the fluid more transparent. The aggregometer then measures the increased light transmission through the specimen. Some aggregometers measure platelet aggregation of whole blood. These instruments use two electrodes that measure impedance (resistance to current flow). When platelet aggregation occurs, the platelets collect at the electrode surface, increasing the impedance at the electrode.

Some inherited platelet disorders that can be differentiated by the aggregation response to different agonists include Glanzmann's thrombasthenia, von Willebrand's disease, and Bernard-Soulier disease. Glanzmann's thrombasthenia is an autosomal dominant condition. The platelet count is normal, but the bleeding time is prolonged. Aggregation is normal with ristocetin, but is abnormal with all the other agonists. Von Willebrand's disease is the most common inherited bleeding disorder. It is associated with an increased bleeding and clotting time and is caused by a deficiency of two coagulation factors, factor VIII and von Willebrand factor. The platelet count may be normal or low. It may be inherited as autosomal dominant or autosomal recessive forms. The aggregation profile in von Willebrand's disease is the reverse of that seen in Glanzmann's thrombasthenia. The aggregation with ADP, collagen, thrombin, epinephrine, and arachidonic acid is normal, but is abnormal with ristocetin. Bernard-Soulier disease is an autosomal recessive condition associated with large platelets and an abnormal bleeding time. The platelet count may be normal or low. It produces the same profile as von Willebrand's disease, but the abnormal aggregation with ristocetin cannot be reversed by addition of von Willebrand factor.

Preparation

The test requires a blood sample collected in sodium citrate. The patient should either avoid food and drink altogether for eight hours before the test, or eat only nonfat foods. High levels of fatty substances in the blood can affect test results.

Because the use of aspirin and/or aspirin compounds can directly affect test results, the patient should avoid these medications for at least one week before the test. The test should be completed within three hours of specimen collection. Specimens that sit at room temperature for four hours or more may lose the ability to aggregate.

Aftercare

Because the platelet aggregation test is ordered when some type of bleeding problem is suspected, the patient

---

KEY TERMS

Aggregation—The blood cell clumping process that is measured in the platelet aggregation test.

Agonist—A chemical that is added to the blood sample in the platelet aggregation test to stimulate the clumping process.

Platelets—Small, round, anucleate disk-shaped blood cells that are involved in clot formation. The platelet aggregation test measures the clumping ability of platelets.

Turbidity—The cloudiness or lack of transparency of a solution.

von Willebrand's disease (vWD)—An autosomal dominant inherited lifelong bleeding disorder caused by a defective gene. The gene defect results in a decreased blood concentration of a substance called von Willebrand factor (vWF). Tests for vWF (and coagulation Factor VIII) are used along with platelet aggregation tests to diagnose this disorder.

---

should be cautioned to watch the puncture site for signs of additional bleeding.

Complications

Risks for this test are minimal in normal individuals. Patients with bleeding disorders, however, may have prolonged bleeding from the puncture wound, or the formation of a bruise (ecchymosis) or blood clot (hematoma) in or under the skin where the blood was withdrawn.

Results

The platelet aggregation test produces a graph in which the x-axis is time and the y-axis is percent transmission. The platelet aggregation curve will vary depending upon the reaction conditions (e.g., pH of the platelet-rich plasma), agonist used, and agonist concentration. The typical aggregation curve is biphasic. It is characterized by an initial increase in light transmission (primary wave) followed by a plateau and a second steeper increase in light transmission (secondary wave) caused by irreversible platelet clumping. An exception to this is aggregation with collagen, which produces a single steep increase in light transmission preceded by a lag phase. An abnormal response can be a decreased or absent primary wave, secondary wave, or both.

Abnormal platelet aggregation can be found in such inherited disorders as von Willebrand's disease, as well as in some connective tissue disorders. Abnormal aggregation can also occur in leukemia or myeloma; with medications taken during recent heart/lung bypass or **kidney dialysis**; and after taking certain other drugs.

Health care team roles

The physician orders the test. The specimen will be drawn by a nurse or phlebotomist, and transported to the laboratory. The clinical laboratory scientist/medical technologist will perform the test. The results are interpreted by a hematopathologist.

Resources

BOOKS

Majerus, Philip W. "Platelets" In *The Molecular Basis of Blood Diseases,* edited by George Stamatoyannopoulos et al. Philadelphia: W. B. Saunders Company, 2001.

Miller, Jonathan L. "Blood Platelets" In *Clinical Diagnosis and Management by Laboratory Methods,* edited by John B. Henry. Philadelphia: W. B. Saunders Company, 2001.

Pagana, Kathleen Deska, and Timothy James Pagana. *Mosby's Diagnostic and Laboratory Test Reference.* St. Louis: Mosby-Year Book, Inc., 1998.

Practical Diagnosis of Hematologic Disorders, 5th ed. Edited by Carl R. Kjeldsberg, MD. Chicago, IL: ASCP Press, 2010.

Mark A. Best

Platelet count *see* **Complete blood count**

Platelet function disorders

Definition

Platelets are cells within the bloodstream that recognize and cling to damaged areas inside **blood vessels**. When they do this, the platelets trigger a series of chemical changes that result in the formation of a **blood** clot. There are certain hereditary disorders that affect platelet function and impair their ability to start the process of blood clot formation. One result is the possibility of excessive bleeding from minor injuries or from menstrual flow.

Description

Platelets are formed in the **bone** marrow—a spongy tissue located inside the long bones of the body—as fragments of a large precursor cell (a megakaryocyte).

These fragments circulate in the bloodstream and form the first line of defense against blood escaping from injured blood vessels.

Damaged blood vessels release a chemical signal that increases the stickiness of platelets in the area of the injury. The sticky platelets adhere to the damaged area and gradually form a platelet plug. At the same time, the platelets release a series of chemical signals that prompt other factors in the blood to reinforce the platelet plug. Between the platelet and its reinforcements, a sturdy clot is created that acts as a patch while the damaged area heals.

There are several hereditary disorders characterized by some impairment of the platelet's action. Examples include von Willebrand disease, Glanzmann's thrombasthenia, and Bernard–Soulier syndrome. Vulnerable aspects of platelet function include errors in the production of the platelets themselves or errors in the formation, storage, or release of their chemical signals. These defects can prevent platelets from responding to injuries or from prompting the action of other factors involved in clot formation.

Causes and symptoms

Platelet function disorders can be inherited, but they may also occur as a symptom of acquired diseases or as a side effect of certain drugs, including aspirin and **nonsteroidal anti-inflammatory drugs** (NSAIDS). The most common inherited bleeding disorder is von Willebrand disease, a relatively minor condition, which is thought to affect as many as one in every 1,000 people. There are several variants of this disorder.

Symptoms of platelet function disorders vary in severity depending on the etiology of the condition and can include bleeding from the nose, gums, vagina, or anus; pinpoint bruises and purplish patches on the skin; and abnormally heavy menstrual bleeding.

Diagnosis

In diagnosing platelet function disorders, specific tests are needed to determine whether the problem is caused by low numbers of platelets or impaired platelet function. A blood smear, a platelet count, and bleeding time are common screening tests. If these tests confirm that the symptoms are due to impaired platelet function, further tests are done—such as platelet aggregation or an analysis of the platelet proteins—that pinpoint the exact nature of the defect.

Treatment

Treatment is intended to prevent bleeding and stop it quickly when it occurs. For example, patients are advised

KEY TERMS

Anemia—A condition in which inadequate quantities of hemoglobin and red blood cells are produced.

Bone marrow—A spongy tissue located within the body's flat bones, including the hip and breast bones and the skull. Marrow contains stem cells, the precursors to platelets and red and white blood cells.

Hemoglobin—The substance inside red blood cells that enables them to carry oxygen.

Megakaryocyte—A large bone marrow cell with a lobed nucleus that is the precursor cell of blood platelets.

Platelets—Fragments of a large precursor cell (a megakaryocyte) found in the bone marrow. These fragments adhere to areas of blood vessel damage and release chemical signals that direct the formation of a blood clot.

to be careful when they brush their teeth to reduce damage to the gums. They are also warned against taking medications that interfere with platelet function. Some patients may require **iron** and folate supplements to counteract potential anemia. Some patients diagnosed with immune or idiopathic platelet disorders can be treated with **corticosteroids**. Platelet transfusions may be necessary to prevent life–threatening hemorrhaging in some cases. Hormone therapy is useful in treating heavy menstrual bleeding. Von Willebrand's disease can be treated with desmopressin (DDAVP, Stimate).

Prognosis

Outcome depends on the specific disorder and the severity of its symptoms. Platelet function disorders range from life–threatening conditions to easily treated or little–noticed problems.

Prevention

Inherited platelet function disorders cannot be prevented except by **genetic counseling**; however, some acquired function disorders may be guarded against by avoiding substances that trigger the disorder.

Resources

PERIODICAL

Nichols, W.L., et al. "Clinical and Laboratory Diagnosis of von Willebrand Disease: A Synopsis of the 2008 NHLBI/NIH Guidelines." *American Journal of Hematology.* 84(6) (June 2009): 366–70.

OTHER

Thiagarajan, P. "Platelet Disorders." eMedicine. June 9, 2009. http://www.emedicine.medscape.com [cited September 14, 2010]

Julia Barrett
Melinda Granger Oberleitner, RN, DNS, APRN, CNS

Pleural effusion

Definition

Pleural effusion occurs when too much fluid collects in the pleural space (the space between the two layers of the pleura). It is commonly known as "water on the lungs." It is characterized by shortness of breath, chest **pain**, gastric discomfort (dyspepsia), and **cough**.

Description

There are two thin membranes in the chest, one (the visceral pleura) lining the **lungs**, and the other (the parietal pleura) covering the inside of the chest wall. Normally, small **blood vessels** in the pleural linings produce a small amount of fluid that lubricates the opposed pleural membranes so that they can glide smoothly against one another during breathing movements. Any extra fluid is taken up by **blood** and lymph vessels, maintaining a balance. When either too much fluid forms or something prevents its removal, the result is an excess of pleural fluid–an effusion. The most common causes are disease of the **heart** or lungs, and inflammation or **infection** of the pleura.

Pleural effusion itself is not a disease as much as a result of many different diseases. For this reason, there is no "typical" patient in terms of age, sex, or other characteristics. Instead, anyone who develops one of the many conditions that can produce an effusion may be affected.

There are two types of pleural effusion: the transudate and the exudate. This is a very important point because the two types of fluid are very different, and which type is present points to what sort of disease is likely to have produced the effusion. It also can suggest the best approach to treatment.

Transudates

A transudate is a clear fluid, similar to blood serum, that forms not because the pleural surfaces themselves are diseased, but because the forces that normally produce and remove pleural fluid at the same rate are out of balance. When the heart fails, pressure in the small blood vessels that remove pleural fluid is increased and fluid "backs up" in the pleural space, forming an effusion. Or, if too little protein is present in the blood, the vessels are less able to hold the fluid part of blood within them and it leaks out into the pleural space. This can result from disease of the **liver** or **kidneys**, or from malnutrition.

Exudates

An exudate—which often is a cloudy fluid, containing cells and much protein—results from disease of the pleura itself. The causes are many and varied. Among the most common are infections such as bacterial **pneumonia** and **tuberculosis**; blood clots in the lungs; and connective tissue diseases, such as **rheumatoid arthritis**. **Cancer** and disease in organs such as the **pancreas** also may give rise to an exudative pleural effusion.

Special types of pleural effusion

Some of the pleural disorders that produce an exudate also cause bleeding into the pleural space. If the effusion contains half or more of the number of red blood cells present in the blood itself, it is called hemothorax. When a pleural effusion has a milky appearance and contains a large amount of fat, it is called chylothorax. Lymph fluid that drains from tissues throughout the body into small lymph vessels finally collects in a large duct (the thoracic duct) running through the chest to empty into a major vein. When this fluid, or chyle, leaks out of the duct into the pleural space, chylothorax is the result. Cancer in the chest is a common cause.

Causes and symptoms

Causes of transudative pleural effusion

Among the most important specific causes of a transudative pleural effusion are:

- Congestive heart failure. This causes pleural effusions in about 40% of patients and is often present on both sides of the chest. Heart failure is the most common cause of bilateral (two-sided) effusion. When only one side is affected it usually is the right (because patients usually lie on their right side).

- Pericarditis. This is an inflammation of the pericardium, the membrane covering the heart.

- Too much fluid in the body tissues, which spills over into the pleural space. This is seen in some forms of kidney disease; when patients have bowel disease and absorb too little of what they eat; and when an excessive amount of fluid is given intravenously.

- Liver disease. About 5% of patients with a chronic scarring disease of the liver called cirrhosis develop pleural effusion.

Causes of exudative pleural effusions

A wide range of conditions may be the cause of an exudative pleural effusion:

- Pleural tumors account for up to 40% of one-sided pleural effusions. They may arise in the pleura itself (mesothelioma), or from other sites, notably the lung.

- Tuberculosis in the lungs may produce a long-lasting exudative pleural effusion.

- Pneumonia affects about three million persons each year, and four of every ten patients will develop pleural effusion. If effective treatment is not provided, an extensive effusion can form that is very difficult to treat.

- Patients with any of a wide range of infections by a virus, fungus, or parasite that involve the lungs may have pleural effusion.

- Up to half of all patients who develop blood clots in their lungs (pulmonary embolism) will have pleural effusion, and this sometimes is the only sign of embolism.

- Connective tissue diseases, including rheumatoid arthritis, lupus, and Sjögren's syndrome may be complicated by pleural effusion.

- Patients with disease of the liver or pancreas may have an exudative effusion, and the same is true for any patient who undergoes extensive abdominal surgery. About 30% of patients who undergo heart surgery will develop an effusion.

- Injury to the chest may produce pleural effusion in the form of either hemothorax or chylothorax.

Symptoms

The key symptom of a pleural effusion is shortness of breath. Fluid filling the pleural space makes it hard for the lungs to fully expand, causing the patient to take many breaths so as to get enough oxygen. When the parietal pleura is irritated, the patient may have mild pain that quickly passes or, sometimes, a sharp, stabbing pleuritic type of pain. Some patients will have a dry cough. Occasionally a patient will have no symptoms at

KEY TERMS

Culture—A test that exposes a sample of body fluid or tissue to special material to see whether bacteria or another type of microorganism is present.

Dyspepsia—A vague feeling of being too full and having heartburn, bloating, and nausea. Usually felt after eating.

Exudate—The type of pleural effusion that results from inflammation or other disease of the pleura itself. It features cloudy fluid containing cells and proteins.

Pleura or pleurae—A delicate membrane that encloses the lungs. The pleura is divided into two areas separated by fluid–the visceral pleura, which covers the lungs, and the parietal pleura, which lines the chest wall and covers the diaphragm.

Pleural cavity—The area of the thorax that contains the lungs.

Pleural space—The potential area between the visceral and parietal layers of the pleurae.

Pneumonia—An acute inflammation of the lungs, usually caused by bacterial infection.

Sclerosis—The process by which an irritating material is placed in the pleural space in order to inflame the pleural membranes and cause them to stick together, eliminating the pleural space and recurrent effusions.

Thoracentesis—Placing a needle, tube, or catheter in the pleural space to remove the fluid of pleural effusion. Used for both diagnosis and treatment.

Transudate—The type of pleural effusion seen with heart failure or other disorders of the circulation. It features clear fluid containing few cells and little protein.

all. This is more likely when the effusion results from recent abdominal surgery, cancer, or tuberculosis. Tapping on the chest will show that the usual crisp sounds have become dull, and on listening with a **stethoscope** the normal breath sounds are muted. If the pleura is inflamed, there may be a scratchy sound called a "pleural friction rub."

Diagnosis

When pleural effusion is suspected, the best way to confirm it is to take chest x rays, both straight-on and from the side. The fluid itself can be seen at the bottom of the lung or lungs, hiding the normal lung structure. If **heart failure** is present, the x-ray shadow of the heart will be enlarged. An ultrasound scan may disclose a small effusion that caused no abnormal findings during chest examination. A computed tomography scan is very helpful if the lungs themselves are diseased.

In order to learn what has caused the effusion, a needle or catheter is often used to obtain a fluid sample, which is examined for cells and its chemical make-up. This procedure, called a **thoracentesis**, is the way to determine whether an effusion is a transudate or exudate, giving a clue as to the underlying cause. In some cases–for instance when cancer or bacterial infection is present–the specific cause can be determined and the correct treatment planned. Culturing a fluid sample can identify the **bacteria** that cause tuberculosis or other forms of pleural infection. The next diagnostic step is to take a

tissue sample, or pleural biopsy, and examine it under a **microscope**. If the effusion is caused by lung disease, placing a viewing tube (bronchoscope) through the large air passages will allow the examiner to see the abnormal appearance of the lungs.

Treatment

The best way to clear up a pleural effusion is to direct treatment at what is causing it, rather than treating the effusion itself. If heart failure is reversed or a lung infection is cured by **antibiotics**, the effusion will usually resolve. However, if the cause is not known, even after extensive tests, or no effective treatment is at hand, the fluid can be drained away by placing a large-bore needle or catheter into the pleural space, just as in diagnostic thoracentesis. If necessary, this can be repeated as often as is needed to control the amount of fluid in the pleural space. If large effusions continue to recur, a drug or material that irritates the pleural membranes can be injected to deliberately inflame them and cause them to adhere close together–a process called sclerosis. This will prevent further effusion by eliminating the pleural space. In the most severe cases, open surgery with removal of a rib may be necessary to drain all the fluid and close the pleural space.

Prognosis

When the cause of pleural effusion can be determined and effectively treated, the effusion itself will reliably clear up and should not recur. In many other cases, sclerosis will prevent sizable effusions from recurring. Whenever a large effusion causes a patient to be short of breath, thoracentesis will make breathing easier, and it may be repeated if necessary. To a great extent, the outlook for patients with pleural effusion depends on the primary cause of effusion and whether it can be eliminated. Some forms of pleural effusion, such as that seen after abdominal surgery, are only temporary and will clear without specific treatment. If heart failure can be controlled, the patient will remain free of pleural effusion. If, on the other hand, effusion is caused by cancer that cannot be controlled, other effects of the disease probably will become more important.

Prevention

Because pleural effusion is a secondary effect of many different conditions, the key to preventing it is to promptly diagnose the primary disease and provide effective treatment. Timely treatment of infections such as tuberculosis and pneumonia will prevent many effusions. When effusion occurs as a drug side-effect, withdrawing the drug or using a different one may solve the problem. On rare occasions, an effusion occurs because fluid meant for a vein is mistakenly injected into the pleural space. This can be prevented by making sure that proper technique is used.

Resources

PERIODICALS

Anderson, Paul B., and Emmet E. McGrath. "Diagnosis of pleural effusion: a systematic approach." *American Journal of Critical Care* 20.2 (2011): 119.

Maskell, Nick A. "Treatment options for malignant pleural effusions." *JAMA, The Journal of the American Medical Association* 307.22 (2012): 2432.

"Treatment of Malignant Pleural Effusion: A Cost-Effectiveness Analysis." *Annals of Thoracic Surgery* (August 2012): 374.

ORGANIZATIONS

American Lung Association, 1301 Pennsylvania Ave. NW, Suite 800, Washington, DC 20001, ((202)) 758-3355, Fax: ((202)) 452-1805, ((800)) 548-8252, info@lungusa.org, http://www.lungusa.org

National Heart Lung and Blood Institute Health Information Center, P.O. Box 30105, Bethesda, MD 20824-0105, ((301)) 592-8573, Fax: ((240)) 629-3246, http://www.nhlbi.nih.gov.

David A. Cramer, MD

Pleural fluid analysis *see* **Thoracentesis**

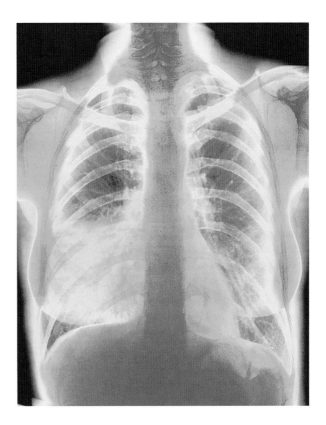

(Colored x-ray of a patient's chest and lungs, lobar pneumonia (blue area), lower lobe, patient's right lung, photograph. Science Photo Library / Photo Researchers, Inc.)

Pneumonia

Definition

Pneumonia is a serious inflammatory lung disorder in which the alveoli—tiny air-filled sacs in the **lungs** that ordinarily absorb oxygen from the air—fill with fluid or pus. As a result of this inflammation, the person cannot get enough oxygen into the bloodstream to meet the needs of body tissues. In addition, the disease organisms responsible for most cases of pneumonia can spread from the lungs into the bloodstream and infect other vital organs, thus causing the person's death. Lobar pneumonia is a form of pneumonia affects one section, or lobe, of the lung; bronchial pneumonia, or bronchopneumonia, affects scattered areas of either lung.

Pneumonia is not a single disease; it has at least 30 different causes. Although most cases of pneumonia are caused by **bacteria**, **viruses**, or other disease organisms, the illness can also be caused by chemical injuries to the lungs, food or saliva accidentally getting into the airway, or even by dust. It is possible for a patient to have bacterial and viral pneumonia at the same time.

Pneumonia is sometimes classified by the ways in which people can acquire it. Some common types of pneumonia include:

- Nosocomial pneumonia: Nosocomial refers to infections acquired by hospital patients. This type of pneumonia can be very serious, partly because hospitalized people are already ill or weak from surgery, and partly because the bacteria found in hospitals are often antibiotic-resistant.

- Ventilator-associated pneumonia: Patients who must be placed on a ventilator to help them breathe are at increased risk of developing pneumonia.

- Community-acquired pneumonia (CAP): CAP refers to pneumonia caused by disease organisms in people who have not been recently hospitalized. This form of pneumonia is frequently seen in patients who present to emergency departments.

- Aspiration pneumonia: Aspiration is the medical term for getting saliva, food particles, or liquids into the airway and lungs. Aspiration pneumonia is common in the elderly, patients with Parkinson disease, and others who may have trouble swallowing normally. The materials that get into the lungs can cause pneumonia either by chemical irritation or by carrying bacteria that cause inflammation.

- Opportunistic pneumonia: Opportunistic infections are caused in people with weakened immune systems by organisms that do not ordinarily cause disease in people with healthy immune systems. People with AIDS are vulnerable to a particular type of pneumonia called PCP, which stands for *Pneumocystis jirovecii* pneumonia. *Pneumocystis jirovecii* is a human-specific fungus.

- Chemical pneumonia. Breathing in certain irritant chemicals, particularly pesticides, can cause pneumonia.

- Walking pneumonia: Walking pneumonia is an older term for pneumonia that does not make patients sick enough to stay in bed; that is, they are well enough to go about their ordinary activities in spite of coughing and headaches. Most cases of walking pneumonia are caused by mycoplasma or by viruses.

- Zoonotic pneumonia: A zoonosis (plural, zoonoses) is a disease that can be transmitted from animals to humans or from humans to other animals. Some forms of pneumonia, particularly those involving chlamydia or parasites, can be transmitted to humans from parrots, cats, dogs, and poultry.

- Emerging diseases. Some emerging diseases, such as severe acute respiratory syndrome (SARS) and avian influenza (bird flu) can cause pneumonia in otherwise healthy people.

Description

Pneumonia has been known and diagnosed since ancient times. One of the earliest descriptions of the disease was written by Hippocrates (c. 460 BC—370 BC), the "Father of Medicine," It was not until 1875, however, that a German bacteriologist named Edwin Klebs (1834–1913) first identified bacteria in the lung secretions of a patient who had died of pneumonia; and it was not until 1884 that scientists recognized that the disease could be caused by more than one bacterium or other pathogen. At the turn of the twentieth century, mortality from pneumonia was about 30% even in the developed countries, but such twentieth-century developments as the discovery of **antibiotics**, improved surgical techniques, and the development of pneumonia vaccines caused the death rate to drop dramatically.

Demographics

Pneumonia is a widespread health problem in the general population as well as hospital inpatients and those in **nursing homes**. According to the Centers for Disease Control and Prevention (CDC), between 1.1 and 1.4 million people in the United States are treated in hospitals each year for pneumonia, with an average stay of 5 days. About 2 percent of nursing home residents are treated for pneumonia in an average year. In 2009, more than 50,000 Americans died from the disease. As of 2012, pneumonia is the seventh leading cause of death in the United States.

Pneumonia is most common in the United States and Canada in the winter months. It affects males more often than females, and African Americans more often than members of other racial or ethnic groups.

In developing countries, pneumonia is a common cause of death among children. The World Health Organization (WHO) estimates that between 1.5 and 2 million children die each year around the world, and that one in three deaths among newborn babies results from pneumonia.

Anatomy of the lung

To better understand pneumonia, it is important to be familiar with the basic anatomic features of the **respiratory system**. The human respiratory system begins at the nose and mouth, where air is breathed in (inspired) and out (expired). The air tube extending from the nose is the nasopharynx. The tube carrying air breathed in through the mouth is the oropharynx. The nasopharynx and the oropharynx merge into the larynx. The oropharynx also carries swallowed substances, including food, water, and salivary secretion, which must pass into the esophagus and then the **stomach**. The larynx is protected by a trap door called the epiglottis, which prevents substances that have been swallowed, as well as those that have been regurgitated (thrown up), from heading down into the larynx and toward the lungs.

The larynx flows into the trachea, which is the broadest part of the respiratory tree. The trachea divides into two limbs, the right and left bronchi. Each one of these branches off into multiple smaller bronchi that penetrate the lung tissue. Each bronchus divides into tubes of smaller and smaller diameter, finally ending in the terminal bronchioles. The air sacs of the lung, in which oxygen-carbon dioxide exchange actually takes place, are clustered at the ends of the bronchioles like the leaves of a tree. They are called alveoli.

The tissue of the lung, which serves only in a supportive role for the bronchi, bronchioles, and alveoli, is known as lung parenchyma.

Function of the respiratory system

The main function of the respiratory system is to provide oxygen, the most important energy source for the body's cells. Inspired air (the air that is breathed in) contains oxygen and travels down the respiratory tree to the alveoli. The oxygen moves out of the alveoli and is sent into circulation throughout the body as part of the red **blood** cells. The oxygen in the inspired air is exchanged within the alveoli for carbon dioxide, the waste product of the human metabolic process. The air that is breathed out contains the gas carbon dioxide. During expiration, carbon dioxide leaves the alveoli. As one breathes in oxygen, one breathes out carbon dioxide.

Respiratory system defenses

Bacteria and viruses do not normally reside in significant numbers inside the lung, part of the upper respiratory system. This relative sterility is in contrast to parts of the gastrointestinal system, where bacteria dwell even in a healthy state. There are multiple safeguards along the path of the respiratory system designed to keep organisms from invading and leading to **infection**.

The first line of defense against infection includes the hairs in the nostrils, which serve as a filter for larger particles. The epiglottis is a "trap door" designed to prevent food and other swallowed substances from entering the larynx and the trachea. Sneezing and coughing, both provoked by the presence of irritants within the respiratory system, help to clear such irritants from the respiratory tract.

Mucus produced through the respiratory system also serves to trap dust and infectious organisms. Tiny hair-like projections (cilia) from cells line the respiratory tract and beat constantly, moving debris trapped by mucus upwards and out of the respiratory tract. This mechanism of protection is called the mucociliary escalator.

The cells that line the respiratory tract produce several types of immune substances that protect against various organisms. Other cells (macrophages) along the respiratory tract actually ingest and kill invading organisms.

Thus the organisms that cause pneumonia are usually carefully kept from entering the lungs by virtue of the host's defenses. However, when an individual encounters a large number of organisms at once, the usual defenses may be overwhelmed, and infection may occur. This may occur either when contaminated air droplets are inhaled, or when aspiration of organisms that inhabit the upper airways occurs.

Risk factors

In addition to exposure to sufficient quantities of causative organisms, certain conditions may make an individual more likely to have pneumonia. Certainly, the lack of normal anatomical structure could result in an increased risk of pneumonia. There are certain inherited defects of cilia that can result in less effective protection. Cigarette smoke, inhaled directly by a smoker or secondhand by an innocent bystander, interferes significantly with ciliary function and inhibits macrophage (a large white blood cell [WBC] that ingests particles and infectious microorganisms) function.

Stroke, seizures, alcohol, and various drugs interfere with the function of the epiglottis. This can lead to a leaky seal on this "trap door," with possible contamination by swallowed substances and/or regurgitated stomach contents. Alcohol and some drugs may also interfere with the normal **cough** reflex. An inadequate cough reflex further decreases the success of clearing unwanted debris from the respiratory tract.

Viruses or such other invasive microorganisms as bacteria may interfere with ciliary function and lead to access to the lower respiratory tract. One of the most invasive viruses is HIV (human **immunodeficiency** virus), the causative virus in **AIDS** (acquired immunodeficiency syndrome). In recent years, this virus has resulted in a significant increase in the incidence of pneumonia. Because AIDS results in a general decreased efficiency of many protective mechanisms of the host's **immune system**, a patient with AIDS may be susceptible to all kinds of pneumonia. This vulnerability includes some parasitic types considered rare prior to the emergence of AIDS in the 1980s. These rare **parasites** are incapable of causing illness in an individual with a normal immune system.

The elderly have a less effective mucociliary escalator, as well as changes in their immune system that compromise their ability to fight infection. These factors cause this age group to be at greater risk for the development of pneumonia.

Various chronic conditions predispose a person to infection with pneumonia. These conditions include **asthma**, **cystic fibrosis**, and neuromuscular diseases, which may interfere with the seal of the epiglottis. Esophageal disorders may result in stomach contents passing upwards into the esophagus. This increases the risk of aspiration into the lungs of stomach contents (with their normally resident bacteria). Diabetes, sickle cell anemia, **lymphoma**, leukemia, and **emphysema** also predispose a person to pneumonia.

Pneumonia is one of the most frequent infectious complications of all types of surgery. Many drugs used during and after surgery may increase the risk of aspiration, impair the cough reflex, and cause a patient to under fill his or her lungs with air. **Pain** after surgery also discourages a patient from breathing deeply enough, and from coughing effectively.

Causes and symptoms

Causes

Pneumonia can have more than 30 different causes, but the five main causes are:

- Bacteria. Bacteria are the most common single class of agents that cause pneumonia, with *Streptococcus pneumoniae* identified in 50% of cases,, *Haemophilus influenzae* in 20%, *Chlamydophila pneumoniae* in 13%, and *Staphylococcus aureus* in 3%. Pneumonia caused by *Chlamydophila pneumoniae* is most common in adults over 65. Other bacteria that may cause pneumonia include *Moraxella catarrhalis* and *Legionella pneumophila*.

- Viruses. Viruses account for about 33% of cases of pneumonia in adults. The most common viruses identified in pneumonia patients are rhinoviruses, coronaviruses, the influenza virus, parainfluenza viruses, respiratory syncytial virus, and adenoviruses.

- Mycoplasmas. Pneumonia caused by mycoplasmas may be accompanied by a skin rash.

- Other infectious pathogens, like fungi (including *Pneumocystis*) and parasites. *Pneumocystis jirovecii* is an extremely important cause of pneumonia in patients with immune problems (such as patients being treated for cancer with chemotherapy, or patients with AIDS). Classically considered a parasite, the organism appears to be more related to fungi. Other parasites that may cause pneumonia include *Toxoplasma gondii*, a protozoon that also infects cats; and *Strongyloides stercoralis*, a threadworm found in soil or water contaminated by feces.

- People who come into contact with bird droppings, such as poultry workers, are at risk for pneumonia caused by the organism *Chlamydia psittaci*. Other *Chlamydia* species include *Chlamydia pneumoniae*, and *Chlamydia trachomatis*. These bacteria are small Gram-negative, obligate intracellular organisms. All three species can cause pneumonia in humans.

- Some irritant chemicals.

Symptoms

Pneumonia can come on either suddenly or gradually. Its major symptoms include chest pain, **fever**, severe coughing, and greenish or pus-colored sputum. The early stages of pneumonia are sometimes mistaken for a cold or flu. The severity of the symptoms depends on the organism causing the illness and the person's age and basic level of health.

Bacterial pneumonia often comes on suddenly with sweating, severe chest pain, high fever (up to 105°F), chills, and a cough that produces greenish or yellowish sputum. It can develop by itself or following a viral infection like a cold or the flu.

Some cases of viral pneumonia are mild. In other cases, the person has symptoms resembling those of **influenza**: fever, aching muscles, **headache**, and **weakness**. Within 12 to 36 hours, however, the patient becomes much sicker, may start gasping for breath, and their cough becomes worse. Patients with viral pneumonia sometimes develop a secondary bacterial pneumonia.

Pneumonia caused by mycoplasma is usually mild and develops gradually. It is common among children and young adults because it spreads rapidly in day care centers, college dormitories, military barracks, prisons, homeless shelters, and overcrowded housing. The most noticeable symptoms of mycoplasmal pneumonia are a dry cough and whitish sputum. Some patients also experience nausea and **vomiting** or **diarrhea**.

Other symptoms that some people with pneumonia experience include:

- Rapid but shallow breathing.
- Loss of appetite.
- Mental confusion and disorientation. This symptom is more common in the elderly.
- Unusual tiredness.
- Heavy sweating and clammy skin.

Diagnosis

The diagnosis of pneumonia is made by a combination of the patient's history (including occupation, recent travel, and exposure to animals or sick people); a **physical examination**; and appropriate laboratory and imaging tests. The doctor will need to know when the symptoms started, whether the patient has been recently hospitalized, whether he or she has had a cold or flu, and similar questions. The physical examination will include listening to the patient's breathing through a **stethoscope** as well as taking the temperature and pulse. Patients with pneumonia typically have abnormal rubbing, crackling, or other harsh sounds that the doctor can hear. In addition, the number of breaths per minute is usually high. Pneumonia is suspected in the patient who is febrile, has a cough, chest pain, and shortness of breath. Fever with a shaking chill is even more suspicious. Many patients cough up clumps of sputum. These secretions are produced in the alveoli during an infection or other inflammatory condition. They may appear streaked with pus or blood.

Severe pneumonia results in the signs of oxygen deprivation. These include a blue appearance of the nail beds or lips (**cyanosis**). The invading organism causes these symptoms in part by provoking an overly strong **immune response** in the lungs. Thus the immune system, which should help fight off infections, kicks into high gear and damages the lung tissue, making it more susceptible to infection. The small **blood vessels** in the lungs (capillaries) become leaky, and protein-rich fluid seeps into the alveoli. This process results in a reduced functional area for oxygen-carbon dioxide exchange. The patient becomes relatively oxygen-deprived while retaining potentially damaging carbon dioxide. The patient breathes faster and faster in an effort to inhale more oxygen and exhale more carbon dioxide.

Mucus production is increased, and the leaky capillaries may tinge the mucus with blood. Mucus plugs actually further decrease the efficiency of **gas exchange** in the lung. The alveoli fill further with fluid and debris from the large number of white blood cells (WBCs) being produced to fight the infection.

Consolidation, a feature of bacterial pneumonia, occurs when the alveoli become solid due to quantities of fluid and debris. Viral pneumonia and mycoplasma pneumonia do not result in consolidation. These types of pneumonia primarily infect the walls of the alveoli and the parenchyma of the lung.

A chest x-ray will usually be ordered. X-ray examination of the chest may reveal certain abnormal changes associated with pneumonia. Localized shadows obscuring areas of the lung may indicate a bacterial pneumonia, while streaky- or patchy-appearing changes in the x-ray picture may indicate viral or mycoplasma pneumonia. Other tests include:

- A complete blood count (CBC), An unusually high number of white blood cells is a common sign of an infection.

- A sputum test. The doctor can collect a sample of the patient's sputum and send it to a laboratory to identify the organisms that may be causing the infection.

- A computed tomography (CT) scan of the chest.

- Thoracentesis. This is a procedure to remove fluid from the space between the lungs and the chest wall. The pleural fluid can be cultured to identify the disease organism that is causing the pneumonia.

- Pulse oximetry. This noninvasive test is done to measure the amount of oxygen in the patient's bloodstream. It is performed by attaching a sensor to the patient's fingertip or earlobe.

- Bronchoscopy. Bronchoscopy is a procedure in which the doctor passes a long flexible tube called a bronchoscope through the nose or mouth and into the airways in order to see whether and where a blockage is present.

Treatment

Treatment depends on the cause of the pneumonia. Pneumonia caused by bacteria or mycoplasma is treated with a 7–10-day course of antibiotics. Community-acquired pneumonia is typically treated with one or more of the following: tigecycline, doxycycline, a quinolone antibiotic, or ceftriaxone. Viral infections cannot be treated by antibiotics; in some cases, the doctor may prescribe antiviral medications like rimantadine, which is used to treat some types of flu. Most patients can care for themselves at home by taking the prescribed medication and by getting plenty of rest, drinking fluids, and taking over-the-counter pain relievers to reduce fever and headaches. It is important for people recovering at home not to return to work or a normal schedule of activities too quickly, as the pneumonia can recur. Recurrences can be more severe than the initial infection.

People who are severely ill and having difficulty breathing are hospitalized, given pure oxygen to breathe, and given intravenous antibiotics. They will be given a follow-up x-ray by the doctor after they are well enough to leave the hospital.

Prognosis

Prognosis varies according to the type of organism causing the infection, the patient's age, and the time elapsed between diagnosis and treatment. Young people who are diagnosed and treated early may recover in about 10 days. Middle-aged adults may take several weeks to recover fully. Mycoplasmal pneumonia takes somewhat longer than either bacterial or viral pneumonia to go away—sometimes as long as 6 weeks. Recovery following pneumonia with *Mycoplasma pneumoniae* is nearly 100%. *Staphylococcus pneumoniae* has a death rate of 30–40%. Similarly, infections with a number of gram-negative bacteria (such as those in the

KEY TERMS

Alveoli (singular, alveolus)—The small air sacs clustered at the ends of the bronchioles in the lungs, in which oxygen-carbon dioxide exchange takes place.

Aspiration—A condition that occurs when solids or liquids that should be swallowed into the stomach are instead breathed into the respiratory system, or when substances from the outside environment are accidentally breathed into the lungs.

Cilia—Hair-like projections from certain types of cells.

Community-acquired—Referring to a contagious disease acquired from others in the general population rather than during hospitalization.

Cyanosis—A bluish tinge to the skin that can occur when the blood oxygen level drops too low.

Mycoplasma—A very small bacterium that causes a mild but long-lasting form of pneumonia.

Nosocomial—Referring to a disease that a person gets while hospitalized.

Opportunistic infection—An infection that occurs only in people with weakened immune systems.

Parenchyma—A term used to describe the supportive tissue surrounding a particular structure. An example is the tissue that surrounds and supports the actually functional lung tissue.

Sputum—Mucus and other matter that is coughed or brought up from the lungs or throat.

Zoonosis (plural, zoonoses)—Any infectious disease that can be transmitted from animals to humans or from humans to other animals.

gastrointestinal tract, which can cause infection following aspiration) have a high death rate—25–50%. *Streptococcus pneumoniae*, the most common organism causing pneumonia, has a death rate of about 5%. More complications occur in the very young, or in elderly individuals who may have infections in multiple areas of the lung simultaneously. Individuals with such other chronic illnesses as **cirrhosis** of the **liver** or congestive **heart failure**; those without a functioning spleen; or those who have other diseases that result in a weakened immune system may experience complications. Patients with immune disorders, various types of **cancer**, transplanted organ(s) or tissue(s) transplants, or AIDS also may experience complications.

The prognosis for recovery is poor for people who develop ventilator-associated pneumonia (about 50 percent will die) or those with bacterial pneumonia that spreads into the bloodstream (about 20 percent will die). Doctors sometimes use a rule called the pneumonia severity index or PSI to estimate a specific patient's chances of recovery. The PSI is based on age, sex, **vital signs**, and laboratory test results.

Health care team roles

In most cases, a diagnosis of pneumonia is made in a physician's office, a general medical clinic, or emergency room by a primary care practitioner. Children and adolescents with pneumonia are most likely to be diagnosed by their primary care physician or pediatrician.

Both registered nurses (RNs) and licensed practical nurses (LPNs) must complete a prescribed course in nursing and pass a state examination. RNs typically have a degree in nursing. Both RNs and LPNs are often the specialists who deal the most with pneumonia patients, both in general hospitals, homes, or other healthcare facilities. Good nursing care and observation are primary requirements. These include monitoring vital signs, including oxygen saturation (the amount of oxygen circulating in the blood), encouraging the patient to move, breathe deeply, cough, and get out of bed with assistance (if indicated) to facilitate good lung expansion. The nurse should also provide education to the patient about the importance of coughing, breathing deeply, and taking in adequate fluid.

Clinical laboratory scientists have specialized training and must pass a state examination. These are the staff members who analyze blood samples or test urine/sputum specimens that reflect the presence of pneumonia at the outset, and as it resolves. These tests are typically ordered by physicians to diagnose and assess the progress of the infection.

Radiologic technologists have specialized training and must pass a state examination. Their responsibility is to take chest x rays to visualize and monitor the course of the pneumonia.

Prevention

Basic preventive measures include washing the hands carefully, particularly during cold and flu season, using hand sanitizers, and frequently cleaning countertops and other hard surfaces that people touch frequently.

Because many bacterial pneumonias occur in patients who are first infected with the influenza virus (the flu), yearly **vaccination** against influenza can decrease the risk of pneumonia in certain patients. This

QUESTIONS TO ASK YOUR DOCTOR

- What should I do to protect my elderly parents against community-acquired pneumonia?

- What is your opinion of the newer pneumococcal conjugate vaccines? Are they safe as well as effective?

- How can I tell the difference between the symptoms of influenza and those of pneumonia?

- What antibiotics do you prescribe most often for pneumonia in children? In adults?

- How many cases of pneumonia do you see and treat in an average year?

is particularly true of the elderly and those afflicted with such chronic diseases as asthma, cystic fibrosis, other lung or **heart** diseases, **sickle cell disease**, diabetes, kidney disease, and some cancers. Another important measure that anyone can take to lower their risk of pneumonia is to quit **smoking** (or not start in the first place).

A specific vaccine against *Streptococcus pneumoniae* and another vaccine (Pneumovax) developed in the early 2000s against *Pneumococcus* are very protective, and should also be administered to people over 65 years of age as well as to smokers and patients with chronic illnesses.

Newer vaccines against pneumococcal pneumonia are called pneumococcal conjugate vaccines (PCVs) because they are made to protect against several different serotypes of the pneumococcus. Prevnar is made from 7 different serotypes; Synflorix from 10 serotypes; and Prevnar 13 from 13 serotypes. Prevnar 13 was approved by the Food and Drug Administration (FDA) for use in the United States in February 2010. The original Prevnar must be used in children under the age of two.

Hib vaccine, which protects against *Haemophilus influenzae* type b, is recommended to be given to all children in the United States below the age of 6. It can safely be given to infants as young as 2 months.

Resources

BOOKS

Hasleton, Philip, and Douglas B. Flieder, eds. *Spencer's Pathology of the Lung*, 6th ed. New York: Cambridge University Press, 2012.

Sethi, Sanjay, ed. *Respiratory Infections*. New York: Informa Healthcare, 2010.

Suarez, Micaela L., and Steffani M. Ortega, eds. *Pneumonia: Symptoms, Diagnosis and Treatment*. New York: Nova Science Publishers, 2011.

PERIODICALS

Almond, M.H., et al. "Influenza-related Pneumonia." *Clinical Medicine* 12 (February 2012): 67–70.

Cohen, A.L., et al. "Integrating Pneumonia Prevention and Treatment Interventions with Immunization Services in Resource-poor Countries." *Bulletin of the World Health Organization* 90 (April 1, 2012): 289–294.

Kontoyiannis, D.P. "Invasive Mycoses: Strategies for Effective Management." *American Journal of Medicine* 125 (January 2012): S25–S38.

Lobdell, K.W., et al. "Hospital-acquired Infections." *Surgical Clinics of North America* 92 (February 2012): 65–77.

Morris, A., and K.A. Norris. "Colonization by *Pneumocystis jirovecii* and Its Role in Disease." *Clinical Microbiology Reviews* 25 (April 2012): 297–317.

Nassisi, D., and M.L. Oishi. "Evidence-based Guidelines for Evaluation and Antimicrobial Therapy for Common Emergency Department Infections." *Emergency Medicine Practice* 14 (January 2012): 1–28.

Principi, N., and S. Esposito. "Use of the 13-valent Pneumococcal Conjugate Vaccine in Infants and Young Children." *Expert Opinion on Biological Therapy* 12 (May 2012): 641–648.

Sachdev, G., and L.M. Napolitano. "Postoperative Pulmonary Complications: Pneumonia and Acute Respiratory Failure." *Surgical Clinics of North America* 92 (April 2012): 321–344.

Wonodi, C.B., et al. "Evaluation of Risk Factors for Severe Pneumonia in Children: the Pneumonia Etiology Research for Child Health Study." *Clinical Infectious Diseases* 54 (April 2012): Suppl. 2: S124–S131.

WEBSITES

American Lung Association (ALA). Pneumonia Information Home Page. http://www.lung.org/lung-disease/pneumonia/ (accessed April 25, 2012).

Centers for Disease Control and Prevention (CDC). CDC Feature: "Pneumonia Can Be Prevented—Vaccines Can Help." http://www.cdc.gov/Features/Pneumonia/ (accessed April 25, 2012).

Mayo Clinic. "Pneumonia." http://www.mayoclinic.com/health/pneumonia/DS00135 (accessed April 25, 2012).

Medscape. "Community-Acquired Pneumonia." http://emedicine.medscape.com/article/234240-overview (accessed April 25, 2012).

Medscape. "Nosocomial Pneumonia." http://emedicine.medscape.com/article/234753-overview (accessed April 25, 2012).

National Heart, Lung, and Blood Institute (NHLBI). "What Is Pneumonia?" http://www.nhlbi.nih.gov/health/health-topics/topics/pnu/ (accessed April 25, 2012).

ORGANIZATIONS

American College of Chest Physicians (ACCP), 3300 Dundee Road, Northbrook, IL United States 60062-2348, (847) 498-1400, Fax: (847) 498-5460, http://www.chestnet.org/accp/

American Lung Association (ALA), 1301 Pennsylvania Ave. NW, Suite 800, Washington, DC United States 20004, (202) 785-3355, Fax: (202) 452-1805, info@lung.org, http://www.lung.org/#

Centers for Disease Control and Prevention (CDC), 1600 Clifton Road, Atlanta, GA United States 30333, (800) CDC-INFO (232-4636), cdcinfo@cdc.gov, www.cdc.gov

National Heart, Lung, and Blood Institute (NHLBI), Health Information Center, P.O. Box 30105, Bethesda, MD United States 20824-0105, (301) 592-8573, Fax: (240) 629-3246, nhlbiinfo@nhlbi.nih.gov, http://www.nhlbi.nih.gov/index.htm

National Institute of Allergy and Infectious Diseases (NIAID), 6610 Rockledge Drive, MSC 6612, Bethesda, MD United States 20892-6612, (301) 496-5717, Fax: (301) 402-3573, (866) 284-4107, ocpostoffice@niaid.nih.gov, http://www.niaid.nih.gov/Pages/default.aspx

World Health Organization (WHO), Avenue Appia 20, 1211 Geneva 27, Switzerland, + 41 22 791 21 11, Fax: + 41 22 791 31 11, info@who.int, http://www.who.int/en/.

Ken R, Wells
Rebecca J. Frey, Ph.D

Pneumonitis *see* **Pneumonia**

Pneumothorax

Definition

Pneumothorax is a collection of air or gas in the chest or pleural space that causes part or all of a lung to collapse.

Description

Normally, the pressure in the **lungs** is greater than the pressure in the pleural space surrounding the lungs. However, if air enters the pleural space, the pressure in the pleura then becomes greater than the pressure in the lungs, causing the lung to collapse partially or completely. Pneumothorax can be either spontaneous or due to trauma.

If a pneumothorax occurs suddenly or for no known reason, it is called a spontaneous pneumothorax. This condition most often strikes tall, thin men between the ages of 20 to 40. In addition, people with lung disorders, such as **emphysema**, **cystic fibrosis**, and **tuberculosis**, are at higher risk for spontaneous pneumothorax.

Traumatic pneumothorax is the result of accident or injury due to medical procedures performed to the chest cavity, such as **thoracentesis** or **mechanical ventilation**. Tension pneumothorax is a serious and potentially life-threatening condition that may be caused by traumatic injury, chronic lung disease, or as a complication of a medical procedure. In this type of pneumothorax, air enters the chest cavity, but cannot escape. This greatly increased pressure in the pleural space causes the lung to collapse completely, compresses the **heart**, and pushes the heart and associated **blood vessels** toward the unaffected side.

Causes and symptoms

The symptoms of pneumothrax depend on how much air enters the chest, how much the lung collapses, and the extent of lung disease. Symptoms include the following, according to the cause of the pneumothorax:

• Spontaneous pneumothorax. Simple spontaneous pneumothorax is caused by a rupture of a small air sac or fluid-filled sac in the lung. It may be related to activity in otherwise healthy people or may occur during scuba diving or flying at high altitudes. Complicated spontaneous pneumothorax, also generally caused by rupture of a small sac in the lung, occurs in people with lung diseases. The symptoms of complicated spontaneous pneumothorax tend to be worse than those of simple pneumothorax, due to the underlying lung disease. Spontaneous pneumothorax is characterized by dull, sharp, or stabbing chest pain that begins suddenly and becomes worse with deep breathing or coughing. Other symptoms are shortness of breath, rapid breathing, abnormal breathing movement (that is, little chest wall movement when breathing), and cough.

• Tension pneumothorax. Following trauma, air may enter the chest cavity. A penetrating chest wound allows outside air to enter the chest, causing the lung to collapse. Certain medical procedures performed in the chest cavity, such as thoracentesis, also may cause a lung to collapse. Tension pneumothorax may be the immediate result of an injury; the delayed complication of a hidden injury, such as a fractured rib, that punctures the lung; or the result of lung damage from asthma, chronic bronchitis, or emphysema. Symptoms of tension pneumothorax tend to be severe with sudden onset. There is marked anxiety, distended neck veins, weak pulse, decreased breath sounds on the affected side, and a shift of the mediastinum to the opposite side.

Diagnosis

To diagnose pneumothorax, it is necessary for the health care provider to listen to the chest

KEY TERMS

Electrocardiagram—A test that provides a typical record of normal heart action.

Mediastinum—The space between the right and left lung.

Pleural—Pleural refers to the pleura or membrane that enfolds the lungs.

Thoracentesis—Also called a pleural fluid tap, this procedure involves aspiration of fluid from the pleural space using a long, thin needle inserted between the ribs.

(auscultation) during a **physical examination**. By using a **stethoscope**, the physician may note that one part of the chest does not transmit the normal sounds of breathing. A **chest x ray** will show the air pocket and the collapsed lung. An electrocardiogram (ECG) will be performed to record the electrical impulses that control the heart's activity. **Blood** samples may be taken to check for the level of arterial **blood gases**.

Treatment

A small pneumothorax may resolve on its own, but most require medical treatment. The object of treatment is to remove air from the chest and allow the lung to re-expand. This is done by inserting a needle and syringe (if the pneumothorax is small) or **chest tube** through the chest wall. This allows the air to escape without allowing any air back in. The lung will then re-expand itself within a few days. Surgery may be needed for repeat occurrences.

Prognosis

Most people recover fully from spontaneous pneumothorax. Up to half of patients with spontaneous pneumothorax experience recurrence. Recovery from a collapsed lung generally takes one to two weeks. Tension pneumothorax can cause death rapidly due to inadequate heart output or insufficient blood oxygen (hypoxemia), and must be treated as a medical emergency.

Prevention

Preventive measures for a non-injury related pneu-mothorax include stopping **smoking** and seeking medical attention for respiratory problems. If the pneumothorax occurs in both lungs or more than once in the same lung, surgery may be needed to prevent it from occurring again.

ORGANIZATIONS

American Association for Respiratory Care, 9425 N. MacArthur Blvd, Suite 100, Irving, TX 75063-4706, (972) 243-2272, Fax: (972) 484-2720, info@aarc.org, http://www.aarc.org.

American Lung Association, 1301 Pennsylvania Ave. NW, Suite 800, Washington, DC 20001, (202) 758-3355, Fax: (202) 452-1805, (800) 548-8252, info@lungusa.org, http://www.lungusa.org.

Lorraine Steefel, RN

Podiatry *see* **Foot care**

Poisoning

Definition

Poisoning is the state produced by the introduction of a toxic substance—that is, any substance that produces an injurious or fatal effect, into the body. Poisoning may be accidental or intentional.

Description

Poisoning commonly involves the introduction of poisonous elements from outside the body. The term also can apply to noxious material produced within the body that, because of a disease condition such as kidney or **liver** failure, cannot be removed; or toxins produced by **bacteria**, as in the case of food poisoning. Poisons can enter the body from multiple external sources. They can be swallowed; injected; inhaled, as in the case of carbon monoxide or aerosol compounds; or they can enter via the skin, as in snake or insect bites and even radiation from the sun that we call sun poisoning. Some question exists regarding whether electromagnetic fields (EMFs) also produce damaging effects within the body.

Poisoning is a common occurrence, and costs the United States about $35 billion each year in treatments and lost productivity. An estimated 10 million cases of poisoning occur in the United States each year, with 830,000 visits to hospital emergency departments. In 2010, 2.4 million exposures to poisonous substances were reported to United States Poison Control.

Common household, industrial, and agricultural products containing toxic substances

Alcohol (rubbing)	Fuel
Antifreeze	Floor/furniture polish
Arsenic	Gasoline
Art and craft supplies	Glues/adhesives
Automotive fluids	Hemlock
Batteries, automotive	Kerosene
Batteries, household	Mercury
Building products	Metal primers
Cleaning products	Metalworking materials
Cosmetics/personal care products	Mothballs
Cyanide	Oven cleaners
Daffodil bulbs	Paint strippers/thinners
Dieffenbachia	Paints, oil-based or alkyds
Disinfectants/air fresheners	Paints, water-based or latex
Drain openers	Pesticides, flea collars, insect repellents
English nightshade	Stains/finishes
Ethanol (found in alcoholic beverages)	Strychnine
Foxglove	Wood preservatives

In 50% of the cases, the victim is a child under the age of five. The most common toxic substances taken in are cosmetics and personal care products, followed by home cleaning products, medications, and plants. Most poisonings, nearly 89%, occur in the home, and are accidental. About 42,000 Americans die each year from poisoning, with 76% of these deaths considered unintentional.

About 71,000 children are taken to emergency departments in the United States each year because of accidental poisoning. Curiosity, inability to read warning labels, a desire to imitate adults, and inadequate supervision lead to childhood poisonings. Children are twice as likely to be poisoned by taking adults' medications as by swallowing cleaning products or other household chemicals. They are also likely to be poisoned by chewing on or swallowing tobacco products. The elderly are the second most likely group to be poisoned. Mental confusion, poor eyesight, and the use of multiple prescription drugs are the leading reasons why this group has a high rate of accidental poisoning. Among people 25 to 64 years old, unintentional poisoning causes more deaths than motor vehicle accidents. A substantial number—approximately 11% of all poisonings—occur as suicide attempts.

Poisons taken internally are common in the home and workplace. There are two major basic types. One group consists of products that were never meant to be safely ingested or inhaled, such as shampoo, hand lotions and sanitizers, paint thinner, pesticides, houseplant leaves, and carbon monoxide. The other group contains products that can be ingested in small quantities but are harmful if taken in large amounts. These include pharmaceuticals, medicinal herbs, or alcohol. Prescription painkillers (methadone, hydrocodone, and oxycodone), are the drugs most commonly involved in poisonings in the home, followed by **cocaine** and heroin. Other types of poisons include the bacterial toxins that cause food poisoning, such as *Escherichia coli*; heavy metals, such as the lead found in the paint on older houses; and the venom found in the **bites and stings** of some animals and insects. The staff at a poison control center and emergency room doctors have the most experience diagnosing and treating poisoning cases.

Causes and symptoms

The effects of poisons are as varied as the poisons themselves. The exact mechanisms of only a few are understood. Some poisons interfere with the **metabolism**. Others destroy the liver or **kidneys**, such as heavy metals and some **pain** relief medications, including acetaminophen (Tylenol) and **nonsteroidal anti-inflammatory drugs** (Advil, ibuprofen). A poison may severely depress the **central nervous system**, leading to **coma** and eventual respiratory and circulatory failure. Potential poisons in this category include anesthetics (e.g. ether and chloroform); opiates (e.g. morphine and codeine); and barbiturates. Some poisons directly affect the respiratory and circulatory systems. Carbon monoxide causes death by binding with hemoglobin that would normally transport oxygen throughout the body. Certain corrosive vapors trigger the body to flood the **lungs** with fluids, effectively drowning the person. Cyanide interferes with respiration at the cellular level. Another group of poisons interferes with the electrochemical impulses that travel between **neurons** in the nervous system. Another group, including cocaine, ergot, strychnine, and some snake venoms, causes potentially fatal seizures.

Severity of poisoning symptoms can range from **headache** and nausea to convulsions and death. The type of poison; the amount and time of exposure; and the age, size, and health of the victim are all factors that determine the severity of symptoms and the chances for recovery.

Plant poisoning

There are more than 700 species of poisonous plants in the United States. Plants are second only to medicines in causing serious poisoning in children under age five. The appearance of a plant offers no determination of its poison. Some plants, such as the yew shrub, are almost entirely toxic: needles, bark, seeds, and berries. In other plants, only certain parts are poisonous. The bulb of the hyacinth and daffodil are toxic, but the flowers are not. It is the flowers of the jasmine plant that are poisonous. Some plants are confusing because portions of them are eaten as food while other parts are poisonous. For example, the fleshy stem (tuber) of the potato plant is nutritious; however, its roots, sprouts, and vines are poisonous. The leaves of tomatoes are poisonous, while the fruit is not. Rhubarb stalks are good to eat, but the leaves are poisonous. Apricots, cherries, peaches, and apples all produce healthful fruit, but their seeds contain a form of cyanide that can kill a child if chewed in sufficient quantities. One hundred milligrams (mg) of moist, crushed apricot seeds can produce 217 milligrams of cyanide.

Common indoor houseplants that contain some poisonous parts include:

- aloe
- amaryllis
- Boston ivy
- caladium
- cyclamen
- dumbcane (also called *Dieffenbachia*)
- philodendron

Common outdoor plants that contain some poisonous part include:

- azalea
- bird-of-paradise flower
- black cherry
- buttercup
- calla lilly
- castor bean
- chinaberry tree
- caffodil
- delphinium
- English ivy
- eucalyptus
- foxglove
- holly
- horse chestnut
- hydrangea
- iris
- jack-in-the-pulpit
- jimsonweed (also called thornapple)
- larkspur
- lily-of-the-valley
- morning glory
- nightshade (several varieties)
- oleander
- potato
- rhododendron
- rhubarb
- sweet pea
- tomato
- wisteria
- yew

Symptoms of plant poisoning range from irritation of the skin or mucous membranes of the mouth and throat to nausea, **vomiting**, convulsions, irregular heartbeat, and even death. It is often difficult to tell if a person has eaten a poisonous plant because there are no telltale empty containers and no unusual lesions or odors around the mouth.

Fungi

Mushrooms are the most common type of fungus that can cause poisoning, known as mycetism. People who collect wild mushrooms should learn to distinguish carefully between edible and poisonous mushrooms. Of the thousands of wild mushroom species native to Canada and the United States, about 250 are known to be poisonous to humans, and 32 are known to cause death if ingested.

Most poisonous mushrooms cause simple gastrointestinal upset, usually nausea and vomiting—which may, however, be severe enough to require hospitalization. Long-term damage to health from these species is rare, however. The most deadly mushrooms belong to the genus *Amanita* and include the death cap (*Amanita phylloides*), the destroying angel (*A. virosa*) and the fool's mushroom (*A. verna*). These species contain a compound called alpha-aminitin, which can cause liver failure within 1 to 3 days after ingestion. Other deadly mushrooms belong to the genus *Cortinarius* and contain a toxic alkaloid called orellanine, which can cause kidney failure.

Household chemicals

Many products used daily in the home are poisonous if swallowed. These products often contain strong acids or strong bases (alkalis). Toxic household cleaning products include:

- ammonia
- bleach
- dishwashing liquids
- drain openers
- floor waxes and furniture polishes
- laundry detergents, spot cleaners, and fabric softeners

- mildew removers
- oven cleaners
- toilet bowl cleaners

Personal care products found in the home can also be poisonous. These include:

- deodorant
- hair spray
- hair straighteners
- nail polish and polish remover
- perfume
- shampoo

Signs that a person has swallowed one of these substances include evidence of an empty container nearby; nausea or vomiting; and **burns** on the lips and skin around the mouth if the substance is a strong acid or alkali. The chemicals in some of these products may leave a distinctive odor on the breath.

Pharmaceuticals

Both over-the-counter and prescription medicines can help the body heal if taken as directed. When taken in large quantities or with other drugs where there may be an adverse interaction, they can subsequently act as poisons. Drug overdoses, both accidental and intentional, are the leading cause of poisoning in adults. Medicinal herbs should be treated like pharmaceuticals and taken only in designated quantities under the supervision of a knowledgeable person. Herbs that have healing qualities when taken in small doses can be toxic in larger doses.

Homicidal poisoning

Not all cases of poisoning are accidental or self-inflicted (suicide). About 3300 cases of poisoning in the United States each year (8% of the total) are classified as undetermined, but several hundred of them are later found to be of criminal intent. Although poisoning accounts for only 3% to 6% of murders in Canada and the United States, it often goes undetected because it leaves no visible signs of trauma. According to the Federal Bureau of Investigation (FBI), the most common poisons used by criminals are strychnine, arsenic, cyanide, ethylene glycol (automobile antifreeze), and thallium. About 36% of homicides by poison involve family members.

Diagnosis

Initially, poisoning is suspected if the victim shows changes in behavior and the signs or symptoms previously described. Evidence of an empty container or information from the victim or bystanders may be helpful in determining exactly what substance has caused the poisoning. A recent history of travel or hiking may be helpful, as some poisonous outdoor plants and mushrooms have delayed effects and symptoms may not appear for several days or even weeks after ingestion. Some acids and alkalis leave burns on the mouth. Such petroleum products as lighter fluid or kerosene leave a distinctive odor on the breath. Vomitus may be tested to determine the exact composition of the poison. Once the patient is hospitalized, **blood** and urine tests may be done to determine his or her metabolic condition.

Treatment

Treatment for poisoning depends on the poison swallowed or inhaled. Contacting a poison control center or hospital emergency room is the first step in getting proper treatment. The poison control center's telephone number is often listed with emergency numbers on the inside cover of the telephone book, or can be reached by dialing 911 or the operator. The poison control center will ask for specific information about the victim and the poison, then give appropriate **first aid** instructions. If the patient is to be taken to a hospital, a sample of vomitus and the poison container should be taken along, if they are available.

Most cases of plant poisoning are treated by inducing vomiting, if the person is fully conscious. Vomiting can be induced by taking syrup of **ipecac**, an over-the-counter product available at any pharmacy.

Mushroom poisoning should be identified and treated as quickly as possible to prevent kidney or liver damage. If possible, samples of the mushroom or vomitus should be given to emergency personnel.

For acid, alkali, or petroleum product poisonings, the patient should not be made to vomit. Acids and alkalis can burn the esophagus if they are vomited, and petroleum products can be inhaled into the lungs during vomiting, resulting in aspiration **pneumonia**.

Once under medical care, doctors have the option of treating the patient with a specific remedy to counteract the poison (antidote) or with **activated charcoal** to absorb the substance inside the patient's **digestive system**. In some instances, pumping the **stomach** may be required. Medical personnel will also provide supportive care as needed, such as intravenous fluids or **mechanical ventilation**.

Prognosis

The outcome of poisoning varies from complete recovery to death, and depends on the type and amount of the poison; the age and general health of the victim; the route of administration; and the speed with which medical care is obtained. In the case of *Amanita* mushrooms, patients who receive immediate treatment have a 10% mortality rate, while those who receive treatment 60 hours after ingestion have a 50% to 90% mortality rate.

Health care team roles

In most cases, a poisoning victim will initially be discovered by a family member or friend. Once the health care staff has been engaged at the request of those involved, it can include:

• Staff at local poison control centers. These are people specially trained regarding the properties and treatment of poisons. Staff may include physicians and nurses who are especially skilled at obtaining necessary information regarding the poison and providing the needed facts in regard to treatment.

• Emergency medical technicians (EMTs), specially trained in providing emergency care to people outside of hospitals. Often under the supervision of an emergency room physician, EMTs are frequently the first to provide medical intervention. They work from ambulances, providing the initial care often in the home, or place where the poisoning took place.

• If the poisoning victim is transported to a hospital emergency room, a licensed physician trained in emergency medicine will either begin or take further measures to negate the effect of the poison.

• Both registered nurses (RNs), and licensed practical nurses (LPNs) work in hospital emergency rooms, and are often located in poison control centers. In emergency rooms, both RNs and LPNs will be responsible for monitoring vital signs, obtaining specimens of vomitus, administering medications such as activated charcoal or ipecac, or providing assistance in carrying out procedures such as gastric lavage (pumping the stomach). Providing reassurance to frightened patients and families, and offering information regarding poisons, especially to the families of children that have been poisoned, are both critical elements of care.

• Clinical laboratory scientists have specialized training and must pass a state examination. They draw blood samples or test urine to do toxic screens for various drugs, or other tests that determine what toxic substance has been ingested.

• Radiologic technologists have specialized training and must pass a state examination. They may be called upon to take a chest x ray to ensure that the person has not aspirated (had foreign material such as vomit enter the lungs), causing aspiration pneumonia.

KEY TERMS

Acid—A chemical substance that contains the element hydrogen and has a pH above seven, which is considered neutral. Acids are generally described as sour or biting in character.

Alkali—A chemical substance that has the ability to neutralize acid. It has a pH below seven, which is considered neutral, and is generally described as caustic in nature.

Aspiration pneumonia—Fluid entering the lungs through choking or vomiting, and leading to infection of the lung.

Gastric lavage—Insertion of a tube into the stomach for the purpose of washing out and removing toxic material.

Ipecac—A medication made from the dried root of a plant native to Brazil, often used to induce vomiting.

Mycetism—The medical term for mushroom poisoning.

Vomitus—The medical term for vomited matter.

• Law enforcement may be involved when criminal poisoning is suspected. Cyanide poisoning, for example, leaves a telltale bitter almond odor on the victim's breath. In some cases, there may be a history of episodes of vomiting or other gastrointestinal symptoms that were previously misdiagnosed as food poisoning or "stomach flu."

Prevention

Most accidental poisonings are preventable. The number of deaths of children from poisoning in the United States has declined from about 450 per year in the 1960s to about 50 each year in the 1990s. This decline has occurred primarily due to better packaging of toxic materials, and to better public education.

Actions to prevent poisonings include:

• removing plants that are poisonous

• keeping medicines and household chemicals locked and in a place inaccessible to children

• keeping medications in child-resistant containers

• never referring to medicine as "candy"

• teaching children to ask an adult before putting anything in their mouth

---

QUESTIONS TO ASK YOUR DOCTOR

- What precautions should I take to prevent accidental poisoning in an elderly parent who takes a number of prescription medications?

- What antidotes would you recommend keeping in the home medicine chest in case of accidental poisoning?

- What should I teach my children about medicines and other household substances that they might put in their mouths?

- What should I know about first aid for suspected poisoning?

• keeping cleaners, bleach, and other poisons in their original containers

• disposing of outdated prescription medicines

• learning to identify poisonous outdoor plants and mushrooms before collecting them

Resources

BOOKS

Holstege, Christopher P., Thomas Neer, Gregory B. Saathoff, and R. Brent Furbee. *Criminal Poisoning: Clinical and Forensic Perspectives.* Burlington, MA: Jones and Bartlett Learning, 2011.

Holstege, Christopher P., and Carol Ann Turkington. *Deadly Daffodils, Toxic Caterpillars: The Family Guide to Preventing and Treating Accidental Poisoning Inside and Outside the Home.* New York: Stewart, Tabori and Chang, 2006.

Magnani, Barbarajean, Michael G. Bissell, and Tai C. Kwong, eds. *Clinical Toxicology Testing: A Guide for Laboratory Professionals.* Northfield, IL: College of American Pathologists, 2011.

Nelson, Lewis S., ed. *Goldfrank's Toxicologic Emergencies,* 9th ed. New York: McGraw-Hill Medical, 2011.

PERIODICALS

Appleton, S. "Frequency and Outcomes of Accidental Ingestion of Tobacco Products in Young Children." *Regulatory Toxicology and Pharmacology* 61 (November 2011): 210–214.

Beno, J.M., et al. "Homicidal Methanol Poisoning in a Child." *Journal of Analytical Toxicology* 35 (September 2011): 524–528.

Centers for Disease Control and Prevention (CDC). "Community-based Opioid Overdose Prevention Programs Providing Naloxone—United States, 2010." *Morbidity and Mortality Weekly Report* 61 (February 17, 2012): 101–105.

Centers for Disease Control and Prevention (CDC). "Drug Overdose Deaths—Florida, 2003–2009." *Morbidity and Mortality Weekly Report* 60 (July 8, 2011): 869–872.

Coulter, C.V., et al. "Methanol and Ethylene Glycol Acute Poisonings—Predictors of Mortality." *Clinical Toxicology (Philadelphia)* 49 (December 2011): 900–906.

Darke, S. "Oxycodone Poisoning: Not Just the 'Usual Suspects.'" *Addiction* 106 (June 2011): 1035–1036.

Gormley, N.J., et al. "The Rising Incidence of Intentional Ingestion of Ethanol-containing Hand Sanitizers." *Critical Care Medicine* 40 (January 2012): 290–294.

Marcus, S.M. "Poison Prevention: Engineering in Primary Prevention." *Clinical Toxicology (Philadelphia)* 50 (March 2012): 163–165.

Mollison, L.C. "Mushroom Poisoning: A Personal Vignette." *Medical Journal of Australia* 195 (December 19, 2011): 720–721.

Westveer, Arthur E., et al. "Homicidal Poisoning: The Silent Offense." *FBI Law Enforcement Bulletin* 73 (August 2004): 1–8. Available online at http://www.fbi.gov/stats-services/publications/law-enforcement-bulletin/2004-pdfs/aug04leb.pdf.

WEBSITES

American Association of Poison Control Centers (AAPCC). "Out-of-Hospital Patient Management Guidelines." http://www.aapcc.org/dnn/PatientManagement.aspx (accessed April 23, 2012). This is a menu of treatment guidelines for 18 of the most common household medications and other chemicals involved in accidental poisonings.

Centers for Disease Control and Prevention (CDC). "Poisoning in the United States: Fact Sheet." http://www.cdc.gov/homeandrecreationalsafety/poisoning/poisoning-factsheet.htm (accessed April 22, 2012).

Centers for Disease Control and Prevention (CDC). "Public Health Grand Rounds: Prescription Drug Overdoses: An American Epidemic." http://www.youtube.com/watch?v=-zryKuf7-kI&feature=BF&list=PLAAB7866D2D8A-CAAE&index=15 (accessed April 23, 2012). Produced in 2011, this is an hour-long video presentation by the director of the CDC about the recent increase in prescription drug poisonings in the United States.

Fischer, David. "A Detailed Look at America's Poisonous Mushrooms." http://americanmushrooms.com/toxicms.htm (accessed April 23, 2012).

Food and Drug Administration (FDA). Poisonous Plant Database. http://www.accessdata.fda.gov/scripts/plantox/index.cfm (accessed April 23, 2012).

University of North Carolina. "Chemical Terrorism Agents and Syndromes." http://img.medscape.com/pi/emed/ckb/emergency_medicine/756148-812410-814287-814390.pdf (accessed April 23, 2012). Includes information about cyanide and poisonous plants and mushrooms.

ORGANIZATIONS

American Association of Poison Control Centers (AAPCC), (800) 222-1222, info@aapcc.org, http://www.aapcc.org/dnn/Home.aspx

Centers for Disease Control and Prevention (CDC), 1600
    Clifton Road, Atlanta, GA United States 30333, (800)
    CDC-INFO (232-4636), cdcinfo@cdc.gov, www.cdc.gov
Food and Drug Administration (FDA), 10903 New Hampshire
    Avenue, Silver Spring, MD United States 20993, (888)
    INFO-FDA (463-6332), http://www.fda.gov/default.htm
National Toxicology Program (NTP), P.O. Box 12233, MD
    K2-05, Research Triangle Park, NC United States 27709,
    (919) 541-3419, http://ntp.niehs.nih.gov/

Joan M. Schonbeck
Rebecca J. Frey, Ph.D.

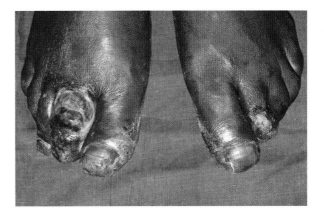

(Leprosy alcoholic neuropathy ulcers on human feet, photograph. Ansary/Custom Medical Stock Photo, Inc. Reproduced by permission.)

Polyneuropathies

Definition

Polyneuropathies encompass a wide range of disorders in which the nerves outside of the **brain** and spinal cord—peripheral to the central nervous system—have been damaged. Polyneuropathy is also referred to as peripheral neuritis or polyneuritis.

Description

Polyneuropathy is a common disorder with many underlying causes. Some of these causes occur frequently, such as diabetes, and others are extremely rare, such as acrylamide **poisoning** and certain inherited disorders. The most common worldwide cause of polyneuropathy is leprosy. Leprosy is caused by the bacterium *Mycobacterium leprae*, which attacks the peripheral nerves. According to statistical data from the World Health Organization, an estimated 1.15 million people suffer from leprosy worldwide.

Leprosy is extremely rare in the United States, where diabetes is the most commonly known cause of polyneuropathy. It has been estimated that more than 17 million people in the United States and Europe suffer from diabetes-related polyneuropathy. Many neuropathies are idiopathic, meaning that no known cause can be found. The most common inherited polyneuropathy in the United States is Charcot-Marie-Tooth disease, which affects approximately 125,000 persons.

Another of the better known polyneuropathies is Guillain-Barré syndrome (GBS, acute idiopathic demyelinating polyneuropathy); it is a complication of viral illnesses, such as cytomegalovirus, Epstein-Barr virus, and human **immunodeficiency** virus (HIV) or bacterial **infection**, including *Campylobacter jejuni* and Lyme disease. The worldwide incidence rate is approximately 1.7 cases per 100,000 people annually. Other well-known causes of polyneuropathies include chronic **alcoholism**, infection, varicella-zoster virus, botulism, and poliomyelitis. Polyneuropathy may develop as a primary symptom, or it may be due to another disease. For example, polyneuropathy is only one symptom of diseases such as amyloid neuropathy, certain cancers, or inherited neurologic disorders. Such diseases may affect the peripheral nervous system (PNS) and the **central nervous system** (CNS), as well as other body tissues.

To understand polyneuropathy and its underlying causes, it may be helpful to review the structures and arrangement of the PNS.

Nerve cells and nerves

Nerve cells are the basic building block of the nervous system. In the PNS, nerve cells can be threadlike—their width is microscopic, but their length may be measured in feet. The long, spidery extensions of nerve cells are called axons. When a nerve cell is stimulated—by touch or **pain**, for example—the message is carried along the axon, and neurotransmitters are released within the cells. Neurotransmitters are chemicals within the nervous system that direct nerve cell communication.

Certain nerve cell axons, such as those in the PNS, are covered with a substance called myelin. This myelin sheath may be compared to the plastic insulation coating electrical wires—it both protects the cells and prevents interference with the signals being transmitted. Protection is also given by Schwann cells, special cells within the nervous system that wrap around both myelinated and unmyelinated axons.

Nerve cell axons leading to the same areas of the body may be bundled together into nerves. Continuing the comparison to electrical wires, nerves may be compared to an electrical cord—the individual components being coated in their own sheaths and then encased together inside a larger protective sheath.

The nervous system is classified into two parts: the CNS and the PNS. The CNS is the brain and the **spinal cord**, and the PNS is composed of the nerves that lead to or branch off from the CNS.

Peripheral nervous system

The peripheral nerves handle a diverse array of functions in the body. This diversity is reflected in the major divisions of the PNS—the afferent and the efferent divisions. The afferent division conveys sensory information from the body to the CNS. When afferent nerve cell endings, called receptors, are stimulated, they release neurotransmitters. These neurotransmitters relay a signal to the brain, which interprets it and reacts by releasing other neurotransmitters.

Some of the neurotransmitters released by the brain are directed at the efferent division of the PNS. The efferent nerves control voluntary movements, such as moving the arms and legs; and involuntary movements, such as making the **heart** pump **blood**. The nerves controlling voluntary movements are called motor nerves, and the nerves controlling involuntary actions are referred to as autonomic nerves. The afferent and efferent divisions continually interact with one another.

Neuropathy

NERVE DAMAGE. When a patient suffers from a polyneuropathy, nerves of the PNS have been damaged. Nerve damage can arise from a number of causes, such as disease, physical injury, poisoning, or malnutrition. These agents may affect either afferent or efferent nerves. Depending upon the cause of damage the nerve cell, axon, its protective myelin sheath, or both may be injured or destroyed.

CLASSIFICATION. There are hundreds of polyneuropathies. Reflecting the scope of PNS activity, symptoms may involve sensory, motor, or autonomic functions. To aid in diagnosis and treatment, symptoms are classified into principal neuropathic syndromes, based on the type of affected nerves and how long symptoms have been developing. Acute development refers to symptoms that have appeared within days, and subacute refers to those that have evolved over a number of weeks. Early chronic symptoms are those that take from months to a few years

to develop, and late chronic symptoms are those that have been present for several years.

The classification system is composed of six principal neuropathic syndromes, which are subdivided into more specific categories. By narrowing the possible diagnoses in this way, specific medical tests can be used more efficiently and effectively. The six syndromes and a few associated causes are:

- Acute motor paralysis accompanied by variable problems with sensory and autonomic functions: Neuropathies associated with this syndrome are mainly accompanied by motor nerve problems, but the sensory and autonomic nerves may also be involved. Associated disorders include Guillain-Barré syndrome, diphtheritic polyneuropathy, and porphyritic neuropathy.

- Subacute sensorimotor paralysis: The term sensorimotor refers to neuropathies that are mainly characterized by sensory symptoms but also have a minor component of motor nerve problems. Poisoning with heavy metals (e.g., lead, mercury, and arsenic), chemicals, or drugs are linked to this syndrome. Diabetes, Lyme disease, and malnutrition are also possible causes.

- Chronic sensorimotor paralysis: Physical symptoms may resemble those in the above syndrome but the time frame for symptom development is prolonged. This syndrome encompasses neuropathies arising from cancers, diabetes, leprosy, inherited neurologic and metabolic disorders, and hypothyroidism.

- Neuropathy associated with mitochondrial diseases: Mitochondria are organelles (structures within cells) responsible for handling a cell's energy requirements. When mitochondria are damaged or destroyed, the cell's energy requirements are not met and it can die.

- Recurrent or relapsing polyneuropathy: This syndrome covers neuropathies that affect several nerves and may come and go, such as Guillain-Barré syndrome, porphyria, and chronic inflammatory demyelinating polyneuropathy.

- Mononeuropathy or plexopathy: Nerve damage associated with this syndrome is limited to a single nerve or a few closely associated nerves. Neuropathies related to physical injury to the nerve, such as carpal tunnel syndrome and sciatica, are included in this syndrome.

Causes and symptoms

Typical symptoms of neuropathy relate to the type of affected nerve. If a sensory nerve is damaged, common symptoms include numbness, tingling in the area, a prickling sensation, or pain. Pain associated with neuropathy can be quite intense and may be described as cutting, stabbing, crushing, or burning. In some cases a normally nonpainful stimulus may be perceived as excruciating, or pain may be felt even in the absence of a stimulus. Damage to a motor nerve is usually indicated by **weakness** in the affected area. If the problem with the motor nerve has persisted, then atrophy (muscle wasting) or lack of muscle tone may be noticeable. Autonomic nerve damage is most noticeable when a patient stands upright and experiences problems such as light-headedness or changes in **blood pressure**. Other indicators of autonomic nerve damage are lack of sweat, tears, and saliva; constipation; urinary retention; and impotence. In some cases heart rhythm irregularities and respiratory problems may develop.

Symptoms may appear over days, weeks, months, or years. Their duration and the ultimate outcome of the neuropathy are linked to the cause of the nerve damage. Potential causes include diseases, physical injuries, poisoning, and malnutrition or alcohol abuse. In some cases neuropathy is not the primary disorder but a symptom of an underlying disease.

Disease

Diseases that cause polyneuropathies may be acquired or inherited; in some cases it is difficult to make the distinction. The diabetes-polyneuropathy link has been well established. A typical pattern of diabetes-associated neuropathic symptoms includes sensory effects that first begin in the feet. The associated pain or pins-and-needles, burning, crawling, or prickling sensations, form a typical "stocking" distribution in the feet and lower legs. Other diabetic neuropathies affect the autonomic nerves and have potentially fatal cardiovascular complications.

Several other metabolic diseases have a strong association with polyneuropathy. Uremia (**chronic kidney failure**) carries a 10%-90% risk of eventually developing neuropathy, and there may be an association between **liver** failure and polyneuropathy. **Atherosclerosis** (accumulation of **lipids** inside **blood vessels**) can impair blood supply to certain peripheral nerves. Without oxygen and nutrients the nerves slowly die. Mild polyneuropathy may develop in patients with hypothyroidism (low thyroid hormone levels). Individuals with acromegaly (abnormally enlarged skeletal extremities caused by an excess of growth hormone) may also develop mild polyneuropathy.

Neuropathy can also result from vasculitis, a group of disorders in which blood vessels are inflamed. When the blood vessels are inflamed or damaged, blood supply to the nerve can be affected, injuring the nerve.

Both viral and bacterial infections have been implicated in polyneuropathy. Leprosy is caused by the **bacteria** *M. leprae*, which directly attacks sensory nerves. Other bacterial illnesses may set the stage for an immune-mediated attack on the nerves. For example, one theory about Guillain-Barré syndrome involves complications following infection with *Campylobacter jejuni*, a bacterium commonly associated with food poisoning. This bacterium carries a protein that closely resembles components of myelin. The **immune system** launches an attack against the bacteria; but, according to the theory, the immune system confuses the myelin with the bacteria in some cases and attacks the myelin sheath as well. The underlying cause of neuropathy associated with Lyme disease is unknown; the bacteria may either precipitate an immune-mediated attack on the nerve or inflict damage directly.

Infection with certain **viruses** is associated with extremely painful sensory neuropathies. **Shingles** is an example of such a neuropathy. After a case of chickenpox the causative virus, varicella-zoster virus, becomes inactive or latent in sensory nerves. Years later the virus may be reactivated and, once reactivated, attacks and destroys axons. Infection with HIV is also associated with polyneuropathy, but the type of neuropathy that develops can vary. Some HIV-linked neuropathies are noted for myelin destruction rather than axonal degradation. Also, HIV infection is frequently accompanied by other infections, both bacterial and viral, that are associated with neuropathy.

Several types of polyneuropathies are associated with inherited disorders. These inherited disorders may primarily involve the nervous system, or the effects on the nervous system may be secondary to an inherited metabolic disorder. Inherited neuropathies fall into several of the principal syndromes because symptoms may be sensory, motor, or autonomic. The inheritance patterns also vary depending upon the specific disorder. The development of inherited disorders is typically prolonged over several years and may herald a degenerative condition—that is, a condition that becomes progressively worse over time. Even among specific disorders there may be a degree of variability in inheritance patterns and symptoms. For example, Charcot-Marie-Tooth disease is usually inherited as an autosomal dominant disorder; however, it can be autosomal recessive or, in rare cases, linked to the X chromosome. Its estimated frequency is approximately one in 2,500 people. Age of onset and sensory nerve involvement can vary between cases. The main symptom is a degeneration of the motor nerves in legs and arms with resultant muscle atrophy. Other inherited neuropathies have a distinctly metabolic component. For example, in familial amyloid polyneuropathies, protein components that make up the myelin are constructed and deposited incorrectly.

Physical injury

Accidental injuries during sports and recreational activities are common causes of polyneuropathy. The common types of injuries in these situations occur from placing too much pressure on the nerve, exceeding the nerve's capacity to stretch, blocking adequate blood supply of oxygen and nutrients to the nerve, and tearing the nerve. Pain may not always be immediately noticeable, and obvious signs of damage may take a while to develop.

These injuries usually affect one nerve or a group of closely associated nerves. For example, a common injury encountered in contact sports such as football is the "burner," or "stinger," syndrome. Typically, a stinger is caused by overstretching the main nerves that span from the neck into the arm. Immediate symptoms are numbness, tingling, and pain that travels down the arm, lasting only a minute or two. A single incident of a stinger is not dangerous, but recurrences can eventually cause permanent motor and sensory loss.

Poisoning

The poisons, or toxins, that cause polyneuropathy include drugs, industrial chemicals, and environmental toxins. Neuropathy that is caused by drugs usually involves sensory nerves on both sides of the body, particularly in the hands and feet; and pain is a common symptom. Neuropathy is a rare side effect of prescription medications. A few drugs that have been linked with polyneuropathy include metronidazole, an antibiotic; phenytoin, an anticonvulsant; and simvastatin, a cholesterol-lowering medication.

Certain industrial chemicals are neurotoxic (poisonous to nerves) following work-related exposures. Chemicals such as acrylamide, allyl chloride, and carbon disulfide have been strongly linked to development of polyneuropathy. Organic compounds, such as N-hexane and toluene, are also encountered in work-related settings, as well as in glue-sniffing and solvent abuse. Either route of exposure can produce severe sensorimotor neuropathy that develops rapidly.

Heavy metals are the third group of toxins that cause polyneuropathy. Lead, arsenic, thallium, and mercury usually are not toxic in their elemental form, but rather as components in organic or inorganic compounds. The types of metal-induced neuropathies vary widely. Arsenic poisoning may mimic Guillain-Barré syndrome; lead affects motor nerves more than sensory nerves; thallium produces painful sensorimotor neuropathy; and the effects of mercury are seen in both the CNS and PNS.

Malnutrition and alcohol abuse

Burning, stabbing pains and numbness in the feet, and sometimes in the hands, are distinguishing features of alcoholic neuropathy. The level of alcohol consumption associated with this variety of polyneuropathy has been estimated as approximately 3 liters of beer or 300 milliliters of liquor daily for three years. However, it is unclear whether alcohol alone is responsible for the neuropathic symptoms, because chronic alcoholism is strongly associated with malnutrition.

Malnutrition refers to an extreme lack of nutrients in the diet. It is unknown precisely which nutrient deficiencies cause polyneuropathies in alcoholics and famine and starvation victims, but it is suspected that the B **vitamins** have a significant role. For example, **thiamine** (vitamin B$_1$) deficiency is the cause of beriberi, a neuropathic disease characterized by **heart failure** and painful polyneuropathy of sensory nerves. **Vitamin E** deficiency seems to have a role in both CNS and PNS neuropathy.

Diagnosis

Clinical symptoms can indicate polyneuropathy, but an exact diagnosis requires a combination of medical history, medical tests, and possibly a process of exclusion. Certain symptoms may suggest a diagnosis, but more information is commonly needed. For example, painful, burning feet may be a symptom of alcohol abuse, diabetes, HIV infection, or an underlying malignant tumor, among other causes. Without further details effective treatment would be difficult.

During the history and **physical examination**, the physician obtains detailed information about the location, nature, and duration of symptoms to exclude some causes or even pinpoint the actual problem. The patient's medical history may also provide clues as to the cause, because certain diseases and medications are linked to specific polyneuropathies. A medical history should also include information about diseases that run in the family, because some polyneuropathies are genetically linked. Information about hobbies, recreational activities, alcohol consumption, and workplace activities can uncover possible injuries or exposures to poisonous substances.

The evaluation of a patient with polyneuropathy also includes laboratory tests, such as blood levels of glucose and creatinine, to detect diabetes and kidney problems, respectively. A **complete blood count** (CBC) is also done to determine levels of different blood cell types.

Iron, vitamin B$_{12}$, folic acid, and other factors may be measured to rule out malnutrition. More specific tests, such as an assay for heavy metals or poisonous substances, or tests to detect vasculitis, are not typically performed unless there is reason to suspect a particular cause. Routine and specialized blood tests are generally performed by a laboratory technologist.

An individual with neuropathy may be referred to a neurologist (physician specializing in nervous system disorders). By considering the results of the physical examination and observing information supplied by the referring primary care physician, the neurologist may be able to narrow down the possible diagnoses. Additional tests, such as nerve conduction studies and **electromyography**, which tests muscle reactions, can confirm that nerve damage has occurred and may also be able to indicate the nature of the damage. For example, if the neuropathy is caused by destruction of the myelin, damage is shown by slowed nerve conduction. If the axon itself has suffered damage, the nerve conduction may be slowed but will also be diminished in strength. Electromyography (performed by technologists often known as electromyographers or EMG technicians) adds further information by measuring nerve conduction and muscle response, which determine whether the symptoms are due to a neuropathy or a muscle disorder.

In approximately 10% of polyneuropathy cases a nerve biopsy may be helpful. In this test the physician surgically removes a small part of the nerve for examination under a **microscope**. This procedure is usually performed to confirm a suspected diagnosis rather than as an initial diagnostic procedure.

Treatment

Treat the cause

Attacking the underlying cause of the neuropathy can prevent further nerve damage and may allow for better recovery. For example, in cases of bacterial infections such as leprosy or Lyme disease, **antibiotics** may be given to destroy the infectious bacteria. Viral infections are more difficult to treat because antibiotics are not effective against them. Neuropathies associated with drugs, chemicals, and toxins are treated in part by stopping exposure to the damaging agent. Chemicals such as ethylenediaminetetraacetic acid (EDTA) are used to help the body concentrate and excrete some toxins. Diabetic neuropathies may be treated by gaining better control of blood sugar levels, but chronic kidney failure may require dialysis or even kidney transplant to prevent or reduce nerve damage. In some cases, such as compression injury or tumors, surgery may be considered to relieve pressure on a nerve.

In a crisis situation, as in the onset of Guillain-Barré syndrome, plasma exchange, intravenous immunoglobulin, and steroids may be prescribed. Intubation and **mechanical ventilation** may be required to support the **respiratory system**. Treatment may focus more on symptom management than on combating the underlying cause, at least until a definitive diagnosis has been made.

Supportive care and long-term therapy

Some polyneuropathies cannot be resolved or may require considerable time for resolution. In these cases long-term monitoring and supportive care are necessary. Medical tests may be repeated to chart the progress of the neuropathy. If autonomic nerve involvement is a concern, regular monitoring of the **cardiovascular system** may be performed.

Because pain is associated with many neuropathies, **pain management** is an important aspect of treatment, especially if the pain becomes chronic. As in any chronic disease narcotics are best avoided. Agents that may relieve neuropathic pain include amitriptyline, carbamazepine, and capsaicin cream. **Physical therapy** and physician-directed exercises can help maintain or improve function. When motor nerves are affected, braces and other supportive equipment can aid patients' ability to move about.

Prognosis

The outcome for polyneuropathy depends heavily upon the underlying cause. Polyneuropathy ranges from a reversible problem to a potentially fatal complication. In the best cases a damaged nerve regenerates. Though nerve cells cannot be replaced if they are killed, they are capable of recovering from damage. The extent of recovery depends upon the extent of the damage and the patient's age and general health status. Recovery can take weeks to years because **neurons** grow very slowly. Full recovery may not be possible, and it may not be possible to determine the prognosis at the outset.

If the neuropathy is a degenerative condition, such as Charcot-Marie-Tooth disease, then the patient's condition will worsen although there may be periods when the disease seems to plateau. Cures have not yet been discovered for many degenerative diseases. For patients with incurable neuropathies, continued symptoms with a potential to worsening to disabilities, are to be expected.

A few polyneuropathies are eventually fatal. Fatalities from polyneuropathies have been associated with some cases of diphtheria, botulism, and other causes. Some diseases associated with neuropathy may also be

KEY TERMS

Afferent—Refers to peripheral nerves that transmit signals to the spinal cord and the brain. These nerves carry out sensory function.

Autonomic—Refers to peripheral nerves that carry signals from the brain and control involuntary actions in the body such as the beating of the heart.

Autosomal dominant or autosomal recessive—Refers to the inheritance pattern of a gene on a chromosome other than X or Y. Genes are inherited in pairs—one gene from each parent. However, the inheritance may not be equal, and one gene may overshadow the other in determining the final form of the encoded characteristic. The gene that overshadows the other is called the dominant gene; the overshadowed gene is the recessive one.

Axon—A long, threadlike projection that is part of a nerve cell.

Central nervous system (CNS)—The part of the nervous system that includes the brain and the spinal cord.

Efferent—Refers to peripheral nerves that carry signals away from the brain and spinal cord. These nerves carry out motor and autonomic functions.

Electromyography—A medical test that assesses nerve signals and muscle reactions. It can determine if there is a disorder with the nerve or if the muscle is not capable of responding.

Inheritance pattern—Refers to dominant or recessive inheritance.

Motor—Refers to peripheral nerves that control voluntary movements, such as moving the arms and legs.

Myelin—The protective coating on axons.

Nerve biopsy—A medical test in which a small portion of a damaged nerve is surgically removed and examined under a microscope.

Nerve conduction—The speed and strength of a signal being transmitted by nerve cells. Testing these factors can reveal the nature of nerve injury, such as damage to nerve cells or to the protective myelin sheath.

Neurotransmitter—Chemicals within the nervous system that transmit information from or between nerve cells.

Peripheral nervous system (PNS)—Nerves that are outside of the brain and spinal cord.

Sensory—Refers to peripheral nerves that transmit information from the senses to the brain.

fatal, but the ultimate cause of death is not necessarily related to the neuropathy—such as with **cancer**.

Health care team roles

The composition of the health care team treating patients with polyneuropathies will necessarily vary depending upon the underlying cause of the condition. For example, patients suffering from diabetes may be managed by physicians specializing in **internal medicine** and/or **endocrinology**. Cancer patients are often managed by oncologists, and patients with degenerative neurological disorders are treated by neurologists. Nearly all patients will also be cared for by laboratory technologists, radiological technologists, and nurses—the latter providing education about the disorder and management of the patient at home, and home safety assessments.

Patients requiring **rehabilitation** services may be seen by physiatrists (physician specialists in physical medicine), as well as physical and occupational therapists. Patients with diabetes and other metabolic or endocrine disorders also may receive counseling from registered dieticians and nutritionists to assist them to better manage these chronic diseases.

Prevention

Polyneuropathies are preventable only to the extent that the underlying causes are preventable. Primary prevention includes vaccines against diseases that cause neuropathy, such as polio and diphtheria. Timely treatment for physical injuries may help prevent permanent or worsening damage to nerves. Precautions when using certain chemicals and drugs are well advised in order to prevent exposure to neurotoxic agents. Control of chronic diseases such as diabetes may also reduce the risk of developing polyneuropathy.

Although not a preventive measure, genetic screening can serve as an early warning for potential problems. Genetic screening is available for some inherited conditions, but not all. In some cases presence of a particular gene does not necessarily mean the person will develop the disease because environmental and other components may be involved.

Resources

BOOKS

Adams, Raymond D, Maurice Victor, and Allan H. Ropper. *Adams & Victor's Principles of Neurology, 9th ed.* New York, McGraw Hill Professional, 2009.

Humes, H. David, ed. *Kelley's Textbook of Internal Medicine.* Philadelphia: Lippincott Williams & Wilkins, 2000, 2764-2765.

ORGANIZATIONS

American Diabetes Association. 1660 Duke St., Alexandria, VA 22314. (800) DIABETES. http://www.diabetes.org.

Charcot-Marie-Tooth Association. Crozer Mills Enterprise Center. 601 Upland Ave., Upland, PA 19015. (800) 606-2682. http://www.charcot-marie-tooth.org.

Guillain-Barré Syndrome Foundation International. P.O. Box 262, Wynnewood, PA 19096. (610) 667-0131. http://www.webmast.com/gbs.

The Myelin Project. 1747 Pennsylvania Ave., NW, Ste. 950, Washington, DC 20006. (202) 452-8994. http://www.myelin.org.

The Neuropathy Association. 60 E. 42nd St., Suite 942, New York, NY 10165. (800) 247-6968. http://www.neuropathy.org/association.html.

Barbara Wexler

Polysomnography

Definition

Polysomnography is a set of tests performed while a patient sleeps. It is done to diagnose and evaluate **sleep disorders**, and examines at a minimum **brain** wave patterns, the movements of both eyes, and the tone of at least one skeletal muscle.

Purpose

Polysomnography is used to diagnose and evaluate many types of sleeping disorders, including disorders of initiating or maintaining sleep (dissomnias) and disorders during sleep (parasomnias), including medical, psychiatric, and dental disorders that have symptoms during sleep. A relatively common dissomnia is **sleep apnea**, a disorder most prevalent in middle-aged and elderly obese men, in which the muscles of the soft palate in the back of the throat relax and close off the airway during sleep. Sleep apnea may cause the patient to snore loudly and gasp for air at night, and to be excessively sleepy and doze off during the day.

Another dissomnia often evaluated by polysomnography is narcolepsy. Narcoleptics suffer from excessive daytime sleepiness, sudden attacks of muscle **weakness** (cataplexy), and hallucinations at sleep onset. Some parasomnias that can be detected using polysomnography include disorders of arousal or rapid-eye-movement (REM) sleep problems, such as nightmares. Medical conditions including sleep-related **asthma**, depression, and panic disorder can be evaluated. Teeth-grinding (**bruxism**) or neurological problems such as restless leg syndrome show up during polysomnography. Finally, the tests can also be used to detect or evaluate seizures of sleep-related epilepsy that occur in the middle of the night, when the patient and his or her family are unlikely to be aware of them.

Precautions

Polysomnography is completely safe, and no special precautions need to be taken.

Description

Polysomnography is performed during an overnight stay in a sleep laboratory. While the patient sleeps, a wide variety of tests can be performed.

One form of monitoring is **electroencephalography** (EEG), in which electrodes are attached to the patient's scalp in order to record his or her brain wave activity. The electroencephalograph records brain wave activity from different parts of the brain and charts them on a graph. The EEG not only helps doctors establish what stage of sleep the patient is in, but may also detect seizures. Standard tests have at least one central electrode attached to the scalp and one reference electrode attached to the ear. Other electrodes can be added in order to pinpoint the area of the brain where abnormal activity is occurring.

Another form of monitoring is continuous electrooculography (EOG), which records eye movement and is useful in determining when the patient is going through a stage of REM sleep. Both EEG and EOG can be helpful in determining sleep latency (the time that transpires between lights out and the onset of sleep), total sleep time, the time spent in each sleep stage, and the number of arousals from sleep.

The air flow through the patient's nose and mouth is measured by heat-sensitive devices called thermistors. This measurement can help detect episodes of apnea (stopped breathing), or hypopnea (inadequate breathing). Another test, called pulse oximetry, measures the amount of oxygen in the **blood** and can be used to assess the

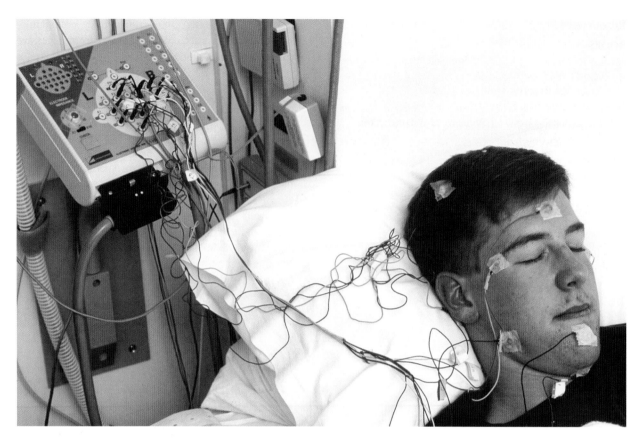

(Male patient with electrodes attached to his face and neck, wires lead to a machine, photograph. Hank Morgan / Photo Researchers, Inc.)

degree of oxygen starvation during episodes of hypopnea or apnea.

The electrical activity of the patient's **heart** is also measured using **electrocardiography** (ECG or EKG). Electrodes are affixed to the patient's chest and pick up electrical activity from various areas of the heart. They help detect cardiac arrythmias (abnormal heart rhythms), which may occur during periods of sleep apnea. **Blood pressure** is also measured as episodes of sleep apnea sometimes dangerously elevate blood pressure.

A final standard measurement is the tone of at least one skeletal muscle, often a muscle of the chin (mentalis or submentalis). This is done using **electromyography** (EMG), which involves placing an electrode on the muscle to record its contractions. If normal, measurements will indicate the general atonia present during REM sleep. Other EMG channels can be placed, particularly on the leg (anterior tibialis), to indicate movement during sleep.

Depending on the suspected disorder, polysomnography can also include sound monitoring to record **snoring**; video monitoring to document body positions; core body temperature readings; incident light intensities; penile swelling (tumescence); and pressure and pH at various levels of the esophagus.

One test that is often performed in conjunction with polysomnography is a Multiple Sleep Latency Test (MSLT). This test is also performed in a sleep laboratory and involves the recording of the sleep of several naps during the day after the overnight test. The MSLT is particularly important for a complete diagnosis of narcolepsy.

Preparation

Patient preparation is necessary to ensure that the night or nights in the sleep laboratory are as close as possible to an unmediated night in the patient's own home. Patients should bring suitable sleepwear and make sure their hair is clean and free from gels or sprays that may interfere with electrode functioning. They should be advised to maintain usual awake-sleep cycles and avoid sleeping pills, alcohol, stimulants, and strenuous **exercise** before the test.

KEY TERMS

Cataplexy—A condition characterized by sudden loss of muscle tone brought on by emotions, often associated with narcolepsy.

Electrocardiography (ECG)—Recording of the electrical activity from various regions of the heart muscle.

Electroencephalography (EEG)—Recording of the electrical activity from various regions of the brain.

Electrooculography (EOG)—Recording of the electrical activity of the muscles that control eye movement.

Narcolepsy—A sleep disorder characterized by attacks of sleep, cataplexy, sleep paralysis, or hallucinations with the onset of sleep.

Sleep apnea—A sleep disorder characterized by lapses in breathing during sleep.

Sleep latency—The time it takes to fall asleep once the lights are out.

Aftercare

Once the test is over, the monitors are detached from the patient. No special measures need to be taken after polysomnography.

Complications

The greatest limitation to polysomnography are the differences between the recording conditions and those that are present in the patient's home. The differences between the sleep laboratory and home have the highest effect on the first night of testing. Detection and elimination of this "first night effect" can be accomplished by the rather costly step of recording for multiple nights. Multiple night recordings are also sometimes necessary to obtain information about problems that only appear sporadically.

Results

Standard analysis still involves the tedious and time-consuming review and scoring of either paper tracings or recordings projected on a computer monitor. However, automatic, computer-based systems are becoming more and more common in clinical and research settings.

Results are interpreted in light of recorded overnight parameters such as the times of lights on/off, total time in bed, and total sleep time. The overnight recording is divided into time periods of approximately 30 seconds. The standard EEG, EMG, and EOG recordings are evaluated, and the predominant stage of sleep, according to the manual of Rechtschaffen and Kales, is assigned to the entire time period.

This data is used to calculate total time and relative proportion of the night spent in each of the six stages of sleep, including REM and non-REM. Latencies to REM and slow-wave sleep (SWS) are also recorded.

Special note is made of such neurophysiologic events as epileptic events, intrusion of alpha-type brain waves into sleep, or periodic activity of the tibialis anterior. Respiratory activities, including apneic or hypopneic episodes and oxygen saturation, are correlated with sleep stages. Other parameters that are being measured, such as body position, gastroesophageal reflux, bruxism, and penile tumescence, are recorded.

If a sleep apnea syndrome is diagnosed, primarily through a showing of periodic breathing stoppage and effects on the pulse and heart, a trial of continuous positive airway pressure or a trial of an oral appliance may be undertaken, either in a partial-night or second-night polysomnography recording.

Health care team roles

Polysomnography is often performed by a specially trained technician called a polysomnographic technologist. Training programs for this position can involve one-to-two-year programs in training as an electrodiagnostic technologist, with additional time for the polysomnography courses. Some typical courses in this area include:

- fundamentals of polysomnography
- sleep disorders
- infant and pediatric polysomnography
- polysomnography instrumentation
- polysomnography recording and monitoring
- polysomnography record scoring

Registration in polysomnography is available from the Board of Registered Polysomnography Technologists. The certification requires passing a written test.

Resources

BOOK

Misulis, Karl E. "Polysomnography Basics." In *Essentials of Clinical Neurophysiology.* Boston: Butterworth–Heinemann, 1997.

PERIODICAL

Grandjean, Cynthia and Susanne Gibbons. "Assessing Ambulatory Geriatric Sleep Complaints." *The Nurse Practitioner* (September 2000).

ORGANIZATIONS

Association of Polysomnographic Technologists. PO Box 14861, Lexena, KS, 66285. (913) 541-1991 ext. 477. http://www.aptweb.org.

National Sleep Foundation. 1522 K St. NW, Suite 500, Washington, DC 20005. (202) 347-3471. http://www.sleepfoundation.org.

Michelle L. Johnson, M.S., J.D.

Porphyrias

Definition

The porphyrias are a group of rare disorders that affect heme biosynthesis. Heme is an essential component of hemoglobin as well as of many enzymes throughout the body.

Description

Biosynthesis of heme is a multistep process that starts with simple molecules and ends with a large, complex heme molecule. Each step of the biosynthesis pathway is directed by its own enzyme (a task-specific protein). As a heme precursor molecule moves through each step, an enzyme modifies it in some way. If the precursor is not modified, it cannot proceed to the next step.

The main characteristic of the porphyrias is a defect in one of the enzymes of the heme biosynthesis pathway. The defect prevents protoporphyrins or porphyrin (heme precursors) from proceeding further along the pathway. Symptoms may be debilitating or life-threatening in some cases. Porphyria is an inherited condition, but it may be acquired after exposure to poisonous substances.

Heme

Heme is primarily synthesized in the **liver** and **bone** marrow. Heme synthesis for immature red **blood** cells, namely the erythroblasts and the reticulocytes, occurs in the bone marrow.

Although production is concentrated in the liver and bone marrow, heme is used in various capacities in virtually every tissue in the body. In most cells, it is a key building block in the construction of factors that oversee **metabolism** as well as transport of oxygen and energy. In immature red blood cells, heme is a featured component of hemoglobin. Hemoglobin is the red pigment that gives red blood cells the ability to transport oxygen as well as their characteristic color.

Heme biosynthesis

The heme molecule is composed of porphyrin and an **iron** atom. Much of the heme biosynthesis pathway is dedicated to constructing the porphyrin molecule. Porphyrin is a large molecule shaped like a four-leaf clover. An iron atom is placed at its center during the last step of heme biosynthesis.

The production of heme may be compared to a factory assembly line. The heme "assembly line" is an eight-step process, requiring eight different—and properly functioning—enzymes:

- Step 1: delta-aminolevulinic acid synthase.
- Step 2: delta-aminolevulinic acid dehydratase.
- Step 3: porphobilogen deaminase.
- Step 4: uroporphyrinogen III cosynthase.
- Step 5: uroporphyrinogen decarboxylase.
- Step 6: coproporphyrinogen oxidase.
- Step 7: protoporphyrinogen oxidase.
- Step 8: ferrochelatase.

The control of heme biosynthesis is complex. There are various chemical signals that can trigger increased or decreased production. These signals can affect the enzymes themselves or their production, starting at the genetic level.

Porphyrias

Under normal circumstances, when heme concentrations are at an appropriate level, precursor production decreases. However, a malfunction in the biosynthesis pathway—represented by a defective enzyme—means that heme biosynthesis does not reach completion. Because heme levels remain low, the synthesis pathway continues to churn out precursor molecules in an attempt to make up the deficit.

The net effect of this continued production is an abnormal accumulation of precursor molecules and development of some type of porphyria. Each type of porphyria corresponds to a specific enzyme defect and an accumulation of the associated precursor. Although there are eight steps in heme biosynthesis, there are only seven types of porphyrias; a defect in ALA synthase activity does not have a corresponding porphyria.

The porphyrias are divided into two general categories, depending on the location of the deficient enzyme. Porphyrias that affect heme biosynthesis in the liver are called hepatic porphyrias. The porphyrias that affect heme biosynthesis in immature red blood cells are called erythropoietic porphyrias. (Erythropoiesis is the process through which red blood cells are produced.)

Incidence of porphyria varies widely between types and occasionally by geographic location. Although certain porphyrias are more common than others, their greater frequency is only relative to other types; all porphyrias are considered rare disorders.

The hepatic porphyrias, and the heme biosynthesis steps at which enzyme defects occur, are:

• ALA dehydratase deficiency porphyria (step 2). This porphyria type is extraordinarily rare; only six cases have ever been reported in the medical literature. The inheritance pattern seems to be autosomal recessive, which means a defective enzyme gene must be inherited from both parents for the disorder to occur.

• Acute intermittent porphyria (step 3). Acute intermittent porphyria (AIP) is also known as Swedish porphyria, pyrroloporphyria, and intermittent acute porphyria. AIP is inherited as an autosomal dominant trait, which means only one copy of the defective gene needs to be present for the disorder to occur. However, simply inheriting this gene does not necessarily mean that a person will develop the disease. Approximately five to 10 per 100,000 persons in the United States carry the gene, but only 10% of carriers ever develop AIP symptoms.

• Porphyria cutanea tarda (step 5). Porphyria cutanea tarda (PCT) is also called symptomatic porphyria, porphyria cutanea symptomatica, and idiosyncratic porphyria. PCT may be acquired, typically as a result of disease (especially hepatitis C), drug or alcohol abuse, or exposure to certain poisons. PCT may also be inherited as an autosomal dominant disorder, but most people with the inherited form remain latent—that is, symptoms never develop. It is the most common of the porphyrias, but the incidence is not well defined.

• Hereditary coproporphyria (step 6). Hereditary coproporphyria (HCP) is inherited in an autosomal dominant manner. As with all porphyrias, it is an uncommon ailment. By 1977, only 111 cases were recorded; in Denmark, the estimated incidence is two in 1 million people.

• Variegate porphyria (step 7). Variegate porphyria (VP) is also known as porphyria variegata, protocoproporphyria, South African genetic porphyria, and Royal malady (supposedly King George III of England and Mary, Queen of Scots, suffered from VP). VP is inherited in an autosomal dominant manner and is especially prominent in South Africans of Dutch descent. Among that population, the incidence is approximately three in 1,000 persons, and it is estimated that there are 10,000 cases of VP in South Africa. Interestingly, it seems that the affected South Africans are descendants of two Dutch settlers who came to South Africa in 1680. Elsewhere, the incidence is estimated to be one to two cases per 100,000 persons.

The erythropoietic porphyrias, and the steps of heme biosynthesis at which they occur, are:

• Congenital erythropoietic porphyria (step 4). Congenital erythropoietic porphyria (CEP) is also called Günther's disease, erythropoietic porphyria, congenital porphyria, congenital hematoporphyria, and erythropoietic uroporphyria. CEP is inherited in an autosomal recessive manner and occurs very rarely. Onset of symptoms usually occurs in infancy, but may be delayed until adulthood.

• Erythropoietic protoporphyria (step 8). Also known as protoporphyria and erythrohepatic protoporphyria, erythropoietic protoporphyria (EPP) is more common than CEP; more than 300 cases have been reported. In these cases, the onset of symptoms typically occurred in childhood.

In addition to the above types of porphyria, there is a very rare type, called hepatoerythopoietic porphyria (HEP), that affects heme biosynthesis in both the liver and the bone marrow. HEP results from a defect in uroporphyrinogen decarboxylase activity (step 5), but strongly resembles congenital erythropoietic porphyria. Only 20 cases of HEP have been reported worldwide; it seems to be inherited in an autosomal recessive manner.

Causes and symptoms

General characteristics

The underlying cause of all porphyrias is a defective enzyme somewhere along the heme biosynthesis pathway. In virtually all cases, the defective enzyme is a genetically linked factor. Therefore, porphyrias are inheritable conditions. However, an environmental trigger—such as diet, drugs, or sun exposure—may be necessary before any symptoms develop. In many cases, symptoms do not develop, and individuals may be completely unaware that they have a gene for porphyria.

All of the hepatic porphyrias—except porphyria cutanea tarda—follow a pattern of acute attacks interspersed with periods of complete symptom remission. For this reason, they are often referred to as the acute porphyrias. The erythropoietic porphyrias and porphyria cutanea tarda do not follow the same pattern and are considered chronic conditions.

The specific symptoms of each porphyria depend on the affected enzyme and whether it occurs in the liver or in the bone marrow. The severity of symptoms can vary widely, even within the same porphyria type. When the porphyria becomes symptomatic, the common factor between all types is an abnormal accumulation of protoporphyrins or porphyrin.

ALA dehydratase porphyria (ADP)

ADP is characterized by a deficiency of ALA dehydratase. Of the few cases on record, the prominent symptoms were **vomiting**; **pain** in the **abdomen**, arms, and legs; and neuropathy. (Neuropathy refers to nerve damage that can cause pain, numbness, or paralysis.) As a result of neuropathy, the arms and legs may be weak or paralyzed and breathing can be impaired.

Acute intermittent porphyria (AIP)

AIP is caused by a deficiency in porphobilogen deaminase, but symptoms usually do not occur unless an individual with the deficiency encounters a biological trigger. Triggers can include hormones (for example oral contraceptives, menstruation, **pregnancy**), drugs, and dietary factors. However, most people with the deficiency never develop symptoms.

Attacks occur after **puberty** and commonly feature severe **abdominal pain**, nausea and vomiting, and constipation. Muscle **weakness** and pain in the back, arms, and legs are also typical symptoms. During an attack, the urine takes on a deep reddish color. The **central nervous system** may also be involved, as demonstrated by hallucinations, confusion, seizures, and mood changes.

Congenital erythropoietic porphyria (CEP)

CEP arises from a deficiency in uroporphyrinogen III cosynthase. Symptoms are often apparent in infancy and include reddish urine and possibly an enlarged spleen. The skin is unusually sensitive to light and blisters easily if exposed to sunlight. (Sunlight induces changes in protoporphyrins in the plasma and skin. These altered molecules can damage the skin.) Increased hair growth is common. Damage from recurrent blistering and associated skin infections can be severe; in some cases facial features and fingers are lost to recurrent damage and **infection**. Deposits of protoporphyrins sometimes occur in the teeth and bones.

Porphyria cutanea tarda (PCT)

PCT is caused by deficient uroporphyrinogen decarboxylase; it may be an acquired or inherited condition. The acquired form usually does not appear until adulthood. The inherited form may appear in childhood, but often demonstrates no symptoms. Early symptoms include blistering on the hands, face, and arms following minor injuries or exposure to sunlight. Lightening or darkening of the skin may occur along with increased hair growth or loss of hair. Liver function is abnormal but the signs are mild.

Hepatoerythopoietic porphyria (HEP)

HEP is linked to a deficiency of uroporphyrinogen decarboxylase in both the liver and the bone marrow. The symptoms resemble those of CEP.

Hereditary coproporphyria (HCP)

HCP is similar to AIP, but the symptoms are typically milder; the disorder is caused by a deficiency in coproporphyrinogen oxidase. The greatest difference between HCP and AIP is that people with HCP may have some skin sensitivity to sunlight. However, extensive damage to the skin is rarely seen.

Variegate porphyria (VP)

VP is caused by deficient protoporphyrinogen oxidase, and, like AIP, symptoms only occur during attacks. Major symptoms of this type of porphyria involve neurologic problems and sensitivity to light. Areas of the skin that are exposed to sunlight are susceptible to burning, blistering, and scarring.

Erythropoietic protoporphyria (EPP)

Owing to deficient ferrochelatase, the last step in the heme biosynthesis pathway—the insertion of an iron atom into a porphyrin molecule—cannot be completed. The major symptoms of this disorder are related to sensitivity to light—including both artificial and natural light sources. Following exposure to light, a patient with EPP experiences burning, **itching**, swelling, and reddening of the skin. Blistering and scarring may occur but are neither common nor severe. EPP may result in the formation of gallstones as well as liver complications. Symptoms can appear in childhood and tend to be more severe during the summer when exposure to sunlight is more likely.

Diagnosis

Depending on the array of symptoms presented, the possibility of porphyria may not immediately come to the physician's mind. In the absence of a family history of porphyria, some symptoms of porphyria, such as abdominal pain and vomiting, may be attributed to other disorders. Neurological symptoms, including confusion and hallucinations, may lead to an initial suspicion of psychiatric illness rather than a physical disorder. Diagnosis may be aided in cases in which these symptoms appear in combination with neuropathy, sensitivity to sunlight, or other factors. Certain symptoms, such as urine the color of port wine, are hallmarks of porphyria.

A common initial test measures protoporphyrins in the urine. However, if skin sensitivity to light is a symptom, a blood plasma test is indicated. If these tests reveal abnormal levels of protoporphyrins, further tests are performed to measure heme precursor levels in the stool and in red blood cells. The presence and estimated quantity of porphyrin and protoporphyrins are easily detected in biological samples using spectrofluorometric testing. This procedure involves the use of a laboratory instrument called a spectrofluorometer, which directs light of a specific strength at a fluid sample. Certain molecules in the sample—such as heme precursors—absorb the light energy and fluoresce. When molecules fluoresce, they emit light at a different strength from the absorbed light. The fluorescence can be detected and quantified by the spectrofluorometer. Not all molecules fluoresce, but among those that do, the intensity and quality of the fluorescence is an identifying characteristic. Diagnostic laboratory work, including analysis of blood, urine and stool samples is performed by laboratory technologists.

Heme precursors in the blood, urine, or stool give some indication of the type of porphyria, but more detailed biochemical testing is required to determine their exact identity. Making this determination yields a strong indicator of which enzyme in the heme biosynthesis pathway is defective, which in turn allows a diagnosis of the particular type of porphyria.

Biochemical tests rely on the color, chemical properties, and other unique features of each heme precursor. For example, a screening test for acute intermittent porphyria (AIP) is the Watson-Schwartz test. In this test, a special dye is added to a urine sample. If one of two heme precursors—porphobilinogen or urobilinogen—is present, the sample turns pink or red. Further testing is necessary to determine whether the precursor is porphobilinogen or urobilinogen—only porphobilinogen is indicative of AIP.

Other biochemical tests rely on the fact that heme precursors become less water soluble (able to be dissolved in water) as they progress further through the heme biosynthesis pathway. For example, to determine whether the Watson-Schwartz urine test is positive for porphobilinogen or urobilinogen, a measure of chloroform is added to the test tube. Chloroform is a water-insoluble substance, and even after vigorous mixing, the water and chloroform separate into two distinct layers. Whether the chloroform layer or the water layer becomes pink indicates which heme precursor is present. Porphobilinogen tends to be water soluble, and urobilinogen is slightly water insoluble. Since like mixes with like, porphobilinogen mixes more readily in the water than chloroform; therefore, if the water layer is pink, an AIP diagnosis is probable.

As a final test, measuring specific enzymes and their activities may be done for some types of porphyrias; however, such tests are not done for screening purposes. Certain enzymes, such as porphobilinogen deaminase (the defective enzyme in AIP), can be easily extracted from red blood cells; however, other enzymes are less readily collected or tested. Basically, an enzyme test involves adding a measure of the enzyme to a test tube containing the precursor it is supposed to modify. Both the production of modified precursor and the rate at which it appears are measured in the laboratory. If a modified precursor is produced, the test indicates that the enzyme is doing its job. The rate at which the modified precursor is produced can be compared to a standard to measure the enzyme's efficiency.

Treatment

Treatment for porphyria revolves around avoiding acute attacks, limiting potential effects, and treating symptoms. However, treatment options vary depending on the type of porphyria that has been diagnosed. Given the rarity of ALA dehydratase porphyria (six reported cases), definitive treatment guidelines have not been developed.

Acute intermittent porphyria, hereditary coproporphyria, and variegate porphyria

Treatment for acute intermittent porphyria, hereditary coproporphyria, and variegate porphyria follows the same basic regime. A patient diagnosed with one of these porphyrias can prevent most attacks by avoiding precipitating factors, such as certain drugs that have been identified as triggers for acute porphyria attacks. Individuals must maintain adequate **nutrition**, particularly in respect to **carbohydrates**. In some cases, an attack can be stopped by increasing carbohydrate consumption or by receiving carbohydrates intravenously.

When an attack occurs, medical attention is needed. Pain is usually severe, and narcotic **analgesics** are the best option for relief. Phenothiazines can be used to counter nausea, vomiting, and **anxiety**; and chloral hydrate or diazepam is useful for sedation or to induce sleep. Intravenously administered hematin may be used to curtail an attack. This drug seems to work by signaling the heme biosynthesis pathway to slow production of precursors. Women, who tend to develop symptoms more frequently than men in response to hormonal fluctuations, may find hormone therapy that inhibits ovulation to be helpful.

Congenital erythropoietic porphyria

The key points of congenital erythropoietic porphyria treatment are avoiding exposure to sunlight and preventing trauma to and infections of the skin. Liberal use of sunscreens and taking beta-carotene supplements can provide some protection from sun-induced damage. Medical treatments such as removing the spleen or administering red blood cell transfusions can have short-term benefits, but do not offer a cure. Oral doses of **activated charcoal** may offer the potential of remission.

Porphyria cutanea tarda

As with other porphyrias, the first line of defense is the avoidance of precipitating factors, especially alcohol. Regular blood withdrawal is a proven therapy for pushing symptoms into remission. For patients who are anemic or cannot have blood drawn for other reasons, chloroquine therapy may be used.

Erythropoietic protoporphyria

Avoiding sunlight, using sunscreens, and taking beta-carotene supplements are typical treatment options for erythropoietic protoporphyria. The drug cholestyramine may reduce the skin's sensitivity to sunlight as well as the accumulated heme precursors in the liver. Liver transplantation has been used in cases of liver failure, but it has not effected a long-term cure of the porphyria.

Prognosis

Even in the presence of a genetic inheritance for a porphyria, symptom development depends on a variety of factors. In the majority of cases, an individual remains asymptomatic throughout life. Porphyria symptoms are rarely fatal with proper medical treatment, but they may be associated with temporarily debilitating or permanently disfiguring consequences. Measures to avoid these consequences are not always successful, regardless of how diligently they are pursued. Although pregnancy has been known to trigger porphyria attacks, it is not as great a danger as was once thought.

KEY TERMS

Autosomal dominant—An inheritance pattern in which a trait is determined by one gene in a pair (genes are inherited in pairs; one copy from each parent).

Autosomal recessive—An inheritance pattern in which a trait is expressed only if both genes in a pair code for that particular characteristic (genes are inherited in pairs; one copy from each parent).

Enzyme—A protein molecule that catalyzes a chemical reaction.

Erythropoiesis—The process through which new red blood cells are created; it begins in the bone marrow.

Erythropoietic—Referring to the creation of new red blood cells.

Gene—A portion of DNA (deoxyribonucleic acid) that codes for a specific product, such as an enzyme.

Hematin—A drug that is administered intravenously to halt an acute porphyria attack. It inhibits heme biosynthesis, preventing the further accumulation of heme precursors.

Heme—A large complex molecule contained in hemoglobin and a number of important enzymes throughout the body. Through these factors, it plays a vital role in metabolism and oxygen and energy transport. Heme is composed of porphyrin and an iron atom.

Hemoglobin—A molecule composed of heme and protein that enables red blood cells to transport oxygen throughout the body. Hemoglobin gives red blood cells their characteristic color.

Hepatic—Referring to the liver.

Neuropathy—A condition characterized by nerve damage. Major symptoms can include weakness, numbness, paralysis, or pain in the affected area.

Porphyrin—A large molecule shaped somewhat like a four-leaf clover. Combined with an iron atom, it forms a heme molecule.

Protoporphyrin—A precursor molecule to the porphyrin molecule.

Health care team roles

Patients diagnosed with porphyrias are cared for by an interdisciplinary treatment team that may include primary care physicians, hematologists, and dermatologists. Laboratory technologists are involved during the diagnostic process, and nurses, health educators, and genetic counselors provide instruction about how to recognize triggers and prevent attacks or flares of the condition.

Prevention

For the most part, the porphyrias are attributable to inherited genes; such an inheritance cannot be prevented. However, symptoms can be prevented or limited by avoiding factors that trigger development.

When there is a family history of porphyria, individuals should consider testing to determine whether they carry the associated gene. Even if symptoms are absent, it is useful to know about the presence of the gene to assess the risks of developing the associated porphyria. This knowledge also reveals whether the individual's offspring may be at risk. Theoretically, it is possible to perform prenatal tests. However, these tests would not indicate whether the child would develop porphyria symptoms; only that they might have the genetic predisposition to develop symptoms.

Resources

PERIODICALS

Fodinger, M. and Sunder-Plassman, G. "Inherited Disorders of Iron Metabolism." *Kidney International Supplement* 55, no. 69 (March 1999): S22-S34.

Murphy, G.M. "The Cutaneous Porphyrias: A Review." *British Journal of Dermatology* 140, no. 4 (April 1999): 573-581.

Nordmann, Y. et al. "The Porphyrias." *Journal of Hepatology Supplement* 30, no. 1 (1999): 12-16.

ORGANIZATION

American Porphyria Foundation. P.O. Box 22712, Houston, TX 77227. (713) 266-9617. http://www. enterprise.net/apf/.

Barbara Wexler

Portable defibrillators *see* **Defibrillators, portable**

Positron emission tomography (PET)

Definition

Positron emission tomography (PET) is a non-invasive scanning technique that utilizes small amounts of radioactive positrons (positively charged particles) to visualize body function and **metabolism**.

Purpose

PET is the fastest growing nuclear medicine tool in terms of increasing acceptance and applications. It is useful in the diagnosis, staging, and treatment of **cancer** because it provides information that cannot be obtained by other techniques such as computed tomography (CT) and **magnetic resonance imaging** (MRI).

PET scans can be performed at medical centers equipped with a small cyclotron. Smaller cyclotrons and increasing availability of certain radiopharmaceuticals are making PET a more widely used imaging modality.

Physicians first used PET to obtain information about **brain** function and to study brain activity in various neurological diseases and disorders, including **stroke**, epilepsy, **Alzheimer's disease**, **Parkinson's disease**, and Huntington's disease; and in psychiatric disorders such as **schizophrenia**, depression, obsessive-compulsive disorder, attention-deficit/hyperactivity disorder, and Tourette syndrome. More and more, PET is being used to evaluate patients for head and neck, **lymphoma**, **melanoma**, lung, colorectal, and esophageal cancers. PET also is used to evaluate **heart** muscle function in patients with **coronary artery disease** or **cardiomyopathy**.

Precautions

There is always a slight risk when radioactive material is injected into the body. However, because the radioactive tracers used are short-lived and clear the body quickly, they are considered safe. The radiation dose received is only slightly more than that received in a **chest x ray**. Still, pregnant women should not have a PET scan.

Description

PET involves injecting a patient with a radiopharmaceutical similar to glucose. An hour after injection of this tracer, a PET scanner images a specific metabolic function by measuring the concentration and distribution of the tracer throughout the body.

When it enters the body, the tracer courses through the bloodstream to the target organ, where it emits positrons. The positively charged positrons collide with negatively charged electrons and gamma rays are produced. The gamma rays are detected by photomultiplier-scintillator combinations positioned on opposite sides of the patient. These signals are then processed by the computer and images are generated.

PET provides an advantage over CT and MRI because it can determine if a lesion is malignant. The two other modalities provide images of anatomical structures but often cannot provide a determination of malignancy. Recently PET has been used in combination with CT and MRI to identify abnormalities with more precision and indicate areas of most active metabolism. This additional information allows for more accurate evaluation of cancer treatment and management.

Health care team roles

Personnel for a PET facility should include a physicist for technical support, calibration, and software; a physician for medical interventions and reading; and administrative staff for scheduling, paperwork, and billing. A trained technologist performs the PET scans. A positron emission tomography technologist performs PET procedures on clinical and research subjects referred for neurologic, oncologic, cardiac, or other conditions.

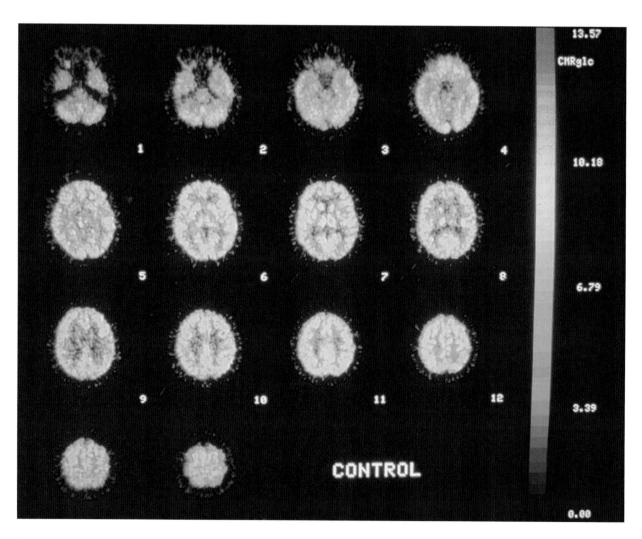

(Positron Emission Tomography (PET) scan control study, photograph by Jon Meyer. Custom Medical Stock Photo. Reproduced by permission.)

The technologist also ensures appropriate patient care, acquires data, and performs analysis according to protocols. A technologist needs training in nuclear medicine. State licensure is required as a nuclear medicine technologist.

Resources

BOOKS

Eisenberg, Ronald L., and Alexander R. Margulis. *A Patient's Guide to Medical Imaging.* New York: Oxford University Press, 2011.

Hillman, Bruce J., and Jeff Charles Goldsmith. *The Sorcerer's Apprentice: How Medical Imaging Is Changing Health Care.* New York: Oxford University Press, 2011.

Khalil, Magdy M, ed. *Basic Sciences of Nuclear Medicine.* New York: Springer, 2011.

PERIODICALS

Garcia, Ernest V. "Physical Attributes, Limitations, and Future Potential for PET and SPECT." *Journal of Nuclear Cardiology* 19, suppl 1 (2012): 19–29.

Gennari, Alessandra, et al. "Whither the PET Scan? The Role of PET Imaging in the Staging and Treatment of Breast Cancer." *Current Oncology Reports* 14, 1 (2012): 20–26.

Hunter, Jill V., et al. "Emerging Imaging Tools for Use with Traumatic Brain Injury Research." *Journal of Neurotrauma* 29, 4 (2012): 654–671.

OTHER

Brain Scans that Spy on the Senses. Howard Hughes Medical Institute. http://www.hhmi.org/senses/e110.html (accessed April 3, 2012).

Fact Sheet: What Is PET?. SNM Advancing Molecular Imaging and Therapy. http://interactive.snm.org/index.cfm?PageID=11123 (accessed April 3, 2012).

Mayo Clinic Staff. *Positron Emission Tomography (PET) Scan.* Mayo Clinic. http://www.mayoclinic.com/health/pet-scan/MY00238 (accessed April 3, 2012).

What Is a PET Scan? How Does a PET Scan Work?. Medical News Today. http://www.medicalnewstoday.com/articles/154877.php (accessed April 3, 2012).

Dan Harvey

Positron emission tomography (PET) unit

Definition

The **positron emission tomography (PET)** unit is a device used to produce images of the body that reflect biochemical changes taking place in the body. Among the body imaging technologies used in medicine, the **PET** unit is characterized by its use of positron-emitting tracer substances. Because of its use of short-lived positron emitting tracers, the PET unit can provide images of biochemical processes. This feature of PET technology distinguishes it from computer tomography (CT) and **magnetic resonance imaging** (MRI) technologies, which can provide only images of the structure of the body.

Purpose

The purpose of the PET unit is to provide images reflecting biochemical changes occurring within the body. The PET unit can also, when used in conjunction with mathematical models of organ systems, quantify biochemical activity (e.g. **blood** flow, metabolic activity in tissue).

Because the PET unit can provide information on biochemical function, it is particularly helpful in assessing tissue viability and biological processes related to tissue health. The PET unit is used for these purposes most often in the fields of **neurology** (study of the **brain**), cardiology (study of the **heart**), and **oncology** (**cancer**).

In neurology, the PET unit is used to diagnose and differentiate among different types of epilepsy, **dementia**, and cerebrovascular disease. Because the regions of the brain that are affected by these abnormalities have blood flow and glucose utilization patterns that are different from healthy parts of the brain, the PET unit can—by using tracers that follow cerebral blood flow, glucose pathways, and oxygen metabolism—identify areas of the brain that are affected. During epileptic seizures, blood flow and glucose use increase in the area of the epileptogenic focus (site originating the seizure). PET scans are used to identify these foci in patients with drug-resistant epilepsy so that surgical intervention can target these seizure-prone areas. In dementia, the PET unit is used to distinguish **Alzheimer's disease** from other types of dementia, because each type of dementia has a characteristic glucose utilization pattern in the brain. The PET unit is also used to evaluate and monitor treatments for **stroke** patients by measuring cerebral blood flow, glucose **metabolism**, and oxygen levels.

In cardiology, the PET unit is used to assess the metabolism and function of myocardial tissue. Blood flow and fatty acid metabolism are measured by the PET unit, and areas that are affected by **coronary artery disease** are easily identified. The state of the myocardial tissue, as reflected in the PET scan, also helps the cardiologist determine the best intervention, e.g. an angiogram rather than a heart bypass.

In oncology, the PET unit has had a long history of being used for the diagnosis and localization of brain tumors. Because tumors have greater blood flow directed to them than normal brain cells, the PET scan can identify where the tumor is localized by pinpointing the area with abnormally high blood flow. More broadly, the PET unit can be used in many parts of the body to grade the severity of tumors and identify metastatic processes. Moreover, because PET identifies variations in metabolic activity, the scans are particularly useful in assessing the effectiveness of radiological treatment of cancer; unlike other types of imaging, PET scans can distinguish between (non-viable) scar tissue caused by the radiological treatment of tumors, and viable tumor cells that might have been missed by the treatment.

Description

Standard components

The components of the PET unit are best understood in the context of the procedures required for **positron emission tomography**.

The first step in the PET process is the creation of the radioisotope (radioactive version of a chemical element) that is to be used in the tracer compound. The creation of the radioisotope takes place in a device called the cyclotron. The cyclotron is a particle accelerator that speeds up a particle so quickly that it strips electrons from the particle. In most PET units, the particle used is hydrogen, and the resulting stripped particle is a proton (represented as H+). A beam of protons created in this way is then used to bombard a stable isotope (non-radioactive version of a chemical element). The bombardment of the stable version of a chemical element with H+ produces a radioactive version of the element.

The most common radionuclides created by a PET cyclotron are C-11 (carbon), N-13 (nitrogen), O-15 (oxygen), and F-18 (flourine). These elements are popular because many of the compounds in the human body are based on these elements or on analogs of these elements, so that a biochemical compound the body naturally uses can be created from these radionuclides. Note that, because these positron-emitting radionuclides decay in a short amount of time (depending on the element, 2–110 minutes), the radionuclide must be produced by a cyclotron within a short distance from the location of the other PET procedures.

Once the radionuclide is generated by the cyclotron, it enters the biosynthesizer unit, where it is used to create radioactive biochemical compounds. Examples of compounds synthesized are 15-C (to measure blood volume), 13-N-glutamine (to measure myocardial metabolism), 15-O_2 (to measure oxygen metabolism), and 18-F-deoxyglucose (to measure glucose metabolism).

The patient is then injected with or inhales the radioactive labeled tracer and is positioned in the gantry of the PET scanner. The scanner consists of a ring of detectors designed to find the location of and quantify the photon emissions from positron-electron reactions. Note that although the decaying radioactive compounds emit positrons, the positrons do not leave the body. Instead, the positrons emitted by the compounds go a short distance within the body before colliding with electrons. In the annihilation reaction that results from this positron-electron collision, high-energy photons are released, and it is these photons that pass through the body and are detected by the PET scanner. The two released photons, in an annihilation reaction, go in exactly opposite directions (180 degrees from each other), so that the PET scanner is able to reconstruct the three-dimensional spatial distribution of the compound by reconstructing the paths of photons and pinpointing the reaction site.

Since the photons released are not detectable visually, the detector ring in the scanner uses scintillation compounds (compounds that detect the photon flashes from the reaction) that convert the detected photon energy into visible forms. The scanner then uses sophisticated mathematical programs to construct coherent PET images from the visible data. When quantitative information is needed, a tracer kinetic model (mathematical model of tracer behavior) is used in conjunction with the PET data to quantify metabolic and functional processes.

The PET scanner is controlled by a computer monitor that allows for entry of text and commands.

The images are previewed on an image monitor, which can be separate from or on the same screen as the control monitor. Because clinicians are often reluctant to diagnose using solely the image monitor, many PET systems allow for the conversion of these images to sheet film that can then be viewed on a standard lightbox. Many systems also have an archival system that saves image data for future retrieval.

Variations of equipment

Because PET facilities differ in their imaging needs and financial resources, there may be variations in the features of cyclotrons and scanners among facilities. For radiotracer production, two different systems are often seen—the remote semiautomated system and the remote automated system. The remote semiautomated system allows the operator to determine the order and timing of the reactions and visually monitor the radionuclide synthesis. The semiautomated system is less expensive than the automated system, and is popular in research settings that do not have a standard set of radiotracers to be routinely produced. In clinical settings, where there is a regular flow of patients, the more costly automated system is used because automated synthesis requires less personnel time and production time, and there is less variation in the radionuclides required.

Cyclotrons are available as "Proton Only" devices or "Dual Particle" devices. Although "Proton Only" machines are cheaper, they restrict the chemical synthesis options through which particular radionuclides can be produced. Large quantities of O-15 used for brain research, for example, would be infeasible with "Proton Only" machines because of the prohibitive costs of the source materials required to synthesize O-15 with this type of machine. In general, institutions that have both clinical and research groups using the PET unit (and thus a broad range of radionuclide needs) use "Dual Particle" devices.

Some cyclotrons have what is called dual irradiation capacity, which allows them to produce two different radioisotopes at the same time. These cyclotrons can also, if both ion beams are used to produce the same type of radioisotope, produce large amounts of a single isotope. Dual irradiation cyclotrons are more expensive than single irradiation cyclotrons and are generally found in institutions with both clinical and research demands.

Although many PET scanners are single-ring scanners, multiple-ring scanners are emerging at advanced research and clinical institutions. These multiple-ring scanners allow for the simultaneous imaging of contiguous cross-sections. These types of scanners allow for faster scanning and more dynamic visualization of body processes.

Settings

Because of the high cost of the PET devices, the PET unit is used primarily in research institutions and advanced clinical (tertiary care) settings. In 1992, Michel Ter-Pergossian, a prominent researcher in PET technology, noted that there were 50-80 PET centers internationally.

Operation

Partly because of radiation safety regulations strictly governing the use and disposal of radioactive materials, radiotracer production and cyclotron operation is mostly automated. The nuclear medicine technologist, typically through a menu-driven computer control unit, designates the specific radiotracer to be synthesized and selects the chemical processes desired. Because the cyclotron is shielded, either in a protected room with concrete walls or behind a shield accompanying the cyclotron unit, the technologist is exposed to very little radiation.

After the radiotracer is produced, quality control (QC) testing is conducted daily. The technologist transfers the materials (in a lead container) from the biosynthesizer unit to the radiochemistry area for QC testing. The compounds are tested for radiochemical purity, radionuclidic purity, correct pH, and sterility. As the pharmacist performs the spectrometry and chromatography tests, he or she stands behind lead shielding. A monitor in the QC testing area indicates the level of radiation exposure in the area to allow the pharmacist to gauge his/her exposure. Staff periodically check their gloves for radioactive contamination, and contaminated items (such as gloves, shoe covers, and syringes) are immediately placed in protected radioactive waste containers.

The scanner operator brings the patient to the scanning room and aligns the patient in a relatively immobile position on the gantry. In the radiochemistry room, he or she or another technologist measures the appropriate patient dose for the radiotracer, and the radiotracer is placed into a Lucite-shielded syringe. The syringe is placed in a lead container, and the technologist carries the lead container to the scanning room, where he or she administers the radiotracer to the patient.

In the control room—an attached room with a window through which the patient can be viewed throughout the entire scan—the technologist controls the scanning and image processing at the control computer. He or she selects the appropriate scanning

KEY TERMS

Annihilation reaction—Reaction between electron and positron in which both are destroyed and each particle's mass is converted into photon energy.

Electron—Negatively charged particle of an atom.

Gantry—Frame in which patient is placed, over which the PET scanner moves.

Photon—High-energy light waves.

Positron—Negatively charged electrons, often symbolized as H+.

Proton—Positively charged particle of an atom.

Radionuclide—A radioactive element.

Radiotracer—A tracer compound with a radioactive element.

Tracer—Substance that can be followed through the course of a biochemical process.

procedure for the area of interest and enters parameters related to image processing. When all parameters have been verified and entered, the technologist enters the commands to execute the scan. Depending on the nature of the question that the scan seeks to answer, the scan may take 10-90 minutes. The technologist assesses the quality of the images, and should be able to identify artifacts from problems arising in the PET detector or image processor. If the PET images are acceptable, they are stored for the physician or researcher to review at a later date.

Health care team roles

A typical team directly involved with using the PET unit consists of a radiochemist, a pharmacist, two nuclear medicine technologists (a scanner operator and a cyclotron operator), and a medical physicist. The radiochemist oversees the radiochemistry facility and supervises all radiotracer production. He or she is the primary cyclotron operator. The pharmacist performs quality control on the radiotracers. He or she can also operate the cyclotron and administer radiotracers to patients. Both nuclear medicine technologists assist in preparing patients for the PET scan. In addition, the scanner operator and cyclotron operator perform quality control on their respective devices. The medical physicist is the radiation safety officer of the facility. He or she ensures that the facility meets the legal safety requirements for dealing with radioactive materials, and

makes sure that personnel are properly trained and monitored.

Nurses and nuclear medicine radiologists are also involved with the PET process. Nurses prepare the patients for the PET scan, monitor patients through the process, and may take blood samples as needed. Nuclear medicine radiologists are the physicians reviewing and interpreting the PET images in the course of patient work-up.

Training

Nuclear medicine technologists, researchers, and physicians who will be using the PET computer stations typically take a week-long course, offered by the makers of the PET unit, to learn how to operate the control computers. Technologists also require a more advanced course in the physics and instrumentation of PET, in radiation safety, and in quality control during image processing. Clinicians who interpret the scans require nuclear medicine training through fellowships or continuing education.

Resources

BOOKS

Granov, Anatoliy, and Leonid Tiutin, Thomas Schwarz, eds. *Positron Emission Tomography*. Springer, 2013.

Juweid, Malik E., and Otto S. Hoekstra, eds. *Positron Emission Tomography*. Humana Press, 2011.

Genevieve Pham-Kanter

Post-traumatic stress disorder

Definition

Post-traumatic stress disorder (PTSD) is primarily caused by human reactions to events outside the realm of ordinary life experience. Domestic and criminal violence, natural disasters, and transportation accidents are major categories of incidents associated with PTSD. Once thought to be experienced primarily by war veterans, PTSD is now known to occur in survivors of sexual, physical, or emotional abuse, and in persons who have witnessed a traumatic event.

PTSD may result from long-term experiences of trauma as well as from time-limited violent events. It is now recognized that repeated traumas or such traumas of long duration as **child abuse**, domestic violence, stalking, cult membership, and hostage situations may also produce the symptoms of PTSD in survivors.

Description

After a traumatic event, the person who suffered the trauma, as well as others who witnessed it or were involved as emergency workers, may experience a range of symptoms. These may include physical **pain**; change in bowel function, such as **diarrhea** and/or constipation; change in sleep patterns, such as sleeping more or less than before the trauma; **heart** palpitations, sweating, being easily startled or becoming hypervigilant; becoming increasingly susceptible to illness.

As the individual struggles to cope with life after the event, ordinary events or situations that resemble the trauma in certain respects often trigger frightening, vivid memories or flashbacks. For example, one survivor of a plane crash would have flashbacks of the crash whenever he smelled something burning. A Vietnam veteran would have flashbacks whenever he heard a car backfire.

Causes and symptoms

Causes

While it is not clear why some people develop PTSD following a trauma and others do not, experts suspect that it may be influenced both by the severity of the event, by the person's personality and genetic make-up, and by whether or not the trauma was expected. In addition, occupational factors play a role; persons who work as fire fighters, police officers, emergency room staff, or in similar high-risk occupations have a higher rate of PTSD than the general population. Lastly, the nature of the trauma itself is a factor; as a rule, traumas resulting from intentional human behavior (rape, torture, genocide, domestic violence, etc.) are experienced as more stressful than traumas resulting from accidents, natural disasters, or animal attacks.

Symptoms

The *Diagnostic and Statistical Manual of Mental Disorders*, 4th edition (DSM-IV), specifies six diagnostic criteria for PTSD:

- Traumatic stressor: The patient has been exposed to a catastrophic event involving actual or threatened death or injury, or a threat to the physical integrity of the self or others. During exposure to the trauma, the person's emotional response was marked by intense fear, feelings of helplessness, or horror.

- Intrusive symptoms: The patient experiences flashbacks, traumatic daydreams, or nightmares, in which he or she relives the trauma as if it were recurring in the present. Intrusive symptoms result from an abnormal process of memory formation.

- Avoidant symptoms: The patient attempts to reduce the possibility of exposure to anything that might trigger memories of the trauma, and to minimize his or her reactions to such memories. This cluster of symptoms includes dissociative symptoms (derealization and depersonalization), psychic numbing, and avoidance of places, persons, or things associated with the trauma. Patients with PTSD are at increased risk of substance abuse as a form of self-medication to numb painful memories.

- Hyperarousal: Hyperarousal is a condition in which the patient's nervous system is always on "red alert" for the return of danger. This symptom cluster includes hypervigilance, insomnia, difficulty concentrating, general irritability, and an extreme startle response.

- Duration of symptoms: The symptoms must persist for at least one month.

- Significance: The patient suffers from significant social, interpersonal, or work-related problems as a result of the PTSD symptoms. A common social symptom of PTSD is a feeling of disconnection from other people (including loved ones); from the larger society; and from God or other sources of meaning.

The symptoms of PTSD usually begin within three months of the trauma, although sometimes PTSD does not develop until years after the initial trauma occurred. Once the symptoms begin, they may fade away again within six months. Others suffer with the symptoms for far longer; and in some cases, the problem may become chronic.

PTSD in children

PTSD in children may trigger the onset of learning disabilities, self-mutilation or other destructive behaviors, sleep terrors, and a variety of conduct disorders. Children may also develop abnormally close attachments to their primary caretakers or other dependency behaviors in their attempts to cope with the traumatic experience.

Treatment

A diagnosis of PTSD does not indicate personal weakness or mental illness. It is a perfectly natural and normal reaction to one or more abnormal events. Just like a perfectly healthy **bone** will break if placed under enough stress, a perfectly healthy person placed under sufficient stress can develop PTSD.

KEY TERMS

Benzodiazepines—A class of drugs that have a hypnotic and sedative action, used mainly as tranquilizers to control symptoms of anxiety.

Cognitive-behavioral therapy—A type of psychotherapy used to treat anxiety disorders (including PTSD) that emphasizes behavioral change as well as alteration of negative thought patterns.

Dissociation—The splitting off of certain mental processes from conscious awareness. Many PTSD patients have dissociative symptoms.

Flashback—An abnormally vivid, often recurrent, recollection of a traumatic event.

Hyperarousal—A condition of abnormally intense nervous excitement. Some symptoms of PTSD are classified as symptoms of hyperarousal.

Hypervigilance—A condition of abnormally intense watchfulness or wariness. Hypervigilance is one of the most common symptoms of PTSD.

Selective serotonin reuptake inhibitors (SSRIs)—A class of antidepressants that work by blocking the reabsorption of serotonin in the brain, raising the levels of serotonin. SSRIs include Prozac, Zoloft, and Paxil.

It is important to understand that not every person who experiences a traumatic event will experience PTSD. There is some evidence that an approach known as critical incident stress debriefing, or CISD, may lower the incidence of PTSD in survivors of a large-scale civilian disaster or war zone trauma. CISD should be offered to survivors within 48 hours of the traumatic event. In general, persons who are experiencing some of the symptoms of PTSD should consult a mental health professional. He or she will diagnose the condition if the symptoms of stress last for more than a month after a traumatic event. While a formal diagnosis of PTSD is made only in the wake of a severe trauma, it is possible to have a mild PTSD-like reaction following less severe stress.

Medication

The most helpful treatment of PTSD appears to be a combination of medication along with supportive and cognitive-behavioral therapies. Effective medications include anxiety-reducing medications and antidepressants, especially the selective serotonin reuptake inhibitors (SSRIs) such as fluoxetine (Prozac). Sleep problems can be lessened with brief treatment with an anti-anxiety drug, such as a benzodiazepine like alprazolam (Xanax), but long-term usage can lead to disturbing side effects, such as increased anger.

Psychotherapy

Therapy can help reduce negative thought patterns and self-talk, in that many PTSD patients blame themselves for the traumatic event, their reactions to it, or both. Cognitive-behavioral therapy focuses on changing specific actions and thoughts with the help of **relaxation** training and breathing techniques. Group therapy with other PTSD sufferers and **family therapy** can also be helpful.

Alternative and complementary approaches

Patients diagnosed with PTSD may benefit from such complementary approaches as **meditation** and mindfulness training, which appear to be useful in reducing the number of flashbacks. **Yoga**, bodywork, and **massage therapy** help to reduce the muscle soreness and tension associated with PTSD. Lastly, some patients find martial arts training useful in restoring a sense of personal competence and safety.

Prognosis

The severity of PTSD depends in part on the predictability of the trauma; its severity; its duration and chronicity; the role of human intention in inflicting the trauma; and the patient's personality style, overall state of health, and genetic predisposition.

With appropriate medication, emotional support, and counseling, most people show significant improvement. On the other hand, prolonged exposure to severe trauma—such as experienced by victims of prolonged physical or sexual abuse and survivors of the Holocaust—may cause permanent psychological scars.

Health care team roles

It is essential for all treatment team members to know their roles and execute them properly throughout the treatment and recovery phases of this disorder. Depending on whether outpatient or inpatient treatment is being provided, the team leaders may include psychiatrists, psychologists, nursing staff, behavior specialists and other medical/behavioral staff. In some cases it may be appropriate to include the patient's religious or spiritual advisor as a member of the team, in that increasing numbers of clergy have taken advanced training in trauma therapy.

Regular meetings are important so that all persons involved can provide input. Family members involved in patient care should be reaffirmed as to their need to provide consistency and adherence to the plan of care. Psychological evaluations will provide a base for the rest of the team to compose and/or update the treatment plan.

During treatment planning phases, needs and strengths are assessed, as well as progress from prior plans. The treatment team leader, normally a behavior specialist, a psychologist or a psychiatrist, will then compose a plan of care that will describe goals for the next phase of care, interventions and other information needed to initiate or continue care.

Resources

BOOKS

Friedman, Matthew J. *Post-Traumatic and Acute Stress Disorders,* 5th edition. Jones & Bartlett Learning, 2010.

McLay, Robert N. *At War with PTSD: Battling Post Traumatic Stress Disorder with Virtual Reality.* The Johns Hopkins University Press, 2012.

Shiromani, Peter, and Terrence Keane, Joseph E. LeDoux, eds. *Post-Traumatic Stress Disorder: Basic Science and Clinical Practice.* Humana Press, 2009.

PERIODICALS

Grieger, Thomas A. "Veterans with post-traumatic stress disorder are at increased risk of developing dementia." *Evidence-Based Mental Health* (February 2011): 12.

Lavin, Joanne. "Surviving postraumatic stress disorder." *Nursing* (September 2011): 41

Lewis-Smith, Andrew. "Post Traumatic Stress Disorder: Cognitive Therapy with Children and Young People." *Child and Adolescent Mental Health* 16.1 (2011): 64.

Skorga, Phyllis, and Charlotte Young. "Acute traumatic stress treatment." *Nursing Times* (8 November 2011): 17.

ORGANIZATIONS

American Psychiatric Association. 1400 K St., NW, Washington, DC 20005.

Anxiety Disorders Association of America. 11900 Parklawn Dr., Ste. 100, Rockville, MD 20852. (301) 231-9350.

National Alliance for the Mentally Ill. 2101 Wilson Blvd. No. 302, Arlington, VA 22201. (703) 524-7600.

National Anxiety Foundation. 3135 Custer Dr., Lexington, KY 40517. (606) 272-7166.

National Institute of Mental Health. Rm 15C-05, 5600 Fishers Lane, Rockville, MD 20857.

National Mental Health Association. 1021 Prince St., Alexandria, VA 22314. (703) 684-7722.

Society for Traumatic Stress Studies, 60 Revere Dr., Ste. 500, Northbrook, IL 60062. (708) 480-9080.

Jacqueline N. Martin, M.S.

Postmortem care

Definition

Postmortem care is the care provided to a patient immediately after death.

Purpose

Postmortem care serves several purposes, including:

• preparing the patient for viewing by family

• ensuring proper identification of the patient prior to transportation to the morgue or funeral home

• providing appropriate disposition of patient's belongings.

• maintaining vital organs, if donation is planned

Precautions

Government regulations at both state and federal level require hospitals to establish policies and procedures to certify death, to identify potential donors, and to care for a body after death. If **organ donation** is anticipated, respiratory and circulatory support must be maintained until vital organs can be harvested. It must be clearly communicated to the family that the devices used to maintain organ perfusion no longer keep the patient alive, but are merely supporting the organs in anticipation of transplant.

Vital organs requiring support are:

• heart

• liver

• lungs

• kidneys

• pancreas

Non-vital tissues such as the cornea, skin, long bones, and middle ear bones do not require support after death.

If the patient had an **infectious disease**, the body must be labeled in accordance with established policy.

Before rigor mortis develops, the nurse should position the body in a normal alignment and close the eyelids and mouth, inserting dentures if necessary. Because of the reduction in body temperature and loss of skin tone (algor mortis) after death, it is important to gently remove all tape and dressings to prevent tissue damage. The skin or body parts should never be pulled on. The head of the bed should be elevated to prevent purplish discoloration (livor mortis) of the face. The body must be stored in a cool place to slow bacterial formation after death.

Description

Equipment

A commercial morgue pack, if available, will contain gauze or string ties, chin straps, a shroud, and three identification tags. In addition to these items, the nurse should gather the following:

- gloves
- ABD pads
- cotton balls
- adhesive bandages to cover wounds or punctures
- plastic bag for belongings
- bath basin with water
- soap
- towels
- washcloths
- clean sheets
- stretcher or morgue cart

Preparation

Before placing the body in a supine position with arms at sides and head on a pillow, the nurse should put on clean gloves. The head of the bed should be slightly elevated. At this time, the nurse can insert the patient's dentures, if worn, and then close the mouth. By placing a fingertip on each eye, the nurse should gently close the patient's eyes. If the eyes will not remain closed, moistened cotton balls can be placed on the eyelids for several minutes, and then a repeated attempt to close the eyes can be made. A folded towel should be placed under the chin to keep the mouth closed. All catheters, tubes, and tape can be removed, but adhesive bandages should be applied to puncture sites.

At the time of death, the patient's survivors become the focus of concern, and the nurse must then be able to offer comfort and support to the living. All the patient's belongings can be gathered for the family to take. If a ring cannot be removed, the nurse can cover the ring with gauze, tape it securely, and tie the gauze to the wrist to prevent loss.

Before the family views the patient, the body is cleansed using soap, water, and washcloths. To absorb any rectal drainage, one or more ABD pads is placed between the buttocks. The body is covered up to the chin in a clean sheet, with the arms placed outside of the sheet, if possible. Then the room must be prepared for receiving the family and friends by removing all trash and providing lower light in the room. If there are unpleasant odors present in the room, a room deodorizer can be used before allowing the family to return.

The nurse can then offer family members the opportunity to view the body, but not force them, letting them know that either viewing or not viewing is acceptable. This is the time to ask family members if they prefer that any jewelry be left on the body. The nurse should clearly document whether personal items are remaining with the body, or to whom the items were given. The nurse can allow survivors privacy in viewing the body, but not leave them alone until it is ascertained that they are comfortable remaining with the body. The nurse can encourage the family to touch and talk as a way to say goodbye to the deceased.

When the family has left, the towel can be removed from under the chin, placing an ABD pad under the chin and wrapping chin straps under the chin, with the straps tied loosely on top of the head. Padding the wrists with an ABD pad prevents bruising, and then the nurse ties the wrists together with gauze or soft string ties; the ankles should be padded and tied in the same manner. It will be necessary to fill out three identification tags with the deceased's name, room, and bed number; date and time of death; and the physician's name. One tag will be tied to the big toe, hand, or foot. Another identification tag must be attached to the shrouded body, and the third identification tag attached to the personal belongings. The nurse must ensure that the patient's identification bracelet is not removed.

Aftercare

A family member should take all the patient's personal belongings. The body will be transported to the morgue or funeral home.

Complications

If organ donation is planned, failure to maintain support for vital organs will mean that organs cannot be harvested.

Results

The patient's family will have the opportunity to view the body, if they wish, in order to begin the grief process. Emotional support of the survivors will be provided by trained staff members.

Health care team roles

Physicians must certify the death. If the death occurred in unusual circumstances, an **autopsy** may be requested. Staff members, pastoral care, or other personnel should remain with the family during preparation of the patient's body for viewing. Nursing is responsible for coordination of all postmortem care. Trained staff members will provide information to the family regarding organ donation.

Resources

BOOKS

Ambrose, Marguerite, and Frances Quinless. "Fundamental Procedures." In *Nursing Procedures,* 3rd ed. Springhouse, PA: Springhouse Corporation, 2000.

Potter, Patricia. *Fundamentals of Nursing,* 5th ed. St Louis, MO: Mosby, 2001.

ORGANIZATIONS

American Academy of Hospice and Palliative Medicine (AAHPM). 4700 W. Lake Avenue, Glenview, IL 60025-1485. (847) 375-4712. http://www.aahpm.org.

Hospice and Palliative Nurses Association. Penn Center West One, Suite 229, Pittsburgh, PA 15276. (412) 787-9301. http://www.hpna.org/.

Hospice Net. Suite 51, 401 Bowling Ave., Nashville, TN 37205. http://www.hospicenet.org/.

Last Acts National Program Office. Partnership for Caring, 1620 Eye Street NW, Suite 202, Washington, DC 20006. (202) 296-8071. http://www.lastacts.org/.

Maggie Boleyn, R.N., B.S.N.

Postoperative care

Definition

Postoperative care is the management of a patient after surgery. This includes care given during the immediate postoperative period, both in the operating room and the postanesthesia care unit (PACU), as well as during the days following the surgery.

Purpose

The goal of postoperative care is to prevent complications such as **infection**, to promote healing of the surgical incision, and to return the patient to a state of health.

Precautions

Thorough postoperative care is crucial to ensuring positive outcomes for patients who have had surgery. There are no contraindications to providing this care. However, skill and careful monitoring are needed to prevent complications and to restore the patient to health as soon as possible.

Description

Postoperative care involves assessment, diagnosis, planning, intervention and outcome evaluation. The extent of postoperative care required by each patient depends on the original health status of the patient, type of surgery, and whether the surgery was performed in a day-surgery setting or in the hospital. Patients who have procedures done in a day-surgery center usually require only a few hours of care by health care professionals before they are discharged to go home. If postanesthesia or postoperative complications occur within these hours, the patient must be admitted to the hospital. Patients who are admitted to the hospital may require days or weeks of postoperative care by hospital staff before they are discharged.

Postanesthesia care unit (PACU)

After the surgical procedure, and anesthesia reversal and extubation if necessary, the patient is transferred to the PACU. The length of time the patient spends there depends on the length of surgery, the type of surgery, the status of regional anesthesia (for example, spinal anesthesia), and the patient's level of consciousness. Rather than being sent to the PACU, some patients may be transferred directly to the critical care unit instead. For example, patients who have had coronary artery bypass grafting (CABG) are sent directly to the critical care unit.

In the PACU, the anesthesiologist or the **nurse anesthetist** reports on the patient's condition, the type of surgery performed, the type of anesthesia given, estimated **blood** loss, and total input and output during the surgery. The receiving nurse should also be made aware of any complications during the surgery, including any variations in hemodynamic stability.

Assessment of the patient's airway patency, **vital signs**, and level of consciousness are the first priorities upon admission to the PACU. The following is a list of other assessment categories:

- surgical site (check that dressings are intact and there are no signs of overt bleeding)
- patency of drainage tubes/drains
- body temperature (hypothermia/hyperthermia)
- patency/rate of IV fluids
- circulation/sensation in extremities after vascular or orthopedic surgery
- level of sensation after regional anesthesia
- pain status
- nausea/vomiting

The patient is discharged from the PACU when they meet established criteria for discharge, as determined by use of a scale. An example is the Aldrete scale, which scores the patient on mobility, respiratory status, circulation, consciousness, and pulse oximetry. Depending on the type of surgery and the patient's condition, the patient may be admitted to either a general surgical floor or the intensive care unit. Since the patient may still be sedated from anesthesia, safety is a primary goal. The patient's call light should be in the hand and all side rails should be up. Patients in a day-surgery setting are either discharged from the PACU to the unit to their home, or are directly discharged home after they have voided, ambulated, and tolerated a small amount of oral intake.

First 24 hours

After the hospitalized patient transfers from the PACU, the receiving nurse should assess the patient again, using the same previously mentioned categories. If the patient reports "hearing" or feeling **pain** during surgery (under anesthesia) the observation should not be discounted. The anesthesiologist or nurse anesthetist should discuss the possibility of an episode of awareness under anesthesia with the patient. Vital signs, respiratory status, pain status, the incision, and any drainage tubes should be monitored every one to two hours for at least the first eight hours. Body temperature must be monitored, since patients are often hypothermic after surgery and may need a warming blanket or warmed IV fluids. Respiratory status should be assessed frequently, including auscultation of lung sounds, assessment of chest excursion, and presence of adequate **cough**. Fluid intake and urine output should be monitored every one to two hours. If the patient doesn't have a urinary catheter, the bladder should be assessed for distension and the patient monitored for inability to void. If they have not voided six to eight hours after surgery, the physician should be notified. If the patient had a vascular or neurological procedure performed, circulatory status or neurological status should be assessed as ordered by the surgeon, usually every one to two hours. The patient may require medication for nausea and/or **vomiting**, as well as for pain.

Patients with a **patient-controlled analgesia** (PCA) pump may need to be reminded how to use it. If the patient is too sedated immediately after the surgery, the nurse may push the button to deliver pain medication for them. The patient should be asked to rate their pain on a pain scale in order to determine their acceptable level of pain. Every attempt should be made by the nurse to keep the patient's pain under control. This often means that the nurse must offer pain medication every hour or two—many times before the patient requests it. Controlling pain is crucial so that the patient may perform coughing, deep breathing exercises, may be able to turn in bed, sit up, and, eventually, ambulate.

Effective preoperative teaching has a positive impact on the first 24 hours postoperatively. If patients understand that they must perform respiratory exercises to prevent **pneumonia**; and that movement is imperative for preventing blood clots, encouraging circulation to the extremities, and keeping the **lungs** clear; then they will be much more likely to perform these tasks. Understanding the need for movement and respiratory exercises also underscores the importance of keeping pain under control. Respiratory exercises (coughing, deep breathing and incentive spirometry) should be done every two hours. The patient should be turned every two hours, and should at least be sitting on the edge of the bed by eight hours after surgery, unless contraindicated (for example, after hip replacement). These patients will have sequential compression devices on their legs until they are able to ambulate. The sequential compression devices are stockings that inflate with air in order to simulate the effect of walking on the calf muscles and return blood to the **heart**. The patient should be encouraged to splint chest and abdominal incisions with a pillow to decrease the pain caused by coughing and moving. Patients should be kept NPO (nothing by mouth) if ordered by the surgeon, at least until their cough and gag **reflexes** have returned. Patients often have a dry mouth following surgery, which can be relieved with oral sponges dipped in ice water or by applying lemon ginger in mouth swabs.

Patients who are discharged home after a day-surgery procedure are given prescriptions for their pain medications and are responsible for their own pain control and respiratory exercises. Their families (or caregivers) should be included in preoperative teaching so that a caregiver can assist the patient at home. The patient should be reminded to call their physician if they have any complications or uncontrolled pain. These patients are often managed at home on a follow-up basis by a hospital-connected visiting nurse or **home care** service.

After 24 hours

After the initial 24 hours, vital signs can be monitored every four to eight hours if the patient is stable. The incision and dressing should be monitored for the amount of drainage and signs of infection; the surgeon may order the dressing to be changed during the first postoperative day. Postoperative dressing changes should be done using sterile technique. For home-care patients this technique must be emphasized. The hospitalized patient should be sitting up in a chair at the bedside and ambulating with assistance by this time period. Respiratory exercises should continue to be performed every two hours and incentive spirometry values should improve. Bowel sounds should be monitored and the patient's diet gradually increased as tolerated, depending on the type of surgery and the physician's orders.

The patient should be monitored for any evidence of potential complication, such as leg **edema**, redness, and pain (**deep vein thrombosis**), shortness of breath (**pulmonary embolism**), dehiscence (separation) of the incision, or ileus. If any of these occur, the surgeon should be notified immediately. If dehiscence occurs, sterile saline-soaked dressing packs should be placed on the wound. The patient and the family should be updated on the evaluation of the patient, the patient's condition, and any teaching as often as necessary.

Preparation

Postoperative care involves many procedures and teaching topics. Preparation for procedures includes having all needed supplies at the bedside. Pain medication should be offered prior to any procedure that is likely to cause discomfort. Preparation for teaching includes having resources available. Many hospitals have **patient education** materials such as handouts and video tapes that can be used to assist in teaching the patient what to expect during the postoperative time period.

KEY TERMS

Deep vein thrombosis (DVT)—Potentially life-threatening blood clot in one of the deep veins of the body, and often in the legs secondary to immobility after surgery. Symptoms include pain, warmth, swelling, and redness.

Dehiscence—Separation of a surgical incision or rupture of a wound closure.

Ileus—Obstruction in or immobility of the intestines. Symptoms include nausea and vomiting, absent bowel sounds, abdominal pain, and abdominal distension.

Incentive spirometer—Device that is used postoperatively to prevent lung collapse and promote maximum inspiration. The patient inhales until a preset volume is reached, then sustains the volume by holding their breath for three to five seconds.

PACU—The post-anesthesia care unit, where the patient is cared for after surgery.

Patient-controlled analgesia pump (PCA pump)—A pump which the patient uses to self-administer medication to control pain.

Pulmonary embolism (PE)—Potentially life-threatening blockage of a pulmonary artery by fat, air, or a blood clot that originated elsewhere in the body. Symptoms include acute shortness of breath and sudden chest pain.

Aftercare

Aftercare includes ensuring that patients are comfortable, either in bed or in a chair, and that they have their call lights accessible. After dressing changes, blood-soaked dressings should be properly disposed of in a biohazard container. Again, pain medication should be offered before any procedure that might cause discomfort. After teaching a patient, or the caregiver, aftercare includes answering all of their questions, and, in some cases, having them demonstrate the techniques they will be using.

Complications

Postoperative care is indicated for all patients who have had an invasive procedure, regardless how minor. However, improper care can lead to complications. For example, changing a surgical dressing without sterile technique can lead to infection. Failure to monitor a patient closely, or failing to assist them with respiratory exercises and ambulation, can lead to pneumonia or deep vein thrombosis, and potentially pulmonary embolus. Patients who have not had thorough teaching on what to expect may resist attempts to assist them, leading to complications and anger on the part of the patient or family.

Results

The goal of postoperative care is to ensure that patients have good outcomes after surgical procedures. A good outcome includes recovery without complications and adequate **pain management**. Another objective of postoperative care is to assist patients in taking responsibility for regaining good health.

Health care team roles

Almost every member of the health care team has a role in postoperative care. The surgeon performs the surgery and manages the patient's postoperative care. The patient's primary care doctor often helps manage the care of hospitalized patients as well. Nurses are at the bedside 24 hours a day, so they monitor the patient for complications, assist the patient with respiratory exercises and regaining mobility, provide postoperative teaching, and generally care for the patient. Respiratory therapists also provide instruction and assistance with respiratory exercises, and monitor the patient's respiratory status. **Radiology** personnel take x-rays that are ordered by the physician, and laboratory personnel draw blood samples and perform blood tests. All team members must communicate with one another and with the patient to provide the best possible postoperative care.

Resources

BOOKS

Bailey, Elizabeth. *The Patient's Checklist: 10 Simple Hospital Checklists to Keep you Safe, Sane & Organized.* New York, NY: Sterling, 2012.

Melnyk, Bernadette M., and Ellen Fineout-Overholt. *Evidence-Based Practice in Nursing & Healthcare: A Guide to Best Practice,* 2nd ed. New York, NY: Lippincott Williams & Wilkins, 2010.

Stewart, Brent., MD, MBA. *Need Surgery? Now What?: A Patient's Guide to Anesthesia.* Tampa, FL: Southern Medical Publishing, 2012.

PERIODICAL

Burns, S. "Revisiting Hypothermia: A Critical Concept." Critical Care Nurse vol. 21 no. 2 (2001): 83-86.

ORGANIZATIONS

American Society of PeriAnesthesia Nurses (ASPAN). 90 Frontage Road, Cherry Hill, NJ 08034-1424. Telephone: (877) 737-9696. http://www.aspan.org/

Association of periOperative Registered Nurses. 2170 South Parker Rd, Suite 400, Denver, CO 80231. Telephone: (800) 755-2676. http://www.aorn.org/.

Abby Wojahn, RN, BSN, CCRN
Laura Jean Cataldo, RN, Ed.D.

Postpartum care

Definition

Postpartum care encompasses management of the mother, newborn, and infant during the postpartal period. This period usually is considered to be the first few days after delivery, but technically it includes the six-week period after **childbirth**, up to the mother's postpartum check-up with her health care provider.

Purpose

Immediately following childbirth, a woman experiences profound physical and emotional changes. She may stay in the hospital or birthing center a very short time, as little as 24–48 hours after delivery. The physical and emotional care a woman receives during the postpartum period can influence her for the remainder of her life.

Precautions

During the postpartum period the mother is at risk for such problems as **infection**, hemorrhage, pregnancy-induced **hypertension**, **blood** clot format-ion, the opening up of incisions, breast problems, and **postpartum depression**.

Description

Postpartum care in the hospital

The initial phase of the postpartum period encompasses the first one to two hours after delivery. It takes place most often in the birthing room or in a recovery room. Once this initial phase is over, the woman has passed through the most dangerous part of childbirth. Assessments of **pain**, the condition of the uterus, vaginal discharge, the condition of the perineum, and the presence/absence of bladder distension (followed by appropriate interventions) are part of the initial postpartum evaluation, and should be done every 15 minutes for the first hour, then generally every 30 minutes for the second hour, and every 4–8 hours thereafter depending on facility policy.

PAIN/DISCOMFORT. The degree of pain and discomfort from incisions, lacerations, and uterine cramping (afterbirth pains) is assessed by hospital staff. The woman may also complain of muscle pain after a prolonged labor. If the level of pain warrants it, analgesic medications are given, usually orally. Women who have undergone cesarean births may have more pain than women who have given birth vaginally, and may need injectable **analgesics**. If a woman complains of pain in her calf, she should be evaluated for thrombophlebitis (swelling caused by a blood clot). Also, if a woman complains of a **headache**, her **blood pressure** should be checked to rule out the presence of pregnancy-induced hypertension. A woman who received **epidural anes-thesia** during delivery may develop a "spinal headache." A spinal headache is due to the loss of cerebrospinal fluid from the subarachnoid space that may occur during the administration of the spinal anesthesia. Spinal headaches should be treated by the anesthesiologist or nurse-anesthetist. Treatment for this type of headache typically includes keeping the patient flat in bed, encouraging increased fluid intake, and administering pain medication.

Breast engorgement is characterized by low-grade **fever** and the absence of systemic symptoms. It is usually bilateral; the breasts feel warm to the touch and appear shiny. Pain from breast engorgement can be minimized for the breastfeeding mother by mild analgesics, the application of warm packs, and frequent nursing. For the mother who is not breastfeeding, this pain can be minimized by mild analgesics and the application of cold packs. A nursing mother may find that the use of a lanolin-based preparation or a nipple shield (although controversial) provides relief for sore or cracked nipples. Changing positions for the nursing baby also can help in reducing irritation and minimizing **stress** on sore spots.

A plugged duct can also cause breast pain. Breast pain caused by a plugged duct is distinguished from breast engorgement by the fact that it usually is confined to one breast and the breast is not warm to the touch. This pain may be relieved by heat packs, gentle massage of the breast toward the nipple, and changing positions for nursing the baby.

FUNDUS. The condition of the uterus is assessed by evaluating the height and consistency of the fundus (the part of the uterus that can be palpated abdominally). Immediately after delivery, uterine contractions begin triggering involution. Involution is the process whereby the uterus and other reproductive organs return to their state prior to **pregnancy**. To properly palpate the uterus, the woman is positioned flat on her back (supine). The health care provider places one hand at the base of the uterus above the symphysis pubis (the interpubic joint of the pelvis) in a cupping manner (to support the lower uterine ligaments). Then, she presses in and downward with the other hand at the umbilicus until she makes contact with a hard, globular mass. If the uterus is not firm, light massaging usually results in tightening. Massaging of the uterus should not be so vigorous as to cause the mother pain. A mother who has had a cesarean delivery should be medicated, if possible, prior to assessment of the fundus, and the health care provider should use the minimal amount of pressure necessary to locate her fundus. The height of the fundus after the first hour following delivery is at the umbilicus or above it. Every day the fundal height decreases by approximately the width of one finger (one cm).

The fundal height may be palpated off of midline because of a distended bladder. If possible, the woman should be encouraged to empty her bladder prior to assessment of the fundus. A full bladder can prevent uterine involution.

A woman sometimes receives the medication oxytocin (Pitocin) after the delivery of the placenta. Oxytocin causes the uterus to contract and can decrease the amount of postpartum bleeding. The health care provider should assess the condition of the uterus frequently and may need to massage the uterus gently to encourage its clamping down on itself, especially when oxytocin has not been given. If the uterus does not firm to gentle massage, then a clot may be present inside. Gentle pressure on the uterus following massage, and while simultaneously supporting the base of the uterus, may expel the clot.

If massaging the uterus does not result in a firming of the fundus, then the physician or nurse-midwife should be contacted immediately. The existence of severe atony or a retained fragment of placenta may result in excessive loss of blood.

VAGINAL DISCHARGE (LOCHIA). The color and amount of vaginal discharge (lochia) is assessed by frequently removing the perineal pad and checking the flow of lochia after delivery. An excessive amount could be a sign of a complication such as clot formation or a retained portion of the placenta. The vaginal discharge is red for one to three days following delivery and is called *lochia rubra*. Between days two and 10, the discharge changes to a pink or brownish color and is called *lochia serosa*. The last phase occurs when the vaginal discharge turns white. This vaginal discharge is referred to as *lochia alba* and may occur from 10–14 days postpartum. The spotting can continue for another six weeks. It is common in mothers who breastfeed their babies. A constant trickling of blood or the soaking through of a perineal pad in an hour or less is not normal and should be further evaluated.

PERINEUM. The condition of the perineal area is assessed for an episiotomy or laceration repair. An episiotomy is the surgical procedure whereby the physician or nurse-midwife extends the vaginal outlet immediately prior to delivery of the baby. The incision is repaired with sutures after delivery.

Generally an episiotomy will be 1–2 inches (2.5–5 cm) in length. By 24 hours postpartum, the edges of the episiotomy should be fused together. An episiotomy may be covered over with edematous tissue and not easily visible, so the examination must the done carefully. If the laceration or episiotomy is infected, it appears red and swollen, and discharges pus. Treatment depends on the severity of the infection and may include sitz baths, application of an antibiotic cream to the wound, oral **antibiotics**, or opening the wound, cleansing the site, and resuturing it.

When the perineal area is examined, the patient should also be checked for the presence of a hematoma (a round area filled with blood) that is caused by the rupturing of small **blood vessels** on the surface of the perineum. After observing the perineum, the rectal area also is evaluated for **hemorrhoids**, making note of their size, character, and number.

The following measures are effective in providing relief of perineal discomfort:

- Application of cold packs to the perineum for the first 24 hours after delivery.

- Application of warm packs to the perineum after the first 24 hours.

- Rinsing of the perineal area with warm water after every void and/or bowel movement. (This is also helpful in preventing infection and in promoting healing.)

- Use of anesthetic sprays and creams. Cleaning the area with witch hazel pads (Tucks) is also soothing.

- Sitting in a sitz bath—a small basin that fits on top of the toilet through which warm water flows—three or four times a day. After discharge, a woman may use her bathtub at home for this purpose.

BLADDER DISTENTION. In the first 48 hours after delivery, it is normal to have an increase in the formation and secretion of urine (postpartum diuresis). A full bladder can cause the uterus to shift upward and not contract effectively. An overdistended bladder can even cause injury to the **urinary system**. A woman should be encouraged to void within her first hour postpartum, and her bladder should be checked after voiding, since urinary retention can be a problem. If the woman had a **cesarean section** and has a Foley catheter in place in her bladder, then the output is checked every hour during the initial postpartum period. The Foley catheter is likely to be removed approximately eight hours after surgery. The health care provider needs to assess for voiding after removal of the Foley catheter.

Postpartum care after hospital discharge

Ideal postpartum care would include several home visits by health care providers in the one to two weeks following delivery to assess the status of the mother and her family. This rarely happens in the United States, but follow-up phone calls by health care providers during the first week and a visit by the mother and baby to her physician or nurse-midwife one to two weeks after the birth are desirable.

Several problems that may arise during the postpartum period do not typically develop until after the new mother is discharged from the hospital. These include **mastitis**, endometritis, and postpartum depression.

MASTITIS. Mastitis is an inflammation of the breast usually caused by streptococcal or staphylococcal infection. It can develop any time a woman is breastfeeding, but usually does not occur before the tenth postpartum day. Symptoms of mastitis often mimic those of the flu and include body aches and a fever of 101 °F (38.6 °C) or more. Mastitis is treated with a course of antibiotics, and women should begin to feel better within 24 hours of beginning antibiotic treatment. If this does not happen, the woman may need to be hospitalized for intravenous antibiotics.

KEY TERMS

Perineum—The area between the rectum and the outlet of the vagina.

Pregnancy-induced hypertension—Vasospasm occurring during pregnancy resulting in such symptoms as hypertension, swelling, and protein in the urine. If not treated, it can sometimes result in a seizure.

Thrombophlebitis—Blood clot formation resulting in inflammation of the lining of a blood vessel.

Umbilicus—Navel; depression in the center of the abdomen where the umbilical cord was attached.

Other measures that may help the mother feel better include bed rest for at least 24 hours, moist heat on the infected breast every two to three hours (when awake), acetaminophen for pain and fever relief, increased fluid intake, and going without a bra for several days. Mastitis does not contaminate the breast milk, and the baby should continue to nurse from both breasts. If nursing from the affected breast is too painful, use of a breast pump or manual expression of milk may be needed to prevent engorgement and facilitate continued milk production.

ENDOMETRITIS. Endometritis is an inflammation of the endometrium, the mucous membrane lining the uterus. It is usually caused by a bacterial infection. Symptoms of this infection include fever, **abdominal pain**, and foul-smelling vaginal discharge. **Physical examination** of the patient reveals a tender uterus. Endometritis is treated with a course of antibiotics and other care, including bed rest, acetaminophen for pain and fever relief, and increased fluid intake. Severe cases may require hospitalization.

POSTPARTUM DEPRESSION. Postpartum depression may appear at any time during the first year after a baby's birth. It ranges in severity from mild, postpartum "blues" that last only a few days shortly after birth, to intense, suicidal, depressive **psychosis**. Not only does postpartum depression cause distress for the new mother and her partner, but it can also interfere with the new mother's ability to bond with her baby and to relate to any other children she may have.

Symptoms of postpartum depression include **anxiety**, mood swings, feelings of guilt, shame or worthlessness, lack of interest in usual activities, decreased appetite, and suicidal thoughts. Any new mother exhibiting signs of postpartum depression should be referred to mental health professionals, support groups, and/or new mother groups. Treating postpartum depression quickly can significantly shorten its duration and improve outcomes.

Postpartum psychosis has symptoms that include hallucinations, agitation, desire to hurt oneself or one's baby, and bizarre feelings or behavior. Postpartum psychosis is a medical emergency and should be addressed by a medical professional immediately. Psychotropic medication is often helpful, as is **psychotherapy**. About 10% of cases of postpartum depression are caused by postpartum thyroiditis, a temporary inflammation of the **thyroid gland** that usually clears up spontaneously in one to four months. Whenever postpartum depression occurs, thyroid function should be tested to rule out hyperthyroidism or hypothyroidism as the cause of symptoms.

Six-week postpartum check-up

Although this postpartum check-up is traditionally scheduled six weeks after delivery, it may be done any time between four weeks and eight weeks after delivery. It usually includes a breast examination, a pelvic examination, any necessary laboratory tests, and a health education component covering such areas as breastfeeding, birth control, and weight reduction. This checkup is also an opportunity to review the pregnancy and birth experience, to discuss problems and assess for depression, to provide emotional support, to answer questions, and to consider if any further referrals are necessary for the new mother.

Health care team roles

The new mother is given instruction on how to hygienically care for her perineal area. She is encouraged to change her perineal pad frequently and to wash her hands afterwards. The presence of a wet pad against sutures is an excellent medium for the development of an infection that could potentially spread to the uterus. The woman is also instructed not to use tampons for six weeks after delivery, since tampon use can cause infection or even toxic **shock** syndrome.

New mothers may be overwhelmed by the degree of discomfort after giving birth and may be frustrated by their desire to interact with their new baby while at the same time being limited by pain, discomfort, and exhaustion. The health care team member can help the new mother by providing perineal care for her until she is able to get out of bed, and by administering pain medications as ordered.

QUESTIONS TO ASK THE DOCTOR

1. Are my current emotional symptoms normal feelings for the postpartum period or might they be symptoms a more serious problem like postpartum depression?

2. When will I safely be able to have intercourse again?

3. What birth control options are appropriate for me? Will they affect my ability to breastfeed safely?

4. If I notice any signs of problems such as infections, who should I call. What if it is after hours or on the weekend?

Other important things health care providers can do for postpartum women include:

- Evaluate pulse, respiratory rate, and blood pressure every 15 minutes during the first hour postpartum, every 30 minutes for two hours, and then every eight hours. Evaluate the woman's temperature at the end of the first hour postpartum and then every four hours for the first two to 12 hours postpartum.

- Help the woman take a shower as soon as she is allowed to, while monitoring her for lightheadedness.

- Place a warm blanket over the mother after delivery if she experiences shaking and chills.

- Provide emotional support to the mother and family through explanations about childbirth and how it can be a highly emotional and psychologically overwhelming time.

- Promote adequate rest.

- Encourage a generous intake of nutrients and fluids.

- Ask if the woman has had a bowel movement prior to discharge and offer medication to soften stools if desired.

- Monitor the woman's voiding and ensure the woman is not having difficulty. Catheterization is sometimes required.

- Assist with ambulation until the woman is steady on her feet.

- Review laboratory tests for signs of anemia, infection, and electrolyte imbalance.

- Teach the woman muscle-strengthening exercises.

- Prepare the mother and family for discharge through discharge teaching.

- Arrange for a home visit if this is provided for through the facility and/or patient's insurance.

Resources

BOOKS

Ladewig, Patricia A. Wieland, London, Marcia L., and Davidson, Michele R. *Clinical Handbook for Olds' Maternal-Newborn Nursing and Women's Health Across the Lifespan,* 9th ed. Boston: Pearson, 2012.

Shields, Sara G., and Candib, Lucy M., eds. *Woman-Centered Care in Pregnancy and Childbirth.* New York: Radcliffe Publishing, 2010.

Thomson, Gill, Dykes, Fiona, and Downe, Soo, eds. *Qualitative Research in Midwifery and Childbirth Phenomenological Approaches.* New York: Routledge, 2011.

PERIODICALS

Leahy-Warren, Patricia, and McCarthy, Geraldine. "Maternal Parental Self-Efficacy in the Postpartum Period." *Midwifery,* (December 2011) 27(6):802–810.

McCaul, Anthony, and Stokes, Jayne. "Perinatal Support to Protect Maternal Mental Health." *Nursing Times,* (December 6–12 2011) 107(48): 16–18.

Weir, Sharada, et al. "Predictors of Prenatal and Postpartum Care Adequacy in a Medicaid Managed Care Population." *Womens Health Issues,* (July-August 2011) 21(4):277–285.

OTHER

"Postpartum Care." Medline Plus. [accessed April 9, 2012] http://www.nlm.nih.gov/medlineplus/postpartumcare.html.

"Postpartum Care: What to Expect After a Vaginal Delivery." The Mayo Clinic. [accessed April 9, 2012] http://www.mayoclinic.com/health/postpartum-care/PR00142

ORGANIZATIONS

American College of Nurse-Midwives, 8403 Colesville Road, Suite 1550, Silver Spring, MD 20910, (240) 485-1800, Fax: (240) 485-1818, www.midwife.org

American Congress of Obstetricians and Gynecologists, PO Box 70620, Washington, DC 20024-9998, (202) 638-5577, (800) 673-8444, resources@acog.org, www.acog.org

Association of Women's Health, Obstetric and Neonatal Nurses, 2000 L Street, NW, Suite 740, Washington, DC 20036, (202) 261-2400, (800) 673-8499, Fax: (202) 728-0575, customerservice@awhonn.org, www.awhonn.org.

Nadine M. Jacobson
Tish Davidson, AM

Postpartum depression

Definition

Postpartum depression (PPD) is a major depressive episode that occurs after **childbirth**. There are conflicting data regarding the time of onset. The *Diagnostic and Statistical Manual of Mental Disorders IV-TR* supports the theory that PPD occurs within four weeks of childbirth. Other clinical investigations report its occurrence up to 12 weeks post-delivery; yet others state that PPD can occur from six to 12 months after delivery. Reports suggest that PPD may last up to one year.

Description

The beginning of PPD tends to be gradual and may persist for many months. There can be a second episode if there is a subsequent **pregnancy**. About 85% of women experience some mood disturbance or disorder during the period immediately following childbirth, however the majority of these cases are mild and resolve without treatment. According to *The Journal of the American Medical Association*, PPD affects approximately 13% of women who have recently given birth. Younger mothers are at an increased risk for PPD compared to those who give birth later in life. Other factors that increase the risk a woman will experience PPD after giving birth include financial troubles, relationship problems with a spouse or partner, physical abuse, and tobacco use.

Mild cases of PPD are sometimes unrecognized by women themselves. Yet PPD is a serious problem that disrupts women's lives and can have negative effects on the baby, other children, the new mother's partner, and other significant relationships. The father's risk of becoming depressed increases significantly during the postpartum period as well.

Postpartum depression is often divided into two types: early onset and late onset. An early-onset depression most often presents as "baby blues," a brief experience during the first days or weeks following birth. During the first week after the birth of their child, up to 80% of mothers may experience the "baby blues." This period is characterized by feelings of oversensitivity, unexpected bouts of crying, irritability, **anxiety**, and mood changes. Symptoms tend to peak between three and five days after childbirth, and normally disappear within a few days.

In short, it is normal for new mothers to experience some anxiety, tiredness, and sadness after giving birth. However when these symptoms do not resolve within a few days, or become very severe, the mother may be experiencing PPD.

Late-onset PPD appears several weeks after the birth. This may involve a growing feeling of sadness, grief, lack of energy, chronic fatigue, inability to sleep, changes in appetite, significant weight loss or gain, difficulty caring for the baby, and sometimes, thoughts of harming the baby.

Causes and symptoms

Experts are not positive about the causes of PPD. It may be caused by factors that vary from person to person. Pregnancy and birth are accompanied by sudden hormonal shifts that can cause a range of emotions. Additionally, the 24-hour responsibilities involved in caring for a newborn present major psychological and lifestyle adjustments for most new mothers. These physical and emotional stresses are usually aggravated by not getting adequate rest until the baby's routine stabilizes.

Experiences of new mothers experiencing PPD vary considerably, but may include the following.

Feelings:

• persistent low mood
• inadequacy, failure, hopelessness, helplessness
• exhaustion, emptiness, sadness, teariness
• guilt, shame, worthlessness
• confusion, anxiety, and panic
• fear for the baby and of the baby
• fear of being alone or going out

Behaviors:

• lack of interest or pleasure in usual activities
• insomnia or excessive sleep; nightmares
• changes in appetite
• decreased energy and motivation
• withdrawal from social contact
• poor self-care
• inability to cope with routine tasks

Thoughts:

• inability to think clearly and make decisions
• lack of concentration and poor memory
• inability to deal with stressful situations
• fear of being rejected by partner
• worry about harming herself, her partner, or her baby
• suicidal ideation

Presence of some symptoms may not indicate a severe problem. However, persistent low mood or loss of interest or pleasure in activities, along with four other symptoms occurring at the same time, may signal a problem. If these symptoms persist for at least two weeks, a clinical depression may be occurring, and professional intervention may be required.

There are several important risk factors for PPD, including:

• stress
• loss of pleasure or interest in living

- lack of sleep (sleep deprivation)
- poor nutrition
- lack of support from one's partner, family, or friends
- family history of clinical depression
- complications for mother or baby during labor and delivery
- premature or postmature delivery
- poor newborn health
- separation of mother and baby
- a difficult baby (i.e., problems with temperament, feeding, sleeping, or settling)
- preexisting neurosis or psychosis
- previous depressive episode

Diagnosis

There is no specific diagnostic test for PPD. However, it is important to understand that PPD is a bona fide illness and that it has specific symptoms, the same as a physical condition. **Blood** tests to measure thyroid hormone levels can rule out postpartum thyroiditis, which can mimic PPD.

It is important to note that a small percentage of women experience postpartum **psychosis**, a rare disorder. This is the most severe, but least common, postpartum depressive condition. Occurring in only 1–2 births per 1,000, postpartum psychosis appears between 48–72 hours and several weeks after delivery. Symptoms may include elated mood, mood changeability, disorganized behavior, insomnia, religious preoccupation, agitation, suicide attempts or suicidal ideation, bizarre feelings or behavior, and hallucinations. Postpartum psychosis is a serious condition that requires immediate psychiatric intervention and possible hospitalization. Without treatment, the mother may seriously harm the baby or herself.

Other psychiatric conditions, such as panic disorder and obsessive-compulsive disorder (OCD), are possible manifestations of PPD.

Complications

If PPD is misdiagnosed or remains untreated, a severely depressed woman may attempt or complete suicide. On a lesser but significant level, untreated PPD can lead to continued depression, anxiety, or postpartum psychosis.

Treatment

Several treatment options exist for mild-to-moderate PPD; these are psychiatric therapies that include interpersonal therapy (IPT) and cognitive-behavior therapy

---

KEY TERMS

Cognitive behavioral therapy—A type of psychotherapy in which people learn to recognize and change negative and self-defeating patterns of thinking and behavior.

Depression—A mental condition in which a person feels extremely sad and loses interest in life. A person with depression may also have sleep problems and loss of appetite and may have trouble concentrating and carrying out everyday activities. Severe depression may instigate a suicide attempt.

Selective serotonin reuptake inhibitors (SSRIs)—A class of antidepressants that work by blocking the reabsorption of serotonin in brain cells, raising the level of the chemical in the brain. SSRIs include Prozac, Zoloft, Luvox, and Paxil.

Serotonin—5-Hydroxytryptamine; a substance that occurs throughout the body with numerous effects including neurotransmission. Low serotonin levels are associated with mood disorders, particularly depression and obsessive-compulsive disorder.

(CBT). Some researchers recommend bright-light therapy for treating PPD. Clinical studies have reported that pregnant, depressed women and postpartum, depressed women, respectively, experienced antidepressant effects when bright-light therapy is administered. Another effective treatment combines antidepressant medication with counseling. Antidepressants generally become effective several weeks after a patient has begun taking them. Medication must be prescribed carefully if the mother is breastfeeding, as it can pass to the baby in the mother's breast milk. It is important for women to inform their physicians if they are breastfeeding. The results of several short-term studies point to relative safety (i.e., lack of toxicity, minimal exposure to the maternal dose, or few adverse effects) in the use of selective serotonin reuptake inhibitor (SSRI) antidepressants by nursing mothers.

Postpartum depression also may be treated with "talk" therapy and participation in a support group. The mother needs to feel cared for, and that her feelings are respected. Nursing staff and allied health professionals can positively affect the treatment course by providing the mother with supportive one-on-one therapy, whereby the therapist listens to the woman's specific concerns and fears.

Alternative treatment measures, such as **homeopathy**, may be helpful, since they are meant to address mental, physical, and spiritual states—all of which are affected by PPD. **Acupuncture**, Chinese and Western herbs may also help by balancing mood and hormone levels. However, caution is strongly advised when taking herbs because they are unregulated. Toxicity studies have not been conducted to evaluate the safety of these substances. Seeking help from a homeopathic practitioner, however, does provide the new mother with an opportunity to discuss specific nutritional needs or mood problems.

Fortunately, there are useful things that a new mother can do for herself, including:

- making each day as simple as possible
- asking for help from supportive friends and family members whenever possible
- avoiding extra pressures or unnecessary tasks
- involving her partner more intensively in the care of the baby from the beginning
- discussing with her partner how both can share the household chores and responsibilities
- scheduling frequent outings, such as walks and short visits with friends
- having the baby sleep in a separate room so that she can sleep more restfully
- sharing her feelings with her partner or another good listener
- talking with other mothers to keep problems in perspective
- sleeping or resting when the baby is sleeping
- taking care of her health and well-being
- allowing others care for the baby when possible
- taking time for herself to do activities she enjoys

Prognosis

With appropriate support from friends and family, many mild cases of PPD go away by themselves. If depression becomes severe, a patient should not attempt to care for herself or the baby; in some cases, psychiatric hospitalization may be necessary. However, a three-pronged approach, consisting of supervised medication, psychiatric counseling, and support from family and friends, may relieve even severe depression in three to six months.

Health care team roles

Nursing staff and allied health professionals can assist in the diagnosis of postpartum depression by observing the patient for symptoms. Since PPD can present as a mood disorder, anxiety state, or

QUESTIONS TO ASK YOUR DOCTOR

1. Are my symptoms normal for the period after childbirth, or could they be symptoms of PPD?
2. Do you know of any support groups for new mothers in this area?
3. How much experience do you have treating PPD?
4. Can you recommend a therapist who has experience treating this kind of issue?
5. Can you recommend any actions I can take at home to help alleviate my symptoms?

psychotic episode, it is critical that nursing staff and allied health professionals understand the warning signs.

During the treatment phase, nursing staff and allied health professionals can help a new mother by providing her with appropriate **patient education** materials, and referrals for ongoing supportive therapy or group **psychotherapy**, if applicable.

Prevention

Regular **exercise** and good **nutrition** can help enhance a new mother's emotional well-being. New mothers should also cultivate good sleeping habits and rest if possible when physically or emotionally tired. It is important for the health professional to teach the patient how to recognize the signs of fatigue and to make time for herself.

Psychotherapy or the use of antidepressant medication can also help to prevent future episodes of postpartum or ongoing clinical depression.

Resources
BOOKS

Kendall-Tackett, Kathleen A. *Depression in New Mothers: Causes, Consequences, and Treatment Alternatives,* 2nd ed. New York: Routledge, 2010.

Langwith, Jacqueline, ed. *Postpartum Depression.* Detroit: Greenhaven Press, 2012.

Zittel, Kimberley. *Postpartum Mood Disorders: A Guide for Medical, Mental Health, and Other Support Providers.* Washing DC: National Association of Social Workers, 2010.

PERIODICALS

Milgrom, Jeannette, et al. "Treating Postnatal Depressive Symptoms in Primary Care." *BMC Psychiatry,* (2011) 11:95.

Sofronas, Marianne, et al. "Obstetric and Neonatology Nurses' Attitudes, Beliefs, and Practices Related to the Management of Symptoms of Maternal Depression." *Issues in Mental Health Nursing,* (2011) 32(12):735–744.

OTHER

"Postpartum Depression." PubMed Health. [accessed April 7, 2012.] http://www.ncbi.nlm.nih.gov/pubmedhealth/PMH0004481/

"Postpartum Depression." The Mayo Clinic. [accessed April 7, 2012.] http://www.mayoclinic.com/health/postpartum-depression/DS00546

ORGANIZATIONS

American Psychiatric Association, 1000 Wilson Boulevard, Suite 1825, Arlington, VA USA 22209, (703) 907-7300, (888) 35-PSYCH (357-7924), apa@psych.org, http://www.psych.org

Postpartum Support International, 6706 SW 54th Avenue, Portland, OR 97219, (503) 894-9453, (800) 944-4PPD (4773), Fax: (503) 894-9452, support@postpartum.net, www.postpartum.net.

Bethanne Black
Tish Davidson, AM

Postural drainage *see* **Chest physical therapy**

Postural evaluation

Definition

Posture can be defined as the position of the body in any environment or mode. Some examples of specific postures are sitting, standing, walking, or leaning forward. Posture is based on the position of the spine and all the joints in the musculoskeletal system. Postural evaluation or analysis consists of evaluating a patient's posture through a series of appropriate tests and measurements. It is part of the branch of **physical therapy** called kinesiology, which includes the study of the **anatomy** and **physiology** of body movement.

Good or normal posture is defined as an imaginary straight line that connects the earlobe, cervical vertebrae, acromion (bony outgrowth on the shoulder blade), lumbar vertebrae, and a set of points behind the hip and slightly in front of the knee and ankle. In an actual postural evaluation, the patient may be asked to stand by a vertical plumb line so that the examiner can visualize any deviations from normal alignment.

Purpose

Good posture in humans is the end product of a complex combination of mechanical, neurological, and psychological factors, including muscular strength and flexibility, **vision**, touch, balance, self-esteem, kinesthetic (a sense of the location and movement of muscles and joints) awareness, and a properly functioning vestibular (inner ear) system. Because of the number of bidy parts and functions involved in good posture, a postural evaluation may serve a variety of purposes:

• As part of the musculoskeletal assessment of a balance evaluation. Postural abnormalities frequently affect an elderly person's sense of balance and his or her ability to react quickly to loss of balance.

• As a step in the differential diagnosis of chronic pain syndromes. Chronic neck and back pain in particular often result from poor posture, which causes muscles to contract, changes the amount of blood flow to the spine, and leads to deformation of the connective tissues in the spine and neck area.

• As part of a physical examination in sports medicine. Deviations from normal posture increase the risk of certain types of athletic injuries, and may interfere with athletic performance.

• In the evaluation of work-related postural problems and repetitive stress injuries (RSI). Some physical therapists now visit work places in order to assess the physical demands of certain jobs—especially jobs that require sitting at desks in front of computers for long periods. These assessments are sometimes called ergonomic evaluations, which means that the design of equipment and other physical features of the workplace is coordinated with the physical requirements of the workers.

Precautions

Postural evaluation is noninvasive and should not cause the patient physical discomfort under normal circumstances. Care should be taken, however, to perform the evaluation in an appropriate examination room to protect the patient's modesty. The room should be kept at a comfortable temperature.

Description

Postural evaluation typically begins with a visual assessment of the patient's posture while he or she is standing by a vertical plumb line. The person's posture is then scored according to check lists for the back view and the side view. Deviations from good posture are rated according to severity, in which a slight deviation is scored as 1 point, a moderate deviation as 2, and a severe deviation as 3 points. The total number of points from both back and side views is then calculated. A score of 12 points or higher is considered poor posture. Some therapists prefer to use posture photographs for a postural evaluation, while other practitioners may order x rays, on the grounds that these imaging modalities yield more accurate results than simple viusal examination.

Visual assessment of posture also includes the clinician's careful visual observation of the patient's positioning during walking, sitting, and weight transfers.

Manual **muscle testing** is an important part of postural analysis. The clinician uses his or her hands to evaluate the various muscles for atrophy (wasting away from disuse), misalignment, overstretching, or constriction and shortening. Manual testing also allows the clinician to determine the extent as well as the presence of muscular imbalance.

Preparation

Accurate evaluation of patients with postural dysfunction requires careful history-taking. This includes family and social history as well as medical history. In most cases changes in posture are due to such anomalies as excessive weight gain, poor postural habits, traumatic injuries, uneven development of the musculature, or congenital defects. A family history may yield information about hereditary disorders that affect posture as well as family members' attitudes toward the patient. In some cases, people develop poor posture in response to physical or emotional abuse.

Results

An accurate postural evaluation provides the physical therapist with necessary information in devising a treatment plan. The goal of **rehabilitation** is to isolate the cause(s) of postural abnormalities and provide appropriate treatment through postural correction exercises and **patient education**. Other treatments can include such modalities as heat, ice, and massage; flexibility exercises; strengthening programs; and cardiovascular conditioning.

Health care team roles

Postural evaluations may be performed by physical therapists, physicians, nurses, and chiropractors. It is

KEY TERMS

Acromion—A bony prominence on the shoulder blade that articulates with the clavicle, forming the acromioclavicular (AC) joint.

Atrophy—The wasting away of muscle tissue from disuse.

Kinesiology—The branch of physical therapy that deals with the anatomy and physiology of body movement.

Osteoarthritis—A degenerative disorder of the cartilage and bone in the joints.

Osteoporosis—A condition characterized by decrease in bone mass and density, and enlargement of bone spaces.

important that physicians—especially pediatricians—nurses, and other allied health professionals routinely evaluate patients' posture in an effort to minimize further complications of various diseases and disorders. Most health care facilities have screening clinics that offer postural assessment free of charge. It is also imperative that individuals with spinal **osteoarthritis**, **osteoporosis**, Marfan's syndrome, and other conditions that affect the spine be properly educated on the importance of good posture. The elderly and others who may have developed **balance problems** should have their posture evaluated as part of an overall balance evaluation.

Resources

BOOKS

Hall, C.M., and L.T. Brody. *Therapeutic Exercise Moving Toward Function.* Philadelphia: Lippincott, Williams & Wilkins, 1999.

Kendall, F.P., E.K. McCreary, and P.G. Provance. *Muscles: Testing and Function.* Baltimore, MD: Williams & Wilkins, 1993.

Lehmkuhl, L. D., and L. K. Smith. *Brunnstrom's Clinical Kinesiology.* Philadelphia: F.A. Davis Co., 1996.

Magee, D. J. *Orthopedic Physical Assessment.* Philadelphia: W. B. Saunders Co., 1997.

ORGANIZATION

National Rehabilitation Information Center and ABLE-DATA (database). 8455 Colesville Road, Suite 935, Silver Spring, MD 20910. (800) 346-2742 or (800) 227-0216.

Mark Damian Rossi, Ph.D., P.T.

Posturography *see* **Balance and coordination tests**

Potassium hydroxide test *see* **KOH test**

Potassium test *see* **Electrolyte tests**

Power of attorney

Definition

Power of attorney, also known as durable medical power of attorney, is a legal mechanism that empowers a designated person to make medical decisions for a patient should the patient be unable to make the decisions due to incapacitation.

Purpose

Power of attorney assures that a patient's wishes are acknowledged in the medical setting. Along with other legal documents such as a living will and a do not resuscitate (DNR) order, the power of attorney designates the agent or person who is legally authorized to act for the patient in the medical setting. All three mechanisms are a part of what is known as advanced medical directives. The purpose of advanced directives is to have the patient's wishes for medical care carried out even when the patient is incapacitated and can no longer make his or her wishes known.

Description

The patient's agent is the person appointed by the patient to represent him or her in medical situations where decisions must be made. This surrogate, through the power of attorney authorization, has all of the rights that the patient has with respect to deciding on medical procedures. These include the rights to refuse treatment, to agree to treatment, or to have treatment withdrawn.

Guided by a living will, which is a document developed in advance that reflects the patient's wishes, the agent acts on behalf of the patient with providers, administrators, and other legal agents. In most states, surrogates can act for the patient on any medical procedure, including a decision to refuse **life support** procedures such as resuscitation. States differ, however, on whether health agents can invoke a DNR order.

In the difficult times that families experience with a seriously ill or terminally ill family member, health agents play a major role in making decisions and stipulating what the patient's wishes are with respect to

his or her treatment or palliative care needs. Health agents can work with or without a living will. The crucial feature of the power of attorney is that it empowers the patient's agent to respond to changes in the patient's health and to make flexible decisions. It is the health agent, rather than the patient, who must be apprised of all medical options, weigh the risk and benefits, and make a decision based on the specific situation.

Preparation

The person who has the medical power of attorney for a patient is only as good as his or her level of understanding of the patient and level of respect for the patient's wishes. There are some specific steps that can be taken to prepare the health care agent for power of attorney responsibilities. These steps include:

- The patient must think about medical treatments he or she would or would not like to have in different medical situations such as accidents, acute and life-threatening injuries, nursing home care, etc.

- If possible, the patient should write down his or her medical wishes and have these developed into a living will.

- The patient will want to convey these medical wishes to family and friends, as well as the identity of the person who will have power of attorney.

- Whether a written document is drafted or not, it is important that the patient have discussions with the designated agent so that his or her wishes can be carried out if the need arises. Not all elements of the medical decisions required can be known in advance. Hence, it is very important that the health agent knows the patient, knows the patient's wishes and rationale, and understands fully what is of value to the patient. Family and health providers should also be informed of the patient's wishes.

Medical decisions likely to be faced in severe health emergencies include options for **cardiopulmonary resuscitation (CPR)**, diagnostic tests, administration of drugs, surgery, the use of life-supporting technologies, and organ and tissue use. However, there are also other decisions that can may require decisions from the agent. These may include family members, and how much say they will have in decision making, issues of visitation, and other issues only somewhat related to the medical care. It is important that the agent understand and honor the wishes of the patient in all of these areas.

Once the initial steps for the advanced instructions are in place, an official medical power of attorney form for the state of residence or health care must be filled out. These may be two different states. It is important to have a medical power of attorney for any and all states in which medical care might be provided.

Normal results

All medical directives, whether the living will, power of attorney, or do not resuscitate order, are respected by all health personnel in whatever medical setting the chosen state stipulates. These generally include hospitals, emergency rooms, emergency vehicles, and short- or long-term care facilities such as **hospice** care. Many states also include the home. The medical directives become a part of the patient's medical record and must be honored by any and all health personnel involved in the patient's treatment or care.

Resources

BOOKS

Cebuhar, Jo Kline. *Last Things First, Just in Case . . .: the Practical Guide to Living Wills and Durable Powers of Attorney for Health Care.* West Des Moines, IA: Murphy Pub., 2006.

Doukas, David John and William Reichel. *Planning for Uncertainty: Living Wills and Other Advance Directives for You and Your Family*, 2nd Ed. Baltimore, MD: Johns Hopkins University Press, 2007.

Haman, Edward A. *Power of Attorney Handbook*, 5th Ed. Naperville, IL: Sphinx Pub., 2004.

PERIODICALS

Make Medical and Financial Preparations. *USA Today* 136.2749 (Oct 2007): 11-12.

Stephenson, Correy E. "Caution: Use Power of Attorney Wisely." *Minnesota Lawyer* (January 21, 2008).

Nancy McKenzie, PhD
Robert Bockstiegel

PPD skin test *see* **Tuberculin skin test**

Prealbumin test

Definition

Formally called the transthyretin test, the prealbumin test (abbreviated the PA test) is a specific clinical indicator of nutritional risk for patients suffering from such diseases as **cancer**, CHF (congestive **heart failure**), diabetes, COPD (chronic obstructive lung disease), HIV/AIDS (human **immunodeficiency** virus/ acquired immune deficiency syndrome), **pneumonia**, and renal disease. The PA test is also used to monitor patients at risk for poor **nutrition** and malnutrition.

Purpose

Prealbumin is considered an important protein found in **blood**. The concentration of prealbumin (also called tryptophan-rich prealbumin (TRPA) and thyroxine-binding prealbumin [TBPA]) in blood plasma or serum is a reliable way to assess the nutritional status of patients (see **nutritional assessment**). The prealbumin test uses the well-established technique called turbidimetric immunoassay to measure the concentration of prealbumin in blood plasma or serum. The technique involves mixing a blood sample with assay reagents. The prealbumin binds specifically with an anti-human prealbumin antibody to produce an insoluble aggregate. The results produce increased turbidity (cloudiness) in the mixture. The degree of turbidity is directly proportional to the prealbumin concentration in the sample. The turbidity can then be measured with an clinical analyzer.

The prealbumin test is commonly used to measure the nutritional status of hospitalized patients because its results are reliable, fast, and accurate. Specifically, a patient should be given the prealbumin test when the physician suspects malnourishment due to poor diet, disease, being fed with intravenous nutrition, or being on hemodialysis. External signs of malnutrition include: inability to think or speak clearly, fainting spells, unusually large weight loss, declining resistance to **infection**, brittle, dry, and sometimes falling out hair, dry or yellowish skin, deteriorating muscles, stunted growth in a child, and stopped menstrual periods in women (amenorrhea). Patients who are more likely to receive the PA test are those who:

• are newly-admitted to a medical facility (especially scheduled for surgery)

• over 65 years of age

- unable to swallow or ingest food for five days
- chronically ill
- present with certain serious diseases and conditions
- have a history of loss of over 20% of body weight
- have a serum albumin level of less than 3.2 mg/dL
- hare placed on total or partial parenteral nutrition or external support.

The test also helps physicians diagnose specific problems with protein-energy malnutrition (PEM). In this condition, which according to recent studies can affect 30–50% of hospitalized patients, the body breaks down muscles, **proteins**, and body fats. This type of malnutrition, when not treated promptly, can lead to serious complications and death.

Proper nutrition before surgery helps to minimize complications such as pneumonia and infection after surgery. Numerous scientific studies have shown that malnutrition can lead to reduced quality of care in patients, higher mortality and morbidity, reduced wound healing, weakened mechanisms for fighting infections, and increased medical and pharmaceutical costs. Nutritional testing on incoming patients to hospitals can help to increase their quality of care. The prealbumin test is a proven and reliable way to test for nutrition.

Precautions

There are no precautions necessary before taking the prealbumin test.

Description

The PA test is a simple blood test. A health professional takes a blood draw with a needle from the patient's vein in the arm or wrist.

The test is given to measure levels of prealbumin. Prealbumin has a half-life of about 1.9 days, which means that the amount diminishes rapidly in the body. This short period helps doctors to quickly acquire a series of readings of a patient's nutrition with respect to the level of prealbumin in the blood. Physicians can monitor the patient much more effectively with the use of this test because they see results within two days, as opposed to 21 days (for example) with albumin, another nutritional marker. The PA test should be given two to three times per week. The results should be reviewed by the patient's physician and a dietitian.

Preparation

The patient should inform the health professional, before the test is performed, about any inflammation present in the body. Inflammation can cause the PA test

to be lower than normal. Drugs such as amiodarone, estrogen drugs, and oral contraceptives (birth control pills) can also produce lower-than-normal results. Hemodialysis patients generally receive inaccurate results.

Aftercare

There is no aftercare with the prealbumin test.

Complications

There are no complications expected with the prealbumin test.

Results

A normal reading for the prealbumin test indicates a normal state of nutrition for the patient. A normal range is from 177–40 mg/dL. The maximum value is usually no more than 60 mg/dL. If prealbumin is low, various proteins and other substances in the blood may be low. If the test indicates an extremely low reading, then the patient may be extremely malnourished, prompting immediate medical care. Abnormally low levels are strong indications of severe or chronic illnesses such as digestive disorders, hyperthyroidism, **liver** disease, or serious infections. Abnormally high readings from the PA test indicate patients with high-dose corticosteroid therapy, high-dose non-steroidal anti-inflammatory medications, Hodgkin's disease, or hyperactive **adrenal glands**.

The accuracy of the PA test is less affected (when compared with other testing methods) by changes in hydration of the patient, along with being less dependent on liver and renal function.

Health care team roles

A health professional will administer the blood draw on the patient. The patient's physician will advise the patient as to the results of the test and a dietician, if necessary, may recommend special dietary measures.

In a medical center or hospital, a nutritional support team should consist of one or more of the following professionals: laboratory technicians, dietitians, pharmacists, nurses, and physicians. This team should be on staff to determine and ensure the nutritional health of its patients.

Resources

BOOKS

Shannon, Joyce Brennfleck, editor. *Medical Tests Sourcebook: Basic Consumer Health Information about Medical Tests.* Detroit, MI: Omnigraphics, 1999.

Shtasel, Philip. *Medical Tests and Diagnostic Procedures: A Patient's Guide to Just What the Doctor Ordered.* New York: HarperPerennial, 1991.

OTHER

Lab Tests Online®, American Association for Clinical Chemistry. "Prealbumin." May 18, 2004. http://www.labtestsonline.org/understanding/analytes/prealbumin/test.html (December 5, 2005).

William Arthur Atkins

Preconception counseling

Definition

Preconception counseling is a form of **patient education** that helps a woman to make lifestyle changes before conception that will assist in promoting a healthy **pregnancy** and a healthy baby.

Although preconception counseling is important for women, it is beneficial for men as well, because there are many lifestyle issues, chronic illnesses, genetic disorders, and overall health concerns that affect men's fertility and their emotional readiness to be good fathers.

Purpose

Various health, lifestyle, and environmental factors can increase the rate of abnormalities, referred to as **birth defects**, seen in babies at birth. Examples of these abnormalities are such conditions as cleft palate/lip, congenital **heart** disease, or spina bifida (opening of the spine). Some abnormalities are hereditary. Birth defects

---

Obstetric history data

Pregnancies and births (term, preterm, abortions, living)
Date of each birth (month and year)
Outcome of each birth:
    Gestational age at birth
    Type of delivery
    Length of labor
    Birth weight
    Gender
    Complications during pregnancy, at delivery, postpartum
Any depression during the year after birth
Present health
Names and location of children
Feelings about previous pregnancies, birthing experiences, parenting
Feelings about any perinatal loss or other losses in which children were involved.

SOURCE: Wheeler, L. *Nurse-Midwifery Handbook: A Practical Guide to Prenatal and Postpartum Care.* Philadelphia: Lippincott-Raven Pub., 1997.

---

are known to occur in 3–6% of all newborns; they are the single largest cause of infant deaths in the United States as of 2012, accounting for 20% of all deaths during the first year of life.

Pregnancy can worsen some chronic maternal diseases, such as **hypertension** or diabetes, or increase the risk of poor neonatal outcome. In addition, alcohol, drugs of abuse, tobacco, and some prescription medications used by the pregnant woman may cause developmental problems in the fetus. Last, preconception counseling can lower the risk of an adverse outcome (**miscarriage**, stillbirth, or preterm delivery) in a future pregnancy in women who have had such an outcome in a previous pregnancy. In 2006 the Centers for Disease Control and Prevention (CDC) made a formal recommendation that all women who have had an adverse outcome in pregnancy receive preconception counseling before trying to conceive again.

Precautions

Not all women visit a health care provider during the critical early weeks of pregnancy. Thus, as a part of patient education, health care professionals should provide preconception counseling in all encounters with women of childbearing age.

Description

Preconception counseling should address the following areas:

Nutrition

DIET. The importance of a well-balanced and nutritious diet should be emphasized in preconception counseling. A woman who is underweight for her height or weighs less than 100 pounds when she conceives may have a small baby (small babies are more likely to have problems during labor and immediately after delivery). A woman who is overweight is at increased risk of developing elevated **blood pressure** and **gestational diabetes** during pregnancy. Women should be informed that trying to lose weight during pregnancy is not advised because it could rob a developing baby of essential nutrients. It is best to lose weight before trying to conceive.

FOLIC ACID SUPPLEMENTATION. Even though many grains and other products are fortified with **folic acid** (a B vitamin), the level may not be high enough to increase the folic acid intake of most childbearing-age women to the recommended level of 400 micrograms (mcg) per day. Therefore, most women of childbearing age should consume 400 mcg (0.4 milligrams, or mg) of folic acid per day. Women with a previous child with a **neural tube defect** and women on antiseizure medication need extra folic acid. Folic acid is thought to help prevent certain birth abnormalities, including spina bifida, other neural-tube defects, and possibly heart abnormalities. Folic acid may also reduce the likelihood of colon **cancer** and coronary heart disease.

Women taking methotrexate (MTX), a drug used to treat cancer, **rheumatoid arthritis**, and other autoimmune diseases, should ask their doctors about the safety of using it during pregnancy because it interferes with the **metabolism** of folic acid. Methotrexate is also used to treat ectopic pregnancies, and is known to cause birth defects in normal pregnancies misdiagnosed as ectopic.

MULTIVITAMIN SUPPLEMENTATION. To ensure an adequate daily intake of **vitamins** and **minerals**, women of reproductive age should take a multivitamin supplement that contains folic acid. Women planning on a pregnancy should be cautious to avoid an excess intake of **vitamin A**, however. It has been chemically associated with a class of retinoids recognized to cause birth abnormalities. Vitamin A doses larger than 10,000 international units (IU) have been linked to a nearly five-fold increase in the occurrence of congenital heart malformations.

OTHER DIETARY ISSUES. Women considering pregnancy should avoid eating fish that are high in mercury, such as shark, swordfish, king mackerel and tilefish. It is safe, however, to eat as much as 12 ounces per week of fish or seafood with low mercury content, such as shrimp, salmon, pollock, catfish, and canned light tuna.

It is also important to make sure that all meat, including beef and pork as well as poultry, is cooked thoroughly before eating. Undercooked meat may carry **parasites** that can cause birth defects.

Women diagnosed with or at risk of anemia may be advised to take an **iron** supplement in addition to multivitamins before attempting to conceive.

Immunizations

RUBELLA (GERMAN MEASLES). All women of childbearing age should be immunized against to rubella. Contracting rubella during pregnancy can result in numerous severe birth abnormalities, including deafness, heart defects, **cataracts**, and mental retardation. Conception is not recommended for at least three months after receiving an immunization for rubella, and the immunization may not be given during pregnancy.

VARICELLA (CHICKENPOX). A woman who has not had varicella should be immunized for it prior to conception. Varicella **infection** can result in serious maternal and fetal complications. For example, 9 percent of women who contract varicella in pregnancy will develop varicella **pneumonia**. The varicella immunization should not be given during pregnancy.

Risk reduction and lifestyle issues

Women contemplating pregnancy should be counseled concerning the following lifestyle behaviors and their potential implications. A woman may not even be aware that she is pregnant for the first few weeks and may engage in dangerous lifestyle behaviors during a critical period of embryonic development. If conception is a possibility, women should try to maintain a healthy lifestyle so that their babies will have the best odds of a good outcome at birth and later on in life. Another consideration is the spacing of pregnancies. As a general rule, it is best to space pregnancies at least 18 months apart. This time frame allows the mother's body to prepare physically for another pregnancy; it also reduces the risk of premature birth in the later pregnancy.

Preconception counseling should also address such matters as the emotional and financial issues related to pregnancy. Many young people are not prepared for the amount of time parenting requires, the changes it brings about in their relationship, and the effects it may have on their education and other future plans. In addition, many young people are surprised by the high expenses involved in having a baby.

Mental health

It is important for men as well as women contemplating pregnancy to be screened for depression, as undiagnosed and untreated depression can be worsened by pregnancy and delivery. In addition, women who are taking medications for **anxiety** (particularly

KEY TERMS

Abruptio placentae—Premature separation of the placenta from the uterine wall after 20 Weeks' gestation. It is an obstetrical emergency.

Folic acid—A water-soluble form of vitamin B_9, essential for the synthesis and repair of DNA. Adequate intake of folic acid before and during pregnancy protects against neural tube defects in the fetus, low birth weight in the infant, and preterm delivery.

Ectopic pregnancy—A complication of pregnancy in which the embryo implants in the fallopian tubes or abdomen outside the uterine cavity.

Gestational diabetes—A condition in which a woman without previously diagnosed diabetes develops high blood glucose levels during pregnancy, especially during the third trimester.

Perinatal—Refers to the period shortly before and after birth, generally from around the 20th week of pregnancy to one to four weeks after birth.

Perinatologist—A specialist in the branch of obstetrics that deals with the high-risk pregnant woman and her fetus. Perinatologists are also known as specialists in maternal-fetal medicine.

Placenta previa—Implantation of the placenta over or close to the internal opening of the cervix.

Preconceptional—Referring to the time period before pregnancy, i.e., conception, occurs.

Preeclampsia—A medical condition that occurs during pregnancy characterized by high blood pressure together with elevated levels of protein in the urine. Other symptoms of preeclampsia may include headaches, rapid weight gain, and swelling of the hands and feet.

Teratogen—Any agent that can cause malformation or disturbed development of an embryo or fetus. Teratogens may be biological or environmental.

diazepam), **bipolar disorder** (particularly lithium), or **seizure disorder** (particularly phenytoin and valproic acid) should consult their doctor before becoming pregnant, as these medications can be teratogenic.

ALCOHOL. Consumption of alcohol during pregnancy can lead to **fetal alcohol syndrome** (FAS), a condition resulting in several physical and behavioral problems in affected children. Even the intake of lower levels of alcohol can cause neurological and behavioral problems in children of women who drink during pregnancy. Studies have found that children of women who consumed alcohol during pregnancy had lower birth weights, were shorter, and had smaller head circumferences.

DRUGS. Infants of pregnant drug users are at risk for prematurity, low birth weight, and perinatal death. Women who abuse drugs should be offered support and referred to groups that can help with drug addiction.

TOBACCO. Women who smoke during pregnancy have an increased risk for abruptio placentae, **placenta previa**, and **preeclampsia**. Their babies may be born prematurely, be smaller, have congenital abnormalities, be at increased risk for sudden infant death syndrome (SIDS), and possibly have developmental delays.

Medical conditions and pregnancy

DIABETES MELLITUS. Women with **diabetes mellitus** should try to attain stability in their **blood** sugar levels prior to conception. Some oral medications for diabetes are contraindicated during pregnancy, so planning is necessary for conception. Complications of diabetes mellitus include large or small babies.

OTHER COMPLICATIONS. Women with medical conditions who are contemplating pregnancy should be counseled as to the risks of pregnancy for themselves and their babies. For example, a woman who has epilepsy should consult with her physician or nurse practitioner about the toxicity of the current medication she is taking to control seizures; a less toxic medication may be recommended for the period of preconception and pregnancy.

REDUCING EXPOSURE TO TERATOGENS. Exposure to various substances can be teratogenic (capable of causing birth defects). Teratogenic hazards include **anticancer drugs**, and such occupation-related teratogens as organic solvents, pesticides, radiation, and anesthetic gases.

Some teratogens can even cause birth defects when the exposure took place prior to conception. The father's exposure to occupational toxins can also contribute to miscarriages, preterm deliveries, and birth defects.

Genetic counseling

Couples may wish to have **genetic counseling** if there is a family history of a child with a genetic abnormality, because of ethnically associated genetic diseases, or for advanced maternal/paternal age (age 34 or 35 in women, 40 or older in men).

QUESTIONS TO ASK YOUR DOCTOR

- Do you offer preconception counseling?
- What factors in my medical history and lifestyle should I take into account before becoming pregnant?
- Should women who are not planning to become pregnant receive preconception counseling anyway?
- What are the benefits of preconception counseling for women? For men?

Other issues

Preconception counseling may include discussions of several other health-related issues:

- contraception
- domestic violence
- exercise
- gynecological screening
- HIV infection
- safe use of prescription and over-the-counter medications
- general health
- safe sex
- sibling concerns

Preparation

Insertion of a form in the patient's chart addressing issues related to preconception counseling can guide the health care provider in performing a thorough assessment and providing appropriate interventions.

Many physicians will also order blood and urine tests in order to check for the presence of anemia, infections, and abnormally high levels of protein in the woman's urine.

Results

Preconception counseling can result in healthier pregnancies, culminating in good birth outcomes.

Health care team roles

The opportunity to provide preconception counseling exists at any time a health care provider is assessing or educating a woman of childbearing age. Such providers include nurses, nurse practitioners, obstetricians, perinatologists (also known as specialists in maternal-fetal medicine), dietitians, **substance abuse** counselors, social workers, geneticists, radiologists, and **radiology** technicians. Health care professionals who are not trained to provide genetic counseling should be prepared to provide support related to **genetic testing**.

Resources

BOOKS

American Academy of Pediatrics and the American Congress of Obstetricians and Gynecologists. *Guidelines for Perinatal Care*, 7th ed. Elk Grove Village, IL: AAP, 2012.

Goodwin, T. Murphy, et al., eds. *Management of Common Problems in Obstetrics and Gynecology*, 5th ed. Hoboken, N.J.: Wiley-Blackwell, 2010.

Hawkins, Joellen W., Diane M. Roberto-Nichols, and J. Lynn Stanley-Haney.*Guidelines for Nurse Practitioners in Gynecologic Settings*, 10th ed. New York: Springer, 2012.

PERIODICALS

Finocchario-Kessler, S., et al. "Discussing Childbearing with HIV-infected Women of Reproductive Age in Clinical Care: A Comparison of Brazil and the US." *AIDS and Behavior* 16 (January 2012): 99–107.

Ford, J.H. "Preconception Risk Factors and SGA Babies: Papilloma Virus, Omega 3 and Fat Soluble Vitamin Deficiencies." *Early Human Development* 87 (December 2011): 785–789.

Hyoun, S.C., et al. "Teratogen Update: Methotrexate." *Birth Defects Research, Part A: Clinical and Molecular Teratology* 94 (April 2012): 187–207.

Kennedy, D., and G. Koren. "Identifying Women Who Might Benefit from Higher Doses of Folic Acid in Pregnancy." *Canadian Family Physician* 58 (April 2012): 394–397.

Lanik, A.D. "Preconception Counseling." *Primary Care* 39 (March 2012): 1–16.

Mathiesen, E.R., et al. "Pregnancy Management of Women with Pregestational Diabetes." *Endocrinology and Metabolism Clinics of North America* 40 (December 2011): 727–738.

Saravelos, S.H., and L. Regan. "The Importance of Preconception Counseling and Early Pregnancy Monitoring." *Seminars in Reproductive Medicine* 29 (November 2011): 557–568.

Shallcross, R., et al. "Prenatal Exposure to Anti-epileptic Drugs: The Need for Preconception Counselling." *Practising Midwife* 14 (December 2011): 20–21.

Squires, K.E., et al. "Health Needs of HIV-infected Women in the United States: Insights from the Women Living Positive Survey." *AIDS Patient Care and STDs* 25 (May 2011): 279–285.

Wade, G.H., et al. "A Preconception Care Program for Women in a College Setting." *American Journal of Maternal-Child Nursing* 37 (May 2012): 164–170.

WEBSITES

American Congress of Obstetricians and Gynecologists (ACOG). "FAQs: Good Health before Pregnancy:

Preconception Care." http://www.acog.org/~/media/For% 20Patients/faq056.pdf (accessed May 19, 2012).

Centers for Disease Control and Prevention (CDC). Preconception Health and Health Care Home Page. http://www.cdc.gov/preconception/index.html (accessed May 19, 2012).

Centers for Disease Control and Prevention (CDC). Preconception Information for Men. http://www.cdc.gov/preconception/men.html (accessed May 19, 2012).

March of Dimes. "Preconception Health Care." URL HERE (accessed)

Merck Manual for Health Care Professionals. "Prenatal Genetic Counseling." http://www.merckmanuals.com/professional/gynecology_and_obstetrics/prenatal_genetic_counseling_and_evaluation/prenatal_genetic_counseling.html (accessed May 19, 2012).

National Institute of Child Health and Human Development (NICHD). "Preconception Care." http://www.nichd.nih.gov/health/topics/preconception_care.cfm (accessed May 19, 2012).

ORGANIZATIONS

American Congress of Obstetricians and Gynecologists (ACOG), P.O. Box 70620, Washington, DC United States 20024-9998, (202) 638-5577, (800) 673-8444, http://www.acog.org/

Association of Women's Health, Obstetric and Neonatal Nurses (AWHONN), 2000 L Street, NW, Suite 740, Washington, DC United States 20036, (202) 261-2400, Fax: (202) 728-0575, (800) 673-8499, http://www.awhonn.org/awhonn/

National Institute of Child Health and Human Development (NICHD)., P.O. Box 3006, Rockville, MD United States 20847, Fax: (866) 760-5947, (800) 370-2943, NICHDInformationResourceCenter@mail.nih.gov, http://www.nichd.nih.gov/

Society for Maternal-Fetal Medicine (SMFM), 409 12th Street, SW, Washington, DC United States 20024, (202) 863-2476, Fax: (202) 554-1132, smfm@smfm.org, https://www.smfm.org/Default.cfm,

Nadine M. Jacobson, R.N.
Rebecca J. Frey, Ph.D.

Prednisone *see* **Corticosteroids**

Preeclampsia and eclampsia

Definition

Preeclampsia and eclampsia are hypertensive disorders of **pregnancy** that occur in 2–6% of pregnancies in the United States with higher rates (up to 18%) reported in developing countries. In developing countries, hypertensive disorders of pregnancy are the single most common cause of death in **childbirth**. Preeclampsia is defined by the presence of three elements: **hypertension**, proteinuria (protein in the urine), and **edema** (fluid retention). If seizures develop following the appearance of the first three factors, the condition is called eclampsia. Untreated preeclampsia progresses to eclampsia in about 1 of 200 cases.

Description

The cause of preeclampsia is unknown, but is thought to be an immunologic disorder possibly related to intolerance to certain fetal or placental **proteins**. Preeclampsia is more likely to develop in primigravidas (women in their first pregnancy); Other risk factors include a family history of preeclampsia; age extremes in the mother (younger than 20 years or older than 40); pre-existing kidney disease or hypertension; diabetes; **multiple pregnancy**; five or more previous pregnancies; African American descent; **obesity**; pre-existing autoimmune disease, **sickle cell disease** or polycystic ovary disease; conception through in vitro fertilization, and genetic abnormalities in the fetus.

Hypertensive disorders of pregnancy affect six major systems or sites in the body: the **central nervous system** (CNS), **kidneys**, **liver**, the **blood**, the **blood vessels**, and the fetus and placenta. In severe cases, the mother may suffer liver failure, rupture of the liver, or pulmonary edema (fluid in the **lungs**); the fetus may die. About one-quarter of cases of preeclampsia are considered severe.

Classification of hypertensive disorders of pregnancy

The most common classification used to define hypertensive disorders of pregnancy is the one recommended by the American College of Obstetricians and Gynecologists (ACOG) and endorsed by the NIH Working Group on High **Blood Pressure**:

• Chronic hypertension, defined as blood pressure greater than or equal to 140 mm Hg systolic or 90 mm Hg diastolic present prior to pregnancy or before the 20th week of pregnancy. During pregnancy, the hypertension remains, but proteinuria does not occur. Women who develop hypertension during pregnancy, without proteinuria or seizures, and whose blood pressure remains elevated after pregnancy are also diagnosed with chronic hypertension.

• Gestational hypertension, defined as elevated blood pressure greater than or equal to 140 mm Hg systolic or 90 mm Hg diastolic that arises after midpregnancy with no proteinuria. Blood pressure returns to normal by 12 weeks postpartum. Final diagnosis of this condition is delayed until the postpartum period. If the patient does not develop preeclampsia, and her blood pressure returns to normal, the final diagnosis is transient hypertension of pregnancy. If her blood pressure remains elevated, a diagnosis of chronic hypertension is given.

• Preeclampsia and eclampsia. Preeclampsia is characterized by blood pressure greater than or equal to 140 mm Hg systolic or 90 mm Hg diastolic occurring after midpregnancy (20 weeks gestation), and accompanied by proteinuria. Preeclampsia may be further categorized as mild or severe. A woman is considered to have severe preeclampsia when her blood pressure reading is 160+ mm Hg systolic or 110+ mm Hg diastolic; her proteinuria is equal to or greater than 5 mg of protein in the urine per 24 hours; or other organ systems are involved. She may have headache, visual disturbances, or other CNS symptoms; pulmonary edema, cyanosis, or other cardiovascular symptoms; and abdominal pain.

• Preeclampsia superimposed on chronic hypertension. Pregnant women with preexisting chronic hypertension may develop preeclampsia. Superimposed preeclampsia is suspected when proteinuria develops or increases suddenly, when previously controlled hypertension exhibits a sudden increase, or when the patient develops thrombocytopenia or elevated liver enzyme levels. Women with preeclampsia superimposed on chronic hypertension have a poorer prognosis than women with either condition alone.

Measurement of blood pressure

For purposes of accuracy and standardization, health professionals should take blood pressure measurements in pregnant women with the patient seated rather than lying on her side, because substantial differences exist between the blood pressures in the upper and lower arms when the patient is lying on her side. In addition, the National Institutes of Health (NIH) recommends that the diastolic pressure reading should be taken at Korotkoff 5, with the disappearance of sound—not at Korotkoff 4, when sound becomes muffled. To meet strict criteria for hypertension, the patient's readings must be elevated on at least two separate occasions at least six hours apart.

Causes and symptoms

As previously mentioned, the initial cause of preeclampsia/eclampsia is not known but is thought to be immunologic. The relationship among the three factors that define preeclampsia appears to be as follows. First, the normal increase in blood plasma volume and decrease in peripheral vascular resistance that occur

during an uncomplicated pregnancy are absent. The patient's blood vessels allow fluid to leak from the vessels into the surrounding tissue, which results in edema. The seizures that characterize eclampsia result from edema of the **brain**. The patient's kidneys are under stress because of diminished blood flow through the kidneys and decreased filtration. This process allows protein molecules to spill over into the urine. Damage to the kidneys lowers urine output and increases the levels of sodium in body tissues. Higher concentrations of sodium result in increased fluid retention. Protein lost through the urine also affects the movement of fluid into the tissues, further increasing fluid retention.

Symptoms of preeclampsia usually occur after week 20 of pregnancy. The patient may complain of:

• edema (swelling) of the hands and feet

• sudden weight gain

• headache

• nausea and vomiting

• abdominal pain

• shoulder pain

• changes in vision

The HELLP syndrome

A liver condition related to hypertension in pregnancy is called the HELLP syndrome. HELLP stands for *h*emolysis, *e*levated *l*iver enzymes, and *l*ow *p*latelet count. Normal liver functioning is altered in the HELLP syndrome as a result of vascular damage related to preeclampsia. Researchers believe that the fetus and mother share a defect in processing fatty acids that leads to destruction of red blood cells, inflammation of the liver, and decreased platelet count. HELLP syndrome is associated with disseminated intravascular coagulation (DIC), **placental abruption** (sudden tearing), acute renal failure, and pulmonary edema. About 30% of pregnancy-related cases of HELLP develop in the postpartum period.

Disseminated intravascular coagulation

Preeclampsia and eclampsia may also be associated with the serious condition known as disseminated intravascular coagulation, or DIC. DIC is a disorder characterized by both bleeding and thrombosis (the formation of intravascular clots). Maternal hemorrhage is a risk in patients with preeclampsia who develop DIC. About 15% of hypertension-related deaths in pregnancy are associated with DIC.

Diagnosis

The diagnosis of preeclampsia is complicated by the fact that the signs of hypertension in pregnancy can be easily confused with the symptoms of chronic hypertension, **gallbladder** and pancreatic diseases, and other disorders. Since prevention of maternal and fetal morbidity and mortality is of the utmost priority, however, the NIH recommends overdiagnosis of preeclampsia rather than underdiagnosis to ensure careful management. Pregnant women should have their weight, blood pressure, and urine checked at every prenatal visit. Regular prenatal visits are extremely important, as the early symptoms of preeclampsia cause no discomfort. The NIH guidelines suggest that women who develop an increase of 30 mmHg systolic or 15 mmHg diastolic over their prenatal baseline measurements should be closely monitored, especially if their protein or uric acid levels are elevated. Early detection of preeclampsia allows for proper management of the condition.

Treatment

Pre-delivery management

Delivery is the definitive treatment of preeclampsia. Even mild preeclampsia that develops at 36 weeks of gestation or later is managed by delivery. Prior to 36 weeks, severe preeclampsia requires delivery of the fetus. Mild to moderate preeclampsia between 20 and 36 weeks is treated with bed rest. Rest increases central blood flow to the patient's **heart**, kidneys, placenta, and other organs. Bed rest at home is an option for some patients with mild preeclampsia and stable home situations. Patients with severe eclampsia or unstable family situations require hospitalization. Monitoring of fetal heart rate and lung maturity is an important part of the management of preeclampsia.

Medications

Medication for preeclampsia is usually directed toward preventing convulsions rather than controlling blood pressure. **Magnesium** sulfate is the drug of choice for controlling seizures during pregnancy. Prophylactic magnesium sulfate administration may continue into the postpartum period.

Emergency care

The primary concern in emergency treatment of convulsions is to assure the patient's safety. The patient is placed on her side to allow any secretions in the mouth to drain, thus decreasing the risk of aspiration. In addition, this position improves blood flow to the

---

KEY TERMS

Cyanosis—A bluish color to the skin that indicates poor circulation and poor oxygenation of the blood and tissues.

Disseminated intravascular coagulation (DIC)—A disorder of blood coagulation characterized by both bleeding and thrombosis (intravascular clotting).

Edema—Abnormal accumulation of fluid in the tissues, cavities, or joint capsules of the body. It is one of three important indications of preeclampsia.

HELLP—A syndrome related to liver dysfunction that develops in some patients with preeclampsia. The letters stand for Hemolysis, Elevated Liver enzyme levels, and Low Platelet count.

Placental abruption—Sudden rupture or tearing of the placenta. The convulsions that characterize eclampsia increase the risk of placental abruption.

Proteinuria—A significant amount of protein in the urine. It is also sometimes called albuminuria.

Thrombocytopenia—A blood platelet count below 100,000 cells/mm^3.

---

placenta and fetus. Delivery of the fetus usually follows as soon as possible after the convulsion to minimize the risk of placental abruption.

Vaginal delivery is preferred to caesarean delivery in order to avoid the additional stress of surgery on the patient's organ systems. The NIH recommends a trial of labor induction, regardless of the condition of the patient's cervix. Magnesium sulfate may be given as an anticonvulsant. Antihypertensive medication is restricted to use for sudden elevations of blood pressure, or if the patient's diastolic pressure reaches 105 to 110 mm Hg.

Prognosis

Risks to the fetus from preeclampsia include intrauterine growth retardation and low birth weight, placental abruption, and stillbirth. The fetus may be delivered prematurely if the condition of the mother deteriorates. Preeclampsia risks to the mother include vascular organ damage. Additional risks of eclampsia include convulsions and accompanying oxygen deprivation, hemorrhage in the brain, temporary blindness, permanent neurological damage, liver or kidney damage, cerebrovascular and cardiovascular complications, and even death. The prognoses for both the fetus and mother increased diuresis. Magnesium sulfate may be given to lessen the risk of convulsions.

QUESTIONS TO ASK YOUR DOCTOR

1. I already have high blood pressure. How will that affect the likelihood that I will develop preeclampsia?

2. How severe is my preeclampsia?

3. Why must I have complete bed rest? What if I am not in a family situation where this is possible?

4. What signs would indicate that my mild preeclampsia is worsening?

5. Is my preeclampsia severe enough to warrant delivery of my baby this early in pregnancy?

6. I had mild preeclampsia in my first pregnancy? Am I likely to have preeclampsia with a second pregnancy and is it likely to be the same or more severe?

Resources

BOOK

Lyall, Fiona and Michael Belfort. *Pre-eclampsia: etiology and Clinical Practice,* re-issue edition New York: Cambridge University Press, 2010.

OTHER

About Preeclampsia. Preeclampsia Foundation 2012 [accessed April 15, 2012]. http://www.preeclampsia.org/health-information/about-preeclampsia

Lim, Kee-Hak. Preeclampsia. Medscape Reference November 10, 2011 [accessed April 15, 2012]. http://emedicine.medscape.com/article/1476919-overview

Preeclampsia and Eclampsia. WebMD March7, 2010 [accessed April 15, 2012]. http://www.webmd.com/baby/guide/preeclampsia-eclampsia

Ross, Michael G. Eclampsia. Medscape Reference November 15, 2011 [accessed April 15, 2012]. http://emedicine.medscape.com/article/253960-overview

ORGANIZATIONS

American College of Obstetricians and Gynecologists, P.O. Box 70620, Washington, DC 20024-9998, (800) 673-8444, (202)638-5577, http://www.acog.org

Association of Women's Health, Obstetric, and Neonatal Nurses, 2000 L St., NW, Suite. 740, Washington, DC (202) 261-2400, (800) 673-8499. Toll free in Canada (800) 245-0231, Fax: (202) 728-0575, customerservice@awhonn.org, http://www.awhonn.org

Preeclampsia Foundation, 6767 N Wickham Road, Suite 400, Melbourne, FL 32940, (321) 421-6957, (800) 665-9341, Fax: (321) 821-0450, info@preeclampsia.org, http://www.preeclampsia.org.

Esther Csapo Rastegari, R.N., B.S.N., Ed.M.
Tish Davidson, AM

Pregnancy-induced hypertension *see* **Preeclampsia and eclampsia**

are excellent in mild preeclampsia (about 75% of cases). If blood pressure readings are within normal limits after several weeks postpartum, the mother may still be at increased risk of hypertension later in life, and should have her blood pressure checked yearly.

The long-term prognosis for children weighing born to preeclamptic mothers weighing is unclear. These individuals do, however, appear to be at increased risk of chronic disease in adult life.

Health care team roles

The responsibilities of nursing staff in the management of preeclampsia and eclampsia include **patient education** and monitoring of patient compliance with the physician's instructions as well as assisting with emergency care. Patients resting at home should be visited and assessed periodically by a home health nurse. These functions are essential to good management of high-risk patients. Providing emotional support to patients with complications during pregnancy is also a critical function. If the patient requires hospitalization, a calm and quiet environment can help decrease the risk of seizure.

Prevention

Since the cause of preeclampsia is unclear, prevention focuses on early detection and management to avoid progression. Bed rest improves blood flow to the placenta and to maternal organs. Lying on the side increases sodium excretion and decreases fluid retention through

Pregnancy

Definition

Pregnancy is the condition of having a developing embryo or fetus in the body. The union of an egg (ovum) with sperm is called fertilization, or conception, and it is this union that produces the embryo. Pregnancy includes the period from conception to birth of the fetus, and usually lasts 10 lunar months (40 weeks/280 days), or nine calendar months as measured from the first day of the last menstrual period (LMP). It is also referred to as a

FDA categories for drugs during pregnancy

Category A   Adequate and well-controlled (AWC) studies in pregnant women have failed to demonstrate a risk to the fetus in the first trimester of pregnancy (and there is no evidence of a risk in later trimesters).

Category B   Animal reproduction studies have failed to demonstrate a risk to the fetus and there are no AWC studies in humans, AND the benefits from the use of the drug in pregnant women may be acceptable despite its potential risks. OR animal studies have not been conducted and there are no AWC studies in humans.

Category C   Animal reproduction studies have shown an adverse effect on the fetus, there are no AWC studies in humans, AND the benefits from the use of the drug in pregnant women may be acceptable despite its potential risks. OR animal studies have not been conducted and there are no AWC in humans.

Category D   There is positive evidence of human fetal risk based on adverse reaction data from investigational or marketing experience or studies in humans, BUT the potential benefits from the use of the drug in pregnant women may be acceptable despite its potential risks (for example, if the drug is needed in a life-threatening situation or serious disease for which safer drugs cannot be used or are ineffective).

Category X   Studies in animals or humans have demonstrated fetal abnormalities OR there is positive evidence of fetal risk based on adverse reaction reports from investigational or marketing experience, or both, AND the risk of the use of the drug in a pregnant woman clearly outweighs any possible benefit (for example, safer drugs or other forms of therapy are available).

SOURCE: U.S. Food and Drug Administration.

gestation period that consists of three trimesters. The trimesters are not equal, but are defined by different stages of a baby's development. The first trimester includes the first 13 weeks of pregnancy. The second trimester consists of weeks 14–26, and the third trimester is weeks 27–40.

Description

At the time of sexual intercourse, a man ejects millions of sperm into the woman's vagina. The sperm travel in all directions, propelled by their whiplike tails, and many swim through the cervix toward the uterus. A very small number of them may survive as long as 48 hours, but only one has to make it to the fallopian tube to meet the egg that has been released from an ovary. It takes approximately 30 minutes following intercourse for the sperm to meet the egg. One sperm penetrates the egg and its tail is shed, while the remainder of the sperm provides one-half of the genetic material of the future fetus—the other half provided by the egg. The fertilized egg then travels along the fallopian tube, arriving in the uterus four to five days later. Fluid secreted by the tube lining provides it with **nutrition** during its travels. After

two to three days in the uterine cavity, the fertilized egg implants into the thick lining of the uterus. Implantation occurs at about day 22 of a normal menstrual cycle. If the fertilized egg were visible to the naked eye, it would appear to be covered with fine hairs, called villi. These villi become the densest where the **blood** supply is richest, and eventually form the placenta. The mother's blood moves slowly around these villi, permitting them to absorb food and oxygen, and to eliminate waste products. The placenta is completely formed and functioning by 10 weeks after fertilization. Between 12 and 20 weeks gestation, the placenta weighs more than the fetus, because the fetal organs are not sufficiently developed to deal with the processes needed for nutrition.

First month

At week four of pregnancy, the embryo is about one-eighth of an inch (0.275 cm) long, and weighs about 1/32 of an ounce (3 g). A formed yolk sac is present.

Second month

During the next four weeks, the embryo will grow to be about one inch long (2.5 cm) and weigh about 5/16 of an ounce (8.7 g). The umbilical cord will form, and the pulsation of the **heart** can be noted. The head and tail of the embryo are formed, and sex glands are determined, although the external genitals cannot be visibly identified as male or female. Limbs are well formed, and toes and fingers are present. The development of a skeleton and the formation of **bone** cells begin. Facial features begin to form, as does the external portion of the ear. The eyelids are fused throughout this period. By this stage, the fetus has a distinctly human appearance, and the beginnings of all the main organ systems are established. Since the structures of the **brain**, heart, **liver**, limbs, ears, nose, and eyes develop by the end of eight weeks, this is considered the most critical period of development. Any exposure to medications, alcohol, or illicit drugs during this time may cause defects, or anomalies, in the fetus.

Third month

Approximately nine weeks after conception, the baby has developed the features of a human being, and is called a fetus, not an embryo. Limb movements first occur at the end of the embryo stage, although they are not coordinated and cannot be felt. At 12 weeks of pregnancy, the fetus is 1–3 inches (7.5 cm) long from head to heel, and weighs about one ounce (28 g). The formation of red blood cells has already occurred in the liver, but now the spleen takes over making them. Urine formation begins between the ninth and twelfth weeks, and is discharged into the amniotic fluid. The fetus can reabsorb some of this fluid after swallowing it. Waste products are now transferred to the mother's circulatory system by crossing the placenta.

Fourth month

Growth is very rapid during this period, and limb movements become coordinated, although it is difficult for the mother to feel them. An ultrasound reveals the bones of the fetal skeleton, which are clearly visible. Their development continues as the limbs lengthen. Scalp hair patterning is also determined during this period, and slow eye movements can occur at about 14 weeks. External genitals can be recognized by 14 weeks, and the external ears stand out from the head. The fetus is now about 6 inches (15 cm) long and weighs about 4 ounces (112 g).

Fifth month

"Quickening" is the mother's feeling the baby move for the first time; it usually occurs during this period. The average time between a mother's first detection of fetal movements and delivery is 147 days, with a deviation between plus or minus 15 days. The baby's skin is now covered with a greasy, cheese-like material called "vernix caseosa," and it protects the delicate fetal skin from cuts, chapping, and hardening, all of which could occur from exposure to the amniotic fluid. Eyebrows and head hair are also visible at 20 weeks, and the fetus is usually completely covered with fine, downy hair (the lanugo), which helps to hold the vernix on the skin. Brown fat forms during this period to prepare for heat production when the baby is born. By 18 weeks, a female fetus has a formed uterus, and the opening for the vagina has begun. Many egg-forming follicles are also forming in the ovaries. By 20 weeks in a male fetus, the testes have begun to descend, but they are still located inside the abdominal wall. The fetus now weighs about one pound (454 g) and is 10 inches (25 cm) long.

Sixth month

There is a substantial weight gain this month. The skin, usually wrinkled, appears clear, and is pink to red because blood is visible in the capillaries. At 21 weeks, rapid eye movements (REMs) begin, and blink-startle responses are visible on ultrasound following a loud noise. Fingernails are present by 24 weeks, and the cells in the lung have begun to secrete a substance necessary to develop the alveoli of the **lungs**. In most medical practices, a fetus born before 24 weeks is not considered viable or capable of living, but if born at 24 weeks,

attempts will be made for survival. The chances of a good outcome are, however, very poor. The fetus now weighs about 1.5 pounds (730 g), and is about 13 inches (32 cm) long.

Seventh month

By 26 weeks, the eyes are partially open and eyelashes are present. At 28 weeks, the eyes are wide open and a good head of hair is often present. At this age, a fetus can often survive even if born prematurely, presuming it is given intensive care. The lungs and **blood circulation** are developed, and can provide a better exchange of oxygen. Also, the **central nervous system** is now more mature, and can manage rhythmic breathing movements as well as assist in controlling body temperature. Toenails are present and more fat is deposited, smoothing the wrinkly skin. At 28 weeks, the bone marrow takes over the red blood cell-making work of the spleen, becoming the major site of this process. At 30 weeks, a light reflex of the eyes can be obtained. The skin is pink and smooth, and the limbs have a chubby appearance. The fetus might weigh as much as 3 lbs (1.3 kg), and is about 14–15 inches (35-37.5 cm) long. The fetus can be observed on ultrasound; it is sucking its thumb and practicing breathing movements. The mother may experience hiccups as rhythmic movements when the baby is practicing its breathing.

Eighth month

Fetuses 32 weeks and older usually survive if born prematurely. At 32 weeks, the fingernails reach the fingertips. At 35 weeks, fetuses have a firm grasp and show a spontaneous orientation to light. Growth continues, but slows as the baby begins to take up most of the room in the uterus. Now weighing between 3.5–4.5 lbs (1.7–2.3 kg), and measuring 16–18 inches (40–45 cm) long, the fetus may prepare for delivery by moving into the head-down position.

Ninth month

At 36 weeks, the body appears plump. The hair covering the body is almost gone. Toenails reach toe tips and the limbs are flexed. A full-term baby is one born anywhere from 37–40 weeks gestation. A baby born before 37 weeks is considered premature. Between 1990 and 2006 the rate of premature births in the United States increased by more than 20% with more than 10% of babies born prematurely in the late 2000s. A baby born after 41 weeks is considered postdate. Adding 0.5 lb (227 g) a week as the due date approaches, the fetus drops lower into the mother's **abdomen** and prepares for the onset of labor, which may begin any time between the

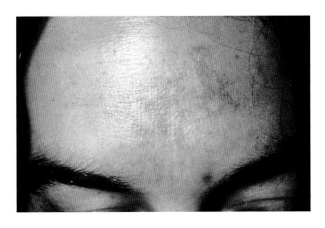

(Forehead of pregnant women with chloasma. NMSB/CMSP)

37th and 41st week of gestation. The expected date of delivery (EDD) of a fetus is 266 days, or 38 weeks after fertilization (i.e., 280 days or 40 weeks after the LMP). Prolongation of pregnancy occurs in 5–6% of women. If the pregnancy continues past 41–42 weeks, the physician will order fetal monitoring to determine the status of the baby. Since the mortality rate increases significantly after two to three weeks postdate, labor is often induced. Most healthy babies will weigh 6–8 lbs (2.7–3.6 kg) at birth, and will be about 19–21 inches (47-52 cm) long.

Causes and symptoms

The first sign of pregnancy is usually a missed menstrual period. A little bleeding or spotting may occur, due to implantation of the fertilized egg. Some women experience no early symptoms of pregnancy during the first few weeks, while others may experience all of them. A woman's breasts usually seem larger and feel tender as the mammary glands prepare for eventual breastfeeding. Nipples begin to enlarge and the veins over the surface of the breasts become more noticeable. Morning sickness (i.e., nausea and **vomiting**) is somewhat common, and can happen at any time—day or night. Extreme sensitivity to **smell** may worsen nausea. It is normal to feel bloated and more tired than usual. Frequent urination is common, and the pregnant woman may find herself getting up during the night to urinate. There may be a creamy white discharge from the vagina; that is normal. Food cravings may occur. Most women gain about 2–4 pounds (0.7–1.8 kg) by the end of the first trimester (0–13 weeks), and their clothes begin to feel tight.

In the second trimester (14–26 weeks), morning sickness usually ends and a woman's appetite may increase. There is a weight gain of about 12–15 pounds (5.4–6.75 kg) during this trimester. Most women begin to look pregnant and feel more energetic. Heart rate increases, as does the volume of blood in the body. This may cause a woman to feel flushed and warm at times. Some women experience constipation, **heartburn** and indigestion, backache, sleeplessness, or swollen feet during the second trimester. Physical activity, such as swimming and walking, will help constipation as well as drinking plenty of fluids (i.e., at least eight glasses of water a day) and eating high-fiber foods (i.e., fruits, vegetables, and whole grains). For backaches, it is important to maintain good posture, avoid lifting very heavy objects, and wear low-heeled shoes. Eating smaller amounts of food more frequently and avoiding fried or spicy foods will help to relieve heartburn or indigestion. When the woman sits down to rest, her feet should be elevated to prevent swelling of the ankles. Pregnant women should try not to stand for long periods of time.

By the third trimester (27–40 weeks), many women begin to experience a range of common symptoms. As the baby grows larger and begins to press against internal organs, a woman may feel somewhat breathless at times. Lying on her left or right side, not on her back, and using pillows to lean on in a semi-propped position can relieve this. Leaking of urine may occur with coughing or sneezing, and frequent urination begins again. As the pelvis widens and the joints become looser, discomfort may be felt in the pelvic joints. Some women feel as if their legs cannot support their weight. This is the body's way of preparing for birth. The joints are loosening so that the baby can fit through the pelvis. Stretch marks may develop on the abdomen, breasts, and thighs, and a dark line may appear from the navel to the pubic hair. A thin fluid called "colostrum" may be expressed from the nipples. **Hemorrhoids** may develop. Gums may become sensitive and bleed more easily, and eyes may dry out, making **contact lenses** uncomfortable to wear. Pica (a craving to eat substances other than food) may occur. **Varicose veins** may be a problem in the second half of pregnancy. This can be alleviated to a certain degree by wearing support hose, not standing for long periods of time, and resting with the feet up. Chloasma (a brown pigment) may appear on the face. This is due to the hormones of pregnancy and will disappear some time after delivery. Weak, irregular, painless tightenings of the uterus become more intense as the body practices for labor. These are called Braxton-Hicks contractions, and feel as if the baby is balling up. In most women, genuine labor consists of regular contractions that increase in intensity. Kicks from an active baby may cause sharp pains, and lower backaches are common. It is important for women in the third trimester to rest often and avoid straining themselves. When resting or sleeping, it may be more comfortable to lie on the left or right side with one leg bent, placing pillows under the **stomach** and between the knees. Weight gain will continue as it did in the second trimester.

In a woman's first pregnancy (later in repeat pregnancies), the baby's head drops down low into the pelvis by the last four weeks. This may relieve pressure on the upper abdomen and the lungs, allowing a woman to breathe more easily. This new position, however, does place more pressure on the bladder.

Total weight gain recommended in pregnancy is 25–35 pounds (12-16 kg) for women of normal weight for their height. Underweight women should possibly gain up to 40 pounds (18 kg), and overweight women should limit weight gain to 15–25 pounds (7–11 kg). Increased fluid volume makes up 2–3 pounds (0.9–1.4 kg); breast enlargement provides 1–2 pounds (0.45–0.9 kg); 2 pounds (0.9 kg) comes from enlargement of the uterus; and amniotic fluid is about 2 pounds (0.9 kg). At term, an infant weighs about 6–8 pounds (2.7–3.6 kg), and the placenta weights 1–2 pounds (0.45–0.9 kg). Usually 4–6 pounds (1.8ndash;2.7 kg) are due to maternal stores of fat and protein that are important for breastfeeding.

While many of the symptoms mentioned are considered normal, there are others that may indicate the presence of complications. A pregnant woman experiencing any of the following should contact her doctor or midwife *immediately*:

• abdominal pain
• rupture of the amniotic sac or fluid leaking from the vagina
• bleeding from the vagina
• no fetal movement for 24 hours (after the sixth month)
• continuous headaches
• marked, sudden swelling of eyelids, hands, or face
• dim or blurry vision
• persistent heartburn (unrelieved by antacids) or a burning sensation in the chest area
• persistent vomiting

Diagnosis

Many women discover they are pregnant after a positive home **pregnancy test**. Urine tests check for the presence of human chorionic gonadotropin (hCG), which is produced by the placenta. The newest home tests can detect pregnancy six to nine days after a missed menstrual period—sometimes earlier. The manufacturers of these tests claim an accuracy rate of 96–99%; but some factors, such as taking medications, sunlight, heat, and medical conditions can affect the test. A negative result followed by no menstrual period within a week

indicates the need to repeat the pregnancy test. While home tests are very accurate, they are less accurate than a pregnancy test performed in a lab. For this reason, women may want to consider having a second test at their doctor's or midwife's office to verify the accuracy of the result.

Blood tests to determine pregnancy are generally used when a very early diagnosis of pregnancy is needed. This more expensive test, which also looks for hCG, can produce a result within nine to 12 days after conception.

Approximately 1 in 33 live-born infants have a birth defect. There are tests that can be performed to determine many of these. As of 2012, there was a prenatal diagnostic screening test for determining the risk of neural tube defects, abdominal wall defects, **Down syndrome**, and trisomy 18. The triple-marker screening test measures levels of alpha fetoprotein (AFP), human chorionic gonadotropin (hCG), and unconjugated estriol. AFP is a protein produced in the fetal yolk sac during the first trimester and later by the fetal liver. Abnormally high levels of this protein are associated with severe neural tube defects. Human chorionic gonadotropin (hCG) is a hormone produced and secreted by the placenta. During early normal pregnancy, the level of this hormone rises rapidly, then begins to decline between the 10th and 20th week of gestation. High levels of hCG during the second trimester are associated with Down syndrome. Unconjugated estriol is produced by the placenta, the fetal **adrenal glands**, and the liver. It rises as normal pregnancy progresses, and its values are often lower with Down syndrome. A woman must have her blood sample drawn between the 15th and 20th week of gestation in order for this test to be accurate.

Other tests are recommended for women who are at higher risk for having a child with a birth defect. This includes women who have previously given birth to a child with a defect, or who have a family history of **birth defects**; women who have been exposed to certain drugs or high levels of radiation; and women 35 years of age or older. The presence of any of these risk factors warrants not only **genetic counseling**, but consideration of an ultrasound by a specialist, chorionic villi sampling (CVS), and/or **amniocentesis**.

First prenatal visit

During a woman's first prenatal visit, the following diagnostic tests are usually performed:

• complete blood count (CBC), for anemia
• blood type, Rh, and antibody screen
• syphilis (VDRL)

KEY TERMS

Alpha-fetoprotein—A substance produced by a fetus's liver that can be found in the amniotic fluid and in the mother's blood. Abnormally high levels of this substance suggests there may be defects in the fetal neural tube, a structure that will include the brain and spinal cord when completely developed. Abnormally low levels suggest the possibility of Down syndrome.

Alveolus/Alveoli—A little hollow space in the thin-walled chambers of the lungs which is surrounded by capillaries for the exchange of carbon dioxide and oxygen.

Amniotic fluid—The fluid or 'bag of waters' that the fetus floats in and maintains a constant body temperature. It is normally clear.

Anomaly—A marked deviation from normal.

Braxton-Hicks contractions—Short, fairly painless uterine contractions during pregnancy that may be mistaken for labor pains. They allow the uterus to grow and help circulate blood through the uterine blood vessels.

Cervix—The narrow lower end of the uterus.

Chloasma—A skin discoloration common during pregnancy, also known as the "mask of pregnancy." The blotches may appear on the forehead, cheeks, and nose, and may merge into one dark mask. Chloasma usually fades after pregnancy, but it may become permanent or recur with subsequent pregnancies.

Diffusion—The process of being widely spread.

Embryo—An unborn child during the first nine weeks of development following conception (fertilization with sperm). For the rest of pregnancy, the embryo is known as a fetus.

Fallopian tube—Either of two slender tubes, one on each side of the uterus, where fertilization takes place.

Fetus—An unborn child from the end of the ninth week after fertilization until birth.

Gestation—The period of development of an embryo and fetus or the duration of a pregnancy in a human.

Human chorionic gonadotropin (hCG)—A hormone produced by the placenta during pregnancy.

Osmosis—The diffusion of a substance across a membrane.

Placenta—The organ that develops in the uterus during pregnancy that links the blood supplies of the mother and baby.

Rhythm method—The oldest method of contraception, with a very high failure rate, in which partners periodically refrain from having sex during ovulation. Ovulation is predicted on the basis of a woman's previous menstrual cycle.

Uterus—The hollow muscular organ in females in which the fertilized egg becomes embedded and develops into an embryo and then a fetus.

Villus/Villi—A small protrusion or projection from the surface of a membrane.

• rubella titer (German measles)

• hepatitis B virus (HBV)

• urinalysis and culture

• Pap smear

• cervical cultures for gonorrhea and chlamydia

• recommendation of HIV antibody test, with counseling

A screening test for **gestational diabetes** is performed between 24 and 28 weeks gestation by giving the woman a 50 g glucose drink, then drawing a blood sample one hour later to check the glucose level. A normal value is less than 130–140 mg/dL. A woman with a family history of diabetes, however, should be tested on her first visit to the obstetrician/gynecologist or nurse-midwife.

Treatment

Women with heart disease, diabetes, lupus, and some hereditary conditions should consult a health professional before getting pregnant, as these conditions increase the risk of morbidity and mortality for both the mother and child.

Prenatal care is vitally important for the health of the unborn baby. During the first trimester, the woman should receive at least 400 micrograms of **folic acid** daily to reduce the chance of neural tube defects. Ideally, this daily dose of folic acid should begin at least three months prior to conception. Generally, requirements for all **vitamins** are increased during pregnancy. Prenatal vitamins prescribed by a physician or midwife usually contain the recommended amount of folic acid, and some contain a stool softener to offset the constipating effects of **iron**. Following delivery, vitamins are also recommended for the breast-feeding woman. Most pregnant women need at least 2,300 calories a day; these should come from good sources of protein, green leafy vegetables, fresh fruit, and breads and cereals. Small meals may be eaten frequently throughout the day.

Since most medications can pass from the mother to the baby, no medication (not even a nonprescription drug) should be taken except under medical supervision. No drug should be considered completely safe (especially during early pregnancy), although many physicians and nurse-midwives approve their patients' use of some drugs, including acetaminophen. Drugs taken during the first three months of a pregnancy may interfere with the normal formation of a baby's organs, leading to birth defects. Drugs taken later on in pregnancy may slow the baby's growth rate, or they may damage specific fetal tissue (such as developing teeth).

To increase the chance of having a healthy baby, a pregnant woman should avoid the following:

- smoking
- alcohol
- street drugs
- large amounts of caffeine (more than one cup of coffee per day)
- more than 5,000 U of vitamin A

Prognosis

Pregnancy is a natural condition and not a disease. If a woman takes good care of herself, plans her pregnancy with medical counseling, maintains optimal health, and obtains good prenatal care, the pregnancy and birth experience will be joyful events. In choosing a caregiver, the pregnant woman must consider what she wants for herself and her baby. The standard hospital experience, despite the homey decorations and presence of family members, frequently demands that the woman in labor remain in bed attached to a fetal monitor. Bed rest and hydration by IV slow down labor, even when normal. The ability to walk and change position during labor can alleviates some of the discomfort felt during contractions.

Many health care facilities are now using nurse-midwives to attend births; their approach permits fewer interventions. Nurse-midwives are nurses who have received additional training in order to care for women having normal pregnancies and birth. If any complications should arise, they are well trained to detect them early, and they will call in the physician with whom they work. The pregnant woman and her partner should make a birth plan for their experience and present it to their

---

QUESTIONS TO ASK YOUR DOCTOR

1. How often should I come in for prenatal care?
2. Who should I call if there is a problem and this office is closed?
3. Can you recommend any parenting classes in this area?
4. Do I currently engage in any behaviors that might put me or my baby at risk?
5. Are the medications I am currently taking safe for my baby?
6. What will the conditions be like in the hospital where I will deliver the baby?

---

caregiver early in the pregnancy to determine if the individual meets their expectations. The American College of Nurse-Midwives can provide the pregnant woman with a list of midwives in her area.

Childbirth education classes for the woman and her partner are extremely important in helping a couple prepare for labor and delivery. Pregnant women should be made aware of the options for the location and circumstances for birth. women have their babies in their own homes or in birthing centers, as opposed to a traditional hospital setting. Many medical professionals recommend against home births, as complications during delivery can arise quickly and the woman and baby may not be able to be taken to the hospital in time to prevent serious consequences including permanent disability and death.

Prevention

There are many methods of **contraception** available to prevent pregnancy. In order of least to most effective, these include:

- spermicide alone
- natural (rhythm) method
- diaphragm or cervical cap
- condom alone
- diaphragm with spermicide
- condom with spermicide
- intrauterine device (IUD)
- contraceptive pill
- sterilization (either man or woman)
- abstinence

Resources

BOOKS

Harms, Roger, and Wick, Myra, eds. *Mayo Clinic Guide to a Healthy Pregnancy.* Intercourse, PA: Good Books, 2011.

Hawkins, Joellen, W., Roberto-Nichols, Diane M., and Stanley-Haney, J. Lynn. *Guidelines for Nurse Practitioners in Gynecologic Settings,* 10th ed. New York: Springer Publishing, 2012.

Murray, Linda J., ed. *Pregnancy: From Preconception to Birth.* New York: DK Publishing, 2010.

PERIODICALS

Denison, Fiona C., and Chiswick, Carolyn. "Improving Pregnancy Outcomes in Obese Women." *Proceedings of the Nutrition Society,* (November 2011) 70(4):457–464.

Saravelos, Sotirios H., and Regan, Lesley. "The Importance of Preconception Counseling and Early Pregnancy Monitoring." *Seminars in Reproductive Medicine,* (November 2011) 29(6):557–568.

OTHER

"Pregnancy Week by week." The Mayo Clinic. [accessed April 19, 2012] http://www.mayoclinic.com/health/pregnancy-week-by-week/MY00331

"Prenatal Care Fact Sheet?" WomensHealth.Gov, The United States Department of Health and Human Services Office on Women's Health. [accessed April 19, 2012] http://www.womenshealth.gov/publications/our-publications/fact-sheet/prenatal-care.cfm

ORGANIZATIONS

American College of Nurse-Midwives, 8403 Colesville Road, Suite 1550, Silver Spring, MD 20910, (240) 485-1800, Fax: (240) 485-1818, www.midwife.org

American College of Obstetricians and Gynecologists, PO Box 70620, Washington, DC 20024-9998, (202) 638-5577, (800) 673-8444, resources@acog.org, www.acog.org

Association of Women's Health, Obstetric and Neonatal Nurses, 2000 L Street, NW, Suite 740, Washington, DC 20036, (202) 261-2400, (800) 673-8499, Fax: (202) 728-0575, customerservice@awhonn.org, www.awhonn.org

Linda K. Bennington
Tish Davidson, AM

Pregnancy massage

Definition

Pregnancy massage is the prenatal use of **massage therapy** to support the physiologic, structural, and emotional well-being of both mother and fetus. Various forms of massage therapy, including Swedish, deep tissue, neuromuscular, movement, and Oriental-based

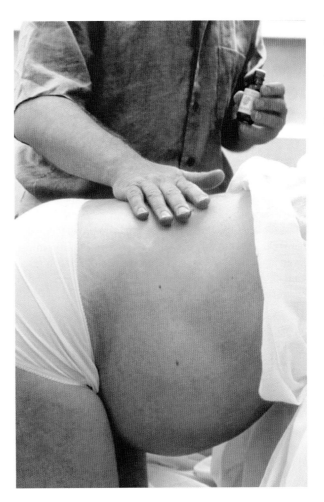

(Masseuse hand massages an aromatherapy oil into the back of a full-term pregnant woman, photograph. Hattie Young / Photo Researchers, Inc.)

therapies, may be applied throughout pregnancy as well as during labor and the postpartum period.

Origins

Cultural and anthropological studies indicate that massage and movement during the childbearing experience were and continue to be a prominent part of many cultures' health care. Indian Ayurvedic medical manuals detail therapists' instructions for rubbing specially formulated oils into pregnant patients' stretched abdominal skin. Traditional sculptures depict Eskimo fathers supporting and lovingly stroking their laboring wives' backs. In certain Irish hospitals laboring women are held and touched by a doula (labor assistant) or midwife through most of their notably short, uncomplicated labors. For billions of women, over thousand of years, midwives' highly developed hands-on skills have provided loving support and eased childbearing discomforts. As massage therapy resumes its place within Western health care methods, pregnancy massage is becoming one of its fastest-growing specialized applications.

Benefits

Profound physiologic, functional, emotional, relational, and lifestyle changes occur during gestation and labor, often creating high **stress** levels. Too much stress can negatively affect maternal and infant health, resulting in reduced uterine **blood** supply and higher incidence of **miscarriage**, prematurity, and other complications. Massage therapy can help a woman approach her due date with less **anxiety** as well as less physical discomfort. Even apart from easing specific aches, massage can act as an overall tonic and increase the expectant mother's body awareness.

Massage therapy can address the various physical challenges of pregnancy: **edema**; foot, leg, or hand discomforts; and **pain** in the lower back, pelvis, or hips. Swedish massage may facilitate gestation by supporting cardiac function, placental and mammary development, and increasing cellular respiration. It can also reduce edema and high **blood pressure** as well as contribute to sympathetic nervous system sedation. Deep tissue, trigger point, and both active and passive movements alleviate stress on weight-bearing joints, muscles, and fascial tissues to reduce neck and **back pain** caused by poor posture and strain on the uterine ligaments. During labor, women whose partners use basic massage strokes on their backs and legs have shorter, less complicated labors. After the baby's birth, massage therapy can gently facilitate the body's return to its pre-pregnancy state, alleviate pain, foster a renewed sense of body and self, and help maintain flexibility despite the physical stresses of infant care. For post-cesarean mothers, specific therapeutic techniques can also reduce scar tissue formation and facilitate the healing of the incision and related soft tissue areas.

Description

When nestled with pillows or other specialty cushions into a side-lying or semi-reclining position, most women are more comfortable for the 30–60 minutes of a typical massage session. A pregnant woman can expect to enjoy many of the same techniques, draping, and professional demeanor offered all massage therapy clients. The lower back, hips, and neck benefit from sensitively applied deep tissue, neuromuscular, and **movement therapy**. Edema in the legs and arms may be relieved with the gliding and kneading strokes of Swedish or lymphatic drainage massage. Pregnant

women should expect a thorough health and prenatal intake interview with their therapists. Cost, procedures, and insurance coverage are similar to those for other massage client populations.

Preparations

In addition to the preparations listed in the massage therapy entry, some expectant women will be asked to secure a release from their maternity health care provider, especially those with complications or high-risk factors.

Precautions

In addition to those listed in the massage therapy entry, the following other precautions are prudent:

- The abdomen should be touched only superficially with a flat, gentle hand.
- Any pressure applied to the inner leg should also be superficial.
- Women who must be on bed rest for any complication are at higher risk of blood clots forming in their legs; therefore, most massage of the legs should be avoided.
- Massage is safest when a woman is either lying on the side or propped semi-sitting at a 45–70 degree angle rather than lying on her back or belly.
- Because there are many other specific body areas and types of techniques that must be avoided or modified according to an individual woman's health condition, advanced specialized training of the therapist and consultation with the expectant woman's physician or midwife are highly recommended. It is better to avoid massage if the woman has vaginal bleeding, abdominal pain, or diarrhea.

Side effects

There are no known side effects to receiving appropriate prenatal massage therapy.

Research and general acceptance

Current research on the benefits of touch is providing a contemporary basis for its reintroduction into maternity care. Scientists have found that rats restricted from cutaneous self-stimulation had poorly developed placentas and 50% less mammary gland development. Their litters were often ill, stillborn, or died shortly after birth due to poor mothering skills. Women who are nauseated and/or **vomiting** prenatally experienced a decrease in these discomforts when they applied finger pressure to a specific **acupuncture** point (**acupressure**) on their forearm several times each day. Pregnant women massaged twice weekly for five weeks

KEY TERMS

Doula—A woman who assists an expectant mother with physical and emotional support during labor.

Edema—An abnormal accumulation of fluid in specific parts of the body, causing swelling of the area. Many women experience edema of the wrists and ankles during pregnancy.

experienced less anxiety, leg, and back pain. When compared with control groups who practiced **relaxation** exercises only, the women who had had massage reported better sleep and improved moods; and their labors had fewer complications, including fewer premature births. Studies show that when women receive nurturing touch during later pregnancy, they touch their babies more frequently and lovingly. During labor the presence of a doula, a woman providing physical and emotional support, including extensive touching and massage, reduces the length of labor and number of complications, interventions, medications, and cesarean sections.

Training and certification

Some massage therapy schools include comprehensive courses in pregnancy massage therapy. More often, however, therapists receive only introductory guidance in maternity applications during their 500–1000 hours of basic training. They then pursue specialization certification in pre- and perinatal massage therapy. Several nationwide programs offer such advanced training in 24–34 hour workshop programs.

Resources

BOOKS

Curties, Debra. *Breast Massage.* Moncton, New Brunswick, Canada: Curties-Overzet Publications Inc., 1999.

Goldsmith, Judith. *Childbirth Wisdom.* New York: Congdon and Weed, 1984.

Klaus, Marshall H., M.D., John H. Kennell, M.D., and Phyllis H. Klaus, M.Ed. *Mothering the Mother.* New York: Addison-Wesley Publishing Company, 1993.

Osborne-Sheets, Carole. *Pre- and Perinatal Massage Therapy: A Comprehensive Practitioners' Guide to Pregnancy, Labor, and Postpartum.* San Diego: Body Therapy Associates, 1998.

Rich, Laurie. *When Pregnancy Isn't Perfect.* New York: Dutton, 1991.

Samuels, Mike, and Nancy Samuels. *The New Well Pregnancy Book.* New York: Fireside, 1996.

Yates, John, PhD. *A Physician's Guide to Therapeutic Massage: Its Physiological Effects and Their Application to Treatment.* Vancouver, BC: Massage Therapists' Association of British Columbia, 1999.

ORGANIZATION

National Association of Pregnancy Massage Therapy. (888) 451-4945.

Carole Osborne-Sheets

Pregnancy test

Definition

Pregnancy is detected by measuring the concentration of human chorionic gonadotropin (hCG) in serum or urine. Human chorionic gonadotropin is a hormone produced by the placenta that supports the corpus luteum after fertilization of the ovum. Production of hCG begins at the time of implantation, and hCG can usually be detected in serum and urine within 10 days after fertilization. The level of hCG in serum and urine is usually above 25 mIU/mL, the cutoff for a positive pregnancy test, before the next expected period. Therefore, pregnancy can be detected reliably within two to three days following the first missed menses using a qualitative hCG test. Many home pregnancy tests claim to be accurate in detecting pregnancy a day after the first missed period or even before. To avoid false positives, it is best to wait until a week after the first missed period or if an earlier test is done, to retest at this time.

In addition to diagnosis of pregnancy, the test is used in emergency departments to rule out pregnancy in circumstances in which x ray and other procedures are contraindicated by pregnancy. The test is also used to rule out pregnancy in females with acute **abdominal pain** that suggests the possibility of ectopic pregnancy (i. e., pregnancy outside the uterus).

Quantitative measurements of hCG are used as an aid to the diagnosis of ectopic pregnancy and trophoblastic tumors. Serial measurements may be used to monitor treatment and recurrence of tumors that secrete hCG. Measurement of hCG is also part of the triple marker screening procedure performed on maternal serum between weeks 15 to 20 to assess the fetal risk of **Down syndrome**.

Description

Chorionic gonadotropin is a hormone consisting of two polypeptide chains or subunits designated alpha and beta. The alpha chain is identical to the alpha chain of luteinizing hormone (LH), follicle-stimulating hormone (FSH), and thyroid stimulating hormone (TSH). The beta chain is identical to that of LH except for the C-terminal end, which contains an additional 24 amino acids. **Antibodies** made against the alpha subunit will cross-react with LH, FSH, and TSH, but antibodies can be made to the beta subunit that are hCG specific. All tests for pregnancy use antibodies to both subunits, which makes the pregnancy test highly specific for hCG. Chorionic gonadotropin is produced at an exponential rate through week 12 of gestation, often reaching in excess of 100,000 mIU/mL. In a normal pregnancy, the production of hCG doubles approximately every two days during this period. The level falls off sharply after the first trimester to approximately 20,000 mIU/mL, and is maintained at this level throughout a normal pregnancy. Following a normal delivery, the hCG can be detected in serum and urine for three to four weeks. This period may be longer following an aborted pregnancy, especially if a trophoblastic tumor was present.

All pregnancy tests are double antibody sandwich immunoassays. The most commonly used platform, called immunochromatography, consists of a disposable device containing a membrane on which an antibody to one hCG subunit is immobilized. The membrane also contains an antibody to the other hCG subunit that is mobile. The mobile antibody is conjugated to an enzyme, dyed latex particle, or colloidal gold particle. The sample is added to the device and is drawn by capillary action onto the membrane, where it mixes with the mobile antibody. If hCG molecules are present, they bind to the mobile antibodies, forming antibody-antigen complexes. These migrate along the membrane to the region containing the immobilized antibody. The immobilized antibody binds to the other hCG subunit forming an antibody-hCG-antibody sandwich that remains fixed to the membrane in the reaction zone region. At this point, the dye or gold particles are focused in the reaction zone and produce color, usually in the form of a plus sign or other visible indicator of a positive test. If an enzyme-conjugated antibody is used, a substrate solution is added, which is hydrolyzed by the enzyme to produce a colored product at the reaction zone.

Precautions

In order to achieve accurate results for home pregnancy tests, the manufacturer's instructions must be followed precisely. When pregnancy tests using urine are performed correctly, they have been found to have an error rate of approximately 2%. Home pregnancy tests may have a significantly higher error rate if the manufacturer's instructions are not followed precisely. Diluted urine may cause a false-negative result. False-positive results may be caused by heterophile antibodies, medications containing mouse **monoclonal antibodies**, autoantibodies, and hyperlipemia. In very early pregnancy, the color reaction may be difficult to interpret. In such cases, the test should be repeated after waiting at least 48 hours. If serum is to be used, standard precautions for the prevention of transmission of **blood** borne pathogens should be followed.

Preparation

No preparation is generally required for a pregnancy test. However, if urine is used, the first morning urine is the specimen of choice because the urine will be more concentrated after an overnight fast. If serum is to be used the area should be thoroughly disinfected before blood is drawn.

Aftercare

No special care is required after a urine test for hCG. If blood is drawn, discomfort or bruising may occur at the puncture site or the person may feel dizzy or faint. Pressure to the puncture site until the bleeding stops reduces bruising; warm packs relieve discomfort. Women who feel faint should be observed until the condition goes away.

Complications

Tests for hCG levels pose no direct risk to a woman's health. The main risk with a home pregnancy test is obtaining a false-negative result, which may be lessened by following the manufacturer's instructions carefully and waiting at least several days after the expected menstrual period before performing the test. A false-negative result can cause a delay in seeking **prenatal care**, which can pose a risk to both the woman and her fetus. For some women a blood draw may cause bruising or redness and discomfort at the site.

Results

HCG levels below 25 mIU/mL will give a negative pregnancy test result for all pregnancy test methods. Home test kits use a cutoff of 50 mIU/mL and will be negative below this level. Following **miscarriage** or **abortion**, the pregnancy test may remain positive for four weeks or longer. An hCG test performed during this time may be positive in the absence of pregnancy.

The upper limit of normal for a quantitative hCG test is approximately 5 mIU/mL. In rare circumstances, such

Ectopic pregnancy—A pregnancy that develops outside the mother's uterus. Ectopic pregnancies often cause severe pain in the lower abdomen and are potentially life-threatening because of the massive blood loss that may occur as the developing embryo/fetus ruptures and damages the tissues in which it has implanted.

Embryo—In humans, the developing individual from the time of implantation to about the end of the second month after conception. From the third month to the point of delivery, the individual is called a fetus.

Hormone—A chemical produced by a specific organ or tissue of the body that is released into the bloodstream in order to exert an effect in another part of the body.

Human chorionic gonadotropin (hCG)—A hormone produced by the placenta of a developing pregnancy.

Hydatidiform mole—A rare, generally benign grape-like mass that grows in the uterus from the remains of an abnormally developed embryo and surrounding tissue. In extremely rare cases, the mole develops into a choriocarcinoma, a malignant tumor that can invade the wall of the uterus.

Implantation—The attachment of the fertilized egg or embryo to the wall of the uterus.

Menstrual cycle—A hormonally regulated series of monthly events that occur during the reproductive years of the human female to ensure that the proper internal environment exists for fertilization, implantation, and development of a baby. Each month, a mature egg is released from the follicle of an ovary. If an egg is released, fertilized, and implanted, the expanded lining of the uterus is maintained. If fertilization and/or implantation does not occur, the egg and all of the excess uterine lining are shed from the body during menstruation.

Miscarriage—Loss of the embryo or fetus and other products of pregnancy before the middle of the second trimester. Often, early in a pregnancy, if the condition of the baby and/or the mother's uterus are not compatible with sustaining life, the pregnancy stops, and the contents of the uterus are expelled. For this reason, miscarriage is also referred to as spontaneous abortion.

Placenta—The organ that unites the fetus to the mother's uterus. The placenta produces hCG, among other hormones, to help maintain the pregnancy. It transfers nutrients and antibodies to the fetus, and waste products from the fetus. After delivery, the placenta, known at this point as the afterbirth, is expelled.

---

as pelvic inflammatory disease, the hCG level in nonpregnancy may be greater than 5 mIU/mL. Persons with trophoblastic tumors, molar pregnancies, and choriocarcinoma will have greatly elevated levels of hCG. HCG may be found in persons with testicular **cancer** and other malignancies that secrete hCG or alpha and/or beta subunits. Quantitative hCG measurement is useful in detecting hCG-secreting tumors. Periodic measurements are useful in evaluating treatment and monitoring patients for recurrence. Maternal serum hCG levels are increased by approximately 25% above normal for the gestational age in Down syndrome pregnancies and in some other trisomy syndromes. In ectopic pregnancy, hCG levels are lower than normal, and the hCG doubling time is less than expected. Minimum hCG increases between timed hCG measurements in the first trimester are:

- two measurements one day apart: 29% increase

- two measurements two days apart: 66% increase

- two measurements three days apart: 114% increase

- two measurements four days apart: 175% increase

- two measurements five days apart: 255% increase

Recovery of a lower than expected increase is evidence of ectopic pregnancy. Decreases in hCG are seen in spontaneous abortion.

Health care team roles

If serum is used, a phlebotomist or nurse collects the blood specimen. A laboratory scientist, nurse, physician assistant, or physician can perform the pregnancy test. The result should be reported to the physician who orders the test. Quantitative hCG tests are ordered and interpreted by a physician and performed by a clinical laboratory scientist, CLS (NCA)/medical technologist, MT(ASCP) or clinical laboratory technician CLT(NCA)/medical laboratory technician MLT(ASCP).

Resources

BOOKS

Kee, Joyce LeFever. *Laboratory and Diagnostic Tests with Nursing Implications,* 8th ed. Upper Saddle River, NJ: Pearson, 2010.

Professional Guide to Signs and Symptoms, 6th ed. Philadelphia: Wolters Kluwer/Lippincott Williams and Wilkins.

Shannon, Joyce Brennfleck, ed. *Medical Tests Sourcebook,* 4th ed. Detroit, MI: Omnigraphics, 2011.

PERIODICALS

Cole, Laurence A. "The Utility of Six Over-The-Counter Home Pregnancy Tests." *Clinical Chemistry and Laboratory Medicine,* (August 2011) 49(8):1317–1322.

Furtado, Larissa V., et al. "Should the Qualitative Serum Pregnancy Test Be Considered Obsolete?" *American Journal of Clinical Pathology,* (February 2012) 137(2):194–202.

OTHER

"Home Pregnancy Tests: Can You Trust the Results?" The Mayo Clinic. [accessed April 19, 2012]. http://www.mayoclinic.com/health/home-pregnancy-tests/PR00100

"Pregnancy Test." Medline Plus. [accessed April 19, 2012]. http://www.nlm.nih.gov/medlineplus/ency/article/003432.htm

ORGANIZATIONS

American Clinical Laboratory Association, 1100 New York Avenue NW, Suite 725 West, Washington, DC 20005, (202) 637-9466, www.acla.com

American College of Obstetricians and Gynecologists, PO Box 70620, Washington, DC 20024-9998, (202) 638-5577, (800) 673-8444, resources@acog.org , www.acog.org

Association of Women's Health, Obstetric and Neonatal Nurses, 2000 L Street, NW, Suite 740, Washington, DC 20036, (202) 261-2400, (800) 673-8499, Fax: (202) 728-0575, customerservice@awhonn.org, www.awhonn.org.

Victoria E. DeMoranville
Tish Davidson, AM

Premature infants

Definition

A premature infant is defined as one born before 37 weeks of gestation (**pregnancy**) without regard to birth weight. The length of a full-term pregnancy ranges from 37 to 42 weeks, measuring from the first day of the last menstrual period. "Preterm" is a word that is sometimes used instead of "premature." Extremely premature infants are defined as those born between 23 and 28 weeks of gestation. As of 2012, babies born at 22 weeks of gestation or less have little chance of survival.

In the United States, about 12% of all infants are born prematurely. African American babies are more likely to be premature and extremely low birth weight (ELBW) babies than Caucasian or Hispanic babies. The rates of survival of premature infants in the developed world have increased dramatically over the last four decades; however, prematurity accounts for more than three-quarters of all of perinatal deaths. In spite of advances in medical technology, these children remain at higher risk of **birth defects**, weakened immune systems, and a variety of chronic medical and developmental disorders. Many require long-term follow-up care.

Description

Chances for survival

The most important factor affecting survival in extremely premature infants is gestational age at the time of birth, which is defined as the estimated time elapsed since conception. Another term for gestational age is postconceptional age. The likelihood of a preterm infant's survival at specific gestational ages in the United States has not changed much since the late 1990s. In the 2010s the chance of preterm survival is as follows:

- 21 weeks or less: 0% survival rate
- 22 weeks: 0–10% survival rate
- 23 weeks: 10–35% survival rate
- 24 weeks: 40–70% survival rate
- 25 weeks: 50–80% survival rate
- 26 weeks: 80–90% survival rate
- 27 weeks and beyond: greater than 90%

The baby's chances of survival increase 3–4% per day between 23 and 24 weeks of gestation, and 2–3% per day between 24 and 26 weeks.

In addition to gestational age, the baby's weight at birth, the presence of breathing problems, the presence of birth defects, and the presence of severe **infection** are important factors influencing survival. Birth weight in

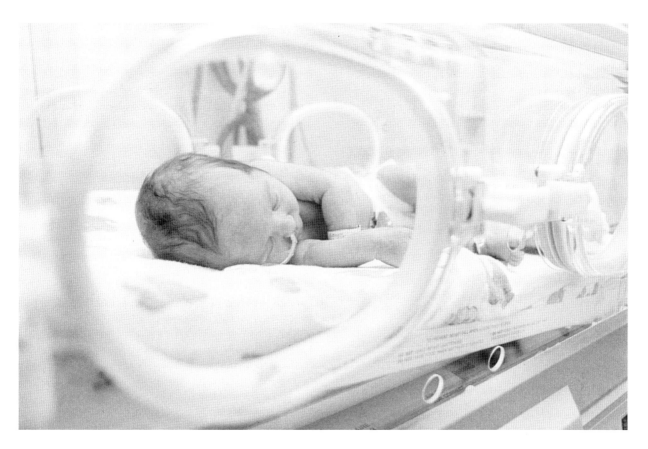

(Premature infant in incubator, photograph. © George Disario/Corbis)

premature infants is categorized as follows: birth weight below 5 lb 8 oz (2500 g) is defined as low birth weight (LBW); weight below 3 lb 5 oz (1500 g) is very low birth weight (VLBW); and weight below 2 lb 3 oz (1000 g) is extremely low birth weight (ELBW).

Other factors affecting survival

Other factors that influence the rate of organ development or the fetal oxygen supply also influence a premature infant's chances for survival. These factors include:

- rupture of the amniotic sac with loss of amniotic fluid before 24 weeks of gestation

- male sex (male infants are slower to mature)

- race (African American infants have slightly better chances of survival than Caucasian infants of the same birth weight)

- uncontrolled diabetes in the mother (slows organ development in the fetus)

- severe hypertension before the eighth month of pregnancy (slows delivery of nutrients and oxygen to the fetus)

Causes and symptoms

Causes of preterm labor

Labor that begins before the 37th week of pregnancy is called premature or **preterm labor**. It is responsible for about 85% of illnesses and deaths in newborns in the United States. Premature labor is sometimes induced because of the mother's or the infant's condition. Preeclampsia/eclampsia is the most common reason for inducing labor; other reasons include fetal distress or bleeding. Common causes of spontaneous premature labor include:

- abruptio placentae, or detachment of the placenta from the uterine wall

- premature rupture of the amniotic sac

- incompetent (too easily dilated) cervix

- multiple pregnancy

- abdominal or cervical surgery during the current pregnancy

- placenta previa (the placenta lies between the baby and the birth canal)

Factors that increase the mother's risk of preterm labor include:

- history of preterm delivery
- history of abortions or miscarriages
- heavy smoking (more than 10 cigarettes per day)
- history of drug abuse
- exposure to diethylstilbestrol (DES), a synthetic estrogen given to treat estrogen deficiency conditions
- urinary tract infection
- malnutrition
- height below 5 ft (1.5 m)
- weight below 100 lb (45 kg)
- age below 18 years

Common medical problems in premature infants

The most common problems in premature infants include **jaundice**, apnea (a pause in breathing lasting longer than 15–20 seconds), and inability to breast-feed or bottle-feed. Apnea in premature infants is accompanied by the baby's turning pale or bluish (cyanotic), and by a slowing-down of its **heart** rate (bradycardia). These problems are particularly likely to affect infants born more than four to six weeks early.

More serious medical problems that are relatively frequent in premature infants are described in the next four subsections.

RESPIRATORY DISTRESS SYNDROME (RDS). Respiratory distress syndrome (RDS) is the most common lung disorder in preterm infants. It is caused by a lack of surfactant in the **lungs**. Surfactant is a surface-active substance produced by the body that coats the lungs and keeps them from collapsing. Babies with RDS typically breathe rapidly, with flaring nostrils and grunting sounds. RDS is usually treated by giving the baby extra oxygen under pressure. Sometimes the baby is also given additional surfactant by intubation.

TRANSIENT TACHYPNEA OF THE NEWBORN (TTNB). Transient tachypnea of the newborn is a disorder lasting for several hours or a few days characterized by rapid, grunting breathing. TTNB is thought to be caused by slow reabsorption of fetal lung fluid. It is also treated with supplemental oxygen.

PATENT DUCTUS ARTERIOSUS (PDA). A patent ductus arteriosus refers to an opening in the **blood** vessel that connects the aorta and the pulmonary artery. In full-term infants, this blood vessel closes in the first few days after birth. In preterm infants, it may remain open, thus allowing too much blood to flow into the baby's lungs. PDAs are treated with indomethacin or ibuprofen to close the blood vessel, or diuretics to decrease the amount of fluid that collects in the baby's lungs. If the medications do not close the ductus, it can be closed surgically.

RETINOPATHY OF PREMATURITY (ROP). Retinopathy of prematurity, or ROP, is the abnormal growth of **blood vessels** in the eyes. ROP is most common in infants who are more than 12 weeks premature. It often resolves on its own, but sometimes requires treatment. Treatment consists of killing the inner lining of the eye at the ends of the abnormal blood vessels to prevent further growth.

Less common but severe medical conditions

The next five subsections briefly describe serious disorders that may affect premature infants.

AIR LEAKS. Air leaks refer to several conditions in preterm infants, all characterized by air leaking from the air sacs in the lungs. The air may be trapped between the chest wall and the lung, trapped in the middle part of the chest, leaked into the **abdomen**, or leaked into the spaces between the tiny air sacs. Premature infants are vulnerable to air leaks because their lungs are not yet fully developed. In milder cases, the air is gradually reabsorbed by the baby's body. In severe cases, the baby may be treated by placement of a **chest tube**, or be placed on a ventilator.

NECROTIZING ENTEROCOLITIS (NEC). Necrotizing enterocolitis (NEC) is an inflammatory disorder in which part of the bowel lining or part of the bowel itself is destroyed. It is not always clear why a specific infant may develop NEC. The baby may vomit, have a swollen or abnormally reddish abdomen, or pass blood in the stool. NEC is usually treated with **antibiotics**. If a section of the bowel itself has been destroyed, surgery may be necessary.

BRONCHOPULMONARY DYSPLASIA (BPD). Bronchopulmonary dysplasia, or BPD, is a long-term lung disease that is most likely to develop in infants who were extremely premature, had severe RDS, or developed infections of the lungs. BPD is diagnosed if the baby's chest x-rays remain abnormal and the baby still needs oxygen by the time it is 36 weeks of gestational age (a month before its full-term due date). Babies with BPD are treated with supplemental oxygen, sometimes for as long as a year after they develop BPD. They may also be given steroids or diuretics.

INTRAVENTRICULAR HEMORRHAGE (IVH). Intraventricular hemorrhage (IVH) is a **brain** disorder in which blood seeps into the ventricles (a series of connecting cavities) of the brain. IVH develops because the blood vessels in the brain of a premature infant are fragile and break open easily. The preterm babies at highest risk for IVH are those weighing less than 2 lb 4 oz (1000 g). There is no specific treatment for IVH, but the condition can be monitored by ultrasound. In mild cases of IVH, the blood in the ventricles is slowly reabsorbed by the body. Babies with **hydrocephalus** (abnormal amounts of cerebrospinal fluid collecting in the ventricles of the brain), which is a possible complication of IVH, are at risk for permanent brain injury.

PERIVENTRICULAR LEUKOMALACIA (PVL). Periventricular leukomalacia (PVL) refers to a softening of the white matter of the brain surrounding the ventricles, caused by the death of brain tissue in these areas. The precise causes of PVL are still not fully understood. PVL often develops in babies with IVH. There is no specific treatment for PVL; moreover, infants with this disorder are at very high risk for motor (movement) and developmental disabilities as they mature.

Diagnosis

Many of the problems associated with prematurity depend on the degree of prematurity and the baby's birth weight. The gestational age of the fetus may be calculated from the date of the mother's last menstrual period or by using ultrasound imaging to observe **fetal development**. After the baby is born, such physical assessment scales as the Dubowitz Maturity Scale may be used to estimate gestational age. The Dubowitz scale bases its determination on the infant's physical and neuromuscular maturity.

Once the baby's gestational age and weight are determined, further tests and electronic monitoring may be used to diagnose problems or to track the baby's condition. A heart monitor or cardiorespiratory monitor may be attached to the baby's chest, abdomen, arms, or legs with adhesive patches to monitor breathing and heart rate. A **thermometer** probe may be taped on the skin to monitor body temperature. Blood samples may be taken from a vein or artery. A radiologic technologist may perform x rays or ultrasound imaging to examine the heart, lungs, and other internal organs.

Treatment

Treatment depends on the types of complications that are present and often occurs in a neonatal intensive care unit. The infant may be placed in a heat-controlled unit (an incubator) to maintain body temperature. Infants that are having trouble breathing on their own may need oxygen either pumped into the incubator, administered through small tubes placed in their nostrils (nasal cannula), or through a respirator or ventilator that pumps air through an endotracheal tube inserted into the airway. Oxygen may be delivered under pressure by continuous positive airway pressure (CPAP) or positive end expiratory pressure (PEEP).

Medications and surgery

The infant may require fluids and nutrients to be administered through an intravenous line inserted into a vein in the hand, foot, arm, leg, or scalp. If the baby needs medications to treat infections, to close a patent ductus, or to increase urinary output, they may also be administered through the intravenous line. Surgery may be required in the treatment of PDA, NEC, or IVH. If hydrocephalus develops as a complication of IVH, it may be treated by surgical placement of a shunt, which is a tube connecting one of the ventricles in the brain to a longer tube under the skin that allows the excess cerebrospinal fluid to be absorbed in the abdomen.

Environmental considerations

Premature infants require special attention to their physical and social environment as well as to the symptoms of any disorders they may have. Some modifications are necessary because the nervous systems of preterm infants are not as fully developed as those of full-term infants.

PHYSICAL ENVIRONMENT. Premature infants experience loud noises and bright lights as stressful. In addition, they are more disturbed by frequent handling than full-term infants. Parents and other caregivers should be advised to position the infant on its side in a flexed position; because premature infants do not have the muscle strength to move against gravity, they tend to lie with arms and legs in an extended position. Over a period of time, this extended position can delay the baby's motor development.

SOCIAL ENVIRONMENT. Neonatal intensive care units, or NICUs, complicate the premature infant's social environment by exposing him or her to many more clinical staff members than the full-term infant, and at the same time keep him or her away from the parents more than the full-term infant. For this reason, skin-to-skin contact with parents, sometimes called kangaroo care, and gentle massage are encouraged as promoting infant and parent well-being. Parents should be encouraged to have early contact with the premature baby to facilitate parent-infant bonding.

Prognosis

The prognoses of premature infants vary widely, depending on gestational age, birth weight, the reasons

KEY TERMS

Apnea—A pause in breathing of more than 15–20 seconds. In premature infants, apnea usually causes a change in the baby's color and a slowing of the heartbeat.

Bronchopulmonary dysplasia (BPD)—A chronic lung disorder that sometimes develops in premature infants who have had severe respiratory distress syndrome or lung infections.

Chronologic or birth age—The infant's age as measured by the time elapsed since birth.

Gestational age—The infant's age as measured by the estimated time since conception; sometimes called postconceptional age.

Hydrocephalus—An abnormal buildup of cerebrospinal fluid in the ventricles of the brain. In premature infants, it is often a complication of IVH.

Intraventricular hemorrhage (IVH)—A condition in which fragile blood vessels within the brain burst and bleed into the hollow chambers (ventricles) of the brain and into the tissue surrounding them.

Kangaroo care—A form of skin-to-skin contact in which either parent of a premature infant holds the baby under the blouse or shirt, against the skin. It is thought to help the infant's development as well as its bonding with the parents.

Necrotizing enterocolitis (NEC)—A condition that sometimes occurs in premature infants in which the lining of the bowel or a section of the bowel itself dies.

Neonatology—The study of the development and disorders of newborn children. A physician who specializes in this field is called a neonatologist.

Patent ductus arteriosus (PDA)—An opening in the blood vessel that connects the aorta and the pulmonary artery. In full-term infants, this opening closes shortly after birth, but in premature infants, it may remain open and allow blood to collect in the infant's lungs.

Periventricular leukomalacia (PVL)—A brain disorder in which some of the white matter of the brain near the ventricles is softened because of the death of tissue in these areas.

Preeclampsia/eclampsia—Complications of pregnancy related to high blood pressure in a woman whose blood pressure was normal before pregnancy. Preeclampsia and eclampsia are common reasons for inducing premature labor.

Preterm—Another word for premature.

Respiratory distress syndrome (RDS)—A condition in which a premature infant lacks a sufficient amount of surfactant, a protective film that helps air sacs in the lungs to stay open.

Retinopathy of prematurity (ROP)—A condition in which the blood vessels in the retina of the eye display abnormal growth.

Surfactant—A protective film that helps air sacs in the lungs to stay open.

Tachypnea—Rapid breathing. Some premature infants develop rapid breathing for a few hours or days. This condition is known as transient tachypnea of the newborn (TTNB).

for premature delivery, and the many other factors discussed above.

Health care team roles

Premature infants receive routine care and monitoring in the NICU from nurses. A neonatologist, who is a physician specializing in care of the newborn, may be consulted if a medical intervention seems necessary. A radiologist may be consulted for radiographic or ultrasound studies, and a surgeon may be called in if an operation is required.

Other health professionals involved in the premature infant's care are the respiratory therapist, who monitors the care of infants requiring supplemental oxygen or **ventilators**; the social worker, who helps families adjust emotionally and provides referrals to hospital and community resources; and the occupational therapist, who evaluates the baby's progress and plans a program of developmental therapy if necessary.

After discharge from the hospital, the infant's growth and development will be monitored by a pediatrician or family physician. This doctor will reinforce the parents' education about caring for their baby, review the hospital records, and give the baby its first immunizations (most can be given at the usual chronological age). Most doctors recommend office

QUESTIONS TO ASK YOUR DOCTOR

1. Are there any factors that make me at high risk for a premature delivery?

2. What facilities does my hospital have to care for very premature babies?

3. What can I do to prevent or delay preterm labor?

4. Do you know of any support groups for parents of very premature babies?

visits every one or two weeks until the infant has adapted satisfactorily to the home environment and is gaining an appropriate amount of weight.

Prevention

Some of the risks and complications of premature delivery can be reduced if the mother receives good **prenatal care**, follows a healthy diet, avoids alcohol consumption, and refrains from cigarette **smoking**. In some cases of premature labor, the mother may be placed on bed rest or given drugs that can postpone labor for days or weeks, giving the fetus more time to develop before delivery. The physician or nurse-midwife may prescribe a steroid medication to be given to the mother if a premature birth is expected, to assist the baby's lung development.

Resources

BOOKS

Gunter, Jennifer. *The Preemie Primer: A Complete Guide for Parents of Premature Babies.* Cambridge, MA: Da Capo Press, 2010.

Linden, Dana Wechsler, Emma Trenti Paroli, and Mia Wechsler Doron. *Preemies: The Essential Guide for Parents of Premature Babies,* 2nd ed. New York: Gallery Books, 2010.

PERIODICALS

McDonald S.D., et al. "High Gestational Weight Gain and The Risk of Preterm Birth and Low Birth Weight: A Systematic Review and Meta-Analysis." *Journal of Obstetrics and Gynaecology Canada.* (Dec 2100) 33(12): 1223–33.

Korja, R., R. Latva, and L. Lehtonen. "The Effects of Preterm Birth on Mother-Infant Interaction and Attachment During The Infant's First Two Years." *Acta Obstetricia et Gynecologica Scandinavica.* (Feb 2012) 91(2):164–73

OTHER

Furdon, Susan A. Prematurity. Medscape Reference January 24, 2012 [accessed April 17, 2012]. http://emedicine. medscape.com/article/975909-overview

Premature Babies. MedlinePlus. April 13, 2012 [accessed April 17, 2012]. http://www.nlm.nih.gov/medlineplus/prematurebabies.html

Subramanian. Siva K. N. Extremely Low Birth Weight Babies. Medscape Reference March 27, 2012 [accessed April 17, 2012]. http://emedicine.medscape.com/article/979717-overview

ORGANIZATIONS

American Academy of Pediatrics, 141 Northwest Point Boulevard, Elk Grove Village, IL 60007-1098, (847) 434-4000, Fax: (847) 434-8000, http://www.aap.org

Association of Women's Health, Obstetric and Neonatal Nurses, 2000 L Street, NW, Suite 740, Washington DC 20036, (202) 261-2400, (800) 673-8499, Fax: (202) 728-0575, customerservice@awhonn.org, www.awhonn.org

National Institute of Child Health and Human Development (NICHD), P.O. Box 3006, Rockville, MD 20847, (800) 370-2943 (800)320-6942, Fax: (866) 760-5947, NICHDInformationResourceCenter@mail.nih.gov, http://www.nichd.nih.gov.

Nadine M. Jacobson, R.N.
Tish Davidson, AM

Premature labor *see* **Preterm labor**

Prenatal care

Definition

Prenatal care is that health care given to a pregnant woman and to the developing fetus until the time of delivery.

Purpose

The purpose of prenatal care is to:

• Establish a baseline for vital signs and current health status.

• Identify women at risk for pregnancy-related complications.

• Minimize pregnancy-related complications through prevention techniques, anticipatory action, and intervention as soon as a complication is recognized.

• Offer education to the woman about possible lifestyle and work-related dangers to her and the developing fetus.

• Provide routine evaluation of the growth and development of the fetus.

• Educate the pregnant woman about normal and abnormal conditions in pregnancy.

Prenatal visit schedule recommended by womenshealth.gov

Consistent prenatal care can help keep you and your baby healthy, spot problems if they occur, and prevent problems during delivery. Typically, routine checkups occur:

Weeks 4–28	Once each month
Weeks 28–36	Twice each month
Weeks 38–birth	Once each week

Women with high-risk pregnancies need to see their doctors more often.

SOURCE: U.S. Department of Health and Human Services Office on Women's Health, 2010.

• Teach the woman to recognize the signs of impending labor.

• Assist in connecting the pregnant woman to childbirth- and or parenting-education classes.

Precautions

Practitioners of prenatal care need to be aware of the possibility of domestic abuse, since such violence may begin with a **pregnancy**. About half of women who are abused prior to becoming pregnant will continue to be abused during the pregnancy. Questions about abuse should be included at the first prenatal visit, and periodically thereafter if suspicion of it arises.

Description

The prenatal period lasts about 38 weeks from conception to delivery, or 40 weeks from the last menstrual period (LMP). It may also be referred to as the antenatal period. While some women come for their first prenatal visit shortly after missing a menstrual period, others may not come for prenatal care until later.

The first prenatal visit is usually the longest, as it includes a complete **health history**, **physical examination** (including pelvic and bimanual exams), and **blood** and urine testing. A recommended schedule for prenatal visits is:

• Once a month until 28 weeks' gestation.

• Every two weeks from week 28 to week 36.

• Every week from week 36 until delivery.

Women with certain health conditions and those who are pregnant later in life may be scheduled for more frequent prenatal visits.

The pregnancy is confirmed at the first prenatal visit. A urine or blood test may be done as well as a physical examination. A woman may have taken a home **pregnancy test** after a missed period and may already be experiencing some nausea, **vomiting**, or breast tenderness. Practitioners should assess the woman's feelings about the pregnancy and assist in appropriate referrals if she needs further counseling.

The complete health history should record the following information:

• The first day of the woman's last menstrual period. The LMP date will be used to calculate the estimated date of delivery, referred to as the due date. Calculation of the due date uses a formula called Naegele's rule: subtract three months from the date of the woman's LMP. Then add one week and one year. Most women deliver within two weeks before or after their due date.

• Previous gynecologic and obstetric history. Practitioners should not assume that this is the woman's first pregnancy. A woman may not divulge her complete history if her partner is present and there are aspects of her history that she has not yet shared. This history should include contraceptive choices and prior exposure to sexually transmitted diseases. If she is Rh-negative, did she receive RHOgam with a previous pregnancy, even if it was terminated early?

• Personal medical history. This should include childhood diseases, allergies, side effects or allergies to medications, chronic diseases such as high blood pressure and diabetes, medications currently being taken, vaccinations, surgeries, and eating disorders. Past conditions may become reactivated during a pregnancy. Women with prior eating disorders may have difficulty gaining weight during a pregnancy. Women should be asked about medication taken before the pregnancy was suspected, as well as any unprotected exposure to x rays. The form of contraception at the time of conception needs to be established, and women should be asked if an intrauterine device (IUD) is in place.

• Family medical history, including ethnicity. Women may need screening if there is a family history of sickle cell disease, Tay-Sachs, cystic fibrosis, or thalassemia. Sometimes there is no family history but testing is still important if suggested by ethnic heritage. Women should be asked if there is a family history of retardation, developmental delay, reproductive loss, or other issues.

• Information about work, lifestyle, and hobbies. This information can be helpful in understanding potential

Common prenatal tests

Test	What it is	How it is done
Amniocentesis (AM-nee-oh-sen-TEE-suhss)	This test can diagnosis certain birth defects, including: • Down syndrome • Cystic fibrosis • Spina bifida It is performed at 14 to 20 weeks. It may be suggested for couples at higher risk for genetic disorders. It also provides DNA for paternity testing.	A thin needle is used to draw out a small amount of amniotic fluid and cells from the sac surrounding the fetus. The sample is sent to a lab for testing.
Biophysical profile (BPP)	This test is used in the third trimester to monitor the overall health of the baby and to help decide if the baby should be delivered early.	BPP involves an ultrasound exam along with a nonstress test. The BPP looks at the baby's breathing, movement, muscle tone, heart rate, and the amount of amniotic fluid.
Chorionic villus (KOR-ee-ON-ihk VIL-uhss) sampling (CVS)	A test done at 10 to 13 weeks to diagnose certain birth defects, including: • Chromosomal disorders, including Down syndrome • Genetic disorders, such as cystic fibrosis CVS may be suggested for couples at higher risk for genetic disorders. It also provides DNA for paternity testing.	A needle removes a small sample of cells from the placenta to be tested.
First trimester screen	A screening test done at 11 to 14 weeks to detect higher risk of: • Chromosomal disorders, including Down syndrome and trisomy 18 • Other problems, such as heart defects It also can reveal multiple births. Based on test results, your doctor may suggest other tests to diagnose a disorder.	This test involves both a blood test and an ultrasound exam called nuchal translucency (NOO-kuhl trans-LOO-sent-see) screening. The blood test measures the levels of certain substances in the mother's blood. The ultrasound exam measures the thickness at the back of the baby's neck. This information, combined with the mother's age, help doctors determine risk to the fetus.
Glucose challenge screening	A screening test done at 26 to 28 weeks to determine the mother's risk of gestational diabetes. Based on test results, your doctor may suggest a glucose tolerance test.	First, you consume a special sugary drink from your doctor. A blood sample is taken one hour later to look for high blood sugar levels.
Glucose tolerance test	This test is done at 26 to 28 weeks to diagnose gestational diabetes.	Your doctor will tell you what to eat a few days before the test. Then, you cannot eat or drink anything but sips of water for 14 hours before the test. Your blood is drawn to test your "fasting blood glucose level." Then, you will consume a sugary drink. Your blood will be tested every hour for three hours to see how well your body processes sugar.
Group B streptococcus (STREP-tuh-KOK-uhss) infection	This test is done at 36 to 37 weeks to look for bacteria that can cause pneumonia or serious infection in newborn.	A swab is used to take cells from your vagina and rectum to be tested.
Maternal serum screen (also called quad screen, triple test, triple screen, multiple marker screen, or AFP)	A screening test done at 15 to 20 weeks to detect higher risk of: • Chromosomal disorders, including Down syndrome and trisomy 18 • Neural tube defects, such as spina bifida Based on test results, your doctor may suggest other tests to diagnose a disorder.	Blood is drawn to measure the levels of certain substances in the mother's blood.

[continued]

risks for the pregnancy, such as alcohol, tobacco, or drug use, work- and hobby-related risks of chemical exposure or physical hazards, exercise patterns, possible exposure to Lyme disease, and nutritional intake. Does the woman's work require heavy lifting or continually standing in one place? Could she be exposed to chemicals that could be teratogenic to the fetus? Does the woman have cats or work in a veterinary office? (Toxoplasmosis is spread through soil, undercooked meat, and cat stool. Pregnant women should avoid contact with used cat litter, sand, or soil.)

• Information about exercise habits. Exercise during pregnancy helps with stress and anxiety, and most women can maintain their prepregnancy exercise routines during pregnancy. However, they need to avoid overheating, as this is harmful to the fetus.

Common prenatal tests

Test	What it is	How it is done
Nonstress test (NST)	This test is performed after 28 weeks to monitor your baby's health. It can show signs of fetal distress, such as your baby not getting enough oxygen.	A belt is placed around the mother's belly to measure the baby's heart rate in response to its own movements.
Ultrasound exam	An ultrasound exam can be performed at any point during the pregnancy. Ultrasound exams are not routine. But it is not uncommon for women to have a standard ultrasound exam between 18 and 20 weeks to look for signs of problems with the baby's organs and body systems and confirm the age of the fetus and proper growth. It also might be able to tell the sex of your baby. Ultrasound exam is also used as part of the first trimester screen and biophysical profile (BPP). Based on exam results, your doctor may suggest other tests or other types of ultrasound to help detect a problem.	Ultrasound uses sound waves to create a "picture" of your baby on a monitor. With a standard ultrasound, a gel is spread on your abdomen. A special tool is moved over your abdomen, which allows your doctor and you to view the baby on a monitor.
Urine test	A urine sample can look for signs of health problems, such as: • Urinary tract infection • Diabetes • Preeclampsia If your doctor suspects a problem, the sample might be sent to a lab for more in-depth testing.	You will collect a small sample of clean, midstream urine in a sterile plastic cup. Testing strips that look for certain substances in your urine are dipped in the sample. The sample also can be looked at under a microscope.

SOURCE: U.S. Department of Health and Human Services Office on Women's Health. womenshealth.gov, 2010.

Overheating includes the use of saunas, hot tubs, and tanning beds. Exercise with potential trauma to the abdomen should be avoided. Exercise may be contraindicated in the case of intrauterine growth retardation, once the membranes have ruptured, vaginal bleeding, or for women at increased risk for preterm labor.

• Social factors and support structure. The extent of the woman's support network should also be assessed. Does she have other children? Is she the primary caregiver for an ailing parent? Does she have a partner who will be able to help her during the pregnancy?

• A verbal review of body systems, from head to toe. These questions may prompt a woman to remember or include information that she otherwise may have discounted as unimportant. It also establishes a baseline of her medical condition, especially if she develops symptoms later on in the pregnancy.

• Physical exam. The physical exam on the first visit will include a head-to-toe assessment in order to establish the presence of any abnormal or unusual findings, along with height, weight, and blood pressure. Women might be encouraged to continue, or begin, monthly breast self-exams for signs of lumps, and to report any physical changes such as thyroid enlargement or the development of varicose veins.

• Pelvic exam. The pelvic exam begins with an assessment of the external genitalia for any signs of redness, infection, vaginal discharge, or lesions. It will include a Pap smear for cervical cancer, as well as an assessment of the vaginal walls and cervix, checking for any growths, lesions, or signs of infection. The pregnancy will be confirmed by checking for changes in the uterine size. A bimanual exam allows the practitioner to check the uterus as well as the ovaries. A rectal exam checks for any rectal masses. The presence of hemorrhoids will also be noted. Cultures may be taken to check for infection or an undiagnosed sexually transmitted disease (STD), such as gonorrhea or chlamydia. Left untreated, these infections can be harmful to the mother and fetus. During the first visit, the practitioner may also evaluate the adequacy of the pelvic size and shape for vaginal delivery.

• Fetal heart tones can be heard by 10 to 12 weeks' gestation. The normal fetal heart rate is 120 to 160 beats per minute. The fundal height will be measured at each visit to chart the growth pattern of the uterus.

• Laboratory work may include a urinalysis, complete blood count, rubella antibody titer, and blood type with Rh factor. Testing for hepatitis B is common. Women should be offered the option of HIV screening, as early detection can provide the opportunity of using medication to decrease the risk of transmission to the fetus. Additional screening may be done for toxoplasmosis, cytomegalovirus, herpes simplex, or group B streptococci.

Normal physical changes to expect during pregnancy should be discussed. The pregnant woman should also be given the emergency number to call when the health facility is closed, along with guidelines about when it is appropriate to call. Teaching about the use of over-the-counter medications should be done, as many people are not aware that nonprescription drugs can be harmful to the developing fetus. Before leaving from the first prenatal visit, the next appointment should be scheduled, to encourage ongoing care.

Subsequent prenatal visits are considerably shorter, unless complications arise. A routine visit includes a urine check for protein, glucose, and possibly ketones; a weight and blood-pressure check; and measurement of fundal height. At each visit the woman should be asked if she is experiencing any of the common discomforts of pregnancy, such as ankle **edema** (swelling), leg cramps, Braxton-Hicks contractions, fatigue, backache, nausea or vomiting, constipation, or shortness of breath. In the first trimester, and again toward the end of pregnancy, the uterus applies pressure on the bladder, possibly resulting in the need for frequent urination. If frequency is accompanied by burning or **pain** with urination, a urinary tract **infection** should be ruled out.

While nausea and vomiting are common until the fourth or fifth month of pregnancy, excessive vomiting can result in **dehydration** and electrolyte imbalance. Sometimes hospitalization is required. The new mother should also be educated about signs that might indicate a developing problem, such as **abdominal pain** (perhaps indicative of an ectopic pregnancy), edema in the face (**preeclampsia**), headaches, blurred **vision**, vaginal bleeding, continual vomiting, decrease in fetal movement, or presence of vaginal fluid (rupture of the amniotic membranes).

An opportunity should be provided to answer any questions the woman might have. Attendance at **childbirth** and/or parenting classes, and access to classes for older siblings, should be discussed. The pregnant woman should also be assessed for signs of depression. As the pregnancy progresses, lying supine can cause the uterus to compress the vena cava, impeding blood flow to the **heart**. This may be experienced as an irregular heart rate or a feeling of **anxiety**. Lying on the left side resolves this problem.

Pregnant women should be encouraged to eat a wide variety of nutritious foods. Women whose prepregnancy weight is within an appropriate range for height should expect to gain about 25–35 pounds (11–16 kg) over the course of the pregnancy. Those who are overweight should gain less, but not try to diet while pregnant. Pica, or the desire to eat nonfood substances, may not cause harm to the fetus if the substances themselves are not harmful and the woman otherwise is eating a balanced diet. Questions to assess for pica should be part of routine visits. A woman's financial situation can affect her ability to purchase nutritious foods. This need should be assessed at the first visit so that an appropriate referral can be made for food stamps, the Women, Infants and Children (WIC) supplemental food program, or other assistance programs. The use of megavitamins should be evaluated, as high doses of fat-soluble **vitamins** can be harmful. Intake of high doses of **vitamin A** is associated with **birth defects**.

At 10 to 18 weeks, **genetic counseling** may be provided for women with a family history of congenital, chromosomal, or neural-tube anomalies, or for women above age 35. Chorionic villi sampling (CVS) may be done between 10 and 12 weeks, while **amniocentesis** may be performed between 14 and 18 weeks. Ultrasound may be done between 12 and 24 weeks to confirm dating of the pregnancy or to check fetal **anatomy**.

A **triple marker screen test** that evaluates maternal serum alpha-fetoprotein, human chorionic gonadotropin (hCG), and unconjugated estriol levels is usually run on a blood sample between 16 and 20 weeks to screen for neural-tube defects. Inadequate intake of **folic acid** is associated with neural-tube defects, such as spina bifida. Elevated levels of alpha fetoprotein may indicate a neural-tube defect, but can also be due to a **multiple pregnancy**, inaccurate dates, or fetal death. The test can also indicate if the fetus has Down's syndrome. As with other laboratory tests, false positives can occur.

At 20 to 22 weeks, women should be aware of the danger of premature rupture of the membranes and **preterm labor**. Fundal height should be at the umbilicus.

Screening for **gestational diabetes** is done around 26 to 28 weeks. The first screening test does not require fasting, and blood is drawn once, an hour after a drink containing 50 gm of glucose is ingested. If the result is abnormal in any way, a three-hour glucose tolerance test (GTT) will be administered. This test is usually done in the morning, after the woman has fasted for eight hours. A sample for the FBS (fasting blood sugar) test is drawn, glucose is given, and blood is then drawn hourly over the next three hours. Babies of mothers with gestational diabetes are at risk of excessive intrauterine growth, and blood sugar abnormalities after birth. While gestational diabetes (GDM) usually resolves when the pregnancy terminates, women with GDM are at increased risk—about 60%—of developing diabetes within the next 16 years.

From 28 weeks to 34 weeks onward, fetal presentation (position) will be checked at each visit.

After 36 weeks the physician may choose to conduct a sterile internal exam to evaluate the condition of the cervix for labor and delivery.

From 40 to 42 weeks fetal well-being and the amount of amniotic fluid may be monitored more closely. Too little or too much may indicate problems. Induction of labor will be considered.

Preparation

In coming to the first prenatal visit, it is helpful for the woman to bring in:

• Medical records from a previous pregnancy not easily accessible by the current practitioner or facility, especially if complications arose.

• Information on family medical history as well as personal medical history.

• Date of last menstrual period.

• Names and dosages of any medications currently being taken (both prescription and over-the-counter products, including any herbal remedies and dietary supplements).

• A list of any questions she may have.

At the first visit, a physical exam will be performed. In preparation, the woman will need to undress, put on a gown, and empty her bladder. (The pelvic exam puts pressure on the bladder, creating discomfort if full.) This may be the first pelvic exam for some women; they should be told what to expect before anything is done. Proper draping can help ease discomfort. For the pelvic exam, the woman will need to lie on her back, with her feet in stirrups. Warming the speculum prevents the woman from tensing as the speculum is inserted.

If an ultrasound is to be done, the woman will need to drink about a quart of water one to two hours prior to the test, without voiding, in order to better visualize the fetal structures. Later in the pregnancy, when there is more amniotic fluid, this will not be necessary. While the ultrasound is painless, having a full bladder can become quite uncomfortable. The nurse or **radiology** technician

---

KEY TERMS

Braxton-Hicks contractions—Irregular tightening of the uterus that begins in the first trimester of pregnancy. The contractions increase in frequency and strength as the pregnancy progresses and may be confused for labor contractions toward the end of the pregnancy. They are sometimes referred to as "false labor pains."

Fundal height—Measured by a tape measure from the top of the symphysis pubis, over the arch of the growing uterus, to the top of the fundus.

Gestation—The length of the pregnancy, from fertilization until birth.

Sickle cell disease—A form of anemia characterized by crescent-shaped red blood cells containing an abnormal form of hemoglobin. Physical symptoms of crisis include fever, joint pain, and weakness. It is most common in people of African American, Mediterranean, Latin American, and Native American descent.

Tay-Sachs disease—A genetic disorder resulting in the progressive degeneration of the central nervous system. It is found primarily in individuals of Eastern European Ashkenazi Jewish descent.

Thalassemia—A genetic-based anemia in which the red blood cells are easily destroyed and release iron into the blood system, which then deposits it in the skin and internal organs. Thalassemia is most commonly found in individuals of Mediterranean, Middle Eastern, and Asian descent.

---

should ensure that the test can begin on time whenever possible.

If a woman is considering an amniocentesis or chorionic villi sampling, she should understand the risks accompanying these procedures (which include a slightly increased chance of **miscarriage**), the information that can be expected, and the options available if abnormal results are found.

Aftercare

After a woman has an internal exam, she should be given a tissue to remove lubricant used for the exam. A sanitary pad may be offered if spotting

QUESTIONS TO ASK YOUR DOCTOR

1. How often should I come in for prenatal care?

2. Who should I call if there is a problem and this office is closed?

3. Can you recommend any parenting classes in this area?

4. Do I currently engage in any behaviors that might put me or my baby at risk?

5. Are the medications I am currently taking safe for my baby?

6. Would you suggest that I receive genetic counseling?

occurred. If abnormal results have been reported, the woman or her partner may need additional time to ask questions, receive appropriate referral information, or be consoled.

Complications

At each visit, weight, **blood pressure**, and urine are checked. A rapid weight gain, increased blood pressure, and proteinuria signal the development of preeclampsia. Vaginal bleeding at any time during pregnancy needs evaluation. Third-trimester bleeding may indicate **placenta previa** or **placental abruption**, two conditions that put the fetus at risk. Sharp abdominal pain may indicate an ectopic pregnancy; the woman needs to be evaluated right away should such pain occur. An ectopic pregnancy can result in rupture of the fallopian tube and internal bleeding. A gush of fluid from the vagina can signal the rupture of the amniotic membranes. If the rupture occurs at the end of pregnancy, it may indicate that labor is about to begin. However, once the membranes have ruptured, the uterus is more easily exposed to infection. Without adequate amniotic fluid, the umbilical cord can prolapse, reducing the oxygen flow to the fetus. Loss of fluid needs to be evaluated to determine if it was due to ruptured membranes or **stress** incontinence.

Results

The goal of prenatal care is the delivery of a healthy baby at term, from a healthy mother prepared to handle the challenges of parenthood.

Health care team roles

Nurses, dieticians, social workers, childbirth educators, midwives, nurse practitioners, obstetricians, and perinatologists play important roles in prenatal care, through careful listening both to what is said and what may be omitted, thorough assessment and documentation, and education and referral. Radiology technicians will see the woman during ultrasound, amniocentesis, and chorionic villi sampling, at a time when she may be anxious about the test being performed. Laboratory technicians may see the woman at the end of a difficult visit, perhaps after she has received bad news or is anxious about an upcoming test. If the pregnant woman is dehydrated, venous access is more challenging to obtain. Providing an understanding, reassuring, and calm environment, and utilizing one's experience to perform the task at hand with the greatest of skill, can minimize any further sense of trauma.

Resources

BOOKS

Harms, Roger, and Wick, Myra, eds. *Mayo Clinic Guide to a Healthy Pregnancy.* Intercourse, PA: Good Books, 2011.

Hawkins, Joellen, W., Roberto-Nichols, Diane M., and Stanley-Haney, J. Lynn. *Guidelines for Nurse Practitioners in Gynecologic Settings,* 10th ed. New York: Springer Publishing, 2012.

Murray, Linda J., ed. *Pregnancy: From Preconception to Birth.* New York: DK Publishing, 2010.

PERIODICALS

Denison, Fiona C., and Chiswick, Carolyn. "Improving Pregnancy Outcomes in Obese Women." *Proceedings of the Nutrition Society,* (November 2011) 70 (4):457–464.

Saravelos, Sotirios H., and Regan, Lesley. "The Importance of Preconception Counseling and Early Pregnancy Monitoring." *Seminars in Reproductive Medicine,* (November 2011) 29(6):557–568.

OTHER

"Group Prenatal Care: Consider the Options. Mary M. Murry (The Mayo Clinic)." [accessed April 16, 2012] http://www.mayoclinic.com/health/group-prenatal-care/MY01336

"Prenatal Care Fact Sheet?" WomensHealth.Gov, The United States Department of Health and Human Services Office on Women's Health. [accessed April 16, 2012]. http://www.womenshealth.gov/publications/our-publications/fact-sheet/prenatal-care.cfm

ORGANIZATIONS

American College of Nurse-Midwives, 8403 Colesville Road, Suite 1550, Silver Spring, MD 20910, (240) 485-1800, Fax: (240) 485-1818, www.midwife.org

American College of Obstetricians and Gynecologists, PO Box 70620, Washington, DC 20024-9998, (202) 638-5577, (800) 673-8444, resources@acog.org, www.acog.org

Association of Women's Health, Obstetric and Neonatal Nurses, 2000 L Street, NW, Suite 740, Washington, DC 20036, (202) 261-2400, (800) 673-8499, Fax: (202) 728-0575, customerservice@awhonn.org, www.awhonn.org.

Esther Csapo Rastegari, R.N., B.S.N., Ed.M.
Tish Davidson, AM

Prenatal nutrition

Definition

Maternal **nutrition** during **pregnancy** affects both the health of the mother and the growing fetus. Requirements for calories and specific nutrients are increased for the baby's growth and proper development. These needs can be met by increasing healthful food consumption and specific nutrient supplementation.

Purpose

Proper prenatal nutrition helps ensure a healthy start for a new baby and promotes the mother's well-being during and after pregnancy. Nurses and other allied health professionals can play a role in educating pregnant women about sufficient weight gain, the importance of a healthy diet, and the following recommendations for supplementation.

Precautions

Maternal weight gain during pregnancy is an important predictor of a baby's birth weight. The height and weight of the mother before pregnancy should be taken into account when assessing maternal nutrient needs. Both underweight and excessively overweight women need special attention. Underweight women are more likely to give birth to premature or low birth-weight infants, while overweight women have an increased risk of developing pregnancy-related complications. Other high-risk groups for low birth-weight babies include women younger than 15 and those older than 35. Women whose pregnancies are fewer than 12 months apart are also at higher risk.

Description

Maternal weight gain is a measure often used to assess how well a pregnancy is progressing. Normal weight gain is considered to be 25–35 pounds (11–16 kg), although individual needs should also be taken into account. Women who are underweight to start with may benefit from gaining more (28–40 pounds; 13–18 kg), while overweight women may try to gain less (15–25 pounds; 7–11 kg). Even for overweight women, however, weight gain is important to allow for proper growth of the fetus.

Nutrient needs during pregnancy depend on physical activity and **metabolism** of the mother. For most women, energy needs increase to about 300 extra calories per day during the second and third trimesters. Protein needs increase to allow for new tissue growth and maintenance; deficiency can result in a lower birth weight. An extra 10 to 12 grams of protein per day is recommended during the last half of pregnancy.

Vitamin and mineral requirements are also increased during pregnancy. To meet those needs, most women in the United States are advised to take a multivitamin supplement with **minerals** while they are pregnant. Eating a well-balanced diet with plenty of fruits, vegetables, and whole grains will also help provide the needed **vitamins**. **Iron** and **calcium** are two minerals of special concern. The fetus acquires most of these minerals during the last trimester of the pregnancy. Doctors recommend daily supplementation of 30 mg of iron in the form of ferrous sulfate to avoid **iron deficiency anemia**, which can cause excessive tiredness in the mother. Calcium intake should be 1,200–1,500 mg per day, which can be obtained through diet or supplementation. Adequate calcium is important so that the mother does not lose **bone** mass during pregnancy. There is also some evidence that calcium supplementation reduces the risk of pregnancy-induced **hypertension**, also known as **preeclampsia**, for women who are at high risk for this condition.

Folate (**folic acid**) is an extremely important vitamin, not only during pregnancy, but before pregnancy as well. Folate is crucial to the development of new cells, and deficiency during pregnancy has been associated with the development of congenital malformations known as neural tube defects (NTDs). The most serious NTDs include spina bifida and anencephaly. Spina bifida is characterized by gaps in the spine, typically resulting in serious lifelong disability. An infant with anencephaly lacks **brain** formation and dies shortly after birth. Because NTDs arise early in pregnancy, before most women know they are pregnant, the United States **Public Health** Service recommends that all women of childbearing age consume 400–800 micrograms of folic acid daily. Adequate amounts of folate can be obtained from the diet, but in practice, most women do not consume enough. To help address this problem, in 1996 the United States Food and Drug Administration (FDA) approved folate fortification of flour, breads, cereal, and rice.

Complications

Good nutrition is especially important for certain conditions during pregnancy. Diabetes, a disease of poor **blood** sugar regulation, is one common problem requiring special attention to diet. Some women develop it only during pregnancy, when it is termed **gestational diabetes**. It can lead to multiple complications, including abnormally enhanced growth of the fetus, a condition called macrosomia. Such babies need special care at birth until blood sugar levels can be brought under control. Control of gestational diabetes includes careful attention to diet so that maternal blood sugar levels are kept as normal as possible throughout pregnancy. Women should eat frequent small meals, select foods high in fiber and complex **carbohydrates**, and avoid highly refined foods and simple sugars.

Another common problem is nausea and **vomiting** in early pregnancy. Because hunger seems to exacerbate the problem, suggestions to alleviate nausea include eating small, frequent meals of easily digestible foods, and having dry crackers near the bed to eat immediately upon awakening. Some women have severe enough symptoms that they are in danger of weight loss, **dehydration**, and electrolyte disturbances. This condition, termed hyperemesis gravidarum, may require hospitalization or medications to treat it if simple nutritional measures cannot control it.

Phenylketonuria (PKU) is a more unusual condition, but it is one in which the importance of maternal nutrition is paramount. PKU and the related condition, hyperphenylalanemia (HPA), are genetic disorders involving the impairment of the ability to digest phenylalanine, an essential amino acid found in protein. Before the disease was recognized, people with PKU developed severe mental retardation in childhood. Since routine screening and early dietary treatment has been instituted, people with PKU now can develop normally. However, women with these conditions may be advised not to become pregnant because of the high risk of mental retardation and congenital defects in the developing fetus. Women who desire

---

KEY TERMS

Congenital malformations—Deformities that occur at birth.

Gestational diabetes—A disorder occurring in pregnancy involving insensitivity to insulin, causing poor blood sugar regulation.

Hyperemesis gravidarum—Excessive vomiting during pregnancy.

Macrosomia—An abnormally large body. Macrosomia of the newborn is a common complication of gestational diabetes.

Phenylketonuria (PKU)—A congenital deficiency of an enzyme that aids in the breakdown of an amino acid, leading to the development of severe mental retardation. PKU can be controlled with a strict diet, which is especially critical during pregnancy of a mother with PKU to avoid physical and mental defects in the fetus.

Pica—A desire that sometimes arises in pregnancy to eat nonfood substances, such as dirt or clay.

Preeclampsia—A syndrome of high blood pressure that develops during pregnancy. The chief danger of preeclampsia is that it will progress to eclampsia, which is a life-threatening condition characterized by seizures.

---

pregnancy should discuss their plans with health personnel in a clinic that specializes in the treatment of these disorders well before becoming pregnant, so that strict dietary measures can be taken before conception and throughout pregnancy.

An abnormal food behavior that sometimes occurs in pregnant women is pica, which involves the consumption of nonfood items such as cornstarch, dirt, hair, cigarette ashes, or coffee grounds. Pica is sometimes associated with iron deficiency, and some think that the consumption of these substances may relieve the nausea and vomiting associated with pregnancy. Although many of these substances are not inherently harmful, there is a concern that such habits may displace the intake of nutritious foods during pregnancy.

Alcohol consumption during pregnancy can result in **fetal alcohol syndrome** (FAS), characterized by varying degrees of numerous physical and mental problems, including mental retardation, facial

QUESTIONS TO ASK YOUR DOCTOR

- How far before trying to conceive should I start taking a folic acid supplement?

- How much weight on average should I gain in each trimester?

- Since I have diabetes, what specific alterations should I mane in my diet and insulin use?

- Will any of the medications I take interfere with the uptake of nutrients during pregnancy?

abnormalities, and **heart** and skeletal defects. Because of the unpredictable effects of even small amounts of alcohol, women are advised to drink no alcohol at any time during pregnancy.

Quitting **smoking** and avoiding second-hand smoke is especially important during pregnancy. Exposure to tobacco smoke increases the risk of a low birth-weight infant.

The effect of food additives is controversial, but some doctors recommend that sugar substitutes, including saccharin and aspartame, be used in moderation if at all. **Caffeine** consumption during pregnancy is another debatable issue. Pregnant women are cautioned not consume excessive amounts of caffeine, as levels above about 300 mg/day have been linked with low birth weight and **miscarriage**. Caffeine occurs in a range of food and drinks such as coffee, tea, soft drinks, and chocolate. In the UK, the Food Standards Agency recommends that pregnant women should not drink more than the equivalent of around four average cups of coffee a day. Many physicians in the United States recommend limiting caffeine to the equivalent of one or two cup of coffee daily.

Especially for teenagers and young women, eating disorders may be of concern. **Anorexia nervosa**, **bulimia nervosa** (characterized by episodes of binge eating and vomiting), use of **laxatives**, or excessive exercising pose a serious risk to the mother and the fetus. Poor weight gain during pregnancy may indicate the presence of an eating disorder.

Results

Good nutrition and adequate weight gain in pregnancy increase the likelihood that the mother will feel her best during pregnancy and that a healthy baby will be born with a normal birth weight. Specific nutrient deficiencies can lead to **birth defects**, as is well documented for folic acid; or health consequences to the mother (e.g., calcium deficiency's possible role in preeclampsia). In addition, nutritional intervention is the treatment of choice for several conditions, including gestational diabetes, nausea and vomiting in pregnancy, and maternal PKU.

Health care team roles

Dietetic professionals, nurse practitioners, nurse midwives, and physicians play an important role in the **prenatal care** of pregnant women. Dietitians can provide the nutrition counseling and education necessary to ensure the normal growth and development of the fetus. They can warn women about the dangers of improper food intake and the outcome it may have on pregnancy. Physicians are primarily responsible for determining that the fetus is growing properly and for detecting and monitoring medical conditions. In uncomplicated pregnancies, nurse practitioners and nurse midwives may play a more prominent role in prenatal care.

Resources

BOOKS

Agricultural Research Service. *Report of the Dietary Guidelines Advisory Committee on the Dietary Guidelines for Americans, 2010.* US Department of Agriculture, U.S. Department of Health and Human Services, 2010.

Peterson, Wendy Jo and Michael Bushong. *Pregnancy Cooking and Nutrition For Dummies.* Indianapolis, IN: Wiley Pub., 2011.

Ward, Elizabeth M. and the American Dietetic Association. *Expect the Best: Your Guide to Healthy Eating Before, During, and After Pregnancy.* Hoboken, NJ: Wiley, 2009.

OTHER

Center for Nutrition Policy and Promotion. January 26, 2012 [accessed February 13, 2012]. http://www.cnpp. usda.gov

March of Dimes. Your Healthy Diet During Pregnancy. MarchofDimes.com September 2009 [accessed February 13, 2012]. http://www.marchofdimes.com/pregnancy/ nutrition_indepth.html

Mayo Clinic Staff. Pregnancy Diet: Focus on These Essential Nutrients. May 21, 2011 [accessed February 13, 2012]. http://www.mayoclinic.com/health/pregnancy-nutrition/ PR00110

United States Department of Agriculture. MyPlate. October 21, 2011 [accessed February 13, 2012]. http://www. choosemyplate.gov

ORGANIZATIONS

American Dietetic Association, 120 South Riverside Plaza, Suite 2000, Chicago, IL 60606-6995, (800) 877-1600, http://www.eatright.org

British Nutrition Foundation, High Holborn House, 52-54 High Holborn, London, United Kingdom WC1V 6RQ, 020 7404 6504, Fax: 020 7404 6747, postbox@nutrition. org.uk, http://www.nutrition.org.uk

National Women's Health Network, 1413 K Street, NW, 4th floor, Washington.

Lisa M. Gourley
Tish Davidson, AM

Preoperative care

Definition

Preoperative care is the preparation and management of a patient prior to surgery. It includes both physical and psychological preparation.

Purpose

Patients who are physically and psychologically prepared for surgery tend to have better outcomes after surgery. Preoperative teaching meets the patient's need for information regarding the surgical experience, which in turn may alleviate any fear that the patient is experiencing. Knowing what to expect after the surgery, and enlisting the patient's input about goals and expectations, often helps the patient cope better with postoperative **pain** and decreased mobility. Preoperative care is extremely important prior to any invasive procedure, regardless of whether the procedure is minimally invasive or major surgery.

Precautions

There are no contraindications to preoperative care. Even in an emergent situation, the patient must be physically prepared and should be prepared psychologically to the degree possible, as indicated by the patient's physical status. If the patient is unresponsive, emotional and psychological preparation should be focused on the family.

Preoperative teaching must be individualized for each patient, since some people want as much information as possible while others only want the minimum. For some patients, receiving too much information increases their **anxiety**. Patients have different capabilities in understanding medical procedures; if printed materials are used for teaching, the nurse must ascertain the patient's literacy level in order to provide appropriate material. The health care professional must maintain a balance between relaying essential information and meeting the patient's information needs.

Description

Preoperative care involves many components and may be done the day before surgery, in the hospital, or during the weeks before surgery on an outpatient basis. Many surgical procedures are now performed in a day-surgery setting and the patient is never admitted to the hospital.

Physical preparation

Physical preparation should include obtaining a complete history and physical, including the patient's surgical and anesthesia history. It should be determined if the patient has ever had an adverse reaction to anesthesia (such as anaphylactic **shock**), or if there is a family history of malignant hyperthermia. Laboratory tests such as CBC, electrolytes, prothrombin time, activated partial thromboplastin time, or **urinalysis** may be done. An EKG should be done if the patient has a history of cardiac disease or is over 50 years of age. A chest X-ray should be taken if the patient has a history of respiratory disease. The patient should be assessed for risk factors that might impair healing, such as nutritional deficits, steroid use, radiation or **chemotherapy**, drug or alcohol abuse, or metabolic diseases such as diabetes. The patient should also provide a list of all medications, **vitamins**, and herbal or food supplements that they use. Supplements are often overlooked, but some can cause adverse effects when used with general anesthetics (e.g. St John's wort, valerian root) and others can prolong bleeding time (e.g. garlic, gingko biloba).

Latex allergy merits mention because it is becoming a **public health** concern. Latex is found in most sterile surgical gloves and is a common component in other medical supplies, including **general anesthesia** masks, tubing, and multi-dose medication vials. It is estimated that 1–6% of the general population and 8–17% of health care workers have this allergy. At least 50% of children with spina bifida are latex sensitive as a result of early, frequent surgical exposure. There is currently no cure available for latex allergy, and research has found that up to 19% of all anaphylactic reactions during surgery may be a result of latex allergy. The best treatment is prevention, but immediate symptomatic treatment is required if the allergic response occurs. Every patient should be assessed for a potential latex reaction. Patients with latex sensitivity should have their chart flagged with a caution label. Latex-free gloves and supplies must be used for anyone with a documented latex allergy.

Bowel clearance may be ordered if the patient is having surgery of the lower gastrointestinal (GI) tract. The patient should start the bowel preparation early in the evening to prevent interrupted sleep during the night. Some patients may benefit from a sleeping pill the night before surgery.

Often skin preparation is ordered for the night before surgery. Skin preparation can take the form of scrubbing with a special soap (i.e., Hibiclens), or hair removal from the surgical area. However, shaving hair is no longer recommended because studies show that shaving the area may increase the chance of **infection**. Instead, adhesive barrier drapes can contain hair growth on the skin around the incision.

Psychological preparation

Patients are often fearful or anxious about having surgery. Health care workers can help decrease anxiety by listening to the patient's concerns, validating their legitimacy, and answering the patient's questions honestly. This process can be especially beneficial for patients who are critically ill or who are having a high-risk procedure. The family needs to be included in psychological preoperative care as much as the patient. In the hospital, pastoral care can be offered. If the patient expresses a fear of dying during surgery, this concern should not be discounted. The surgeon should be notified. In some cases, the procedure may be postponed until the patient feels more secure.

Children may be especially fearful. They should be allowed to have a parent with them as much as possible, as long as the parent is not demonstrably fearful and contributing to the child's apprehension. Children should also be encouraged to bring a favorite toy or blanket with them on the day of surgery.

Preparing the patient and family psychologically helps them to cope better with the patient's postoperative course. Preparation leads to superior outcomes, since the goals of recovery are known ahead of time and the patient is able to manage postoperative pain more effectively.

Informed consent

Obtaining the patient's or guardian's written consent for the surgery is a vital portion of preoperative care. By law, the physician who will perform the procedure must explain the risks and benefits of the surgery, along with other treatment options. However, the nurse is often the person who actually witnesses the patient's signature on the consent form. The nurse should verify that the patient

understands everything the physician told them by asking the patient to explain what they have been told.

Patients who are mentally impaired, heavily sedated, or critically ill are not considered legally able to give consent. In this situation, the next of kin (spouse, adult child, adult sibling, or person with medical **power of attorney**) may act as a surrogate and sign the consent form. Children under age 18 must have a parent or guardian sign.

Preoperative teaching

Preoperative teaching includes teaching about the preoperative period, the surgery itself, and the postoperative period.

Instruction about the preoperative period deals primarily with where the patient should go on the day of surgery, the time they should arrive, and how they should prepare for surgery. For example, they should be told how long they should be NPO (nothing by mouth), which medications to take prior to surgery, and the medications that should be brought with them (such as inhalers for patients with **asthma**).

Instruction about the surgery itself includes informing the patient about what will be done during the surgery and how long it is expected to take. The patient should be told where the incision would be. Children having surgery should be allowed to "practice" on a doll or stuffed animal. It may be helpful to demonstrate procedures on the doll prior to doing them on the child. It is also important to tell the family (or other concerned parties) where they can wait during the surgery, when they can expect progress information (and from whom), and how long it will be before they can see the patient.

Informing the patient about what to expect during the postoperative period is one of the best ways to improve the patient's outcome. Instruction about expected activities can also increase compliance and help prevent complications. This includes the opportunity for the patient to practice coughing and deep breathing exercises, use an incentive spirometer, and practice splinting the incision. Additionally, the patient should be informed about early ambulation, The patient should also be taught that the respiratory interventions decrease the occurrence of **pneumonia** and that early leg exercises and ambulation decrease the risk of **blood** clots.

Patients hospitalized postoperatively should be informed about the tubes and equipment that they will have. These may include multiple IV lines, drainage tubes, dressings, and monitoring devices. In addition, they may have sequential compression stockings on their legs to prevent blood clots until they start ambulating.

Pain management is the primary concern for many patients having surgery. Preoperative instruction should include information about the pain management method that they will utilize postoperatively. Patients should be encouraged to ask for or take pain medication before the pain becomes unbearable, and should be taught how to rate their pain on a pain scale. This instruction allows the patients, and others who may be assessing them, to evaluate the pain consistently. If they will be using a **patient-controlled analgesia** (PCA) pump, they should be taught how to use it during the preoperative period. Use of alternative methods of pain control (distraction, imagery, positioning, mindfulness **meditation**, **music therapy**) may also be presented.

Finally, long-term goals should be discussed, such as when the patient will be able to eat solid food, when they will be discharged if they are hospitalized, and when they will be able to drive a car or return to work.

Preparation

Preparation for preoperative care involves ensuring that all supplies for physical preparation are accessible. To prepare for teaching, any applicable patient handouts or videos should be gathered and offered to the patient. The consent form should be ready for the patient to sign, with the name of the physician and the procedure filled in. A sufficient amount of time should be scheduled so that the patient does not feel rushed, and the patient should understand that they have the right to add or strike

QUESTIONS TO ASK YOUR DOCTOR

- Can you tell me more about my upcoming surgical procedure?
- What are the risks and benefits of having my surgical procedure?
- What will happen during my preoperative care?
- How should I continue my care after I get home?

out items on the generic consent form that they do not wish to agree to. For example, a patient who is about to undergo a **tonsillectomy** might choose to strike out (and initial) an item that indicates sterility might be a complication of the operation.

Aftercare

The only aftercare required is to ensure that the patient understands the surgery and that all of their questions are answered.

Complications

Complications can result from improper preoperative care. For example, surgery may be done on the wrong side of the body if the incorrect body part is marked during physical preparation. Hospitalized patients may be given the wrong preoperative medications, or sedatives may be inadvertently given before **informed consent** is obtained.

Results

The anticipated outcome of preoperative care is a patient who is informed about their surgical course and able to cope with it successfully. The goal is to decrease complications and promote recovery.

Health care team roles

As mentioned above, the physician is legally responsible for discussing the risks and benefits of the procedure and for obtaining the patient's informed consent. However, the nurse is often the one who witnesses the patient's signature. If the nurses were not present for the physicians' discussions with the patients, the nurses must ensure that the patients understand the risks and benefits of the surgery by having the patients relate what they were told by their physician. The nurse is usually responsible for preoperative instruction, although a respiratory therapist often teaches about the postoperative respiratory exercises, especially in a hospital setting. Laboratory personnel may draw blood samples and perform laboratory tests. **Radiology** personnel perform the **chest x ray** if one is ordered.

Resources

BOOKS

Bailey, Elizabeth. *The Patient's Checklist: 10 Simple Hospital Checklists to Keep you Safe, Sane & Organized.*New York, NY: Sterling, 2012.

Melnyk, Bernadette M., and Ellen Fineout-Overholt. *Evidence-Based Practice in Nursing & Healthcare: A Guide to Best Practice,*2nd ed. New York, NY: Lippincott Williams & Wilkins, 2010.

Stewart, Brent., MD, MBA.*Need Surgery? Now What?: A Patient's Guide to Anesthesia.*Tampa, FL: Southern Medical Publishing, 2012.

PERIODICALS

Barnes, S. "Preparing for Surgery: Providing the Details." Journal of Perianesthesia Nursing 16, no. 1 (2001): 31-32.

Flanagan, K. "Preoperative Assessment: Safety Considerations for Patients Taking Herbal Products." Journal of Perianesthesia Nursing 16, no. 1 (2001): 19-26.

Olsen-Chavarriaga, D. "Informed Consent: Do You Know Your Role?" Nursing 2000 30, no. 5 (2000): 60-61.

ORGANIZATIONS

American Society of PeriAnesthesia Nurses (ASPAN). 90 Frontage Road, Cherry Hill, NJ 08034-1424. Telephone: (877) 737-9696. http://www.aspan.org/

Association of periOperative Registered Nurses. 2170 South Parker Rd, Suite 400, Denver, CO 80231. Telephone: (800) 755-2676. http://www.aorn.org/.

Abby Wojahn, RN, BSN, CCRN
Laura Jean Cataldo, RN, Ed.D.

Presbyopia

Definition

The term presbyopia means "older eye," and is a **vision** condition involving the loss of the eye's ability to focus on close objects.

Description

Presbyopia is a condition that occurs as a part of normal **aging**. The condition develops gradually over a number of years. Symptoms are usually noticeable by age

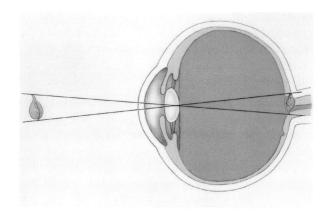

(June Hill Pedigo/CMSP)

40 to 45, and continue to develop until the process stabilizes some 10 or 20 years later. Presbyopia occurs without regard to other eye conditions.

Causes and symptoms

In the eye, the crystalline lens is located just behind the iris and the pupil. Tiny ciliary muscles pull and push the lens, adjusting its curvature, and thereby adjusting the eye's ability to bring objects into focus. As individuals age, the lens becomes less flexible and elastic, and the muscles become less powerful. Because these changes result in inadequate adjustment of the lens of the eye for various distances, objects that are close will appear blurry. The major cause of presbyopia is loss of elasticity of the lens of the eye. Loss of ciliary muscle power and loss of elasticity of the zonules that connect the ciliary muscle to the lens, however, are also believed to contribute to the problem.

Symptoms of presbyopia result in the inability to focus on objects close at hand. As the lens hardens, it is unable to focus the rays of light that come from near objects. Individuals typically have difficulty reading small print, such as that in telephone directories and newspaper advertisements, and may need to hold reading materials at arm's length. Symptoms include **headache** and eyestrain when doing close work, blurry vision, and eye fatigue. Symptoms may be worse early in the morning or when individuals are fatigued. Dim lighting may also aggravate the problem.

Diagnosis

Presbyopia is officially diagnosed during an **eye examination** conducted by optometrists (O.D.s) or ophthalmologists (M.D.s).

O.D.s or M.D.s, with the help of ophthalmic assistants, should perform a comprehensive eye exam to diagnose the condition. The assistant should take a detailed patient history prior to the exam. This is especially important when diagnosing premature presbyopia.

The optometrist or ophthalmologist, or in some cases a highly trained assistant, will begin the ocular examination by testing visual acuity and refraction. During the exam the clinician also will determine ocular motility and alignment, nearpoint of convergence, near fusional vergence amplitudes, relative accommodation measurements, accommodative amplitude and facility of accommodation.

To further determine presbyopia, the clinician should perform near retinoscopy and intermediate distance testing, which can be performed with a phoropter or trial lens.

There are five different types of presbyopia:

• Incipient presbyopia is the earliest stage in which symptoms are documented. Usually the patient has trouble reading small print, but may perform well on testing and may actually reject a near vision prescription.

• Functional presbyopia is the point at which patients usually notice the difficulties with near vision. The age when this occurs varies and depends on environment, task requirements, nutrition, and general health.

• Absolute presbyopia is the result of continuous gradual decline in accommodation, and is the next phase after functional presbyopia. At this stage, little accommodative ability remains.

• Premature presbyopia is the appearance of the disease at an earlier age than expected because of nutritional, environmental, or disease-related causes. Pharmaceuticals may also be a cause of premature presbyopia.

• Nocturnal presbyopia occurs when accommodation decreases in low-light conditions.

Treatment

Presbyopia cannot be cured, but physicians can help patients compensate for it by prescribing reading, bifocal, or trifocal eyeglasses. A convex lens is used to make up for the lost automatic focusing power of the eye. Half-glasses can be worn, which leave the top open and uncorrected for distance vision. Bifocals achieve the same goal by allowing correction of other refractive errors (improper focusing of images on the retina of the eye).

In addition to glasses, **contact lenses** can be useful in the treatment of presbyopia. Contact lens technicians need to take the patient's medical history to ensure the patient is a good candidate for contact lenses. Some lenses require a greater care commitment, so each patient's expectations need to be discussed before any lens is prescribed.

The two common types of contact lenses prescribed for presbyopia are bifocal and monovision contact lenses.

Bifocal lenses come in two designs, simultaneous vision and alternating vision. Soft and rigid lenses are available in the simultaneous vision design, but only RGP lenses are available in the alternating vision design. Alternating vision lenses behave more like bifocal eyeglasses than the simultaneous design. This alternating lens allows patients to look through two distinct visual zones and adjust their gaze for distance vision or for reading. To prevent rotation while in the eye, bifocal contact lenses use a specially manufactured type of lens. Good candidates for bifocal lenses are those patients who have a good tear film (moist eyes), good binocular vision (ability to focus both eyes together) and visual acuity in each eye, and no disease or abnormalities of the eyelids. The bifocal contact lens wearer must be motivated to invest the time it requires to maintain contact lenses and be involved in occupations that do not impose high visual demands. Further, bifocal contact lenses may limit binocular vision. Bifocal contact lenses are relatively expensive, in part due to the time it takes the patient to be accurately fitted.

An alternative to wearing eyeglasses or bifocal contact lenses is monovision contact lenses. Monovision fitting provides one contact lens that corrects for near vision and a second contact lens for the alternate eye that corrects for distance vision. If distance vision is normal, the individual wears only a single contact lens for near vision. Monovision works by having one eye focus for distant objects while the other eye becomes the reading eye. The **brain** learns to adapt to this and will automatically use the correct eye depending on the location of material in view. Advantages of monovision lenses are patient acceptability, convenience, and lower cost.

Several problems exist with the use of contact lenses in the treatment of presbyopia. Health care professionals need to ask patients to report any headache, fatigue, or decrease in visual acuity during the adjustment period. Monovision contact lenses usually result in a small reduction in high-contrast visual acuity and reduced depth perception as compared with bifocal contact lenses. In addition, since monovision corrects one eye for distance and one for eye for near vision, intermediate distances are often out of focus, especially in absolute presbyopia.

Some ophthalmologists are performing laser thermal keratoplasty (LTK) on presbyopic patients. The LTK

KEY TERMS

Accommodation—The ability of the eye to change its focus from near to distant objects.

Binocular vision—Using both eyes at the same time to see an image.

Ciliary muscles—The small muscles that permit the lens to change its shape in order to focus on near or distant objects.

Lens (or crystalline lens)—The eye structure behind the iris and pupil that helps focus light on the retina.

Visual acuity—Sharpness or clearness of vision.

procedure was approved to treat **hyperopia** in mid-2000, but some surgeons are treating presbyopia as an "off-label" procedure. The LTK procedure takes three seconds per eye and involves no cutting or removal of corneal eye tissue. Instead, the surgeon uses a holium:YAG laser to direct eight simultaneous spots of laser energy to the periphery of the cornea to shrink the corneal collagen. The laser heats the corneal collagen and steepens its shape, improving its refractive (focusing) power. Presbyopes receiving this treatment should be advised of regression after possibly just a few years.

Laser-assisted in-situ keratomileusis (LASIK) is another option for presbyopes. Surgeons correct one of the patient's eyes to achieve a monovision effect. This technique allows for good intermediate vision that facilitates reading menus or putting on makeup, but it can cause reduction in binocular distance vision and depth perception.

In preparatory interviews with patients, physicians and ophthalmic assistants should stress that with whatever surgical treatment the patient chooses, there will be regression. The aging process continues and therefore advancing presbyopia is unavoidable.

Prognosis

The changes in vision due to aging usually start in a person's early 40s and continue for several decades. At some point, there is no further development of presbyopia, as the ability to accommodate is virtually gone.

Health care team roles

Nurses, ophthalmic assistants, and well-trained technicians can perform a number of tasks previously required of an ophthalmologist or optometrist. Technicians can assist in diagnosing presbyopia by performing the first-level testing of refraction, as well as taking medical and lifestyle history, retinal photography, automated refractometry, automated keratometry, and corneal topography.

Allied health professionals also play an important role in performing the contact lens examination. Before prescribing contact lenses, technicians take a written and oral interview of the patient to determine if the patient is a suitable contact lens candidate. The technician must assess the technical aspects of the patient's ocular status. Next, the technician must discuss the patient's needs and expectations and evaluate all the information to make the correct lens choice. This is especially important for presbyopic patients choosing monovision, as this modality requires a larger commitment from patients.

The physician, or sometimes a contact lens technician, selects the lens material and design, then determines which trial lens is needed. A technician determines the lens parameters by using the results from the trial lens insertion. The patient's palpebral aperture and visual iris diameter are measured to determine the appropriate diameter for the contact lens. The technician will review the findings and make the recommendation to the prescribing physician for the proper contact lenses.

Before the patient is sent home with the lenses, the technician will give a detailed demonstration of inserting, removing, and cleaning the lenses.

Nurses and assistants also prepare patients for surgery by taking history, **blood pressure** and inserting eyedrops. They also may be involved in preparing the surgical areas, especially if surgery is performed in an ambulatory surgery center. Ophthalmic nurses are specially trained to assist in ocular surgeries.

Patient education

Doctors should emphasize with patients the challenges of choosing monovision and bifocal contact lenses to treat presbyopia. Doctors also should stress that surgical procedures are not permanent, and that patients may have to be retreated if regression occurs.

Prevention

There is no known way to prevent presbyopia.

Resources

BOOK

Pallikaris, Ioannis, and Sotiris Plainis, W. Neil Charman. *Presbyopia: Origins, Effects, and Treatment.* Slack Incorporated, 2012.

PERIODICALS

Charters, Lynda. "Presbyopia: strategies in use; corneal approach; guidelines can be adapted to everyday practice with high rate of satisfaction among patients." *Ophthalmology Times* (1 November 2011): 25.

Cunningham, Derek N. "Surgical options for presbyopes: the presbyopic population continues to expand every year. But, you can help your patients select the best corrective procedure to fit their visual needs." *Review of Optometry* (15 December 2011): 38.

Krader, Cheryl Guttman. "Near vision results stable: minimally invasive: presbyopia correction safe and sustained after femtosecond laser intrastromal procedure." *Ophthalmology Times* (1 October 2011): 20.

ORGANIZATIONS

American Academy of Ophthalmology. P.O. Box 7424, San Francisco, CA 94120-7424. (415) 561-8500. http://www.eyenet.org.

American Optometric Association. 243 N. Lindbergh Boulevard, St. Louis, MO 63141. (314) 991-4100. AmOptNEWS@aol.com.

Contact Lens Association of Ophthalmologists, 721 Papworth Avenue, Suite 206, Metairie, LA 70005, (504) 835-3937, http://www.clao.org.

Lighthouse National Center for Vision and Aging. 111 E. 59th Street, New York, NY 10022. (800) 334-5497. http://www.lighthouse.org.

National Eye Institute. 2020 Vision Place, Bethesda, MD 20892-3655. (301) 496-5248; Publications: (800) 869-5248. http://www.nei.nih.gov.

Mary Bekker

Presenile dementia *see* **Alzheimer's disease**

Pressure ulcer

Definition

Pressure ulcers, also commonly known as bedsores, decubitus ulcers, and pressure sores, are among the most serious skin injuries. These tender or inflamed patches develop when skin covering a weight-bearing part of the body is squeezed between **bone** and another body part or some other hard object. The ulceration results from the loss of **blood** flow and oxygen (ischemic hypoxia) to the tissues owing to prolonged pressure on a body part.

Description

Pressure ulcers are most likely to occur in people who have decreased mobility, including the frail, elderly, or seriously ill. People who have **atherosclerosis** (artery disease), diabetes, **heart** disease, incontinence, malnutrition, **obesity**, **paralysis**, and **spinal cord** injuries are all at high risk for developing pressure ulcers. This often-painful condition usually begins with shiny red skin that quickly blisters and deteriorates into open sores that can harbor life-threatening infections. These ulcerations are most likely to develop on the:

- ankles
- back of the head
- heels
- hips
- knees
- spine
- shoulder blades

Pressure ulcers usually develop over bony prominences and are graded, or staged, to classify the amount of tissue damage that is observed. These stages are:

- Stage I. The skin is reddened, and the damage may be superficial. The first sign of skin ulceration occurs when pressure squeezes the tiny blood vessels that supply the skin with nutrients and oxygen. The area does not return to its normal appearance after the source of pressure is removed.

- Stage II. There is partial-thickness skin loss involving the epidermis (outer layer), the dermis (inner layer), or both. The skin is blistered, peeling, or has a shallow crater, though the damage is still minor.

- Stage III. There is full-thickness skin loss involving damage to, or necrosis (death) of, the subcutaneous (under the skin) tissue. It may extend down to, but not through, the underlying fascia (connective tissue). This type of ulcer usually appears as a deeper crater. Drainage may be seen.

- Stage IV. Full-thickness skin loss is present, with extensive tissue destruction and damage to muscle, bone, or the supporting structures such as tendons. This stage of ulceration is associated with high morbidity.

Causes and symptoms

The primary risk factors leading to the formation of a pressure ulcer include all of the following:

- Pressure. Very intense pressure, even if it occurs for a short time, may cause a pressure ulcer. Less intense pressure that lasts over a long period of time may also cause ulceration.

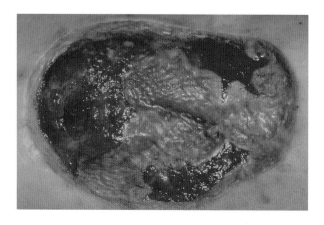

(Bed sore, photograph by Michael English. Custom Medical Stock Photo. Reproduced by permission.)

- Friction. This phenomenon occurs when two forces move against each other. When a patient's skin is dragged or pulled over bed sheets, friction occurs, with possible tissue injury resulting. The friction injury often happens when a patient is pulled, instead of lifted, up in bed.

- Shear. Deeper than a friction injury, shear happens when the skin located over a bony prominence slides over a hard surface. The skin and surrounding structures remain in one position because pressure keeps the skin stuck to a surface such as bed sheets. The shearing literally tears at the skin, the subcutaneous layer, and the muscle as well. Deep tissue injury and vascular damage may occur.

- Tissue maceration. Prolonged moisture on the skin can decrease the skin's resiliency and alter its pH (the measure of acidity and alkalinity).

Pressure ulcers usually develop in six stages:

- erythema
- erythema, swelling of tissue, and possible peeling of the outer layer of skin
- dead skin, draining wound, and an exposed layer of subcutaneous tissue
- tissue necrosis through the skin and subcutaneous layers, into the muscle
- inner fat and muscle necrosis
- destruction of bone, local infections, and potential for sepsis

Diagnosis

Physical examination, medical and nursing history, and patient and caregiver observation are the basis of diagnosis. Special attention must be paid to any physical or mental impairment such as incontinence or confusion that could complicate a patient's recovery. Staging is done based on the wound's characteristics and depth of soft tissue damage. Correct staging can only be done after all necrotic (dead) tissue has been removed, allowing for complete inspection of the wound bed (area). According to the National Pressure Ulcer Advisory Panel, once a particular stage (I, II, III, or IV) has been assigned to a pressure ulcer, it will always remain at that stage. Although pressure ulcers will heal to progressively more shallow depths, they do not replace the lost muscle, fat, or dermis. Instead, the ulcer is filled in with scar tissue. Therefore, when a Stage IV ulcer has healed, it should be classified as a healed Stage IV ulcer, not a Stage 0 ulcer.

Treatment

The desired outcomes of pressure ulcer treatment are to protect the remaining healthy cells, heal the ulcer completely, and prevent the formation of other pressure ulcers. If addressed promptly, surface pressure ulcers can be prevented from developing into more serious **wounds**.

Pressure ulcer management contains four basic components:

- Debridement. This is a procedure that involves the removal of dead tissue or other debris from the wound. Debridement can be done by a sharp method, where the tissue is actually cut out with a scalpel or other sharp instrument, and is usually performed by a physician, physician's assistant, or an advanced practice nurse. Another method is mechanical debridement, which utilizes wet-to-dry dressings, wound irrigation, and dextranomers (beads placed into the wound bed to absorb drainage). Enzymatic debridement utilizes certain topical debriding agents to help remove the dead tissue. Autolytic debridement uses synthetic dressings that help the involved tissue self-digest from enzymes that are contained in wound fluids. This last method should not be used for infected pressure ulcers.

- Cleansing. Normal saline is the recommended solution for cleansing wounds because it does not harm the wound bed, and it adequately cleanses the majority of wounds. Solutions such as hydrogen peroxide, povidone iodine, iodophor, and acetic acid are cytotoxic (toxic to cells), and should not be used. There are several commercially prepared wound cleansers containing surfactants (surface-active substances) and other ingredients, but these may also have some toxic effects on the cells. In order to minimize wound damage during cleansing, appropriate irrigation methods should be used. Too little pressure, such as that produced with a bulb syringe, yields poor results; while too much pressure will cause damage to healthy tissue. Irrigating the ulcer using a 35-ml syringe with a 19-gauge

KEY TERMS

Cytotoxic—The characteristic of being destructive to cells.

Ischemia—The temporary deficiency of blood flow to a tissue or organ.

Necrotic—Relating to the death of a portion of tissue.

angiocatheter will usually provide enough pressure to get rid of eschar (scabs), bacteria, and other debris. In addition, the use of daily whirlpool treatments may help facilitate the removal of necrotic tissue.

- Infection management. Because of the various factors that may affect a patient's resistance to infection, the patient should be closely monitored for any signs of infection in the wound so that antibiotics can be initiated promptly. These signs include a sudden deterioration of the ulcer, changes in the color or texture of the granulation (new capillaries formed on the surface of a wound in healing) tissue, or alterations in the amount or appearance of the wound drainage. In addition, any increase in redness, edema, or tenderness of the ulcerated area should be reported to the physician.

- Dressings. When selecting a dressing for a pressure ulcer, the most important factor is the ability of the dressing to keep the wound bed moist and the surrounding healthy, intact skin dry. There are numerous types of dressings available; and selection should be determined based on the preference of the physician and nurse, the time available to perform wound care, and the specific conditions of each wound.

Other adjunctive treatments that promote healing include electrical stimulation, ultrasound, hyperbaric (high pressure) oxygen, and laser irradiation. If there is extensive tissue necrosis, or if there are signs of **infection**, the physician may order topical and/or systemic antibiotic treatment. Very deep ulcers that do not respond to treatment may require skin grafts or **plastic surgery**.

Many patients are interested in complementary or alternative treatments, and several have been suggested in the treatment of pressure ulcers. **Zinc** and **vitamins** A, C, E, and B complex help skin repair injuries and stay healthy, but large doses of vitamins or **minerals** should not be used without consulting a physician. Various herbal remedies, including a tea tree oil rinse and an herbal tea made from the calendula plant, may act as

antiseptic agents. Again, the physician or health care professional should be consulted when considering any of these treatments.

Prognosis

With prompt, appropriate treatment, pressure ulcers should begin to heal in two to four weeks. If the ulcer exhibits no signs of progress in three weeks, the treatment plan should be reevaluated. The National Pressure Ulcer Advisory Panel recommends that if a non-healing wound is clean, then the ulcer should be treated with topical **antibiotics**. If the bedsore still does not respond within two weeks, then other factors need to be explored.

Health care team roles

Several members of the health care team are important when treating the patient with a pressure ulcer. The physician orders treatment and performs any necessary surgical interventions. The nurse plays a primary role in assessing the wound and administering treatment, consulting with the physician on **wound care** decisions, and providing **patient education**. Physical therapists may also participate in pressure ulcer care by providing whirlpool treatments.

Prevention

It is usually possible to prevent pressure ulcers from forming and/or worsening. A variety of measures can be taken to accomplish this goal. At-risk individuals should be identified. These individuals include those with a history of previous pressure ulcers, since healed full-thickness pressure ulcers have only 80% of the strength of non-injured skin. A systematic skin assessment should be performed daily on all patients at risk for ulcer formation. Because a health care professional may not be available to assess homebound patients, the family or other caregivers should be educated on the symptoms of early skin breakdown and on when to notify their health care professional.

Other methods of pressure ulcer prevention are:

- Always cleanse the skin of incontinent patients at the time of soiling.

- Moisturize dry skin to keep it well hydrated.

- Turn and reposition the patient at least every two hours. Keep a turning schedule posted at the bedside.

- Utilize proper patient positioning, lifting, and transferring methods to avoid friction and shear. Use a lift sheet when moving the patient.

- Use pillows or cushions to pad bony prominences and support limbs.

- Consider using an alternating pressure mattress or other support surface designed to reduce pressure on the skin.

- Do not massage bony prominences, as this could cause deep tissue damage.

- Encourage adequate consumption of protein, calories and fluids.

- Maintain or improve the patient's activity level. Perform range of motion exercises, if possible.

- Instruct the patient, family, and any other caregivers regarding appropriate preventive care.

Resources

BOOK

Ignatavicius, Donna D., et al. *Medical-Surgical Nursing Across the Health Care Continuum.* Philadelphia: W.B. Saunders Company, 1999.

PERIODICALS

Calianno, Carol. "Assessing and Preventing Pressure Ulcers." *Advances in Skin and Wound Care* (October 2000): 244.

Cervo, Frank A., et al. "Pressure Ulcers—Analysis of Guidelines for Treatment and Management." *Geriatrics* (March 2000): 55.

ORGANIZATION

National Pressure Ulcer Advisory Panel. 11250 Roger Bacon Drive, Suite 8, Reston, VA 20190-5202. (703) 464-4849. http://www.npuap.org.

Deanna M. Swartout-Corbeil, R.N.

Preterm labor

Definition

Preterm labor is characterized by contractions or irritability of the uterus between weeks 20–36 of gestation that cause effacement and/or dilatation of the cervix.

Description

The usual length of a human **pregnancy** is from 37 to 42 weeks after the first day of the last menstrual period. The baby is more likely to survive and be healthy if it remains in the uterus for the full term of the pregnancy. Between 8% and 10% of births in the United States are preterm births. Preterm labor is the greatest cause of newborn illness and death in the United States.

Causes and symptoms

The causes of preterm labor are often not identifiable. Women with a previous history of preterm labor have the highest risk of developing it again, between 17 and 37%. Other risk factors are: low socioeconomic status, non-white race, maternal age less than 18 or greater than 40, premature rupture of membranes (bag of waters), multiple gestation (twins, triplets, etc.), harmful maternal behaviors (**smoking**, drug use, alcohol use, no **prenatal care**), uterine abnormalities (fibroid tumor, abnormally shaped uterus, incompetent cervix, exposure to diethylstilbestrol—their mothers took DES when they carried them), infectious causes (**infection** of the uterus, kidney infection), fetal causes (intrauterine fetal death, intrauterine growth retardation, **birth defects**), and abnormal implantation of the placenta.

The symptoms of preterm labor can include contractions of the uterus or tightening of the **abdomen** occurring every 10 minutes or more often. The uterine contractions of preterm labor, sometimes painful, will usually increase in frequency, duration, and intensity. Other symptoms associated with preterm labor can include menstrual-like cramps; abdominal cramping with or without **diarrhea**; pressure or **pain** in the pelvic region; low backache; or a change in the color or amount of vaginal discharge. As labor progresses the cervix, the opening of the uterus, will open (dilate) and the tissue around it will become thinner (efface). Premature rupture of membranes (when the water breaks) may also occur.

An occasional contraction can occur anytime during pregnancy and does not necessarily indicate that labor is starting. Premature contractions are sometimes confused with Braxton-Hicks contractions, which can occur throughout the pregnancy. Braxton-Hicks contractions do not cause the cervix to open or efface and are considered "false labor."

Diagnosis

The health care provider will conduct a pelvic examination and ask about the timing and intensity of the contractions. A physician or nurse will conduct a vaginal examination and determine if the cervix has started to dilate or efface. An ultrasound technician may proceed with a transvaginal ultrasound (ultrasound of the vagina by use of a probe that is inserted into the vagina), to measure cervical length. A cervical length of less than 0.98–1.18 in (2.5–3.0 cm) is associated with preterm labor.

Urine may be collected to screen for infection. A cervical culture or a wet smear may also be done to look for infection. Presence of fetal fibronectin in vaginal and cervical secretions, between 24 and 24 weeks gestation, may indicate impending preterm labor. Fibronectin is a substance that functions as an adhesive between the fetal membranes and the underlying decidua.

A fetal **heart** monitor is placed on the mother's abdomen to record the heartbeat of the fetus and to time the contractions. Occasionally the woman will have home monitoring of contractions and fetal activity.

A fetal ultrasound may be performed to determine the age and weight of the fetus, the condition of the placenta, and to see if there is more than one fetus present. Another test, **amniocentesis**, may be done to determine if the baby's **lungs** are mature. During an amniocentesis, a needle-like tube is inserted through the mother's abdomen into the uterus to draw out some of the fluid surrounding the fetus (amniotic fluid). Analysis of the amniotic fluid can determine if the baby's lungs are mature. A baby with mature lungs is much more likely to survive outside the uterus.

Treatment

The goal of treatment is to stop preterm labor and to prevent the fetus from being delivered prior to term. A first recommendation may be for the woman with premature contractions to lie down and to drink water or other fluids. If contractions continue or increase, medical attention should be sought. In addition to bed rest, medical care may include intravenous fluids. Sometimes, this extra fluid is enough to stop contractions.

In some cases, oral or injectable drugs, like terbutaline sulfate (Bricanyl), ritodrine (Yutopar), **magnesium** sulfate, nifedipine (Procardia), or indomethacin (Indocin) are administered to delay delivery. When used to treat preterm labor, these medications are called tocolytic agents. Unfortunately, no study has conclusively demonstrated that the use of tocolytic drugs has significantly improved neonatal outcome. Medications used to treat preterm labor can have maternal and fetal side effects. Magnesium sulfate can lead to pulmonary **edema**, profound muscular **paralysis**, and respiratory depression. Terbutaline and Ritodrine can cause **arrhythmias** and **hypoglycemia** as well as pulmonary edema. Pregnant women who are treated with these medications need to be monitored closely in a hospital environment.

An advantage of tocolysis is in delaying delivery so that drugs that will enhance fetal lung maturity can be administered. A delay in delivery also allows for transfer to a tertiary facility that is equipped to care for premature babies. The preferred drugs to stimulate lung maturity are dexamethasone and betamethasone, **corticosteroids** that promote the fetal production of surfactant after 24 hours of administration. The benefit of these corticosteroids

will last up to seven days, at which time the medications can be readministered.

If a vaginal or urinary tract infection is detected, antibiotic therapy is usually indicated. **Antibiotics** may briefly prolong the pregnancies of women who have ruptured their membranes.

Prognosis

Once symptoms of preterm labor occur during the pregnancy, the mother and fetus need to be monitored regularly. If the preterm labor cannot be stopped or controlled, the infant will be delivered prematurely. These infants that are born prematurely have an increased risk of health problems, including birth defects, lung problems, mental retardation, blindness, deafness, and developmental disabilities. If the infant is born too early, its body systems may not be mature enough for it to survive. Evaluating the infant's lung maturity is one of the keys to determining its chances of survival.

Health care team roles

Prior to initiating tocolytic medications, it is important to obtain such baseline laboratory test results as **hematocrit**, serum glucose, potassium, sodium chloride, and carbon dioxide levels. An electrocardiogram is frequently ordered because tocolytic drugs can cause an increased heart rate (tachycardia) and sometimes arrhythmias. An external uterine and fetal monitor should be put in place and often monitors of maternal **vital signs** are also applied. Accurate fluid intake and output measurements are important in detecting the development of pulmonary edema (fluid in the lungs).

Other potentially serious complications of tocolytic therapy include: low **blood pressure (hypotension)**, cardiac arrest, respiratory depression, low potassium, high **blood** sugar, maternal death, kidney failure, hepatitis, and gastrointestinal bleeding.

Ritodrine is a drug that is sometimes used in the management of preterm labor. To administer the medication accurately, it should be delivered as a piggyback to a main intravenous solution that goes through an infusion pump and a microdrip tubing set. To avoid hyperglycemia, a potential side effect, the woman should receive few IV solutions containing dextrose. The ritodrine drip is increased gradually, usually every 10 minutes until uterine contractions cease, the maximum dose is reached, and/or side effects become too intense. The nurse should assess the patient's vital signs every 15 minutes during titration, and then every 30 minutes until uterine contractions stop. Ask the patient to inform the health care provider if she starts to experience any

KEY TERMS

Braxton Hicks contractions—Tightening of the uterus or abdomen that can occur throughout pregnancy. These contractions do not cause changes to the cervix and are sometimes called false labor or practice contractions.

Cervix—The opening at the bottom of the uterus, which dilates or opens in order for the fetus to pass into the vagina or birth canal during the delivery process.

Contraction—A tightening of the uterus during pregnancy. Contractions may or may not be painful and may or may not indicate labor.

Decidua—The part of the lining of the uterus that sloughs off during menstruation.

chest pain or shortness of breath. The health care provider should listen to the lungs for any abnormal breath sounds that could indicate the development of pulmonary edema. A heart rate greater than 120 beats per minute (bpm), a blood pressure lower than 90/60, and any cardiac arrhythmias should be reported immediately. Continue to monitor laboratory values every four hours. The fetal response to contractions and medication administration should be monitored continuously. Closely monitor daily weights to assess for possible pulmonary edema resulting from fluid retention. If therapy with ritodrine is successful in halting uterine contractions, then oral administration of ritodrine or terbutaline will often be ordered. Other tocolytic medications that are delivered in a similar manner are magnesium sulfate, subcutaneous terbutaline, nifedipine, and indomethacin.

Patient education

Health care professionals should educate all pregnant women about the signs and symptoms of preterm labor, ensuring an understanding of even the more subtle symptoms. Pregnant women should be alert for symptoms that could be indicative of preterm labor, such as constant, dull, low **back pain**; vaginal spotting; pelvic pressure and/ or tightening of the abdomen; cramping; increased vaginal discharge; and intestinal-like cramping.

Pregnant women who are at home on bed rest should be given the following instructions:

- Stay on bed rest except to get up to use the bathroom.

- Drink eight to ten glasses of liquids a day.

- Do not engage in such activities as nipple stimulation that could trigger contractions.

- Do not engage in sexual activities, including masturbation.

- Promptly inform the health care provider if the membranes rupture (sudden gush of vaginal fluid) or if there is any vaginal bleeding.

- Communicate to the health care provider any symptoms of a urinary tract infection (burning on urination and frequent urination) or of a vaginal infection (vaginal burning, itching, or discomfort).

Prevention

Smoking, poor **nutrition**, and drug or alcohol abuse can increase the risk of premature labor and early delivery. Smoking, drug and alcohol use should be stopped. A healthy diet and prenatal vitamin supplements (prescribed by the health care provider) are important for the growth of the fetus and the health of the mother. Pregnant women are advised to see a health care provider early in the pregnancy and to receive regular prenatal examinations throughout the pregnancy. The health care provider should be informed of any medications that the mother is receiving and any maternal health conditions.

Resources

BOOKS

Hisley, Shelton M. *The Women's Health Companion to Maternal-Child Nursing Care: Optimizing Outcomes for Mothers, Children, and Families.* F.A. Davis Company, 2011.

Pillitteri, Adele. *Maternal and Child Health Nursing: Care of the Childbearing and Childrearing Family,* 6th edition. Lippincott Williams & Wilkins, 2009.

ORGANIZATION

The March of Dimes Resource Center. (888) 663-4637 (888-MODIMES). http://www.modimes.org.

Nadine M. Jacobson, R.N.

Preventive dentistry

Definition

Preventive dentistry is the area of dentistry that focuses on those procedures and life practices that help people to prevent the beginning or progression of oral disease. It includes at-home dental care performed by patients, as well as dental care and education by professional dental staff in the office or clinic.

Purpose

Preventive dentistry includes two aspects of dental care, both performed to help patients avoid dental disease or to catch it in its early, more treatable stages. In part, it is the **oral hygiene** care performed by the patient at home. Preventive dentistry also encompasses what is done by the dental staff in their offices to help patients maintain healthy teeth and gums. In either case, the objective is to stop the development of oral disease or to find it at an early stage. Dental health professionals most often look for early signs of periodontal disease, dental decay, and other changes in the soft tissue of the mouth that could lead to **oral cancer**.

Precautions

Preventive dentistry should always be prescribed and not harm patients when done correctly. At times, dentists do need to take precautions when someone has a medical condition that would be affected by some of the procedures. Dentists need to be aware of certain medical conditions, such as mitral valve prolapse, which need to be treated with prophylactic **antibiotics**. **Allergies** to any of the medications or materials used in preventive dentistry are rare.

Description

Preventive care in a dental office includes **prophylaxis**, or the cleaning of the teeth, which removes accumulations of calculus. It includes examination of the teeth and soft tissue, using visual and tactile exams, radiographic examination, such as x rays, and oral **cancer** screening. Newer techniques to diagnose periodontal or gum disease include computerized measurement devices that measure the bacterial content in the mouth. Sometimes, dentists prescribe medications to help prevent dental disease. These include anti-inflammatory mouthwashes to prevent periodontal problems.

Preventive procedures often performed by dentists for children include the use of fluoride supplements and applications. Dentists apply dental sealants to children's teeth, forming a barrier between tooth crevasses and **bacteria** to help ward off dental decay. Dental health professionals also look for malocclusions and might refer patients to a dental specialist, such as an orthodontist, to correct a patient's bad bite. Experts state that children should be evaluated by an orthodontist by age seven.

An important part of preventive dentistry performed by dental professionals is educating patients about at-home care, **nutrition**, and **smoking cessation**. At-home procedures performed by patients that help ward off dental disease include regular and proper brushing, flossing, and use of mouth rinses and at-home fluoride applications, if necessary. Dentists and their staff explain proper brushing and flossing techniques. Proper brushing includes use of a soft, nylon toothbrush with round-ended bristles. Patients should place the bristles along the gum line at a 45-degree angle to cover the tooth surface and gum line. The brushing technique should be gentle and in a rolling back-and-forth motion, with two to three teeth being brushed at a time. Patients should brush the inner surfaces of their teeth and tilt the brush vertically to brush the front teeth. Ideally, patients should use a back-and-forth motion to brush the biting surface of the teeth and the tongue. Flossing removes plaque from between teeth and at the gum line. It should be done with an 18-inch strip of floss wrapped around the middle fingers of each hand. The remaining 1–2 in (2–5 cm) of floss that is inserted between the teeth should be directed by the thumbs. By keeping the floss taut, patients can use their index fingers to guide the floss between the lower teeth with a gentle zig-zag motion, while contouring the floss around the sides of the teeth. They should floss each tooth with a clean section of the floss and ensure that the floss goes under the gum line.

Preventive dental care should begin within the first year of life before teeth first appear, and continue throughout life. Even before teeth erupt, parents can clean infants' gums after feeding. Preventive care in adolescence includes brushing and flossing, as well as wearing custom-made mouth guards to protect the teeth during contact sports. Considering that 75% of Americans have some form of dental disease, regular dental visits are particularly important for adults. Seniors often benefit from training in proper techniques of **denture care** and cleaning, which include brushing the replacement teeth. Those who have problems moving their hands because of arthritis, for example, also benefit from tips for adapting toothbrushes for easier handling.

Results

The results of good preventive dental care are healthy teeth and gums throughout one's life and the early detection of oral disease. Preventive procedures, such as fluoride applications and sealants, can prevent tooth decay. Regular dental checkups and oral cancer screenings can catch oral cancer at its most treatable stages. Dental checkups and consistent at-home preventive dental care can stave off caries (tooth decay) and periodontal disease, which can lead to tooth loss. An estimated 75% of adults have periodontal disease. Regular dental checkups can reduce the risk of permanent tooth and gum damage, and expensive treatment in the future. As a result of preventive dental care, people tend to keep their original teeth throughout life and don't

KEY TERMS

Calculus—A hard deposit formed plaque hardens on the teeth.

Dental decay—The destruction of the tooth enamel.

Fluoride—A naturally occurring mineral in all water sources, which effectively prevents and reverses the early signs of tooth decay.

Malocclusion—Condition in which the bite (the way the teeth meet) is misaligned.

Periodontal disease—Disease of the areas surrounding the teeth, primarily the gums, ligaments, and bones.

Plaque—The thin, sticky film of bacteria that grows on teeth.

Prophylaxis—In dentistry, prevention of dental disease by regular cleanings.

need as much restorative dental work. Preventive dental examinations also ensure that a dentist will notice any oral signs of systemic disease. A dental checkup might reveal a lesion in the mouth that could lead to a referral to a physician for further investigation.

Treatments resulting from preventive dental procedures are designed to stop the process of the disease. Restorative dentistry, including the placement of fillings, crowns, and dental work, addresses tooth decay and tooth loss that can result from periodontal disease. Periodontal treatments help restore healthy gums and can prevent tooth loss.

Health care team roles

The dentist oversees the process of examination, diagnosis, treatment planning, and education. The allied dental personnel include the **dental hygienist** and dental assistant. Dental hygienists sometimes perform preventive techniques, including cleaning, fluoride and sealant application, and **patient education**. The dental assistant in some states, depending on state licensing, can perform many of the same procedures as the hygienist, assist the dentist during checkups, and provide patient guidance and education.

Resources

BOOKS

Harris, Norman, and Franklin Garcia-Godoy, Christine N. Nathe. *Primary Preventive Dentistry*, 8th edition. Prentice Hall, 2013.

Limeback, Hardy, ed. *Comprehensive Preventive Dentistry.* Wiley-Blackwell, 2012.

ORGANIZATIONS

American Dental Association. 211 E. Chicago Ave., Chicago, IL 60611. (312) 440-2806. http://www.ada.org.

American Dental Hygienists' Association. 444 North Michigan Avenue, Suite 3400, Chicago, IL 60611. (312) 440-8900. http://adha.org.

Lisette Hilton

Preventive medicine

Definition

Preventive medicine is a branch of medicine that focuses on developing policies and programs to promote and maintain the health of individuals, communities, and other defined populations.

Description

Although all physicians practice preventive to some degree—for example, counseling patients to stop **smoking** or prescribing prenatal **vitamins** to pregnant women—, in the United States, preventive medicine is a medical specialty recognized by the American Board of Medical Specialties. This article discusses preventive medicine within the context of a board certified medical specialty.

Preventive medicine involves less hands-on patient care than many medical specialties and has a strong **public health**, policy, and research component. Preventive medicine physicians can work setting health policy for governmental organizations at the federal, state, and local level. They also can work for the military, corporations and nonprofit organizations, and academic and research institutions.

Preventive medicine physicians study ways to prevent disease and disability in specific populations, and, when prevention is not possible, to develop effective responses to health crises. For example, they may develop policies to protect the public water supply, guide state health care agencies on immunization programs, respond to a bioterrorist incident, identify and moderate workplace hazards, prevent disease outbreak among military service members, and deliver preventive services to underserved populations such as the homeless.

Preventive medicine has several subdivisions.

- Occupational medicine deals with preventing and eliminating physical, chemical, biological, and mental health workplace hazards. From 1955–2012, 3,961 physicians were board certified in occupational.

- Public health and general preventive medicine involve managing the health of communities and specific populations. Between 1949 and 2012, 5,025physicians were board certified in public health and/or general preventive medicine.

- Aerospace medicine is a small specialty that concerns research about and care of passengers and crew of airplanes and space vehicles. It examines both physiological and psychological stress of those populations. Many aerospace physicians work for NASA and the military. From 1953–2102, 1,519 physicians were board certified in aerospace medicine.

Preventive medicine also recognizes two subspecialties, medical **toxicology** and undersea and hyperbaric medicine, that require additional training. Hyperbaric medicine deals with exposure to gasses under greater than normal atmospheric pressure. Between 1995 and 2012, only 19 physicians were certified in medical toxicology and from 1993–2012 439 physicians were certified in undersea medicine and hyperbaric medicine.

Origins

Preventive medicine as a board certified medical specialty is relatively new in the United States. It has its origins in the formation of the American Board of Preventive Medicine and public health founded in 1948. In 1952, the board changed its name to the American Board of Preventive Medicine, by which it is known today. The following year, aviation medicine, now called aerospace medicine, was added as a specialty. In 1989, undersea medicine, now known as undersea and hyperbaric medicine, was added as a subspecialty, followed by medical toxicology in 1992.

Purpose

The purpose of preventive medicine is to maintain health, prevent illness, and prevent disability in specific populations. This is done primarily by setting policy and doing research and teaching rather than through clinical practice.

Training and certification

Preventive medicine physicians require less hands-on patient experience and more academic experience. Core competencies required to become board certified in preventive medicine include biostatistics, epidemiology, management, administration and policy, clinical preventive medicine and occupational and environmental health.

To become board certified in preventive medicine, one must graduate from an accredited medical school and become a licensed physician. Additional requirements for people who have graduated from medical school since 1984 include one year of postgraduate clinical experience that must include at least six months of hands-on patient care. This is followed by academic course work and practical experience to complete a master's in public health (MPH) degree and at least one additional year of residency in preventive medicine and passing of appropriate examinations. Subspecialty certification requires additional residency.

Alternative certification procedures are open to individuals who graduated from medical school before 1984. In addition, continuing education and re-certification are required every 10 years to remain board certified.

Resources

BOOKS

Jekel, James F., and David L. Katz, Dorothea Wild, Joann G. Elmore. *Epidemiology, Biostatistics and Preventive Medicine.* Saunders, 2007.

Varkey, Prathibha. *Mayo Clinic Preventive Medicine and Public Health Board Review.* Oxford University Press, USA, 2010.

OTHER

American Association Medical Colleges. Careers in Medicine: Specialty Information—Preventive Medicine. 2012 [accessed August 24, 2012]. https://www.aamc.org/students/medstudents/cim/specialties/63670/cim_pub_preventivemed.html

American Board of Preventive Medicine. What is Preventive Medicine? [accessed August 24, 2012]. https://www.theabpm.org/aboutus.cfm

ORGANIZATIONS

American Board of Preventive Medicine, 111 West Jackson Boulevard, Suite 1110, Chicago, IL 60604, (312) 939-ABPM [2276], Fax: (312) 939-2218, abpm@theabpm.org, https://www.theabpm.org

American College of Hyperbaric Medicine, 6737 W. Washington Street, Ste 3265, West Allis, WI 53214, (414) 918-9300, Fax: (414) 918-9301, admin@achm.org, http://www.achm.org

American College of Preventive Medicine, 455 Massachusetts Avenue NW, Suite 200, Washington, DC 20001, (202) 466-2044, Fax: (202) 466-2662, info@acpm.org, http://www.acpm.org.

Tish Davidson, AM

Primary tooth development *see* **Tooth development, primary**

Private insurance plans

Definition

Private insurance plans include all forms of health insurance that are not funded by the government. These plans are intended to protect their beneficiaries from the high costs that may be incurred for health care. Most private insurance plans in the United States are employment-based; of the 194 million Americans who were covered by private health insurance in 1999, 172 million, or 89%, were enrolled in employment-based plans.

Description

Private health insurance plans may be purchased on an individual or a group basis. Most group plans are offered by large employers, although some are offered by voluntary associations. Individual policies are usually more expensive than group policies; they may also have additional coverage restrictions.

There are several major categories of private health insurance in the United States.

Indemnity plans

Indemnity plans are private insurance plans that allow beneficiaries to choose any physician or hospital when they need medical care. Most indemnity plans have a deductible, or amount that the policyholder must pay before the plan will pay any benefits. After the deductible, indemnity plans pay a co-insurance percentage, most often 70–90% of the charges. The beneficiary pays the remainder of the bill.

Preferred Provider Organization (PPO) plans

PPO plans are like indemnity plans in that they usually have both a deductible and a co-insurance percentage. Unlike indemnity plans, however, PPOs offer beneficiaries a list of physicians and hospitals from which they must select in order to receive the plan's maximum benefit. PPOs tend to be less expensive than indemnity plans because health care providers are often willing to reduce their fees in order to participate in these plans. Many large companies have moved their insured employees into PPOs because of their cost effectiveness.

A person enrolled in a PPO can choose to go "out of network" and continue under the care of their present physician. They may also propose their physician for membership in the PPO so that continuity of service can be provided.

Health Maintenance Organization (HMO) plans

HMOs usually have no deductibles; the beneficiary is charged a small co-payment, typically $5 or $10, per visit, and the plan covers all other charges. Beneficiaries are, however, usually offered a much smaller list of health care providers from which to choose. In most HMOs, each beneficiary selects a primary care doctor who is responsible for all health care needs. Referrals to specialists must be made through the primary care doctor. Like PPOs, HMOs are usually able to charge lower premiums because their health care providers agree to substantially reduced fees.

Long-term care (LTC) insurance

Long-term care insurance, or LTC, is a type of private health insurance intended to cover the cost of custodial or nursing **home care**. It can be very expensive, and persons considering this form of insurance should not purchase it if the premiums would cause financial hardship in the present.

Medigap insurance plans

Medigap insurance plans are private plans intended to supplement **Medicare** coverage, because Medicare does not offer complete health insurance protection. There are ten standard Medigap benefit "packages," identified by the letters A through J, that are available in most states, United States territories, and the District of Columbia. Medigap policies pay most or all of the co-insurance amounts charged by Medicare, and some Medigap policies cover Medicare deductibles.

Medical savings accounts

Medical savings accounts (MSAs) are not health insurance plans in the strict sense, but offer a partial alternative to expensive individual private insurance plans. MSAs are similar to Individual Retirement Accounts (IRAs) and have been considered a significant tax break for self-employed individuals. They were created as a four-year pilot project by the Health Insurance Portability and Accountability Act (**HIPAA**) of 1996. The federal government issued an extension on these accounts for two years, effective December 31, 2000. The government will not revoke these accounts once they have been opened.

An MSA must be combined with a qualified high-deductible private health plan. Without an MSA, a self-employed individual can deduct qualified medical expenses only under the itemized deductions of a 1040 tax form and the expenses must exceed 7.5% of the adjusted gross income.

Viewpoints

The high cost of health insurance

The cost of private health insurance has risen steadily over the past two decades, largely because of the rising cost of health care in the United States. Between 1980 and 1995, the total amount spent on health care in the United States rose from $247.2 billion to $1.04 trillion, more than a 400% increase. The reasons for the escalating costs include the following:

• Increased longevity. The life expectancy of most Americans is around 75 years. When older people join an insured group, the whole group's health care risks and costs rise.

• Advances in medical technology. New technology is often expensive.

• Increased use of health care. Between 1991 and 1996, the average number of visits to doctors' offices rose from 2.7 per person to 3.4.

The rising costs of health insurance over the past thirty years have caused many employers to curtail or drop health insurance as an employee benefit. The cost of health insurance premiums increased from $16.8 billion in 1970 to $310 billion in 1995. Some employers have increased the amount of money that employees are expected to contribute toward their health care. Others, particularly smaller businesses, do not offer insurance at all. A 1997 study found that only 34% of workers in smaller businesses were covered through their employers, whereas 82% of employees in the largest companies were covered. Workers in large-employer health insurance plans are also more likely to have policies that cover more health services, policies with lower deductibles, and more opportunities to enroll in HMOs.

The uninsured

The U. S. Census Bureau reported in 1997 that 43.4 million people in the United States, or 16.1% of the population, had no health insurance coverage. Between 1998 and 1999, both the number and the proportion of uninsured Americans declined slightly, to 42.6 million and 15.5% respectively.

Some workers do not have health insurance because they cannot afford it. In the 1950s, employer-based health insurance served most American families reasonably well because many workers were employed by large firms and remained with them for life. Over the past two decades, however, more and more people are employed by small firms that do not offer health insurance as a benefit, and more workers move from company to company every few years. Most uninsured workers are either self-employed, work only part-time, or work in low-wage jobs that do not give them access to lower-cost employer-sponsored group plans. At the same time, workers in these three categories do not qualify for coverage by government programs for low-income people.

The other major category of uninsured people includes those who cannot purchase private insurance at affordable rates because they are likely to need expensive medical services. Those who have a high risk of developing **cancer** or are HIV-positive may not be able to obtain coverage from any insurance company. Some insurance companies began introducing so-called "preexisting condition" clauses in their policies as early as the 1980s that denied private insurance to anyone already diagnosed with a serious medical condition. The Health Insurance Portability and Accountability Act of 1996 was intended to help workers who could not change their jobs because they had family members with serious health problems. They would be denied health insurance by the preexisting condition clauses in the plan offered by their new employer. HIPAA requires employer-sponsored insurance plans to accept transfers from other plans without imposing preexisting condition clauses.

An individual private health insurance plan can be expensive and restrictive. It may, however, be the only choice for a consumer who is not employed; is self-employed; or is a new hire at a company and must wait for several months or more before the company's coverage takes effect.

Tax credit proposals

One approach to the rising costs of private health insurance that is gaining bipartisan political support is to offer tax credits that would allow more Americans to purchase health insurance. The present federal tax code favors workers who already have employer-sponsored health insurance. Supporters of the tax credit approach maintain that it would give workers a wider choice of health plans; create greater portability of health insurance; and encourage groups other than employment-based populations (e.g., church groups, unions, fraternal organizations, etc.) to sponsor insurance plans for their members.

KEY TERMS

Co-insurance—The percentage of health care charges that an insurance company pays after the beneficiary pays the deductible. Most co-insurance percentages are between 70% and 90%.

Deductible—An amount of money that an insured person is required to pay on each claim made on an insurance policy.

Indemnity plans—Private health insurance plans that allow the policyholder to choose any physician or hospital when health care is needed.

Long-term care (LTC) insurance—A type of private health insurance intended to cover the cost of long-term nursing home care or home health care.

Medigap—A group of ten standardized private health insurance policies intended to cover the coinsurance and deductible costs that Medicare does not cover.

Portability—A feature that allows employees to transfer health insurance coverage or other benefits from one employer to another when they change jobs.

Preferred provider organizations (PPOs)—Private health insurance plans that require beneficiaries to select their health care providers from a list approved by the insurance company.

Premium—The amount paid by an insurance policyholder for insurance coverage. Most health insurance policy premiums are payable on a monthly basis.

Resources

BOOK

Morrisey, Michael A. *Health Insurance.* Health Administration Press, 2007.

WEBSITE

"The Affordable Care Act; Read the Law." HealthCare.gov. http://www.healthcare.gov/law/full/index.html (accessed November 9, 2012).

ORGANIZATIONS

Health Insurance Association of America. 555 13th Street, NW, Suite 600, East Washington, DC 20004-1109. (888) 844-2782. http://www.hiaa.org.

United States Census Bureau, Housing and Household Economics Statistics Division. (301) 457-3242. http://www.census.gov/hhes.

United States Department of Health and Human Services. 200 Independence Avenue, S.W. Washington, D.C. 20201.

Jacqueline N. Martin, M.S.

PRK *see* **Refractive eye surgeries**

Proctosigmoidoscopy *see* **Sigmoidoscopy**

▌ Professional-patient relationship

Definition

The professional-patient relationship is a bond of trust between the patient and the medical professional who is performing treatment.

Description

The relationship established between patients and health care providers is fiduciary in nature, which means that it is based on trust. In this respect it is similar to the relationships between lawyers and clients or between clergy and their congregations. The professional trusts the patient or client to disclose all the information that may be relevant to his or her condition or illness, and to be truthful while disclosing it. In return, the patient or client trusts the health care professional to maintain high standards of competence; to protect the confidentiality of private information; and to carry out his or her work in the best interests of the patient rather than taking advantage of the patient's vulnerability.

Ethical principles

Health care professionals are obligated to act according to ethical and legal standards. Ethical guidelines refer to the moral standards that are considered to govern health care. The fundamental ethical principles underlying Western medical practice have not changed since they were first enunciated by Hippocrates (460–377 BC). These principles include:

- Honesty: The professional does not withhold necessary information from the patient or lie to the patient about the nature or seriousness of his or her condition.

- Beneficence (doing good): The professional uses his or her knowledge and skills to balance good results and potential harms, and act in the patient's best interests.

- Justice. The professional does not refuse treatment on the basis of a patient's race, religion, nationality, income, or other personal characteristic.

- Avoiding conflicts of interest. This principle means that the professional must not benefit personally from his or her professional actions or influence. For example, a physician should prescribe a particular medication because it is the best choice for the patient, not because the professional owns stock in the company that manufactures the drug.

- Pledging to do no harm. This principle means that the professional must avoid actions detrimental to the patient.

All major organizations of health care providers, including the American Hospital Association, the American Medical Association, the American Dental Association, and the American Nurses Association have formal ethical guidelines for professional-patient relationships. These ethical policy statements are based on the ancient Hippocratic oath.

Legal obligations

In the United States and Canada, the legal obligations of health care providers are based on and presuppose the traditional ethical standards of good medical practice. These legal obligations include accepting federal and state examination and licensure standards; government regulation of **medical records**; court orders regarding reporting or disclosure of a patient's medical records; and a number of other obligations.

The legal obligations and liabilities of health care professionals have become increasingly complex over the last 30 years. This development is partly the result of technological advances that pose new questions to the legal system. For example, the safe operation of **medical lasers** depends on proper engineering and maintenance procedures as well as on the surgeon's skill and training in using the laser. A patient injured by a malfunctioning laser might decide to sue the manufacturer and the **hospital administration** as well as the surgeon. In addition, however, the growing complexity of health care legislation is part of a larger trend toward resolving social issues through litigation rather than through public debate or other means.

Viewpoints

Historical background

Prior to the second half of the twentieth century, the patient-physician relationship was strictly hierarchical. The physician was assumed to know what was best for the patient, and the patient was expected to follow "doctor's orders." After World War II, however, patients in the developed countries began to take a more active role in their health care. This change was related to the larger proportion of high-school students going on to college, and to the rapid spread of medical information via television and health care books written for the general public. Patients who were employed in other fields requiring specialized training, or who read widely, were less impressed by the physician's educational credentials and more likely to question his or her advice.

The social context of contemporary health care

In addition to the rise in education level among the general population in Europe and North America, several other factors have helped to reshape patient-professional relationships. The most important factors are the following:

- The loss of a social consensus regarding moral issues. At one time, health care professionals could be fairly sure that they and their patients agreed on the major moral issues that were likely to arise in health care situations. Today, however, there is widespread disagreement within the professions as well as in the general population about such questions as abortion, euthanasia, organ donation, limitations on medical research, and others. A patient who disagrees with his or her health care provider on the moral implications of a procedure is now generally allowed to refuse the procedure.

- The high-pressure education of health care professionals. Over the past thirty years, the training of physicians, nurses, dentists, pharmacists, and other health care professionals has become much more demanding. One factor is the sheer accumulation of scientific knowledge; today's medical, dental, or nursing student must master a much larger body of information than students of previous generations. Another factor is the increased tendency toward professional specialization, which makes it more difficult for health care providers to see patients as whole human beings.

- Managed care. Managed care has changed physician-patient relationships by requiring patients to choose their doctor from a list of providers approved by the managed care organization. In many instances patients have left physicians who were trusted and who had cared for them for years. In other instances managed care organizations have terminated physicians on short notice, thus disrupting continuity of patient care. Some observers have remarked that patients' attitudes toward physicians have become increasingly adversarial because they think doctors are more concerned with pleasing insurance companies than to provide good care.

• Changes in communications technology. The widespread use of computers in managed care and health insurance organizations to store databases of patient information has raised questions about preserving confidentiality. In addition, the increasing popularity of e-mail for communication between patients and professionals opens up concerns about the security and privacy of electronic files.

• Multicultural issues. Hospitals and medical or dental offices have been increasingly confronted with the complications that can arise in cross-cultural professional-patient relationships. Different ethnic and racial groups in the United States have widely varying customs and attitudes toward such matters as expressing physical pain or grief; undressing in front of a professional of the opposite sex; asking questions about their diagnosis and treatment; and other issues that arise in medical settings.

Professional implications

Now, at the beginning of the twenty-first century, the major emphasis of the professional-patient relationship is on the medical professional and the patient as partners making a a joint decision about the patient's treatment. Patients have requested and been given more rights concerning their medical treatment. Medical professionals should encourage patients to learn about their medical problems, weigh the benefits of different treatments, and make choices based on their own beliefs and values.

Some specific issues

Recent changes in professional-patient relationships have tended to cluster around several specific issues.

INVOLVEMENT OF FAMILY MEMBERS IN PROFESSIONAL/PATIENT RELATIONSHIPS. Although discussions of professional-patient relationships often proceed as if the relationship concerns only two people, the care provider and the patient, in many cases family members are also involved. In the cases of children and elderly patients, family members may be needed to describe the patient's symptoms or provide care at home. With regard to the elderly, different family members may

have sharp disagreements about the level of health care that is necessary, which can complicate the professional's work.

CONFIDENTIALITY. The computerization of patient information, combined with the increasing involvement of federal and state governments in health care, has led some observers to ask whether present security measures are adequate. Both trends—the use of computers and the expansion of government regulation—increase the number of people who have access to patient records and private information.

In the United States and Canada, the courts generally recognize two limitations on the professional's obligation to preserve confidentiality. The first is a court order that requires the physician to deliver confidential information about a patient. The second limitation concerns situations in which a patient is endangering his or her own life or the lives of others.

SEXUAL MISCONDUCT. The most explosive issue in recent years has been the rise in the number of reported incidents of sexual harassment or abuse of patients on the part of health professionals. The two specialties that have studied the issue most carefully are psychiatry and obstetrics-gynecology. Most such incidents (about 85%) involve male professionals and female patients; another 12% involve male professionals and male patients. The remaining 3% involve female professionals.

Studies of sexual misconduct on the part of professionals have reported the following findings:

• The greater degree of patient participation in medical decision-making does not do away with a basic inequality in professional-patient relationships. The patient is dependent on the professional's knowledge and authority, and the professional is obligated not to exploit that advantage.

• People who are seriously ill are emotionally vulnerable. They are less able to protect themselves against violation of their physical or psychological boundaries. Thus they cannot be regarded as "consenting" to a sexual relationship with a health care provider.

• Many adult patients were abused as children and find it difficult to protect themselves in adult life even apart from health crises. In particular, many women have been trained in childhood to be passive and compliant in the face of aggressive or exploitative behavior from men. These patients should not be accused of inviting or "asking for" sexual abuse.

• Some medical procedures appear to be fertile ground for poor communication or misunderstanding between the professional and patient.

KEY TERMS

Boundaries—The limits that define a human being's personal space. Boundaries may be physical, psychological, emotional, or spiritual.

Confidentiality—The protection and maintenance of strict privacy and secrecy in relationships between professionals and their patients or clients.

Ethics—The rules of conduct recognized as governing a particular group, as medical professionals.

Hippocratic Oath—The ethical pledge attributed to Hippocrates that is used as a standard for care by physicians worldwide.

Rapport—The relation between professional and patient, particularly one that is harmonious and empathic.

Most medical, dental, and nursing schools in the United States and Canada now include courses in professional ethics, communication skills, and understanding of the social context of professional-patient relationships. Students are taught that mutual respect and clear communication between professionals and patients are the most effective safeguards against abuse.

Resources

BOOK

Rutter, Peter, M.D. *Sex in the Forbidden Zone: When Men in Power—Therapists, Doctors, Clergy, Teachers, and Others—Betray Women's Trust.* Los Angeles, CA: Jeremy P. Tarcher, Inc., 1989.

PERIODICAL

Fitzsousa, Michael, ed. "Doctor-Patient Relationship." *Yale Medicine: Alumni Bulletin of the Yale University School of Medicine* 35, no. 2 (Spring, 2001): 20-41.

OTHER

American Academy of Pediatrics, Committee on Bioethics. Appropriate Boundaries in the Pediatrician-Family-Patient Relationship. Policy Statement, adopted August 1999.

Canadian Medical Association. The patient-physician relationship and the sexual abuse of patients. Policy summary approved by the CMA Board of Directors, June 1, 1994.

ORGANIZATIONS

American Hospital Association. One North Franklin, Chicago, IL 60606-3421. http://www.aha.org.

American Medical Association. 515 N. State Street, Chicago, IL 60610. (312) 464-5000. http://www. ama-assn.org.

American Nurses Association. 600 Maryland Avenue, SW, Suite 100 West, Washington, DC 20024. (202) 651-7000. http://www.ana.org.

Canadian Medical Association. 1867 Alta Vista Drive, Ottawa ON K1G 3Y6. (613) 731-8610x2307 or (888) 855-2555. Fax (613) 236-8864. cmamsc@cma.ca.

Peggy Elaine Browning

Progesterone assay *see* **Sex hormones tests**
Prolactin test *see* **Pituitary hormone tests**
Prolapsed disk *see* **Herniated disk**

Prophylactic antibiotic premedication

Definition

Prophylactic antibiotic premedication is the practice of prescribing limited antibiotic therapy to dental patients who are at risk of contracting microbial disease as a result of invasive dental procedures.

Purpose

Oral **bacteria** can enter the bloodstream during dental procedures and are normally destroyed by the body's **immune system**. In certain cases, however, bacteria may settle on abnormal **heart** valves or tissue that has been weakened by surgery or an existing heart problem. Infective **endocarditis**, an **infection** of the endocardium or heart valves, can be the result. Prophylactic premedication with approved**antibiotics** manages and reduces the risk of infection.

A study published in November 2000 called into question whether antibiotic **prophylaxis** is necessary for dental treatment. Such treatment, the study concluded, does not seem to be a risk factor for infective endocarditis. The American Dental Association (ADA) and American Heart Association have stated that their current recommendations are valid, although further research is warranted. The ADA's Council on Scientific Affairs continues to monitor, analyze, and assess research in prophylactic premedication with antibiotics.

The use of prophylactic premedication in oral health care has undergone many changes since its inception. Dosages have been decreased, and the conditions requiring premedication have changed. Premedication for patients who are recipients of large joint prostheses is no longer universally recommended. Some associations of orthopedists, for instance, state that routine antibiotic coverage is not necessary for patients who have joint prostheses and are undergoing dental procedures. It is recognized, however, that decisions regarding premedication should be made on an individual basis.

Precautions

According to the American Heart Association, endocarditis rarely occurs in people with normal hearts. Certain preexisting heart conditions are susceptible to bacteremia, however. These include:

- an artificial (prosthetic) heart valve
- a history of previous endocarditis
- heart valves damaged (scarred) by conditions such as rheumatic fever
- congenital heart or heart valve defects
- mitral valve prolapse with a murmur
- hypertrophic cardiomyopathy

Description

Procedures affected

Dental procedures for which antibiotic premedication is indicated include those in which bleeding is likely. They include:

- dental extractions
- periodontal procedures, including surgery, scaling and root planing, probing, and periodontal maintenance
- dental implant placement and reimplantation of avulsed (torn-out) teeth
- endodontic (root canal) instrumentation or surgery— only beyond the apex
- subgingival placement of antibiotic strips
- initial placement of orthodontic fibers
- intraligamentary local anesthetic injections
- prophylactic cleaning of teeth or implants where bleeding is anticipated
- restorative dentistry with or without retraction cord
- local anesthetic injections
- intracanal endodontic treatment, post-placement and buildup
- placement of rubber dams
- postoperative suture removal
- placement of removable prosthodontic/orthodontic appliances
- taking of oral impressions, fluoride treatments
- taking of oral radiographs, orthodontic appliance adjustment

- shedding of primary teeth

Dosages recommended

The American Heart Association recommends the following standard regimens for dental treatment in patients at risk of bacterial endocarditis.

- General adult patients: 2 grams amoxicillin (children, 50 mg/kg) given orally one hour before procedure.
- Adult patients unable to take oral medications: 2 grams ampicillin (children, 50 mg/kg) given intramuscularly or intravenously within 30 minutes before procedure.
- Adult patients allergic to amoxicillin, ampicillin, or penicillin: 600 mg clindamycin (children, 20 mg/kg) given orally one hour before procedure. Alternatively, use 2 grams cephalexin or cefadroxil (children, 50 mg/kg) given orally one hour before procedure. Cephalosporins should not be used in patients with immediate-type hypersensitivity reaction to penicillins. Another alternative is 500 mg azithromycin or clarithromycin (children, 14 mg/kg) given orally one hour before procedure.
- Adult patients allergic to amoxicillin, ampicillin, or penicillin who are unable to take oral medications: 600 mg clindamycin (children, 20 mg/kg) intravenously within 30 minutes before procedure. Alternatively, use 1 gram cefazolin (children, 25 mg/kg) intramuscularly or intravenously within 30 minutes before procedure.

Preparation

Antibiotic premedication is given to the patient either one hour (oral) or 30 minutes (intramuscular and intravenous) prior to the procedure.

Complications

When prophylactic premedication is prescribed for dental treatment, prior use of antibiotics should be considered. Resistant organisms may develop, especially if the proposed dental treatment closely follows prior antibiotic exposure. In that case, it is recommended that dentists consult with the patient's physician on the drug chosen and its dosage.

Possible allergic reactions to antibiotics must also be considered. Careful attention to the patient's **health history** is indicated to determine any prior allergy.

Patients who have difficulty swallowing may be given antibiotics intravenously or intramuscularly.

KEY TERMS

Bacteremia—Presence of bacteria in the blood.

Cardiomyopathy—Chronic disorder of the heart muscle that may involve hypertrophy and obstructive damage to the heart.

Endocardium—Membrane lining the chambers of the heart and covering the cusps of the various valves.

Infective endocarditis—A systemic disease characterized by focal bacterial infection of the heart valves, with formation of bacteria-laden vegetation.

Mitral valve prolapse—Downward displacement of the valve between the left atrium and ventricle of the heart.

Results

Prophylactic antibiotic premedication manages and reduces the risk of infective endocarditis as a result of dental treatment.

Health care team roles

Dentists prescribing prophylactic antibiotic premedication should consult with the patient's physicians, both general and specialty. When treating a patient with heart problems, for instance, the dentist would contact the patient's cardiologist. In determining whether a patient with a large joint prosthesis should be premedicated, the dentist should confer with the patient's orthopedic specialist.

Every member of the dental team must be aware of the risks of infective endocarditis to their patients. Health questionnaires should be scrutinized at the initial visit to identify patients at risk. On follow-up visits, health histories should be updated.

Resources

PERIODICALS

"Antibiotic prophylaxis and prevention of endocarditis." *Journal of the American Dental Association* (September 2011): 1062.

Lockhart, Peter B. "Antibiotic prophylaxis for dental procedures: are we drilling in the wrong direction?" *Circulation* (3 July 2012): 11–12.

ORGANIZATIONS

American Dental Association. 211 East Chicago Ave., Chicago, IL 60611. (312) 440-2500. http://www.ada.org.

American Heart Association. 7272 Greenville Ave., Dallas, TX 75231. (800) 242-8721. http://www.americanheart.org.

Cathy Hester Seckman, R.D.H.

Prophylaxis

Definition

A prophylaxis is a measure taken to maintain health and prevent the spread of disease. Antibiotic prophylaxis is the focus of this article and refers to the use of **antibiotics** to prevent infections.

Purpose

Antibiotics are well known for their ability to treat infections. But some antibiotics also are prescribed to *prevent* infections. This usually is done only in certain situations or for people with particular medical problems. For example, people with abnormal **heart** valves have a high risk of developing heart valve infections after even minor surgery. This happens because **bacteria** from other parts of the body get into the bloodstream during surgery and travel to the heart valves. To prevent these infections, people with heart valve problems often take antibiotics before having any kind of surgery, including dental surgery.

Antibiotics also may be prescribed to prevent infections in people with weakened immune systems, such as people with **AIDS** or people who are having **chemotherapy** treatments for **cancer**. But even healthy people with strong immune systems may occasionally be given preventive antibiotics—if they are having certain kinds of surgery that carry a high risk of **infection**, or if they are traveling to parts of the world where they are likely to get an infection that causes **diarrhea**, for example.

In all of these situations, a physician should be the one to decide whether antibiotics are necessary. Unless a physician says to do so, it is not a good idea to take antibiotics to prevent ordinary infections.

Because the overuse of antibiotics can lead to resistance, drugs taken to prevent infection should be used only for a short time.

Description

Among the drugs used for antibiotic prophylaxis are amoxicillin (a type of penicillin) and fluoroquinolones

KEY TERMS

AIDS—Acquired immunodeficiency syndrome. A disease caused by infection with the human immunodeficiency virus (HIV). In people with this disease, the immune system breaks down, opening the door to other infections and some types of cancer.

Antibiotic—A medicine used to treat infections.

Chemotherapy—Treatment of an illness with chemical agents. The term is usually used to describe the treatment of cancer with drugs.

Immune system—The body's natural defenses against disease and infection.

such as ciprofloxacin (Cipro) and trovafloxacin (Trovan). These drugs are available only with a physician's prescription and come in tablet, capsule, liquid, and injectable forms.

Recommended dosage

The recommended dosage depends on the type of antibiotic prescribed and the reason it is being used. For the correct dosage, check with the physician or dentist who prescribed the medicine or the pharmacist who filled the prescription. Be sure to take the medicine exactly as prescribed. Do not take more or less than directed, and take the medicine only for as long as the physician or dentist says to take it.

Precautions

If the medicine causes nausea, **vomiting**, or diarrhea, check with the physician or dentist who prescribed it as soon as possible. Patients who are taking antibiotics before surgery should not wait until the day of the surgery to report problems with the medicine. The physician or dentist needs to know right away if problems occur.

For other specific precautions, see the entry on the type of drug prescribed such as penicillins or fluoroquinolones.

Side effects

Antibiotics may cause a number of side effects. For details, see entries on specific types of antibiotics. Anyone who has unusual or disturbing symptoms after taking antibiotics should get in touch with his or her physician.

Interactions

Whether used to treat or to prevent infection, antibiotics may interact with other medicines. When this happens, the effects of one or both of the drugs may change or the risk of side effects may be greater. Anyone who takes antibiotics for any reason should inform the physician about all the other medicines he or she is taking and should ask whether any possible interactions may interfere with drugs' effects. For details of **drug interactions**, see entries on specific types of antibiotics.

Resources

PERIODICALS

Amodio, Emanuele, et al. "Perioperative antibiotic prophylaxis in plastic surgery: A prospective study of 1100 adult patients." *Journal of Plastic, Reconstructive & Aesthetic Surgery* 65.5 (2012): 601.

"Antibiotic prophylaxis and prevention of endocarditis." *Journal of the American Dental Association* (September 2011): 1062.

Bowe, Edwin A., Joseph Conigliaro, and Brenda G. Fahy. "Perioperative antibiotic process improvement reaps rewards." *American Journal of Medical Quality* 26.3 (2011): 185.

Lockhart, Peter B. "Antibiotic prophylaxis for dental procedures: are we drilling in the wrong direction?" *Circulation* (3 July 2012): 11-12.

Misra, U. "Antibiotic prophylaxis for caesarean section." *Anaesthesia* 67.9 (2012): 1046.

Nancy Ross-Flanigan

Proprioceptive neuromuscular facilitation

Definition

Proprioceptive neuromuscular facilitation (PNF) is a **rehabilitation** technique that was initiated over 50 years ago. It is used to stimulate the neuromuscular system in an effort to excite proprioceptors (sensory organs in muscles, tendons, bones, and joints) in order to produce a desired movement.

Purpose

An individual with a neuromuscular disorder may have dyscoordinated movement, that is, movement that is jerky or unsteady. PNF is a specific treatment approach that attempts to make movement more efficient and to improve function during activities of daily living.

Precautions

When using PNF, care must be taken during the movements. Injuries to tendons, muscles, or ligaments can occur if movement is not indicated or is too aggressive.

Description

PNF involves many combinations of motions. The goal is to incorporate postural and righting **reflexes**, which are important for maintaining balance. Usually during PNF motions or patterns, resistance is given, first during the stronger part of the range and followed by the weakest part of the range. Other techniques in PNF have the patient isometrically contract the involved muscle or muscle group (agonist), followed by immediately contracting the muscle or muscle group opposite the involved group (antagonist). This technique is called rhythmic stabilization. Another technique incorporates rhythmic stabilization alternately. Contraction of agonist and antagonist in an alternating fashion is called slow reversal.

PNF is based on flexion and extension, but is performed in diagonal patterns. This practice maximizes neuromuscular facilitation by lengthening the muscle or muscle group as much as possible, thus incorporating the stretch reflex.

There are various types of movement patterns in PNF, including unilateral and bilateral patterns. Unilateral patterns are usually based on one limb, either upper or lower, and can incorporate head and trunk movement. Bilateral patterns are done on either both upper or lower limbs at the same time. There are other techniques within the scope of PNF that are used to facilitate. Facilitatory techniques used to stimulate the neuromuscular system include stretch, traction, approximation, and maximal resistance. Other techniques that require significant participation by the patient are rhythmic stabilization, contract-relax, hold-relax, slow reversal, and repeated contractions.

Complications

Which PNF technique is used in therapy depends on a patient's needs. For example, it would not be advisable to apply a stretch technique to an area of known muscle tearing or around a fracture area. Overstretching a limb with known hypertonicity may cause significant muscle or tendon damage. Care must be taken to minimize stresses placed on muscle, tendon, or joints when known pathology is present.

Results

The goal of PNF is to restore neuromuscular function to an individual who presents with impairment to the neuromuscular system. By restoring neuromuscular function, the individual can improve gait, mobility, and self-care. Thus, the goal of PNF is to restore movement, control posture and body awareness, improve coordination, and improve muscle function.

Health care team roles

PNF techniques are typically used by physical and occupational therapists. Nurses and other allied health care professionals must realize that PNF alone does not restore neuromuscular function. Activities of daily living (ADL) must be integrated within the total construct of rehabilitation, that is, during self-care, recreation, and socialization. Nurses and other allied health care professionals must provide an environment that facilitates this integration of rehabilitation with other activities.

Resources

BOOKS

Adler, Susan S., Dominiek Beckers, and Math Buck. *PNF in Practice: An Illustrated Guide,* 3rd edition. Springer, 2007.

Sharma, Krishna N. *Handbook of Proprioceptive Neuromuscular Facilitation: Basic Concepts and Techniques.* LAP LAMBERT Academic Publishing, 2012.

Mark Damian Rossi, Ph.D, P.T., C.S.C.S.

Prostaglandins *see* **Uterine stimulants**

Prostate-specific antigen test *see* **Tumor marker tests**

Prostate biopsy

Definition

Prostate biopsy is a surgical procedure to remove small samples of prostate tissue for microscopic examination. The prostate gland lies just below the urinary bladder and surrounds the urethra. The gland

KEY TERMS

Agonist—The muscle that contracts to create movement or tension. For example, the quadriceps muscles are the agonists in knee extension.

Antagonist—The muscle that opposes the movement being completed. The hamstrings are antagonists to the quadriceps during knee extension.

Dyscoordinated—Movement that is asynchronous, jerky, and unsteady.

Extension—The act of straightening a joint to bring the bones more in line, e.g., straightening the knee or elbow.

Flexion—Bending of a joint, such as bending or flexing the knee.

Postural—Pertaining to the position of the head, neck, trunk and lower limbs in relation to the ground and the vertical.

Proprioceptors—Sensory organs in muscle, tendon, bone, and joint that provide information to the brain about the surrounding environment, such as position.

Righting—The ability to maintain one's head and center of gravity within one's base of support. For example, while standing on a moving bus, an individual adjusts to maintain an upright posture as the bus comes to a stop.

produces enzyme-rich secretions that contribute to the seminal fluid via ducts that enter the urethra.

Purpose

A prostate biopsy is usually performed to determine whether the patient has **prostate cancer**. Occasionally, it may also be used to diagnose a condition called benign prostatic hypertrophy (BPH), a progressive enlargement of the prostate that may cause obstruction of urine flow in older males.

A prostate biopsy is ordered when other tests have indicated a need to visualize samples of prostate tissue for abnormalities. These tests are the digital rectal examination (DRE) and the prostate-specific antigen (PSA) **blood** test. The DRE is a routine screening test performed by the physician to feel for any enlargement or nodular growth of the patient's prostate. Higher than normal levels of the protein marker PSA can be an indicator of prostate **cancer**. If either the DRE or PSA results are abnormal, the physician may order additional

tests, including a prostate biopsy. **Computed tomography scans**, **magnetic resonance imaging**, and ultrasonograms provide detailed pictures of the prostate and can also be used to determine the extent and spread of prostate disease. However, a prostate biopsy (examination of the cells of the gland under a **microscope**) remains the most definitive test for diagnosing and staging prostate cancer.

Precautions

A prostate biopsy is ordered only when the physician has used prior diagnostic tools that indicate an abnormal prostate. Prostate biopsies are usually performed by a urogenital system specialist (urologist). Special precautions will be required before the biopsy if the patient has a history of abnormal bleeding or is currently taking a blood-thinning medication.

Description

According to the American Cancer Society, next to skin cancer, prostate cancer continues to be the most commonly diagnosed cancer in American men. Prostate biopsies are usually performed in one of two ways. They can be performed by inserting a needle through the wall of the rectum or by inserting a needle through the perineum (the area between the base of the penis and the rectum). The patient may be given a sedative to help him relax. In preparation for the biopsy the patient will have an **enema**, and will begin antibiotic therapy to prevent an **infection**.

Needle biopsy via the rectum

This procedure, called a transrectal ultrasound-guided biopsy, is the most commonly performed type of prostate biopsy, and can usually be performed in the physician's office without **general anesthesia**. The patient is asked to lie on his side or on his back with his legs in stirrups. Local anesthetic is administered, and the urologist uses a thin needle attached to a spring-loaded gun directed by ultrasound to collect samples from the prostate. The gun is able to insert and remove the needle into the prostate tissue rapidly, creating less discomfort and trauma for the patient. The procedure can often be completed within 30 minutes. Usually the tissue samples are obtained by fine-needle aspiration, as opposed to larger core tissue samples that create more discomfort for the patient.

Needle biopsy via the perineum

If the chances of a complication for the patient are too great for the transrectal ultrasound-guided biopsy, the urologist may choose another route through the perineum for access to the prostate. The skin of the perineum is thoroughly cleansed and a local anesthetic is injected at the site where the biopsy is to be performed. Once the area is numb, the physician makes a small (1 in/2.5 cm) incision in the perineum. The physician places one finger in the rectum to guide the placement of the biopsy needle, and the needle is then inserted into the prostate. A small amount of tissue is collected, and the needle is withdrawn. The needle is then reinserted into another part of the prostate and another sample of tissue is collected. In this manner, samples are collected from several areas. After the procedure, pressure is applied at the biopsy site to stop bleeding. The patient usually experiences only slight discomfort and the procedure can often be completed within 30 minutes.

Preparation

Before scheduling the biopsy, the physician, nurse, or physician assistant completes a thorough medical history of the patient to include all medications that the patient is taking, a list of any medications to which the patient is allergic, and a history of any bleeding problems. The patient may be given an antibiotic shortly before the test to reduce the risk of infection. Usually an enema is required prior to the biopsy procedure, and the patient will be given instructions on administration of the enema.

Aftercare

The physician, nurse, or physician assistant should monitor the patient for any complications, excessive bleeding, or **pain** from the procedure. After the procedure, the patient commonly experiences minor rectal bleeding, blood in urine or feces, and sometimes blood in the semen. These side effects usually last only for a few days. Often, the physician will prescribe **antibiotics** to guard against potential infection. The patient should drink fluids to help reduce any burning sensation and the chances of a urinary tract infection.

Complications

Prostate biopsy performed with a bioptic gun is a low-risk procedure. The possible complications include abnormal bleeding, urinary tract infection, or an inability to urinate. These complications are treatable, and the patient should notify the physician promptly if symptoms occur. If the patient develops a high **fever**, chills, or unusual pain or bleeding after the procedure, he should notify the physician immediately.

Results

The prostate tissue is fixed, stained, and prepared on glass slides for microscopic analysis by a pathologist who will examine the samples for the presence of cancerous cells. If the prostate tissue samples show no sign of inflammation, and if no cancerous cells are detected, the results are normal. If malignant cells are present, the pathologist grades them, in order to estimate the aggressiveness of the tumor. The most commonly used grading system is called the Gleason system; the higher the Gleason score, the more likely it is that the cancer is fast-growing and may have already spread to other areas (metastasized).

Health care team roles

Training

The urologist and several non-physician health care providers are involved in the biopsy process. The urologist has received specialized training in ultrasound-guided biopsy procedures. The additional health care team members have obtained specialized training to assist the urologist by preparing the patient for the procedure and monitoring the patient during the procedure. They also ensure that the urologist has all of the instruments and equipment required before, during, and after the procedure. A health care provider properly packages and labels the specimens for transport to the pathology laboratory.

Patient education

The health care provider can be an important resource for patients who require a prostate biopsy. Health care professionals should make men aware of certain risk factors that can increase their chances of developing prostate cancer. Three important risk factors are age greater than 50, family history of prostate cancer, and African American descent. A health care provider should explain in detail the procedure to be performed and the possible complications associated with the biopsy.

The health care provider will instruct the patient in self-administering an enema. Following a needle biopsy, the health care providers should tell the patient that he may experience some minor discomfort, and that he should avoid strenuous activities for the remainder of the day. The health care provider should also inform that patient that he may notice a small amount of blood in his urine or minor bleeding from his rectum for two or three days after the test. The provider should emphasize to the patient that he or she should call the physician immediately when experiencing

KEY TERMS

Benign prostatic hypertrophy (BPH)—A noncancerous condition of the prostate that causes growth of the prostate tissue, thus enlarging the prostate and obstructing urination.

Biopsy—The surgical removal and microscopic examination of living tissue for diagnostic purposes.

Computed tomography (CT) scan—A medical procedure in which a series of x rays is taken at different angles and reconstructed by a computer in order to form detailed pictures of areas inside the body.

Digital rectal examination—A routine screening test that is used by physicians to detect any enlargement in the prostate gland or any hardening or other abnormality of the prostate tissue. The doctor inserts a gloved and lubricated finger (digit) into the patient's rectum, which lies just behind the prostate. Typically, since a majority of tumors develop in the posterior region of the prostate, they can be detected through the rectum.

Magnetic resonance imaging (MRI)—An imaging procedure that creates a detailed computer-constructed image of the target tissue based upon its deflection of a magnetic field produced by a powerful magnet. The magnetic field deflection is measured using radio waves (not x rays).

Pathologist—A doctor who specializes in the diagnosis of diseases by studying cells and tissues removed by biopsy.

Ultrasonogram—An image produced by high-frequency sound waves that cannot be heard by human ears. The sound waves are deflected by internal organs and tissues. These sound waves produce a pattern of echoes that are then used by the computer to create pictures of areas inside the body.

unusual bleeding, pain, fever, or an inability to urinate for 24 hours. The health care provider should provide the patient with the results of the test as soon as they are available.

Resources

BOOKS

Blum, Ralph, and Mark M.D. Scholz. *Invasion of the Prostate Snatchers: An Essential Guide to Managing Prostate Cancer for Patients and their Families.* Other Press, 2011.

Epstein, Jonathan I., and George J. Netto. *Biopsy Interpretation of the Prostate,* 4th edition. Lippincott Williams & Wilkins, 2007.

McHugh, John C. *The Decision: Your prostate biopsy shows cancer. Now what?: Medical insight, personal stories, and humor by a urologist who has been where you are now.* Jennie Cooper Press, 2010.

ORGANIZATIONS

American Cancer Society. 1599 Clifton Road NE, Atlanta, Georgia 30329. (800) 227-2345. http://www.cancer.org.

American Urological Association. 1120 N. Charles Street, Baltimore, MD 21201. (410) 727-1100. http://www.auanet.org.

National Prostate Cancer Coalition. 1300 19th Street NW, Suite 400, Washington, DC 20036. (202) 842-3600 ext. 214. http://www.pcacoalition.org.

Linda D. Jones, B.A., PBT (ASCP)

Prostate cancer

Definition

Prostate **cancer** is a disease in which the cells of the prostate (a gland found in the **male reproductive system**) become abnormal and start to grow uncontrollably, forming tumors. Tumors that can spread to other parts of the body are called malignant tumors or cancers. Tumors that are not capable of spreading in this way are said to be benign.

Description

The prostate is a gland that produces the fluid (semen), which contains sperm. The prostate is about the size of a walnut and lies just beneath the urinary bladder. Usually prostate cancer is slow growing, but it can grow faster in some instances. As a prostate cancer grows, some of the cells may break off and spread to other parts of the body through the lymphatic or the **blood** systems. This process is known as metastasis. The most common sites of spreading are the lymph nodes and various bones in the spine and the pelvic region.

The **lymphatic system** is composed of ducts that transport extracellular fluid from distant areas of the body to the **heart**. Fluid enters lymph ducts and travels toward the heart. Any fluid collected is mixed with the blood. Any excess fluid is eliminated from the blood by the **kidneys**. Along the lymph system are clusters of specialized tissue called lymph nodes. These nodes act as strainers and retain cellular debris to prevent it from entering the blood stream. Lymph nodes also retain

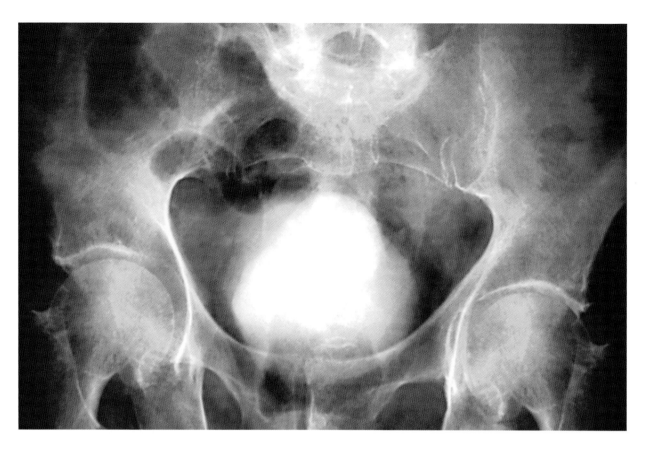

(Colored x-ray of the pelvis of a male patient showing enlarged prostate gland, photograph. GJlp / Photo Researchers, Inc.)

cancer cells that escape from tumors. For this reason, surgeons often remove some lymph nodes for analysis to determine the extent that a cancer may have spread beyond its original (primary) site.

The cause of prostate cancer is not clear; however, several risk factors are known. The average age at diagnosis of prostate cancer is approximately 67 years. In fact, two-thirds of prostate cancer cases occur in men over the age of 65. As men grow older, the likelihood of developing prostate cancer increases. Hence, age appears to be a risk factor for prostate cancer. Race may be another contributing factor. African Americans have the highest rate of prostate cancer in the world while the rate in Asians is one of the lowest. However, although the rate of prostate cancer in native Japanese men is low, the rate in Japanese Americans is closer to that of white American men. This finding suggests that environmental factors also play a role in prostate cancer.

There is some evidence to suggest that diets high in red meat, **calcium** and/or high-fat dairy products increase the risk of prostate cancer. **Obesity** has been linked in some studies to the development of a more aggressive form of prostate cancer. Studies also suggest that nutrients such as soy isoflavones, **vitamin E**, selenium, **vitamin D** and carotenoids (including lycopene, the red color agent in tomatoes and beets) may decrease prostate cancer risk. These substances contain particularly high levels of molecules called antioxidants, which seem to oppose the formation of cancer cells. Workers in industries, such as welding, with exposure to the metal cadmium, appear to have a higher than average risk of prostate cancer. Male sex hormone levels also may be linked to the rate of prostate cancer. Presence of inflammation of the prostate, also known as prostatitis, is being actively researched to determine if there is a link to prostate cancer development.

Genetic profile

An estimated 5–10% of prostate cancer is due to hereditary causes. Among men with early prostate cancer, a hereditary cause is likely in up to a third of cases before age 60 and in almost half of men diagnosed with prostate cancer at age 55 or less. Studies have found around a two- to three-fold increased rate of prostate cancer in close relatives of men with the disease. Hereditary prostate cancer is likely in a family if there are three cases of prostate cancer in close relatives, three affected generations (either mother's or father's side), or two relatives with prostate cancer before age 55.

Demographics

Prostate cancer is the most common cancer among men in the United States, and is the second leading cause of cancer deaths. The American Cancer Society estimates that in 2012, 241,740 new cases of prostate cancer will be diagnosed, and it will cause 28,170 deaths. One in six men in the United States will be diagnosed with prostate cancer at some point in their lives. Prostate cancer affects black men about twice as often as it does white men, and the mortality rate among African Americans is also higher. African Americans have the highest rate of prostate cancer in the world. The prostate cancer rate varies considerably around the world. The highest rates are in North America and Western Europe, whereas the rates are moderate in Africa and lowest in Asia. It is unclear what roles genetics, diet, economics, and health care access play in these rates.

Although incidence rates of prostate cancer are high, it is important to note that for most men, prostate cancer is a very treatable disease. As of 2012, the number of men alive after a diagnosis of prostate cancer is rapidly approaching three million men.

Causes and symptoms

Frequently, prostate cancer has no symptoms, and the disease is diagnosed when a man goes for a routine screening examination. However, when the tumor is larger or the cancer has spread to nearby tissues, the following symptoms may be seen:

• weak or interrupted flow of urine

• frequent urination (especially at night)

• difficulty starting urination

• inability to urinate

• pain or burning sensation when urinating

• blood in the urine (hematuria)

• persistent pain in the lower back, hips, or thighs (bone pain)

• difficulty having or keeping an erection (impotence)

Diagnosis

Although prostate cancer may be very slow-growing, it can be quite aggressive, especially in younger men. When the disease is slow growing, it often may go undetected. Because it may take many years for the cancer to develop, many men with the disease are likely to die of other causes rather than from the cancer.

Prostate cancer is frequently curable when detected early. However, because the early stages of prostate cancer may not have any symptoms, it often goes undetected until a man goes for a routine **physical examination**. Diagnosis of the disease is made using some or all of the following tests.

Digital rectal examination (DRE)

In order to perform this test, a physician puts a lubricated, gloved finger (digit) into the rectum to feel for any lumps in the prostate. The rectum lies just behind the prostate gland, and a majority of prostate tumors begin in the posterior region of the prostate. The posterior portion of the prostate is most accessible to a physician's examining finger. If the physician does detect an abnormality, additional tests may be ordered to confirm these findings.

Blood tests

Blood tests are used to measure the amounts of certain protein markers, such as prostate-specific antigen (PSA), found circulating in the blood. The cells lining the prostate generally make this protein and a small amount can normally be detected in the bloodstream. However, prostate cancers typically produce large amounts of this protein, and it can be easily detected in the blood. Hence, when PSA is found in the blood in higher than normal amounts (for a man's age group), cancer may be present. Occasionally, other blood tests also are used to help with the diagnosis.

Transrectal ultrasound

A small sound-producing device (transducer) is placed in the rectum and sound waves are released from it. These sound waves bounce off the prostate tissue, and an image is created by a computer using the reflected sound waves. Since normal prostate tissue and prostate tumors reflect the sound waves differently, the test can be used to detect tumors. Though the insertion of the transducer into the rectum may be slightly uncomfortable, the procedure is generally painless and only takes about 20 minutes.

PROSTATE BIOPSY. If cancer is suspected from the results of any of the above tests, a physician will remove a small piece of prostate tissue with a hollow needle. This sample is then analyzed under a **microscope** for the presence of cancerous cells. **Prostate biopsy** is the most definitive diagnostic tool for prostate cancer.

If cancer is detected during the microscopic examination of the prostate tissue, a pathologist will grade the tumor. This means that the tumor will be scored on a scale of two to 10 to indicate how aggressive it is. Tumors with a lower score are less likely to grow and spread than are tumors with higher scores. This method of grading tumors is called the Gleason system. This is different from staging of the cancer. When a physician stages a cancer, a number is assigned. The number indicates whether it has spread and the extent of spread of the disease. In Stage I, the cancer is localized in the prostate in a single area, while in the last stage, Stage IV, the cancer cells have spread to other parts of the body.

X rays and imaging techniques

X-ray studies may be ordered to determine whether the cancer has spread to other areas. Imaging techniques (such as computed tomography [CT] scans and **magnetic resonance imaging** [MRI]), in which a computer is used to generate a detailed picture of the prostate and adjacent areas, may be undertaken to get a clearer view of the internal organs. A **bone** scan may be used to check whether the cancer has spread to bones. A ProstaScint scan may be used to check for prostate cancer cells in the body in tissues such as lymph nodes and other soft tissue organs.

Controversy continues to exist related to need, frequency and types of tests used to screen for prostate cancer. The American Cancer Society advocates that men 50 years and older who are not at high risk for the development of prostate cancer discuss options for screening with a health care provider. Men who are at higher risk should begin these discussions prior to age 45. Research has not yet conclusively determined that the benefits of screening for prostate cancer outweigh the cons associated with testing and with subsequent treatment which may be ordered. The frequency of testing should be determined by PSA levels.

Treatment

A physician and patient will decide on a treatment after considering many factors. For example, the man's age, the stage of the tumor, his general health, and the presence of any coexisting illnesses have to be considered. In addition, a man's personal preferences and the risks and benefits of each treatment method are also taken into account before any decision is made.

Surgery

For early-stage prostate cancer (Stage I and Stage II), surgery is frequently considered for men who are in good health. Radical prostatectomy involves complete removal of the prostate. During the surgery, some of the lymph nodes near the prostate may be removed to determine whether the cancer has spread beyond the prostate gland. Because the seminal vesicles (the glands where seminal fluid is made) are removed along with the prostate, **infertility** is often a side effect of this type of surgery. In order to minimize the risk of impotence (inability to have an erection) and incontinence (inability to control urine and/or stool flow), a procedure known as a nerve-sparing prostatectomy is used. However, some men will experience varying degrees of impotence and urine and/or **fecal incontinence** even after the nerve-sparing procedure.

In a different surgical method, known as the transurethral resection procedure or TURP, only the cancerous portion of the prostate is removed, by using a small wire loop that is introduced into the prostate through the urethra. This technique is most often used in men who cannot have a radical prostatectomy due to age or other illness, and it is infrequently recommended.

Radiation therapy

Radiation therapy involves the use of high-energy x-rays to kill cancer cells or to shrink tumors. It can be used instead of surgery for early-stage cancer. The radiation can either be administered from a machine outside the body (external beam radiation), or small radioactive pellets can be implanted in the prostate gland in the area surrounding a tumor (interstitial brachytherapy). Brachytherapy is usually reserved for the treatment of men with prostate cancers which are small and confined to the prostate and whose Gleason scores and PSA levels are low.

Hormone therapy

Hormone therapy is commonly used when the cancer is in an advanced stage and has spread to other parts of the body. Prostate cells need the male hormone testosterone to grow. Decreasing the levels of this hormone or inhibiting its activity may cause the cancer to shrink or stop growing. Hormone levels can be decreased in several ways. Orchiectomy is a surgical procedure that involves complete removal of the testicles, leading to a decrease in the levels of testosterone. Alternatively, drugs (such as LHRH agonists or anti-androgens) that bind to the male hormone testosterone and block its activity can be given. Luteinizing hormone releasing hormone (LHRH) agonists stimulate the **pituitary gland** in the **brain** to release luteinizing hormone. This release results in a decreased level of testosterone. Another approach involves administering the female hormone estrogen. When estrogen is given, the body senses the presence of a sex hormone and stops making the male hormone testosterone. However, there

KEY TERMS

Anti-androgen drugs—Drugs that block the activity of male hormones.

Benign—A term for a tumor that does not metastasize and is not life-threatening.

Benign prostatic hyperplasia (BPH)—A non-cancerous condition of the prostate that causes growth of prostatatic tissue, thus enlarging the prostate and blocking urination.

Biopsy—The surgical removal and microscopic examination of living tissue for diagnostic purposes.

Chemotherapy—Treatment of the cancer with synthetic drugs that destroy the tumor either by inhibiting the growth of the cancerous cells or by killing the cancer cells.

Estrogen—A female sex hormone.

Hematuria—Blood in the urine.

Hormone therapy—A treatment for prostate cancer that involves reducing the levels of the male hormone testosterone so that the growth of the prostate cancer cells is inhibited.

Lymph nodes—Small, bean-shaped structures that are scattered along the lymphatic vessels. These nodes serve as filters and retain any bacteria or cancer cells that are traveling through the system.

Malignant—A tumor that is capable of spreading to other organs and poses a serious threat to a person's life.

Metastasis—The spreading of cancer from the original site to other locations in the body.

Prostatectomy—The surgical removal of the prostate gland.

Radiation therapy—Treatment using high-energy radiation from x-ray machines, cobalt, radium, or other sources.

Rectum—The last 5–6 in (12–15 cm) of the large intestine that leads to the anus.

Semen—A whitish, opaque fluid released at ejaculation.

Seminal vesicles—Tubes above the prostate that make seminal fluid.

Testicles—Two egg-shaped glands that produce sperm and male sex hormones.

Testosterone—A male sex hormone produced mainly by the testicles.

Transrectal ultrasound—A procedure in which a probe is placed in the rectum. High-frequency sound waves that cannot be heard by humans are sent out from the probe and reflected by the prostate. These sound waves produce a pattern of echoes that are then used by the computer to create sonograms or pictures of areas inside the body.

---

are some side effects to hormone therapy. Men may have "hot flashes," enlargement and tenderness of the breasts, or impotence and loss of sexual desire—as well as blood clots, heart attacks, and strokes, depending on the dose of estrogen.

Chemotherapy

Chemotherapy is the use of drugs to kill cancer cells. The drugs can either be taken in pill form or injected into the body through a needle that is inserted into a blood vein. This type of treatment is called systemic treatment because the drug enters the blood stream, travels through the whole body, and kills cancer cells that are outside the prostate. Chemotherapy is sometimes used to treat prostate cancer that has recurred after other treatment. Research is ongoing to find more drugs that are effective for the treatment of prostate cancer.

Watchful waiting

Watchful waiting, also referred to as active surveillance or careful observation without immediate active treatment, means that no immediate treatment is recommended, but physicians keep the man suspected of having prostate cancer under careful observation. This option is generally used among older men when the tumor is not very aggressive and they have other, more life-threatening illnesses. Prostate cancer in older men tends to be slow-growing. Therefore, the risk of a man dying from prostate cancer, rather than from other causes, is relatively small.

Prognosis

According to the American Cancer Society, the survival rate for all stages of prostate cancer combined has increased dramatically over the last 30 years. Due to

QUESTIONS TO ASK YOUR DOCTOR

- Is my prostate cancer still confined to the prostate?
- Will treatment be required? If so, what type of treatment will be conducted?
- How will I know if my cancer is responding to treatment?
- How long do you anticipate treatment will last?
- What short- and long-term side-effects can I expect from my treatments?
- What resources are available in this community for men diagnosed with prostate cancer?

early detection and better screening methods, nearly 60% of the tumors are diagnosed while they are still confined to the prostate gland. Overall 5 year, 10 year, and 15 year survival rates (all stages) for men diagnosed with prostate cancer are 99%, 98%, and 91% respectively.

Health care team roles

A family physician or internist often makes an initial diagnosis of prostate cancer. A urologist often confirms the diagnosis and supervises treatment. A cancer oncologist may administer radiation or chemotherapy treatments. A surgeon may excise a tumor of the prostate. Nurses provide care throughout hospitalization. Nurses also provide education to the patient and family according to the physician's orders, as well as **home care**.

Prevention

There is no known way to prevent prostate cancer. Some experts feel that dietary modifications may delay the onset of prostate cancer. This view is not universally shared. Individuals with a family history of prostate cancer should be undergo screening to detect prostate cancer as recommended by the most current screening guidelines.

Resources

BOOK

Nelson, W.G., Carter, H.B., DeWeese, T.L., et al "Prostate Cancer." In Clinical Oncology, 4th ed. Edited by Abeloff, M.D., Armitage, J.D., Lichter, A.S., et al. Philadelphia: Elsevier, 2008, 1653-99.

PERIODICALS

Abarado,C. & Mahon, S.M. "Androgen-Deprivation Bone Loss in Patients with Prostate Cancer." Clinical Journal of Oncology Nursing (April, 2010); 14(2): 191-8.

DeSousa, A., Sonavane, S., & Mehta, J. "Psychological Aspects of Prostate Cancer." Prostate Cancer Prostatic Dis 92012); 15(2): 120-7.

Doyle-Lindrud, S. "Managing Side Effects of the Novel Taxane Cabazitaxel in Castrate-Resistant Prostate Cancer." Clinical Journal of Oncology Nursing (June, 2012); 16(3): 286-91.

Galbraith, M., Hays, L., & Tanner, T. "What Men are Saying About Surviving Prostate Cancer: Complexities Represented in a Decade of Comments." Clinical Journal of Oncology Nursing (Feb, 2012); 16(1); 65-72.

Howlett, K., Koetters, T., Edrington, J., West, C., et al "Changes in Sexual Function on Mood and Quality of Life in Patients Undergoing Radiation Therapy for Prostate Cancer." Oncology Nursing Forum (Jan, 2010); 37(1): E58-E66.

Marroquin, J.M. "To Screen or Not to Screen: Ongoing Debate in the Early Detection of Prostate Cancer." Clinical Journal of Oncology Nursing (Feb, 2011); 15(1): 97-8.

Violette, P.D., & Saad, F. "Chemoprevention of Prostate Cancer." J Am Board Fam Med (2012); 25(1):111-9.

ORGANIZATIONS

American Cancer Society, 250 Williams Street NW, Atlanta, Georgia United States 30303, www.cancer.org

American Society of Clinical Oncology, 2318 Mill Road, Suite 800, Alexandria, Virginia United States 22314, (571) 4831300, www.asco.org

American Urological Association, 1000 Corporate Blvd., Linthicum, Maryland United States 21090, (866) 7464282, http://www.auanet.org

National Cancer Institute, 6116 Executive Boulevard, Suite 300, Bethesda, Maryland United States 20892-8322, (800) 4226237, www.cancer.gov

National Comprehensive Cancer Network, 275 Commerce Drive, Suite 300, Fort Washington, Pennsylvania United States 19034, (215) 690-0300, www.nccn.org

Oncology Nursing Society, 125 Enterprise Drive, Pittsburgh, Pennsylvania United States 25275, (866) 2574667, www.ons.org

Prostate Cancer Foundation, 1250 Fourth Street, Santa Monica, California United States 90401, (800) 7572873, www.pcf.org

Us Too Prostate Cancer Education and Support, 5003 Fairview Avenue, Downers Grove, Illinois United States 60515, (800) 8087866, http://www.ustoo.org

L. Fleming Fallon, Jr., MD, DrPH
Melinda Oberleitner, R.N., D.N.S.

Prostate ultrasound

Definition

A prostate ultrasound is a diagnostic test used to detect potential problems with a man's prostate. An ultrasound test involves very high-frequency sound waves that pass through the body. The pattern of reflected sound waves, or "echoes," shows the outline of the prostate. This test can show whether the prostate is enlarged, and whether an abnormal growth that might be **cancer** is present.

Purpose

The prostate is a chestnut-shaped organ surrounding the beginning of the urethra in men. It produces a milky fluid that is part of the seminal fluid discharged during ejaculation. Prostate disorders are common in men over 50. In cases of **prostate cancer**, ultrasound is often crucial, since early detection, when the lesion is localized and curable, can lead to effective therapy.

A doctor may decide to do a prostate ultrasound following a digital rectal examination (DRE) that reveals any prostate abnormalities such as lumps or an **enlarged prostate**, or following a **blood** test that reveals abnormal levels of a substance called prostate-specific antigen (PSA), a normal protease produced by the prostate epithelium. Currently, testing for PSA is the best available tumor marker. Abnormal levels of PSA may indicate the presence of cancer. However, the PSA test is non-specific, and PSA can be elevated without the presence of prostate cancer.

The ultrasound procedure involves a special probe inserted into the rectum that sends sound waves to the prostate gland. The waves bounce off the prostate surface and are translated by computer as an image on a screen.

If cancer is suspected, the doctor will want to take a tissue sample (**prostate biopsy**) to test it to see if it is cancerous. An ultrasound can show the location on the prostate from which the sample should be taken. It can also reveal if the cancer has begun to spread to other locations.

Ultrasound is also used in treatment of prostate cancer. If a doctor decides to treat the cancer with a surgical freezing procedure, ultrasound is used as an aid in the procedure. Doctors are also experimenting with a procedure that uses heat to kill cancerous prostate tissue. During this procedure, called high-intensity focused ultrasound (HIFUS), an ultrasound probe first creates an image of the prostate, then high energy ultrasound beams target specific areas, generating heat that destroys cancerous tissue.

Ultrasound also can reveal other types of prostate disease, such as prostatitis.

Precautions

A prostate ultrasound study is generally not performed on men who have recently had surgery on their lower bowel. This is because the test requires placing an ultrasound probe about the size of a finger into the rectum.

Description

The prostate ultrasound technique performed is called transrectal **ultrasonography**. This technique not only allows for visualization of the prostate; it is used to position the needle if a biopsy is performed. During the procedure, the cylinder-shaped ultrasound probe, or transducer, is gently placed in the rectum as the patient lies on his left side with the knees bent. This position allows for more comfort and easier insertion. The probe is rocked back and forth to obtain images of the entire prostate. Pictures of the prostate are produced and measurements are taken. The procedure takes about 15–25 minutes to perform. After the test, the patient's doctor can be notified right away, and usually he or she will have a written report within 36 hours.

During a biopsy, a small needle is inserted very rapidly into the prostate gland. Sample tissue is taken and sent to a pathology lab for preparation. Transrectal ultrasound-guided core biopsy of the prostate is regarded as the most effective determinant of the grade, volume, and localization of a tumor and of its distribution within the prostate. Usually, six to eight biopsies are taken.

Recently, in an effort to improve prostate cancer diagnosis, physicians have performed experiments with ultrasound contrast-agent enhanced color Doppler imaging. By revealing increased vascularity associated with prostate cancer, the procedure can allow for more targeted biopsies, thus reducing the number of biopsies needed.

Preparation

Patients are instructed to have an **enema** two to four hours before an exam. Feces or gas could impede the progress of the rectal probe. Patients also are instructed not to urinate for one hour before the test. If biopsies may be done, the doctor will prescribe an antibiotic that usually is taken in four doses starting the night before the biopsy, the morning of the test, the evening after the test, and the following morning.

Aftercare

For the most part, transrectal ultrasound is a painless procedure. The patient may be warned that there could be some discomfort as the probe is inserted. Generally, the patient is allowed to leave after a radiologist or urologist has reviewed the results. There may be some mucus or a small amount of bleeding from the rectum after the ultrasound. Some patients notice a small amount of blood in the urine for up to two days after the test. Blood may also be present in the semen. As long as the amount of blood is small and resolves after one to two days, there is no cause for concern.

Complications

There are no serious risks from a prostate ultrasound study. **Infection** is rare and probably is a result of biopsy rather than the sonogram itself. If the ultrasound probe is moved too vigorously, some bleeding may continue for a few days.

Results

Modern ultrasound techniques can display both the smooth-surfaced outer shell of the prostate and the core tissues surrounding the urethra. The entire volume of the prostate should be less than 20 milliliters, and its outline should appear as a smooth echo-reflecting (echogenic) rim. Some irregularities within the substance of the gland and **calcium** deposits are normal findings.

An enlarged prostate with dimmed echoes may indicate either prostatitis or benign enlargement of the gland, called benign prostatic hypertrophy (BPH). A distinct focal lump of tissue more likely means cancer. Cancer also often appears as an irregular area within the gland that distorts the normal pattern of echoes. In either case, a biopsy should clarify the diagnosis.

Health care team roles

The procedure is performed by a specially trained diagnostic medical sonographer. The sonographer assists the physician and radiologist in gathering sonographic data necessary to diagnose prostate cancer. Sonographers can have extensive, direct patient contact that may include performing some invasive procedures. The sonographer obtains and records patient history; performs diagnostic procedures and obtains diagnostic images; analyzes technical information; and provides an oral and written summary of technical findings to the physician for medical diagnosis. A urologist or radiologist performs the biopsy.

Training

Medical sonography programs vary in length from one to four years depending on the program design and degree or certificate awarded. Program entry requirements vary as well, and range from a high-school diploma to specific qualifications in a clinically related health profession. Graduation from an accredited program is followed by a qualifying exam administered by the American Registry of Diagnostic Medical Sonographers (ARDMS). Continuing education is required.

Resources

BOOKS

Hagen-Ansert, Sandra L. *Textbook of Diagnostic Ultrasonography,* 5th ed. St. Louis, MO: Mosby, 2000.

Salmans, Sandra. *Prostate: Questions You Have . . . Answers You Need.* Allentown, PA: People's Medical Society, 1996.

ORGANIZATION

Prostate Health Council. American Foundation for Urologic Disease. 1128 N. Charles St., Baltimore, MD 21201. 800-242-AFUD.

Daniel J. Harvey

Prostheses, lower limb *see* **Lower limb prostheses**

Prostheses, upper limb *see* **Upper limb prostheses**

Prosthetics

Definition

Prosthetics is the art or science of making and adjusting artificial parts to the human body. A prosthesis (plural, prostheses) is a human-made product used to augment a damaged or replace a missing body part. The word *prosthesis* comes from two Greek words that mean "to place at" or "to add." The branch of prosthetics that deals with missing teeth or other **dental prostheses** is called prosthodontics.

A related field is orthotics, which is concerned with the design and fitting of devices intended to strengthen or correct the function of the torso or a limb. An orthosis (plural, orthoses) is an orthopedic device intended to compensate for the **weakness** of or damage to a limb as the result of disease or trauma. The word *orthosis* comes from a Greek verb that means "to align" or "to straighten." Health care professionals with specialized training in this field are called orthotists.

Description

Prosthetics is a multidisciplinary profession that includes surgeons, nurses, prosthetists, and physical therapists. Others involved in a patient's treatment can include a prosthetics technician, prosthetics assistant, **rehabilitation** counselor, and social worker. The rapid and ongoing development of robotic and other externally powered prosthetic limbs since the 1980s means that engineers and materials experts are also involved in contemporary prosthetics.

The goal of prosthetics is to replace all or part of a missing limb so that a patient can function. The loss may be congenital (present at birth), traumatic, or the result of a disease process that requires amputation, such as diabetes or **gangrene**. This replacement can involve fitting a man with an artificial leg so that he can walk, or equipping a woman with an artificial hand so that she can hold objects. Other examples of prostheses include artificial **heart** valves, artificial eyes, and dentures.

Guide for preprosthetic evaluation

Item to be evaluated	Observe for:
Activities of daily living	Transfers; ambulatory status; home (including hazards and barriers); self-care
Medical status	Cause of amputation; associated diseases/symptoms; medications
Neurologic	Sensation; neuroma; phantom pain; mental status
Psychological	Emotional status; family and work situations; prosthetic goals
Range of motion	Hips; knee; ankle
Residuum length	Bone length; soft-tissue, redundant-tissue length
Residuum shape	Cylindrical, conical, hourglass, "dog-ears," bulbous, above-knee adductor roll
Skin	Scar; open lesions; sensation; grafts
Vascularity (both limbs if vascular disease is cause of amputation)	Pulses; color; temperature; edema; pain; trophic changes

SOURCE: Sanders, G.T. *Lower Limb Amputation: A Guide to Rehabilitation*. Philadelphia: F.A. Davis Co., 1986.

Historical background

The use of prostheses was known in ancient times, as Egyptian mummies that are at least three thousand years old have been discovered with prosthetic wooden toes and feet. Pliny the Elder (23–79 AD), a Roman naval commander who died during the disastrous first-century eruption of Vesuvius, recorded the case of a Roman general who had an iron arm fashioned to replace one lost in battle. In the fifteenth century, steel and **copper** began to be used along with iron and wood to make prostheses. René-Robert de La Salle (1643–1687), the French explorer who traveled across the Great Lakes region and the Mississippi Valley, is reported to have had an iron hand.

Functional prostheses were introduced in the sixteenth century. Gotz von Berlichingen, a German mercenary sometimes known as Gotz of the Iron Hand, devised a pair of prosthetic iron hands that could be moved with a set of springs and catches. Ambroise Paré (1510–1590), the "father of battlefield medicine," was a French surgeon who invented a leg prosthesis that had a knee lock control and could be moved into a kneeling as well as a standing position. These early functional prostheses were all human-powered.

The development of functional prosthetics was advanced in the twentieth century by the needs of

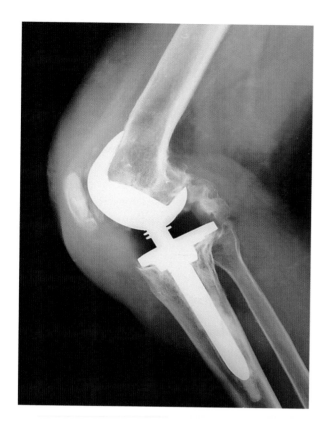

(Colored x-ray of the prosthetic knee (white), patient with osteoarthritis, photograph. Zephyr / Photo Researchers, Inc.)

and construct prosthesis that fit the patient as accurately as possible. The patient's measurements can be scanned into the computer by a handheld wand or a laser. Electronic knee joint prostheses can now be constructed with a computer chip programmed to meet the needs and lifestyle of the individual patient.

Demographics

Patients requiring prosthetic care range from children born with missing limbs to elderly adults requiring hip joint replacement surgery. Such traumas as automobile accidents or combat injuries in the military may cause the loss of a limb, and such vascular conditions as diabetes may lead to the amputation of a limb. According to the Amputee Coalition, there are 2 million Americans as of 2012 who are amputees. There are 185,000 amputations each year in the United States. Of these, 54% are due to vascular disease (including diabetes), 43% to trauma, and 2% to **cancer**. African Americans are more likely to require amputations than members of other racial or ethnic groups, and men are more likely to require amputations than women.

The costs of prostheses are high, ranging in price from $6,000 for some lower-limb prostheses to as much as $36,000 for an upper limb prosthesis. In addition, limb prostheses must be replaced every three to four years because of wear and tear.

wounded veterans of World War I (1914–1918) and World War II (1939–1945). Doctors and biomedical engineers began to use aluminum, plastics, fiberglass, and other lighter-weight materials to design prostheses that were easier to use and longer-lasting. The development of silicone and polyvinyl chloride (PVC) also made it possible to design prostheses with lifelike "skin" and other features that enable the artificial limbs to look as lifelike as possible. Prostheses of this type are known as cosmeses (singular, cosmesis) after the Greek word for "ornament."

The nest development came in the 1980s and 1990s with the introduction of externally powered prostheses. The first microprocessor-powered prosthetic knee was introduced in the early 1990s, followed by a prosthetic leg in 1997 (the C-Leg) that is powered by a lithium-ion battery and uses hydraulic cylinders to flex or rotate the knee joint. Another newer form of prosthesis is the myoelectric upper limb prosthesis, which uses electrical signals from the patient's voluntary muscles in the remaining part of the limb to control the motions of an electrically powered hand, elbow, or wrist. As of 2012, computer-aided design (CAD) and computer-aided manufacturing (CAM) are increasingly used to design

Contemporary prosthetic practice

The prosthetic health care team

Patients are seen by a prosthetics health care team, which can include a surgeon, nurse, prosthetist, prosthetics technician, prosthetics assistant or fitter, and physical therapist. An orthotist may also be a member of the team if the patient requires braces or similar support devices as well as a prosthesis.

Prosthetists may supervise several staff members. In some workplaces, the prosthetics assistant assists the prosthetist and may fabricate, repair, and maintain artificial appliances. However, prosthetics may be made by the prosthetics technician, an allied health worker who takes direction from the prosthetist and the prosthetics assistant. The technician also repairs and maintains prostheses. In some settings, the technician may have no contact with patients.

Work settings

Members of the prosthetics health care team work in hospitals, rehabilitation facilities, medical centers, medical schools, colleges, and universities. Prosthetics

technicians may work in those settings or in labs and facilities that manufacture prostheses.

The prosthetist designs and fits prostheses. When surgery is planned, the prosthetist consults with the surgeon about the point at which a limb is to be amputated. The prosthetist's input includes recommendations about fitting the prosthesis after surgery.

Pre- and postoperative care

For some members of the health care team, patient contact begins before surgery. The doctor examines the patient to determine if more treatment is needed. If amputation is required, those who counsel the patient may include the doctor, nurse, and social worker. They will try to help the patient prepare emotionally and physically for surgery and rehabilitation. Questions for the patient and doctor to think about together in choosing a prosthesis include:

• The level of amputation.
• The shape and contour of the residual limb.
• The type of function the prosthesis will be expected to perform.
• The patient's level of cognition.
• The patient's occupation and hobbies.
• The importance of the device's external appearance (cosmesis).
• The patient's financial resources.

After surgery, the patient may be seen by the surgeon or primary care doctor. During the rehabilitation phase, the prosthetist and therapist will help the patient adjust to the prosthetic. The nurse and social worker may provide **patient education** and support. If needed, the patient may be referred to a rehabilitation counselor or a vocational counselor. In addition, the patient will see the prosthetist, prosthetics assistant, or prosthetics technician if the prosthetic needs adjusting.

The early stages of all prosthetic treatment usually involves the prosthetist working with the physical therapist. The therapist can evaluate such factors as the patient's strength and ability to wear a prosthetic.

Education and training

Such members of the health care team as surgeons, nurses, physical therapists, and social workers may receive training in the use of prosthetics while studying for their respective professions. Prosthetists must complete a four-year bachelor of science degree that includes specialized prosthetic training. They also serve a clinical residency and may continue their education at the master's degree level.. Programs for prosthetics

KEY TERMS

Congenital—Present at birth.

Cosmesis (plural, cosmeses)—A prosthesis designed to look as lifelike as possible.

Orthosis (plural, orthoses)—An orthopedic device intended to compensate for the weakness of or damage to a limb as the result of disease or trauma.

Prosthesis (plural, prostheses)—A human-made product used to augment a damaged or replace a missing body part.

assistants and technicians range from six months to two years. In addition, people working in these allied health professions can receive certification through the American Academy of Orthotists and Prosthetists (AAOP). Board certification is based on education, employment, completion of certification of program modules (continuing education courses), and membership in the academy.

According to the Academy, a prosthetist's scope of practice includes the following:

• Assessment of the patient's prosthetic (and/or orthotic) needs. This assessment includes a review of the patient's history and a through examination of the patient's physical health and cognitive abilities.
• Formulation of a comprehensive orthotic/prosthetic treatment plan.
• Implementation of the treatment plan. This step may include fabrication of the prosthesis as well as measuring and preparing the patient for the device, evaluating the prosthesis for safety and functionality after delivery, and instructing the patient in the proper care and maintenance of the device.
• Follow-up treatment. This stage includes assessment of the patient's psychological and physical health, the fit of the device, any necessary adjustments, the patient's adherence to the treatment plan, and careful documentation of all the patient's records.
• Promotion of competency. Prosthetists are encouraged to take continuing education courses and contribute to the education of other health care professionals.

Advanced education and training

The name of the American Academy of Orthotists and Prosthetists reflects the close relationship between the fields of orthotics and prosthetics. While orthotics usually focuses on temporary treatment with a brace,

QUESTIONS TO ASK YOUR DOCTOR

- Have you ever had to treat a patient with a prosthesis?
- Can you recommend a prosthetist in our local area?
- Have you ever taken any continuing education courses on amputation and the needs of amputees?
- What kinds of financial assistance are available for people who need prostheses?

prosthetics involves permanent replacement of a body part with an artificial appliance. However, some patients require both prosthetics and orthotics, so schools offer degrees and certificates in both disciplines. Allied health professionals with education and experience in both disciplines will be twice as employable as those with degrees or certificates in only one of the professions. Education is the key to career advancement for an allied health employee with only one specialty. A prosthetics technician can advance to assistant and then prosthetist by completing more classes.

The American Academy of Orthotists and Prosthetists offers continuing education courses and forums so that allied health workers remain knowledgeable about new developments in their professions.

Future outlook

The need for prosthetists, prosthetics assistants, and prosthetics technicians is expected to increase with the **aging** of the so-called baby boomer generation. According to the AAOP, employment for professionals in the field is 100% as of 2012. Salaries in 2012 range from about $95,000 per year for board-certified prosthetists with 15 years' experience to $39,000 for a fitter with six years' experience. The existence of a rapidly growing senior population is a global trend, and prosthetics care should be in increasing demand worldwide. Among the needs for older populations are hip replacement, knee replacement, and replacement of limbs amputated because of diabetes and other conditions.

Another population that will require the services of prosthetists is military veterans of Iraq and Afghanistan. The types of injuries resulting from improvised explosive devices (IEDs) and other types of blasts often result in limb loss.

Resources

BOOKS

Matthijs, Silvia, and Raphae? l Sidransky, eds. *Amputations: Types, Procedures, and Risks.* Hauppauge, NY: Nova Science Publishers, 2011.

May, Bella J., and Margery A. Lockard. *Prosthetics and Orthotics in Clinical Practice: A Case Study Approach.* Philadelphia: F.A. Davis, 2011.

Weiss, Lyn, Jay Weiss, and Thomas Pobre, eds. *Oxford American Handbook of Physical Medicine and Rehabilitation.* New York: Oxford University Press, 2010.

PERIODICALS

Behrend, C., et al. "Update on Advances in Upper Extremity Prosthetics." *Journal of Hand Surgery* 36 (October 2011): 1711–1717.

Fleming, M., et al. "Dismounted Complex Blast Injuries: Patterns of Injuries and Resource Utilization Associated with the Multiple Extremity Amputee." *Journal of Surgical Orthopaedic Advances* 21 (Spring 2012): 32–37.

Huband, M. "Prosthetic Rehabilitation." *Dermatologic Clinics* 29 (April 2011): 325–330.

Kent, J., et al. "Biomechanical Models in the Study of Lower Limb Amputee Kinematics: A Review." *Prosthetics and Orthotics International* 35 (June 2011): 124–139.

Latlief, G., et al. "Patient Safety in the Rehabilitation of the Adult with an Amputation." *Physical Medicine and Rehabilitation Clinics of North America* 23 (May 2012): 377–392.

Resnik, L., et al. "Advanced Upper Limb Prosthetic Devices: Implications for Upper Limb Prosthetic Rehabilitation." *Archives of physical Medicine and Rehabilitation* 93 (April 2012): 710–717.

Schultz, A.E., and T.A. Kuiken. "Neural Interfaces for Control of Upper Limb Prostheses: The State of the Art and Future Possibilities." *PM and R: The Journal of Injury, Function, and Rehabilitation* 3 (January 2011): 55–67.

Shih, J.J., et al. "Brain-Computer Interfaces in Medicine." *Mayo Clinic Proceedings* 87 (March 2012): 268–279.

WEBSITES

Amputee Coalition. "Prosthetics." This is a gateway portal with a menu of specific topics related to prosthetics, such as function, maintenance, cosmesis, and insurance issues. http://www.amputee-coalition.org/limb-loss-resource-center/resources-by-topic/prosthetics/index.html (accessed May 8, 2012).

Medscape. "Lower Limb Prosthetics." http://emedicine.medscape.com/article/317358-overview (accessed May 8, 2012).

Medscape. "Prosthetic Knees." http://emedicine.medscape.com/article/1983871-overview (accessed May 8, 2012).

Medscape. "Upper Limb Prosthetics." http://emedicine.medscape.com/article/317234-overview (accessed May 8, 2012).

Orthotists and Prosthetists. "Education Pathways." This is a gateway portal to the training required to become a

prosthetist, assistant, fitter, or technician. http://www.opcareers.org/education_pathways/ (accessed May 8, 2012).

Orthotists and Prosthetists. "O and P Technology." This is an overview of recent advances in the bioengineering and computerization of prosthetics and orthotics. http://www.opcareers.org/op_technology/ (accessed May 8, 2012).

ORGANIZATIONS

American Academy of Orthotists and Prosthetists (AAOP), 1331 H Street, NW, Suite 501, Washington, DC United States 20005, (202) 380-3663, Fax: (202) 380-3447, http://www.oandp.org/

American Orthotic and Prosthetic Association (AOPA), 330 John Carlyle Street, Suite 200, Alexandria, VA United States 22314, (571) 431-0876, Fax: (571) 431-0899, info@AOPAnet.org, http://www.aopanet.org/

American Physical Therapy Association (APTA), 1111 North Fairfax Street, Alexandria, VA United States 22314, (703) 684-APTA (2782), Fax: (703) 684-7343, (800) 999-2782, http://www.apta.org/

Amputee Coalition, 900 East Hill Avenue, Suite 290, Knoxville, TN United States 37915-2566, (888) 267-5669, http://www.amputee-coalition.org/index.html

International Society for Prosthetics and Orthotics (ISPO), 22-24 Rue du Luxembourg, Brussels, Belgium B-1000 Brussels, +322 213.13.79, Fax: +322 213.13.13, ispo@ispoint.org, http://www.ispoint.org/

Liz Swain
Rebecca J. Frey, Ph.D.

Prosthodontics *see* **Dental specialties**

Protein-modified diet *see* **Diet therapy**

Protein C test *see* **Thrombosis risk tests**

Protein components test *see* **Hypercoagubility tests**

Protein electrophoresis test

Definition

Electrophoresis is a technique used to separate the different components (fractions) of a mixture, such as **proteins** in a biological sample. Separation is based on differences in the charge (and sometimes size) of the molecules, which determines their rate of movement in an electric field. Serum protein electrophoresis is a screening test that measures the major **blood** proteins. Protein electrophoresis testing can also be performed on urine and cerebrospinal fluid (CSF) samples.

Purpose

Protein electrophoresis testing is used to evaluate, diagnose, and monitor a variety of diseases and conditions through examination of the amounts and types of protein in a blood, urine, or CSF specimen.

Precautions

Certain other diagnostic tests or prescription medications can affect the results of protein electrophoresis tests. The administration of a contrast dye used in some other tests may falsely elevate apparent protein levels. Drugs that can alter results include aspirin, bicarbonates, chlorpromazine (Thorazine), **corticosteroids**, isoniazid (INH), and neomycin (Mycifradin). The total serum protein concentration may also be affected by changes in the patient's posture or by the use of a tourniquet during venipuncture.

Protein is less concentrated in urine and CSF than in blood. Urinary and CSF proteins must be concentrated before analysis, and the added sample handling can lead to contamination and erroneous results. In the collection of a CSF specimen, it is important that the sample not be contaminated with blood proteins that would invalidate the CSF protein measurements.

Description

Proteins are biologically important organic molecules—polymers of amino acids—that contain the elements carbon, hydrogen, nitrogen, and oxygen. Certain proteins may also contain sulfur, **phosphorus**, **iron**, iodine, selenium, or other trace elements. There are twenty-two amino acids commonly found in all proteins. The human body is capable of producing fourteen of these amino acids; the remaining eight so-called essential amino acids must be obtained from food. Proteins are found in muscles, blood, skin, hair, nails, and the internal organs and tissues. Enzymes, hemoglobin, and **antibodies** are proteins, as are many hormones.

Protein mixtures can be fractionated into individual component proteins by a variety of techniques, including precipitation, chromatography, ultracentrifugation, or electrophoresis.

A serum protein electrophoresis test is used to determine the percentage of each protein in the blood by separating them into five distinct classes: albumin, alpha$_1$-globulin, alpha$_2$-globulin, beta-globulin, and gamma-globulins (immunoglobulins). High-resolution protein electrophoresis uses a higher current to separate the major proteins comprising the alpha$_1$-globulin,

Protein electrophoresis

Electrophoresis results	Disease

Total protein:
  6.4–8.3 g/dl (64.0–83.0 g/L)
Albumin:
  3.5–5.0 g/dl (35–50 g/L)
Alpha$_1$ globulin:
  0.1–0.3 g/dl (1–3 g/L)
Alpha$_2$ globulin:
  0.6–1.0 g/dl (6–10 g/L)
Beta globulin:
  0.7–1.1 g/dl (7–11 g/L)
	Normal results

Decreased albumin Increased alpha$_2$ globulin	Acute infections, tissue necrosis, burns, surgery, stress, myocardial infarction
Slightly decreased albumin Slightly increased gamma gobulin Normal alpha$_2$ globulin	Chronic infection, granulomatus diseases, cirrhosis, rheumatoid-collegen diseases
Greatly decreased albumin Greatly increased alpha$_2$ globulin Normal increase in beta globulin	Nephrotic syndrome
Decreased albumin Increased gamma globulin Incorporation of beta and gamma peaks	Far-advanced cirrhosis
Greatly increased gamma globulin	Cirrhosis, chronic infection, globulin with a broad peaksarcoidosis, tuberculosis, endocarditis, rheumatoid-collagen disease
Decreased gamma globulin with normal other globulin levels	Light-chain multiple myeloma
Thin spikes in gamma globulin	Myeloma, macroglobulinemia, gammopathies

SOURCE: Pagana, K.D. and T.J. Pagana. *Mosby's Diagnostic and Laboratory Test Reference.* 3rd ed. St. Louis: Mosby, 1997.

alpha$_2$-globulin, and beta-globulin fractions. This procedure produces nine or more bands, including alpha$_1$ antitrypsin, alpha$_2$ macroglobulin, haptoglobulin, transferrin, and complement proteins.

In addition to standard protein electrophoresis, the **immunofixation electrophoresis** test (IFE) may be used to assess the blood levels of specific immunoglobulins. An IFE test is usually ordered if a serum protein electrophoresis test shows an unusually high amount of protein in the gamma-globulin fraction. The IFE tests determine whether the increase in the gamma-globulin fraction is caused by excess immunoglobulins (antibodies) and whether it is polyclonal or monoclonal in nature. Polyclonal increases are caused by infections, **allergies**, and inflammatory diseases, while monoclonal increases are caused by malignant or benign proliferations of the antibody-producing cells (plasma cells).

Serum proteins

The total serum protein concentration may be used to assess a patient's hydration state: **dehydration** leads to high total serum protein concentration. Further, the levels of different blood proteins rise or fall in response to such disorders as **cancer**, intestinal or kidney protein-wasting syndromes, disorders of the **immune system**, **liver** dysfunction, impaired **nutrition**, and chronic fluid-retaining conditions.

ALBUMIN. Albumin, which is produced in the liver, is the most abundant blood protein. It makes a major contribution to the osmotic pressure that regulates the movement of water between the tissues and the bloodstream. Albumin binds **calcium**, thyroid hormones, fatty acids, and many drugs, maintaining them in the circulation and preventing filtration in the **kidneys**. Low serum albumin levels can be indicative of pathology, and can increase free therapeutic drug levels and decrease total calcium levels. Albumin levels can play a role in the efficacy and toxicity of therapeutic drugs, and in **drug interactions**.

GLOBULINS. Serum globulins are present in protein electropherograms as four main fractions: alpha$_1$-, alpha$_2$-, beta-, and gamma-globulins.

• The major alpha$_1$-globulin is the "acute-phase" protein alpha$_1$-antitrypsin, a protease inhibitor produced by the lungs and liver. Alpha$_1$-antitrypsin deficiency is a marker of an inherited disorder characterized by an increased risk of emphysema.

• Alpha$_2$-globulins include serum haptoglobin, alpha$_2$-macroglobulin, and ceruloplasmin. Haptoglobin is an acute-phase protein that binds free hemoglobin released from red blood cells during hemolysis. Haptoglobin binding prevents excretion of free hemoglobin by the kidneys. In addition to hemolysis, low haptoglobin levels can indicate chronic liver disease, tumor metastasis, or severe sepsis. Alpha$_2$-macroglobulin, a broad-spectrum protease inhibitor, accounts for about one-third of the alpha$_2$-globulin fraction: its concentration is increased during nephrosis. Ceruloplasmin is an acute-phase protein involved in the storage and transport of copper and iron: its concentration is increased during pregnancy and decreased in Wilson's disease.

• Beta-globulins include transferrin, low-density lipoproteins (LDL), and complement components. Transferrin transports dietary iron to the liver, spleen, and bone marrow. LDL (also referred to as beta lipoprotein) is the major carrier of cholesterol in the blood: high levels are associated with atherosclerosis. Complement is a system of blood proteins required for antibody-mediated cell lysis and involved in the inflammatory response.

- The gamma-globulin fraction contains the immunoglobulins, a family of proteins that function as antibodies. Antibodies, produced in response to infection, allergic reactions, and organ transplants, recognize and bind antigens to facilitate destruction by the immune system. The immune response is regulated by a large number of antigen-specific gamma-globulins that fall into five main classes called IgG, IgA, IgM, IgO, and IgE. Immunoglobulin deficiency due to inherited disorders can range from partial or complete loss of a single immunoglobulin class to complete absence of all immunoglobulins. An abnormally high level of immunoglobulins is generally found in acute and chronic infections, and is an indicator of autoimmune disease. When the serum protein electrophoresis test demonstrates a significant deviation from the normal gamma-globulin levels, an IFE test should be ordered to determine the polyclonal or monoclonal nature of the specific globulin(s) involved.

Quantification of each immunoglobin class and each of the proteins mentioned above may be performed by a procedure called immunonephelometry. This technique uses an antibody specific for the protein to be measured. When the antibody binds to the protein, an immune complex is formed that increases the amount of light scattered by the sample.

Deviations in serum proteins levels from reference levels are considered in conjunction with symptoms and results from other diagnostic procedures.

Urinary proteins

Protein electrophoresis is performed on urine samples to classify disorders that cause protein loss via the kidneys. Hemoglobin and myoglobin are found in the urine of trauma and burn victims, and in patients with **infection** or hemolysis. Protein electrophoresis of urine is most often performed in order to detect the presence of light chain fragments of immunoglobulins. These protein fragments are sufficiently small to filter through the kidneys and are excreted in the urine. They are called Bence-Jones proteins, and are found in patients who have **multiple myeloma**, a malignant proliferation of antibody-producing cells. Bence-Jones proteins may also be found in other variants of multiple myeloma, such as light chain disease, and in patients with systemic autoimmune diseases that result from degradation of immune complexes.

Cerebrospinal fluid (CSF) proteins

An increase in total protein concentration in the CSF is often found in bacterial and fungal **meningitis** and with **central nervous system** (CNS) tumors. The main use of CSF protein electrophoresis testing is in the diagnosis of **multiple sclerosis**.

The protein electrophoresis test method

In a clinical protein electrophoresis test, proteins are separated on the basis of how fast they move on a medium in an electrical field. In a standard electrophoresis test, a small amount of sample is applied to a cellulose acetate strip or gel made of agarose or polyacrylamide. The strip or gel is positioned between the apparatus electrodes, and a voltage is applied across it. Under the conditions of the test, the proteins in the sample are negatively charged and migrate toward the positive electrode at different rates. The migration rate is mainly dependent on the charge of the protein molecules; however, on polyacrylamide gel it is also dependent on size. When electrophoresis is complete, the gel is treated with a dye to stain the proteins, and the intensity of stain in the bands is measured and recorded by a densitometer. In a capillary electrophoresis test, samples are automatically transferred from the collection tubes to the head of a fluid-filled glass capillary tube: the electrophoretic separation occurs during the transport of the proteins through the capillary, and the individual proteins are detected and quantified on-line by absorption of ultraviolet light. Both gel and capillary electrophoresis procedures produce a recording of each protein fraction as a peak. The area under the peak is used to calculate the percentage of the fraction. This is multiplied by the total protein concentration (determined by chemical analysis) to give the concentration of each fraction. The levels of proteins thus determined are compared with reference levels to ascertain whether a disease state is present.

Standard electrophoresis systems

High-throughput and semi-automated protein electrophoresis testing is available in most laboratories through the use of integrated systems of gels, reagent kits, and densitometers.

Capillary electrophoresis systems

In 1998, the introduction of fully automated clinical capillary electrophoresis instruments was introduced. The advantages of the capillary electrophoresis methodology include direct sampling of a minimal volume from the primary collection tube, automated detection of proteins without staining, rapid sample throughput, and improved accuracy and reproducibility. Agarose and capillary systems are also used to separate DNA, an increasingly important technology.

KEY TERMS

Acute-phase proteins—Proteins produced during the acute-phase response, a set of physiological changes that occur in response to trauma conditions.

Albumin—A blood protein produced in the liver that helps to regulate water distribution in the body.

Antibodies—Immunoglobulin protein molecules produced by B cells and plasma cells during the immune response. Each antibody-binding site can bind part of an antigen to trigger immune defenses.

Antigen—Foreign body that triggers immune response.

Bence-Jones protein—The Ig light chain, part of an immunoglobulin, that is detected by urine protein electrophoresis in the case of multiple myeloma.

Complement—A group of complex proteins of the beta-globulin type in the blood that bind to antibodies during anaphylaxis. In the complement cascade, each complement component interacts with another in a cascade that causes cell membrane damage, leading to lysis.

Electropherogram—The pattern of stained proteins on an electrophoresis gel, or a graph showing peaks of proteins separated by electrophoresis.

Electrophoresis—A technique used to separate the proteins in a biological sample on the basis of charge and size as they migrate under the influence of an applied electric field.

Globulins—Plasma or serum proteins other than albumin, so named because of their globular shape. Four globulin fractions can be measured by electrophoresis in order to diagnose or monitor a variety of serious illnesses.

Paraprotein—An immunoglobulin produced by a clone of identical B-cells. Also called monoclonal protein.

Protein—Proteins, such as enzymes and antibodies, are biologically important polymers of amino acids that contain the elements carbon, hydrogen, nitrogen, and oxygen. Certain proteins may also contain sulfur, phosphorus, iron, iodine, selenium, or other trace elements.

Preparation

The sample for the serum protein electrophoresis test is obtained by venipuncture. No anticoagulant should be used. It is usually not necessary for the patient to restrict food or fluids before the test; a 12-hour fast is requested before drawing blood for lipoprotein testing. The urine protein electrophoresis test requires either an early morning urine sample or a 24-hour urine sample according to the physician's request. CSF is collected by **lumbar puncture** performed in a hospital setting; because of risks associated with the procedure, the patient must sign a consent form. Any factors that might affect test results, such as whether the patient is taking any medications, should be noted.

Complications

Risks posed by the venous puncture are minimal but may include slight bleeding from the puncture site, fainting or lightheadedness after the sample is drawn, or the development of a small bruise at the puncture site.

Lumbar puncture can lead to leakage of cerebrospinal fluid from the puncture site, **headache**, infection, symptoms of meningitis, nausea, **vomiting**, or difficulty urinating. Rarely, pre-existing intracranial pressure can

lead to **brain** herniation resulting in brain damage and/or death. The patient must be kept lying flat in the hospital under observation for at least six to eight hours after the procedure.

Results

The following serum protein electrophoresis reference values are representative; some variation among laboratories and specific methods is to be expected. The values were obtained by standard electrophoresis on agarose gels.

- total protein: 6.4 to 8.3 g/dL (about 0.5 g/dL lower in nonambulatory patients)

- albumin: 3.5 to 5.0 g/dL

- $alpha_1$-globulin: 0.1 to 0.3 g/dL

- $alpha_2$-globulin: 0.6 to 1.0 g/dL

- beta-globulin: 0.7 to 1.2 g/dL

- gamma-globulin: 0.7 to 1.6 g/dL

Albumin levels are increased in dehydration and decreased in malnutrition, **pregnancy**, liver disease, inflammatory diseases, and protein-losing states such as **malabsorption syndrome** and certain kidney disorders.

Alpha$_1$-globulins are increased in inflammatory diseases and decreased or absent in juvenile pulmonary **emphysema**, a hereditary disease.

Alpha$_2$-globulins are increased in acute and chronic inflammation and nephrotic syndrome; decreased values may indicate hemolysis.

Beta-globulin levels are increased in conditions of high **cholesterol** (hypercholesterolemia), in multiple myeloma, and in **iron deficiency anemia**; and decreased in disorders associated with complement depletion.

Gamma-globulin levels are increased in chronic inflammatory disease and autoimmune conditions such as **rheumatoid arthritis** and systemic lupus erythematosus, **cirrhosis**, in acute and chronic infection, and in multiple myeloma. The gamma-globulins are decreased in a variety of genetic immune disorders, in secondary immune deficiency related to steroid use, leukemia, or severe infection.

Detection of a discrete (monoclonal) band in the gamma region of the electropherogram indicates the presence of a paraprotein. Type IgG or IgA paraproteins associated with multiple myeloma may be found by serum protein electrophoresis testing; however, the tumor may produce only Ig light chains that are removed from the blood by the kidneys. The Ig light chain (Bence-Jones protein) can be detected by urine protein electrophoresis.

In CSF, the total protein concentration is normally 0.015 to 0.045 g/dL, with gamma-globulin accounting for 3–12%. Increased gamma-globulin indicates multiple sclerosis, bacterial or fungal meningitis, neurosyphilis, or Guillain-Barré syndrome. Detection of monoclonal bands in CSF plays an important role in the diagnosis of multiple sclerosis.

In urine, normally no globulins and less than 0.050 g/dL albumin are present. Abnormal results indicate disruption of kidney function or acute inflammation. The presence of the Bence-Jones protein indicates multiple myeloma.

Health care team roles

Nurses are involved in the collection of blood samples by venipuncture, in patient support during and after lumbar puncture, and in instructing patients in the procedure for midstream collection of urine samples. A lumbar puncture is generally performed by a physician. Medical laboratory workers are responsible for preparation of samples for electrophoresis testing.

Training

The preparation of urine and CSF samples for electrophoresis testing often involves concentration and,

in the case of urine samples and some CSF samples, centrifugation. Electrophoresis is classified as a high-complexity test and is performed by laboratory personnel with special training, most often by a clinical laboratory scientist (CLS) or medical technologist (MT).

Resources

BOOKS

Burtis, C. A., and E. R. Ashwood. *Tietz Fundamentals of Clinical Chemistry,* 5th ed. Philadelphia: W. B. Saunders, 2001.

Cahill, Matthew, ed. *Handbook of Diagnostic Tests.* Springhouse, PA: Springhouse Corporation, 1995.

Marshall, W. J. *Clinical Chemistry,* 4th ed. Edinburgh, London, New York, Philadelphia, St. Louis, and Toronto: Mosby, 2000.

Pagana, K. D., and T. J. Pagana, eds. *Mosby's Diagnostic and Laboratory Test Reference.* St. Louis: Mosby-Year Book, Inc., 1998.

Shintani, H., and J. Polonsky, eds. *Handbook of Capillary Electrophoresis Applications.* London: Blackie Academic and Professional, 1998.

OTHER

Beckman Coulter Clinical Electrophoresis website. 2001. http://www.beckmancoulter.com/beckman/clindiag/prodinfo/electrophoresis/.

HealthWide website. 2000 Healthwide.com, Inc. http://www.healthwide.com/ency.

Patricia L. Bounds

Protein metabolism

Definition

Protein **metabolism** is the chemical cycle of breaking down protein (catabolism) and using the components to synthesizing (anabolism) new molecules to be used in the body. The process is also known as proteometabolism.

Description

Proteins, fats, and **carbohydrates** (called macronutrients) are part of a complex metabolic cycle that is essential to life. During digestion food containing these nutrients is chemically broken down into its basic components and absorbed for use in the body. Protein molecules are split into their basic building blocks, called amino acids, which are then chemically re-arranged to synthesize new proteins that the body needs. Fats are broken down into fatty acids and **cholesterol**, and carbohydrates are split into simple sugars such as glucose and fructose, which provide most of the energy to drive chemical reactions in the body. These smaller, simpler molecules are absorbed in the **small intestine** and enter the circulatory system. They then pass through the **liver** where some of these "building block molecules" are synthesized into more complex compounds needed by the body.

In order for cellular metabolism to occur, two reactions happen continuously. Small molecules are build up into larger molecules, a process called anabolism or constructive metabolism, while large molecules are broken down into their component parts during a process called catabolism or destructive metabolism. This building up and breaking down is regulated by a complex set of hormones and enzymes, themselves proteins. For an individual to remain healthy, the processes of anabolism and catabolism must remain in balance.

Catabolism, or the breakdown of nutrients obtained from food, releases energy that drives all metabolic activities in the body. For example, glucose is broken down to provide energy for cellular respiration that allows functions such as muscle movement. Proteins are broken into amino acids then re-synthesized into hormones and enzymes to regulate chemical reactions in the cell, and molecules used for tissue growth and repair. Carbohydrates and fats are the preferred sources of energy for cellular metabolism. When the supply of fats and carbohydrates is insufficient to meet the body' needs, proteins can be broken down to supply energy. This accounts for the loss of muscle seen in prolonged cases of starvation.

Protein is a nitrogen-containing compound found in all plants and animals. There is a continuous need for protein to make hormones, enzymes, **antibodies**, and to produce new tissue (growth) and repair damaged tissues (maintenance). About 75% of human body tissue is made of protein. From 1–2% of the body's total protein is broken down each day into amino acid and recycled into new proteins. About 60–70% of the amino acids the body needs come from this recycling process. The rest must be supplied by diet.

A complex molecule

Proteins are complex nitrogen-containing molecules formed by a combination of about 20 amino acids. These twenty amino acids can be connected in thousands of different combinations to form all the different proteins in the body. During protein formation (anabolism) the amino acids are connected in long chains called polypeptides that fold into three-dimensional shapes.

The combinations of amino acids produce proteins with unique shapes that perform specific functions in the body such as catalyzing metabolic reactions, repairing tissue, or stimulating glands to produce other proteins.

The body can synthesize 11 amino acids naturally. The remaining nine must be obtained from dietary protein. The nine amino acids that cannot be synthesized by the body are called essential amino acids. It is an absolute requirement for health that diet include foods that contain an adequate amount of these essential amino acids. Foods that contain all the essential amino acids are called complete proteins. Examples of complete proteins are all meats and fish, eggs, and dairy products. Foods that lack one or more essential amino acid are called incomplete proteins. Most plant proteins are incomplete proteins. Dried beans, lentils, and rice are examples of incomplete proteins. Although some excess amino acids are converted into fat and stored as a future energy source, the body cannot not store amino acids for use in making future proteins. As a result, humans need a steady supply of protein in their diets. Individuals whose diet is completely or primarily vegetarian must make sure to eat combinations of foods that provide all the essential amino acids, for example red beans and rice or corn tortillas and beans.

Digestion of protein

The digestion of proteins begins in the **stomach** where the hormone pepsin is secreted by the stomach. Pepsin breaks the long polypeptide molecules into smaller peptides. The mechanical churning of the stomach assists digestion by mixing food with gastric (stomach) secretions. When the contents of the stomach reach a certain degree of acidity, the pyloric sphincter, a muscle that separates the stomach from the small intestine, opens. The stomach contents, called chyme, flow into the duodenum, or upper part of the small intestine. As chyme moves through the small intestine, enzymes break the chemical bonds in the peptides, reducing the proteins to their component amino acids. (Breakdown of fats and carbohydrates is occurring simultaneously under the direction of different hormones and enzymes). In the small intestine, intestinal cells and **blood vessels** are in close proximity, separated only by **cell membranes**. Amino acids molecules are small enough that they can move though the intestinal wall and into **blood** where they (along with glucose, fatty acids, and the other products of digestion) are carried by a large blood vessel to the liver.

The liver is at the **heart** of protein metabolism. It has both anabolic and catabolic functions. In the liver, amino acids are synthesized into larger proteins that circulate

KEY TERMS

Calcium—A substance mineral found in bones and teeth.

Cholesterol—A soft, waxy, and fatty substance (lipid) found in animal tissue and fat.

Cell—The basic structural unit of all living organisms, such as animals and plants.

Cirrhosis—A condition where healthy liver cells are replaced by scar tissue. The condition is most often caused by alcoholism.

Enzyme—A protein that helps regulate the speed pf a chemical reaction.

Glucose—A simple of sugar that can be used by the body.

Nitrogen—A chemical element found in all proteins.

Triglycerides—Fatty compounds consisting of three fatty acids and one glycerol molecule.

through the body performing a huge variety of tasks including stimulating production of other proteins. The liver also breaks down proteins, for example, hemoglobin found in dead red blood cells. The liver cleanses the blood by removing cellular debris and processing excess nitrogen that is produced by chemical reactions within cells. This excess nitrogen is initially in the form of ammonia (NH_3. If allowed to remain in the blood, it would rapidly become toxic to the body. The liver converts ammonia to non-toxic urea that is removed from the body in urine. This lost nitrogen must then be replaced through diet.

Function

Protein metabolism consists of a cycle of breaking down proteins, synthesizing new ones and removing nitrogenous waste products that result from these reactions. The amount of protein needed to balance this cycle changes throughout an individual' life. Growing children who are creating new muscle and **bone**, for example, have higher protein needs than adults.

Role in human health

The Daily Reference Intake (DRI) for protein changes with age. The DRI is a United States government-determined measure of the amount of a nutrient an individual should consume daily and replaces the recommended daily amount (RDA) measurement.

Current DRI guidelines call for children ages 1–3 to consume 1.1 grams of protein per kilogram of body weight (g/kg body weight) or roughly 17 g/day. Children ages 4–13 should receive 0.95 g/kg body weigh, and children 14–18 should receive 0.85 g/kg body weight. For reference, 3 ounces of lean beef provide about 30 grams of protein; milk provides about 1 g/ounce or 8 grams per cup; an egg contains about 6 grams of protein. Adolescent boys have higher protein requirements than adolescent girls, and pregnant women have higher protein requirements than non-pregnant women.

A negative nitrogen balance occurs when a person loses (through excretion) more protein than is provided through diet. Negative nitrogen balance is often associated with inadequate caloric intake (starvation) and not just inadequate protein intake. However, malnutrition can occur a person's diet does not include food with all of the essential amino acids. This can be a particular problem individuals who eat no animal products. Negative nitrogen balances also may occur after surgery and during advanced stages of **cancer**.

Common diseases and disorders

Health conditions related to protein metabolism are generally caused by the amount of dietary protein consumed. Inadequate protein intake is rarely an issue in the United States because most people routinely eat food containing far more than the recommended protein DRI. People who eat too much protein are at risk of gaining weight since excess protein is converted to fat. Meat, a good source of protein, also contains fat and cholesterol. A diet with too much protein from fatty meat can result in high cholesterol, and an increased risk for heart disease.

In addition, excessive protein consumption increases the amount of **calcium** excreted in urine. Calcium is crucial to bone health, so bone strength may be affected by a prolonged high-protein diet. Excess dietary protein can also damage the liver and **kidneys**. Furthermore, recommended daily intake of protein for healthy individuals is harmful to people with **cirrhosis** of the liver, therefore, people with liver or kidney damage may be placed on low-protein diets.

Inadequate protein intake can inhibit growth, reduce muscle mass weaken the **immune system**. Over time, it can strain the heart and cause death. Severe lack of protein, known as protein energy malnutrition, can be caused by eating disorders such as anorexia and bulimia.

Starvation is another cause of low-protein intake. Starvation (intake of inadequate calories) may be the result of a famine, economic conditions, or caregiver abuse. In poor countries, severe protein malnutrition causes a disorder called kwashiorkor. This condition primarily affects children between the ages of 1 and 3. Once these children are weaned and no longer receiving breast milk, their diets consist of foods containing little protein. Symptoms of this condition include impaired growth, a swollen stomach, and fatigue. Treatment consists of slowly reintroducing a balanced, higher calorie diet. If not treated, kwashiorkor can result in liver damage and death.

Resources

BOOKS

Garrison, Jr., Robert and Elizabeth Somer. *The Nutrition Desk Reference* New York: McGraw-Hill, 1998.

Tortora, Gerard, and Sandra Reynolds Grabowski. *Introduction to the Human Body* New York: John Wiley & Sons, 2001.

PERIODICALS

Davis, Carla. "A Question of Protein." *Vegetarian Times* 331 (May 2005): 26.

Hrastar, Laura M. "New Amines on the Block: Synthetic Amino Acids Aid Understanding of Large Protein Complexes." *The Scientist* 19 i11 (June 6, 2005): 34.

ORGANIZATION

American Dietetic Association. 120 South Riverside Plaza, Suite 2000, Chicago, IL 60606-6995. (800) 877-1600. http://www.eatright.org

Liz Swain

Protein S test *see* **Thrombosis risk tests**

Proteins

Definition

Proteins are linear chains of amino acids connected by chemical bonds between the carboxyl group of each amino acid and the amine group of the one following. These bonds are called peptide bonds, and chains of only a few amino acids are referred to as polypeptides rather than proteins.

Description

Proteins are all around us. Much of the body's dry weight is protein; even bones are about one-quarter protein. The animals we eat and the microbes that attack us are likewise largely protein. The leather, wool, and silk clothing that we wear are nearly pure protein. The insulin that keeps diabetics alive and the "clot-busting" enzymes that may save **heart** attack patients are also proteins. Proteins can even be found working at industrial sites—protein enzymes produce not only the high-fructose corn syrup that sweetens most soft drinks, but also fuel-grade ethanol (alcohol) and other gasoline additives.

Within our bodies and those of other living things, proteins serve many functions. They digest foods and turn them into energy; they move our bodies and move molecules about within our cells; they let some substances pass through **cell membranes** while keeping others out; they turn light into chemical energy, making both **vision** and photosynthesis possible; they allow cells to detect and react to hormones and toxins in their surroundings; and, as **antibodies**, they protect our bodies against foreign invaders. There are simply too many proteins—possibly more than 100,000—to even consider mentioning them all.

Proteins are made up of separate compounds called amino acids. It is these amino acids that our bodies actually need, not the entire protein molecule. Some amino acids are essential—they must be obtained from diet because they cannot be synthesized by humans in adequate amounts. There are nine essential amino acids. Others are nonessential, because they can be made in the body from precursors (components) of other amino acids. There are eleven nonessential amino acids.

Protein structure

Many proteins have components other than amino acids. For example, some may have sugar molecules chemically attached. Exactly which types of sugars are involved and where on the protein chain attachment occurs will vary with the specific protein. In a few cases, it may also vary among different people. The A, B, and O **blood** types, for example, differ in precisely which types of sugar are or are not added to a specific protein on the surface of red blood cells.

Other proteins may have fat-like (lipid) molecules chemically bonded to them. These sugar and lipid molecules are always added after synthesis of the protein's amino acid chain is complete. Such molecules can significantly affect the protein's properties.

Many other types of molecules may also be associated with proteins. Some proteins, for example, have specific metal ions associated with them. Others carry small molecules that are essential to their activity. Still others associate with nucleic acids in chromosomal or ribosomal structures.

Scientists have traditionally addressed protein structure at four levels: primary, secondary, tertiary, and quaternary. Primary structure is simply the linear sequence of amino acids in the peptide chain.

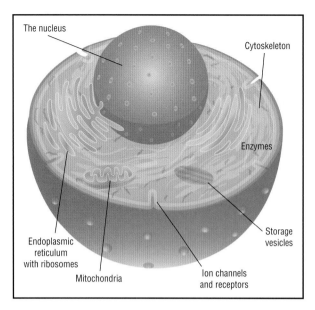

The nucleus

Cytoskeleton

Enzymes

Storage vesicles

Endoplasmic reticulum with ribosomes

Mitochondria

Ion channels and receptors

(Diagram of the structure of a protein. Illustration by GGS Information Services, Inc. The Gale Group.)

It determines the protein's shape. Secondary and tertiary structure both refer to the three-dimensional shape into which a protein chain folds. The distinction is partly historical: secondary structure refers to certain highly regular arrangements of amino acids that scientists could detect as long ago as the 1950s, while tertiary structure refers to the complete three-dimensional shape. Tertiary structure determines the function of the protein. Determining a protein's tertiary structure can be difficult even today, although researchers have made major strides within the past decades.

The tertiary structure of many proteins shows a "string of beads" organization. The protein includes several compact regions known as domains, separated by short stretches in which the protein chain assumes an extended, essentially random configuration. Some scientists believe that domains were originally separate proteins that, over the course of evolution, have come together to perform their functions more efficiently.

Quaternary structure refers to the way in which protein chains—either identical or different—associate with each other. For example, a complete molecule of the oxygen-carrying protein hemoglobin includes four protein chains of two slightly different types. Simple laboratory tests usually allow scientists to determine how many chains make up a complete protein molecule.

PRIMARY PROTEIN STRUCTURE: PEPTIDE-CHAIN SYNTHESIS. Proteins are made (synthesized) in living things according to "directions" given by DNA and carried out by RNA and proteins. The synthesized

protein's linear sequence of amino acids is ultimately determined by the linear sequence of DNA bases—or of base triplets known as codons—in the gene that codes for it. Each cell possesses elaborate machinery for producing proteins from these blueprints.

The first step is copying the DNA blueprint, essentially fixed within the cell nucleus, into a more mobile form. This form is messenger ribonucleic acid (mRNA), a single-stranded nucleic acid carrying essentially the same sequence of bases as the DNA gene. The mRNA is free to move into the main part of the cell, the cytoplasm, where protein synthesis takes place.

Besides mRNA, protein synthesis requires ribosomes and transfer ribonucleic acid (tRNA). Ribosomes are the actual "factories" where synthesis takes place, while tRNA molecules are the "trucks" that bring amino acids to the ribosome and ensure that they are incorporated at the right spot in the growing chain.

Ribosomes are extremely complex assemblages. They comprise almost 70 different proteins and at least three different types of RNA, all organized into two different-sized subunits. As protein synthesis begins, the previously separate subunits come together at the beginning of the mRNA chain; all three components are essential for the synthetic process.

Transfer RNA molecules are rather small, only about 80 nucleotides long. (Nucleotides are the fundamental building blocks of nucleic acids, as amino acids are of proteins.) Each type of amino acid has at least one corresponding type of tRNA (sometimes more). This correspondence is enforced by the enzymes that attach amino acids to tRNA molecules, which "recognize" both the amino acid and the tRNA type and do not act unless both are correct.

Transfer RNA molecules are not only trucks but translators. As the synthetic process adds one amino acid after another, they "read" the mRNA to determine which amino acid belongs next. They then bring the proper amino acid to the spot where synthesis is taking place, and the ribosome couples it to the growing chain. The tRNA is then released and the ribosome then moves along the mRNA to the next codon, that is, the next base triplet specifying an amino acid. The process repeats until the "stop" signal on the mRNA is reached, upon which the ribosome releases both the mRNA and the completed protein chain and its subunits separate to seek out other mRNAs.

SECONDARY STRUCTURE. The two major types of secondary structure are the alpha helix and the beta sheet, both discovered by Linus Pauling and R. B. Corey in 1951.

In an alpha helix, the backbone atoms of the peptide chain—the carboxyl carbon atom, the a-carbon atom (to which the side chain is attached), and the amino nitrogen atom—take the form of a three-dimensional spiral. The helix is held together by hydrogen bonds between each nitrogen atom and the oxygen atom of the carboxyl group belonging to the fourth amino acid up the chain.

Beta sheets feature several peptide chains lying next to each other in the same plane. The stabilizing hydrogen bonds are between nitrogen atoms on one chain and carboxyl-group oxygen atoms on the adjacent chain. Since each amino acid has its amino group hydrogen-bonded to the chain on one side and its carboxyl group to the chain on the other side, sheets can grow indefinitely.

TERTIARY STRUCTURE. Within seconds to minutes of their synthesis on ribosomes, proteins fold up into an essentially compact three-dimensional shape—their tertiary structure. Ordinary chemical forces fully determine both the steps in the folding pathway and the stability of the final shape. Some of these forces are hydrogen bonds between side chains of specific amino acids. Others involve electrical attraction between positively and negatively charged side chains. Perhaps most important, however, are what are called hydrophobic interactions—a scientific restatement of the observation that oil and water do not mix.

Some amino acid side chains are essentially oil-like (hydrophobic—literally, "water-fearing"). They accordingly stabilize tertiary structures that place them in the interior, largely surrounded by other oil-like side chains. Conversely, some side chains are charged or can form hydrogen bonds. These are hydrophilic, or "water-loving," side chains. Unless they form hydrogen or electrostatic bonds with other specific side chains, they will stabilize structures in which they are on the exterior, interacting with water.

The forces that govern a protein's tertiary structure are simple. With thousands or even tens of thousands of atoms involved, however, the interactions can be extremely complex. Today's scientists are only beginning to discover ways to predict the shape a protein will assume and the folding process it will go through to reach that shape.

Digestion, metabolism, and elimination

Food in the human diet consists of proteins, **carbohydrates**, fats, **vitamins**, and **minerals**. The majority of minerals and vitamins pass through to the bloodstream without the need for further digestive changes, but other nutrient molecules must be broken down to simpler substances before they can be absorbed and used. Foods in the **stomach** are broken down by the action of the gastric juice containing hydrochloric acid and a protein-digesting enzyme called pepsin. Gastric juice is needed mainly for the digestion of protein by pepsin. If a hamburger and bun reach the stomach, there is no need for extra gastric juice for the bun (carbohydrate), but the hamburger (protein) will require a much greater supply of gastric juice. The gastric juice already present will begin the breakdown of the large protein molecules of the hamburger into smaller molecules: polypeptides and peptides.

From the time a protein-containing food is eaten, to its breakdown and subsequent use or excretion, many complicated processes and steps take place in the body. These processes are part of **metabolism**, in which a series of metabolic pathways are involved in the breakdown of the foods. Proteins are initially degraded into constituent amino acids, which may be converted to compounds called pyruvic acid or acetyl-CoA before being passed into the metabolic pathway known as the Krebs cycle; or they may enter the Krebs cycle directly after being converted into one of the metabolites of this metabolic pathway.

Proteins contain substantial amounts of nitrogen. When dietary protein is broken down into amino acids, nitrogen is produced and is eliminated in the urine in the form of urea, and in smaller amounts as uric acid, ammonia, and creatinine. Unabsorbed protein is excreted in the feces, but only about 10 grams per day because protein is used very efficiently in the body. Amino acids may be recycled many times for different functions. There are minute losses of protein as skin, or in menstrual blood, semen, and hair.

Function

After water, protein makes up the greatest percentage of human body weight. This key nutrient provides the building blocks children and adults need for growing, maintaining, and repairing worn-out cells. Without protein, human bodies could not regulate fluids and immune systems would shut down. In fact, if not for protein there would be no hormones or enzymes—the protein compounds that take part in every single physical function. The role of protein in the diet is mainly as a source of amino acids, some of which are essential because they cannot be produced in the body. Others are referred to as nonessential because they can be made in the body from simple precursors. Amino acids are central to every human bodily function with every chemical reaction that occurs. Some of the uses of amino acids are:

- synthesizing of substances called purines and pyrimidines, important for deoxyribonucleic acid (DNA)

- producing creatine in skeletal muscle; creatine is needed for subsequent production of creatinine
- building and maintaining muscle and tissues
- maintaining proper cellular function
- controlling chemical reactions through enzymes.

There are also circulating proteins in the plasma of the blood that vary depending on the levels in the diet. Some examples of plasma proteins with important functions in the body are serum albumin, retinal binding protein, fibrinogen, etc. If the protein intake is low, these proteins will be reduced in the blood and therefore their functions in the body may be affected.

Approximately 300 grams of protein is produced per day in the body with a dietary intake of about 100 grams. Some of the protein needed is acquired from endogenous sources (in the body from protein breakdown) and is released into the intestinal lumen; it is estimated at about 70 grams per day.

Role in human health

The human body, minus water, is mostly composed of amino acids. Almost all of the hormones are amino acids. Regulation of **protein metabolism** is necessary to maintain proper bodily function, therefore, it is important to eat protein-rich foods. Protein is also important for building body tissue and synthesizing enzymes. Twenty amino acids are used for protein synthesis. Animals and plants are quick and available sources of what are termed "essential" amino acids; they are called essential because the body cannot internally build them. Normal growth and health are dependent upon these essential amino acids. These essential amino acids are histidine, tryptophan, lysine, methionine, phenylalanine, threonine, valine, leucine, isoleucine, and possibly arginine. Tyrosine and cysteine are produced in the body from phenylalanine and methionine respectively. The "nonessential" amino acids include alanine, glycine, serine, glutamic acid, aspartic acid, asparagine, glutamine, and proline. They are considered nonessential because the body can produce them with simple precursors.

Protein requirements

On a per kilogram basis, protein requirements in humans are highest in infancy and gradually decline throughout life, except in circumstances such as **pregnancy**, **lactation**, and illness. The Recommended Daily Allowance (RDA) suggests protein requirements based on age incrementally. The amount of protein needed also depends on body weight, but it is not a linear relationship. A person who weighs 400 lbs (181.43 kg) does not need four times as much protein as a person weighing 100 lbs (45.35 kg). From birth to three months, protein needs are at their highest (2.2 grams per kilogram of body weight). The requirement for adult males and females is 0.8 g/kg. This amount is equal to about 63 grams of dietary protein for a male aged 25-50 years who weighs 174 lbs (79 kg), and 50 grams for a female aged 25-50 years who weighs 139 lbs (63 kg). The average Western diet contains ample amounts of protein. In fact, most people in industrialized countries eat more protein than they need. In the United States, true protein deficiency is rare except when excess protein is lost and protein requirements are increased, as in cases of:

- burns
- fever
- fractures
- surgery
- wasting and/or cachexia associated with cancer (Approximately half of all cancer patients experience cachexia, a wasting syndrome that induces metabolic changes leading to a loss of muscle and fat.)
- chronic renal failure, when the patient is undergoing hemodialysis or peritoneal dialysis

Protein requirements may also be increased in training athletes because of greater muscle mass during training season.

In general, consequences of inadequate protein intake may include a faster loss of muscle mass from the body, higher risks of **infection**, and reduced protein reserves for use during periods of trauma or infection. In addition, protein breakdown is rapid when a person is fasting or bedridden.

Dietary sources of protein

Meat, milk, eggs, poultry, and seafood are considered high-quality, "complete" proteins because they have all the essential amino adds (protein's building blocks) in just the right proportion. Those sources are considered more complete than vegetable protein, such as beans, peas, and grains, also considered a good— even if not complete—source of amino acids. Except for soy, plant sources—nuts, beans, seeds, and grains— are deficient in one or more of the essential amino acids. But plant foods contain other vital nutrients (such as phytochemicals and fiber) not found in animal foods. Dietitians recommend that a healthy diet should consist of foods from a variety of sources and should include 10–20% of daily calories from protein (poultry, fish, dairy, soy protein, nuts, legumes, eggs, peanut butter, and vegetable sources).

Dietary guidelines

The food pyramid, developed by nutritionists, provides a visual guide to healthy eating. At its base are those foods that should be eaten numerous times each day, while at its apex are those foods that should be used sparingly. The pyramid suggests a range of servings in each group so that the number of servings can be adjusted to suit each individual's caloric requirements. The daily recommendations (from bottom to top) of the food pyramid include:

• Bread, cereal, rice, and pasta: 6–11 servings.

• Vegetables: 3–5 servings.

• Fruits: 2–4 servings.

• Milk, yogurt, and cheese: 2–3 servings.

• Meat, poultry, fish, dried beans, eggs, and nuts: 2–3 servings.

• Fats, oils, and sweets: use sparingly.

Protein-modified diets

High-protein diets are designed to provide about 1.5 g of protein for each kilogram of a person's body weight. Complex proteins, such as milk and meats, should make up one-half to two-thirds of the daily protein requirement. High-protein diets are recommended for people who:

• Have an increased need for protein due to protein-calorie malnutrition; severe stress; or conditions such as AIDS, cancer, or burns with high metabolic rates that lead to the loss of large amounts of protein

• Have malabsorption syndromes, celiac disease, or other disorders characterized by poor food absorption.

A low-protein diet excludes dairy products and meats, and requires that about three-fourths of the daily allowance of protein come from high-value protein sources. Supplements may be prescribed to prevent amino-acid deficiencies. Low-protein diets are used in treatment of conditions such as **liver cirrhosis** and kidney disease (excluding chronic renal failure patients who have increased protein needs because of losses that occur during dialysis).

Common diseases and disorders

The metabolic pathways in the body for protein metabolism and energy metabolism are interrelated. Certain metabolic conditions distort this relationship, namely diabetes, kidney failure, **fever**, **cancer**, and liver cirrhosis.

Inborn errors of metabolism (also called human hereditary biochemical disorders) have genetic origins; these errors interfere with the synthesis of proteins, carbohydrates, fats, enzymes, and many other substances in the body. Abnormalities in the breakdown, storage, or production of proteins, fats, and carbohydrates, or in the energy cycles of cells are typically the manifestations of this disorder. Disease and death may result from the absence or excess of normal or abnormal metabolites. For example, phenylketonuria (PKU) is a hereditary condition in which phenylalanine (an amino acid) is not properly metabolized. PKU may cause severe mental retardation. Some inborn errors of metabolism require dietary and/or nutrient modification depending on the specific metabolic error. A low-phenylalanine diet is normal treatment for PKU.

Celiac disease, also known as nontropical sprue, gluten enteropathy, or celiac sprue, is an inherited disorder resulting in malabsorption because of an allergic reaction after consumption of a protein called gluten. This intolerance causes patients with celiac disease to suffer weight loss, **diarrhea**, malnutrition, and bloating. By eliminating foods containing gluten from the diet, further damage to the intestines can be prevented, symptoms are relieved, and malabsorption of nutrients is corrected. Gluten is found in wheat, rye, barley, and oats. Registered dietitians and physicians can assist the patient with the diet modifications needed for each disease.

Other conditions that may occur due to protein metabolism or absorption abnormalities include:

• muscle wasting and atrophy, which may occur when there is decreased protein absorption and metabolism due to causes such as malabsorption syndrome

• edema (fluid retention in the body's tissues) due to decreased protein absorption

• malnutrition and weight loss due to decreased fat, carbohydrate, and protein absorption

Protein-calorie malnutrition (or protein-energy malnutrition) is a condition associated most closely with weight loss, starvation, or illness and is common in cancer patients. It occurs when a lack of protein and calories are consumed to sustain body composition. When inadequate calories are consumed, the body's functionality declines, which may lead to illness and perhaps death. Exhaustion, **weakness**, decreased resistance to infection, and a progressive wasting of body muscle and fat stores occur.

Certain conditions may require protein restrictions, for example, acute liver or kidney failure, and uremia (increased urea in the blood).

Powder and tablet forms of amino acids have become popular as health supplements. But their

Alpha helix—A type of secondary structure in which a single peptide chain arranges itself in a three-dimensional spiral.

Beta sheet—A type of secondary structure in which several peptide chains arrange themselves alongside each other.

Cachexia—A condition in which the body weight "wastes" away, characterized by a constant loss of weight, muscle, and fat.

Creatine—A substance found in skeletal muscles; it is produced by other amino acids.

Domain—A relatively compact region of a protein, separated from other domains by short stretches in which the protein chain is more or less extended; different domains often carry out distinct parts of the protein's overall function.

Enzymes—Enzymes are protein catalysts that increase the speed of chemical reactions in the cell without themselves being changed.

Hormones—Hormones are messengers that travel to tissues or organs, where they may stimulate or inhibit specific metabolic pathways.

Messenger ribonucleic acid (mRNA)—A molecule of RNA that carries the genetic information for producing one or more proteins; mRNA is produced by copying one strand of DNA, but is able to move from the nucleus to the cytoplasm (where protein synthesis takes place).

Peptide bond—A chemical bond between the carboxyl group of one amino acid and the amino nitrogen atom of another.

Phenylketonuria (PKU)—A rare hereditary condition in which phenylalanine (an amino acid) is not properly metabolized. PKU may cause severe mental retardation.

Polypeptide—A group of amino acids joined by peptide bonds; proteins are large polypeptides, but no agreement exists regarding how large they must be to justify the name.

Primary structure—The linear sequence of amino acids making up a protein.

Quaternary structure—The number and type of protein chains normally associated with each other in the body.

Protein-calorie malnutrition—A lack of protein and calories are consumed to sustain the body composition, resulting in weight loss and muscle wasting.

Ribosome—A very large assemblage of RNA and protein that, using instructions from mRNA, synthesizes new protein molecules.

Secondary structure—Certain highly regular three-dimensional arrangements of amino acids within a protein.

Tertiary structure—A protein molecule's overall three-dimensional shape.

Transfer ribonucleic acid (tRNA)—A small RNA molecule, specific for a single amino acid, that transports that amino acid to the proper spot on the ribosome for assembly into the growing protein chain.

Wasting—When inadequate calories are consumed, it can lead to "wasting" or depletion of body mass. Wasting results in weight loss in tissues such as skeletal muscle and adipose tissue (fat).

---

prolonged, excessive use can upset the natural amino acid balance and lead to kidney, liver, and nervous system damage. Do not take these supplements without first consulting a registered dietitian or physician.

Resources

BOOKS

Institute of Medicine. *Dietary Reference Intakes: Applications in Dietary Assessment.* Washington, D.C.: National Academy Press, 2001.

Lobley, Gerald E., et al., eds. *Protein Metabolism and Nutrition.* West Lafayette, IN: Purdue University Press, 1999.

Mahan, L. Kathleen, and Sylvia Escott-Stump., eds. *Krause's Food, Nutrition, & Diet Therapy.* London: W.B. Saunders Co., 2000.

Rodwell-Williams, Sue. *Essentials of Nutrition and Diet Therapy (With CD-ROM for Windows and Macintosh).* London: Mosby-Year Book, 1999.

Salway, J.G. *Metabolism at a Glance,* 2nd ed., Oxford: Blackwell Science Inc., 1999.

Welle, Stephen *Human Protein Metabolism.* New York: Springer Verlag, 1999.

White, John S., and Dorothy C. White, eds. *Proteins, Peptides, & Amino Acids Source Book.* Totowa, NJ: Humana Press Inc., 2001.

PERIODICAL

Omran M. L., and J. E. Morley. "Assessment of protein energy malnutrition in older persons, part I: History, examination, body composition, and screening tools." *Nutrition* 16, no. 1 (January 2000): 50-63.

ORGANIZATIONS

American Dietetic Association. 216 W. Jackson Blvd., Chicago, IL 60606-6995. (312) 899-0040. http://www.eatright.org/.

Food and Nutrition Information Center Agricultural Research Service, USDA. National Agricultural Library, Room 304, 10301 Baltimore Avenue, Beltsville, MD 20705-2351. (301) 504-5719. Fax: (301) 504-6409. http://www.nal.usda.gov/fnic/. fnic@nal.usda.gov.

Crystal Heather Kaczkowski, MSc.

Prothrombin time *see* **Coagulation tests**

PSA test *see* **Tumor marker tests**

Psoriasis

Definition

Named for the Greek word *psōra* meaning "itch," psoriasis is a chronic, non-contagious disease characterized by inflamed lesions covered with silvery-white scabs of dead skin.

Demographics

Psoriasis, which affects at least four million Americans, is slightly more common in women than in men. Although the disease can develop at any time, 10%–15% of all cases are diagnosed in children under 10, and the average age at the onset of symptoms is 28. Psoriasis is most common in fair-skinned people and extremely rare in dark-skinned individuals.

Description

Normal skin cells mature and replace dead skin every 28–30 days. Psoriasis causes skin cells to mature in less than a week. Because the body can't shed old skin as rapidly as new cells are rising to the surface, raised patches of dead skin develop on the arms, back, chest, elbows, legs, nails, folds between the buttocks, and scalp.

Psoriasis is considered mild if it affects less than 5% of the surface of the body, moderate if 5%–30% of the skin is involved, and severe if the disease affects more than 30% of the body surface.

Types of psoriasis

Dermatologists distinguish different forms of psoriasis according to what part of the body is affected, how severe symptoms are, how long they last, and the pattern formed by the scales.

PLAQUE PSORIASIS. Plaque psoriasis (psoriasis vulgaris), the most common form of the disease, is characterized by small, red bumps that enlarge, become inflamed, and form scales. The top scales flake off easily and often, but those beneath the surface of the skin clump together. Removing these scales exposes tender skin, which bleeds and causes the plaques (inflamed patches) to grow.

Plaque psoriasis can develop on any part of the body, but most often occurs on the elbows, knees, scalp, and trunk.

SCALP PSORIASIS. At least 50 of every 100 people who have any form of psoriasis have scalp psoriasis. This form of the disease is characterized by scale-capped plaques on the surface of the **skull**.

NAIL PSORIASIS. The first sign of nail psoriasis is usually pitting of the fingernails or toenails. Size, shape, and depth of the marks vary, and affected nails may thicken, yellow, or crumble. The skin around an affected nail is sometimes inflamed, and the nail may peel away from the nail bed.

GUTTATE PSORIASIS. Named for the Latin word *gutta,* which means "a drop," guttate psoriasis is characterized by small, red, drop-like dots that enlarge rapidly and may be somewhat scaly. Often found on the arms, legs, and trunk and sometimes in the scalp, guttate psoriasis can clear up without treatment or disappear and resurface in the form of plaque psoriasis.

PUSTULAR PSORIASIS. Pustular psoriasis usually occurs in adults. It is characterized by blister-like lesions filled with non-infectious pus and surrounded by reddened skin. Pustular psoriasis, which can be limited to one part of the body (localized) or can be widespread, may be the first symptom of psoriasis or develop in a patient with chronic plaque psoriasis.

Generalized pustular psoriasis is also known as Von Zumbusch pustular psoriasis. Widespread, acutely painful patches of inflamed skin develop suddenly. Pustules appear within a few hours, then dry and peel within two days.

Generalized pustular psoriasis can make life-threatening demands on the **heart** and **kidneys**.

Palomar-plantar pustulosis (PPP) generally appears between the ages of 20 and 60. PPP causes large pustules to form at the base of the thumb or on the sides of the heel. In time, the pustules turn brown and peel. The disease usually becomes much less active for a while after peeling.

Acrodermatitis continua of Hallopeau is a form of PPP characterized by painful, often disabling, lesions on the fingertips or the tips of the toes. The nails may become deformed, and the disease can damage **bone** in the affected area.

INVERSE PSORIASIS. Inverse psoriasis occurs in the armpits and groin, under the breasts, and in other areas where skin flexes or folds. This disease is characterized by smooth, inflamed lesions and can be debilitating.

ERYTHRODERMIC PSORIASIS. Characterized by severe scaling, **itching**, and **pain** that affects most of the body, erythrodermic psoriasis disrupts the body's chemical balance and can cause severe illness. This particularly inflammatory form of psoriasis can be the first sign of the disease, but often develops in patients with a history of plaque psoriasis.

PSORIATIC ARTHRITIS. About 10% of partients with psoriasis develop a complication called psoriatic arthritis. This type of arthritis can be slow to develop and mild, or it can develop rapidly. Symptoms of psoriatic arthritis include:

• joint discomfort, swelling, stiffness, or throbbing
• swelling in the toes and ankles
• pain in the digits, lower back, wrists, knees, and ankles
• eye inflammation or pink eye (conjunctivitis)

Causes and symptoms

The cause of psoriasis is unknown, but research suggests that an immune-system malfunction triggers the disease. Factors that increase the risk of developing psoriasis include:

• family history
• stress
• exposure to cold temperatures
• injury, illness, or infection
• steroids and other medications
• race

Trauma and certain **bacteria** may trigger psoriatic arthritis in patients with psoriasis.

Diagnosis

A complete medical history and examination of the skin, nails, and scalp are the basis for a diagnosis of psoriasis. In some cases, a microscopic examination of skin cells is also performed.

KEY TERM

Arthritis—An inflammation of joints.

Blood tests can distinguish psoriatic arthritis from other types of arthritis. **Rheumatoid arthritis**, in particular, is diagnosed by the presence of a particular antibody present in the blood. That antibody is not present in the blood of patients with psoriatic arthritis.

Treatment

Age, general health, lifestyle, and the severity and location of symptoms influence the type of treatment used to reduce inflammation and decrease the rate at which new skin cells are produced. Because the course of this disease varies with each individual, doctors must experiment with or combine different treatments to find the most effective therapy for a particular patient.

Mild-moderate psoriasis

Steroid creams and ointments are commonly used to treat mild or moderate psoriasis, and steroids are sometimes injected into the skin of patients with a limited number of lesions. In mid-1997, the United States Food and Drug Administration (FDA) approved the use of tazarotene (Tazorac) to treat mild-to-moderate plaque psoriasis. This water-based gel has chemical properties similar to **vitamin A**.

Brief daily doses of natural sunlight can significantly relieve symptoms. Sunburn has the opposite effect.

Moisturizers and bath oils can loosen scales, soften skin, and may eliminate the itch. So can adding a cup of oatmeal to a tub of bath water. Salicylic acid (an ingredient in aspirin) can be used to remove dead skin or increase the effectiveness of other therapies.

Moderate psoriasis

Administered under medical supervision, ultraviolet light B (UVB) is used to control psoriasis that covers many areas of the body or that has not responded to topical preparations. Doctors combine UVB treatments with topical medications to treat some patients and sometimes prescribe home **phototherapy**, in which the patient administers his or her own UVB treatments.

Photochemotherapy (PUVA) is a medically supervised procedure that combines medication with exposure to ultraviolet light (UVA) to treat localized or widespread psoriasis. An individual with wide-spread psoriasis that has not responded to treatment may enroll in one of the day treatment programs conducted at special facilities throughout the United States. Psoriasis patients who participate in these intensive sessions are exposed to UVB and given other treatments for six to eight hours a day for two to four weeks.

Severe psoriasis

Methotrexate (MTX) can be given as a pill or as an injection to alleviate symptoms of severe psoriasis or psoriatic arthritis. Patients who take MTX must be carefully monitored to prevent **liver** damage.

Psoriatic arthritis can also be treated with **nonsteroidal anti-inflammatory drugs** (NSAIDs), like acetaminophen (Tylenol) or aspirin. Hot compresses and warm water soaks may also provide some relief for painful joints.

Other medications used to treat severe psoriasis include etrentinate (Tegison) and isotretinoin (Accutane), whose chemical properties are similar to those of vitamin A. Most effective in treating pustular or erythrodermic psoriasis, Tegison also relieves some symptoms of plaque psoriasis. Tegison can enhance the effectiveness of UVB or PUVA treatments and reduce the amount of exposure necessary.

Accutane is a less effective psoriasis treatment than Tegison, but both have similar side effects, including nosebleeds, inflammation of the eyes and lips, bone spurs, hair loss, and **birth defects**. Tegison is stored in the body for an unknown length of time and should not be taken by a woman who is pregnant or planning to become pregnant. A woman should use reliable birth control while taking Accutane and for at least one month before and after her course of treatment.

Cyclosporin emulsion (Neoral) is used to treat stubborn cases of severe psoriasis. Cyclosporin is also used to prevent rejection of transplanted organs, and Neoral, approved by the FDA in 1997, should be particularly beneficial to psoriasis patients who are young children or African Americans, or those who have diabetes.

Other conventional treatments for psoriasis include:

- Capsaicin (*Capsicum frutecens*), an ointment that can stop production of the chemical that causes the skin to become inflamed and halts the runaway production of new skin cells. Capsaicin is available without a prescription, but should be used under a doctor's supervision to prevent burns and skin damage.
- Hydrocortisone creams, topical ointments containing a form of vitamin D called calcitriol, and coal-tar shampoos and ointments can relieve symptoms. Hydrocortisone creams have been associated with such side effects as folliculitis (inflammation of the hair follicles), while coal-tar preparations have been associated with a heightened risk of skin cancer.

Alternative treatment

Nontraditional psoriasis treatments include:

- Soaking in warm water and German chamomile (*Matricaria recutita*) or bathing in warm salt water.
- Drinking as many as three cups a day of hot tea made with one or a combination of the following herbs: burdock (*Arctium lappa*) root, dandelion (*Taraxacum mongolicum*) root, Oregon grape (*Mahonia aquifolium*), sarsaparilla (*Smilax officinalis*), and balsam pear (*Momardica charantia*).
- Taking two 500-mg capsules of evening primrose oil (*Oenothera biennis*) a day. Pregnant women should not use evening primrose oil, and patients with liver disease or high cholesterol should use it only under a doctor's supervision.
- Eating a diet that includes plenty of fish, turkey, celery (for cleansing the kidneys), parsley, lettuce, lemons (for cleansing the liver), limes, fiber, and fruit and vegetable juices.
- Eating a diet that eliminates animal products high in saturated fats, since they promote inflammation.
- Drinking plenty of water (at least eight glasses) each day.
- Taking nutritional supplements including folic acid, lecithin, vitamin A (specific for the skin), vitamin E, selenium, and zinc.

Other helpful alternative approaches include identifying and eliminating food allergens from the diet, enhancing the fuction of the liver, augmenting the hydrochloric acid in the **stomach**, and completing a detoxification program. Constitutional homeopathic treatment, if properly prescribed, may also help resolve psoriasis.

Prognosis

Most cases of psoriasis can be controlled, and most people who have psoriasis can live normal lives.

Some people who have psoriasis are so self-conscious and embarrassed about their appearance that they become depressed and withdrawn. The Social Security Administration grants disability benefits to about 400 psoriasis patients each year, and a comparable number die from complications of the disease.

Prevention

A doctor should be notified if:

- psoriasis symptoms appear or reappear after treatment
- pustules erupt on the skin and the patient experiences fatigue, muscle aches, and fever
- unfamiliar, unexplained symptoms appear

Resources

BOOKS

Ferri, Fred, ed. *Ferri's Clinical Advisor 2010.* Philadelphia: Mosby Elsevier, 2009.

Goldman, L. and Ausiello D., eds. *Cecil Textbook of Internal Medicine.* 23rd ed. Philadelphia: Saunders, 2008.

Habif, T.P. *Clinical Dermatology.* 5th ed. St. Louis: Mosby, 2009.

Rakel, R.E., and Bope, E.T. *Conn's Current Therapy.* 60th ed. Philadelphia: Saunders Elsevier, 2009.

Rakel, R. *Textbook of Family Medicine 2007.* 7th ed. Philadelphia: Saunders Elsevier, 2009.

ORGANIZATIONS

American Academy of Dermatology, 930 N. Meacham Road, P.O. Box 4014, Schaumburg, IL 60168-4014, (847) 330-0230, Fax: (847) 330-0050, http://www.aad.org

American Skin Association, Inc., 150 E. 58th St., 3rd floor, New York, NY 10155-0002, (212) 688-6547, http://www.americanskin.org.

National Psoriasis Foundation, 6600 S.W. 92nd Ave., Suite 300, Portland, OR 97223, (800) 723-9166, http://www.psoriasis.org.

Maureen Haggerty

Psychiatric assisting

Definition

A psychiatric assistant, also known as a psychiatric technician or mental health technician, works in a variety of inpatient psychiatric settings with mentally ill adults and children or those with behavioral disorders.

Description

Psychiatric assistants or technicians work with emotionally disturbed or mentally impaired individuals, usually in psychiatric hospitals or mental health clinics. They work as members of interdisciplinary teams of mental health professionals, such as psychiatrists, psychologists, registered nurses, clinical social workers, and others. In general, psychiatric aides help patients with personal grooming and participation in educational, recreational, and therapeutic activities. They may interact and spend more time with patients than any other treatment team members. Psychiatric assistants usually have some type of formal training or education in the behavioral sciences. These paraprofessionals participate in both the planning and implementing of individual patient treatment plans. They may be given responsibility for interviewing patients, record keeping, assisting in administration of medications, and coordinating therapy and group therapy sessions. Psychiatric assistants must have good observation skills, as their job entails recognizing and reporting changes in the behavior of patients to other team members.

Work settings

Psychiatric assistants or technicians work in a wide variety of settings, including psychiatric hospitals, community general hospitals, community mental health centers, psychiatric clinics, schools for the mentally retarded, social service agencies, geriatric **nursing homes**, child or adolescent centers, and halfway houses. They generally work a 35- to 40-hour week. Because patients need care 24 hours a day, scheduled work hours may include nights, weekends, and holidays. Most of the psychiatric assistants' work time is spent on their feet.

Psychiatric assistants are often confronted with violent patients who must be restrained, which is an emotionally draining and sometimes dangerous task. However, many psychiatric assistants glean satisfaction from assisting those in need of support and encouragement. Individuals in this field should be healthy, tactful, patient, understanding, assertive, emotionally stable, dependable, and have a strong desire to help people. They should also be able to work as part of a team, have good communication skills, and be willing to perform repetitive, routine tasks. Opportunities for advancement within these occupations are limited. To enter other health occupations, psychiatric assistants often need additional formal training. Some employers and unions provide opportunities by simplifying the educational paths to advancement. Working as a psychiatric assistant can also help individuals decide whether to pursue a career in the health care field.

Education and training

Most psychiatric technicians are required to have a least a bachelor's degree and several hours of clinical training on the psychiatric unit. Individual requirements vary from state to state, but many states require specific college coursework credits in nursing science,

KEY TERMS

Interdisciplinary team—A team of professionals from many different disciplines, such as nurses, psychotherapists, social workers, psychologists, occupational therapists, and physicians.

Paraprofessional—A paraprofessional assists professional-level personnel such as nurses, physicians, and therapists in hospitals, medical facilities, and mental health facilities.

mental disorders, developmental disabilities, and **pharmacology**. To help keep psychiatric assistants current with recent advances in their field, some states require employees to complete several hours of continuing education courses every two years in order to maintain their position or certification. Some facilities provide classroom instruction for newly hired assistants, and others rely exclusively on informal on-the-job instruction from a licensed nurse or an experienced team member. Such training may last several days to a few months. From time to time, psychiatric assistants may also attend lectures, workshops, and in-service training.

Advanced education and training

Advanced training and education is not always required of psychiatric assistants. However, some psychiatric assistants choose to pursue a master's degree in clinical social work or psychology to further their career and gain useful clinical expertise. Advanced or "senior" psychiatric assistants may be required to hold a postgraduate degree in some states. The American Association of Psychiatric Technicians offers a voluntary certification exam for psychiatric assistants to test their knowledge of basic psychiatric technology. This certification is a benefit to mental health assistants, psychiatric aides, and related employees in the 46 states that do not have licensed psychiatric technicians, and also to those in the armed forces. The examination is a 201-question, open-book written test that individuals can take at home. Although it tests for basic knowledge about nursing, mental illness and developmental disabilities, it is not nearly as comprehensive as the licensing exams that some states require. National certification allows individuals to put the initials NCPT after their names, which stands for Nationally Certified Psychiatric Technician. In some cases, those who are certified receive better pay and promotional opportunities. In some instances, such as for

mental health workers employed by the Navy, certification is required.

Future outlook

Nationally, employment of psychiatric assistants is predicted to grow more slowly than average through 2008. On one hand, some growth will result from the increasing population of elderly people. Elderly adults may have mental health problems, such as **Alzheimer's disease**, that require care. In addition, outpatient mental health centers will need more aides, because people are often more accepting of treatment for drug abuse and **alcoholism**. Thus, more people will go to these centers, and there will be a greater need for psychiatric assistants. On the other hand, employment in hospitals is predicted to decline. Because hospitals employ about half of all psychiatric assistants, this decline will have a significant effect on the occupation. The main reason for this decline is that hospitals are admitting fewer psychiatric patients because of poor reimbursement rates from insurance companies and government agencies. The turnover rate in this field is high because of low wages and lack of advancement opportunities. Therefore, many jobs are expected to open as workers leave this occupation.

According to the American Association of Psychiatric Technicians, a major area of expansion for psychiatric assistants is the compelling need to provide treatment to thousands of state prison inmates with serious mental illness and developmental disabilities. The Department of Corrections estimates that one out of every 12 inmates suffers from serious mental illness. Because the prison population is expected to grow to more than 240,000 inmates by the turn of the century, a tremendous opportunity exists for psychiatric assistants and tecnicians. Psychiatric assistants function in various aspects of this challenging new program, including crisis intervention, mental health screening, patient assessment, implementation of treatment programs, supervising suicide risks, administering medications, maintaining **medical records**, and quality assurance. Another function involves parole programs that prepare inmates for productive lives after release.

Resources

ORGANIZATIONS

The American Association of Psychiatric Technicians. http://www.psych-health.com/main.htm

Indiana Career and Postsecondary Advancement Center. http://icpac.indiana.edu/career_profiles.

Bethanne Black

Psychiatric rehabilitation

Definition

Psychiatric **rehabilitation** involves helping people with mental illness gain or improve skills while obtaining the necessary resources and support to reach their goals.

Purpose

The purposes of psychiatric rehabilitation include helping individuals cope more effectively with the symptoms of their disorders; preventing or delaying the reemergence of symptoms; assisting the individual in managing or reducing secondary symptoms not relieved by medication, e.g., social withdrawal or apathy; teaching or restoring social and living skills that may never have been learned or that have atrophied during periods of illness or hospitalization; and enhancing support while lessening **stress** in the individual's environment.

Therefore, the goals of rehabilitation professionals are to sustain symptomatic relief, establish or reestablish interpersonal and independent living skills, and help individuals reach a satisfactory quality of life.

Description

The concepts of mental health and mental illness are culturally determined. In the United States mental illness is generally viewed as a maladaptive response to stress, evidenced by thoughts, feelings, and behaviors that interfere with social, occupational, or physical functioning.

Of the estimated 40 million people in the United States who have psychiatric disabilities, approximately five million are considered seriously mentally ill. People with psychiatric disabilities often have limited daily functioning that includes difficulties in relating, problems coping with stress, difficulty concentrating, and a lack of energy or initiative.

Psychiatric rehabilitation takes place in a variety of settings, including mental health centers, hospitals, sheltered workshops, halfway houses, correctional facilities, places of employment, and the individual's home. It most often involves assessment, training, and modification of personal and community environments. Because rehabilitation focuses on adjustment to everyday life, it is important for the individual to participate as much as possible in choosing the objectives.

Complications

Medications prescribed for severe mental illnesses, called neuroleptic drugs, have a number of side effects. Standard drugs prescribed for **schizophrenia**, one of the most debilitating mental illnesses, include Haldol, Thorazine, Trilafon, Mellaril, Serentil, Stelazine, and Prolixin. Side effects include agitation, sleepiness and lethargy, dry mouth, eye problems, allergic reactions, weight gain, menstrual irregularities, and **sexual dysfunction**. Malignant neuroleptic syndrome, a less common but more serious side effect, causes very high body temperatures that can be fatal in some cases if not treated promptly. Hyperprolactinemia or high levels of the female hormone prolactin are common among those taking neuroleptics. This side effect causes menstrual abnormalities while increasing the risk for **osteoporosis** and **breast cancer**.

The most disturbing and common of the side effects are known as extrapyramidal symptoms, which cause movement and coordination difficulties. Women are at higher risk for these symptoms; and the risk increases with the length of time the drug is taken and with age. Nearly every neuroleptic drug can cause extrapyramidal side effects, which occur in up to 70% of patients taking these medications. A condition known as acute dystonia can develop shortly after taking **antipsychotic drugs**, resulting in abnormal muscle spasms, particularly of the neck, jaw, trunk, and eye muscles. The most serious effect of antipsychotic therapy is tardive dyskinesia, which causes repetitive and involuntary movements or tics—most often of the mouth, lips, legs, arms, or trunk.

Results

The effectiveness of medication is determined by the degree to which it helps the individual manage the symptoms of their illness. Effectiveness of treatments that help develop an individual's coping skills are measured are assessed on the basis of how well the individual is able to develop these skills.

Health care team roles

Professionals involved in psychiatric rehabilitation vary according to setting and may include nurses, psychiatric social workers, rehabilitation counselors, clinical psychologists, psychiatrists, recreation therapists, and paraprofessionals.

A psychiatric nurse's responsibilities may include case management, client advocacy, managing medications, facilitating therapy (individual, family, or group), clinical supervision, serving as a liaison, and consulting.

Psychiatric social workers are skilled in assessing family, social, and environmental factors that contribute to dysfunctional behavior in the individual or the family. They are also primary contributors to the planning and implementation of follow-up care.

Rehabilitation counselors most often are involved in case management and in assisting individuals with employment, housing, coping skills, and academic preparation.

Psychologists most directly involved in the diagnosis and treatment of mental illness are called clinical psychologists. Clinical psychologists are concerned with the diagnosis of mental illness and have expertise in diagnosing and assessing treatment effects by using personality inventories and tests, including intelligence tests.

The role of the psychiatrist involves making medical diagnoses, prescribing medications, and administering additional treatments such as electroconvulsive therapy (ECT), commonly known as **shock** treatment.

Recreation or activity therapists provide structured activities designed to help individuals deal with their problems. They assist in diagnostic and personality evaluation through observing clients during activities. Activity therapists often prescribe activities that enable individuals to express emotions and develop skills in relating with others.

Resources

BOOKS

Chitty, Kay. *Professional Nursing: Concepts and Challenges,* 3rd edition. Philadelphia: W. B. Saunders, 2001.

Corrigan, Patrick and Daniel Giffort. *Building Teams and Programs for Effective Psychiatric Rehabilitation.* Jossey-Bass, 1998.

Pratt, Carlos. *Psychiatric Rehabilitation.* Academic Press, 1999.

Stanhope, Marcia, and Jeanette Lancaster. *Community and Public Health Nursing,* 5th edition. St. Louis: Mosby, 2000.

Townsend, Mary. *Essentials of Psychiatric/Mental Health Nursing.* F.A. Davis, 1999.

PERIODICAL

Garske, Gregory. "The challenge of rehabilitation counselors: Working with people with psychiatric disabilities." *Journal of Rehabilitation* (Jan/Feb/Mar 1999).

Bill Asenjo, MS, CRC

Psychological tests

Definition

Psychological tests are written, visual, or verbal evaluations administered to assess the cognitive and emotional functioning of children and adults.

Purpose

Psychological tests are used to assess a variety of mental abilities and attributes, including cognitive skills, motivation, personality traits, and neurological functioning.

Achievement and ability tests

For children, academic achievement, ability, and intelligence tests may be used as tools in school placement, in determining the presence of a learning disability or a developmental delay, in identifying giftedness, or in tracking intellectual development. Intelligence testing may be used with adults to determine vocational ability (e.g., in career counseling) or to assess adult intellectual ability in the classroom.

Personality tests

Personality tests are administered for a wide variety of reasons, from diagnosing psychopathology (e.g., personality disorder, depressive disorder) to screening job candidates. They may be used in an educational or vocational setting to determine personality strengths and weaknesses, or in the legal system to evaluate parolees.

Neuropsychological tests

Patients who have experienced a traumatic **brain** injury, brain damage, or organic neurological problems (for example, **dementia**) are administered neuropsychological tests. Neuropsychological testing evaluates cognitive function, including general intelligence, attention, **memory** span, and judgment; and motor, sensory, and speech ability. Tests can also be used to assess emotional stability, quality of language production, distractibility and other qualities. These tests can document impairments that can be used to diagnose specific neurological illness or damage. In addition, certain neuropsychological measures may be used to screen children for developmental delays and/or learning disabilities.

Precautions

Psychological testing requires a clinically trained examiner to administer the tests. All psychological tests should be administered, scored, and interpreted by a trained and experienced professional—preferably a psychologist or psychiatrist with expertise in the appropriate area.

Psychological tests are only one element of a psychological assessment. They should never be used alone as the sole basis for a diagnosis. A detailed history of the test subject and a review of psychological, medical, educational, or other relevant records are required to lay the groundwork for interpreting the results of any psychological measurement.

Cultural and language differences in the test subject may affect test performance and may result in inaccurate test results. The test administrator should be informed before psychological testing begins if the test taker is not fluent in English and/or belongs to a minority culture. In addition, the subject's motivation and motives may also affect test results.

Description

Psychological tests are formalized measures of mental functioning. Most are objective and quantifiable; however, certain projective tests may involve some level of subjective interpretation. Also known as inventories, measurements, questionnaires, and scales, psychological tests are administered in a variety of settings, including preschools, primary and secondary schools, colleges and universities, hospitals, outpatient healthcare settings, social agencies, prisons, and employment or human resource offices. They come in a variety of formats, including written, verbal, and computer administered.

Achievement and ability tests

Achievement and ability tests are designed to measure the level of an individual's intellectual functioning and cognitive ability. Most achievement and ability tests are standardized, meaning that norms were established during the design phase of the test by administering the test to a large representative sample of the test population. Achievement and ability tests follow a uniform testing protocol, or procedure (i.e., test instructions, test conditions, and scoring procedures), and their scores can be interpreted in relation to established norms. Common achievement and ability tests include the Wechsler intelligence test (WISC-III and WAIS) and the Stanford-Binet intelligence scales.

Personality tests

Personality tests and inventories evaluate the thoughts, emotions, attitudes, and behavioral traits that comprise personality. The results of these tests determine an individual's personality strengths and weaknesses, and may identify certain disturbances in personality, or psychopathology. Tests such as the Minnesota Multiphasic Personality Inventory-2 (MMPI-2) and the Millon Clinical Multiaxial Inventory III (MCMI-III), are used to screen individuals for specific psychopathologies or emotional problems.

Another type of personality test is the projective personality assessment. A projective test asks a subject to interpret some ambiguous stimuli, such as a series of inkblots. The subject's responses provide insight into his or her thought processes and personality traits. The best known projective psychological test is the Rorschach, or inkblot test. The patient is asked to look at each blot and to say what it looks like or what it could be. Because the stimulus is ambiguous, the patient must impose his or her own interpretation. In doing so, thoughts, feelings, and themes, some of which are unconscious, are projected into the material. Projective tests have lower validity and reliability than objective tests. However, the information they provide tends to be richer and more varied. Another projective assessment, the Thematic Apperception Test (TAT), asks the subject to tell a story about a series of pictures. The TAT is often used in a test battery in conjunction with the Rorschach. The TAT purports to provide information about important themes in a person's life or the content of their thinking, whereas the Rorschach provides information about the process and form of a person's thoughts. Although these tests are widely used, research has demonstrated that the examiners' subjective interpretations often affect the outcomes of these tests.

Neuropsychological tests

Many insurance plans cover all or a portion of diagnostic neuropsychological or psychological testing. **Medicare** reimburses for psychological and neuropsychological testing. Billing time typically includes test administration, scoring and interpretation, and reporting.

Preparation

Prior to the administration of any psychological test, the administrator should provide the test subject with information on the nature of the test and its intended use, complete standardized instructions for taking the test (including any time limits and penalties for incorrect responses), and information on the confidentiality of the results. After these disclosures are made, **informed consent** should be obtained from

KEY TERMS

Norms—A fixed or ideal standard; normative or mean score for a particular age group.

Psychopathology—A mental disorder or illness, such as schizophrenia, personality disorder, or major depressive disorder.

Quantifiable—Can be expressed as a number. The results of quantifiable psychological tests can be translated into numerical values, or scores.

Reliability—Capable of producing trustworthy results. Projective tests, such as the Rorschach and Thematic Apperception (TAT) tests, often produce unreliable results because they are easily influenced by the examiner's own assumptions.

Representative sample—A random sample of people that adequately represent the test-taking population in age, gender, race, and socioeconomic standing.

Standardization—The process of determining established norms and procedures for a test to act as a standard reference point for future test results.

Validity—Producing creditable results because of precision of method or adherence to an established norm. Projective tests, such as the Rorschach and Thematic Apperception (TAT) tests, often have questionable validity because they are easily influenced by the examiner's own assumptions.

the test subject before testing begins (except in cases of legally mandated testing, in which consent is not required of the subject).

Results

All psychological and neuropsychological assessments should be administered, scored, and interpreted by a trained professional. When interpreting test results for test subjects, the test administrator will review with subjects: what the test evaluates, its precision in evaluation, any margins of error involved in scoring, and what the individual scores mean in the context of overall test norms and the background of the test subject.

Health care team roles

Nursing staff and allied health professionals can assist in the administration of psychological tests by being familiar with each test and the reason it is being administered. Prior to the administration of psychological tests, nursing staff can provide appropriate **patient education** materials as necessary.

Resources

BOOKS

Gregory, Robert J. *Psychological Testing: History, Principles, and Applications,* 5th edition. Allyn & Bacon, 2006.

Hebben, Nancy, and William Milberg. *Essentials of Neuropsychological Assessment,* 2nd edition. Wiley, 2009.

Strauss, Esther, Elisabeth M. S. Sherman, and Otfried Spreen. *A Compendium of Neuropsychological Tests: Administration, Norms, and Commentary,* 3rd edition. Oxford University Press, 2006.

ORGANIZATIONS

The American Psychological Association. Committee on Psychological Tests and Assessments. 750 First St. NE, Washington, DC 20002-4242. (202) 336-5500. http://www.apa.org/psychnet.

The ERIC Clearinghouse on Assessment and Evaluation. O'Boyle Hall, Department of Education, The Catholic University of America, Washington, DC 20064. (800) 464-3742. http://www.ericae.net.

Bethanne Black

Psychosis

Definition

Psychosis is a symptom or feature of mental illness typically characterized by radical changes in personality, impaired functioning, and a distorted or nonexistent sense of objective reality.

Description

Patients suffering from psychosis have impaired reality testing; that is, they are unable to distinguish personal subjective experience from the reality of the external world. They experience hallucinations and/or delusions that they believe are real, and may behave and communicate in an inappropriate and incoherent fashion. Psychosis may appear as a symptom of a number of mental disorders, including mood and **personality disorders**. It is also the defining feature of **schizophrenia**, schizophreniform disorder, schizoaffective disorder, delusional disorder, and the psychotic disorders (i.e., brief psychotic disorder, shared psychotic disorder, psychotic disorder due to a general medical condition, and substance-induced psychotic disorder).

Causes and symptoms

Psychosis may be caused by the interaction of biological and psychosocial factors, depending on the disorder in which it presents; psychosis can also be caused by purely social factors, with no biological component.

Biological factors that are regarded as contributing to the development of psychosis include genetic abnormalities and substance use. With regard to chromosomal abnormalities, studies indicate that 30% of patients diagnosed with a psychotic disorder have a microdeletion at chromosome 22q11. Another group of researchers has identified the gene G72/G30 at chromosome 13q33.2 as a susceptibility gene for childhood-onset schizophrenia and psychosis not otherwise specified.

With regard to **substance abuse**, several different research groups reported in 2004 that cannabis (**marijuana**) use is a risk factor for the onset of psychosis.

Migration is a social factor that influences people's susceptibility to psychotic disorders. Psychiatrists in Europe have noted the increasing rate of schizophrenia and other psychotic disorders among immigrants to almost all Western European countries. Black immigrants from Africa or the Caribbean appear to be especially vulnerable. The stresses involved in migration include family breakup, the need to adjust to living in large urban areas, and social inequalities in the new country.

Schizophrenia, schizophreniform disorder, and schizoaffective disorder

Psychosis in schizophrenia and perhaps schizophreniform disorder appears to be related to abnormalities in the structure and chemistry of the **brain**, and appears to have strong genetic links, but its course and severity can be altered by social factors such as **stress** or a lack of support within the family. The cause of schizoaffective disorder is less clear cut, but biological factors are also suspected.

Delusional disorder

The exact cause of delusional disorder has not been conclusively determined, but potential causes include heredity, neurological abnormalities, and changes in brain chemistry. Some studies have indicated that delusions are generated by abnormalities in the limbic system, the portion of the brain on the inner edge of the cerebral cortex that is believed to regulate emotions. Delusional disorder is also more likely to develop in persons who are isolated from others in their society by language difficulties and/or cultural differences.

Brief psychotic disorder

Trauma and stress can cause a short-term psychosis (less than a month's duration) known as brief psychotic disorder. Major life-changing events such as the death of a family member or a natural disaster have been known to stimulate brief psychotic disorder in patients with no prior history of mental illness.

Psychotic disorder due to a general medical condition

Psychosis may also be triggered by an organic cause, termed a psychotic disorder due to a general medical condition. Organic sources of psychosis include neurological conditions (for example, epilepsy and cerebrovascular disease), metabolic conditions (for example, porphyria), endocrine conditions (for example, hyper- or hypothyroidism), renal failure, electrolyte imbalance, or **autoimmune disorders**.

Substance-induced psychotic disorder

Psychosis is also a known side effect of the use, abuse, and withdrawal from certain drugs. So-called recreational drugs, such as hallucinogenics, PCP, amphetamines, **cocaine**, marijuana, and alcohol, may cause a psychotic reaction during use or withdrawal. Certain prescription medications such as steroids, anticonvulsants, chemotherapeutic agents, and antiparkinsonian medications may also induce psychotic symptoms. Toxic substances such as carbon monoxide have also been reported to cause substance-induced psychotic disorder.

Shared psychotic disorder

Shared psychotic disorder, also known as *folie à deux* or psychosis by association, is a relatively rare delusional disorder involving two (or more) people with close emotional ties. In the West, shared psychosis most commonly develops between two sisters or between husband and wife, while in Japan the most common form involves a parent and a son or daughter. Shared psychosis occasionally involves an entire nuclear family.

Psychosis is characterized by the following symptoms:

• Delusions. Those delusions that occur in schizophrenia and its related forms are typically bizarre (i.e., they could not occur in real life). Delusions occurring in delusional disorder are more plausible, but still patently untrue. In some cases, delusions may be accompanied by feelings of paranoia.

• Hallucinations. Psychotic patients see, hear, smell, taste, or feel things that aren't there. Schizophrenic

KEY TERMS

Brief psychotic disorder—An acute, short-term episode of psychosis lasting no longer than one month. This disorder may occur in response to a stressful event.

Delirium—An acute but temporary disturbance of consciousness marked by confusion, difficulty paying attention, delusions, hallucinations, or restlessness. Delirium may be caused by drug intoxication, high fever related to infection, head trauma, brain tumors, kidney or liver failure, or various metabolic disturbances.

Delusional disorder—Individuals with delusional disorder suffer from long-term, complex delusions that fall into one of six categories: persecutory, grandiose, jealous, erotomanic, somatic, or mixed.

Delusions—An unshakable belief in something untrue that cannot be explained by religious or cultural factors. These irrational beliefs defy normal reasoning and remain firm even when overwhelming proof is presented to refute them.

Hallucinations—False or distorted sensory experiences that appear to be real perceptions to the person experiencing them.

Paranoia—An unfounded or exaggerated distrust of others, sometimes reaching delusional proportions.

Porphyria—A disease of the metabolism characterized by skin lesions, urine problems, neurologic disorders, and/or abdominal pain.

Schizoaffective disorder—Schizophrenic symptoms occurring concurrently with a major depressive or manic episode.

Schizophrenia—A debilitating mental illness characterized by delusions, hallucinations, disorganized speech and behavior, and inappropriate or flattened affect (a lack of emotions) that seriously hampers the afflicted individual's social and occupational functioning. Approximately 2 million Americans suffer from schizophrenia.

Schizophreniform disorder—A short-term variation of schizophrenia that has a total duration of one to six months.

Shared psychotic disorder—Also known as *folie à deux*, shared psychotic disorder is an uncommon disorder in which the same delusion is shared by two or more individuals.

Tardive dyskinesia—Involuntary movements of the face and/or body that are a side effect of the long-term use of some older antipsychotic (neuroleptic) drugs. Tardive dyskinesia affects 15%-20% of patients on long-term neuroleptic treatment.

hallucinations are typically auditory or, less commonly, visual; but psychotic hallucinations can involve any of the five senses.

- Disorganized speech. Psychotic patients, especially those with schizophrenia, often ramble on in incoherent, nonsensical speech patterns.

- Disorganized or catatonic behavior. The catatonic patient reacts inappropriately to his/her environment by either remaining rigid and immobile or by engaging in excessive motor activity. Disorganized behavior is behavior or activity that is inappropriate for the situation, or unpredictable.

Diagnosis

Patients with psychotic symptoms should undergo a thorough **physical examination** and history to rule out such possible organic causes as seizures, **delirium**, or alcohol withdrawal, and such other psychiatric conditions as dissociation or panic attacks. If a psychiatric cause such as schizophrenia is suspected, a mental health professional will typically conduct an interview with the patient and administer one of several clinical inventories, or tests, to evaluate mental status. This assessment takes place in either an outpatient or hospital setting.

Psychotic symptoms and behaviors are considered psychiatric emergencies, and persons showing signs of psychosis are frequently taken by family, friends, or the police to a hospital emergency room. A person diagnosed as psychotic can be legally hospitalized against his or her will, particularly if he or she is violent, threatening to commit suicide, or threatening to harm another person. A psychotic person may also be hospitalized if he or she has become malnourished or ill as a result of failure to feed, dress appropriately for the climate, or otherwise take care of him- or herself.

Treatment

Psychosis that is symptomatic of schizophrenia or another psychiatric disorder should be treated by a psychologist and/or psychiatrist. An appropriate course of medication and/or psychosocial therapy is employed to treat the underlying primary disorder. If the patient is considered to be at risk for harming himself or others, inpatient treatment is usually recommended.

Treatment of shared psychotic disorder involves separating the affected persons from one another as well as using antipsychotic medications and **psychotherapy**.

Antipsychotic medication such as thioridazine (Mellaril), haloperidol (Haldol), chlorpromazine (Thorazine), clozapine (Clozaril), sertindole (Serlect), olanzapine (Zyprexa), or risperidone (Risperdal) is usually prescribed to bring psychotic symptoms under control and into remission. Possible side effects of antipsychotics include dry mouth, drowsiness, muscle stiffness, and tardive dyskinesia (involuntary movements of the body). Agranulocytosis, a potentially serious but reversible health condition in which the white **blood** cells that fight **infection** in the body are destroyed, is a possible side effect of clozapine. Patients treated with this drug should undergo weekly blood tests to monitor white blood cell counts for the first six months, then every two weeks thereafter.

After an acute psychotic episode has subsided, antipsychotic drug maintenance treatment is typically employed and psychosocial therapy and living and vocational skills training may be attempted.

Prognosis

Prognosis for brief psychotic disorder is quite good; for schizophrenia, less so. Generally, the longer and more severe a psychotic episode, the poorer the prognosis is for the patient. Early diagnosis and treatment are critical to improving outcomes for the patient across all psychotic disorders.

Approximately 10% of America's permanently disabled population is comprised of schizophrenic individuals. The mortality rate of schizophrenic individuals is also high—approximately 10% of schizophrenics commit suicide, and 20% attempt it. However, early diagnosis and long-term follow up care can improve the outlook for these patients considerably. Roughly 60% of patients with schizophrenia will show substantial improvement with appropriate treatment.

Resources

BOOKS

Capps, Donald. *Understanding Psychosis: Issues and Challenges for Sufferers, Families, and Friends.* Lanham, MD: Rowman & Littlefield, 2010.

Porter, Robert S., and Justin L. Kaplan, eds. *The Merck Manual of Diagnosis and Therapy.* 19th ed. Whitehouse Station, NJ: Merck Research Laboratories, 2011.

PERIODICALS

Addington, A. M., et al. "Polymorphisms in the 13q33.2 Gene G72/G30 Are Associated with Childhood-Onset Schizophrenia and Psychosis Not Otherwise Specified." *Biological Psychiatry* 55, no. 10 (May 15, 2004): 976–980.

Sim, M.G., E. Khong, and G. Hulse. "Cannabis and Psychosis." *Australian Family Physician* 33, no. 4 (April 2004): 229–232.

Tolmac, J., and M. Hodes. "Ethnic Variation among Adolescent Psychiatric In-Patients with Psychotic Disorders." *British Journal of Psychiatry* 184 (May 2004): 428–431.

Williams, N. M., and M. J. Owen. "Genetic Abnormalities of Chromosome 22 and the Development of Psychosis." *Current Psychiatry Reports* 6, no. 3 (June 2004): 176–182.

ORGANIZATIONS

American Psychiatric Association, 1000 Wilson Blvd., Suite 1825, Arlington, VA 22209-3901, (703) 907-7300, apa@psych.org, http://www.psych.org

American Psychological Association, 750 1st Street NE, Washington, DC 20002-4242, (202) 336-5500; TDD/TTY: (202) 336-6123, (800) 374-2721, http://www.apa.org

National Alliance on Mental Illness, 3803 North Fairfax Drive, Suite 100, Arlington, VA 22203, (703) 524-7600, Fax: (703) 524-9094, http://www.nami.org

National Institute of Mental Health, 6001 Executive Blvd., Room 8184, MSC 9663, Bethesda, MD 20892-9663, (301) 433-4513; TTY: (301) 443-8431, (866) 615-6464; TTY: (866) 415-8051, Fax: (301) 443-4279, nimhinfo@nih.gov, http://www.nimh.nih.gov.

Paula Anne Ford-Martin
Rebecca Frey, PhD

Psychotherapy

Definition

Psychotherapy can be defined as a means of treating psychological or emotional problems such as **neurosis** or personality disorder through verbal and nonverbal communication. It is the treatment of psychological distress through talking with a specially trained therapist, and learning new ways to cope rather than merely using medication to alleviate the distress. It is done with the immediate goal of aiding the person in increasing self-knowledge and awareness of relationships with others. Psychotherapy is carried out to assist people in becoming more conscious of their unconscious thoughts, feelings, and motives.

Psychotherapy's longer-term goal is making it possible for people to exchange destructive patterns of behavior for healthier, more successful ones.

Different approaches to psychotherapy

The psychodynamic approach was derived from principles and methods of psychoanalysis, and it encompasses psychoanalysis, Jungian analysis, Gestalt therapy, client-centered therapy, and somatic or body therapies, among other forms of psychotherapy. Psychoanalysis is therapy based upon the work of Austrian physician Sigmund Freud (1856–1939), and those who followed—Carl Jung, Alfred Adler, Erich Fromm, Karen Horney, and Erik Erikson. The basis of psychoanalytic therapy is the belief that behavior and personality develop in relation to unconscious wishes and conflicts from childhood. Gestalt therapy, developed by Frederick (Fritz) Perls, emphasizes the principles of self-centered awareness and accepting responsibility for one's own behavior. Client-centered therapy was formulated by Carl Rogers; it introduced the idea that individuals have the resources within themselves for self-understanding and for change. Part of this concept is that the therapist exposes his or her own true feelings and does not adopt a professional posture, keeping personal feelings unclear. Somatic or body therapies include: **dance therapy**, holotropic breathwork, and Reichian therapy.

The behavioral approach to psychotherapy encompasses various behavior modification techniques and theories, including assertiveness training/social skills training, operant conditioning, hypnosis/hypnotherapy, sex therapy, systematic desensitization, and others. Systematic desensitization was pioneered by Joseph Wolpe after he became frustrated with psychoanalysis. This therapy is a combination of deep muscular **relaxation** and emotive imagery exercises, in which the client relaxes and the therapist verbally sets scenes for the client to imagine. These scenes include elements of the client's fears, building from the smallest fear toward the largest fear. The therapist monitors the client and introduces the scenes, working to maintain the client's relaxed state.

The cognitive approach stresses the role that thoughts play in influencing behavior. Rational-emotive therapy and reality therapy are both examples of the cognitive approach. Rational-emotive therapy was pioneered by Albert Ellis in the mid-1950s. This therapy is based on the belief that events in and of themselves don't upset people, but people get upset about events because of their attitudes toward the events. Ellis's therapy set out to change people's attitudes about events through objective, firm direction from the therapist and talk therapy. Reality therapy, developed by William Glasser, is based upon the idea that humans seek to satisfy their complex needs, and the behaviors they adopt are intended to accomplish that satisfaction. In Glasser's theory, some people usually fulfill themselves and are generally happy, while others are unable to fulfill themselves and get angry or depressed.

The family systems approach includes **family therapy** in several forms and attempts to modify relationships within the family. Family therapy views behaviors and problems as the result of family interactions, rather than as belonging to a specific family member. One theory, developed by Murray Bowen, has become its own integrated system with eight basic concepts, including differentiation of self and sibling position. This system attempts to help an individual become differentiated from the family, while remaining in touch with the family system.

In the practical application of these approaches, psychotherapy can take many forms. Some of the most commonly practiced forms include:

• Counseling, the provision of both advice and psychological support, is the most elemental form of psychotherapy. Counseling can be short-term therapy done to assist a person in dealing with an immediate problem such as marital problems or family planning, substance abuse, bereavement, or terminal illness. Or it can be longer-term, more extensive treatment that addresses feelings and attitudes that impair success.

• Group psychotherapy requires less therapist time, and is thus less expensive. In fact, the interactions that occur between members of the group are expected to provide the change and healing each member receives. The therapist functions as a facilitator, or one who encourages and directs the group interchanges. Group therapy provides each member with the additional benefit of sharing and feedback from others experiencing similar emotional problems. This sharing and feedback has been found to be therapeutic; and the group can actually function as a trial social setting, allowing people to try out newly-learned behaviors.

• Family therapy began in the 1930s, when Freudian analyst Alfred Adler used it in working with his patients' entire families. Since the 1950s, it has been a widely used and highly respected modality of therapy based upon the belief that the relationships and interactions within a family have a profound impact upon the patient's mental difficulties. Family therapy generally does not deal with internal conflicts, but rather encourages positive interactions between the various family members.

All forms of psychotherapy require an atmosphere of absolute mutual trust and confidentiality. Without this total safety, no form of therapy will be successful.

Origins

Psychotherapy had its beginnings in the ministrations of some of the earliest psychologists, priests, magicians, and shamans of the ancient world. They attempted to determine the causes of a person's emotional distress by talking, counseling, and educating, and interpreting both behavior and dreams. Many of these practices became suspect as the work of charlatans, and fell into disrepute over the centuries. There was little change or progress in the treatment of mental illness over the centuries that followed.

Austrian physician Franz Anton Mesmer (1734–1815) began using what he termed *magnetism* and both the power of suggestion and hypnosis in 1772. Mesmer's treatments, too, fell into disrepute after his theories were rejected by a medical board of inquiry in 1784. Then, nearly a century later, Mesmer's ideas were rediscovered by French neurologist Jean-Martin Charcot (1825–1893). Dr. Charcot used suggestion and hypnosis for treating psychological difficulties at the Salpêtrière Hospital in Paris in the late nineteenth century. Mesmer is now known as the Father of Hypnosis.

In the late nineteenth and early twentieth century, Austrian physician Sigmund Freud studied Charcot's work, and came to believe that hypnosis was less a treatment for mental illness than a means of determining its underlying cause. Freud used hypnosis as one means of uncovering the often traumatic, not consciously recalled memories of his neurotic patients, just as he used their dreams to evaluate their mental conflicts. He later abandoned hypnosis because he did not induce successful trances in his **neurology** patients. His *The Interpretation of Dreams*, published in 1899, made the point that a person's dreams were actually a window into the inner, unknown mind—the royal road to the unconscious. He used the information he obtained not only to help his patients, but also to collect data that eventually helped verify some of his psychodynamic assumptions.

Sigmund Freud theorized that the human personality is composed of three basic parts, the id, the ego, and the superego. The id is defined as the most elemental part, the one that unconsciously motivates people toward fulfilling instinctive urges. The ego is more related to intellect and judgement. It arbitrates between the internal, usually unrecognized desires all human beings have and the reality of the external world. The superego, unconscious controls dictated by moral or social standards outside of ourselves, is probably most easily described as another name for the conscience.

Freud believed that mental illness was the result of a person's unability to resolve conflict, or inadequate settlement of disharmony among the ego, superego, and id. To deal with these internal psychic conflicts, people develop defense mechanisms, which is normally a healthy response. The defense mechanisms become harmful to mental health when overused, or used inappropriately. Freud further postulated that childhood psychic development is primarily based upon sexuality; he divided the first eighteen months of life into three sex-based phases, oral, anal, and genital.

Freud's earliest students, including Carl Jung and Alfred Adler, came to believe that Freud had over-estimated the influence sexuality has on psychic development, and found other influences that help to shape human personality. In the late 1800s and into the twentieth century, 1904 Nobel Prize winner Ivan Petrovich Pavlov pioneered the research that would later result in behavioral therapies, such as the work of American behaviorist Burrhus Frederic Skinner. And in the 1930s, American psychologist Carl Ransom Rogers began his school of psychology that emphasized the importance of the relationship between the patient (or client, according to Rogers) and the therapist in bringing about positive psychic change.

Primal therapy, developed by Arthur Janov in the 1960s, is based upon the assumption that people must relive early life experiences with all the acuity of feeling that was somehow suppressed at the time in order to free themselves of compulsive or neurotic behavior. Primal therapy was a cathartic approach that many therapists now believe can impede progress because a person can become addicted to the release (even "high") associated with the catharsis and seek to keep repeating it for the momentary satisfaction. Transactional analysis, based on Eric Berne's work, came into favor in the 1970s, and supposes that all people function as either a parent or child at various times. It teaches the person to identify which role he or she is filling at any given time and to evaluate whether this role is appropriate.

Benefits

The generally accepted aims of psychotherapy are:

- Increased insight into or improved understanding of one's own mental state. This can range from simply knowing one's strengths and weaknesses, to understanding that symptoms are signs of a mental illness, to deep awareness and acceptance of inner feelings.

- The resolution of disabling conflicts, or working to create a peaceful and positive settlement of emotional struggles that stop a person from living a reasonably happy and productive life.

- Increasing acceptance of self by developing a more realistic and positive appraisal of the person's strengths and abilities.

- Development of improved and more efficient and successful means of dealing with problems so that the patient can find solutions or means of coping with them.

- An overall strengthening of ego structure, or sense of self, so that normal, healthy means of coping with life situations can be called upon and used as needed.

Though there are no definitive studies proving that all five of these goals are consistently realized, psychotherapy in one form or other is a component of nearly all inpatient and community-based psychiatric treatment programs.

Description

Classic Freudian psychotherapy is usually carried out in 50-minute sessions three to five times per week. The patient lies on a couch while he or she talks with the therapist. Freudian therapy characteristically requires ongoing treatment for several years, though in Freud's era it did not. Most other forms of individual psychotherapy, including Jungian, counseling, humanistic, Gestalt, or behavioral therapies, are carried out on a weekly basis (or more frequently, if necessary), in which the person meets with his or her therapist in the therapist's office, and may or may not continue for longer than a year.

Group therapy is held in a variety of settings. A trained group therapist chooses the people that presumably would benefit and learn from interactions with one another. The size of a group is usually five to 10 people, plus a specially trained therapist who guides the group discussion and provides examination of issues and concerns raised.

Child psychotherapy is done for the same reasons as adult psychotherapy—to treat emotional problems through communication. The obvious difference is that child psychotherapy must acknowledge the child's stage of development. This recognition means that the therapist may use different techniques, including play, rather than only talking to the patient.

A newer direction in the treatment of mental disorders is the use of brief psychotherapy sessions, often combined with medication, to treat neurotic conditions. Another short-term psychotherapy modality is often termed crisis intervention, and is used to aid people in dealing with specific crises in their lives, such as the death of a loved one.

KEY TERMS

Behavioral therapy—A collection of techniques for treating mental disorders based upon changing abnormal behavior rather than attempting to analyze its fundamental basis. It is particularly used in phobic or obsessional disorders, and seeks to eliminate symptoms rather than uncovering the underlying psychological cause.

Magnetism—(Animal magnetism) A discredited theory put forth by Viennese physician Franz Anton Mesmer, stating that all persons possess magnetic forces that can be used to influence magnetic fluid in other people and therefore effect healing. Mesmer opened a clinic in Paris in 1778, and appeared to cure people apparently suffering from hysterical conditions, such as emotionally caused paralysis.

Neurosis—A term commonly used to describe a range of relatively mild psychiatric disorders in which the sufferer remains in touch with reality. Neurotic disorders include mild depression, anxiety disorders (including phobias and obsessive compulsive disorders), somatization disorders, dissociative disorders, and psychosexual disorders.

Personality disorder—A group of conditions characterized by a general failure to learn from experience or adapt appropriately to changes, resulting in personal distress and impairment of social functioning.

Research and general acceptance

Psychotherapy in its many forms has been accepted and used throughout the world for over one hundred years. It is normally covered as a valid treatment of mental disorder by both public and private health insurers. Because the various types of psychotherapy have different aims, and mental illnesses usually do not have absolute measurable signs of recovery, evaluating psychotherapy's effectiveness is difficult. As a general rule, the majority of people who undergo treatment with psychotherapy can expect to make appreciable gains. Studies have revealed, however, that not everyone who goes into therapy will be helped, or helped as much as others, and some will even be harmed.

Training and certification

Though the actual clinical practice of psychotherapy is very much the same among disciplines, therapists

QUESTIONS TO ASK YOUR DOCTOR

- How do I know which form of psychotherapy is most appropriate for the problems I'm currently facing?

- Are any, some, most, or all forms of psychotherapy typically covered by health insurance plans?

- Is it essential or necessary to have other members of the family become involved in counseling when the problem that concerns me is family-based?

- Under what circumstances, if any, is medication a better treatment for psychological problems than "talk therapy"?

- What evidence is there that the type of psychotherapy you are recommending is actually effective?

come from a variety of different fields, including medicine, psychology, social work, and nursing.

Psychiatrists are required to complete four years of medical school and one year of internship, followed by a three-year residency in psychiatry. In order to be a psychoanalyst, a minimum of three years' further training at a psychoanalytic institute is necessary, along with personal ongoing analysis.

Psychologists earn a Ph.D. in clinical psychology followed by a year of supervised practice, and additionally may take specialized training at a specific psychotherapeutic school, including therapy for themselves.

Social workers who specialize in mental health must earn a master's degree or doctorate before being allowed to practice.

Psychiatric nurses generally earn a master's degree and practice in hospitals or community mental health centers.

Most states in the United States require a license to practice as a psychotherapist, and by law in the majority of the states, they are accountable only to the other members of their profession.

Resources

BOOKS

Bach, Sheldon. *The How-to Book for Students of Psychoanalysis and Psychotherapy*. London: Karnac, 2011.

Bateman, Anthony, Dennis Brown, and Jonathan Pedder. *Introduction to Psychotherapy: An Outline of Psychodynamic Principles and Practice*, 4th ed. New York: Routledge 2010.

Corey, Gerald. *Theory and Practice of Counseling and Psychotherapy*. Belmont, CA: Wadsworth, 2013.

Schore, Allan N. *The Science of the Art of Psychotherapy*. New York: W.W. Norton, 2012.

OTHER

Grohol, John M. *Psychotheraphy.* http://psychcentral.com/psychotherapy/ (accessed May 9, 2012).

Mayo Clinic Staff. *Psychotherapy.* http://www.mayoclinic.com/health/psychotherapy/MY00186 (accessed May 9, 2012).

Mental Health and Psychotherapy. WebMD. http://www.webmd.com/anxiety-panic/guide/mental-health-psychotherapy (accessed May 9, 2012).

Types of Psychotherapy (Approaches). http://www.strisik.com/therapy/approaches.htm (accessed May 9, 2012).

Joan Schonbeck

Psyllium preparations *see* **Laxatives**

PTSD *see* **Post-traumatic stress disorder**

Puberty

Definition

Puberty is the period of human development during which physical growth and sexual maturation occur.

Description

Beginning as early as age eight in girls—and two years later on average in boys—the hypothalamus (part of the **brain**) signals hormonal changes that stimulate the pituitary. In turn, the pituitary releases its own hormones called gonadotropins that stimulate the gonads and **adrenal glands**. From these glands comes a flood of sex hormones—androgens and testosterone in the male, estrogens and progestins in the female—that regulate the growth and function of the sex organs. The gonadotropins are the same for males and females, but the sex hormones they induce are different.

In the United States, the first sign of puberty occurs on average at age 11 in girls, with menstruation and fertility following about two years later. Boys lag behind by about two years. Puberty may not begin until age 16 in boys and may continue in a desultory fashion beyond age 20. In contrast to puberty, which triggers physiological changes, adolescence is more of a social/cultural term referring to the interval between childhood and adulthood.

Diagnosis

Puberty has been divided into five Sexual Maturity Rating (SMR) stages by two doctors, W. Marshall and J. M. Tanner. These ratings are often referred to as Tanner Stages 1-5. Staging is based on pubic hair growth, male genital development, and female breast development. Staging helps determine whether development is normal for a given age. Both genders also grow axillary (arm pit) hair and develop pimples. Males develop muscle mass, a deeper voice, and facial hair. Females redistribute body fat. Along with the maturing of the sex organs, there is a pronounced growth spurt averaging 3–4 inches (7.5–9 cm) and culminating in full adult stature. Puberty can be precocious (early) or delayed. It all depends upon the sex hormones.

Puberty falling outside the age limits considered normal for any given population should prompt a search for the cause. As health and **nutrition** have improved over the past few generations, there has been a gradual lowering of the average age for the normal onset of puberty.

- Excess hormone stimulation is the cause of precocious puberty. It can come from the brain in the form of gonadotrophins or from the gonads and adrenals. Overproduction may be caused by functioning tumors or simple glandular overactivity. Brain overproduction can also be the result of brain infections or injury.

- Likewise, delayed puberty is due to insufficient hormone. If the pituitary output is inadequate, so will be the output from the gonads and adrenals. On the other hand, a normal pituitary will overproduce if it senses there are not enough hormones in circulation.

- There are several congenital disorders (polyglandular deficiency syndromes) that include failure of hormone output. These children do not experience normal puberty, but it may be induced by giving them the proper hormones at the proper time.

- Finally, there are abnormalities in hormone production in females that produce male characteristics—so called virilizing syndromes. Should one of these appear during adolescence, it will disturb the normal progress of puberty. Virilizing requires abnormal hormones in a female, while feminizing results from the lack of male hormones. Each embryo starts out life as female. Male hormones transform it into a male if they are present.

Delayed or precocious puberty requires measurement of the several hormones involved to determine which are lacking or which are in excess. There are

KEY TERMS

Adrenals—Glands on top of the kidneys that produce four different types of hormones.

Computed tomography scan (CT)—A method of creating images of internal organs using x rays.

Embryo—The life in the womb during the first two months.

Hormone—A chemical produced in one place that has an effect somewhere else in the body.

Hypothalamus—Part of the brain located deep in the center of the skull and just above the pituitary.

Gonads—Glands that make sex hormones and reproductive cells–testes in the male, ovaries in the female.

Magnetic resonance imaging (MRI)—A method of creating images of internal organs. Magnetic resonance imaging (MRI) uses magnetic fields and radio-frequency signals.

Pituitary—The "master gland" of the body, controlling many of the others by releasing stimulating hormones.

Syndrome—A collection of abnormalities that occur often enough to suggest they have a common cause.

blood tests for each one. If a tumor is suspected, imaging of the suspect organ needs to be done with x rays, **computed tomography scans (CT scans)**, or magnetic resonance imaging(MRI).

Treatment

Puberty can be a period of great **stress**, both physically and emotionally. The psychological changes and challenges of puberty are compounded if its timing is off.

If puberty is early, the offending gland or tumor may require surgical attention, although there are several drugs now that counteract hormone effects. If it is delayed, puberty can be stimulated with the correct hormones. Treatment should not be delayed, because necessary **bone** growth is also affected.

Prognosis

For individuals facing delayed or accelerated puberty, properly administered hormones can restore the normal growth pattern.

Health care team roles

Pediatricians or family physicians usually diagnose abnormalities of puberty. Endocrinologists may assist with assessment and treatment. Therapists and counselors may provide emotional support as needed.

Prevention

As puberty is an entirely normal process, there is neither a way nor a need to prevent it.

Resources

BOOKS

Bryan, Jenny. *Adolescence.* Austin, TX: Raintree/Steck Vaughn, 2000.

Hoffman, Adele, and Donald Graydanus. *Adolescent Medicine,* 3rd ed. New York: McGraw Hill, 1997.

Madaras, Lynda. *What's Happening to My Body? Book for Boys: The New Growing-Up Guide for Parents and Sons,* 3rd Edition. New York, Newmarket Press, 2001.

Madaras, Lynda. *What's Happening to My Body? Book for Girls: The New Growing-Up Guide for Parents and Daughters,* 3rd Edition. New York: Newmarket Press, 2001.

Needleman, Robert E. "Adolescence." In *Nelson Textbook of Pediatrics,* 16th edition. Edited by Richard E. Behrman, et al., Philadelphia: Saunders, 2000, p. 52-57.

Rice, F. Philip, and Kim G. Dolgin. *The Adolescent: Development, Relationships, and Culture,* 10th edition. Needham Heights, MA: Allyn & Bacon, 2001.

Silverstein, Alvin, Virginia Silverstein, and Laura Nunn. *Puberty.* New York: Franklin Watts, 2000.

PERIODICALS

Chemaitilly W., et al. "Central precocious puberty: clinical and laboratory features." *Clinical Endocrinology (Oxford)* 54, no. 3 (2001): 289-294, 2001.

Lazarus, G.M. "Gender-specific medicine in pediatrics." *Journal of Gender Specific Medicine* 4, no. 1 (2001): 50-53.

Ojeda, S.R., and S. Heger. "New thoughts on female precocious puberty." *Journal of Pediatric Endocrinology and Metabolism* 14, no. 3 (2001): 245-256.

ORGANIZATIONS

American Academy of Pediatrics. 141 Northwest Point Boulevard, Elk Grove Village, IL 60007-1098. (847) 434-4000. Fax: (847) 434-8000. http://www.aap.org/default. htm. kidsdoc@aap.org.

American Psychiatric Association. 1400 K Street NW, Washington, DC 20005. (888) 357-7924. Fax: (202) 682-6850. apa@psych.org.

American Psychological Association. 750 First Street NW, Washington, DC, 20002-4242. (800) 374-2721 or (202) 336-5500. http://www.apa.org/.

L. Fleming Fallon, Jr., MD, DrPH

Public health

Definition

Public health is the science and clinical practice of population and community-based efforts to prevent disease and disability, and promote physical and mental health. It considers the health of groups, communities, or populations as opposed to the health of individuals. Public health addresses a variety of medical and social issues including:

• environmental health

• nutrition and food safety

• immunization and infectious diseases

• injury and violence prevention

• maternal, infant, and child health

• substance abuse

• chronic disease prevention and treatment

• access, availability, and affordability of health care

• education, screening, and outreach services

Description

The science of public health is called epidemiology. It is the study of the occurrence of disease in naturally existing populations, such as nations, cities, or communities. The term "epidemiology" comes from the Greek word epidemic, which means "upon the people." The earliest epidemiologists (public health scientists) worked to prevent the spread of epidemics.

Today, epidemiologists gather and analyze information about populations to manage and prevent disease. Epidemiologists are trained in highly specialized research methods: surveillance, investigation, analysis, and evaluation. Surveillance refers to systematic data collection and analysis; it enables the epidemiologists to detect changes that may require investigation. Epidemiological investigation involves observation, detailed descriptions of the problem, documentation of data, and analysis.

Evaluation is the process that helps to answer a question, such as "How often should men between the ages of 40 and 60 be screened for **hypertension** (high **blood pressure**)?"

By analyzing population data, epidemiologists also are able to describe diseases and determine the factors that cause them. Epidemiology is a quantitative science; it measures rates and proportions. Two commonly used rates are prevalence and incidence rates. Prevalence describes the characteristics of a given population at a specific moment in time; it is like a snapshot.

Incidence describes the rate of development of a disease in a given population over a specified time interval. Incidence offers a longer view of population dynamics, like a video, as opposed to the snapshot offered by the prevalence rate. Epidemiologists also analyze other rates, such as morbidity (disease-related illness) and mortality (death).

Public health practitioners rely on the findings of epidemiologists to develop health services, allocate resources, and determine standards of care. The results of epidemiological studies also influence health policy. For example, epidemiological research helps to determine how many health care professionals are needed based on population; the effectiveness of various treatments; and schedules for immunization or screening.

Viewpoints

Historically, public health disease prevention activities focused primarily on sanitation (also referred to as environmental health) and hygiene. Public health measures aimed to ensure the safety of food and water supplies, and to prevent transmission of communicable (capable of being transmitted) diseases. In some developing countries, these same basic public health problems, such as adequate food supplies and potable (fit to drink) water, continue to threaten health and longevity.

During and after World War II, advances in medicine such as the development of **antibiotics**, cardiac surgery, and physical **rehabilitation** changed the emphasis of public health in the United States. Federal, state, and local governments enacted legislation to protect public health. Federal laws aimed at safeguarding public health. Major regulations passed during the twentieth century include:

- the 1938 Food, Drug and Cosmetic Act, which bans distribution of unsafe products and prohibits false advertising

- the 1972 Clean Water Act, which forbids release of pollutants into rivers, streams, and waterways

- the 1974 Safe Drinking Water Acts, which established standards for safe drinking water

- the 1976 Resource Conservation and Recovery Act, which stipulates the safe storage, transport, treatment and disposal of hazardous waste materials

- the 1990 Clean Air Act, which reduced industrial discharge or emission of pollutants into the air and set standards for vehicular emissions

Today, public health practitioners continue to work to prevent disease. However, their efforts are often directed to addressing social issues, such as access to health care, and promoting lifestyle change, such as **smoking cessation**, responsible sexual behavior, and violence prevention.

Frequently, public health professionals must work cooperatively with persons in other disciplines to achieve health promotion objectives. For example, public health practitioners may work with educators and schools to help combat illiteracy, since persons unable to read may be less able to obtain needed health care services. Similarly, they may work with urban planners and housing specialists to identify health hazards such as lead-based paints or asbestos.

The Healthy People 2010 initiative is a national plan to assist states, communities, and professional associations to develop programs to improve health. Coordinated by the Office of Disease Prevention and Health Promotion (ODPHP) of the Department of Health and Human Services, the program's goals are to: increase quality and years of healthy life; and eliminate health disparities. Healthy People 2010 targets ten areas for improving the health standards in the United States. They are:

- physical activity
- overweight and obesity
- tobacco use
- substance abuse
- responsible sexual behavior
- mental health
- injury and violence
- environmental quality
- immunization
- access to health care

The goal of "Healthy People 2010" is not only to increase the quality of life for people and help them to live longer, but also to eliminate any disparity in health care delivery. The life expectancy of Americans has increased more than 30 years since 1900, with many

KEY TERMS

Communicable—Capable of being transmitted.

Disparity—Inequality or lack of similarity; may be associated with differences in care or treatment.

Epidemiology—The study of disease occurrence in human populations.

Evidence-based practice—The process by which health care providers incorporate the best research or evidence into clinical practice in combination with clinical expertise and within the context of patient values.

Incidence—The rate of development of a disease in a given population over time.

Potable—Safe to drink.

Prevalence—The rate describing the characteristics of a given population at a specific moment in time.

older Americans living well into their 70s, 80s, and even 90s. Physical health, as well as mental health, has become more and more important as many older adults want to "age in place," and not be forced to live in long-term-care facilities. Older adults are concerned about their quality of life (QOL). It is with good health education that all individuals can become empowered to take care of themselves.

Helping Americans maintain a good QOL is only part of the "Healthy People 2010" effort. Disparities still exist among minority groups; minorities have not enjoyed the same health improvement progress as other Americans. Minority Americans have higher rates of diabetes, HIV and **AIDS**, infant mortality, and **heart** disease. Life expectancy for these populations is less than that of others, and minority groups living in poverty often do not have access to adequate health care.

The latest "Healthy People" publication, entitled "Healthy People 2020", remains grounded on a **vision** of *a society in which all people live long, healthy lives* and emphasizes ideas health equality for all individuals throughout all stages of life. This latest publication utilizes an interactive website as its main means of communication and offers evidence-based resources to those who access the site.

The Cooperative Actions for Health Program (CAHP) is a collaborative grant program that is co-sponsored by the American Public Health Association and the American Medical Association (AMA). Its purpose is to build, support, and strengthen state and local collaboration between medical and public health professionals to improve the public's health. The program fosters collaboration through grant funding, developing a communication network to share ideas and coordinate policy-making efforts between the APHA and the AMA.

Professional implications

Medical, nursing and allied health professionals and practitioners work in the field of public health. Public health professionals are employed by hospitals, health plans, managed care organizations, clinics, medical relief organizations (e.g., American Red Cross, American Heart Association, American Cancer Society) and schools as well as federal, state, and local government health departments. Careers in public health include:

- public health nursing
- environmental health technologists and specialists
- restaurant and food safety inspectors
- community health educators
- epidemiologists, biostatisticians, and researchers
- administrators
- patient and consumer health advocates

Public health nursing began in the United States during the late 1800s. Public health nurses helped to prevent and manage outbreaks of smallpox, cholera, typhoid, **tuberculosis**, and other communicable diseases. The profession continues to attract nurses interested in community health education and preventive services. Public health nurses (also called community health nurses) work in clinics, schools, voluntary agencies, and provide skilled nursing assessments, visiting nurse services, and **home care**.

Federal government agencies that belong to the U.S. Department of Health and Human Services provide many vital public health services. The agencies devoted to health care include the **Health Care Financing** Administration (HCFA), Office of Development Services, Food and Drug Administration (FDA), National Institutes of Health (NIH) and the Centers for Disease Control and Prevention (CDC).

HCFA administers **Medicare** and **Medicaid**, programs that finance health care services for older adults, persons with disabilities and those unable to afford medical care. The FDA is the agency responsible for ensuring food, drug, and cosmetic safety. It also enforces labeling practices, so that consumers receive accurate, truthful information about the content, benefits, and risks of products.

Each of the 13 institutes of the NIH is involved in organ or disease-specific research activities. The seven centers of the CDC research and track infectious and other diseases in order to identify sources of disease and prevent their spread.

Resources

BOOKS

Barr, Donald A., MD, Ph.D. *Introduction to U.S. Health Policy: The Organization, Financing, and Delivery of Health Care in America.*3rd ed., Baltimore, MD: The Johns Hopkins University Press, 2010.

Gambrill, Eileen.*Critical Thinking in Clinical Practice: Improving the Quality of Judgments and Decisions,*3rd ed. New York, NY: Wiley, 2012.

Mason, Diana J., et al.*Policy &Politics in Nursing and Health Care,*6th ed. New York, NY: Saunders, 2011.

McKenzie, James F., Brad L. Neiger., and Rosemary Thackeray. *Planning, Implementing, & Evaluating Health Promotion Programs.*6th ed., San Francisco, CA: Benjamin Cummings, 2012.

Schimpff, Stephen C., MD.*The Future of Health-Care Delivery: Why It Must Change and How It Will Affect You.* Dulles, VA: Potomac Books Inc, 2012.

Wallace, Robert B., ed. *Public Health & Preventive Medicine,*15th ed. New York, NY: McGraw Hill, 2007.

PERIODICALS

Clark, Noreen M., and Elizabeth Weist. "Mastering the New Public Health." American Journal of Public Health 90, no. 8 (August 2000): 1208-1211.

Meyer, Ilan H., and Sharon Schwartz. "Social Issues as Public Health: Promise and Peril." American Journal of Public Health 90, no. 8 (August 2000): 1189-1191.

OTHER

Partners in Information Access for the Public Health Workforce. http://phpartners.org/.

ORGANIZATIONS

Agency for Healthcare Research and Quality, Office of Communications and Knowledge Transfer, 540 Gaither Road, Suite 2000, Rockville, MD 20850. Telephone: (301) 427-1104. http://www.ahrq.gov

American Public Health Association. 800 I. Street, NW Washington, DC 20001-3710. (202) 777-2532. http://www.apha.org.

Centers for Disease Control and Prevention (CDC). 1600 Clifton Road, Atlanta, GA 30333. http://www.cdc.gov.

U.S. Department of Health and Human Services (USDHHS), HealthyPeople.gov. 200 Independence Avenue, S.W., Washington, DC 20201.http://www.healthypeople.gov/2020/default.aspx.

U.S. Department of Health and Human Services (USDHHS), Office of Disease Prevention and Health Promotion. 1101 Wootton Parkway, Suite LL100, Rockville, MD 20852. (240) 453-8280. http://odphp.osophs.dhhs.gov/Default.asp.

Meghan M. Gourley
Barbara Wexler
Laura Jean Cataldo, RN, Ed.D.

Public health administration

Definition

Public health administration is the aspect of the field of public health that concentrates on management of personnel and programs. Administration is needed on a day-to-day basis to ensure that organizations operate efficiently and successfully, as programs require supervision and guidance. The field of administration is concerned with theories and techniques derived from a variety of fields, including statistics, behavioral psychology, policy analysis, communications, budgeting, and other aspects of organizational management.

Description

The work of a public health administrator is at the same time similar to and different from that of persons engaged in administration in other fields. The administrative elements are similar; they include supervising employees, coordinating programs, preparing budgets, monitoring programs, and evaluating results and outcomes. Aspects that are specific to the field of public health include health and disease prevention programs. Public health administrators conduct educational campaigns and try to maintain the health of the people they serve. Other health professionals have similar aims of maintaining health but often focus on restorative or curative measures rather than preventive programs.

There are 10 core public health functions with which an administrator must be familiar. There is a specialized body of public health law. Data are constantly being generated. These data must be sorted, classified, stored, and interpreted. There are highly sophisticated computer systems and databases to keep track of diseases, vital events, waste materials, insects, pollutants, and a host of other aspects of public health. Data that are collected must be organized, analyzed, and presented to such constituencies as members of the public, governmental agencies, and other health care professionals. The overall health of the public being served must be periodically assessed. Intervention programs must be designed, implemented, and evaluated. Other forms of research are also conducted.

The day-to-day activities of a public health administrator include human resources management, finance, performance measurement and improvement, communications, and marketing, which maintains relations with members of the media and local government. A public health administrator must build relationships with such various constituencies as consumer groups, health care providers, and legislators. Leadership is an important aspect of public health administration.

Work settings

The most common work setting for a public health administrator is an office within a local health department or public health agency. There are approximately 3,300 local boards of health in the United States. Their sizes vary from a single municipality to an entire state. Many consist of one or more counties. Each employs a staff of professionals that provide specialized services. Each provider has a supervisor; larger organizations have more than one layer of supervision. In addition, there are public and private organizations that provide public health services, including nonprofit organizations like the American Red Cross and the American Cancer Society. Governments also employ public health administrators. The number of persons who provide some administrative services within the realm of public health is thus extensive.

Undergraduate education and postgraduate training

Basic preparation for a career in public health administration usually begins with a college degree but does not end at the undergraduate level. It is possible to learn administration from experience on the job but the time required is increasing each year. As of 2012, a master's degree is the functional minimum level of education for admission into the field of public health administration; the different types of master's degrees are described in the next section. The actual field of study at the college level can vary; however, an undergraduate degree in management, public health, nursing, community health, applied health, allied health or a related discipline is useful preparation for graduate work in public health administration. An optimal undergraduate curriculum should include course work

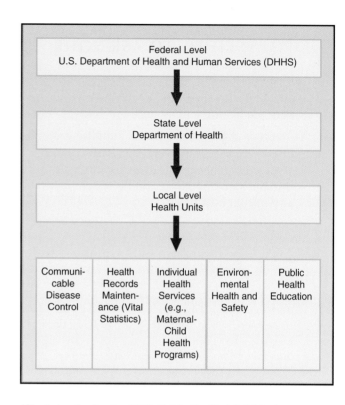

(Chart showing levels of U.S. Public Health Administration, photograph. From Fundamentals of Nursing, Standards and Practices 2nd edition by Delaune/Ladner. © 2002. Reprinted with permission of Delmar Learning: www.thomsonrights.com Fax 800-730-2215.)

in the following subject areas: management, accounting, finance, economics, biology, environmental health or science, marketing, business, health law, and budgeting.

Initial training following completion of the master's degree begins with job orientation. This is relatively similar for most entry-level positions in the field. During orientation, the structure and reporting relationships of an organization are described. Basic laws and other legal requirements are outlined. Job duties of a particular position are explained. Organizational regulations and requirements are reviewed.

A high level of interpersonal and communications skills is vital to public health administrators, as much of their time is spent writing reports and explaining their decisions to other health care professionals and the wider community. With health care budgets shrinking as of 2012, many administrators must also be skilled in writing grant proposals as well as budgeting increasingly scarce funding resources. In addition, public health administrators must acquire competence in cross-cultural

KEY TERMS

Epidemiology—The study of patterns and distribution of disease in large groups of people.

Vital event—An occurrence for which a certificate is typically issued. Examples of vital events include births, deaths, marriages, and adoptions.

communication, as many public health programs at the local level are intended to reach minorities and other under-served populations.

Ongoing training occurs at two levels. The first is specific to a particular working agency or environment. It consists of office and organizational updates, program changes, and information pertaining to other local issues. The second is specific to the field of public health. These updates typically occur at professional conferences and through articles in the secondary literature of public health. They consist of changes in programs that have been proposed or imposed by federal or other funding agencies. They also include new findings related to theories or practice that have been developed by researchers. Changes in reporting procedures fall within this category.

Advanced education and training

There are 49 schools of public health accredited by the Council on Education for Public Health (CEPH) in the United States as of 2012 that offer master's degrees in the field. Master's-level training in public health administration is obtained by completing a formal graduate degree program. The most commonly earned graduate credential is a Master of Public Health (MPH) degree. This degree provides a broad-based curriculum for anyone in the field of public health and is appropriate for persons just entering the field as well as those with experience. Other master's degrees are also useful. These include Master of Business Administration (MBA), Master of Health Services Administration (MHSA), Master of Public Administration (MPA), Master of Hospital Administration (MHA), and Master of Management (MM) degrees. The core requirements of the different degree programs are similar and typically include course work in statistics, economics, management, finance, marketing, issues, law, and human resource administration. Elective courses help to tailor a graduate curriculum to the specific needs of each student.

There are some differences among the degree courses described. These are typically related to the focus afforded by the training. For example, a MPH degree is specifically concentrated on public health. An MBA provides more general training. While both degrees are useful, the MPH

is focused on health. In an analogous manner, MHSA coursework focuses on issues related to managing health service providers and organizations. MPA focuses on administration in a public or not for profit environment. The MHA is geared for hospital administrators, while the MM is very general. MPH degree curriculum includes courses in epidemiology and environmental health. The others typically substitute additional courses in economics, accounting, or labor relations.

Some workers in public health administration require continuing education units to maintain a license or certification. Examples of such workers include nurses, social workers, health officers, sanitarians, and physicians. The rules for many of these professionals are not set by federal or national agencies, but rather may be specific to the state that has issued the credential. Professionals earning continuing education credits may include courses and seminars that cover aspects of public health administration. In this way, they acquire new and updated knowledge. The Association of Schools of Public Health (ASPH) offers both a basic Certified in Public Health (CPH) credential and Certified in Public Health Continuing Education (CPHCE) credits for professionals in public health. The CPH credential, which was first offered in 2008, requires passing an examination; maintaining the credential requires recertification every two years. The cost of the CPH examination as of 2012 is about $400.

All persons seeking to enter the field of public health administration will require professional training and preparation. This requirement will translate into opportunities for teachers of this subject. With demand for trained persons increasing, the demand for teachers is also likely to increase.

Future outlook

The outlook for persons seeking employment in public health administration is ambiguous as of 2012. On the one hand, the Bureau of Labor Statistics (BLS) expects jobs in this field to increase at an above-average rate. With recent rapid changes in managed care and the restructuring of health care delivery, disease prevention and public health have assumed new importance in the mainstream practice of medicine. New emphases in the field of public health since the early 2000s include environmental health, drug abuse and addiction treatment, and women and children's health; startup programs in these areas will require persons with training in public health administration.

In spite of the favorable job outlook, however, entry into the field is increasingly competitive because stiff performance standards have been instituted since the early 2000s. With increased requirements for training and preparation, salaries for public health administrators are likely to increase. As the baby boomer generation ages and retires, the number of agencies and organizations providing services is expected to rise. These demands, too, are likely to drive up salaries for public health administrators. As of 2012, salaries in the field range from $45,000 to $95,000 per year; the salary depends on the applicant's experience and credentials, and the size of the public health department or organization.

The downside of job opportunities in the field, however, is the increasing levels of pressure on public health administrators to accomplish more in less time with fewer support staff as a result of shrinking funding. The economic downturn of 2008 coupled with the ever-increasing cost of health care in general means that public health administrators face numerous financial as well as managerial challenges in meeting their organizations' goals. According to a report published in the spring of 2012, over 23,000 jobs in local health departments were lost between 2008 and 2010 because of the recession and subsequent funding cuts. In addition, a June 2012 editorial in the New England Journal of Medicine noted that the number of health care- and public health-related jobs is not by itself a measure of improved health care: "The key policy goals should be to achieve better health outcomes and increase overall economic productivity, so that we can all live healthier and wealthier lives."

Resources

BOOKS

Levy, Barry S, and Joyce R. Gaufin, eds. *Mastering Public Health: Essential Skills for Effective Practice.* New York: Oxford University Press, 2012.

Novick, Lloyd F., Cynthia B. Morrow, and Glen P. Mays. *Public Health Administration: Principles for Population-based Management,* 2nd ed. Sudbury, MA: Jones and Bartlett, Publishers, 2008.

Rose, Patti Renee. *Cultural Competency for Health Administration and Public Health.* Sudbury, MA: Jones and Bartlett, 2011.

Turnock, Bernard J. *Essentials of Public Health,* 2nd ed. Sudbury, MA: Jones and Bartlett Learning, 2012.

PERIODICALS

Baicker, Katherine, and Amitabh Chandra. "The Health Care Jobs Fallacy." *New England Journal of Medicine* 366 (June 28, 2012): 2433–2435.

Drehobl, P.A., et al. "Public Health Surveillance Workforce of the Future." *Morbidity and Mortality Weekly Report: Surveillance Summaries* 61 (July 27, 2012): Supplement 25–29.

Willard, R., et al. "Impact of the 2008–2010 Recession on Local Health Departments." *Journal of Public Health Management and Practice* 18 (March-April 2012): 106–114.

WEBSITES

"Member Schools." Association of Schools of Public Health. http://www.asph.org/document.cfm?page=200 (accessed October 4, 2012).

"What Is Public Health?" Association of Schools of Public Health. http://www.whatispublichealth.org/what/index.html (accessed October 4, 2012).

ORGANIZATIONS

American Public Health Association (APHA). 800 I Street, NW. Washington, DC 20001-3710. (202) 777-APHA, (202) 777-2534. http://apha.org/.

Association of Schools of Public Health (ASPH). 1900 M Street, NW, Suite 710. Washington. DC 20036. (202) 296-1099, (202) 296-1252. info@asph.org. http://www.asph.org/.

Association of State and Territorial Health Officials (ASTHO). 2231 Crystal Drive, Suite 450, Arlington, VA 22202. (202) 371-9090, (571) 527-3189. http://www.astho.org/.

Council on Education for Public Health (CEPH). 1010 Wayne Avenue, Suite 220, Silver Spring, MD 20910. (202) 789-1060. (202) 789-1895. http://www.ceph.org/.

National Association of County and City Health Officials (NACCHO). 1100 17th Street, NW, Seventh Floor, Washington, DC 20036. (202) 783-5550, (202) 783-1583. info@naccho.org. http://naccho.org/.

National Association of Local Boards of Health (NALBOH). 1840 East Gypsy Lane Road, Bowling Green, OH 43402. (419) 353-7714, (419) 352-6278. http://www.nalboh.org/.

L. Fleming Fallon, Jr., MD, PhD, DrPH

▌Puerperal infection

Definition

Puerperal **infection** is a bacterial infection that occurs following **childbirth**. The diagnostic criteria require that the childbearing woman have a temperature over 100.4 °F (38 °C) on any two of the first 10 postpartum days after day one, or over 101.5 °F (38.6 °C) during the first 24 hours.

Description

The incidence of puerperal infection is 1–8% of the postpartum female population in the United States. The incidence is five to 10 times higher when a woman delivers by **cesarean section**. As most births in the United States occur in hospitals, the majority of puerperal infections are considered nosocomial, or hospital-acquired. With **antibiotics** readily available in industrialized countries, death related to puerperal infection is very rare, at 0.3 in 100,000. In developing nations, the death rate due to puerperal infection is estimated to be 100 times higher. Puerperal infection may occur in the genital tract, breast, urinary tract, **lungs**, **blood** vessel, or wound.

Endometritis—Inflammation of the mucous membrane lining the inner surface of the uterus.

Lochia—Discharge from the uterus of blood, mucus, and tissue during the puerperal peiord.

Mastitis—Inflammation of the breast.

Nosocomial—Pertaining to a hospital or infirmary.

Postpartum—After childbirth.

Puerperal—Period immediately following childbirth.

Causes and symptoms

The usual cause of puerperal infection is a bacterial infection in the genital tract, primarily the uterus. This infection, called endometritis, is associated with prolonged rupture of membranes; difficult vaginal birth which involved the use of forceps or vacuum extractor; multiple vaginal examinations; low socioeconomic status; and the primary predisposing factor of cesarean section delivery, with an incidence of postoperative infection reported at 29–85%.

Symptoms of endometritis include elevated temperature, low **abdominal pain** or tenderness, vaginal discharge, or a heavy, malodorous lochia usually in the first two to seven days postpartum. Endometritis is usually polymicrobial, that is, more than one bacterial species is found upon culture. The mixed species tend to multiply their negative effects. Other symptoms in puerperal infection are dependent on the infected site. **Mastitis** or breast infection can be caused by bacterial contamination from the breastfeeding infant's mouth. Symptoms include elevated temperature, localized inflammation, breast tenderness, general malaise, and muscle aching. Symptoms of a urinary tract infection include elevated temperature, frequent voiding, urgency to void, and **pain** upon voiding. **Back pain**, as well as nausea and **vomiting**, are common with pyelonephritis. Lung infection, or **pneumonia**, may be seen especially in the patient who has received **general anesthesia**. Symptoms include decreased or abnormal breath sounds, **cough**, and chest wall discomfort. An infection in a blood vessel, *phlebitis*, may be caused by the introduction of **bacteria** by a contaminated intravenous needle or at the site of a blood clot, thrombophlebitis. Wound sites in the postpartum woman may include episiotomy or cesarean section incision. These sites, if infected, would have inflammation, swelling, and drainage, and the patient would have an elevated temperature. It is interesting to note that while vaginal secretions contain up to 10 billion organisms per gram of fluid, only 1% of postpartum women develop infection in perineal tears or episiotomies.

Diagnosis

Diagnosis of puerperal infection is made on the basis of the presenting symptoms, which must be thoroughly investigated. In addition, diagnostic testing may include a **complete blood count**, **chest x ray**, **urinalysis**, or **wound culture**. High vaginal or endocervical cultures are not helpful in identifying a uterine pathogen, and transabdominal uterine aspiration is not recommended, as it may only serve to spread the infection. Blood cultures may be done, but they are only positive 8% of the time. Radiologic testing is helpful if symptoms are resistant to initial treatment or if pneumonia is suspected. Ultrasound or computed tomography scan (CT scan) may identify a potential abdominal **abscess** or blood clot. **Magnetic resonance imaging** (MRI) may also be used if symptoms of a blood clot are present.

Treatment

Antibiotic therapy is the mainstay of treatment in puerperal infection. Hospitalization may or may not be necessary. Clindamycin and gentamicin may be used as initial therapy, as they are broad-spectrum antibiotics, that is, covering more than one organism. Ampicillin may be added if symptoms persist. If an abscess has been diagnosed, surgical drainage may be required. In the presence of thrombophlebitis, heparin therapy will be needed to provide anticoagulation.

Prognosis

With access to appropriate antibiotics, the prognosis of rapid recovery from puerperal infection is excellent.

Health care team roles

Physicians and nurses are involved in the prevention, diagnosis, and treatment of puerperal infection. Good **prenatal care** is essential for avoiding the risk of infection after childbirth. Postpartum nurses assess patients for signs and symptoms of infection and educate patients about these signs and symptoms prior to discharge. Home health nurses making follow-up visits assess patients for signs and symptoms of infection. Emergency physicians are seeing an increasing number of postpartum patients presenting with a **fever** or evidence of infection due to earlier discharge from the hospital after childbirth.

Prevention

Identification of risk factors such as premature rupture of membranes or the use of prophylactic antibiotics at the time of an emergent cesarean section will lower the incidence of puerperal infection. The fundamental practice of strict **aseptic technique** is the first line of prevention.

Resources

BOOKS

Charles, Jonathan, and David Charles. "Postpartum Infection." In *Obstetric and Perinatal Infections*, edited by David Charles. St. Louis: Mosby-Year Book, Inc., 1993.

Rivlin, Michel E. "Puerperal Infections." In *Manual of Clinical Problems in Obstetrics and Gynecology*, 4th edition. Edited by Michel E. Rivlin and Rick W. Martin. Boston: Little, Brown and Company, 1994.

PERIODICAL

Aronoff, David M., and Katie L. Mason. "Postpartum Group A Streptococcus Sepsis and Maternal Immunology." *American Journal of Reproductive Immunology* 67.2 (2012): 91.

Janine Diebel, R.N.

Pulmonary artery catheterization *see* **Swan-Ganz catheterization**

Pulmonary embolism

Definition

Pulmonary **embolism** is an obstruction of a **blood** vessel in the **lungs**, usually due to a blood clot, which blocks a coronary artery.

Description

Pulmonary embolism is a fairly common condition that can be fatal. According to the American **Heart** Association, an estimated 600,000 Americans develop pulmonary embolism annually; 60,000 die from it. As many as 25,000 Americans are hospitalized each year for pulmonary embolism, which is a relatively common complication in hospitalized patients. Even without warning symptoms, pulmonary embolism can cause sudden death. Treatment is not always successful.

Pulmonary embolism is difficult to diagnose. Less than 10% of patients who die from pulmonary embolism were diagnosed with the condition. It occurs when emboli block a pulmonary artery, usually due to a blood clot that breaks off from a large vein and travels to the lungs. More than 90% of cases of pulmonary embolism are complications of **deep vein thrombosis**, blood clots from the leg or pelvic veins. Emboli can also be comprised of fat, air, or tumor tissue. When emboli block the main pulmonary artery, pulmonary embolism can quickly become fatal.

Causes and symptoms

Pulmonary embolism is caused by emboli that travel through the blood stream to the lungs and block a pulmonary artery. When this occurs, circulation and oxygenation of blood is compromised. The emboli are usually formed from blood clots but are occasionally comprised of air, fat, or tumor tissue. Risk factors include: prolonged bed rest, surgery, **childbirth**, heart attack, **stroke**, congestive **heart failure**, **cancer**, **obesity**, a broken hip or leg, oral contraceptives, sickle cell anemia, congenital **coagulation disorders**, chest trauma, certain congenital heart defects, and old age.

Common symptoms of pulmonary embolism include:

- labored breathing, sometimes accompanied by chest pain
- a rapid pulse
- a cough that produces bloody sputum
- a low fever
- fluid build-up in the lungs

Less common symptoms include:

- coughing up a lot of blood
- pain caused by movement
- leg swelling
- bluish skin
- fainting
- swollen neck veins

In some cases there are no symptoms.

Diagnosis

Pulmonary embolism can be diagnosed through the patient's history, a physical exam, and diagnostic tests including **chest x ray**, lung scan, pulmonary **angiography**, **electrocardiography**, arterial blood gas measurements, and leg vein **ultrasonography** or venography.

A chest x ray can be normal or show fluid or other signs and rule out other diseases. The lung scan shows poor flow of blood in areas beyond blocked arteries. The patient inhales a small amount of a radiopharmaceutical and pictures of airflow into the lungs are taken with a gamma camera. Then a different radiopharmaceutical is injected into an arm vein and lung blood flow is scanned. A normal result essentially rules out pulmonary embolism. A lung scan can be performed in a hospital or an outpatient facility and takes about 45 minutes.

Pulmonary angiography is the most reliable test for diagnosing pulmonary embolism but it is not used often, because it carries some risk and is expensive,

KEY TERMS

Deep vein thrombosis—A blood clot in the calf's deep vein. This frequently leads to pulmonary embolism if untreated.

Emboli—Clots or other substances that travel through the blood stream and get stuck in an artery, blocking circulation.

Thrombosis—The development of a blood clot inside a blood vessel.

invasive, and not readily available in many hospitals. Pulmonary angiography is a radiographic test which involves injection of a pharmaceutical "contrast agent" to show up the pulmonary arteries. A cinematic camera records the blood flow through the lungs of the patient, who lies on a table. Pulmonary angiography is usually performed in a hospital's **radiology** department and takes 30 minutes to one hour.

An electrocardiograph shows the heart's electrical activity and helps distinguish pulmonary embolism from a heart attack. Electrodes covered with conducting jelly are placed on the patient's chest, arms, and legs. Impulses of the heart's activity are traced on paper. The test takes about 10 minutes and can be performed in a physician's office or hospital lab.

Arterial blood gas measurements can be helpful, but they are rarely diagnostic for pulmonary embolism. Blood is taken from an artery instead of a vein, usually in the wrist and it is analyzed for oxygen, carbon dioxide and acid levels.

Venography is used to look for deep vein thrombosis, the most likely source of pulmonary embolism. It is very accurate, but it is not used often, because it is painful, expensive, exposes the patient to a fairly high dose of radiation, and can cause complications. Venography identifies the location, extent, and degree of attachment of the blood clots and enables the condition of the deep leg veins to be assessed. A contrast solution is injected into a foot vein through a catheter. The physician observes the movement of the solution through the vein with a **fluoroscope** while a series of x rays are taken. Venography takes between 30–45 minutes and can be done in a physician's office, a laboratory, or a hospital. Radionuclide venography, in which a radioactive isotope is injected, is occasionally used,

especially if a patient has had reactions to contrast solutions. Most commonly performed tests are ultrasound and Doppler studies of leg veins.

Treatment

Patients with pulmonary embolism are hospitalized and generally treated with clot-dissolving and clot-preventing drugs. **Oxygen therapy** is often needed to maintain normal oxygen concentrations. For people who can't take anticoagulants and in some other cases, surgery may be needed to insert a device that filters blood returning to the heart and lungs. The goal of treatment is to maintain the patient's cardiovascular and respiratory functions while the blockage resolves, which takes 10–14 days, and to prevent the formation of other emboli.

Thrombolytic therapy to dissolve blood clots is the aggressive treatment for very severe pulmonary embolism. Streptokinase, urokinase, and recombinant tissue plasminogen activator (TPA) are thrombolytic agents. Heparin is the injectable anticoagulant (clot-preventing) drug of choice for preventing formation of blood clots. Warfarin, an oral anticoagulant, is usually continued when the patient leaves the hospital and doesn't need heparin any longer.

Prognosis

About 10% of patients with pulmonary embolism die suddenly within the first hour of onset of the condition. The outcome for all other patients is generally good; only 3% of patients who are properly diagnosed and treated die. In cases of undiagnosed pulmonary embolism, about 30% of patients die.

Prevention

Pulmonary embolism risk can be reduced in certain patients through judicious use of antithrombotic drugs such as heparin, venous interruption, gradient elastic stockings and/or intermittent pneumatic compression of the legs.

ORGANIZATION

American Heart Association National Center, 7272 Greenville Avenue, Dallas, TX 75231, ((800)) 242-8721, Review. personal.info@heart.org

Lori De Milto

Pulmonary function test

Definition

Pulmonary function tests are a group of procedures that measure the function of the **lungs**, revealing problems in the way a patient breathes. These tests can determine the cause of shortness of breath and may help confirm the diagnosis of lung diseases, such as **asthma**, chronic **bronchitis**, or **emphysema**. The tests may also be performed before any major lung surgery to make sure the person will not be at risk of complications because of reduced lung capacity.

Purpose

Pulmonary function tests can help diagnose a range of respiratory diseases that might not otherwise be obvious to the clinician or the patient. These tests are important, since many kinds of lung problems can be successfully treated if detected early.

The tests are also used to measure how a lung disease is progressing, and how serious the lung disease has become. Pulmonary function tests also can be used to assess a patient's response to different treatments.

If a patient shows signs of decreased lung function relative to the normal values for a person of his or her race, sex, age, height, and weight, that person may suffer from a pulmonary disease. There are two causes of abnormal pulmonary function, obstructive lung diseases and restrictive lung diseases.

Obstructive lung diseases are characterized by a decreased ability to get air out of the lungs. A patient with an obstructive lung disease generally does not experience difficulty getting air into his or her lungs. Obstructive lung diseases are most easily remembered with the acronym CABBE: **cystic fibrosis**, asthma, brochiectasis, chronic bronchitis, and emphysema.

Restrictive lung diseases are characterized by a decreased capacity to draw air into the lungs. A patient with a restrictive lung disease generally does not experience difficulty getting air out of his or her lungs. The cause of restrictive lung diseases may be either directly related to a dysfunction of the lungs (intrapulmonary) or not related to a dysfunction of the lungs (extrapulmonary). Intrapulmonary restrictive lung diseases include **pneumonia**, pulmonary fibrosis, and pulmonary **edema**. Extrapulmonary causes of restrictive lung diseases include rib **fractures**, head trauma, and neuromuscular disorders.

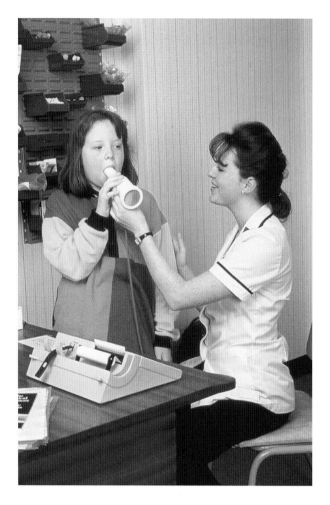

(Pulmonary function test, a cystic fibrosis patient, receiving treatment. Custom Medical Stock Photo. Reproduced by permission.)

Precautions

Before any pulmonary function test is performed by a patient, the clinician ordering the test should be aware of any conditions that the patient may have that may affect the reliability of the test results. Also, because pulmonary function testing requires deep breathing, the test itself may aggravate these same conditions.

Conditions in a patient that contraindicate pulmonary function testing include: the coughing-up of **blood** from the respiratory tract (hemoptysis); a collapsed or partially collapsed lung (**pneumothorax**); an unstable **heart** condition, recent heart attack, or blood clot near the lungs; an abnormal localized bulging of a blood vessel (**aneurysm**) in the chest, **abdomen**, or head; recent surgery of the chest or abdomen; recent eye surgery; and current nausea or **vomiting**. If a patient suffers from one or more of these conditions, pulmonary function tests should be postponed until these conditions are resolved.

The patient should not wear clothing that constricts the chest area. Patients should not have eaten a heavy meal three hours or less before the test. Smokers should provide their **smoking** history and the time of their last cigarette. In order for pulmonary function tests to yield accurate results, the patient must be able to respond to direction; so the tests may not be useful in very young children, uncooperative patients, and physically incapacitated individuals.

Description

One of the most common of the pulmonary function tests is spirometry. This test, which can be given in a hospital or doctor's office, measures how much and how fast the air is moving in and out of the lungs. This test is covered in greater detail in the separate **spirometry tests** entry.

A peak flow meter can determine how much a patient's airways have narrowed. A test of **blood gases** is a measurement of the concentration of oxygen and carbon dioxide in the blood, which shows how efficient the **gas exchange** is in the lungs.

Another lung function test reveals the efficiency of the lungs in absorbing gas from the blood. This efficiency is measured by testing the volume of carbon monoxide a person breathes out after a known volume of the gas has been inhaled.

Preparation

The healthcare provider conducting a pulmonary function test should explain the test and any and all potential side effects to the patient prior to the test being performed. The health care provider should then demonstrate the proper breathing technique for the patient, and the patient should then practice this technique until he or she is able to accurately duplicate the proper technique on two consecutive trials. The health care provider should also indicate that while most side effects of pulmonary function tests are extremely rare, the patient should stop the test if he or she becomes extremely uncomfortable or feels intense **pain** in the head, eye, chest, or abdomen.

Prior to the test, the age, race, and sex of the patient should be recorded, along with a height measurement in stocking feet and a weight measurement. This information will allow each individual's results to be compared to normal values for people in the same demographic category.

Aftercare

There is usually no patient care required after the administration of a pulmonary function test. If a patient feels lightheaded or dizzy, he or she should lie down until the symptoms subside. In rare cases, oxygen may have to be administered to prevent pneumothorax or to restore normal breathing patterns.

Complications

In general, pulmonary function tests are safe procedures that simply require deep breathing. In very rare instances complications can occur. These include pneumothorax; increased fluid pressure between the bones of the **skull** and the **brain** (increased intracranial pressure); loss of consciousness, **dizziness**, and/or lightheadedness; chest pain; uncontrollable coughing; and contraction of an **infection** from the test equipment.

Results

Normal results

Normal test results are based on a person's age, height, weight, race, and gender. Normal results are expressed as a percentage of the predicted lung capacity for a person of the same age, height, weight, race, and sex. Any measurement within 20% of the predicted value is considered a normal result.

Abnormal results

Abnormal results mean that the person's lung capacity is less than 80% of the predicted value. Such findings usually mean that there is some degree of chest or lung disease.

Health care team roles

Pulmonary function tests are generally ordered by a primary care doctor (M.D. or D.O.) or advanced practice nurse, and performed either by a physician, nurse, or respiratory technician under the direction of a doctor specifically trained in pulmonary function testing. When the results of pulmonary function testing are inaccurate, the most frequent reason is inadequate **patient education** and/or technician training. It is recommended that personnel conducting pulmonary function testing have one of the following credentials: certified **respiratory therapy** technician (CRTT); registered respiratory therapist (RRT); certified pulmonary function technologist (CPFT); or registered pulmonary function technologist (RPFT). A doctor specializing in diseases of the lungs (pulmonologist) may be consulted to examine abnormal pulmonary function test results.

Resources

BOOKS

Des Jardins, T. *Cardiopulmonary Anatomy and Physiology: Essentials for Respiratory Care,* 3rd ed. Albany, NY: Delmar Publishers, 1998.

Madama, Vincent C., and Vince Madama. *Pulmonary Function Testing and Cardiopulmonary Stress Testing.* Albany, NY: Delmar Publishing, 1997.

Ruppel, Gregg L. *Manual of Pulmonary Function Testing,* 7th ed. St. Louis, MO: Mosby-Year Book, Inc. 1998.

Wagner, Jack. *Pulmonary Function Testing: A Practical Approach.* Baltimore, MD: Williams and Wilkins, 1996.

ORGANIZATION

National Lung Health Education Program (NLHEP). 1850 High Street, Denver, CO 80218. http://www. nlhep.org/.

Paul A. Johnson

Pulmonary rehabilitation

Definition

Pulmonary **rehabilitation** is a multidisciplinary, individually designed intervention program, including **exercise** and education, that helps patients with chronic lung disorders manage the physiological and psychosocial symptoms of their condition and improve their level of daily functioning and well-being.

Purpose

The purpose of a pulmonary rehabilitation program is to help patients with **chronic obstructive pulmonary disease** (COPD) or other chronic lung conditions manage their condition. Exercise and education are provided to help increase the patient's level of fitness and independent functioning, reduce dyspnea and psychological symptoms (**anxiety**, depression, social isolation), slow down or prevent the progression of disease, and improve quality and possibly length of life.

Pulmonary rehabilitation has not been found to improve pulmonary function, and that is not its goal. Other measures of physiologic improvement such as improved muscle function, cardiac function, and aerobic function have been found, and the main purpose of **cardiac rehabilitation** is to "reverse the deconditioning and psychosocial accompaniments of pulmonary disability." Pulmonary rehabilitation is also increasingly recognized as valuable in preparation for lung transplantation and lung volume-reduction surgery, which require patients to have good physical conditioning.

Precautions

Patients should be examined by a physician before beginning rehabilitation. Certain coexisting medical conditions, especially those that preclude or limit exercise, may contraindicate pulmonary rehabilitation, or require modification and special precautions. Since treatment is individualized, any special needs will be addressed in the exercise prescription and program design. Some particular conditions that may contraindicate participation in pulmonary rehabilitation include acute respiratory **infection**, ischemic cardiac disease, congestive **heart failure**, serious **liver** dysfunction, disabling **stroke**, severe psychiatric or cognitive disorders, acute cor pulmonale, severe pulmonary **hypertension**, and metastatic **cancer**.

Description

Pulmonary rehabilitation is a multidisciplinary, comprehensive program of education, exercise, and

Essentials of pulmonary therapy

Treatment components	Purpose	How to perform	When to use
Breathing exercises	Assists in removing secretions; relaxation; and used to increase thoracic cage mobility and tidal volume	Patient is taught to produce a full inspiration followed by a controlled expiration; use hand placement for sensory feedback	When patients are breathing spontaneously
Coughing	Removal of secretions from the larger airways	Steps: (1) Inspiratory gasp; (2) Closing of the glottis; (3) Contraction of expiratory muscles; (4) Opening of the glottis	When patients are breathing spontaneously
Percussion	Used with postural drainage for mobilization of secretions	Rhythmic clapping of cupped hands over bare skin or thin material covering area of lung involvement; performed during inspiration and expiration	When coughing or suctioning, breathing exercises, and patient mobilization are not adequate to clear retained secretions
Postural drainage	Mobilize retained secretions through assistance of gravity	Patient positioned so that involved segmental bronchus is uppermost	Same as above
Vibration	Used with postural drainage for mobilization of secretions	Intermittent chest wall compression over area of lung involvement; performed during expiration only	Same as above

SOURCE: Mackenzie, C.F., et al. *Chest Physiotherapy in the Intensive Care Unit.* Baltimore: Williams & Wilkins, 1981.

behavior modification, individually designed for patients with lung diseases such as COPD. COPD includes such conditions as chronic **bronchitis** and **emphysema**, which can be progressive and life-threatening. Other chronic lung conditions that may be suitable for pulmonary rehabilitation include **cystic fibrosis**, **asthma**, bronchiectasis, and environmental lung disease, as well as neuromuscular disorders such as **Parkinson's disease** and **multiple sclerosis**.

The rehabilitation program is designed to help patients learn more about their condition and how to manage its symptoms, as well as to take active steps, such as **smoking cessation**, oxygen use, and exercise, in order to improve their level of physical functioning; stop the progression of the disease as much as possible; and learn how to better live with the condition. Improved physical functioning, reduction in physical and psychological symptoms, and ability to perform activities of daily living (ADLs) more easily and independently, can contribute to improved quality of life.

A typical program, which is individually designed but involves group participation, may last up to three hours per session, a few days each week. Programs generally last a few weeks to a few months, and prepare the patient to continue exercise, symptom management, and other skills learned in the program on their own. An in-home follow-up program may also be included.

Patients may participate in rehabilitation as inpatients or outpatients, and will also be encouraged to exercise on their own at home if it is safe for them to do so without monitoring. Some insurance companies cover all or part of the rehabilitation program.

The two main components of the daily program are exercise and education. Exercise is important for maintaining or improving muscle strength, endurance and overall fitness, which may have declined due to inactivity and symptoms of the disease. Decreased physical activity and associated decline in fitness play a large part in causing the physical limitations associated with COPD. A regular exercise program can improve overall fitness and energy, and make performance of ADLs easier.

The exercise program is individually prescribed to meet the physical needs of each patient, and includes a warm-up and cool-down period, and aerobic activity. The warm-up and cool-down periods may include stretching and light strength or resistance training. Exercises involving upper and lower extremities are important for overall fitness and for improvement in function during specific activities. For example, lower body exercise helps with ambulation, stair climbing, and general fitness; and conditioning of the arms facilitates improved functioning in many tasks that require arm and upper body use, such as grooming, cooking, and household tasks. Some of the muscle groups used in arm and upper torso positioning serve respiratory functions, and thus upper extremity conditioning can also have a beneficial effect on ventilation.

The aerobic exercise component comprises activities such as walking or using a stationary bicycle, treadmill, or other equipment. Exercise is monitored by physical therapists, respiratory nurses, or other qualified health care providers. **Blood pressure**, **heart** rate, oxygen saturation, and dyspnea levels are evaluated to determine the appropriate exercise prescription, and may be monitored during exercise sessions. Ventilatory training may also be included in the exercise program for certain patients. This therapy involves controlled breathing exercises; **chest physical therapy** techniques such as postural drainage, chest percussion, directed **cough**, and vibration; and training of the inspiratory muscles.

The educational component of the rehabilitation program consists of classes, reading materials, and counseling or training sessions that cover various specific subjects, procedures, and issues of importance to patients with chronic pulmonary disease. Education is provided by a variety of professionals, including respiratory nurses, respiratory therapists, occupational therapists, physical therapists, social workers, and dieticians. A psychologist or other mental health professional may provide counseling to address depression, anxiety, social isolation, or other psychosocial symptoms related to COPD.

Some of the educational subjects covered include **anatomy** and **physiology** related to pulmonary function and disease, exercise theory, **nutrition**, techniques for using oxygen and inhalers, and ways to conserve energy. Education related to good nutrition and weight management can be helpful, because patients may be undernourished and have muscle wasting of the respiratory muscles, which can make breathing more difficult. If anemia is present, it can decrease oxygen-carrying capacity. Electrolyte imbalances affect cardiopulmonary performance, so these and other deficiencies should be treated in order to improve functioning. If patients are overweight, the extra weight increases oxygen and energy demands and may increase fatigue. Patients who have not yet stopped **smoking** should be strongly encouraged to do so.

Preparation

Examination and referral by a physician are generally required before a patient begins pulmonary rehabilitation. A medical history should be provided to the rehabilitation team. Some tests that may be administered prior to the patient's entry into a rehabilitation

program include pulmonary function tests (PFTs), chest x rays, arterial **blood** gas (ABG) analysis, pulse oximetry, and sputum examination. PFTs are performed with a spirometer to measure lung performance and determine the presence and extent of lung disease. A **chest x ray** can detect emphysema and other lung disease, including **lung cancer**, for which there is increased risk among smokers with COPD. Pulse oximetry measures oxygen in the blood and helps determine when supplemental oxygen is required. Exercise tests may be used to determine the length and intensity of the exercise prescription.

Aftercare

Patients may be able to participate in various follow-up or maintenance programs or support groups, as well as check-ins with their physician, in order to maintain benefits and continue monitoring their condition.

Complications

Risk of complications such as muscle injury or cardiac reactions is always present with exercise, but will be minimized by careful exercise prescription and monitoring. Disease-related complications that should be watched for include **fever**, unusual or extreme shortness of breath, irregular pulse, unanticipated weight changes, gastric complaints, or any other change that is unusual for the patient.

Results

The primary goals of cardiac rehabilitation are to reduce symptoms and respiratory impairment, and to improve the patient's quality of life and possibly prolong their life. Some of the specific changes that affect overall improvement in health, functioning and quality of life include: improvement in pulmonary function, reduction of the work involved in breathing, increased efficiency of energy use, improved exercise performance, increased function in activities of daily living, alleviation of dyspnea, nutritional correction, and improved emotional state. Other possible results are a decrease in frequency and duration of hospital stays and decrease in use of other health care resources.

Health care team roles

The various educational and therapeutic components of a comprehensive pulmonary rehabilitation program are best addressed by a variety of health care professionals. The team may include respiratory nurses; respiratory, physical and occupational therapists; psychologists or other mental health professionals; exercise specialists; and dieticians, as well as a program director. The physical therapist may be involved in exercise prescription and monitoring; providing education in areas related to anatomy, physiology, exercise, and **physical therapy**; and providing other therapeutic treatments, such as chest physical therapy.

Resources

BOOKS

American Association of Cardiovascular and Pulmonary Rehabilitation. *Guidelines for Pulmonary Rehabilitation Programs,* 2nd ed. Champaign, IL: Human Kinetics, 1998.

Brannon, F. J., M. W. Foley, J. A. Starr, and L. M. Saul. *Cardiopulmonary Rehabilitation: Basic Theory and Application,* 3rd ed. Philadelphia: F. A. Davis, 1998.

PERIODICALS

Camp, Pat G. et al. "Quality of Life After Pulmonary Rehabilitation: Assessing Change Using Quantitative and Qualitative Methods." *Physical Therapy* 8, no. 10 (October 2000).

Celli, Bartolome R., MD. "Pulmonary rehabilitation for COPD: A practical approach for improving ventilatory conditioning." *Postgraduate Medicine* 103, no. 4 (April 1998).

ORGANIZATIONS

American Association of Cardiovascular and Pulmonary Rehabilitation (AACVPR). 7600 Terrace Avenue, Suite 203, Middleton, WI 53562. (608) 831-6989. http://www.aacvpr.org/.

American College of Chest Physicians (ACCP). 3300 Dundee Road. Northbrook, IL 60062-2348. (847) 498-1400.

American Physical Therapy Association (APTA). 1111 North Fairfax Street. Alexandria, VA 22314. (703) 684-2782. http://www.apta.org.

Diane Fanucchi, B.A., C.M.T.

Pulmonology

Definition

Pulmonology is a branch of medicine that diagnoses and treats diseases of the **lungs** and lower **respiratory system** (bronchi).

Description

Pulmonology is a subspecialty of **internal medicine**. A physician who specializes in this branch of medicine in the United States is called a pulmonologist. In Canada, the physician is called a respirologist. In other English speaking countries, a pulmonary specialist is called a respiratory physician.

Pulmonologists treat serious chronic lung diseases such as **asthma**, **emphysema**, **chronic obstructive pulmonary disease** (COPD), **tuberculosis**, and the respiratory complications of **cystic fibrosis** and **AIDS**. They also treat acute diseases such as **pneumonia** and work with critical care teams to treat people who are on mechanical **ventilators**. Most treatment involves drug therapy.

Pulmonologists may supervise respiratory therapists and work with other allied health professionals as part of a **pulmonary rehabilitation** team. Pulmonologists may take biopsies of the linings of the airways and lungs, but they do not do major surgery. If chest or lung surgery is needed, it is done by a thoracic (chest) surgeon in consultation with the pulmonologist.

The most common diagnostic tool used by pulmonologists is the bronchoscope. When inserted into the airways, a bronchoscope allows the pulmonologist to see the lining of the airways and take biopsies for examination in the laboratory. While most pulmonologists use the bronchoscope for diagnostic purposes, some pulmonologists specialized in a relatively new area known as interventional pulmonology. Interventional pulmonologists use bronchoscopes equipped with miniature tools and guided by imaging technology to treat rather than diagnose certain conditions.

Origins

Pulmonology was not recognized as a subspecialty of internal medicine until the second half of the twentieth century. Its predecessor was a branch of medicine known as phthisology that involved specialized treatment of tuberculosis. As tuberculosis became more treatable and the number of cases declined, this specialty gradually evolved into treatment of other respiratory diseases and became pulmonology. The American College of Chest Physicians founded in 1935 includes pulmonologists

KEY TERMS

Asthma—A disease in which the air passages of the lungs become inflamed and narrowed.

Biopsy—A procedure in which suspicious tissue is removed and examined by a pathologist for cancer or other disease.

Bronchi (singular bronchus)—Two major airways that branch off the trachea and carry air to and from the lungs

Bronchoscope—A thin, usually flexible, lighted tube that is used to view the air passages in the lungs.

Chronic obstructive pulmonary disease (COPD)—Lung diseases, such as emphysema and chronic bronchitis, in which airflow is obstructed, causing labored breathing and impairing gas exchange.

Pulmonary hypertension—Potentially life-threatening condition in which blood pressure in the pulmonary artery increases to abnormal levels. Primary pulmonary hypertension, which is rare, occurs without any known cause. Secondary pulmonary hypertension is often a complication of lung diseases like emphysema and bronchitis.

only adults. Some physicians do a third year of fellowship and become board certified in both pulmonology and critical care. To become a pediatric pulmonologist, the physician must complete a residency in **pediatrics** and then a three-year fellowship in pulmonology and pass examinations to become board certified.

Resources

OTHER

American College of Physicians. Pulmonology. 2012. http://www.acponline.org/patients_ families/about_internal_medicine/subspecialties/pulmonology [accessed August 23, 2012].

ORGANIZATIONS

American College of Chest Physicians, 3300 Dundee Road, Northbrook, IL 60062-2348, (847) 498-1400, Fax: (847) 498-5460, http://www.chestnet.org.

American Lung Association, 1301 Pennsylvania Ave., NW Suite 800, Washington, DC 20004, (212) 315-8700, (800) LUNG-USA [(800) 548-8252].

European Respiratory Society, 4, Avenue Ste-Luce, CH 1003 Lausanne, Switzerland, +41 21 213 01 01, Fax: + 41 21 213 01 00, http://www.ersnet.org.

National Heart Lung and Blood Institute Health Information Center, P.O. Box 30105, Bethesda, MD 20824-0105, (301) 592-8573; TTY: (240) 629-3255, Fax: (240) 629-3246, :nhlbiinfo@nhlbi.nih.gov, http://www.nhlbi.nih.gov.

Tish Davidson, AM

among its members in the United States. The European Respiratory Society serves to support respiratory physicians and allied health professionals in Europe.

Purpose

The purpose of pulmonology is to diagnose and treat serious respiratory diseases. In the case of chronic disease, the purpose of pulmonology is to supervise a program of pulmonary **rehabilitation** that gives the patient the best possible level of functioning.

Training and certification

To become a pulmonologist, an individual must graduate from an accredited medical school or school of **osteopathy**. Graduation is followed by an internship and three-year accredited residency in internal medicine. Following successful completion of the internal medicine residency, the physician participates in a two-year pulmonary fellowship after which he or she takes specialized examinations to become a board certified pulmonologist. This qualifies the physician to treat

Pulse assessment

Definition

Pulse assessment is the detection of a patient's pulse.

Purpose

Pulse assessment is performed to establish a baseline on a patient's admission (from which to compare any significant changes), and to detect any abnormalities from the healthy state.

Precautions

As there may be no prior knowledge of the patient's previous pulse recordings for comparison, it is important for the nurse or other health professional to know the range of normal values that apply to patients of different ages. Any known medical and surgical history or

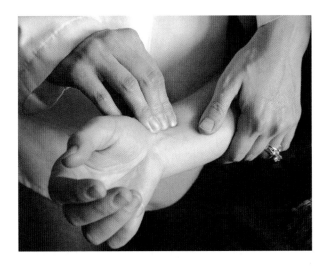

(Copyright © 2005 Kelly A. Quin.)

abnormal readings of any of the **vital signs**, as well as details of any current medication the patient is taking, should be obtained. Exertion, such as climbing stairs, may affect the results. Therefore the patient should have rested prior to having their pulse taken and should have refrained from consuming tobacco, caffeinated drinks, and alcohol 30 minutes prior to the procedure. Of course, these precautions cannot be taken in an emergency situation.

Description

The pulse is checked as one indicator of abnormalities of the **heart** by observing the rate, rhythm, and the strength and tension of the beat against the arterial wall. The pulse may be recorded hourly to every four hours, or p.r.n. (when required), based on the patient's condition. For example, the pulse may be recorded postoperatively every 15 minutes in the recovery room.

Preparation

The equipment required for pulse assessment is a watch with a second hand sweep or a digital readout. The pulse may be read where a surface artery runs over a **bone**, e.g. the radial artery (in the forearm), carotid artery (in the neck), temporal artery (at the temple), popliteal artery (at the back of the knee), or dorsalis pedal artery (at the instep). The radial artery in the wrist is the option used most often. The physician may choose sites such as the carotid artery pulse if atrial or ventricular problems are suspected.

To take the radial pulse, the patient should be sitting or lying comfortably, so that the readings are taken in similar positions each time and that there is little excitement to affect the results. The patient's forearm should not be raised to a level higher than the heart, as this position will change the reading. The nurse should place the index, middle, and ring fingers over the radial artery, which is located above the wrist on the anterior surface of the thumb side of the wrist. Apply gentle pressure to avoid obstructing the patient's **blood** flow. The rate, rhythm, strength, and tension of the pulse should be noted. Using a watch, the pulsations that are felt where the artery rests against the bone are counted for half a minute, and the result doubled to give the beats per minute. However, any irregularities noted within the 30-second count means that the pulse should be recorded for one full minute to avoid any discrepancies.

Aftercare

The nurse should make the patient comfortable and reassure him or her that recording the pulse is part of normal health checks and that it is necessary to ensure the patient's health is being correctly monitored. Any abnormalities in the pulse must be reported in the nurse's notes and relayed to the attending physician.

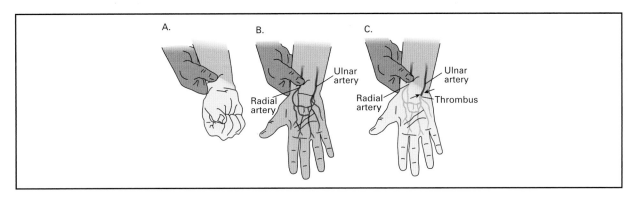

(From Fundamentals of Nursing, Standards and Practices 2nd edition by Delaune/Ladner. © 2002. Reprinted with permission of Delmar Learning: www.thomsonrights.com Fax 800-730-2215.)

KEY TERMS

Amplitude—The fullness of the pulse.

Arteriosclerosis—Hardening and thickening of the walls of the arteries, causing loss of elasticity. It may also include calcium deposits in the arteries.

Bradycardia—A slow heartbeat or pulse below 60 bpm in an adult.

p.r.n.—*pro re nata*, when required.

Pulsus alternans—Alternating weak and strong beats of the pulse.

Tachycardia—A rapid heartbeat or pulse above 100 bpm in an adult.

Thyrotoxicosis—Hyperthyroidism.

Results

The average heart rate for older children and adults can range from 50 to 90 beats per minute (bpm). This is an average; rates vary between males and females, with age, and with the patient's health and level of fitness. It is not abnormal for athletes to display a low pulse rate.

The pulse is an indicator of the health of the heart and the arterial circulation. Factors such as **anxiety**, medication, or pulmonary disease may also cause the heart rate to be faster or slower.

A low-volume, or weak, pulse may be caused by a number of factors, including **myocardial infarction**, **shock**, intracranial pressure, or the use of vasoconstrictor drugs.

Pulse pressure may become raised due to arteriosclerosis, as the heart has to pump harder to promote the flow of blood around the body. This high-pressure pulse is called a bounding pulse, and may also be caused by conditions such as **fever**, **pregnancy**, or thyrotoxicosis. It may also be an indicator that pulmonary disease is present.

Other conditions that can be detected in part by pulse assessment include tachycardia (a heart beat that is too fast) and bradycardia (a heartbeat that is too slow). The nurse would also be able to detect missed heartbeats and pulsus alternans (alternating strong and weak beats).

The pulse is recorded and compared with normal ranges for the patient's age, gender, and medical condition, and a decision is required regarding the interpretation of the results as to whether any further action should be taken.

Health care team roles

Patients may ask questions about specific concerns they have regarding pulse recordings or a particular disease. Nurses should have a thorough knowledge of what pulse irregularities indicate to enable them to answer the patient's questions, or provide counseling on the prevention of illness and injuries, or direct the person to their doctor. Further tests may be performed to evaluate the heart and diagnose abnormalities.

Resources

BOOKS

Guyton, Arthur C., and John E. Hall. *Textbook of Medical Physiology,* 9th edition. Philadelphia: W B Saunders Publishing, 1996, p. 173.

Nettina, Sandra M. *The Lippincott Manual of Nursing Practice,* 6th edition. Lippincott-Raven Publishers, 1996, p. 249.

Tierney, Lawrence M., Stephen J. McPhee, and Maxine A. Papadakis. *Current Medical Diagnosis and Treatment 2000.* 39th edition. New York: Lange Medical Books/ McGraw-Hill Publishing, 2000, p. 353.

ORGANIZATION

American Nurses Association. 600 Maryland Avenue SW, Suite 100 West, Washington, DC 20024. (202) 651-7000.

Margaret A. Stockley, RGN

Pulse oximeter

Definition

The pulse oximeter is a photoelectric instrument for measuring oxygen saturation of the **blood**.

Purpose

A pulse oximeter measures the amount of oxygen present in the blood by registering pulsations within an arteriolar bed. It is a noninvasive method widely used in the hospital, including for newborns, patients with pulmonary disorders, and patients undergoing pulmonary and cardiac procedures. Oxygen levels can be estimated during **exercise**, surgery or medical procedures, or while the patient is asleep.

KEY TERMS

Arteriolar bed—An area in which arterioles cluster between arteries and capillaries.

Arterioles—The smallest branch of arteries.

Capillaries—Tiny blood vessels with a diameter of a red blood cell through which a single layer of cells flows.

Deoxyhemoglobin—Hemoglobin with oxygen removed.

Oxyhemoglobin—Hemoglobin combined with oxygen.

Description

Oximeters are used in hospital settings such as intensive care units, pulmonary units, and in health care centers. Portable hand-held devices are available, and are used for spot-checking patients and for in-home use with a doctor's supervision.

The oximeter consists of a light-emitting diode (LED), a photodetector probe containing a permanent or disposable sensor, alarms for pulse rate and oxygen levels, a display screen, and cables. The device works by emitting beams of red and infrared light that are passed through a pulsating arteriolar bed. Sensors detect the amount of light absorbed by oxyhemoglobin and deoxyhemoglobin in the red blood cells. The ratio of red to infrared light measured by the photodetector indicates the amount of oxygen present in the blood. The sensor is attached to the body over the arteriolar area in the ear, the finger tip, the big toe, or across the bridge of the nose. Clip sensors can be used on fingers and the earlobe.

Operation

Several steps can be taken to enhance accurate readings. If possible, the patient should be instructed not to smoke 24 hours prior to pulse oximetry. Fingernail polish should be removed if the oximeter will be attached to the finger. For patients with poor circulation, hands should be slowly warmed with warm towels before attaching the oximeter. Abnormally high or low temperatures, as well as reduced hemoglobin, can influence the amount of oxygen adhering to the hemoglobin within the red blood cells, altering the reading.

Care should be taken with attaching the sensors and selecting the site for optimum reading levels. The sensor should be wrapped securely around the finger to prevent outside light from interfering with the reading and rendering it invalid. An appropriate site is chosen to monitor the oxygen levels by ensuring that there is strong arterial pulsation, and that the capillary bed fills promptly if squeezed.

The device must not be used near flammable anesthetics.

Maintenance

Older devices may be affected by motion. They should be checked regularly to insure proper function.

Health care team roles

Nurses and allied health professionals attach the pulse oximeter and explain to the patient that it is used for monitoring purposes. Staff monitor the site where the sensor has been applied every four hours for clip sensors and every six hours for wrapped sensors. Any loss of pulsation, swelling, or change in color requires a change of site.

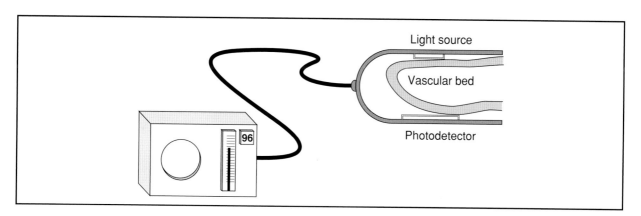

(Oximetry, illustration by Argosy, Inc. Cengage Learning, Gale.)

Training

Staff should be familiar with the device and the department's protocol to ensure standardization in operating the equipment.

Resources

BOOK

Jarvis, Carolyn. *Physical Examination and Health Assessment,* 6th edition. Saunders, 2011.

PERIODICALS

Anderson, Mary Ann, Pamela D. Hill, and Cynthia L. Johnson. "Comparison of pulse oximetry measures in a healthy population." *MedSurg Nursing* (March–April 2012): 70.

Barnett, Emma, Richard Barraclough, and Annette Duck. "Effect of recording site on pulse oximetry readings." *Nursing Times* (10 January 2012): 22–23.

Kang, Sok-Leng, Wilf Kelsall, and Suzanne Tobin. "Neonatal pulse oximetry screening: a national survey." *Archives of Disease in Childhood. Fetal and Neonatal Edition* (July 2011): F312.

King, Alexandra. "Clear benefits of pulse oximetry in neonates–one small step to improving postnatal cardiac care." *Nature Reviews Cardiology* 8.10 (2011).

Margaret A. Stockley, RGN

Punctures *see* **Wounds**

Pyelography *see* **Intravenous urography**

Pyorrhea *see* **Periodontitis**

Qigong

Definition

Qigong (pronounced "chee-gung," also spelled *chi kung*) is translated from the Chinese to mean "energy cultivation" or "working with the life energy." Qigong is an ancient Chinese system of postures, exercises, breathing techniques, and meditations. Its techniques are designed to improve and enhance the body's *qi*. According to traditional Chinese philosophy, qi is the fundamental life energy responsible for health and vitality.

Origins

Qigong originated before recorded history. Scholars estimate qigong to be as old as 5000–7000 years. Tracing the exact historical development of qigong is difficult, because it was passed down in secrecy among monks and teachers for many generations. Qigong survived through many years before paper was invented, and it also survived the Cultural Revolutions in China of the 1960s and 1970s, which banned many traditional practices.

Qigong has influenced and been influenced by many of the major strands of Chinese philosophy. The Taoist philosophy states that the universe operates within laws of balance and harmony, and that people must live within the rhythms of nature—ideas that pervade qigong. When Buddhism was brought from India to China around the seventh century A. D., **yoga** techniques and concepts of mental and spiritual awareness were introduced to qigong masters. The Confucian school was concerned with how people should live their daily lives, a concern of qigong as well. The martial arts were highly influenced by qigong; and many of them, such as **t'ai chi** and kung fu, developed directly from it. Traditional Chinese medicine also shares many of the central concepts of qigong, such as the patterns of energy flow in the body. **Acupuncture** and **acupressure** use the same points on the body that qigong seeks to stimulate. In China, qigong masters have

been renowned physicians and healers. Qigong is often prescribed by Chinese physicians as part of the treatment.

Due to the political isolation of China, many Chinese concepts have been shrouded from the Western world. Acupuncture was only "discovered" by American doctors in the 1970s, although it had been in use for thousands of years. With an increased exchange of information, more Americans have gained access to the once-secret teachings of qigong. In 1988, the First World Conference for Academic Exchange of Medical Qigong was held in Beijing, China, where many studies were presented to attendees from around the world. In 1990, Berkeley, California hosted the First International Congress of Qigong. In the past decade, more Americans have begun to discover the beneficial effects of qigong, which motivate an estimated sixty million Chinese to practice it every day.

Benefits

Qigong may be used as a daily routine to increase overall health and well-being, as well as for disease prevention and longevity. It can be used to increase energy and reduce **stress**. In China, qigong is used in conjunction with other medical therapies for many chronic conditions, including **asthma**, **allergies**, **AIDS**, **cancer**, headaches, **hypertension**, depression, mental illness, strokes, **heart** disease, and **obesity**.

Description

Basic concepts

In Chinese thought, qi, or chi, is the fundamental life energy of the universe. It is invisible but present in the air, water, food and sunlight. In the body, qi is the unseen vital force that sustains life. We are all born with inherited amounts of qi, and we also get acquired qi from the food we eat and the air we breathe. In qigong, the breath is believed to account for the largest quantity of acquired qi, because the body uses air more than any other substance. The balance of our physical, mental, and emotional levels also affect qi levels in the body.

Qi travels through the body along channels called meridians. There are twelve main meridians, corresponding to the twelve principal organs as defined by the traditional Chinese system: the lung, large intestines, **stomach**, spleen, heart, **small intestine**, urinary bladder, kidney, **liver**, **gallbladder**, pericardium, and the "triple warmer," which represents the entire torso region. Each organ has qi associated with it, and each organ interacts with particular emotions on the mental level. Qigong techniques are designed to improve the balance and flow of energy throughout the meridians, and to increase the overall quantity and volume of qi. In qigong philosophy, mind and body are not separated as they often are in Western medicine. In qigong, the mind is present in all parts of the body, and the mind can be used to move qi throughout the body.

Yin and yang are also important concepts in qigong. The universe and the body can be described by these two separate but complementary principles, which are always interacting, opposing, and influencing each other. One goal of qigong is to balance yin and yang within the body. Strong movements or techniques are balanced by soft ones, leftward movements by rightward, internal techniques by external ones, and so on.

Practicing qigong

There are thousands of qigong exercises. The specific ones used may vary depending on the teacher, school, and objective of the practitioner. Qigong is used for physical fitness, as a martial art, and most frequently for health and healing. Internal qigong is performed by those wishing to increase their own energy and health. Some qigong masters are renowned for being able to perform external qigong, by which the energy from one person is passed on to another for healing. This transfer may sound suspect to Western logic, but in the world of qigong there are some amazing accounts of healing and extraordinary capabilities demonstrated by qigong masters. Qigong masters generally have deep knowledge of the concepts of Chinese medicine and healing. In China, there are hospitals that use medical qigong to heal patients, along with herbs, acupuncture, and other techniques. In these hospitals, qigong healers use external qigong and also design specific internal qigong exercises for patients' problems.

There are basic components of internal qigong sessions. All sessions require warm-up and concluding exercises. Qigong consists of postures, movements, breathing techniques, and mental exercises. Postures may involve standing, sitting, or lying down. Movements include stretches, slow motions, quick thrusts, jumping, and bending. Postures and movements are designed to strengthen, stretch, and tone the body to improve the flow of energy. One sequence of postures and movements is known as the "Eight Figures for Every Day." This sequence is designed to quickly and effectively work the entire body, and is commonly performed daily by millions in China.

Breathing techniques include deep abdominal breathing, chest breathing, relaxed breathing, and holding breaths. One breathing technique is called the "Six Healing Sounds." This technique uses particular breathing sounds for each of six major organs. These sounds are believed to stimulate and heal the organs.

Meditations and mind exercises are used to enhance the mind and move qi throughout the body. These exercises are often visualizations that focus on different body parts, words, ideas, objects, or energy flowing along the meridians. One mental exercise is called the "Inner Smile," during which the practitioner visualizes joyful, healing energy being sent sequentially to each organ in the body. Another mental exercise is called the "Microscopic Orbit Meditation," in which the practitioner intently meditates on increasing and connecting the flow of qi throughout major channels.

Discipline is an important dimension of qigong. Exercises are meant to be performed every morning and evening. Sessions can take from 15 minutes to hours. Beginners are recommended to practice between 15–30 minutes twice a day. Beginners may take classes once or twice per week, with practice outside of class. Classes generally cost between $10–$20 per session.

Preparations

Qigong should be practiced in a clean, pleasant environment, preferably outdoors in fresh air. Loose and comfortable clothing is recommended. Jewelry should be removed. Practitioners can prepare for success at qigong by practicing at regular hours each day to promote discipline. Qigong teachers also recommend that students prepare by adopting lifestyles that promote balance, moderation, proper rest, and healthy diets, all of which are facets of qigong practice.

Precautions

Beginners should learn from an experienced teacher, as performing qigong exercises in the wrong manner may cause harm. Practitioners should not perform qigong on either full or completely empty stomachs. Qigong should not be performed during extreme weather, which may have negative effects on the body's energy systems.

KEY TERMS

Martial arts—Group of diverse activities originating from the ancient fighting techniques of the Orient.

Meridians—Channels or conduits through which qi travels in the body.

Qi—Basic life energy, according to traditional Chinese medicine.

Yin/Yang—Universal characteristics used to describe aspects of the natural world.

Menstruating and pregnant women should perform only certain exercises.

Side effects

Side effects may occur during or after qigong exercises for beginners, or for those performing exercises incorrectly. Side effects may include **dizziness**, dry mouth, fatigue, headaches, insomnia, rapid heartbeat, shortness of breath, heaviness or numbness in areas of the body, emotional instability, **anxiety**, or decreased concentration. Side effects generally clear up with rest and instruction from a knowledgeable teacher.

Research and general acceptance

Western medicine generally does not endorse any of the traditional Chinese healing systems that utilize the concept of energy flow in the body, largely because this energy has yet to be isolated and measured scientifically. New research is being conducted using sophisticated equipment that may verify the existence of energy channels as defined by the Chinese system. Despite the lack of scientific validation, the results of energy techniques including qigong and acupuncture have gained widespread interest and respect. Furthermore, qigong masters have demonstrated to Western observers astounding control over many physical functions, and some have even shown the ability to increase electrical voltage measured on their skin's surface. Most of the research and documentation of qigong's effectiveness for medical conditions has been conducted in China, and is slowly becoming more available to English readers. Papers from the World Conferences for Academic Exchange of Medical Qigong are available in English, and address many medical studies and uses of qigong.

Training and certification

In China, qigong has been subject to much government regulation, from banning to increased requirements for teachers. In the United States at this time, qigong has not been regulated. Different schools may provide teacher training, but there are no generally accepted training standards. Qigong teachings may vary depending on the founder of the school, who is often an acknowledged Chinese master. The organizations listed below can provide further information to consumers.

Resources

BOOKS

Lui, Dr. Hong, and Paul Perry. *Mastering Miracles: The Healing Art of Qi Gong as Taught by a Master.* New York: Warner Books, 1997.

MacRichie, Mames. *Chi Kung: Cultivating Personal Energy.* Boston: Element, 1993.

Reid, Daniel. *A Complete Guide to Chi Gung.* Boston: Shambhala, 1998.

Tzu, Lao. *The Tao Te Ching: A New English Version*, translated by Stephen Mitchell. New York: HarperCollins: 1988.

PERIODICALS

Butow, Phyllis, et al. "A critical review of the effects of medical qigong on quality of life, immune function, and survival in cancer patients." *Integrative Cancer Therapies* 11.2 (2012): 101–110.

Garberg, Jodi, et al. "Qigong massage for motor skills in young children with cerebral palsy and Down syndrome." *AJOT: American Journal of Occupational Therapy* 66.3 (2012): 348.

Jancin, Bruce. "Qigong alleviates chronic fatigue symptoms." *Clinical Psychiatry News* (July 2012): 16.

Klotter, Jule. "Qigong and tai chi." *Townsend Letter* (February–March 2011): 37.

Lynch, Mary, et al. "A randomized controlled trial of qigong for fibromyalgia." *Arthritis Research & Therapy* 14 (2012): R178.

ORGANIZATIONS

Chinese National Chi Kung Institute. PO Box 31578. San Francisco, CA 94131. (800) 824-2433.

International Chi Kung/Qi Gong Directory. 2730 29th Street. Boulder, CO 80301. (303) 442-3131.

Qigong Human Life Research Foundation. PO Box 5327. Cleveland, OH 44101. (216) 475-4712.

Douglas Dupler

Quadriplegia *see* **Paralysis**

Radial keratotomy

Definition

Radial keratotomy (RK) is eye surgery performed to correct **myopia** by changing the cornea's shape.

Purpose

RK was introduced in North America in 1978. RK is one of several surgical techniques for reducing or eliminating the need for corrective lenses. It is most successful in patients with low to moderate nearsightedness—people whose eyes require up to -5.00 diopters of correction.

Precautions

RK cannot help patients whose nearsightedness is caused by keratoconus, a condition in which the cornea is cone shaped. The procedure usually is not performed on patients under 18 because their **vision** is unstable. Women who are pregnant, have just given birth, or are breast-feeding should not have RK because hormones may cause temporary corneal changes. **Glaucoma** patients or patients with any disease that interferes with healing should not have RK.

Radial keratotomy weakens the cornea, making it vulnerable to injuries long after surgery. A **head injury** after RK can cause the cornea to tear and can lead to blindness. Sports enthusiasts should be warned of this danger.

RK's success cannot be guaranteed. An ophthalmologist estimates the probability of the surgery's success in correcting vision. In some cases, patients with myopia that has caused their near vision to be clear prior to surgery may need corrective lenses for near vision following surgery. Some patients still require lenses for distance vision. RK does not eliminate **presbyopia** and the eventual need for reading glasses.

Description

With clear vision, light passes through the cornea and the lens of the eye and focuses on the retina. In a myopic patient, the eyeball is usually too long, so that light focuses in front of the retina. RK reduces myopia by flattening the cornea. This flattening reduces the cornea's focusing power, allowing the light to focus further back onto the retina, forming a clearer image.

For RK, a surgeon uses a small diamond-blade knife to make four to eight radial incisions approaching the edge of the cornea. These slits are made in a pattern that resembles the spokes of wheel. As the cornea heals, its center flattens.

Before surgery the patient is given a sedative. A local anesthetic—usually eye drops—is used to numb the eye. The patient remains conscious during the procedure. The surgeon utilizes a surgical **microscope** to magnify the cornea while making the slits. The treatment usually lasts 30 minutes.

Most ophthalmologists perform RK on one eye at a time. Surgeons once thought they could use the results of the first eye to predict how the well the procedure would work on the second eye. However, a study in the *American Journal of Ophthalmology* in 1997 found that this was not the case. The authors cautioned that there might be other reasons not to operate on both eyes at once, such as increased risk of **infection**.

RK's costs depends on the surgeon, but usually range from $1,000 to $1,500 per eye. It is usually not covered by insurance.

Preparation

RK patients should be carefully screened by an ophthalmic assistant or physician before surgery is approved to avoid possible complications. This screening should include a comprehensive eye exam, either by the ophthalmologist or a co-managing optometrist at least a few days before surgery. At this time, the physician or

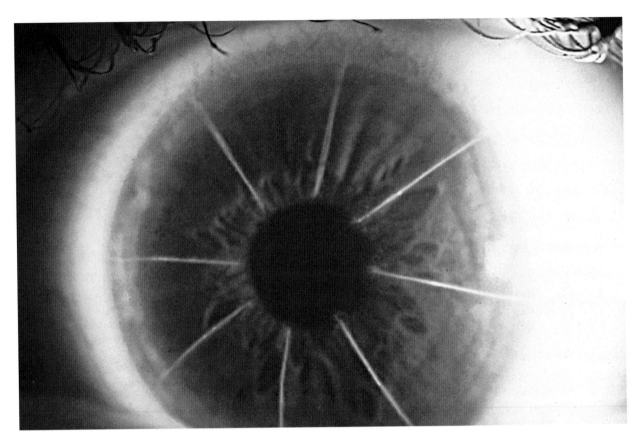

(Radial keratotomy scars on the human eye, photograph by Bob Masini. Phototake NYC. Reproduced by permission.)

ophthalmic assistant should chart any dry eye or any corneal disease that may hinder surgery. They also should perform corneal topography, which creates a map of the patient's eye.

Assistants must advise patients to discontinue wearing **contact lenses** weeks prior to the visual exams to make sure vision is stable; and they must also advise the doctor of contact lens wear.

Before surgery, ophthalmic staff administer eye drops and a sedative to the patient. The physician tests the patient's vision, and the patient rests while waiting for the sedative to take effect. Immediately before the surgery, ophthalmic staff administer local anesthetic eye drops.

Before beginning the procedure, the surgeon measures the cornea's thickness to decide how deep the slits should be, and marks an area in the center of the cornea called the optical zone. This is the part of the cornea in the area over the pupil that the patient sees through. No cuts are made in this region.

Aftercare

After surgery, some patients feel **pain** and are given eye drops and medications to relieve discomfort. For several days the eye may feel scratchy and look red. This is normal. The eye also may water, burn, and be sensitive to light.

Patients should be advised to use eye drops for several weeks to protect against infection. Patients also should be told to protect the head and eyes.

The cornea heals slowly, and full recovery can take months. This is one reason RK has fallen out of favor with surgeons and patients. Laser-refractive surgeries, such as laser-assisted in situ keratomileusis (LASIK), have better results with faster recovery. Such procedures as LASIK and corneal rings have rendered RK virtually obsolete.

While the cornea is healing, patients may experience better eyesight in the morning than in the evening (or vice versa); pain; glare; starburst or halo effects; or a hyperopic shift. As the cornea flattens, vision may become more hyperopic. For this reason, the surgeon may initially undercorrect the patient. This gradual shift may occur over several years. This procedure leaves permanent scars on the cornea.

If RK does not completely correct nearsightedness, corrective lenses may be needed. Presbyopic patients will still require reading glasses.

KEY TERMS

Cornea—The transparent part of the eye that covers the iris and the pupil.

Diopter (D)—Unit describing the amount of focusing power of a lens.

Iris—The colored part of the eye.

Laser-assisted in situ keratomileusis (LASIK)—A type of refractive eye surgery using a laser and microkeratone to change the shape of the cornea.

Local anesthetic—Used to numb an area in which surgery or another procedure is to be done, without causing the patient to lose consciousness.

Myopia—Nearsightedness. People with myopia cannot see distant objects clearly.

Ophthalmologist—A physician who specializes in treating eyes.

Photorefractive keratectomy (PRK)—A type of refractive eye surgery using a laser to change the shape of the cornea.

Pupil—The part of the eye that looks like a black circle in the center of the iris. It is actually an opening through which light passes.

Retina—A membrane lining the back of the eye onto which light is focused to form images.

Patients return to the surgeon for a follow-up exam one day post-operatively. After that, patients may be referred to the co-managing optometrist for the subsequent three or four visits. Patients should be advised to report any pain or nausea immediately to the attending physician.

Complications

Complications from RK include:

• cataract

• infection

• lasting pain

• tears along an incision, especially after being hit in the head or eye

• vision loss

• hyperopic shift

Complications are reduced when an ophthalmologist experienced with RK performs the surgery. Younger patients also tend to heal faster.

Results

The desired result of radial keratotomy is myopia reduction. A study reported by the National Eye Institute in 1994 tracked the success of 374 patients who had RK 10 years earlier. The study found that:

• 85% had at least 20/40 vision.

• 70% did not need corrective lenses for distance vision.

• 53% had 20/20 vision without glasses.

• 30% still needed glasses or contact lenses to see clearly.

• 1–3% had worse vision than before they had RK.

• 40% had a hyperopic shift.

Health care team roles

Allied health professionals help prepare patients for refractive surgery. Advanced and intermediate level ophthalmic technicians perform refractions and help determine the patient's eligibility for surgery. These professionals also may perform corneal topography.

Specially trained ophthalmic nurses assist during surgery. They prepare the operating room and equipment, and administer eye drops. Advanced ophthalmic technologists, who are trained for additional duties such as taking ophthalmic photographs and using ultrasound, may administer eye medications, perform tests, maintain surgical equipment and assist in refractive surgery.

Training

The American Society of Cataract and Refractive Surgery keeps physicians informed of the latest advances in surgery. Optometrists are advised to observe surgeries and attend seminars to learn more about follow-up treatments.

Ophthalmic assistants who want to assist in these surgeries can receive additional training from certified education programs.

Resources

PERIODICALS

Brown, David C., M.D. "How to Diversify." *Ophthalmology Management Online http://www.ophmanagement.com/ archive_results.asp?loc=archive/11119934028pm.html.*

Feldman, Miriam Karmel. "Cataract Warning: RK Patients Need Special Care." *EyeNet Magazine Online http://www. eyenet.org/eyenet_mage/02_00/cataract.html.*

Koffler, Bruce H., M.D. "Post-Op Strategies." *Ophthalmology Management Online http://www.ophmanagement.com/ archive_results.asp?loc= archive/1180041950pm.html.*

OTHER

"Refractive Surgery: New Options in Vision Correction."
American Society of Cataract and Refractive Surgery
Online. http://www.ascrs.org/eye/refract.html.

Snyder, Robert W. "The Differences in Radial Keratotomy
Surgery." The University of Arizona Health Sciences
Center. http://www.ahsc.arizona.edu/opa/crnap/rk.htm.

ORGANIZATIONS

American Academy of Ophthalmology. P.O. Box 7424, San
Francisco, CA 94120-7424. (415) 561-8500. http://www.
eyenet.org.

American Optometric Association. 243 N. Lindbergh Blvd.,
St. Louis, MO 63141. (314) 991-4100. http://www.aoanet.
org/aoanet/.

American Society of Cataract & Refractive Surgery. 4000
Legato Road, Suite 850, Fairfax, VA 22033. (703)
591-2220. http://www.ascrs.org.

Mary Bekker

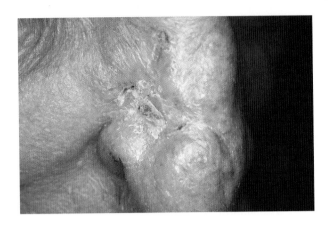

(Radiation injuries, to a person's nose, photograph. Custom Medical Stock Photo. Reproduced by permission.)

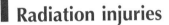

Radiation injuries

Definition

Radiation injuries are caused by ionizing radiation emitted by sources such as the sun, x-ray and other diagnostic machines, tanning beds, and radioactive elements released in nuclear power plant accidents and detonation of nuclear weapons during war and as part of terrorist acts.

Demographics

Anyone has the potential for being injured by radiation, whether it is naturally, such as from a severe sunburn, or artificially, such as from radiation leaked from a nuclear power plant or expelled through a nuclear weapon.

Description

Ionizing radiation is made up of unstable atoms that contain an excess amount of energy. In an attempt to stabilize, the atoms emit the excess energy into the atmosphere, creating radiation. Radiation can either be electromagnetic (in the form of a wave) or particulate.

The energy of electromagnetic radiation is a direct function of its frequency. The high–energy, high–frequency waves that can penetrate solids to various depths cause damage by separating molecules into electrically charged pieces, a process known as ionization. X rays are a type of electromagnetic radiation. Atomic particles come from radioactive isotopes as they decay to stable elements. Electrons are called beta particles when they radiate. Alpha particles are the nuclei of helium atoms—two protons and two neutrons—without the surrounding electrons. Alpha particles are too large to penetrate a piece of paper unless they are greatly accelerated in electric and magnetic fields. Both beta and alpha particles are types of particulate radiation. When over-exposure to ionizing radiation occurs, there is chromosomal damage in deoxyribonucleic acid (DNA). DNA is very good at repairing itself; both strands of the double helix must be broken to produce genetic damage.

Because radiation is energy, it can be measured. There are a number of units used to quantify radiation energy. Some refer to effects on air, others to effects on living tissue. The roentgen, named after German physicist Wilhelm Conrad Röentgen (1845–1923), sometimes spelled Roentgen, who discovered x rays in 1895, measures ionizing energy in air. A rad expresses the energy transferred to tissue. The rem measures tissue response. A roentgen generates about a rad of effect and produces about a rem of response. The gray and the sievert are international units equivalent to 100 rads and rems, respectively. A curie, named after French physicists Marie Curie (1867–1934) and Pierre Curie (1859–1906) who experimented with radiation, is a measure of actual radioactivity given off by a radioactive element, not a measure of its effect. The average annual human exposure to natural background radiation is roughly 3 milliSieverts (mSv).

Any amount of ionizing radiation will produce some damage, as there is radiation everywhere, from the sun (cosmic rays) and from traces of radioactive elements in the air (radon) and the ground (uranium, radium, carbon-14, potassium-40 and many others).

Earth's atmosphere protects humans and other living things from most of the sun's radiation. However, living at 5,000 feet (1,500 m) altitude in Denver, Colorado, approximately doubles exposure to radiation. Further, a flight in a commercial airliner increases it by about 24 times more when lifting humans above 80% of that atmosphere, or at about 32,800 feet (10,000 m) in altitude. Because no amount of radiation is perfectly safe and because radiation is ever present, arbitrary limits have been established to provide some measure of safety for those humans exposed to unusual amounts. Less than 1% of them reach the current annual permissible maximum of 2,000 mrem (20 mSv).

A 2001 ruling by the Federal Court of Australia indicated that two soldiers died from **cancer** caused by exposure to radiation while occupying Hiroshima in 1945. The soldiers were exposed to less than 500 rem (5 Sv) of radiation. The international recommendation for workers, as of 2010 and after more than a century of scientific study, is a safety level of up to 2,000 mrem (20 mSv). Further, according to the U.S. Nuclear Regulatory Commission, the average American nuclear worker receives about 120 mrem (1.2 mSv) per year, while a typical x-ray scan produces about 10 mrem (0.1 mSv).

Many international agencies, such as the International Agency for Research on Cancer (IARC), part of the World Health Organization WHO), suggests that even extremely low doses of radiation can be potentially harmful. For the most part, however, such doses are generally safe for such workers but the potential for harm does exist, as based on internationally recognized scientific studies. Specifically, the IARC conducted an international study of nearly half a million nuclear workers in 15 countries. Their exposure to low levels of radiation was found to be "statistically compatible with the current bases for radiation protection standards."

Ultraviolet (UV) radiation exposure from the sun and tanning beds

UV radiation from the sun (naturally produced by the closest star to earth) and tanning beds and lamps (artificially produced by humans) can cause skin damage, premature **aging**, and skin cancers. Malignant **melanoma** is the most dangerous of skin cancers. Thus, a definite link exists between type UVA exposure used in tanning beds and its occurrence. UVB type UV radiation is associated with sunburn, and while not as penetrating as UVA, it still damages the skin with over exposure. Skin damage accumulates over time, and effects do not often manifest until individuals reach middle age. Light-skinned people who most often burn rather than tan are at a greater risk of skin damage than darker-skinned

individuals who almost never burn. The U.S. Food and Drug Administration (FDA) and the Centers for Disease Control and Prevention (CDC) discourage the use of tanning beds and sun lamps and encourage all people to use sunscreen with at least a sun protection factor (SPF) of 15 or greater. In 2009, the International Agency for Research on Cancer classified tanning beds as "carcinogenic to humans," with carcinogenic meaning that it causes cancer. This classification by the IARC is its highest cancer risk category. In fact, IARC studies that prompted the cancer classification found UVA, UVB, and UVC radiation all cause cancer in laboratory animals.

Over exposure during medical procedures

Ionizing radiation has many uses in medicine, both in diagnosis and in treatment. X rays, CT (computed tomography) scanners, and fluoroscopes use it to form images of the body's insides. Nuclear medicine uses radioactive isotopes to diagnose and to treat medical conditions. In the body, radioactive elements localize to specific tissues and give off tiny amounts of radiation. Detecting that radiation provides information on both **anatomy** and function. During the past 15 years, skin injuries caused by too much exposure during medical procedures have been documented. In 1995, the FDA issued a recommendation to physicians and medical institutions to record and monitor the dosage of radiation used during medical procedures on patients in order to minimize the amount of skin injuries. The FDA suggested doses of radiation not exceed 1 Grey (Gy). (A Grey is roughly equivalent to a sievert.)

As of 2001, the FDA was preparing further guidelines for fluoroscopy, the procedure most often associated with medical-related radiation skin injuries such as rashes and more serious **burns** and tissue death. Injuries occurred most often during **angioplasty** procedures using fluoroscopy. As of September 3, 2010, the FDA is still in the process of issuing updated guidelines for radiation safety performance standards for diagnostic x-ray systems, such as flurorscopic x-ray systems. These updated standards will better parallel with new developments in technology and product usage, along with being more similar to international standards.

CT scans of children have also been problematic. Oftentimes the dosage of radiation used for an adult is not decreased for a child, leading to radiation over exposure. Children are more sensitive to radiation and a February 2001 study indicates 1,500 out of 1.6 million children under 15 years of age receiving CT scans annually will develop cancer. Studies show that decreasing the radiation by half for CT scans of children will effectively decrease the possibility of over exposure while still providing an effective diagnostic image. The benefits to receiving the medical treatment utilizing radiation is still greater than the risks involved, however, more stringent control over the amount of radiation used during the procedures will go far to minimize the risk of radiation injury to the patient. As of the latest information available from the Alliance for Radiation Safety in Pediatric Imaging (ARSPI), its article *What Parents Should Know About CT Scans for Children: Medical Radiation Safety* states, "The estimated increased risk of cancer over a person's lifetime from a single CT scan is controversial but has been estimated to be a fraction of this risk (0.03–0.05%). These estimates for the population as a whole do not represent a direct risk to one child. This information shows that the risk of developing cancer related to a single CT scan is very small, but the available research indicates that there may be some risk and the risk may be cumulative."

The ARSPI's Image Gently Campaign promotes minimizing the risk of medical radiation exposure in children by doing the following:

- only image when there is a definite medical benefit

- use the minimum amount of radiation for adequate imaging based on size of the child

- image only the indicated area

- avoid multiple scans

- use alternative diagnostic studies (such as ultrasound or MRI [magnetic resonance imaging]) when possible

Radiation exposure from nuclear accidents, weaponry, and terrorist acts

Between 1945 and 1987, there were 285 nuclear reactor accidents, injuring over 1,550 people and killing 64. The most striking example was the meltdown of the graphite core nuclear reactor at Chernobyl (in the Ukraine, of the former Soviet Union) in 1986, which spread a cloud of radioactive particles across the entire continent of Europe. Information about radiation effects is still being gathered from that disaster, however 31 people were killed in the immediate accident, and at least 1,800 children have thus far been diagnosed with thyroid cancer. In a study published in May 2001 by the British Royal Society, children born to individuals involved in the cleanup of Chernobyl and born after the accident are 600% more likely to have genetic mutations than children born before the accident. These findings indicate that exposure to low doses of radiation can cause inheritable effects.

Since the terrorist attacks on the World Trade Center and the Pentagon on September 11, 2001, the possibility of terrorist-caused nuclear accidents has been a growing concern. As of 2008, All 104 active nuclear power plants in the United States are on full alert, but they are still vulnerable to sabotage such as bombing or attack from the air. The Federal Aviation Administration (FAA) has established a no-fly zone of 12 miles (19 km), at an altitude of below 18,000 feet (5,500 m), around nuclear power plants. There is also growing concern over the security of spent nuclear fuel—more than 40,000 tons of spent fuel is housed in buildings at closed plants around the country. Unlike the active nuclear reactors that are enclosed in concrete-reinforced buildings, the spent fuel is stored in non-reinforced buildings. Housed in cooling pools, the spent fuel could emit dangerous levels of radioactive material if exploded or used in makeshift weaponry. Radioactive medical and industrial waste could also be used to make "dirty bombs." Since 1993, the Nuclear Regulatory Commission (NRC) has reported 376 cases of stolen radioactive materials.

On March 15, 2011, the Japanese government imposed a 18-mile (30-km) no-fly zone around the Fukushima Daiichi Nuclear Power Plant after it was damaged from a 9.0-magnitude earthquake (commonly called the 2011 Tōhoku earthquake) that hit on March 11, 2011, off the coast of northeastern Japan. At least three nuclear reactors sustained explosions due to the deadly earthquake, which caused a build-up of gas within their containment walls. On March 18, 2011, the International Atomic Energy Agency (IAEA) described the situation as "extremely serious."

Causes and symptoms

Radiation can be caused by accidental exposure to high doses of radiation, such as from a nuclear bomb or an accident from a nuclear power plant. It can also be caused by excessive exposure to radiation from medical equipment, such as in treatments by patients or by improper use of such equipment by medical personnel.

Radiation can damage every tissue in the body. The particular manifestation will depend upon the amount of radiation, the time over which it is absorbed, and the susceptibility of the tissue. The fastest growing tissues are the most vulnerable, because radiation as much as triples its effects during the growth phase. **Bone** marrow cells that make **blood** are the fastest growing cells in the body. A fetus in the womb is equally sensitive. The germinal cells in the testes and ovaries are only slightly less sensitive. Both can be rendered useless with very small doses of radiation. More resistant are the lining cells of the body—skin and intestines. Most resistant are the **brain** cells, because they grow the slowest.

Many signs and symptoms can occur after a person has been exposed to a large amount of radiation. Some of these signs and symptoms from radiation sickness (radiation **poisoning**) include:

- Bleeding of the mouth, gums, nose, and rectum
- Bloody stool
- Bruising of the body
- Burning of the skin
- Dehydration
- Diarrhea
- Fainting and dizziness
- Fatigue, tiredness, and weakness
- Hair loss
- Inflammation of body areas (that were not covered at the time of exposure)
- Mouth ulcers
- Open sores on skin, especially those uncovered at the time of radiation exposure
- Vomiting and nausea
- Ulcers of the mouth
- Ulcers of the esophagus, intestines, and stomach

The length of exposure makes a big difference in what happens. Over time the accumulating damage, if not enough to kill cells outright, distorts their growth and causes scarring and/or cancers. In addition to leukemias, cancers of the thyroid, brain, bone, breast, skin, **stomach**, and lung all arise after radiation. Damage depends, too, on the ability of the tissue to repair itself. Some tissues and some types of damage produce much greater consequences than others.

There are three types of radiation injuries.

- External irradiation: as with x-ray exposure, all or part of the body is exposed to radiation that either is absorbed or passes through the body
- Contamination: as with a nuclear accident, the environment and its inhabitants are exposed to radiation. People are affected internally, externally, or with both internal and external exposure
- Incorporation: dependent on contamination, the bodies of individuals affected incorporate the radiation chemicals within cells, organs, and tissues and the radiation is dispersed throughout the body

Immediately after sudden irradiation, the fate of those affected depends mostly on the total dose absorbed. This information comes mostly from survivors of the two atomic bomb blasts over Japan in 1945.

- Massive doses incinerate immediately and are not distinguishable from the heat of the source
- A sudden whole body dose over 50 Sv (5,000 rem, or 5 mrem) produces such profound neurological, heart, and circulatory damage that patients die within the first two days (100 percent chance of fatalities)
- Doses around 10 to 20 Sv (1,000 to 2,000rem, or 1 to 2 mrem) range affect the intestines, stripping their lining and leading to death within three months from vomiting, diarrhea, starvation, and infection
- Victims receiving around 6 to 10 Sv (600 to 1,000 rem, or 0.6 to 1.0 mrem) all at once usually escape an intestinal death, facing instead bone marrow failure and death within two months from loss of blood coagulation factors and the protection against infection provided by white blood cells
- A dose of from 2 to 6 Sv (200 to 600 rem, or 1 to 2 mrem) gives a fighting chance for survival if victims are supported with blood transfusions and antibiotics (generally no fatalities occur if proper medical procedures are followed)
- People suffering from 1 to 2 Sv (100 to 200 rem, or 0.5 to 1.0 mrem) will have a brief, non-lethal sickness with vomiting, loss of appetite, and generalized discomfort. At this level, victims still receive several thousand times more than an average person does in normal exposure over one year

Diagnosis

Diagosis of a person who has been exposed to a high dose of radiation should seek out immediate assistance from medical personnel. When a known major incident has occurred, medical personnel will be at the site within a short period. In any case, medical personnel will take the necessary steps to measure the amount of radiation absorbed into the body of these victims. The amount of radiation absorbed into the human victims will dictate which treatments will be used and how likely the person will survive over the next few days, weeks, and months.

The following are critical information to acquire in order to provide the best diagnosis and, thus, treatment, for these victims. This vital information is:

- Symptoms: Check for onset of vomiting and other signs and symptoms with respect to the time of initial exposure (generally, the shorter [longer] the time of vomiting from initial exposure, the higher [lower] the radiation dose received)
- Distance from source: Determine the distance the victim was from the radiation source, along with the

KEY TERMS

Computed tomography—A medical imaging method that uses tomography along with computer processing to generate three-dimensional images from a series of two-dimensional x-ray images.

Deoxyribonucleic acid(DNA)—The chemical of chromosomes and hence the vehicle of heredity.

Dirty bomb—A radiological weapon that combines radioactive material and conventional explosives; in other words, a conventional bomb could be exploded near radioactive material causing the area to become contaminated with radioactive material.

Gray—Abbreviated Gy, it is an unit within the International System of Units (SI) that refers to absorbed radiation dose of ionizing radiation. One Gray is defined as the absorption of one joule of ionizing radiation by one kilogram of matter.

Isotope—An unstable form of an element that gives off radiation to become stable. Elements are characterized by the number of electrons around each atom. One electron's negative charge balances the positive charge of each proton in the nucleus. To keep all those positive charges in the nucleus from repelling each other (like the same poles of magnets), neutrons are added. Only certain numbers of neutrons work. Other numbers cannot hold the nucleus together, so it splits apart, giving off ionizing radiation. Sometimes one of the split products is not stable either, so another split takes place. The process is called radioactivity.

Rem—short for roentgen equivalent in man, rem is a dose equivalent radiation. One rem is equal to 0.01 Sievert (Sv).

Sievert—Abbreviated Sv, it is a unit of dose equivalent radiation in the International System of Units (SI). One Sv is equal to 100 rem, or 100,000 millirem (mrem).

Tomography—Any of a number of medical imaging procedures that image sections of a body with the use of various types of penetrating waves, such as x rays.

UVA—Ultraviolet A is a long wave of ultraviolet radiation, with a wavelength of 400 to 315 nanometers and an energy level of 3.10 to 3.94 electron volts.

UVB—Ultraviolet B is a medium wave of ultraviolet radiation, with a wavelength of 315 to 280 nanometers and an energy level of 3.94 to 4.43 electron volts.

UVC—Ultraviolet C is a short wave of ultraviolet radiation, with a wavelength of 280 to 1000 nanometers and an energy level of 4.43 to 12.4 electron volts.

duration of the exposure (generally, the further away from [closer to] the radiation source, the less [more] radiation exposure)

- Blood tests: Take blood tests over several days to determine white blood cell counts and any changes in the DNA of blood cells (which help to verify the amount of bone marrow damage and, thus, the amount of radioactive material in the body)

- Dosimeter: If such a device was exposed to the same radiation event, it can be effectively used to compare the amount absorbed by people

- Geiger counter: A survey-meter device can be scanned across the body of people to determine the amount of radioactive particles on the victim

- Radiation type: A determination as to the type of radiation people have been exposed to can help to treat victims in a more effective manner

Treatment

It is clearly important to have some idea of the dose received as early as possible, so that attention can be directed to those victims in the 2–10 Sv range that might survive with treatment. Blood transfusions, protection from **infection** in damaged organs, and possibly the use of newer stimulants to blood formation can save many victims in this category.

Local radiation exposures usually damage the skin and require careful **wound care**, removal of dead tissue, and skin grafting if the area is large. Again **infection control** is imperative.

One of the best known, and perhaps even mainstream, treatments of radiation injury is the use of *Aloe vera* preparations on damaged areas of skin. It has demonstrated remarkable healing properties even for chronic ulcerations resulting from radiation exposure.

QUESTIONS TO ASK YOUR DOCTOR

- What should I do if I begin to show signs and symptoms from radiation exposure?
- What should I expect from the side effects of radiation? Are there any long-term effects that I should be concerned about?
- How much radiation have I been exposed to?
- What is my prognosis for recovery? What are my chances of surviving? Could I die?
- Are there special medical facilities treat people with radiation exposure? Is so, how do I contact them?

Alternative treatment

There is considerable interest these days in benevolent chemicals called "free radical scavengers." How well they work is yet to be determined, but population studies strongly suggest that certain diets are better than others, and that those diets are full of free radical scavengers, otherwise known as antioxidants. The recommended ingredients are beta-carotene, **vitamins** E and C, and selenium, all available as commercial preparations. Beta-carotene is yellow-orange and is present in yellow and orange fruits and vegetables. **Vitamin C** can be found naturally in citrus fruits. Traditional Chinese medicine (TCM) and **acupuncture**, botanical medicine, and **homeopathy** all have contributions to make to recovery from the damage of radiation injuries. The level of recovery will depend on the exposure. Consulting practitioners trained in these modalities will result in the greatest benefit.

Prognosis

The degree to which one has been exposed to radiation and to the length of time of that exposure will determine the prognosis of individual cases. If people survive ten to fifteen years after the radiation exposure, most illnesses associated with the exposure will have presented themselves. Illnesses involving the endocrine glands, thyroid, nervous system, digestive organs, and sensory organs seem to be especially prevalent in such people.

Prevention

Injuries caused by radiation exposure can be avoided by not working or living around known sources of radiation. If such sites cannot be avoided, then workers should wear badges that consistently measure exposure levels. When being diagnosed or treated with radiation, make sure protective shields are used over the body not be diagnosed or treated. In addition, discuss with your family doctor or other medical professions whenever radiation devices are used to make sure they are essentially needed.

Resources

BOOKS

Adler, Arlene M, and Richard R. Carlton, editors. *Introduction to Radiologic Sciences and Patient Care*. St. Louis: Elsevier Saunders, 2012.

Khalil, Magdy M. *Basic Sciences of Nuclear Medicine*. Berlin: Springer, 2011.

Saha, Gopal B. *Fundamentals of Nuclear Pharmacy*. New York: Springer, 2010.

Yarbro, Connie Henke, Debra Wujcik, and Barbara Holmes Gobel, editors. *Cancer Nursing: Principles and Practice*. Sudbury, MA: Jones and Bartlett, 2011.

OTHER

"How Radioactivity Can Affect You." Oasis LLC. http://www.oasisllc.com/abgx/effects.htm (accessed March 22, 2011).

"Japan Imposes No-Fly Zone Above Crippled Nuclear Plant." NYC Aviation News. (March 15, 2011). http://nycaviation.com/2011/03/japan-imposes-no-fly-zone-above-crippled-nuclear-plant/ (accessed March 22, 2011).

"Japan's crisis extremely serious: IAEA chief." Hindustan Times. (March 18, 2011). http://www.hindustantimes.com/News-Feed/restofasia/IAEA-chief-says-Japan-s-crisis-extremely-serious/Article1-674806.aspx (accessed March 22, 2011).

"Radiation-Emitting Products: Medical Imaging." U.S. Food and Drug Administration. (October 3, 2010). http://www.fda.gov/Radiation-EmittingProducts/RadiationEmittingProductsandProcedures/MedicalImaging/MedicalX-Rays/ucm135572.htm (accessed March 22, 2011).

"Radiation Sickness." Mayo Clinic. (March 17, 2011). http://www.mayoclinic.com/health/radiation-sickness/DS00432 (accessed March 22, 2011).

"Radiation Sickness." MedlinePlus, U.S. National Library of Medicine and National Institutes of Health. (January 8, 2009). http://www.nlm.nih.gov/medlineplus/ency/article/000026.htm (accessed March 22, 2011).

"Radiation Standards and Organizations Provide Safety for Public and Workers." Nuclear Energy Institute. (October 2010). http://www.nei.org/resourcesandstats/documentlibrary/safetyandsecurity/factsheet/radiationstandards/ (accessed March 22, 2011).

"WHO: Tanning Beds Cause Cancer." World Health Organization. (July 28, 2009). http://www.webmd.com/skin-problems-and-treatments/news/20090728/who-tanning-beds-cause-cancer (accessed March 22, 2011).

ORGANIZATION

International Agency for Research on Cancer, 150 Cours Albert Thomas, CEDEX 08, Lyon France 69372, 33 (0)4 72 73 8485, Fax: 33 (0)4 72 73 8575, http://www.iarc.fr/.

Jacqueline L. Longe

Radiation sickness *see* **Radiation injuries**

Radiation treatments *see* **Radiotherapy**

Radioactive iodine uptake test *see* **Thyroid radionuclide scan**

Radioallergosorbent test (RAST) *see* **Allergy tests**

Radioimmunoassay *see* **Immunoassay tests**

Radiologic technology

Definition

Radiologic technology is a general term applied to the allied health profession that encompasses the use of ionizing radiation (x ray), sound or radio waves, radioactive substances to produce an image, and magnetic imaging. These resultant images are used by the radiologist to help in making a diagnosis.

Description

Radiologic technology is a broad-based category that includes general x ray, ultrasound, **mammography**, nuclear medicine, computerized axial tomography (CAT scan), radiation therapy, and **magnetic resonance imaging** (MRI). General x-ray technology is a primary link between the physician and the diagnosis. X rays are often required so that the physician can diagnose and treat the patient based on the patients' complaints or conditions.

The x-ray image is created by the controlled and careful use of radiation through the body part being examined. The image is captured on a film, which is placed under the patient. The x-ray beam passes through the body part being examined, and creates a latent image on the film. The latent image is processed, and then is evaluated by the radiologist, with the written and/or verbal report given to the referring physician. Some examples of subspecialties of medical radiography are contrast studies, **pediatrics**, trauma, surgery, and special procedures (e.g., **angiography** or other interventional procedures).

Mammography is another name for breast imaging and evaluation of breast disease. Mammographers are radiographers who are proficient in screening and diagnostic imaging, as well as interventional procedures such as needle localizations (pre-biopsy), core biopsies, and **breast ultrasound**.

Ultrasonography is the imaging of **anatomy** using high frequency sound waves. The sonographer obtains diagnostic images or patterns that the physician evaluates in the diagnosis of disease. A scan is created by using gel and a transducer, or probe, moving it over the surface of the relevant anatomy. The transducer bounces sound into and back from the anatomic area, and an image is then created on the monitor attached to the machine. This specialty has several distinct areas: **abdominal ultrasound**, adult and pediatric **echocardiography**, obstetrical-gynecological ultrasound, and vascular ultrasound.

Nuclear medicine is very different from medical radiography, because in radiography the x-ray beam from the machine is the source of radiation. It is instantaneous and is controlled by the technical factors selected by the radiographer. In nuclear medicine, the patient becomes the source of radiation, and the radiation itself is constantly emitted. The patient orally ingests or is intravenously injected with a radioactive substance, or radioisotope. The images are 'collected' via the nuclear medicine camera sorting radioactive signals from the patient. The radioactivity levels are different for the body part or organs being imaged. The nuclear medicine technologist has protocols that are followed for selecting the type of radioisotope to inject, based on the exams ordered.

Computerized axial tomography, or CAT scans, are studies that image the body using multiple projections of the x-ray beam to create sectional images of an organ or anatomic region. These axial sections are selected and manipulated by the technologist, using computer programs that direct the protocols for these exams.

The radiation therapy technologist applies therapeutic radiation doses in strictly controlled circumstances to cure or arrest disease. In daily or weekly contact with the **cancer** patient, and working directly with the physician, the technologist assists in the calculation of radiation dosage and operates a variety of sophisticated radiation treatment equipment and instruments, including computers.

MRI (magnetic resonance imaging) uses radio waves and a strong magnetic field rather than ionizing radiation to provide three-dimensional images of the organs or body structures being examined. The technique has

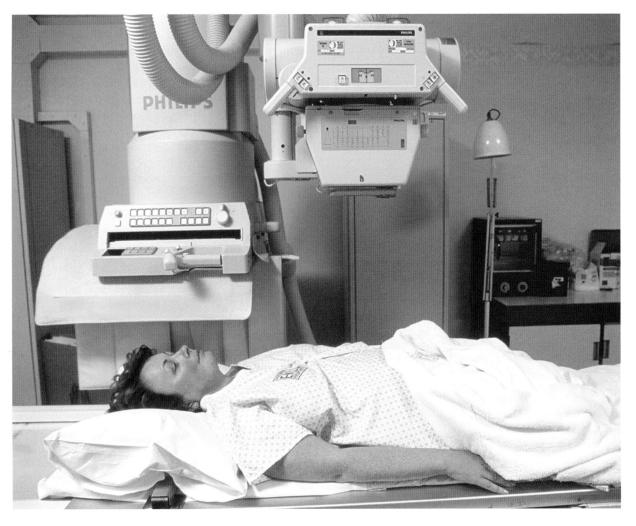

(Woman undergoing urography, or pyelography, x-rays of the urinary tract, photograph. Josh Sher / Photo Researchers, Inc.)

proven critical in diagnosing a variety of conditions throughout the body, including cancer, cardiovascular disease, **stroke**, and **bone** and joint disorders. MRI requires specialized equipment and expertise and allows evaluation of some body structures that may not be as visible with more conventional imaging methods. MRI is highly accurate in showing soft tissue structures near and around bones, the **cardiovascular system**, as well as major organs. Additionally, because it is a non-ionizing modality, it is gaining increasing popularity in imaging the reproductive system.

Work settings

The majority of **radiology** technologists work in a hospital setting. Others are employed in government, health industries, **public health**, mental health, education, private offices and clinics. Those professionals with advanced degrees might also pursue careers in the areas

of management, quality control, equipment maintenance, or application specialties.

Education and training

The radiologic technologist must first complete a two-year accredited radiology technology program. This consists of both classroom and clinical training. Typically, student radiographers will demonstrate their ongoing training in the classroom, and will rotate through each segment of the radiology department. The students will work with the registered technologist, and must show clinical competency prior to working independently. The students will pass clinical tests in order to progress through the training process. Upon completion of the program, the students will be required to take the national registry exam given by the American Registry of Radiologic Technology (ARRT). This is a national registry for technologists

KEY TERMS

Contrast—A substance used by injection or ingestion to demonstrate certain organs or anatomy.

Latent image—The x-ray image created on film, prior to development.

Processing—Film development.

Radioactive—Giving off radiation.

Radioisotope—A chemical element used in injections for nuclear medicine that can be detected in the body by the emission of radiation.

Radiologist—The physician who interprets the films and makes a diagnosis.

mandated. In some cases, both clinical and didactic requirements exist. Some disciplines will require approximately one year beyond the requisite radiography coursework, such as sonography, CAT scan, MRI, and mammography. As a nuclear medicine technologist, it is the standard to obtain a four-year university degree. In each case, the technologist needs recorded hours of clinical experience in the core discipline. The registered technologist (RT) must also document 24 hours of continuing education credits every two years in order to maintain certification and compliance with the ARRT as well as with state and federal agencies that regulate certain areas such as mammography.

Future outlook

Employment opportunities for radiologic technologists continue to expand. These professionals are expected to be increasingly in demand due to technological expansions, and the increased need for faster, more detailed diagnoses. As technology refines, so must the varying disciplines of radiologic technology. With the introduction of digital imaging, and better quality equipment and contrast media, changes continue at breakneck speed. In addition, access to higher technology

who pass and maintain the standards set forth by this organization.

Advanced education and training

For those radiographers that choose to specialize in the previously mentioned areas, further study is

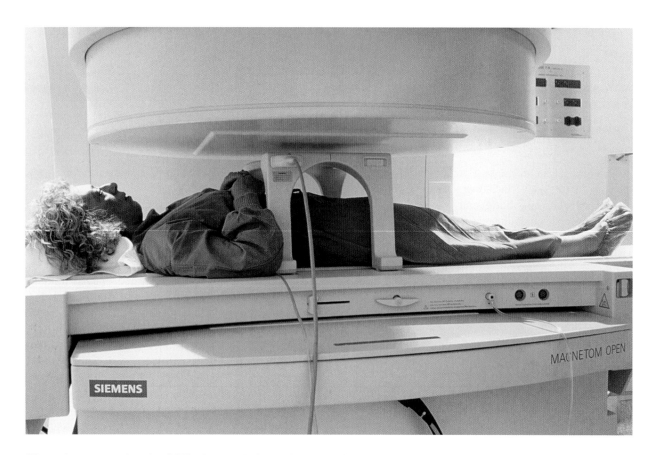

(Magnetic resonance imaging (MRI), photograph. Mauro Fermariello / Photo Researchers, Inc.)

has become more widespread as these newer modalities become the gold standard in some cases. Although this is positive for the profession, there continues to be a shortage of primary x-ray technologists, as those new graduates pursue specialties and bigger salaries. This specialization, while important, has caused serious hardship in many radiology departments, working with staffing shortages and creating tech fatigue, while the demand remains high. This is a challenge that is being addressed industry-wide.

Resources

BOOK

Brant, William E., and Clyde A. Helms, eds. *Fundamentals of Diagnostic Radiology*. Philadelphia: Lippincott, Williams & Wilkins Publishing, 1999.

PERIODICAL

Cruise, Kristi R. L., and James Robert Cruise. "Radiology Administrators' Opinions of Education." *Journal of the American Society of Radiologic Technologists* 72 (March-April, 2001), 314-319.

ORGANIZATIONS

American Society of Radiologic Technologists (ASRT). 15000 Central Ave. SE, Albuquerque, NM 87123-3917. (800) 444-2778 or (505) 298-4500. Fax: (505) 298-5063. http://www.asrt.org.
Radiological Society of North America (RSNA). 820 Jorie Boulevard, Oak Brook, IL 60523-2251. http://www.rsna.org.

Debra Novograd, B.S., R.T.(R)(M)

Radiology

Definition

Radiology is a specialized branch of medicine that uses imaging for diagnosis and treatment.

Description

Radiology uses various types of rays (x rays, radio waves, ultrasound, gamma rays) in conjunction with computer technology to see inside the body. A physician who specializes in this branch of medicine is called a radiologist. The radiologist often is assisted by a radiologist assistant, a radiologic technician, and sometimes a radiologic nurse. However, only a physician can make the official interpretation of images.

There are two main types of radiologists: diagnostic radiologists and interventional radiologists. Diagnostic radiologists look at images and interpret what is occurring in the body as an aid to treatment. Interventional radiologists use guided imagery to perform minimally invasive treatments. Diagnostic radiologists can specialize in certain parts of the body such as breast imaging or cardiovascular (**heart** and **blood vessels**) imaging. Interventional radiologists can specialize in specific procedures (e.g., angiograms or stent placement) or treating specific diseases. (e.g., **oncology** (**cancer**) radiologists).

The most familiar radiologic procedure is the plain x ray. In this procedure, which is painless, a body part is exposed to a safe, low dose or radiation (x rays). The amount of radiation that passes through a material depends on its density. As a result, on a photographic plate or screen located behind the body part being x rayed, **bone**, the most dense material, shows up as white. Muscles and other soft tissue show up as gray. Air shows up as black. So, for example, a broken bone will appear white with a darker line at the site of the break.

Since the 1970s, other imaging techniques developed in tandem with increased computing power. Among the imaging techniques radiologist use today are:

• computed tomography (CT). CT works on the same principle as plain x rays, only an x-ray tube circulates around the body taking hundreds of images that are then combined by a computer

• magnetic resonance imaging (MRI). Instead of x rays, MRI uses a combination of radio waves and strong magnets to produce images that are then processed by a computer. MRI produces better pictures of soft tissue than plain x rays. It is often used to diagnose muscle and joint injuries, heart defects, and brain damage. Because MRI does not use x rays, it is safer for patients, especially children.

• ultrasound. Ultrasound images are created using the echoes of high frequency sound waves. Because no radiation is used, ultrasound images are extremely safe. Ultrasound is often used to examine the development of the fetus in a pregnant woman.

Fluoroscopy is the technique of introducing a contrast material into the body. The contrast material acts as a dye that is visible on x-ray film. When combined with imaging techniques, the contrast material allows the radiologist to see the movement of body fluids in real time. For example, the radiologist can see **blood** flowing through arteries and determine where a blockage occurs. Fluoroscopy is used by interventional radiologists to guide their miniature instruments to the area needing treatment.

Origins

In 1895, German physicist Wilhelm Conrad Roentgen discovered a new type of ray when he passed an electric current through a tube containing a gas at very low pressure. He called these rays x rays (x designating unknown) and observed that they caused fluorescence on a cardboard painted with barium platinocyanide. After more experimentation, he determined that the rays would differentially pass through the body and create an image on a treated screen. It is said that the first radiograph, or what is now commonly called a plain x ray, was of the bones in his wife's hand. Other scientists confirmed his Roentgen's findings, and he was awarded the Nobel Prize in physics in 1901.

The application of x rays to diagnosing damage to the body was immediately apparent, and the science of radiology was born. Initially, the apparatus to create radiographs was large, awkward, and difficult to use. The equipment was first operated by physicians, but as early as 1903, training courses were established to teach nonphysicians how to use x-ray machines. The x-ray technicians, known as radiographers, soon became an important part of the diagnostic process. In 1920 in Great Britain, the Society of Radiographers was founded as a professional organization for x-ray operators.

Over time x-ray machines were refined, and x rays became a common diagnostic tool in hospitals. The machines were not without problems, however. X-ray tubes initially were not shielded, exposing the operator to high levels of radiation that could result in damage or death. Shielding became standard in the 1920s, as the effects of radiation exposure were better understood. Other refinements, including improved photographic plates, the use of lower and safer levels of radiation to create radiographs, and better shielding of patients, occurred throughout the second half of the twentieth century.

For years, x rays were taken using photographic plates that had to be developed. Improved computing power in the 1980s allowed diagnostic x rays to be recorded as digital images. Not only are digital x rays available immediately, they can be stored digitally and transmitted over the internet to physicians in other locations.

In the second half of the twentieth century, other imagining techniques combined with greater computing power produced new ways for radiologists to diagnose and treat the body. Computed tomography, ultrasound imaging, and magnetic resonance have in replaced plain x rays as the diagnostic tool of choice in many situations.

In the mid-1960s, radiologists began to combine guided imaging techniques occurring in real time with minimally invasive treatments. One of the earliest applications of this combination was the angiogram.

KEY TERMS

Angiogram—An x-ray (radiographic) study of the blood vessels. An angiogram uses a radiopaque substance, or contrast medium, to make the blood vessels visible under x ray.

Catheter—A long, thin, flexible tube that can be inserted into a vein and moved through the cardiovascular system.

Stent—A device made of expandable, metal mesh that is placed (by using a balloon catheter) at the site of a narrowing artery; the stent stays in place to keep the artery open.

Contrast material injected into the bloodstream allowed radiologists to see blood vessels and then to guide a catheter through the blood vessel and unblock or repair it. Charles Dotter, a pioneer of this technique, was awarded the Nobel Prize in medicine in 1978.

From Dotter's work developed a subspecialty known as interventional radiology. Interventional radiology allows many patients who would formerly needed open surgery to be treated with minimally invasive techniques using miniature instruments inserted through small incisions in the skin and blood vessels guided by real time imaging. The Society of Interventional Radiologists (originally called the Society of Cardiovascular Radiology) was formed in 1974. Today interventional radiologists continue to pioneer minimally invasive treatments that are safer for patients than open surgery.

Purpose

Radiology serves two purposes: diagnosis and treatment. The type of imaging used depends on the part of the body being examined or treated.

Training and certification

Radiologists are medical doctors (MDs) or doctors of **osteopathy** (DOs) who have completed four years of study at an accredited medical school. In the United States, they also complete a one-year internship and a four-year residency in radiology along with various licensing examinations. Following the residency, a radiologist may enter a one- or two-year fellowship in one of the various radiology subspecialties. A board certified radiologist has passed examinations given by the American Board of Radiology (MDs) or the American Osteopathic Board of Radiology (ODs). Continuing education classes and re-certification examinations are required at specific intervals to maintain certification. Comparable education and training is required in most European countries, although programs and examinations are structured slightly differently.

Radiologist assistants complete a four-year university degree and often a master's degree followed by a clinical internship supervised by a radiologist. Radiologist assistants are certifed by the American Registry of Radiologic Technologists.

Radiologic technologists usually have a two-year academic degree (associate's degree) or two years of formal training in a vocational school. They usually specialize in working with only one type of imaging equipment. Radioligic technologists are certified by the American Society of Radiologic Technologists.

Resources

PERIODICAL

"Global Statement Defining Interventional Radiology." *Journal of Vascular Interventional Radiology.* (2010) 21:1147–1149. http://www.sirweb.org/news/newsPDF/IR_Global_Statement.pdf

OTHER

D'Allesandro, Michael P. RadiologyEducation.com [accessed August 20, 2012]. http://www.radiologyeducation.com.

Radiological Society of North America. RadiologyInfo.org. 2012 [accessed August 20, 2012]. http://www.radiologyinfo.org.

ORGANIZATIONS

American College of Radiology, 1891 Preston White Drive, Reston, VA 20191, (703) 648-8900, http://www.acr.org

Radiological Society of North America, 820 Jorie Blvd, Oak Brook, IL Oak Brook, IL 60523-2251, (630) 571-2670, (800) 381-6660, Fax: (630) 571-7837, http://www.rsna.org

Society of Interventional Radiology, 3975 Fair Ridge Drive, Suite 400 North, Fairfax, VA 22033, (703) 691-1805, Fax: (703) 691-1855, http://www.sirweb.org.

Tish Davidson, AM

Radiotherapy

Definition

Radiotherapy is the use of high-energy penetrating radiation (x rays, gamma rays, proton rays, and neutron rays) to kill **cancer** cells.

Purpose

The primary purpose of radiotherapy is to eliminate or shrink localized cancers. It is also sometimes used to treat metastases—often **brain** metastases—in cases in which surgical treatment would be riskier. The aim of radiotherapy is to kill as many cancer cells as possible, while doing as little damage as possible to healthy tissue. In some cases, the purpose is to kill all cancer cells and effect a cure. In other cases, when cures are not possible, the purpose is to alleviate the patient's **pain** by reducing the size of the tumors that cause pain.

For some kinds of cancers (for example, Hodgkin's disease, non-Hodgkin's **lymphoma**, **prostate cancer**, and laryngeal cancer), radiotherapy alone is often the preferred treatment. Radiation is, however, also used in conjunction with surgery, **chemotherapy**, or both; and survival rates for combination therapy in these cases are often greater than survival rates for any single treatment modality used alone. Radiotherapy is especially useful when surgical procedures cannot remove an entire tumor without damaging the function of surrounding organs. In these cases, surgeons remove as much tumor mass as possible, and the remainder is treated with radiation (irradiated).

Precautions

Radiotherapy has serious side effects; therefore, anyone considering it should be sure that it is the best possible treatment option for their cancer. Cancer treatment research moves so rapidly that some doctors may not be aware of the latest advances in treatments outside their own specialties that might be safer and better. Accordingly, patients who have had radiotherapy recommended to them should consider getting a second opinion.

Description

Radiotherapy is also known as radiation therapy, radiation treatment, x-ray therapy, cobalt therapy, and electron beam or "gamma knife" therapy. Recent advances in medical technology have made it even more useful for patients and have reduced some of its unpleasant side effects. Radioactive implants allow delivery of radiation to localized areas, with less injury to surrounding tissues than radiation from an external source that must pass through those tissues. Proton radiation also causes less injury to surrounding tissues than traditional photon radiation, because proton rays can be tightly focused. Current research with radioimmunotherapy and neutron capture therapy may provide ways to direct radiation exclusively to cancer cells—and in the

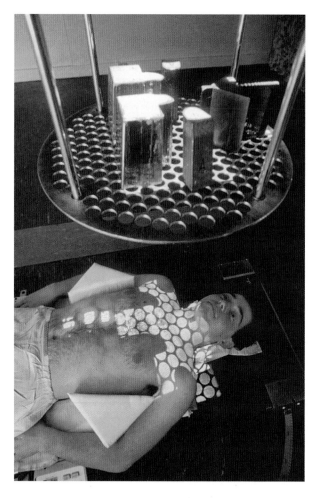

(Patient undergoing radiotherapy on a linear accelerator to treat Hodgkins disease, a cancer of the lymphatic system, photograph. Martin Dohrn / Photo Researchers, Inc.)

case of radioimmunotherapy, to cancer cells that have metastasized (spread to other sites throughout the body).

How radiotherapy works

High-energy radiation kills cells by damaging their DNA and thus blocking their ability to divide and proliferate. Other cytotoxic mechanisms include the production of poisonous OH⁻ free radicals in the cellular cytoplasm.

Radiation kills normal cells about as well as cancer cells, but cells that are undergoing rapid growth and division (such as cancer cells, skin cells, **blood** cells, **immune system** cells, and **digestive system** cells) are the most susceptible to radiation. Fortunately, most normal cells are better able to repair radiation damage than are cancer cells. Accordingly, radiation treatments are parceled into component treatments that are spaced over a given time interval (usually about seven weeks).

The spacing of radiation treatments allows cells to repair themselves during the time between treatments. Since the repair rate of normal cells is greater than the repair rate of cancerous cells, a smaller fraction of the radiation-damaged cancerous cells will have been replaced by the time of the next treatment. This procedure is called fractionation because the total radiation dose is divided into fractions. Fractionation allows cancer cells to be killed more effectively with less ultimate damage to the surrounding normal cells. Ideally all the cancer cells will be gone after the last treatment session.

Types of radiation used to treat cancer

PHOTON RADIATION. Early radiotherapy made use of x rays and gamma rays. X rays and gamma rays are essentially high-energy, ionizing electromagnetic rays composed of massless particles of energy called photons. The distinction between the two is that gamma rays originate from the decay of radioactive substances (like radium and cobalt-60), while x rays are generated by devices that excite electrons (such as cathode ray tubes and linear accelerators). These ionizing rays are part of the electromagnetic spectrum, which also includes ultraviolet, visible, and infrared light; radio waves; and microwaves. Ionizing rays act on cells by disrupting the electrons of atoms within the molecules inside cells. These atomic changes disrupt molecules and hence disrupt cell functions, most importantly their ability to divide and make new cells.

PARTICLE RADIATION. Particle radiation is expected to become an increasingly important part of radiotherapy. Proton therapy has been available since the early 1990s on a limited scale. Proton rays consist of protons, which have mass and charge, in contrast to photons, which have neither mass nor charge. Like x rays and gamma rays, proton rays disrupt atomic electrons in target cells. The advantage of proton rays is that they can be directed to conform to the shape of the tumor more precisely than x rays and gamma rays. Consequently, proton rays cause less injury to surrounding tissue and fewer side effects. They allow physicians to deliver higher radiation doses to tumors without increasing damage to the surrounding tissue. Proton therapy is therefore more effective and requires fewer treatment sessions than conventional x-ray therapy.

Neutron therapy is a second type of particle radiation. Neutron rays are very high-energy rays composed of neutrons, which are particles with mass but no charge. Unlike x rays, gamma rays, and proton rays, they disrupt atomic nuclei rather than electrons; thus the likelihood of cells repairing this kind of intensive damage is very small. Neutron therapy can be more effective at treating larger tumors than conventional radiotherapy. The central part of large tumors lack sufficient oxygen to be susceptible to damage from conventional radiation, which is dependent upon oxygen. Neutron radiation, however, can do its damage in the absence of oxygen, so it can kill cells in the centers of large tumors. Neutron therapy has been shown to be especially effective for the treatment of inoperable salivary gland tumors, **bone** cancers, and some advanced cancers of the **pancreas**, bladder, lung, prostate, and uterus.

Another promising type of neutron therapy, neutron capture therapy, is still in the experimental stage. It has, however, the advantage of being able to deliver high doses of radiation to a very limited area. Neutron capture therapy begins with a medication that binds to tumor cells but not to other cells. The medication is chemically combined with boron and given to the patient. The tumor is then irradiated with neutrons. When the neutrons interact with the boron atoms, the boron nuclei split, creating tiny nuclear fission events just big enough to kill one cell. If the drug does not bind to neighboring noncancerous cells, then only cancer cells will be damaged, and the damage to these cells should be irreversible.

Phototherapy is the newest approach to radiotherapy. In phototherapy, a porphyrin derivative is used to attach to and illuminate the tumor. The tumor can then be targeted for selective uptake of radiation.

Modes of delivery

EXTERNAL BEAM THERAPY. Traditionally, radiotherapy has been delivered from a beam of radiation originating outside the body. This modality is called "external beam therapy." The external beam passes through the body before and after it irradiates the tumor; thus it can injure tissue in its path.

BRACHYTHERAPY. In brachytherapy, the radiation remains inside the body. Brachytherapy uses gamma ray-generating radioactive isotopes such as cesium-137 or iodine-125. The isotope is placed in small tubes and implanted close to or inside the tumor. The patient stays in the hospital for a few days; after that time, the radioactive isotope has either decayed to a low level, or the implant is removed. This form of therapy is especially useful in treating tumors for which surgery or external beam therapy radiation would cause critical damage to tissues surrounding the tumor. Brachytherapy has been effective against prostate cancer and cervical cancer.

RADIOIMMUNOTHERAPY. Until the mid-1990s, the only way to treat cancer that has spread (metastasized) to multiple locations throughout the body has been with traditional chemotherapy, which uses drugs that kill cells that divide and reproduce quickly (proliferate) in a nonspecific way. Recently, cancer vaccines have been used successfully to extinguish metastatic **melanoma**. Vaccine treatment is a form of immunotherapy; it specifically kills melanoma cells and not other cells, even though they may also be proliferating.

Radioimmunotherapy is another form of immunotherapy that is still experimental. Researchers expect that radioimmunotherapy will be able to kill metastatic cancer cells almost anywhere in the body. **Antibodies** are immune system molecules that specifically recognize and bind to only one molecular structure, and they can be designed to bind specifically to a certain type of cancer cell. To carry out radioimmunotherapy, antibodies with the ability to bind specifically to a patient's cancer cells will be attached to an isotope that emits gamma rays when it is injected into the patient's bloodstream. These special antibody molecules will travel around the body until they encounter a cancer cell, and then they will bind to it. Then the gamma rays will kill the cancer cell. It will be difficult, however, for researchers to calculate the correct dose of antibody and isotope that will kill an unknown number of cancer cells and at the same time use isotope levels that won't destroy the antibody molecules before they encounter cancer cells.

Preparation

Before radiotherapy, the size and location of the patient's tumor, as well as the nature of the surrounding tissue in the path of the radiation beam, must be determined as accurately as possible so that the radiation treatment will be maximally effective. **Magnetic resonance imaging** (MRI) and computed tomography (CT) are used to provide detailed images of the tumor. The correct radiation dose, the number of sessions (fractions), the interval between sessions, and whether to give each fraction from the same direction or from different directions to lower the total dose imparted to a given surrounding area, are calculated on the basis of the tumor type, its size, and the sensitivity of the nearby tissues.

Shields are sometimes constructed for the patient to protect certain areas of the body. The patient's skin may be marked with ink or tattoos to help achieve correct positioning for each treatment, or molds may be built to hold tissues in exactly the right place each time.

Three-dimensional conformal external beam therapy

For some types of tumors, including prostate cancer, a beam-shaping technique known as three-dimensional conformal therapy is used to deliver higher doses of

KEY TERMS

Antibody—A protein molecule made by the immune system cells in response to a foreign substance; it recognizes and binds specifically to that substance.

Atom—The smallest part of an element having the chemical properties of the element.

Cancer vaccine—A drug given to induce a patient's immune system to attack his or her cancer.

Fractionation—In radiotherapy, a procedure in which a radiation treatment regimen is divided into many (usually 10–25) treatment sessions over a time span of several weeks.

Gamma rays—Short-wavelength, high-energy electromagnetic radiation emitted by radioactive substances.

Hodgkin's disease—Cancer of the lymphatic system, characterized by lymph node enlargement and the presence of large polyploid cells called Reed-Sternberg cells.

Immunotherapy—A treatment modality that utilizes cells or molecules of the immune system.

Ionizing radiation—High-energy radiation that has enough energy to move atomic electrons out of their orbits and thereby ionize the surrounding medium.

Isotope—One of two or more atom types of the same element that have the same number of protons in their nuclei but different numbers of neutrons.

Melanoma—One of the three most common types of skin cancer; melanoma is the most dangerous type because it frequently metastasizes.

Metastasis (plural, metastases)—A secondary tumor resulting from the spread of cancerous cells from the primary tumor to other parts of the body.

Neutron—A subatomic particle with a charge of zero and a mass slightly greater than that of a proton.

Proton—A subatomic particle with a charge of +1 and a mass about 1836 times that of an electron.

X rays—Short-wavelength, high-energy electromagnetic radiation produced by atom bombardment.

radiation to the tumor site while sparing surrounding tissue to a greater extent than is possible with the nonconformal approach. Three-dimensional conformal therapy requires **CT scans** that allow the radiologist and physicist to accurately plan field shapes and prepare shields appropriately shaped for the treatment plan.

Intensity-modulated radiotherapy (IMRT)

As with three-dimensional conformal therapy, intensity-modulated radiotherapy requires a CT scan prior to dose planning. The information from the CT scan is used to plan the delivery of the radiation. The key difference between three-dimensional conformal therapy and IMRT is that IMRT produces a plan that can be transferred to a floppy or optical disk. The diskette is then used to control a dynamic beam-shaping device called a collimator that is attached to the linear accelerator. The collimator has multiple small fingers about three millimeters wide that move in and out of the radiation field during treatment. The information on the floppy or optical disk controls the movement of the beam-shaping fingers. The beam rotates around the patient in some treatment regimens. The ability of IMRT to precisely shape the beam in very small increments even while it's moving allows the therapist to

deliver even higher doses to the tumor and spare even more of the healthy surrounding tissues than three-dimensional conformal therapy does. For some tumors, like prostate cancer, even greater precision can be attained by using a special ultrasound machine. Prior to each treatment, the ultrasound machine is used to pinpoint the location of the prostate gland relative to the radiation source. The information from the ultrasound scan allows the therapist to position the patient with a degree of precision measured in millimeters before the therapy begins.

Aftercare

Follow-up is important for patients who have received radiotherapy. They should go to their radiation oncologist at least once within the first several weeks after their final treatment to see if their treatment was successful. They should also see an oncologist every six to twelve months for the rest of their lives so they can be checked to see if the tumor has reappeared or spread.

Treatment of symptoms following radiotherapy depends on which part of the body is being treated and the type of radiation. Nevertheless, many patients experience skin burn, hair loss, fatigue, nausea, and **vomiting** regardless of the treatment area.

Affected skin should be kept clean and can be treated like a sunburn, with skin lotion or **vitamin A** and D ointment. Patients should avoid perfume or scented skin products, and protect affected areas from the sun.

Nausea and vomiting are expected when the dose is high or if the **abdomen** or another part of the digestive tract is irradiated. Sometimes nausea and vomiting occur after radiation to other regions, but in these cases the symptoms usually disappear within a few hours after treatment. Nausea and vomiting can be treated with **antacids** or with such antiemetics as Compazine, Tigan, or Zofran.

Fatigue frequently sets in after the second week of therapy and may continue until about two weeks after the therapy is finished. Patients may want to limit their activities, cut back their work hours, or take time off from work. They also may need to take naps and get extra sleep at night.

Patients who receive external beam therapy do not become radioactive and should be assured that they do not pose a danger to others. Some patients who receive brachytherapy, however, do go home with low levels of radioactivity inside their bodies. These patients should be given instructions about any dangers they might pose to children and people of childbearing age, and how long these dangers will last.

Emotional support is an important part of the care for patients undergoing any treatment for cancer. Radiotherapy can cause significant changes in a patient's appearance—particularly hair loss—and many patients fear that their spouses or partners will no longer find them attractive. There are many support groups available for radiotherapy patients and their families, as well as resources to help them cope with the external side effects of radiation treatment.

Complications

Radiotherapy can be highly toxic to patients because it kills normal cells as well as cancerous ones. There are risks of anemia, nausea, vomiting, **diarrhea**, hair loss, skin burn, sterility, and death. The benefits of radiation therapy, however, almost always exceed the risks involved.

Results

The probable outcome of radiation treatment is highly variable depending on the disease. For some diseases like Hodgkin's disease, about 75% of the patients are cured. Moreover, up to 86% of prostate cancer victims treated with both external and internal radiation are symptom-free five years after radiotherapy. On the other hand, radiation therapy is less successful in treating **lung cancer**; only about 9% of lung cancer patients are cured.

Resources

BOOKS

Cukier, Daniel, and Virginia McCullough. *Coping with Radiotherapy: A Ray of Hope.* Chicago: Contemporary Books, 1996.

Radiotherapy. In *The Merck Manual of Diagnosis and Therapy*, edited by Mark H. Beers, MD, and Robert Berkow, MD. Whitehouse Station, NJ: Merck Research Laboratories, 2004.

OTHER

3D-Conformal Radiation Therapy. Kimmel Cancer Center, Radiation Oncology, http://www.kcc.tju.edu/RadOne/crachy/three.htm.

Intensity Modulated Radiation Therapy (IMRT): A Patient-Centered Guide. Oncolink, University of Pennsylvania Cancer Center, http://cancer.med.upenn.edu/specialty/rad_onc/treat/imrt/.

Radiotherapy and You. A Guide to Self-Help During Treatment. Bethesda, MD: National Institutes of Health. National Cancer Institute. http://cancernet.nci.nih.gov/Radiation/radintro.html#anchor632185.

ORGANIZATIONS

American Cancer Society. 1599 Clifton Road NE, Atlanta GA 30329-4251. (800) ACS-2345. http://www.cancer.org.

National Association for Proton Therapy. 7910 Woodmont Avenue, Suite 1303, Bethesda, MD 20814. (301) 913-9360. http://www.protontherapy.org/Default.htm.

Radiological Society of North America, Inc. 820 Jorie Boulevard, Oak Brook, IL 60523-2251. (630) 571-2670. Fax: (630) 571-7837. http://www.rsna.org.

Stephen John Hage, AAAS, RT-R, FAHRA

Range-of-motion exercises *see* **Exercise**

Rapid plasma reagin test *see* **Syphilis tests**

Rapid streptococcus antigen tests

Definition

A rapid streptococcus antigen test is used to quickly diagnose **strep throat**, a contagious **infection** of the pharynx caused by a group A streptococcus (*Streptococcus pyogenes*), commonly referred to as GAS.

Purpose

Rapid streptococcus antigen tests are used to identify a strep throat. While a **throat culture** remains the gold standard for diagnosis of group A streptococcus infection, this procedure takes 24–48 hours for results. A rapid strep test takes only five minutes to perform. Since streptococci are sensitive to penicillin and related drugs, antibiotic therapy can be initiated immediately when the test is positive. A positive test result eliminates the need for bacterial throat culture.

Precautions

An untreated strep throat can increase the patient's risk of developing scarlet or **rheumatic fever**, which is associated with **meningitis**; and diseases affecting the **heart**, skin, **kidneys**, and joints. False-negative results occur with this test with a frequency ranging from four to 39%. Therefore, negative test results should be confirmed by throat culture.

Description

Approximately 10–19% of all sore throats are caused by group A beta-hemolytic streptococci. The majority of strep throat infections occur in children who are between the ages of five and 15, although adults with weakened immune systems are also at risk. The highest incidence of strep throat occurs during the winter and early spring months. Rapid streptococcal tests utilize **antibodies** to detect streptococcal antigens. There are four different direct streptococcal antigen detection platforms available in a wide number of different commercial products. These are latex agglutination, optical immunoassay, double antibody sandwich immunoassay, and immunochromatographic detection. The majority of rapid assays used today are based on double antibody sandwich and/or immunochromatography because these techniques do not require mixing, multiple reagent addition, or washing. An example of a combined double antibody sandwich immunochromatography method is described below.

The first step of a rapid strep test is the extraction of specific group A streptococcal carbohydrate antigen from the swab. The swab is placed in a test tube to which the extracting reagents have been added. The swab is rotated vigorously in the solution while pressing the tip against the sides of the test tube. After all fluid is pressed from the swab, it is discarded and the extract is applied to a nitrocellulose membrane containing both immobilized antibodies and non-immobilized antibodies to different regions of the group A strep antigen. The nonimmobilized antibodies are conjugated to dyed colloidal gold particles. If group A streptococcal carbohydrate antigen is present in the extract, the conjugated antibodies bind to it, forming antigen-antibody complexes. These migrate along the membrane until they reach the reaction zone containing immobilized antibodies to the same group A strep antigen. These antibodies capture the antigen-antibody complexes, forming a colored band or line (usually pink or blue) in the reaction zone area.

Specificity of these tests is approximately 97–98%. Few causes of false positives have been reported. False positives are possible when the patient's throat contains a heavy growth of *Staphylococcus aureus*. False-negative test results are commonly reported and often occur when insufficient antigen is obtained from the swab extraction procedure.

Preparation

All rapid group A strep tests require a sample from the infected patient's throat. The sample is obtained by depressing the tongue and swabbing the back of the throat and tonsils, while avoiding the tongue, saliva and lips. The swab should come in contact with all the inflamed areas, vesicles and pustular tonsils. Swabs made of rayon or Dacron should be used. Swabs containing cotton, calcium alginate, or wooden shafts, or that have been placed in transport medium containing charcoal are not recommended.

Aftercare

There are no aftercare concerns with this test.

Complications

There are no complications associated with this test.

Results

Normal results are negative. However, these assays tend to have low sensitivity, and thus it is recommended that all negative tests be followed by culture of a different throat swab on a **blood** agar plate for the isolation of beta-hemolytic streptococci. A positive result indicates an infection with group A streptococcus, and does not require culture follow-up.

Health care team roles

These tests are usually performed in a doctor's office by a nurse.

Resources

BOOK

Henry, John B. *Clinical Management by Laboratory Methods,* 19th ed. Philadelphia: Saunders, 1996, pp. 1140-3.

OTHER

"Streptococcal screen." MedLine Plus. http://www.nlm.nih.gov/medlineplus/ency/article/003745.htm.

Victoria E. DeMoranville

Rash

Definition

The popular term for a group of spots or red, inflamed skin that is usually a symptom of an underlying condition or disorder. Often temporary, a rash is only rarely a sign of a serious problem.

Description

A rash may occur on only one area of the skin, or it could cover almost all of the body. Also, a rash may or may not be itchy. Depending on how it looks, a rash may be described as:

- blistering (raised oval or round collections of fluid within or beneath the outer layer of skin)
- macular (flat spots)
- nodular (small, firm, knotty rounded mass)
- papular (small solid slightly raised areas)
- pustular (pus-containing skin blister)

Causes and symptoms

There are many theories as to the development of skin rashes, but experts are not completely clear what causes some of them. Generally a skin rash is an intermittent symptom, fading and reappearing. Rashes may accompany a range of disorders and conditions, such as:

- Infectious illness. A rash is symptom of many different kinds of childhood infectious illnesses, including chickenpox and scarlet fever. It may be triggered by other infections, such as Rocky Mountain spotted fever or ringworm.
- Allergic reactions. One of the most common symptoms of an allergic reaction is an itchy rash. Contact dermatitis is a rash that appears after the skin is exposed to an allergen, such as metal, rubber, some cosmetics or lotions, or some types of plants (e.g. poison ivy). Drug reactions are another common allergic cause of rash; in this case, a rash is only one of a variety of possible symptoms, including fever, seizures, nausea and vomiting, diarrhea, heartbeat irregularities, and breathing problems. This rash usually appears soon after the first dose of the course of medicine is taken.

- Autoimmune disorders. Conditions in which the immune system turns on the body itself, such as systemic lupus erythematosus or purpura, often have a characteristic rash.

- Nutritional disorders. For example, scurvy, a disease caused by a lack of Vitamin C, has a rash as one of its symptoms.

- Cancer. A few types of cancer, such as chronic lymphocytic leukemia, can be the underlying cause of a rash.

Rashes in infancy

Rashes are extremely common in infancy, and are usually not serious at all and can be treated at home.

Diaper rash is caused by prolonged skin contact with **bacteria** and the baby's waste products in a damp diaper. This rash has red, spotty sores and there may be an ammonia **smell**. In most cases the rash will respond within three days to drying efforts. A diaper rash that does not improve in this time may be a yeast **infection** requiring prescription medication. A doctor should be consulted if the rash is solid, bright red, causes **fever**, or the skin develops blisters, **boils**, or pus.

Infants also can get a rash on cheeks and chin caused by contact with food and **stomach** contents. This rash will come and go, but usually responds to a good cleaning after meals. About a third of all infants develop "acne" usually after the third week of life in response to their mothers' hormones before birth. This rash will disappear between weeks and a few months. Heat rash is a mass of tiny pink bumps on the back of the neck and upper back caused by blocked sweat glands. The rash usually appears during hot, humid weather, although a baby with a fever can also develop the rash.

A baby should see a doctor immediately if the rash:

- appears suddenly and looks purple or blood-colored
- looks like a burn
- appears while the infant seems to be sick

Diagnosis

A physician can make a diagnosis based on the medical history and the appearance of the rash, where it appears, and any other accompanying symptoms.

KEY TERMS

Purpura—A group of disorders characterized by purple or red brown areas of discoloration visible through the skin.

Scurvy—A nutritional disorder that causes skin bruising and hemorrhages.

Treatment

Treatment of rashes focuses on resolving the underlying disorder and providing relief of the **itching** that often accompanies them. Soothing lotions or oral **antihistamines** can provide some relief, and topical **antibiotics** may be administered if the patient, particularly a child, has caused a secondary infection by scratching. The rash triggered by **allergies** should disappear as soon as the allergen is removed; drug rashes will fade when the patient stops taking the drug causing the allergy. For the treatment of diaper rash, the infant's skin should be exposed to the air as much as possible; ointments are not needed unless the skin is dry and cracked. Experts also recommend switching to cloth diapers and cleaning affected skin with plain water.

Prognosis

Most rashes that have an acute cause, such as an infection or an allergic reaction, will disappear as soon as the infection or irritant is removed from the body's system. Rashes that are caused by chronic conditions, such as **autoimmune disorders**, may remain indefinitely or fade and return periodically.

Prevention

Some rashes can be prevented, depending on the triggering factor. A person known to be allergic to certain drugs or substances should avoid those things in order to prevent a rash. Diaper rash can be prevented by using cloth diapers and keeping the diaper area very clean, breast feeding, and changing diapers often.

Resource

ORGANIZATION

American Academy of Dermatology, P.O. Box 4014, Schaumburg, IL 60168-4014, Fax: (847) 240-1859, (866) 503-SKIN (7546), http://www.aad.org.

Carol A. Turkington

RDS *see* **Respiratory distress syndrome**

Reactive airway disease *see* **Asthma**

Recreation therapy

Definition

Recreation therapy, or therapeutic recreation, strives to improve the functioning and independence of individuals who are ill or disabled. Recreation therapists provide services in clinical facilities and in the community.

Description

Incorporating a variety of interventions to treat individuals with physical, cognitive, and emotional conditions, recreation therapists educate their patients to make them better-informed participants in their own health care. As a result, patients are taught to use activity to cope with the stresses of illness and disability. Therapeutic recreation activities may include, for example, wheelchair sports, **exercise** programs, and social activities—which preserve physical, cognitive, social and emotional health, thereby reducing the need for medical services.

A recreation therapist's responsibilities vary according to the setting and the patients served. Most recreation therapists are involved in the assessment of physical, mental, emotional, and social functioning towards determining the patient's needs, interests, and abilities based on information from standardized evaluations, observations, **medical records**, medical staff, family, and the patients themselves. The role of the recreation therapist is to then develop and implement therapeutic interventions consistent with the individual's needs and interests. For example, patients who place themselves in isolation may be encouraged to play games with others; a person with **paralysis** may be instructed in adaptation and compensatory strategies to throw a ball or swing a racket. Patients may be instructed in **relaxation** techniques to reduce **stress** and tension, correct stretching and limbering exercises, proper body mechanics for participation in recreation activities, pacing and other energy conservation techniques, and individual as well as team activities.

Work settings

Recreation therapists employed in hospitals are typically members of an interdisciplinary treatment team that develops patient treatment plans. Recreation therapists are often responsible for one or more group activities each day. Such activities might include, for example, stress management groups, community outings, family activities, exercise, and leisure education groups. Depending on the needs of the individuals, recreation therapists are responsible for the provision of programs that may include adapted aquatics, wheelchair basketball, social recreation for adults with mental retardation, downhill skiing for individuals with physical disabilities, summer camps, or adapted golf lessons. In addition, the patient may be met by the recreation therapist to conduct an assessment, or for developing a discharge plan. Responsibilities also include documenting the individual's progress in charts and communicating with other professionals, as well as with the patient's family members. Recreation therapists employed in an institution are usually expected to plan evening and weekend activities, special events, and holiday activities. Patients are often encouraged to participate in the creation and organization of these activities. The recreation therapist is also responsible for adapting activities as needed, and for providing adaptive equipment to enable the participation of individuals with disabilities or limitations. These services are designed to help meet the goals identified in the individual's treatment plan.

A variety of agencies and organizations employ recreation therapists. They may hold positions in acute-care hospitals, **rehabilitation** centers, **nursing homes**, psychiatric hospitals, community recreation centers, pediatric hospitals, group homes, senior centers, community mental health centers, public and private schools, correctional facilities, and private practice. Individuals of all ages and walks of life benefit from the services provided by recreation therapists.

The services of community-based recreation therapists are also used in park and recreation departments, special education programs for school districts, or programs for older adults and people with disabilities. In these programs, clients are helped to develop leisure activities. The role of the recreation therapist is to provide them with opportunities for exercise, mental stimulation, creativity, and fun.

In schools, recreation therapists assume an important role in helping counselors, parents, and special education teachers address the special needs of students. Recreation therapists are especially important in helping to ease the transition phase into adult life for children with disabilities. The recreation therapist may work with the client, the client's family, and other professionals to design and implement treatment and education plans.

Many recreation therapists fulfill the role of advocate on behalf of the individual with a disability. This may include addressing issues such as limited transportation resources, inaccessible facilities, and legislation that affects people with disabilities. Participation on advisory committees is a frequent activity of the recreation therapist, whose job also includes consultations with outside agencies to ensure that resources and services are provided for people with disabilities.

Education and training

Most employers require a minimum of a bachelor's degree in therapeutic recreation or in recreation with an option or emphasis in therapeutic recreation. In addition, an associate degree in recreation therapy; training in art, drama, or **music therapy**; or qualifying work experience may be sufficient for employment in nursing homes.

A bachelor's degree in therapeutic recreation is awarded upon successful completion of required course work and a supervised internship. During an internship, students are placed in an agency for a minimum of one semester so that what they have learned in the classroom can be put into practice.

In recent years, professional credentialing has become more important for employment. National certification is available through the National Council for Therapeutic Recreation Certification (NCTRC), an independent credentialing body. The National Council for Therapeutic Recreation Certification awards the title of Certified Therapeutic Recreation Specialist (CTRS) based upon prescribed education and experience requirements and successful performance on a 200-item national examination. Some states have additional requirements for licensure, registration or certification as well. Credentialing helps ensure that the minimum requirements needed to safely provide therapeutic recreation services have been met.

Future outlook

Employment opportunities for recreation therapists are expected to grow. The projected demand is due to the increase in the need for long-term care, and physical and **psychiatric rehabilitation**.

In 1996, there were approximately 38,000 employed recreation therapists. Hospitals have 42% in their employ; nursing homes had 38% employed. Residential facilities, community mental health centers, **adult day care** programs, correctional facilities, community programs for people with disabilities, and **substance abuse** centers had these therapists working for them. One out of every four recreation therapists were self-employed; this vocational path generally involves contracting with long-term care facilities or community agencies to develop and oversee programs.

Resources

OTHER

Resources for the Recreation Therapy Professional. http://www.recreationtherapy.com/.

ORGANIZATIONS

American Therapeutic Recreation Association. http://www.atra-tr.org.

National Therapeutic Recreation Society (NTRS). http://www.nrpa.org/branches/ntrs.htm.

Bill Asenjo, MS, CRC

Rectal cancer *see* **Colorectal cancer**

Rectal medication administration

Definition

Rectal medicines are medications prepared specifically for insertion into the rectum. They are compounded in many forms. Liquid rectal medicine solutions are given by **enema**. Creams, lotions, and ointments are applied externally or inserted internally using an applicator. Suppositories are prepared by mixing medicine with a wax-like substance to form a semi-solid, bullet-shaped form that will melt after insertion into the rectum.

Purpose

Rectal medications are administered for a localized effect on the rectum or for a systemic effect when a patient is **vomiting**, unable to swallow, or unconscious. Rectal medicine is most commonly used as a localized treatment for constipation or as a topical treatment for rectal inflammation or **infection**. Rectal suppositories may be used for the treatment of **fever**, nausea, and **pain**; they may also be prescribed to induce sedation or bronchodilation, or to reduce the nausea and vomiting that can accompany **chemotherapy**. Medicated enemas may be used to cleanse the bowel, to combat **bacteria**, or to kill **parasites**.

Precautions

Rectal medications must be used with caution in the cardiac patient who has **arrhythmias** or has recently had a **myocardial infarction** (i.e., **heart attack**). Insertion of a rectal medicine can cause vagus nerve stimulation and may trigger an arrhythmia—such as bradycardia. Rectal medicines should not be given to the patient with undiagnosed **abdominal pain** because peristalsis of the bowel can cause an inflamed appendix to rupture. Rectal medicines should be used cautiously in patients who have undergone recent surgery on the rectum, bowel, or prostate gland. If the patient has rectal bleeding or a prolapse of rectal tissue from the rectal opening, the medicine should be withheld and the physician consulted before administration. Rectal medicines should not be taken orally, and only medications labeled as rectal preparations should be placed in the rectum.

Description

Administration of rectal medication should be done after the patient is positioned correctly. Lifting the upper buttocks will enable visualization of his or her rectal opening. External lotions, ointments or creams can be applied directly, using a gloved finger or a 4x4 gauze pad. Prior to administering internal rectal medicine, the tip of the suppository, enema catheter, or applicator should be lubricated with a water-soluble lubricant. To insert a rectal suppository, the lubricated, tapered end of the suppository should be placed at the rectal opening and gently pushed into the rectum. The suppository should be pushed continually toward the umbilicus until the full length of the nurse's gloved index finger has been inserted into the rectal opening (i.e., about 3 inches, or 7.5 cm, for an adult patient). When inserting suppositories into children, the suppository should be pushed about 1 inch (2.5 cm) beyond the rectal opening, or up to the first knuckle of the nurses's index finger. When inserting suppositories into infants, the little finger should be inserted one-half inch (1.25 cm) beyond the rectal opening. The buttocks should be released, and the finger removed.

Administration of internal rectal medicated cream or ointment requires placement of the applicator's lubricated tip at the rectal opening, gently pushing the applicator into the rectal opening about 3 inches (7.5 cm) for an adult (or as indicated on the applicator's directions). The correct dosage of medicine should then be squeezed into the rectum. After withdrawal of the applicator tip, the buttocks should be released.

To administer rectal medicine using an enema solution, the lubricated tip of the enema catheter must also be placed at the rectal opening. The tip of the catheter should then be gently advanced into the rectum, about 3 inches (7.5 cm) for an adult (or as indicated on the enema tubing). After the patient is alerted, the enema tubing should be opened, allowing the enema solution to flow into the rectum. A prepared enema should also be administered in this manner.

When all of the solution has been administered, the enema catheter should be removed. Then, the buttocks should be released.

Preparation

Before administering rectal medicine, the door to the room should be closed to assure patient privacy. The patient should be encouraged to empty his or her bladder and bowels before the procedure. After removing lower garments and underwear, the patient should be positioned in bed on his or her left side, with the top knee bent and pulled slightly upward. A waterproof pad should be placed under the patient's hips to protect the bedding, and sheets should be draped over the patient to cover all of his or her body except the buttocks.

After placing a bedpan within quick access, the nurse should explain the procedure to the patient. This explanation should include the importance of breathing slowly through the mouth to enhance **relaxation** of the rectal sphincter and to avoid oppositional pressure. The patient should be made aware that there may be an urge to push the medicine out, but that he or she should try to hold it for at least 10–15 minutes after instillation (30 minutes for suppositories), as most rectal medications need time to be absorbed. It is advisable for the professional to check the medication label each time the medicine is given, to avoid medication errors. It must be the right medicine and the right dose (strength), the right time, the right patient, and the right method. The expiration date on the label should be inspected. If the medicine is outdated, it should not be used.

The nurse should wash his or her hands and put on gloves. The foil wrap should be removed from the rectal preparation or suppository. To prepare internal rectal creams, lotions or ointments, the applicator should be examined so that the nurse can estimate the proper amount to instill after insertion. In preparation for rectal enema instillations, the directions on the package of premixed, disposable enemas should be read. Most premixed disposable enemas come with the tip already lubricated. The cap from the tip should be removed, and air should be expelled from the apparatus before use. If liquid medicine solutions are given using a standard enema bag and tubing, the procedure for enema instillation should be followed.

Aftercare

After administering rectal medicines, the nurse should remain near the patient in case there is a need for assistance with the bedpan, or to walk to the bathroom. If a suppository is expelled within the first

KEY TERMS

Arrhythmia—An irregularity of the heartbeat.

Bradycardia—An abnormal slowing of the heart rate to fewer than 60 beats per minute.

Myocardial infarction—A cardiac condition caused by decreased blood flow and oxygen to the heart muscle; may cause tissue death and heart damage. Commonly known as a heart attack.

Peristalsis—The wave-like muscular contractions of the intestinal walls that move food and refuse through the gastrointestinal system.

Prostate gland—A gland found in males, located below the bladder and around the urethra, that secretes the fluid for semen and controls the release of urine from the bladder.

Rectum—The last portion of the large intestine located just above the anal canal, where stool collects prior to evacuation from the body.

Vagus nerve—One of the paired cranial nerves that supplies motor and sensory enervation to the abdominal and thoracic organs.

few minutes of insertion, the tip should be relubricated and reinserted. Medicated enemas that are expelled immediately may need to be repeated, using fresh solution. Directions provided with a prepared enema should be followed, but the physician may need to be consulted. To assist the patient with retaining the medicine, the nurse can apply gentle pressure to the rectal opening, using a 4x4 gauze pad or by squeezing the buttocks together after rectal medicine instillation. A 4x4 gauze pad should also tucked between the buttocks to collect seepage; this may help the patient feel more secure. After the procedure is completed, the patient should be covered and instructed to remain still for 10–15 minutes (30 minutes if a suppository was inserted). This period will allow time for medication absorption. Items that can be reused, such as enema pouches, tubing, and applicator tips, should be cleaned with warm running water and allowed to air dry. Ointments and creams need to be recapped and returned to the medicine boxes. Disposable items and gloves should be placed in an appropriate trash bag that can be sealed and discarded.

Complications

Rectal medicines can cause tissue irritation or allergic reactions. If irritation, swelling, redness, bleeding or prolapse of the rectal tissue is apparent, or if the patient complains of pain or burning, the medication should be stopped and the physician notified.

Results

When given correctly, rectal medications work within 30–60 minutes to relieve pain, nausea, constipation, or fever. Rectal ointments for swelling and irritation of **hemorrhoids** may reverse the condition within several days. Because of their liquid state, rectal enemas are absorbed quickly and work rapidly. Retention enemas are meant to be held for 30 minutes to achieve full therapeutic effect.

Health care team roles

Rectal medicines are administered by a licensed nurse (R. N. or L. P. N.) in the health care setting. An alert and cooperative patient may be allowed to apply external and internal rectal ointments and suppositories under the direction of the nurse. The nurse, however, should assess the site and the effectiveness of the medicine. The patient or members of the patient's family can be taught to administer rectal medicines in the home setting.

Resources

BOOK

Nurse's Clinical Guide: Medication Administration, Pennsylvania: Springhouse Corporation, 2000.

OTHER

Forms of Medication, Complete Home Medical Guide, Columbia Medical College of Physicians and Surgeons Online, 2001. http://cpmcnet.columbia.edu/texts/guide/hmg34_0003.html.

"Medication Information."Nebraska Health System Clinic Pharmacy Online, September 2000. http://www.unmc.edu/rxweb/genifo.htm.

"Mesalamine (Rectal)." Medline Plus. National Institutes of Health Online, January 2001. http://www.nlm.nih.gov /medlineplus/druginfo/mesalaminerectal202351.html.

"Procedure For Medication Administration, Procedure 61." University of Arkansas Online, December 2000. http://www.uams.edu/nursingmanual/Procedures/procedure61.htm.

"Taking Your Medicine." Rectal Suppositories, Express Scripts. Drug Digest Online, 2000. http://www.drugdigest.org/DD/TakingYourMedicine/MedsDetail/0,4011,2,00.html.

Mary Elizabeth Martelli, R. N., B. S.

Red blood cell indices

Definition

Red **blood** cell (RBC) indices are calculations derived from the **complete blood count** that aid in the diagnosis and classification of anemia. Measurements needed to calculate indices are the red blood cell count, hemoglobin, and **hematocrit**. The hematocrit is the percentage of blood by volume that is occupied by the red cells. The three RBC indices are:

- Mean corpuscular volume (MCV). The average size of the red blood cells expressed in femtoliters. MCV is calculated by dividing the hematocrit (as percent) by the RBC count in millions per microliter of blood, then multiplying by 10.

- Mean corpuscular hemoglobin (MCH). The average amount of hemoglobin inside an RBC expressed in picograms. The MCH is calculated by dividing the hemoglobin concentration in grams per deciliter by the RBC count in millions per microliter, then multiplying by 10.

- Mean corpuscular hemoglobin concentration (MCHC). The average concentration of hemoglobin in the RBCs expressed as a percent. It is calculated by dividing the hemoglobin in grams per deciliter by the hematocrit, then multiplying by 100.

Purpose

Red blood cell indices help classify types of anemia, a decrease in the oxygen carrying capacity of the blood. Healthy people have an adequate number of correctly sized red blood cells containing enough hemoglobin to carry sufficient oxygen to all the body's tissues. Anemia is diagnosed when either the hemoglobin or hematocrit of a blood sample is too low.

The mechanisms by which anemia occurs will alter the RBC indices in a predictable manner. Therefore, the RBC indices permit the physician to narrow down the possible causes of an anemia. The MCV is an index of the size of the RBCs. When the MCV is below normal, the RBCs will be smaller than normal and are described as microcytic. When the MCV is elevated, the RBCs will be larger than normal and are termed macrocytic. RBCs of normal size are termed normocytic. Failure to produce hemoglobin results in smaller than normal cells. This occurs in many diseases, including **iron deficiency anemia**, thalassemia (an inherited disease in which globin chain production is deficient), and **anemias** associated with chronic **infection** or disease. Macrocytic cells occur when division of RBC precursor cells in the **bone** marrow is impaired. The most common causes of macrocytic anemia are **vitamin B$_{12}$** deficiency, folate deficiency, and **liver** disease. Normocytic anemia may be caused by decreased production (e.g. malignancy and other causes of bone marrow failure), increased destruction (hemolytic anemia), or blood loss. The RBC count is low, but the size and amount of hemoglobin in the cells are normal.

A low MCH indicates that cells have too little hemoglobin. This is caused by deficient hemoglobin production. Such cells will be pale when examined under the **microscope** and are termed hypochromic. **Iron** deficiency is the most common cause of a hypochromic anemia. The MCH is usually elevated in macrocytic anemias associated with vitamin B$_{12}$ and folate deficiency.

The MCHC is the ratio of hemoglobin mass in the RBC to cell volume. Cells with too little hemoglobin are lighter in color and have a low MCHC. The MCHC is low in microcytic, hypochromic anemias such as iron deficiency, but is usually normal in macrocytic anemias. The MCHC is elevated in hereditary spherocytosis, a condition with decreased RBC survival caused by a structural protein defect in the RBC membrane.

Cell indices are usually calculated from tests performed on an automated electronic cell counter. However, these counters measure the MCV, which is directly proportional to the voltage pulse produced as each cell passes through the counting aperture. Electronic cell counters calculate the MCH, MCHC, hematocrit, and an additional parameter called the red cell distribution width (RDW). The RDW is a measure of the variance in red blood cell size. It is calculated by dividing the standard deviation of RBC volume by the MCV and multiplying by 100. A large RDW indicates abnormal variation in cell size, termed anisocytosis. The RDW aids in differentiating anemias that have similar indices. For example, thalassemia minor and iron deficiency anemia are both microcytic and hypochromic anemias, and overlap in MCV and MCH. However, iron deficiency anemia has an abnormally wide RDW, but thalassemia minor does not.

Precautions

Certain prescription medications may affect the test results. These drugs include zidovudine (Retrovir), phenytoin (Dilantin), and azathioprine (Imuran). When the hematocrit is determined by centrifugation, the MCV and MCHC may differ from those derived by an electronic cell counter, especially in anemia. Plasma trapped between the RBCs tends to cause an increase in

KEY TERMS

Anemia—A variety of conditions in which a person's blood can't carry as much oxygen as is needed by the tissues.

Hypochromic—A descriptive term applied to a red blood cell with a decreased concentration of hemoglobin.

Macrocytic—A descriptive term applied to a larger than normal red blood cell.

Mean corpuscular hemoglobin (MCH)—A calculation of the average weight of hemoglobin in a red blood cell.

Mean corpuscular hemoglobin concentration (MCHC)—A calculation of the average concentration of hemoglobin in a red blood cell.

Mean corpuscular volume (MCV)—A measure of the average volume of a red blood cell.

Microcytic—A descriptive term applied to a smaller than normal red blood cell.

Normochromic—A descriptive term applied to a red blood cell with a normal concentration of hemoglobin.

Normocytic—A descriptive term applied to a red blood cell of normal size.

Red cell distribution width (RDW)—A measure of the variation in the size of red blood cells.

the hematocrit, giving rise to a somewhat higher MCV and lower MCHC.

RBC indices require 3–5 mL of blood collected by venipuncture. A nurse or phlebotomist usually collects the sample following standard precautions for the prevention of transmission of bloodborne pathogens.

Aftercare

Discomfort or bruising may occur at the puncture site. Pressure to the puncture site until the bleeding stops reduces bruising; warm packs relieve discomfort. Some people feel dizzy or faint after blood has been drawn and should be treated accordingly.

Complications

Other than potential bruising at the puncture site, and/or **dizziness**, there are no complications associated with this test.

Results

Normal results for red blood cell indices are as follows:

- MCV: 80–96 fl (femtoliters)
- MCH: 27–33 pg (picograms)
- MCHC: 33–36%
- RDW: 12–15%

Health care team roles

A phlebotomist, or sometimes a nurse, collects the blood, and a clinical laboratory scientist, CLS(NCA)/medical technologist, MT(ASCP) or clinical laboratory technician CLT(NCA)/medical laboratory technician MLT(ASCP) performs the testing. Results are interpreted by a physician.

Resources

BOOKS

Chernecky, Cynthia C., and Barbara J. Berger. *Laboratory Tests and Diagnostic Procedures,* 3rd ed. Philadelphia, PA: W. B. Saunders Company, 2001.

Kee, Joyce LeFever. *Handbook of Laboratory and Diagnostic Tests,* 4th ed. Upper Saddle River, NJ: Prentice Hall, 2001.

Mosby's Diagnostic and Laboratory Test Reference, 10th ed. Edited by Kathleen Deska Pagana and Timothy James Pagana. St. Louis, MO: Mosby, 2010.

Victoria E. DeMoranville
Robert Harr

Red blood cell test *see* **Hemoglobin test**

Reflex tests

Definition

Reflex tests are simple physical tests of nervous system function.

Purpose

A reflex is a simple nerve circuit. A stimulus, such as a light tap with a rubber hammer, causes sensory **neurons** (nerve cells) to send signals to the **spinal cord**. There, the signals are conveyed both to the **brain** and to nerves that control muscles affected by the stimulus. Without any brain intervention, these muscles may respond to an appropriate stimulus by contracting.

Reflex tests measure the presence and strength of a number of **reflexes**. In so doing, they help to assess the integrity of the nerve circuits involved. Reflex tests are performed as part of a neurological exam, either a "mini-exam" done to quickly confirm integrity of the spinal cord, or a more complete exam performed to diagnose the presence and location of a **spinal cord injury** or neuromuscular disease.

Deep tendon reflexes are responses to muscle stretch. The familiar "knee-jerk" reflex is an example of a reflex. This tests the integrity of the spinal cord in the lower back region. The usual set of deep tendon reflexes tested, involving increasingly higher regions of the spinal cord, includes:

- ankle
- knee
- abdomen
- forearm
- biceps
- triceps
- patellar

Another type of reflex test is called the Babinski test, which involves gently stroking the sole of the foot to assess proper development and function of the spine and cerebral cortex.

Precautions

Reflex tests are entirely safe, and no special precautions are needed.

Description

The examiner uses a reflex hammer or rubber mallet to strike different points on the examinee's body, and observes the response. The points chosen for eliciting reflexes are the tendons of specific muscles. Tapping specific sites is intended to provide a quick stretch to the muscle. Muscle spindles, or receptors, mediate the reflex lying within the muscle—not the site of the hammer strike. The examiner may position, or hold, one of the limbs during testing, and may require exposure of the ankles, knees, **abdomen**, and arms. Reflexes can be difficult to elicit if the individual being examined is paying too much attention to the stimulus. To compensate for this, that person may be asked to perform some **muscle contraction**, such as clenching teeth or grasping and pulling the two hands apart. When performing the Babinski reflex test, the examiner will gently **stroke** the outer soles of the person's feet with the mallet while checking to see whether or not the big toe extends out as a result.

Muscle stretch (deep tendon) reflexes

Reflex	Stimulus	Response
Biceps	Tap biceps tendon	Contraction of biceps
Brachioradialis (periosteradial)	Tap styoid process of radius (insertion of brachioradialis)	Flexion of elbow and pronation of forearm
Jaw (maxillary)	Tap mandible in half-open position	Closure of jaw
Patellar	Tap patellar tendon	Extension of leg at knee
Tendocalcaneus	Tap Achilles tendon	Plantar flexion at ankle
Triceps	Tap triceps tendon	Extension of elbow
Wrist extension	Tap wrist extensor tendons	Extension of wrist
Wrist flexion	Tap wrist flexor tendon	Flexion of wrist

SOURCE: Rothstein, J.M., S.H. Roy, and S.L. Wolf. *The Rehabilitation Specialist's Handbook.* 2nd ed. Philadelphia: F.A. Davis Co., 1998.

Preparation

The examiner positions the person to be examined in a comfortable position, usually seated on the examination table with legs hanging free. There is no other preparation.

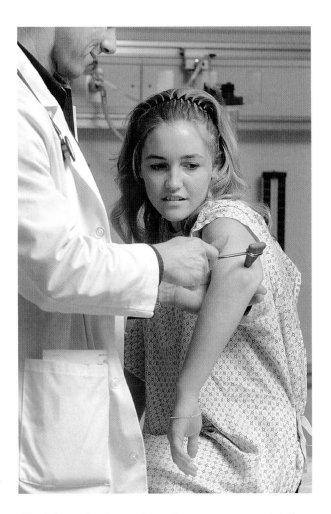

(Physician performing a reflex test on a young woman's left arm, photograph. Photo Researchers, Inc. Reproduced by permission.)

Aftercare

A reflex examination is not invasive. No care after the examination is required.

Complications

The pressure exerted by a reflex hammer is minimal and does not hurt the person being examined. A reflex examination is not invasive. There are no complications from performing the examination.

Results

Normal results

The strength of the response depends partly on the strength of the stimulus. For this reason, an examiner will attempt to elicit the response with the smallest stimulus possible. Learning the range of normal responses requires some clinical training. Responses should be the same on both sides of the body. A normal response to the Babinski reflex test depends upon the age of the person being examined. In children under the age of one and a half years, the big toe will extend out with or without the other toes. This is due to the fact that the fibers in the spinal cord and cerebral cortex have not been completely covered in myelin, the protein and lipid sheath that aids in processing neural signals. In adults and children over the age of one and a half years, the myelin sheath should be completely formed and as a result, all the toes will curl under (plantar flexion reflex).

Abnormal results

Weak or absent response may indicate damage to the nerves outside the spinal cord (**peripheral neuropathy**), damage to the motor neurons just before or just after they leave the spinal cord (motor neuron disease), or muscle disease. Excessive response may indicate spinal cord

KEY TERMS

Lesion—A pathologic change in body tissue.

Myelin—A substance composed largely of fat that constitutes the sheaths of various nerve fibers throughout the body.

Neurology—The study of nerves.

damage above the level controlling the hyperactive response. Different responses on the two sides of the body may indicate early onset of progressive disease, or localized nerve damage, as from trauma. An adult or older child who responds to the Babinski with an extended big toe may have a lesion in the spinal cord or cerebral cortex.

Health care team roles

A reflex examination is usually conducted by a physician. Neurologists (doctors with specialized training in **neurology**) often perform reflex tests. Physician assistants, physical therapists, and nurses may also test reflexes as they examine or evaluate individuals.

Resources

BOOKS

Adams, Raymond D, Maurice Victor, and Allan H. Ropper. *Adams & Victor's Principles of Neurology, 9th ed.* New York, McGraw Hill Professional, 2009.

Aminoff, Michael J. *Neurology and General Medicine,* 4th ed. London: Churchill Livingstone, 2007.

Bickley, Lynn S., Robert A. Hoekelman, and Barbara Bates. *Bates' Guide to Physical Examination and History Taking.* Philadelphia, PA: Lippincott, 1999.

DeGowin, Robert L., and Donald D. DeGowin. *DeGowin's Diagnostic Examination,* 7th ed. New York: McGraw Hill, 1999.

Seidel, Henry M. *Mosby's Guide to Physical Examination,* 4th ed. St. Louis, MO: Mosby Year Book, 1999.

Shwartz, Mark A., and William Schmitt. *Textbook of Physical Diagnosis: History and Examination,* 3rd ed. Philadelphia, PA: Saunders, 1998.

OTHER

Explore Science. http://www.explorescience.com/activities/Activity_page.cfm?ActivityID=38.

King's College (London). http://www.umds.ac.uk/physiology/mcal/sreflex.html.

Loyola University (Chicago). http://www.meddean.luc.edu/lumen/MedEd/medicine/pulmonar/pd/pstep56.htm.

University of Washington. http://faculty.washington.edu/chudler/chreflex.html.

Washington University (St. Louis). http://www.neuro.wustl.edu/neuromuscular/mother/reflex.html.

ORGANIZATIONS

American Academy of Family Physicians. 11400 Tomahawk Creek Parkway, Leawood, KS 66211-2672. (913) 906-6000. http://www.aafp.org/. fp@aafp.org.

American Academy of Neurology. 1080 Montreal Avenue, St. Paul, Minnesota 55116. (651) 695-1940. http://www.aan.com/resources.html. web@aan.com.

American College of Physicians. 190 N Independence Mall West, Philadelphia, PA 19106-1572. (800) 523-1546 x2600 or (215) 351-2600. http://www.acponline.org/cgi-bin/feedback.

L. Fleming Fallon, Jr., MD, PhD, DrPH

Reflexes

Definition

Reflexes are the body's automatic reaction to some type of sensory stimuli. They involve nerve impulses passing from a receptor to a nerve center and then outward to, for example, a nerve or a gland.

Description

Reflexes are classified as unconditioned and conditioned.

Unconditioned reflexes

Unlike most human behaviors, unconditioned reflexes occur without specific learning or experience. They are considered involuntary acts, because a response occurs automatically when a stimulus (for example, a pinprick) takes place.

Unconditioned reflexes that protect us from harm are called nociceptive reflexes. For example, sneezing, coughing, and gagging are automatic responses to **foreign bodies** in the nose and throat. Eye blinking or winking helps protect the eye from harm. Reacting quickly to touching a hot stove is yet another example of a nociceptive reflex.

Most reflex acts are very complicated. However, in simple reflexes four events are involved: reception, conduction, transmission, and response. The stimulation is received by receptors, or sensitive nerve endings. These may be in the eye, ear, nose, tongue, or skin. Energy from the stimulus is changed into nerve impulses and conducted from the receptor to the **central nervous**

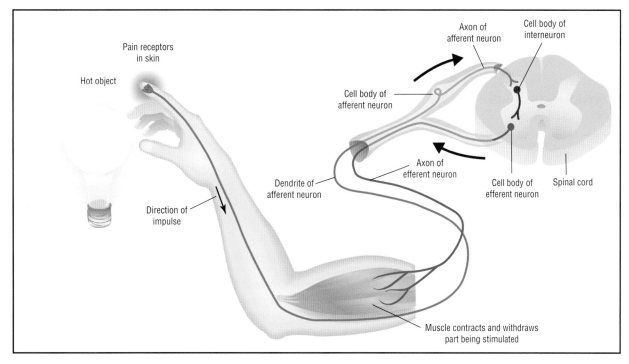

(Path of nerve impulse from fingertip to spinal cord. Illustration by GGS Information Services, Inc. The Gale Group.)

system. From there, the nerve impulses are transmitted to the motor nerves that control muscle action. The motor nerves conduct the impulses to the muscles and glands, causing them to respond or act. For example, touching a hot stove stimulates receptors in the skin of the finger. This creates a nerve impulse that travels along a sensory nerve to the **spinal cord**. In the spinal cord, the sensory nerve fibers interlace with motor nerve fibers. The nerve impulse passes from the sensory fibers to the motor fibers, which relay it to the muscles, causing them to contract. When the muscles contract, the person's hand jerks back.

People have many reflex reactions to emotional stimuli, such as anger or fear, including changes in **blood pressure** and respiration. Lie detectors measure specific physical reactions to emotional stimuli.

Conditioned reflexes

Conditioned reflexes are acquired as the result of experience. When an action is performed repeatedly, the nervous system learns to react automatically. Walking, running, and typing are examples of learned conditioned activities that require a large number of complex muscular coordinations.

Conditioned reflexes work by association. For example, a dog's mouth begins to water when the animal smells food. The Russian physiologist Ivan P. Pavlov showed that the flow of saliva, originally an automatic reaction to the **smell** of food, may become a conditioned reflex. Pavlov rang a bell each time he brought food to a dog. Eventually, the dog's mouth began to water when Pavlov merely rang the bell without food being present. The dog associated the ringing of the bell with the food, just as it associated the odor with the food.

Function

In a simple reflex, a sensory receptor initiates a nerve impulse in an afferent sensory nerve fiber that conducts it to the spinal cord. In the gray matter of the spinal cord, the afferent nerve impulse is fired over the synaptic gap to an efferent motor fiber that passes along the impulse to the appropriate muscle, producing the reflex.

Role in human health

Nerve cells are sensitive to disturbances caused by tumors, trauma, circulatory problems, metabolic disorders, and a host of other diseases that can be diagnosed by determining which reflexes show abnormalities. Abnormal reflexes may suggest the presence of significant central nervous system or peripheral nerve problems.

Reflex tests measure the presence and strength of a number of reflexes to help assess the integrity of the nerve circuits involved. Reflex tests are performed as part

KEY TERMS

Afferent—Conveying impulses toward a nerve center, such as the brain or spinal cord.

Efferent—Conveying nervous impulses outward to nerves or neurons.

Nociceptive—A stimulus that causes pain or injury.

Synaptic gap—The space between neurons across which a nerve impulse is transmitted by a neurotransmitter. Also referred to as a synaptic cleft.

of a neurological exam to quickly confirm the integrity of the spinal cord or to diagnose the presence and location of **spinal cord injury** or neuromuscular disease.

Common diseases and disorders

Some of the more common reflex-related diseases and disorders include **stroke**, traumatic **brain** or spinal cord tumors or injury, **multiple sclerosis**, Wernicke-Korsakoff syndrome, **cerebral palsy**, and diabetic neuropathy.

Stroke

Stroke is a brain disorder involving loss of brain functions due to interruption of the brain's **blood** supply.

Brain and spinal cord injury

Brain and spinal cord injuries most commonly result from motor vehicle accidents, **falls**, **sports injuries**, industrial accidents, gunshot **wounds**, and criminal assault. Damage to the spinal cord affects all nerve function at and below the level of the injury, including muscle control and sensation.

Brain and spinal tumors

Brain and spinal cord tumors are abnormal growths of tissue found inside the **skull** or the spinal column. The word tumor is used to describe both abnormal growths that are new (neoplasms) and those present at birth (congenital).

Multiple sclerosis

Multiple sclerosis involves inflammation within the central nervous system, followed by demyelination, which is a loss of the protective myelin sheaths that surround nerve fibers. When the myelin is damaged, nerve impulses are not transmitted quickly and efficiently. As a result of the inflammatory process, lesions develop in the brain and spinal cord, causing a variety of neurologic symptoms, such as **vision** loss, numbness or tingling, **weakness**, unsteady gait, double vision, fatigue, heat intolerance, partial or complete **paralysis**, and electric **shock** sensations when bending the neck. These symptoms may cease or may persist after an attack. Symptoms may become progressively worse over time. For individuals with progressive forms of multiple sclerosis, these symptoms may gradually worsen over time without rapid or abrupt changes.

Wernicke-Korsakoff syndrome

Wernicke-Korsakoff syndrome usually affects people between 40 and 80 years old. The onset is gradual. The syndrome is actually two disorders that may occur independently or together. Wernicke's disease involves damage to multiple nerves in both the central nervous system and the peripheral nervous system. It may also include symptoms caused by alcohol withdrawal. The cause is generally attributed to malnutrition—especially lack of vitamin B$_1$ (**thiamine**), which commonly accompanies habitual alcohol use or **alcoholism**.

Korsakoff syndrome, or Korsakoff **psychosis**, involves impairment of **memory** and intellectual/cognitive skills such as problem solving or learning, along with multiple symptoms of nerve damage. The most distinguishing symptom is confabulation (fabrication), during which the person makes up detailed, believable stories about experiences or situations to cover the gaps in their memory. Korsakoff psychosis involves damage to areas of the brain.

Cerebral palsy

Cerebral palsy is a persistent qualitative motor disorder caused by nonprogressive damage to the brain. Although manifested primarily by motor dysfunction, the disorder also may involve sensory deficits and impairment of the intellect. The majority of cases are caused during labor and delivery or during the first month of infancy. Cerebral palsy may be caused by premature birth, prolonged labor, or traumatic delivery. Any situation that interferes with fetal oxygen supply can produce brain damage and cerebral palsy.

Diabetic neuropathy

Diabetic neuropathy is a nerve disorder caused by diabetes. Symptoms of neuropathy include numbness and sometimes **pain** in the hands, feet, or legs. Nerve damage caused by diabetes can also lead to problems with internal organs such as the digestive tract, **heart**, and sexual organs, causing indigestion, **diarrhea** or constipation, **dizziness**, bladder infections, and impotence.

Resources

BOOKS

Schwartz, J. H., ed. *Principles of Neural Science.* Stamford, CT: Appleton & Lange, 2000.

Simon, R. *Clinical Neurology.* 4th ed. Stamford, CT: Appleton & Lange, 1998.

ORGANIZATIONS

American Academy of Neurology. 10890 Montreal Avenue, St. Paul, MN 55116. (651) 695-1940. http://www.aan.com/.

National Institute of Neurological Disorders and Stroke. http://www.ninds.nih.gov

National Stroke Association. 9707 E. Easter Lane, Englewood, CO 80112. (800) STROKES. (303) 649-9299. http://www.stroke.org/

Spinal Cord Injury Resource Center. http://www.spinalinjury.net/.

Bill Asenjo, PhD, CRC

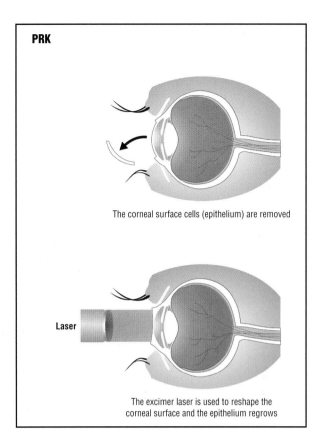

PRK

The corneal surface cells (epithelium) are removed

Laser

The excimer laser is used to reshape the corneal surface and the epithelium regrows

(Diagram showing PRK eye surgery. Illustration by GGS Information Services, Inc. The Gale Group.)

Refractive eye surgeries

Definition

Refractive eye surgeries are medical procedures used to correct refractive errors such as **myopia**, **hyperopia**, and **presbyopia**. The three most widely utilized refractive surgeries approved by the U.S. Food and Drug Administration (FDA) are photorefractive keratectomy (PRK), laser-assisted in-situ keratomileusis (LASIK), and laser thermal keratoplasty (LTK). PRK and LASIK use an excimer laser to correct myopia by reshaping the cornea. The two techniques differ in how the surface layer of the cornea is treated.

Purpose

Refractive surgeries are performed to correct hyperopia, myopia, and presbyopia in patients who do not want to wear eyeglasses or **contact lenses**. After refractive surgery, most patients are able to see well enough to pass a driver's license exam without glasses or contact lenses. Some patients will still need corrective lenses, but the lenses won't need to be as strong or thick.

Precautions

Medical history is important in determining the appropriate refractive surgery patients. Patients for LASIK and PRK must be older than 18 years of age, have healthy corneas, and have **vision** that has been stable for the past year. People who may not be good candidates are pregnant women or women who are breastfeeding, patients with very small or very large refractive errors, those with low contrast sensitivity, people with scarred corneas or macular disease, or those with autoimmune diseases or diabetes. Patients with **glaucoma** should not have LASIK because the intraocular pressure (IOP) of the eye is raised during the procedure. A patient with persistent lid infections (i.e., blepharitis) may not be a good candidate because of an increased **infection** risk.

LTK patients must be at least 40 years old, have stable vision for at least six months, fall in the low-to-moderate range of hyperopia (+0.75–+2.50 diopters), and have no more than 0.75 diopters of **astigmatism**. Pregnant or nursing women, patients with clinically significant corneal dystrophy or scarring in the 6 mm or 7 mm central zone, patients with a history of herpetic keratitis, patients with an autoimmune disease, collagen

Lasek

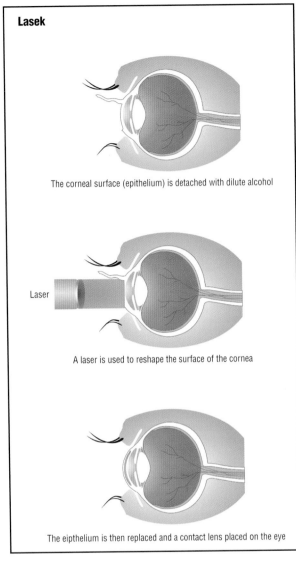

The corneal surface (epithelium) is detached with dilute alcohol

Laser

A laser is used to reshape the surface of the cornea

The eipthelium is then replaced and a contact lens placed on the eye

(Diagram showing lasek eye surgery. Illustration by GGS Information Services, Inc. The Gale Group.)

vascular disease, clinically significant atopic syndrome, insulin-dependent diabetes, or an immuno-compromised status should not have LTK.

Description

Refractive surgeries that correct myopia are similar in nature. PRK and LASIK are both performed with an excimer laser, which uses a cold beam of ultraviolet light to reshape the cornea so that light will focus properly on the retina. In myopia, the cornea is either too steep or the eye is too long for a clear image to be focused on the retina. PRK and LASIK flatten the cornea so that the image will focus more precisely on the retina.

In PRK, the surface of the cornea is removed by the laser. In LASIK, the outer layer of the cornea is sliced,

lifted, and moved aside while the cornea is reshaped with the laser. The outer layer is then replaced to speed healing. For LASIK and PRK, the patient's eye is numbed with anesthetic drops. No injections are necessary.

Before LASIK, the cornea's surface is marked with a dye marker so that the flap of cornea can be precisely aligned when it is replaced. The ophthalmologist places a suction ring from a microkeratome, a lathe-like surgical instrument, on the corneal limbus (where the clear cornea meets the white of the eye). When the device is properly positioned, the surgeon applies suction by using a foot pedal, causing the eye's pressure to elevate to 80 mm Hg from a minimum of 65 mm Hg. During this time, the microkeratome lathes the top 10% of the total corneal thickness, which creates a thin flap of tissue. The thin layer is folded back, the cornea is reshaped with the laser beam, and the flap layer is replaced. Because the flap is not permanently removed, patients have a faster recovery time and experience far less discomfort than with PRK. A physician or ophthalmic assistant administers antibiotic drops, and the eye is patched until the following day's checkup.

In PRK, a small area of the surface layer of the cornea is vaporized. It takes about three days for the surface cells to grow back, and vision will be blurred.

PRK and LASIK take only a few minutes. Patients are usually able to return home immediately after surgery.

The LTK system resembles a slit lamp used in a general eye exam, so it is non-threatening to patients. Before the procedure, an ophthalmic assistant administers three sets of anesthetic eyedrops with three minutes between each set. Ophthalmologists use a retractor to keep the eyelids open, and the other eye is patched. There is a three-minute waiting period after insertion of the laser to evaluate the tear film for irregularities or uneven dry spots on the cornea. The patient focuses on a fixating light, and the 16-spot nomogram for the degree of correction is programmed into the LTK unit's computer. The laser is applied for three seconds.

After the procedure, the ophthalmic assistant or physician will give the patient topical antibiotic drops. There is no postoperative patching. Some patients may experience a foreign-body sensation for a few hours after LTK. It sometimes takes a few weeks for vision to stabilize. Patients are usually seen one day postoperatively.

The cost of refractive surgery can vary with geographic area and the surgeon. In general, the procedure costs $1,350–$2,500 per eye for PRK and about $500 more per eye for LASIK. LTK is slightly

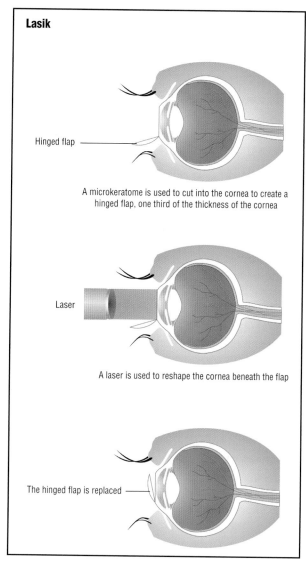

Lasik

Hinged flap

A microkeratome is used to cut into the cornea to create a hinged flap, one third of the thickness of the cornea

Laser

A laser is used to reshape the cornea beneath the flap

The hinged flap is replaced

(Diagram showing lasik eye surgery. Illustration by GGS Information Services, Inc. The Gale Group.)

topography, which creates a topographical map of the patient's eye.

Assistants need to advise patients to discontinue wearing contact lenses prior to the visual exams to make sure vision is stable, and advise the doctor of contact lens wear.

Before surgery, ophthalmic staff administer eye-drops and a sedative to the patient. The physician tests the patient's vision, and the patient rests while waiting for the sedative to take effect. Immediately before the surgery, ophthalmic staff administer local anesthetic eyedrops.

Ophthalmic staff also will check the microkeratome settings before surgery and test their accuracy. Some complications from refractive surgery result from a faulty microkeratome.

Aftercare

The patient returns to the surgeon for a follow-up visit the next day. After that, postoperative treatment may be handled by a co-managing optometrist. The doctor usually prescribes antibiotic and anti-inflammatory eyedrops. PRK patients have a longer recovery time and may need steroidal eyedrops for months. After LASIK, antibiotic and anti-inflammatory drops are prescribed for one week.

LTK patients are treated similarly, with antibiotic drops and an over-the-counter (OTC) **pain** reliever. Patients may have a foreign-body sensation for a few hours. It may take a few weeks for the eye to stabilize.

The attending physician will require the patient to return for a few months so that the patient's eye health and vision stability can be monitored. After that, yearly checkups are recommended.

Complications

There is a risk of under- or over-correction with LASIK and PRK. If vision is under-corrected, a second procedure can be performed to achieve results that may be closer to 20/20 vision. About 5–10% of PRK patients return for an enhancement, as do 10–25% of LASIK patients. Patients with very high myopia (over -15.00 diopters) may experience improvement after LASIK, but are not likely to achieve 20/40 vision or better without glasses.

Severe dry eye syndrome is a possible complication of LASIK, and has been reported more often as the number of procedures performed has increased. The condition may be permanent. Physicians may prescribe

more expensive than LASIK, at about $3,000 per eye. Refractive surgery may not be covered by insurance.

Preparation

Refractive eye surgery patients should be carefully screened by an ophthalmic assistant or physician before surgery is approved to avoid some possible complications. This screening should include a comprehensive eye exam, completed by either the ophthalmologist or a co-managing optometrist at least a few days before the surgery. At this time, the physician or ophthalmic assistant should chart any dry eye or corneal disease that may hinder surgery. They also should perform corneal intensive artificial tear therapy, and the use of punctal plugs or other procedures may be required.

Haze is another possible side effect, and is more likely to occur after PRK. Corneal scarring, halos, glare at night, or an irritating bump on the cornea are other side effects. Infection and vision loss are also possible with these procedures, but are extremely rare.

Most LASIK complications are related to the creation and realignment of the flap. The microkeratome must be in good working order and sharp. LASIK requires surgical skill and the complication rate is related to the experience level of the surgeon. In one study, the rate of LASIK complications declined from 3% for surgeons during their first three months using this technique, to 1% after a year's experience in the technique, to 0% after 18 months of experience.

Because LTK was approved in mid-2000, many of its complications have not yet been identified. Potential complications include corneal infiltrate or ulcer, uncontrolled intraocular pressure, late onset of haze, decrease in best spectacle-corrected visual acuity, or **retinal detachment**. In some cases the procedure is not successful at all.

Results

Most patients experience vision improvement immediately after refractive surgery. Vision tends to become sharper a few days after surgery and then stabilizes. Final visual acuity is achieved within three to six months with LASIK and six to eight months with PRK.

LASIK is more complicated than PRK because of the microkeratome procedure. However, LASIK generally has faster recovery time, less pain, and less chance of halos and scarring than PRK. LASIK can treat higher degrees of myopia (-5.00--25.00 diopters). LASIK also requires less use of steroids.

An LTK patient's vision will be overcorrected (improvement will be initially dramatic) for one to three months. The effect of improved near vision may diminish over time as distance vision improves.

There has been regression noted with LTK. The LTK mean rate of change decreases progressively, reaching only 0.02 diopters per month between 18 and 24 months. If the regression continues at the expected rate, the corrective effect would dissipate no sooner than 11 years after the procedure.

Health care team roles

Allied health professionals play an important role in preparing patients for refractive surgery. Advanced and

---

KEY TERMS

Blepharitis—An inflammation of the eyelid.

Cataract—A condition in which the lens of the eye turns cloudy and interferes with vision.

Cornea—The clear, curved tissue layer in front of the eye. It lies in front of the colored part of the eye (iris) and the black hole in the center of the iris (pupil).

Diopter (D)—A unit of measure of the power or strength of a lens.

Excimer laser—An instrument that is used to vaporize tissue with a cold, coherent beam of light with a single wavelength in the ultraviolet range.

Hyperopia—The inability to see near objects as clearly as distant objects, and the need for accommodation to see objects clearly.

Intraocular lens (IOL) implant—A small, plastic device (IOL), usually implanted in the lens capsule of the eye to correct vision after the lens of the eye is removed. This is the implant that is used in cataract surgery.

Macular degeneration—A condition usually associated with age, in which the area of the retina called the macula is impaired. This condition interferes with vision.

Microkeratome—A precision surgical instrument that can slice an extremely thin layer of tissue from the surface of the cornea.

Myopia—A vision problem in which distant objects appear blurry. Myopia results when the cornea is too steep or the eye is too long and the light doesn't focus properly on the retina. People who are myopic or nearsighted can usually see near objects clearly, but not far objects.

Refractive surgery—A surgical procedure that corrects visual defects.

Retina—The sensory tissue in the back of the eye that is responsible for collecting visual images and sending them to the brain.

---

intermediate-level ophthalmic technicians perform refractions and help determine the patient's eligibility for refractive surgery. These professionals also may perform corneal topography.

Specially trained ophthalmic nurses assist during the surgery. They check the microkeratomes and administer eyedrops. Advanced ophthalmic technologists, who are specially trained for additional duties such as taking ophthalmic photographs and using ultrasound, may administer eye medications, perform ophthalmologic tests, maintain ophthalmic surgical equipment and assist in refractive surgery.

Patient education

Refractive surgeons should carefully screen patients for these procedures and make sure the patients are aware of the possible complications before the procedure begins. Some highly myopic patients expecting "perfect" vision will be disappointed when they discover they still need eyeglasses for distance vision.

Ophthalmic staff also need to stress that while LTK vision improvements may be startling at first, those changes are likely to fade. These patients should be advised they may still need glasses for fine print. **Aging** and the onset of presbyopia will still affect their vision.

Training

Ophthalmologists are advised to observe other surgeons perform these procedures before they begin. Laser companies offer seminars to help doctors perfect their techniques. Other groups, such as the American Society of Cataract and Refractive Surgery, keep physicians informed of the latest advances. Co-managing optometrists are advised to observe surgeries and attend seminars to learn more about follow-up treatments.

Ophthalmic assistants who want to assist in these surgeries can receive additional training from certified education programs.

Resources

PERIODICALS

Brint, Stephen F., et al. "Photorefractive Keratectomy versus Laser in Situ Keratomileusis: Comparison of Optical Side Effects." *Ophthalmology* 107 (2000): 925-933.

Gorman, David, and Arthur M. Cotliar. "Refractive Surgery Options: RK vs PRK vs LASIK." *Newsweek*, 16 June 1997, S38.

OTHER

"Career Cards-Vision Care." East Texas Area Health Education Center. http://www.etxahec.org/hcp/20a.htm.

"Laser Vision Correction Surgery." Your Eye Site. http://www.youreyesite.com/laserrisks.htm.

ORGANIZATIONS

American Academy of Ophthalmology. PO Box 7424, San Francisco, CA 94120-7424 (415) 561-8500. http://www.eyenet.org.

American Society of Cataract and Refractive Surgery. 4000 Legato Road, Suite 850, Fairfax, VA 22033-4055. (703) 591-2220. http://www.ascrs.org.

Food and Drug Administration. 5600 Fishers Lane Rockville, MD 20857. (888) 463-6332. http://www.fda.gov.

Mary Bekker

Regional anesthetic *see* **Anesthesia, local**
Regional enteritis *see* **Crohn's disease**
Registered dietician *see* **Dietetics**

Registered nurse

Definition

Registered nurses, or RNs, are health care professionals who work as part of health care teams to promote health and prevent and treat disease. They are patient advocates and health care educators working to teach not only patients but also families and the community.

Description

With more than 2 million positions in the field, RNs make up the largest health care occupation. More than half of all health professions students are nursing students, and there are four times as many RNs in the United States as physicians. Most nurses are women; only 5–7% of all nurses are men.

Nurses work collaboratively with physicians and other health care providers, although the nursing profession is independent of medicine and other health disciplines. RNs' roles span from direct patient care to case management. Nurses are an integral part of the health care system. In fact, most health care services involve nursing care in some form.

In the area of direct patient care, RNs have many responsibilities:

- They observe, assess, and record patients' symptoms, responses to treatment, and progress.
- They provide assistance to physicians and other health care providers during examinations and treatments.
- They administer medications and take vital signs.
- They help patients to rehabilitate and heal.
- They educate patients and families about appropriate care after treatment, as well as long-term health.
- They develop and manage plans for nursing care.

In hospitals, RNs often work as staff nurses, providing care at the bedside and managing patients' medical needs. In some cases, RNs in hospitals supervise licensed practical nurses and aides.

RNs who work in office settings, for physicians or in clinics, assist administratively in the office and help the medical staff with patient preparation and examination. They administer medications, perform some lab tests and injections, as well as dress **wounds** and incisions. RNs also assist with minor surgery techniques and record taking.

Nurses in the nursing home setting provide a variety of care to elderly or sickly patients who cannot care for themselves because of age or illness. RNs in nursing home settings spend a good deal of their time developing treatment plans and performing other administrative duties, including supervising LPNs and nursing aides. They also provide direct patient care, assessing residents' medical conditions, monitoring treatment, and performing more advanced tasks, such as starting intravenous fluids. Nurses in this setting might concentrate on an area of specialization, such as long-term **rehabilitation**, in which they would care for **stroke** and **head injury** patients.

Home health nurses are often RNs who provide periodic at-home care for patients who might be recovering from illness or suffering from a chronic condition. While home health nurses work independently during their time in the home, the care they provide is prescribed by a physician or nurse practitioner.

RNs in **public health** nursing work in a variety of government and community organizations, including as school nurses and in public health clinics. The focus in this area of nursing is to make health care accessible to populations, including the underserved and those in rural areas. The goal is to improve overall health care in a community. Public health nurses work with community members to plan and implement programs to enhance community health care and educate groups about good health practices, such as disease prevention, child care and **nutrition**. They work in partnership with families, schools and other public organizations to help educate members about health. And these RNs make arrangements for health screenings, such as immunizations and **blood pressure** and **cholesterol** testing.

Occupational health or industrial nurses provide health care services on site in different environments. These nurses might work at a company's headquarters providing nursing care to employees or at a resort providing nursing care to tourists. RNs in this environment provide emergency care, prepare accident reports and make arrangements for any necessary additional care. Especially in the employee environment, they might coordinate health screenings, health counseling and assess work environments for safety.

In 2010, RNs' median annual income was $64,690. The median income that year of RNs working in hospitals was $64,650; home health care services $60,690; offices and clinics run by MDs $62,880; and nursing and personal care facilities $58,180.

The job market has been changing for RNs, making them more in demand. Much of this growth in opportunity is due to changing demographics. As more people become elderly, more will need nursing care and many more will need long-term care. The expansion of managed care has led to an increased emphasis on primary care. Another factor in the growth of the need for RNs is advancing technology, which requires the knowledge of RN or higher-level nurses. Essentially, the world is open to RNs because of opportunity and need now and in the future.

Work settings

The largest group of nurses work in hospitals, where they usually focus on a particular area of care, such as emergency room, intensive care, critical care, maternity, **oncology**, or **pediatrics**; or rotate throughout the hospital.

Nurses also work caring for patients on an outpatient basis in doctors' offices, clinics, surgery centers and emergency medical clinics. Some also work in **nursing homes**; public health facilities, such as government or private agencies and schools; on-site work environments in the occupational health or industrial nursing field; or in administrative positions within a corporate or organizational setting overseeing other nurses.

Nurses who work in hospitals generally work in fast-paced, pressure-filled environments. Many hospitals today are short-staffed due to budget cuts and the nursing shortage. Nurses in these and other environments spend considerable time standing and perform tasks that are hard on the body, such as lifting patients. Nurses often work all types of shifts, including daytime, weekend, and night shifts. Many nurses see the flexibility in scheduling as a positive factor—especially if they juggle childcare responsibilities. Nursing can be a dangerous occupation. They often care for people with infectious diseases, such as hepatitis, and are near radiation, chemicals used for instrument sterilization, and anesthetics. To avoid possible hazards, nurses must adhere to rigid safety guidelines. There is also an emotional toll involved with the job, as nurses often have close, daily contact with patients who are severely ill or dying.

Education and training

RNs must graduate from a nursing program and pass a national examination to become licensed. They must periodically renew their licenses and, depending on which state they workin, must also take continued education courses for license renewal.

There were more than 2,200 entry-level RN programs in the United States in 2004. RNs can pursue one of three educational options. They can complete an associate degree in nursing, which is usually offered at community and junior colleges and is about two years long; a bachelor of science degree in nursing, taken at colleges and universities and usually taking from four to five years; or a diploma program, which is given in hospitals and lasts about two to three years. Licensed graduates at any of these levels usually qualify to start work at the staff nurse level. Most RNs graduate with either an associate's or bachelor's degree. Today an increasing number of nurse executives are saying that they want a majority of their hospital staff nurses to have bachelor's degrees because of the more complex demands of patient care. In 2000, 22% of RNs reported have a diploma, 33% had a bachelor's degree and 34% held an associate's degree. There have been discussions in some states of requiring an RN to obtain a bachelor's degree or higher; however, this trend would not affect current associate degree RNs and would probably take place on a state-by-state basis. Most agree that there are more opportunities for advancement for RNs with bachelor's degrees in nursing. A bachelor's degree is often necessary for administrative positions and is required for admission to graduate nursing programs of all types, including research, consulting, teaching, and clinical specialization.

Students in nursing programs take courses in **anatomy**, **physiology**, **microbiology**, nutrition, psychology, chemistry, nursing, and other behavioral sciences. In addition to classroom instruction, nursing students receive supervised clinical experience in hospitals and other health care facilities. Nursing students receive a variety of clinical experience in settings such as hospital maternity, psychiatric, pediatric and surgical wards. They also gain experience in public health departments, home health agencies, and ambulatory clinics.

Advanced education and training

RNs can go on to become **advanced practice nurses**, which include nurse practitioners, clinical nurse specialists, certified registered nurse anesthetists, and certified nurse-midwives. Advanced practice nurses generally have master's degrees or certificates. Nurse practitioners deliver front-line primary and acute care. They can prescribe medications, and diagnose and treat common acute illnesses and injuries. Nurse practitioners

provide immunizations, conduct physical exams, and provide care to manage chronic diseases, such as diabetes. Certified nurse-midwives are trained to provide prenatal and gynecological care to healthy women. They also deliver babies in all types of settings, including the patient's home, and provide **postpartum care**. Clinical nurse specialists specialize in areas such as cardiology, oncology and pediatrics. Certified registered nurse anesthetists administer anesthetics to patients in inpatient, outpatient, and in-office settings. They are often the sole providers of anesthesia.

RNs can also go on to careers in teaching, research, or administration. These areas require master's degrees in nursing or PhD or doctorate-level degrees. Doctorally prepared RNs tend to go into education or research.

Future outlook

Registered nursing is projected to be among the 10 occupations in the United States to have the largest number of new jobs. Many areas of the country are suffering from severe nursing shortages and the problem is expected to get worse as baby boomers age. In sum, nurses will be able to pick and choose the paths of their careers. It is expected that job growth in nursing will be faster than average, largely because of technical advances in patient care. These advances will diagnose disease earlier and improve upon current treatments. With the median age of nurses over 40, many nurses will be retiring. Many of the positions in the future will come from openings left by these **aging** nurses. Areas that are expected to experience significant growth in nursing are ambulatory care settings, nursing homes, and home health care.

While hospitals will continue to need a tremendous number of nurses, hospitals are expected to grow more slowly than other health care environments. This is because the number of inpatients is expected to remain somewhat steady; patients are being released earlier and more procedures are being done outside hospitals. Nurses will find more opportunity in the hospital's specialty areas, including outpatients services, such as **chemotherapy** and rehabilitation. Home health employment for nursing will probably grow rapidly. A growing number of elderly who need nursing care but do not want to leave their homes will stimulate the expansion of this area of nursing. Nurses who are able to perform complex procedures in the home will be at the forefront of those able to take advantage of the home health opportunity. Nurses who want to work in nursing homes will find much faster than average growth in opportunities, due to the growing number of people who are too old to live on their own.

Resources

OTHER

Occupational Outlook Handbook, 2006-07 Ed. U.S. Department of Labor. Bureau of Labor Statistics. Division of Information Services. 2 Massachusetts Ave., NE., Room 2860. Washington, D.C. 20212. (202) 691-5200. http://stats.bls.gov.

ORGANIZATIONS

American Association of Colleges of Nursing. (202) 463-6980. http://www.aacn.nche.edu.
American Nurses Association. 600 Maryland Avenue, SW, Suite 100 West. Washington, DC 20024. (202) 651-7000. http://www.nursingworld.org.

Lisette Hilton

▌Rehabilitation

Definition

Rehabilitation is a treatment or treatments designed to facilitate the process of recovery from injury, illness, or disease to as normal a condition as possible.

Purpose

The purpose of rehabilitation is to restore some or all of the patient's physical, sensory, and mental capabilities that were lost due to injury, illness, or disease. Rehabilitation includes assisting the patient to compensate for deficits that cannot be reversed medically. It is prescribed after many types of injury, illness, or disease, including amputations, arthritis, **cancer**, cardiac disease, neurological problems, orthopedic injuries, **spinal cord** injuries, **stroke**, and traumatic **brain** injuries. The Institute of Medicine has estimated that as many as 14% of all Americans may be disabled at any given time.

Precautions

Rehabilitation should be carried out only by qualified therapists. Exercises and other physical interventions must take into account the patient's deficit. An example of a deficit is the loss of a limb.

Description

A proper and adequate rehabilitation program can reverse many disabling conditions or can help patients cope with deficits that cannot be reversed by medical care. Rehabilitation addresses the patient's physical, psychological, and environmental needs. It is achieved by restoring the patient's physical functions and/or modifying the patient's physical and social environment. The main types of rehabilitation are physical, occupational, and **speech therapy**.

Each rehabilitation program is tailored to the individual patient's needs and can include one or more types of therapy. The patient's physician usually coordinates the efforts of the rehabilitation team, which can include physical, occupational, speech, or other therapists; nurses; engineers; physiatrists (physical medicine); psychologists; orthotists (makes devices such as braces to straighten out curved or poorly shaped bones); prosthetists (a therapist who makes artificial limbs or protheses); and vocational counselors. Family members are often actively involved in the patient's rehabilitation program.

Physical therapy

Physical therapy helps the patient restore the use of muscles, bones, and the nervous system through the use of heat, cold, massage, whirlpool baths, ultrasound, **exercise**, and other techniques. It seeks to relieve **pain**, improve strength and mobility, and train the patient to perform important everyday tasks. Physical therapy may be prescribed to rehabilitate a patient after amputations, arthritis, **burns**, cancer, cardiac disease, cervical and lumbar dysfunction, neurological problems, orthopedic injuries, pulmonary disease, spinal cord injuries, stroke, traumatic brain injuries, and other injuries/illnesses. The duration of the physical therapy program varies depending on the injury/illness being treated and the patient's response to therapy.

Exercise is the most widely used and best known type of physical therapy. Depending on the patient's condition, exercises may be performed by the patient alone or with the therapist's help, or with the therapist moving the patient's limbs. Exercise equipment for physical therapy could include an exercise table or mat, a stationary bicycle, walking aids, a wheelchair, practice stairs, parallel bars, and pulleys and weights.

Heat treatment, applied with hot-water compresses, infrared lamps, short-wave radiation, high frequency electrical current, ultrasound, paraffin wax, or warm baths, is used to stimulate the patient's circulation, relax muscles, and relieve pain. Cold treatment is applied with ice packs or cold-water soaking. Soaking in a whirlpool can ease muscle spasm pain and help strengthen movements. Massage aids circulation, helps the patient relax, relieves pain and muscle spasms, and reduces swelling. Very low strength electrical currents

KEY TERMS

Orthotist—A health care professional who is skilled in making and fitting orthopedic appliances.

Physiatrist—A physician who specializes in physical medicine.

Prosthetist—A health care professional who is skilled in making and fitting artificial parts (prosthetics) for the human body.

applied through the skin stimulate muscles and make them contract, helping paralyzed or weakened muscles respond again.

Occupational therapy

Occupational therapy helps the patient regain the ability to do normal everyday tasks. This may be achieved by restoring old skills or teaching the patient new skills to adjust to disabilities through adaptive equipment, orthotics, and modification of the patient's home environment. Occupational therapy may be prescribed to rehabilitate a patient after amputation, arthritis, cancer, cardiac disease, head injuries, neurological injuries, orthopedic injuries, pulmonary disease, spinal cord disease, stroke, and other injuries/illnesses. The duration of the occupational therapy program varies depending on the injury/illness being treated and the patient's response to therapy.

Occupational therapy includes learning how to use devices to assist in walking (artificial limbs, canes, **crutches**, walkers), getting around without walking (wheelchairs or motorized scooters), or moving from one spot to another (boards, lifts, and bars). The therapist will visit the patient's home and analyze what the patient can and cannot do. Suggestions on modifications to the home, such as rearranging furniture or adding a wheelchair ramp, will be made. Health aids to bathing and grooming could also be recommended.

Speech therapy

Speech therapy helps the patient correct **speech disorders** or restore speech. Speech therapy may be prescribed to rehabilitate a patient after a brain injury, cancer, neuromuscular diseases, stroke, and other injuries/illnesses. The duration of the speech therapy program varies depending on the injury/illness being treated and the patient's response to therapy.

Performed by a speech pathologist, speech therapy involves regular meetings with the therapist in an individual or group setting and home exercises. To strengthen muscles, the patient might be asked to say words, smile, close his mouth, or stick out his tongue. Picture cards may be used to help the patient remember everyday objects and increase his vocabulary. The patient might use picture boards of everyday activities or objects to communicate with others. Workbooks might be used to help the patient recall the names of objects and practice reading, writing, and listening. Computer programs are available to help sharpen speech, reading, recall, and listening skills.

Other types of therapists

Inhalation therapists, audiologists, and registered dietitians are other types of therapists. Inhalation therapists help the patient learn to use respirators and other breathing aids to restore or support breathing. Audiologists help diagnose the patient's **hearing loss** and recommend solutions. Dietitians provide dietary advice to help the patient recover from or avoid specific problems or diseases.

Rehabiltation centers

Rehabilitation services are provided in a variety of settings including clinical and office practices, hospitals, skilled-care **nursing homes**, sports medicine clinics, and some health maintenance organizations. Some therapists make home visits. Advice on choosing the appropriate type of therapy and therapist is provided by the patient's medical team.

Resources

ORGANIZATIONS

National Rehabilitation Association, 633 S. Washington St., Alexandria, VA 22314, (703) 836-0850,

National Rehabilitation Information Center, 8201 Corporate Drive, Suite 600, Landover, MD 20785, (800) 346-2742, naricinfo@heitechservices.com, http://www.naric.com

Rehabilitation International, 25 East 21st Street, 4th floor, New York, NY 10010, (212) 420-1500, Fax: (212) 505-0871, ri@riglobal.org, http://www.riglobal.org.

Lori De Milto

Rehabilitation technology

Definition

Rehabilitation technology is a profession that uses technology to help people with physical disabilities increase their independence.

Description

The goal of rehabilitation technology is to remove barriers so that people with disabilities are able to live independently. This goal could be achieved by technology ranging from a wheelchair with a customized joystick controller to a computer equipped with voice-recognition software. Those are some of the assistive devices that allow a disabled person to be socially active, for example to work and attend school.

Rehabilitation technology is a team-oriented profession that brings together people with a range of expertise. A rehabilitation technologist may work with a rehabilitation engineer. For example, the technologist evaluates a patient's wheelchair seating needs; the engineer could make necessary modifications.

Rehabilitation is a longtime goal of healthcare. During the 1990s, technological advances increased the scope of equipment and devices for use in the rehabilitation of disabilities. In addition, the **Americans with Disabilities Act** of 1990 banned discrimination against people with physical and mental disabilities. The federal law banned discrimination in the areas of employment, public services like transportation systems, and public accommodations such as restaurants and theaters.

While the law guaranteed rights for individuals with disabilities, the profession of rehabilitation technology provided the tools to help those people improve their quality of life. Sometimes referred to as assistive technology, rehabilitation technology generally involves the areas of: wheeled mobility and seating, computer access, augmentative communication, home and worksite modifications, and environmental controls.

Wheeled mobility and seating

Wheelchairs and scooters are evaluated for factors including the person's capabilities. The sip-and-puff wheelchair is operated by blowing and sucking air into the controller. Another issue for motorized equipment is how the person is seated and positioned in the chair. Modifications could include cushions or a redesign of the equipment.

Adaptive seating is also an issue for people with orthopedic conditions. Accommodations in the workplace and classroom include arranging for chairs that provide support.

Team members working in this area include rehabilitation technologists or physical therapists and rehabilitation engineers.

Computer access

Computer access removes the barriers to computers for people with physical and visual disabilities.

Adaptive devices include items such as a mouth-operated joystick that is used on an onscreen keyboard. A visually impaired person with low **vision** could use large-print software. For the blind person, there is software that utilizes Braille and sound.

Technologists involved in this area include engineers with experience in rehabilitation and computer applications. They work with allied health professionals trained in computer access. The job title for these people may be rehabilitation technologist or occupational therapist.

Augmentative communication

Augmentative communication is also known as alternative communication. Systems in this area provide other means of communication for people with impaired speaking or writing skills. Assistive devices range from letter boards to voice-output computers and electronic augmentative communication devices. On the board are letters that the person points to as a means of communicating. The electronic devices are portable computers programmed with synthesized speech. The person uses the device to speak to others.

The professionals working in this area are licensed speech pathologists trained in augmentative devices. Another job title is augmentative communication specialist.

Home and worksite modifications

Home and worksite modifications are adaptations that allow a person to live independently and earn a living. Modifications in the home and workplace could include the installation of wheelchair ramps and lighting. In the home, doors could be widened for wheelchair access. Other changes might include lowering kitchen counters and installing handrails in the bathroom.

An occupational therapist or rehabilitation engineer would give recommendations about the modifications. The changes would be made by a professional experienced in architecture or industrial design.

Other workplace modifications could include changes to office furniture and tools that give people the ability to perform their jobs. In the home, devices that allow people to live independently include utensils with foam handles. These are easier to hold for people with limited hand function. These adaptive devices are called aids to daily living; they are also referred to as environmental controls.

Environmental controls

Environmental controls are devices or equipment that remove barriers to performing tasks such as grooming, using appliances, turning lights on, and using a telephone or VCR. The controls are available for use in the home, on the job, and in the classroom. Aids include spring-loaded scissors and a device that helps people put socks on. Furthermore, some voice-activated systems control the TV, turn lights and appliances off and on, and open and close doors.

An occupational therapist is among the team members who make recommendations about environmental controls.

Work settings

Rehabilitation technology is a profession that encompasses occupations in health care, technology, science, and engineering. Within those occupations are researchers, people designing or refining equipment, those who sell the equipment and individuals who help people obtain and use equipment.

Employers of rehabilitation technology professionals include rehabilitation facilities operated by private hospitals, health maintenance organizations, and state rehabilitation agencies. Other employers are businesses that design, manufacture and sell equipment. Schools employ special education technology consultants. Occupational therapists and physical therapists with rehabilitation technology experience work in rehabilitation centers, hospitals, and residential- care facilities. Some allied health professionals have education, experience, and the job title of rehabilitation technologist. The degree and profession are sometimes known as assistive technology.

Education and training

Educational requirements vary within the professions associated with rehabilitation technology. Some community colleges offer two-year degrees in areas such as assistive technology. A two-year degree is a requirement for an **occupational therapy** assistant, according to the American Occupational Therapy Association.

Occupational therapists must have a bachelor degree or advanced post-baccalaureate degree. Therapists and assistants must do fieldwork and pass a national certification exam. In addition, states require licensing.

Professional certification

Professional certification was voluntary as of December of 2005. At that time, RESNA offered certification exams for Assistive Technology Provider (ATP), Rehabilitation Engineering Technologist (RET), and Assistive Technology Supplier (ATS). The ATP credential demonstrates knowledge and training in the use of devices. A professional must have that credential before earning RET certification. RET skills include designing and modifying assistive technology devices. The ATS credential is for people involved in the sales and service of assistive technology equipment.

Eligibility for ATP testing was based on years of education and experience in late 2005. A person with a bachelor's degree or higher in a rehabilitation science discipline needed at least two years of direct assistive-technology experience. Requirements varied for the person with a two-year degree in rehabilitation science. A professional needed to work full time for two years in assistive technology service or three years for 20 hours per week.

For the RET certificate, a bachelor's degree was required in engineering, engineering technology, engineering-related disciplines, or computer science. Also required were at least two years of fulltime relevant employment. Furthermore, permission to test could be granted to candidates with degrees from non-accredited programs. Accreditation is granted by the Accreditation Board for Engineering and Technology, Inc.

Advanced education and training

For the allied health professional with work experience or a two-year degree, a four-year degree may be the next step in a career path. Employers sometimes require the additional education.

Advanced education programs are often at the graduate level. These include master's degrees in rehabilitation science and technology. These programs include clinical coursework as well as courses related to science and technology. Some engineering schools also offer graduate degrees in **biomedical engineering** with an emphasis in rehabilitation technology.

Furthermore, continuing education is crucial for all occupations within rehabilitation technology. As technology advances, professionals will need to remain current about new equipment and how to use it.

Future outlook

Employment within occupations that work with rehabilitation technology is projected to increase from 21 to 35 percent through the year 2012, according to the U.S. Department of Labor's Bureau of Labor Statistics "Occupational Outlook Handbook 2004-05." The bureau projected faster than average job growth in the occupations of biomedical engineering, occupational therapy, **physical therapy**, speech-language pathology, and rehabilitation counseling.

Although rehabilitation technology was not listed as a profession in the handbook, the reasons for increased employment would apply to allied-health professionals with expertise in assistive technology and rehabilitation technology. For biomedical engineers and the rehabilitative professions, projected job growth was related to the **aging** population. The number of older people continues to increase as people live longer.

While the bureau forecast increased employment, there was a caution that proposed federal legislation could place a limit on the reimbursement for services. Those changes could have negative effects on the employment of therapists, counselors, and speech pathologists. However, the bureau rated the impact as a short-term effect, and projected that the demand would continue to grow for people in those occupations.

Resources

BOOKS

Bureau of Labor Statistics, U.S. Department of Labor. *Occupational Outlook Handbook, 2004-05 Edition, Cardiovascular Technologists and Technicians. http://www. bls.gov/oco* (cited Nov. 26, 2005).

Scherer, Marcia. *Living in the State of Stuck, 4th ed.* Brookline, MA: Brookline Books, 2005.

PERIODICALS

Cowan, Donna M., and Yasmin Khan. "Assistive Technology for Children with Complex Disabilities." *Current Paediatrics* 15 i3 (June 2005): 207(6).

Gavin-Dreschnack, Deborah. "Wheelchairs: One Size Does Not Fit All." *Nursing Homes* 54 i4 (April 2005): 68(2).

Technology Broadens Options. *Paraplegia News* 58 i8 (August 2004): 21(1).

ORGANIZATIONS

American Occupational Therapy Association. 4720 Montgomery Lane, Bethesda, MD 20824-1220. (301) 652-2682. http://www.aota.org.

Rehabilitation Engineering & Assistive Technology Society of North America. 1700 N. Moore St., Suite 1540, Arlington VA 22209-1903. (703) 524-6686. http://www.resna.org.

Liz Swain

Relaxation

Definition

Relaxation therapy is a broad term used to describe a number of techniques that promote **stress** reduction, the elimination of tension throughout the body, and a calm and peaceful state of mind.

Origins

Relaxation therapy has been around for thousands of years in the forms of transcendental **meditation** (TM), **yoga**, **t'ai chi**, **qigong**, and vipassana (a Buddhist form of meditation meaning insight and also known as mindfulness meditation). Progressive relaxation, a treatment that rids the body of **anxiety** and related tension through progressive relaxation of the muscle groups, was first described by Dr. Edmund Jacobson in his book *Progressive Relaxation*, published in 1929. And in 1975, Dr. Herbert Benson published his groundbreaking work *The Relaxation Response*, which described in detail the stress-reduction mechanism in the body that short-circuits the "fight-or-flight" response and lowers **blood pressure**, relieves muscle tension, and controls **heart** rate. This work gave further credence and legitimacy to the link between mind and body medicine. A number of today's commonly used relaxation techniques, such as cue-controlled relaxation, are a direct result of Benson's work in this area.

Benefits

Stress and tension have been linked to numerous ailments, including heart disease, high **blood** pressure, **atherosclerosis**, **irritable bowel syndrome**, ulcers, anxiety disorders, insomnia, and **substance abuse**. Stress can also trigger a number of distinct physical symptoms, including nausea, **headache**, hair loss, fatigue, and muscle **pain**. Relaxation therapies have been shown to reduce the incidence and severity of stress-related diseases and disorders in many patients.

Description

There are a number of different relaxation methods available. Some of the most widely taught and practiced by health care providers include progressive relaxation, cue-controlled relaxation, breathing exercises, guided imagery, and biofeedback.

Progressive relaxation

Progressive relaxation is performed by first tensing, and then relaxing, the muscles of the body, one group at a time. Muscle groups can be divided a number of different ways, but a common method is to use the following groupings: 1) Hands and arms; 2) head, neck, and shoulders; 3) torso, including chest, **stomach** and back; and 4) thighs, buttocks, legs, and feet. The patient lies or sits in a comfortable position, and then starts with the first muscle group, focusing on the feeling of the muscles and the absence or presence of tension. The patient then tenses the first muscle in the group, holds the tension for approximately five seconds, and releases and relaxes for up to 30 seconds. The contrast allows the individual to notice the difference between feelings of tension and feelings of relaxation. The procedure is repeated with the next muscle in the group, and so on, until the first group is completed. The patient then starts on the next muscle group.

Progressive relaxation can be guided with verbal cues and scripts, either memorized by the patient or provided on instructional audiotapes. The procedure remains the same, but the individual is prompted on which muscles to flex and relax, and given other cues about noticing the difference between the tense and relaxed state. Some individuals may prefer progressive relaxation that is prompted with a tape, because it allows them to completely clear their minds and to just follow the given instructions.

Deep breathing exercises

Individuals under stress often experience fast, shallow breathing. This type of breathing, known as chest breathing, can lead to shortness of breath, increased muscle tension, and inadequate oxygenation of blood. Breathing exercises can both improve respiratory function and relieve stress and tension.

Before starting to learn breathing exercises, individuals should first become aware of their breathing patterns. This can be accomplished by placing one hand on the chest and one hand on the **abdomen**, and observing which hand moves further during breathing. If it is the hand placed on the chest, then chest breathing is occurring and breathing exercises may be beneficial.

Deep breathing exercises are best performed while lying flat on the back, usually on the floor with a mat. The knees are bent, and the body (particularly the mouth, nose, and face) is relaxed. Again, one hand should be placed on the chest and one on the abdomen to monitor breathing technique. The individual takes a series of long, deep breaths through the nose, attempting to raise the abdomen instead of the chest. Air is exhaled through the relaxed mouth. Deep breathing can be continued for up to 20 minutes. After the **exercise** is complete, the individual checks again for body tension and relaxation. Once deep breathing techniques have been mastered, an individual can use deep breathing at any time or place as a quick method of relieving tension.

Release-only relaxation

Like progressive relaxation, release-only relaxation focuses on relieving feelings of tension in the muscles. However, it eliminates the initial use of muscle tensing as practiced in progressive relaxation, focusing instead solely on muscle relaxation. Release-only relaxation is usually recommended as the next step in relaxation therapy after progressive relaxation has been mastered.

In release-only relaxation, breathing is used as a relaxation tool. The individual sits in a comfortable chair and begins to focus on breathing, envisioning tension leaving the body with each exhalation. Once even, deep, abdominal breathing is established, the individual begins to focus on releasing tension in each muscle group until the entire body is completely relaxed.

Cue-controlled relaxation

Cue-controlled relaxation is an abbreviated tension relief technique that combines elements of release-only relaxation and deep breathing exercises. It uses a cue, such as a word or mental image, to trigger immediate feelings of muscle relaxation. The cue must first be associated with relaxation in the individual's mind. This is accomplished by choosing the cue and then using it in breathing and release-only relaxation exercises repeatedly, until the cue starts to automatically trigger feelings of relaxation outside of the treatment sessions. Cues can be as simple as the word "relax," and are frequently used on relaxation audiotapes. They can also be a visual cue, such as a mental image of a white-sand Caribbean beach, a flower-filled meadow, or other relaxing images. Guided imagery also uses such visualization exercises to produce feelings of relaxation.

Guided imagery

Guided imagery is a two-part process. The first component involves reaching a state of deep relaxation through breathing and muscle relaxation techniques. During the relaxation phase, the person closes the eyes and focuses on the slow inhalations and exhalations. Or, he or she might focus on releasing the feelings of tension from their muscles, starting with the toes and working up to the top of the head. Relaxation tapes often feature soft music or tranquil, natural sounds such as rolling waves and chirping birds in order to promote feelings of relaxation.

Once complete relaxation is achieved, the second component of the exercise is the imagery, or visualization itself. Relaxation imagery involves conjuring up pleasant, relaxing images that rest the mind and body. These may be experiences that have already happened, or they may be new situations.

The individual may also use mental rehearsal. Mental rehearsal involves imagining a situation or scenario and its ideal outcome. It can be used to reduce anxiety about an upcoming situation, such as **childbirth**, surgery, or even a critical event such as an important competition or a job interview. Individuals imagine themselves going through each step of the anxiety-producing event and then successfully completing it.

Biofeedback

Biofeedback, or applied psychophysiological feedback, is a patient-guided treatment that teaches an individual to manipulate muscle tension through relaxation, visualization, and other cognitive techniques. The name biofeedback refers to the biological signals that are fed back, or returned, to the patient in order for the patient to develop techniques of controlling them.

During biofeedback, one or more special sensors are placed on the body. These sensors measure muscle tension, **brain** waves, heart rate, and body temperature; and translate the information into a visual and/or audible readout, such as a paper tracing, a light display, or a series of beeps. While the patient views the instantaneous feedback from the biofeedback monitors, he begins to recognize what thoughts, fears, and mental images influence his physical reactions. By monitoring this relationship between mind and body, he can then use thoughts and mental images deliberately to manipulate heart beat, brain wave patterns, body temperature, and other bodily functions, and to reduce feelings of stress. This is achieved through relaxation exercises, mental imagery, and other cognitive therapy techniques.

As the biofeedback response takes place, the patient can actually see or hear the results of his efforts instantly through the sensor readout on the biofeedback equipment. Once these techniques are learned and the patient is able to recognize the state of relaxation or visualization necessary to alleviate symptoms, the biofeedback equipment itself is no longer needed. The patient then has a powerful, portable, and self-administered treatment tool to deal with problem symptoms.

There are dozens of other effective therapies that promote relaxation, including hypnosis, meditation, yoga, aromatherapy, **hydrotherapy**, t'ai chi, massage, **art therapy**, and others. Individuals should choose a type of relaxation therapy based on their own unique interests and lifestyle requirements.

Preparations

If an individual is considering relaxation therapy to alleviate physical symptoms such as nausea, headache, high blood pressure, fatigue, or gastrointestinal problems, he or she should consult a doctor first to make sure there is not an underlying disorder or disease causing the symptoms. A complete **physical examination** and comprehensive medical history will be performed, and even if an organic cause for the symptoms is found, relaxation exercises may still be recommended as an adjunctive, or complementary, treatment to relieve discomfort.

Relaxation therapy should always take place in a quiet, relaxing atmosphere where there is a comfortable place to sit or recline. Some people find that quiet background music improves their relaxation sessions. If an instructional audiotape or videotape is to be used, the appropriate equipment should be available.

The relaxation session, which can last anywhere from a few minutes to an hour, should be uninterrupted. Taking the phone off the hook and asking family members for solitude can ensure a more successful and relaxing session.

Precautions

Most commonly practiced relaxation techniques are completely safe and free of side effects.

Relaxation techniques that involve special exercises or body manipulation such as massage, t'ai chi, and yoga should be taught or performed by a qualified health care professional or instructor. These treatments may not be suitable for individuals with certain health conditions such as arthritis or **fibromyalgia**. These individuals should consult with their health care professional before engaging in these therapies.

Biofeedback may be contraindicated (not recommended) in some individuals who use a pacemaker or other implantable electrical devices. These individuals should inform their biofeedback therapist before starting

KEY TERMS

Qigong—An exercise practice derived from traditional Chinese medicine that is designed to facilitate energy flow throughout the body.

T'ai chi—A martial art that uses exercise to balance the body's energy flow to the body center in order to promote physical well-being.

treatments, as certain types of biofeedback sensors have the potential to interfere with their use.

Relaxation therapy may not be suitable for some patients. Patients must be willing to take a very active role in the treatment process, and to practice techniques learned in treatment at home.

Some relaxation therapies may also be inappropriate for cognitively impaired individuals (e.g., patients with organic brain disease or a traumatic brain injury) depending on their level of functioning. Given the wide range of relaxation therapies available, if one type of relaxation treatment is deemed inappropriate for these patients, a suitable alternative can usually be recommended by a qualified health care professional.

Side effects

Relaxation therapy can induce sleepiness, and some individuals may fall asleep during a session. Relaxation therapy should not be performed while operating a motor vehicle or in other situations where full and alert attention is necessary. Other than this, there are no known adverse side effects to relaxation therapy.

Research and general acceptance

Relaxation therapies have been successfully used in relieving stress and anxiety for many years, and are generally well-accepted by the medical community for this purpose.

Recent research published in 1999 has also indicated that relaxation therapy may be useful in reducing the incidence of **preterm labor** in women at risk for delivering prematurely. The study also found that women who discontinued relaxation exercises, for whatever reasons, delivered earlier and had lower birth weight babies than those who continued the treatment.

Training and certification

Relaxation therapy techniques are used by many licensed therapists, counselors, psychologists, psychiatrists,

and other health care professionals. There are many self-help books, audiotapes, and videos available that offer instruction in relaxation techniques.

Resources

BOOK

Davis, Martha, et al. *The Relaxation & Stress Reduction Workbook.* 4th edition. Oakland, CA: New Harbinger Publications, Inc., 1995.

OTHER

Brennan, Patricia. "Stress First Aid Kit." (Guided imagery audiotape set.) Available from Inside Out Publishing at (888) 727-3296 or http://www.facingthedawn.com.

ORGANIZATION

The American Psychological Association. 750 First St. NE, Washington DC 20002-4242. (800) 374-2721. http://www.apa.org.

Paula Ford-Martin

Renal calculi *see* **Kidney stones**

Renal failure, acute *see* **Kidney failure, acute**

Renal failure, chronic *see* **Kidney failure, chronic**

Renal radionuclide scan *see* **Kidney radionuclide scan**

Renin assay *see* **Plasma renin activity**

Reproductive health

Definition

A person's reproductive health is the maintenance of the health of his or her reproductive system, which include respectively the penis and the testes; and the vagina, uterus, and breasts. The reproductive health spectrum also includes **pregnancy** and **infertility**.

Description

The reproductive systems

The **female reproductive system** comprises ovaries, fallopian tubes, uterus, vagina, breasts, and external genitalia. The ovaries hold the eggs and release them during ovulation. When an egg is fertilized, it travels through the fallopian tubes and is implanted in the uterus. The uterus, through the placenta and umbilical cord, nurtures the fetus for approximately 40 weeks, at which time the woman delivers.

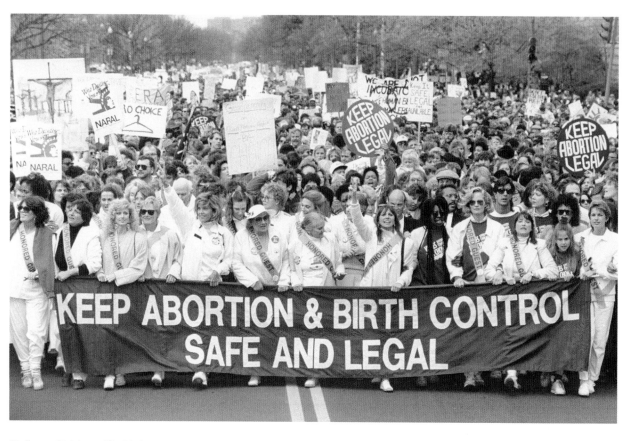

(© Susan Steinkamp/Corbis.)

The **male reproductive system** consists of the testes, epididymis, vas deferens, urethra, seminal vesicles, prostate, and penis. During intercourse, the penis—the copulating organ—becomes engorged with **blood** and becomes erect. Upon ejaculation, mature sperm cells are ejected into the vagina after moving through the vas deferens, passing the seminal vesicles and prostate gland. After the semen is deposited in the vagina, the sperm swim through the cervix, into the uterus, and up into the fallopian tubes. The egg is fertilized in the fallopian tubes, if indeed an egg is present.

Infertility

A person is infertile when he or she is unable to perform the function of reproduction. Infertility is considered a disease and affects about ten million men and women in the United States, according to the Centers for Disease Control and Prevention.

Infertility disorders in men include azoospermia, in which no sperm cells are produced; and oligospermia, in which few sperm cells are produced. Although the number of cases is rare, infertility can be caused by a genetic disorder. Typically, male infertility rests with the testes, responsible for the production of sperm. Disorders

of the thyroid, adrenal and pituitary glands, **liver**, and kidneys—as well as infections and trauma to the testes—can contribute to male infertility.

Further, hazards in a man's workplace can affect his ability to have healthy children. These are called reproductive hazards, and include radiation, chemicals, drugs (legal and illegal), heat, and heavy metals, such as lead. Still, every man does not suffer the effects of workplace hazards; frequency, length, and method of exposure (inhalation, skin contact, ingestion) are a few of the factors that affect whether a man is exposed to any dangerous degree. These hazards, unfortunately, can arrest or slow the production of sperm. If there are fewer sperm to fertilize the egg, there will be fewer chances that the egg will be fertilized; if there are no sperm produced, the man is termed "sterile." If the workplace hazard has prevented sperm from being produced at all, the man is permanently sterile.

In women, infertility can be caused by an ovulation disorder, blocked fallopian tubes, pelvic inflammatory disease (PID), or endometriosis.

The vast majority of individuals suffering from infertility—85 to 90%—can be treated with medication or surgery. The remaining percentage of persons may turn to *in vitro* fertilization, in which conception takes place outside the body and the embryo is implanted in the uterus by a physician.

Viewpoints

Abortion

One of the most explosive and controversial aspects of reproductive health is **abortion**. Issues of morality, religion, and politics are often part of these discussions. Worldwide, it is estimated that nearly half of all human pregnancies are unplanned. Many result from incorrect use or failure of contraceptives. Women also may become pregnant because they do not have access to family planning alternatives or are pressured by a partner not to use contraceptives.

Abortion became legal in the United States in 1973 following the landmark U.S. Supreme Court decision in *Roe vs. Wade.* Since then, the Court has heard at least 20 major cases challenging the law. The Supreme Court, however, has upheld the fundamental principles of *Roe vs. Wade* as of 2012.

Most abortions are performed within the first trimester, or the first three months of pregnancy. Fewer than 9% of abortions are performed in the second trimester, and in only rare cases when there is serious health concern are abortions performed in the final trimester.

Contraception

The purpose of contraceptives is to avoid pregnancy by preventing the likelihood of fertilization or implantation of a fertilized egg. Women can use devices that fit into either the vagina or uterus; these devices are known as barrier methods. There are advantages and disadvantages to each method. Sometimes they can cause serious side effects, such as excessive menstrual bleeding. Barrier contraceptive devices, in addition to preventing pregnancy, also can help prevent sexually transmitted infections (STIs) and the human **immunodeficiency** virus (HIV), the virus that causes acquired immune deficiency syndrome (**AIDS**). Male barrier methods include latex condoms.

Female barrier methods include the diaphragm, female condom, cervical cap, sponge, and intrauterine device (IUD). These devices also can be used with a chemical combination known as a spermicide, which helps to kill sperm during intercourse.

A diaphragm is a dome-shaped flexible barrier with a rim that fits into the vagina and prevents sperm from reaching the cervix. Health professionals recommend that diaphragms be used with spermicide to achieve an 82–94% effectiveness rate against pregnancy. Instruction is required on how to insert and remove the diaphragm. This device, which can be inserted up to six hours before intercourse, must remain in the vagina for six hours after intercourse. There are two disadvantages to the diaphragm. The diaphragm may be dislodged during sex. There is also an increased risk of bladder and urinary tract infections.

The female condom is designed to line the inside of the vagina. Made from polyurethane, unlike male condoms (which are made from latex), and used without a spermicide, the female condom can be inserted up to eight hours before intercourse.

The cervical cap is a small dome, but is not as flexible as the diaphragm. It is placed tightly on the cervix one-half hour to 48 hours prior to intercourse, and is used with spermicide. When used alone, the cervical cap provides an 82–94% effectiveness rate. With spermicide, the cervical cap provides an even greater degree of confidence against unwanted pregnancy. There are several reasons that cervical caps are not widely used. Some women have difficulty with their insertion, which must be done at least one-half hour before intercourse. There is some discomfort when they are being inserted. Cervical caps can also be difficult to remove, and repeated intercourse dictates reapplication of the unit. There is some risk of irritation and allergic reaction. Last, because of the risks of toxic **shock** syndrome (TSS), women should not wear the cervical cap more for more than 48 hours after intercourse.

The contraceptive sponge also acts as a barrier and is used with a spermicide. The sponge is available without a prescription, and the woman does not need training to insert and remove it. However, the spermicide used with the sponge may be irritating and cause allergic reactions. The sponge should not be used more than once, and should be left in the vagina for six hours after intercourse. If left in for more than six hours, the woman is at risk for toxic shock syndrome.

The IUD, inserted by a health professional, blocks the fallopian tubes so that sperm have fewer chances of passing through the tubes to fertilize the woman's egg. In the event that sperm do pass through the tubes and an egg is fertilized, the IUD can prevent the fertilized egg from becoming implanted in the uterus. An IUD, however, can cause cramping and bleeding in women, and can be spontaneously expelled. This device has also been known to increase a woman's risk of developing PID, might increase her menstrual flow, and can cause cramping. The rate of effectiveness with the IUD is greater than 99%.

Birth control pills (also called "combined pills") are more than 99% effective against pregnancy. They do not offer any protection against STIs. While they have some other disadvantages for women, such as possible **dizziness**, nausea, menstruation changes, and weight and mood fluctuations, there are also advantages. These include continuous contraceptive protection, if taken as prescribed. They are reversible. When one stops taking them, the pills stop working, and another method of birth control must be used immediately. Birth control pills must be taken daily, and are contraindicated for smokers over 35 years of age. They also increase blood clot risk.

The minipill, which is progestin only, has a 95% estimated effectiveness rate. It can also cause irregular bleeding, breast tenderness, weight gain, and a slightly increased chance of ectopic pregnancy; it does provide some protection against PID. It is completely ineffective as a barrier to STIs.

With a greater than 99% effectiveness rate and continuous protection against pregnancy for up to five years, the woman who has had a subdermal implant does not need to be bothered remembering to take a pill. An in-office procedure is required, though, to surgically introduce the implant. The patient may suffer from side effects, which may include menstrual bleeding irregularities and weight change.

Another birth control method with a greater than 99% effectiveness rate is the contraceptive injection (medroxyprogesterone acetate). The patient has three months of protection, with no need to remember to do anything related to birth control on a daily basis. The woman requires quarterly injections at the doctor's office by the doctor or nurse. As with the implant, there may be side effects, which also include changes in menstrual bleeding and weight.

Tubal ligation, performed surgically by a physician, is a procedure that is irreversible. After a woman has undergone this procedure, she has a greater than 99% guarantee against becoming pregnant.

Men have far fewer choices in barrier contraceptives, but condoms are the most popular choice. They are easy to obtain and the best means of protection from STIs and HIV. Made from latex, condoms are placed over the penis before intercourse to prevent the ejaculation of sperm into the woman's vagina. They can be used with or without spermicides. Without a spermicide, condoms are 88–98% effective against pregnancy. With spermicide, condoms may provide even higher protection against pregnancy. The disadvantages of using a condom are possibly reduced feeling by the man. There may also

KEY TERMS

Azoospermia—In infertile men, the lack of sperm being produced.

Cervix—The lowest part of the uterus that connects the vagina to the uterus.

Contraceptives—Devices or medications designed to prevent pregnancy by suppressing ovulation, preventing sperm from passing through the cervix to fertilize an egg, or preventing implantation of a fertilized egg.

Diaphragm—A barrier form of contraception that is a flexible, dome-shaped device with a rim that blocks sperm from passing through the cervix.

Endometriosis—The presence and growth of functioning endometrial tissue in places other than the uterus that often results in severe pain and infertility.

Epididymis—Elongated cordlike structure along the posterior border of testes.

Fallopian tubes—Tubes that are part of a woman's reproductive system that extend from the uterus to the ovaries and carry a fertilized egg to the uterus for implantation.

Infertility—The inability of a person to perform the function of reproduction because of a physical, mental, or hormonal problem.

In vitro fertilization—Fertilization of an egg by sperm outside of the body.

Oligospermia—Low sperm count in men.

Ovulation—The discharge of a mature ovum, or egg, from the ovary.

Prostate—A gland made up of muscular and glandular tissue that surrounds the urethra at the bladder in men.

Testes—Male gonads; the paired egg-shaped glands normally located in the scrotum where sperm develop.

Urethra—Membranous canal through which urine is released from the bladder to the outside of the body.

Vas deferens—A duct that carries sperm from the testicles to the urethra.

be less sexual spontaneity—and, of course, condoms can break.

The man also has the option of having a vasectomy. The vasectomy provides continuous contraceptive protection. It is more than 99% effective, and has no side effects.

Spermicide may be used alone, but it must be inserted within one hour before intercourse, requires reapplication for repeated intercourse, must be left in place for six to eight hours afterward, and is often messy. It may give some protection against chlamydia and gonorrhea. Spermicide's effectiveness rate against pregnancy is 79–97% when properly used. It provides a greater measure of safety when used with a condom.

Lastly, there is periodic abstinence, which requires no equipment, foams, or gels. It does, however, necessitate extremely careful planning, motivation, and patience. When a couple is practicing abstinence, intercourse during half of the menstrual cycle is prohibited. If a woman has an irregular cycle, the couple cannot use this method, as fertile periods cannot be determined with any degree of confidence.

Family planning

Couples trying to control their number and rate of pregnancies can do so through family planning. Women may want to increase their chances of getting pregnant or determine the most infertile times to have intercourse so that they can prevent pregnancy. Women may choose to use barrier methods or oral contraceptives to prevent pregnancy, and men may use condoms.

In "natural family planning," women chart their menstruation and ovulation to determine fertile and infertile periods—but without actually having to use artificial **contraception**. Typically, women ovulate on the 14th day of their monthly cycle, which is the best time to become pregnant—although a woman is fertile over a range of days because sperm can remain viable inside the genital tract for up to 48 hours. Basal body temperatures and the texture of cervical mucus should be recorded. These data will aid in the determination of the woman's fertile days.

In 1970, President Richard Nixon signed into law Title X of the **Public Health** Service Act, referred to as "America's family planning program." The program provides funding for low-income women who need contraceptives to prevent pregnancy. The program set a minimum standard of care that requires women to have options among contraceptive methods, and prohibits coercion of women to choose one method over another. Individuals are charged fees for service based on their income and ability to pay. Title X monies do not fund abortions. The program provides for pelvic exams, Pap tests, breast examinations, safe-sex counseling, infertility screening, and referrals to specialized health care when needed.

QUESTIONS TO ASK YOUR DOCTOR

- How can I determine the form of contraceptive that will be best for me to use?
- What are the health and medical risks of having an abortion compared to the risks of childbirth itself?
- What steps can I take to ensure that my reproductive system remains in as healthy a condition as possible at all times?
- If my partner and I are unable to become pregnant, how do we determine the cause of this problem?
- What options for achieving pregnancy are available for a couple of whom one is infertile?

Professional implications

There is a variety of health disciplines that serves the needs of individuals seeking reproductive health services. Gynecologists treat women seeking services that include Pap exams, breast exams, and pelvic exams; obstetricians provide medical care for women who are pregnant and planning to carry their babies to term. These professionals can refer women to specialists for further care as necessary—such as radiologists (who perform mammograms and a variety of ultrasound procedures) and oncologists (in cases of possible or confirmed diagnoses of gynecological cancers). In lieu of an obstetrician, a pregnant woman may consult a midwife. Women may also consult their primary care doctors for basic reproductive health questions. Primary care physicians typically can perform routine Pap and pelvic exams and give advice on contraception.

Similarly, men can consult their primary care doctors for reproductive health care. For further problems and follow-up, however, urologists should be consulted.

For other issues related to reproductive health—particularly those of an emotional nature—licensed social workers, psychologists, psychiatrists, and sex therapists may be helpful.

Resources

BOOKS

Foster, Angel M., and L. L. Wynn, eds. *Emergency Contraception: The Story of a Global Reproductive Health Technology.* New York: Palgrave Macmillan, 2012.

Taylor, Hugh S., et al. *Oxford American Handbook of Reproductive Medicine*. Oxford: Oxford University Press, 2012.

van Look, Paul F. A., Kis Heggenhougen, and Stella R. Quah, eds. *Sexual and Reproductive Health: A Public Health Perspective*. San Diego, CA: Academic Press, 2011.

ORGANIZATIONS

Alan Guttmacher Institute. 125 Maiden Lane, New York, NY 10038. (212) 248-1111. http://www.agi-usa.org.

American Society for Reproductive Medicine. 1209 Montgomery Highway, Birmingham, AL 35216-2809. (205) 978-5000. http://www.asrm.org".

Planned Parenthood Federation of America. 434 West 33rd St., New York, NY 10001. (212) 541-7800. http://www.plannedparenthood.org.

Meghan M. Gourley

Reproductive system, female

Definition

The female reproductive system is composed of organs that produce female eggs (called female gametes or ova), provide an environment for fertilization of the egg by a male sperm (male gamete), and support the development and expulsion of a fetus in **pregnancy** and **childbirth**.

Description

The normal female reproductive system is composed of external and internal genitals (genitalia).

External genitals

The external genitals (together, they are called the "vulva") are composed of the genital structures visible from outside the body: the greater lips (labia majora), the lesser lips (labia minora), the clitoris, and the opening of the vagina to the outside (the other end of the vagina opens inside the body to the uterus). The labia majora are two large lips that protect the other external genitals. The outer surface of these lips is covered with oil-secreting (sebaceous) glands; their inner surface has hair. The lesser lips (labia minora) are found just inside the greater lips and protect the immediate opening to the vagina (this opening is called the "introitus," Latin for "entrance") and the opening to the urethra (which carries urine from the bladder out of the body). The clitoris is a small structure found at the top of the lesser lips; it is very sensitive to stimulation and may become erect. The perineum is the area between the vagina and the anus in the female (in the male, the perineum is the area between the scrotum and the anus). Two glands, one located on either side of the introitus, are called Bartholin's glands. They secrete a mucus that provides lubrication during sexual intercourse.

Internal genitals

The internal genitals are the vagina, the uterus (womb), the fallopian tubes, and the ovaries. The vagina extends approximately 3 to 4 inches (7 to 10 cm) from the outside of the body to the opening of the uterus. The lower third of the vagina (closest to the outside) is encircled by muscles that control its opening and closing. The uterus is the organ found at the top of the vagina and consists of two main parts: the neck (cervix) and the body (corpus). The neck is the opening of the uterus to the vagina that allows sperm to enter the uterus and allows menstrual fluid to exit. The neck is an important means of protecting the body of the uterus from disease-causing germs; a thick mucus normally covers the neck of the uterus but changes in consistency during ovulation to allow sperm to penetrate. The body of the uterus is the main part of the uterus. It can enlarge to hold a developing fetus during pregnancy. The inner lining of the body of the uterus is called the endometrium, which thickens and then sheds menstrual fluid during each menstrual period if fertilization does not occur.

The fallopian tubes (also called the oviducts or uterine tubes) are muscular structures that extend from the upper edges of the uterus to the ovaries. The fallopian tubes facilitate the transfer of a mature egg from one of the two ovaries to the body of the uterus. A fallopian tube is the site of normal fertilization. The ovaries are a pair of small oval-shaped structures and are suspended near the fallopian tubes by ligaments. A human female will not produce any new developing eggs (oocytes) after she is born. Although she is born with approximately two million eggs, only about 300,000 to 400,000 remain at onset of **puberty**, and only about 300 of these will develop fully and enter a fallopian tube for possible fertilization. The eggs start as oocytes and develop in what are called ovarian or Graafian follicles, small spherical sacs that burst when the mature egg (called an ovum) is ready to be released into a fallopian tube for possible fertilization, or for discharge in the menstrual fluid if fertilization does not take place.

The human egg is a round cell that, when mature, is surrounded by a number of protective layers (the oolemma, zona pellucida, and zona radiata). It contains half the number of chromosomes of a human cell that is not egg or sperm (that is, 23 instead of 46 chromosomes)

Female Reproductive System

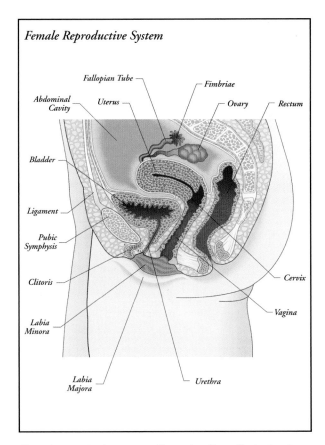

Fallopian Tube
Fimbriae
Abdominal Cavity
Uterus
Ovary
Rectum
Bladder
Ligament
Pubic Symphysis
Clitoris
Cervix
Vagina
Labia Minora
Labia Majora
Urethra

(Female reproductive system, illustration. Kopp Illustration, Inc. Reproduced by permission of The Gale Group.)

and is therefore called a haploid (one-fold) cell. When the egg is fertilized by sperm, the resulting cell will have the full number of 46 chromosomes and will be considered a diploid (two-fold) cell.

Function

Menstruation

The menstrual cycle ranges from 21 to 40 days in most women, with an average cycle lasting 28 days. The first time a girl has a period (the onset of menstruation) is called "menarche"; the permanent cessation of menstruation some decades later is called "menopause" and marks the traditional end of a woman's ability to reproduce. In the 1990s, women past **menopause** have been impregnated with another woman's egg after it has been fertilized by artificial insemination, and these older women have successfully given birth to healthy babies.

Menstruation occurs when the lining of the uterus begins to shed menstrual fluid; the first day of bleeding is the first day of the menstrual cycle. The menstrual cycle has two phases. The follicular phase extends from the first day of the cycle until immediately before a mature egg gets released from the ovary.

In the second phase of the menstrual (ovulatory) cycle, called the "luteal" phase, the mature follicle bursts and releases an egg, a process called ovulation. The second phase of the menstrual cycle lasts approximately fourteen days until the first day of the next period (using as an example the average 28 day menstrual cycle). The ruptured empty follicle collapses to form the corpus luteum.

Fertilization

During the ovulatory phase of the menstrual cycle, the mature egg is released from the ovary and swept into the fallopian tube. If sperm cells are present in the fallopian tube, fertilization may occur. Pregnancy begins at the moment of fertilization (also called conception), when the sperm penetrates the egg. The fertilized egg, also called a zygote, then begins to move down the fallopian tube into the uterus, where it implants itself in the thick tissue of the lining of the uterus. In the uterus, this replicating cluster of cells is called a blastocyst; after two weeks of development, it is called an embryo; eight weeks after conception, it is called a fetus.

Hormones

A complex balance of hormones is required for reproduction. There are two main groups of hormones that are necessary for normal functioning of the female reproductive system.

The first group contains hormones of the **central nervous system** (CNS). A part of the **brain** called the hypothalamus is the main area of hormonal control; it secretes so-called releasing hormones that travel to the **pituitary gland** located at the base of the brain. Gonadotropin-releasing hormone (GnRH) secreted by the hypothalamus triggers the release of gonadotropic hormones from the anterior pituitary gland. Gonadotropin refers to any hormone that stimulates the gonads (the structures capable of producing eggs or sperm, that is, the ovaries or the testicles), regulates their development and their hormone-secreting functions, and contributes to the production of eggs or sperm.

There are two gonadotropic hormones secreted by the anterior pituitary gland: the follicle-stimulating hormone (FSH) and the luteinizing hormone (LH). The development of the ovarian follicles is dependent upon these hormones. FSH (as its name suggests) stimulates the development of several follicles in each cycle. During the first half of the follicular phase, increasing levels of FSH cause maturation of ovarian follicles (only one follicle will mature completely). It is the LH that begins the second phase of the menstrual cycle, when a surge of LH causes the mature follicle to burst and release an egg.

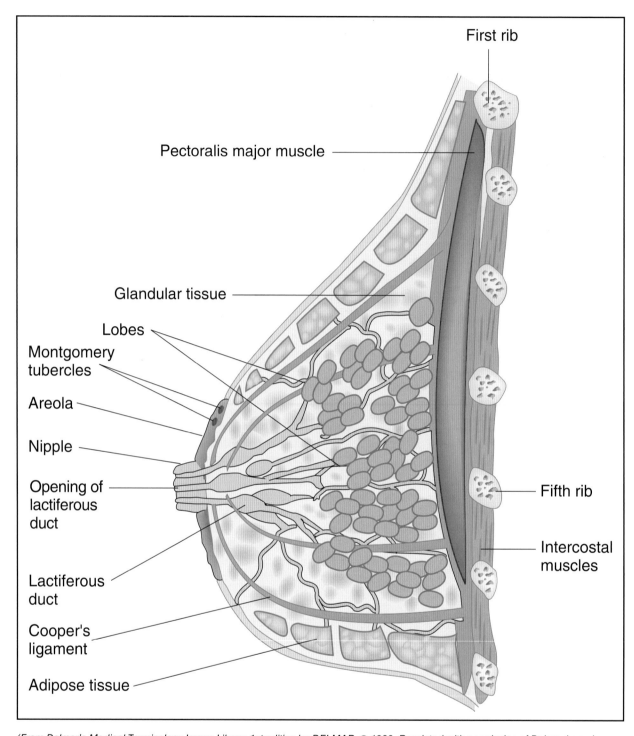

First rib

Pectoralis major muscle

Glandular tissue

Lobes

Montgomery
tubercles

Areola

Nipple

Opening of
lactiferous
duct

Fifth rib

Intercostal
muscles

Lactiferous
duct

Cooper's
ligament

Adipose tissue

FSH and LH also control the production of ovarian hormones (the second group of hormones regulating the female reproductive system).

The ovarian hormones in turn are divided into two groups: ovarian peptide hormones and ovarian steroid hormones.

There are two ovarian peptide hormones, inhibin and relaxin. Inhibin is secreted by the granulosa cells of the follicles. It inhibits the releasing of FSH from the anterior pituitary gland and also inhibits the release of GnRH from the hypothalamus. Thus inhibin has a role in controlling further follicular development. Relaxin is produced near the end of pregnancy by the corpus luteum and promotes **relaxation** of the birth channel.

There are two biologically extremely active ovarian steroid hormones: estrogen and progesterone. Estrogen is produced by the granulosa cells of developing follicles and by the corpus luteum following ovulation. This production of estrogen is dependent upon luteinizing hormone (LH). The most potent estrogenic hormone in human beings is estradiol. It is synthesized and secreted by ovarian follicles, specifically by the theca interna cells (these cells synthesize androstenedione, which is then converted into estradiol and estrone). Estradiol can also be synthesized by the fetoplacental unit and, perhaps, by the adrenal cortex. It has the following biological functions: to promote the growth and maturation of the female secondary sex characters, to induce estrus in conjunction with progesterone to prepare the endometrium for implantation of a fertilized ovum, and to support pregnancy.

Progesterone is a hormone produced by the corpus luteum. (It can also be secreted by the placenta and by the adrenal cortex.) Together with estrogen, it prepares the endometrium for implantation of the fertilized ovum, it maintains the uteroplacentofetal unit, and it promotes the development of the fetus.

Another important endocrine organ secreting the steroid hormones (estrogen and progesterone) is the placenta. It helps maintain the uterine mucosa during pregnancy. The placenta also produces and secretes chorionic gonadotropic hormone. The actions of human chorionic gonadotropin (hCG) resemble those of LH. The presence of hCG in urine in early pregnancy is the basis of most pregnancy tests. Human chorionic gonadotropic hormone maintains the secretory integrity of the corpus luteum.

Common diseases and disorders

Infertility

Infertility is diagnosed when a sexually active couple is unable to get the woman pregnant (or she is unable to carry a pregnancy to a successful childbirth) after one year of attempts. There are numerous reasons why infertility may occur:

- low number or lack of sperm cells produced by the male

- lack of ovulation (no eggs released from ovaries)

- abnormal fallopian tubes

- occurrence of what would normally be the lining of the uterus somewhere else than in the uterus (endometriosis), such as in the fallopian tubes

- problems with thick mucus in the neck of the uterus (Hence, sperm are not able to enter the uterus.)

A number of techniques may be used to assist a couple in getting the woman pregnant. These include fertilization in a dish (in vitro fertilization, IVF; *in vitro* is Latin for "in glass"). Eggs are removed from the woman, placed in a culture dish, and fertilized by sperm, then inserted into the uterus for implantation. An alternate technique is gamete intrafallopian transfer, or GIFT. Male and female reproductive cells are removed from the man and woman and then transferred to the fallopian tube where fertilization may take place naturally.

Cancer

Cancer (uncontrolled and abnormal new growth of cells) may occur in any of the structures of the reproductive system, male or female. Common types of cancer in women include the following:

- Cancer of the uterus (uterine carcinoma). It is the most common cancer of the female reproductive system.

- Cancer of the neck of the uterus (cervical carcinoma). It may be caused by the sexually-transmitted human papillomavirus or HPV.

- Cancer of the ovaries (ovarian carcinoma). It has the highest death rate of all cancers of the female reproductive system.

- Cancer of the external genitals (vulvar carcinoma). It is usually a type of skin cancer.

- Cancer of the vagina (vaginal carcinoma). It may be caused by the sexually-transmitted human papillomavirus (HPV).

- Cancer of the fallopian tubes. It is the rarest cancer of the female reproductive system.

- Tumors that form in the uterus during or after pregnancy (hydatidiform moles).

Other

Amenorrhea is the absence or abnormal stopping of menstrual periods. A number of factors may abnormally stop menstruation. They include abnormal production of LH and FSH, excessive **exercise**, extreme **stress**, and near starvation.

Painful menstruation, that is, menstruation with severe cramps or aches is called dysmenorrhea. It may be caused by excessive production of prostaglandins (the hormones that cause the uterus to contract forcefully at childbirth, thus squeezing the fetus into the vagina) or by diseased genitals.

KEY TERMS

Amenorrhea—Abnormal absence or stopping of menstrual cycles.

Dysmenorrhea—Painful menstruation.

Endometrium—The inner lining of the uterus.

External genitals—The greater lips (labia majora), the lesser lips (labia minora), the clitoris, and the opening of the vagina.

Follicle—A small spherical sac located in an ovary in which an oocyte develops and matures; when the follicle bursts, the mature egg (ovum) is released into the fallopian tube. Only about 300 follicles burst during a woman's lifetime.

Gamete—A one-fold (haploid, that is, having 23 instead of 46 chromosomes) cell involved in sexual reproduction; the male gamete is the sperm; the female gamete is the egg.

Internal genitals—The vagina, uterus, fallopian tubes, and ovaries.

Menarche—The first menstrual cycle in a girl's life.

Menopause—The permanent stopping of menstrual cycles, traditionally marking the end of a woman's ability to reproduce.

Menstruation—The discharge of the lining of the uterus (endometrium) as it sheds during the menstrual cycle when pregnancy does not take place.

Zygote—A two-fold (diploid, that is having 46 chromosomes) cell resulting from fertilization of the female egg by a sperm.

Premenstrual syndrome (PMS) occurs during the luteal phase of the menstrual cycle and is characterized by numerous symptoms. These include changes in mood and behavior, cramps, headaches, fluid retention, and fatigue. Approximately 40% of menstruating women complain of some sort of PMS.

Toxic **shock** syndrome (TSS) is a rare but devastating disease associated with tampon use. Although the exact cause of the disease is not known, it has been linked to **infection** by *Staphylococcus aureus*. If *S. aureus* enters the vagina, it is possible that tampon use could promote the growth of these deadly **bacteria**. *S. aureus* may then secrete poisons (toxins) that enter the bloodstream and lead to TSS. Symptoms start with **fever**, **vomiting**, **diarrhea**, and low **blood pressure**, but may eventually involve multiple organ systems and result in death.

Resources

BOOKS

Fogel, Catherine I. "Common Reproductive Concerns." In *Maternity and Women's Health Care*, edited by Michael S. Ledbetter. St. Louis, MO: Mosby, 2000.

Hart, David M., and Jane Norman. *Gynaecology Illustrated*. London: Harcourt Publishers, 2000.

Shephard, Bruce D., and Carroll A. Shephard. *The Complete Guide to Women's Health*. New York: Penguin Books, 1997.

OTHER

Berkow, Robert, Mark H. Beers, Andrew J. Fletcher, and Robert M. Bogin, eds. "Female Reproductive System." The Merck Manual of Medical Information: Home Edition. 2001. http://www.merck.com/pubs/mmanual_home/sec22/231.htm.

ORGANIZATIONS

American College of Obstetricians and Gynecologists. 409 12th Street SW, P.O. Box 96920, Washington, DC, 20090-6920. http://www.acog.org.

National Association for Women's Health. 300 West Adams Street, Suite 328, Chicago, IL 60606-5101. (312) 786-1468. http://www.nawh.org.

Stéphanie Islane Dionne

Reproductive system, male

Definition

The male reproductive system is composed of organs that work together to produce sperm and deliver them to the female reproductive tract for fertilization of the ovum.

Description

The normal male reproductive system is composed of numerous anatomical structures, including the testis, the excretory ducts, the auxiliary glands, the penis, and the various hormones that control reproductive functions.

Testis

The testis is responsible for the production and maturation of sperm in a process called spermatogenesis. It is also the site of synthesis and secretion of androgens (male sex hormones). The testes (plural) develop in the **abdomen** and descend into the scrotum in the normal male. The scrotum is a muscular sac in which the testes hang from the spermatic cord.

Male Reproductive System

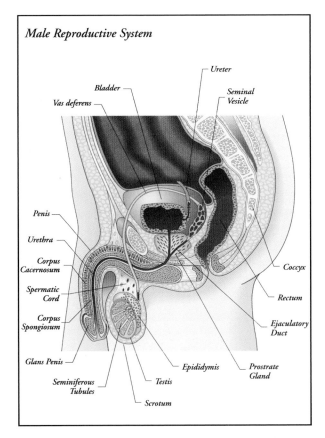

Bladder
Ureter
Vas deferens
Seminal Vesicle
Penis
Urethra
Corpus Cacernosum
Coccyx
Spermatic Cord
Rectum
Corpus Spongiosum
Ejaculatory Duct
Glans Penis
Epididymis
Prostrate Gland
Seminiferous Tubules
Testis
Scrotum

(Male reproductive system, illustration. Kopp Illustration, Inc. Reproduced by permission of The Gale Group.)

The testis is subdivided into the tubular compartment and the interstitial compartment. The tubular compartment is composed of up to 900 seminiferous tubules, which are populated by three main types of cells: germ cells, peritubular cells, and Sertoli cells. Germ cells become mature sperm in the spermatogenic process. Peritubular cells produce various factors that aid in the transportation of mature sperm to the epididymis. Sertoli cells secrete various factors that determine the sperm production and testis size of an adult male.

Androgens are produced in the interstitial compartment of the testis. Leydig cells are responsible for the production and secretion of testosterone. Immune cells such as macrophages and lymphocytes are also found in the interstitial compartment, and aid in the proliferation and hormone production of Leydig cells.

Sperm cells are composed of a head (containing the nucleus and acrosome), the body (containing the mitochondria, or energy-producing organelles), and the tail. The nucleus contains the cell's genetic material (chromatin) while the acrosome contains enzymes that are capable of penetrating the protective layers around the egg. The mitochondria provide energy for tail motility; this is essential for movement of the sperm through the female reproductive tract.

Excretory ducts

The excretory ducts are responsible for the transfer of sperm from the seminiferous tubules of the testis to the urethra and include the epididymis, the vas deferens, and intratesticular ducts. The epididymis is a tubular structure through which sperm exiting the seminiferous tubules pass. Testicular sperm are not fully mature and would not be able to fertilize an ovum (egg). Complete maturation occurs in the epididymis in the two to twelve days that sperm are typically stored before being passed to the vas deferens. The vas deferens functions to carry mature sperm from the epididymis to the urethra; it is also called the ductus deferens. Secretions from the auxiliary glands are mixed with sperm in the vas deferens to form semen.

Auxiliary glands

The auxiliary glands include two bulbourethral glands, one prostate, and two seminal vesicles. These glands contribute the secretions that compose semen. The bulbourethral glands (also called the glands of Cowper) secrete a fluid that lubricates the urethra prior to ejaculation. The prostate secretes a fluid rich in **zinc**, citric acid, choline, and various **proteins**. The secretions of the seminal vesicle are high in fructose (an energy source for sperm) and prostaglandins (fatty acid derivatives).

Penis

The penis is the male organ of sexual reproduction and consists of three elongated bodies that cause erection, the two corpora cavernosa and the corpus spongiosum. These tissues become engorged with **blood** when stimulated by the nervous system during arousal. Blood is supplied by the superficial and deep arterial systems (which carry blood to the penile skin and erectile tissue, respectively). The urethra runs through the corpus spongiosum to the glans penis (distal end of the penis). The organ is covered with loose skin that forms the prepuce (foreskin) over the glans penis.

Function

Endocrine control

Normal reproductive function is dependent on complex interactions between various hormones. A portion of the **brain** called the hypothalamus secretes releasing hormones that travel to the **pituitary gland**, located at the base of the brain. The secretion of gonadotropin-releasing hormone (GnRH) from the hypothalamus triggers the release of luteinizing hormone (LH) and follicle-stimulating hormone (FSH) from the pituitary gland. LH stimulates testosterone production by Leydig cells in the testis, and FSH promotes spermatogenesis.

Male sexual act

The male sexual act can be divided into three main steps: erection, emission, and ejaculation. Erection is the result of increased blood flow to the erectile tissues of the penis; stimulation of the nervous system during arousal causes a release of acetylcholine (a neurotransmitter) that in turn causes vasodilation (increase in the diameter of **blood vessels**). Emission is the passage of sperm and secretions into the urethra mediated by release of the hormone adrenaline. Ejaculation occurs when the sperm are forced from the urethra by contraction of the bulbocavernous muscles. A release of noradrenaline causes the blood vessels in the penis to contract, decreasing blood flow and resulting in detumescence (loss of erection).

Fertilization

In order to fertilize the ovum, ejaculated sperm must move into the vaginal tract, pass through the cervix, survive in the uterus, and enter the fallopian tubes. Usually only healthy, motile sperm will reach the ovum and have the opportunity to fertilize it. Numerous protective layers (including the oolemma, the zona pellucida, and the zona radiata) surround the ovum, and sperm cells must penetrate each of these layers for fertilization to occur. Binding of a sperm cell to the zona pellucida induces the acrosome reaction, which permits the sperm to penetrate the zona pellucida and reach the egg membrane. The sperm and egg membranes fuse to form a zygote, and subsequent reactions prevent the binding of additional sperm cells to the egg membrane.

Common diseases and disorders

Diseases of the male reproductive system are classified based on the localization (e.g., testis, pituitary gland, etc.) and cause (e.g., congential malformation, cancerous tumor, etc.) of the disorder. Some common examples of andrological disorders include:

• Infertility: Male infertility may be the symptom of multiple disorders. A blockage in both of the vas deferentia or a testicular disorder may result in the complete absence of sperm (azoospermia). Low sperm counts might result from a prolonged increase in scrotal temperature—as in the case of a varicocele, a

KEY TERMS

Acrosome—A compartment in the head of the sperm that contains enzymes that allow the sperm to penetrate the protective layers of an egg.

Androgen—A male sex hormone.

Azoospermia—The complete absence of sperm in ejaculate.

Gynecomastia—Enlargement of the male mammary gland; a symptom of hypogonadism.

Hypogonadism—A condition in which there is decreased sexual development and growth of the testes.

Leydig cells—Found in the interstitial compartment of a testis; responsible for the production and secretion of testosterone.

Sertoli cells—Found in the tubular compartment of a testis; aids in the process of spermatogenesis.

Spermatogenesis—The process of the formation of sperm.

Varicocele—An abnormal swelling of veins in the scrotum.

Zygote—The cell resulting from the fusion of the male and female gametes.

disturbance in testicular blood circulation. Retrograde ejaculation is another cause of male infertility; semen travels in the wrong direction, up the urethra to the bladder instead of down toward the penis.

• Hypogonadism: This describes a condition in which there is decreased sexual development and growth of the testes. Hypogonadism may result from tumors, hormone imbalances, or chromosomal abnormalities. Its symptoms (after puberty) include voice alteration, decreased size of testes, gynecomastia (enlargement of mammary glands), an infantile penis, or osteoporosis.

• Erectile dysfunction: It is estimated that the incidence of erectile dysfunction (ED) is twice as high as that of coronary heart disease. ED may result from reduced penile blood flow, low serum levels of testosterone, use of psychotropic drugs, alcohol abuse, metabolic disorders such as diabetes mellitus, or muscle cell impairment.

• Prostate cancer: The prostate surrounds the urethra and secretes seminal fluids. Prostate cancer is the second most common cause of cancer death of men in the United States, and the second most commonly diagnosed form of cancer (after skin cancer).

Resources

BOOKS

Kirby, Roger S., Michael G. Kirby, and Riad N. Farah, eds. *Men's Health*. Oxford, UK: Isis Medical Media, Ltd., 1999.

Nieschlag, E. and H. M. Behre, eds. *Andrology: Male Reproductive Health and Dysfunction*. Berlin: Springer-Verlag, 2001.

OTHER

Berkow, Robert, Mark H. Beers, Andrew J. Fletcher, and Robert M. Bogin, eds. "Infertility." The Merck Manual of Medical Information: Home Edition. 2001.

ORGANIZATION

American Society of Andrology. 74 New Montgomery, Suite 230, San Francisco, CA 94105. (415) 764-4823. http://www.andrologysociety.com.

Stéphanie Islane Dionne

▌Respiratory distress syndrome

Definition

Respiratory distress syndrome (RDS) of the newborn, also known as hyaline membrane disease, is an acute lung disease present at birth. RDS almost exclusively affects premature babies who weigh less than 5.5 lbs (2.5 kg). In these babies, the lack of a pulmonary substance called surfactant allows layers of tissue called hyaline membranes to develop in the **lungs**. This development prevents inhaled oxygen from passing into the **blood vessels** (capillaries) and thereby into the bloodstream. The lungs are said to be airless. Untreated, the infant will die within a few days after birth.

Description

To breathe properly, the alveoli (small air sacs in the lungs) of a newborn infant must remain open so that oxygen in the air can enter the capillaries that surround the alveoli. Normally, during the last months of **pregnancy**, cells in the alveoli produce a substance called surfactant that maintains a low surface tension inside the alveoli. This allows the sacs to expand at the moment of birth, enabling the infant to breathe. Surfactant is produced starting at about 34 weeks of pregnancy and, by the time the fetal lungs mature at 37 weeks, a normal amount is present; after this point, it can be detected in the amniotic fluid.

When an infant is born prematurely without enough surfactant in the alveoli, the lungs may collapse, making it very difficult for the baby to get enough oxygen. Sometimes a layer of glassy, fibrous tissue called a hyaline membrane forms in the air sacs, making it even harder for oxygen to pass through the membrane to the capillaries.

Causes and symptoms

RDS nearly always occurs in **premature infants**, and the earlier the birth. There is a direct relationship between the degree of prematurity and the percentage of newborns that develop RDS. Half of infants born at between 26 and 28 weeks of pregnancy develop RDS, while about 30% of infants born between at 30–31 weeks develop the disorder. The syndrome is also seen in some infants whose mothers have diabetes. Paradoxically, RDS is less likely to occur in the presence of conditions that are equally harmful: abnormally slow fetal growth, toxemia, and early rupture of the amniotic sac. In the United States, RDS occurs in about 1% of pregnancies.

An infant with RDS may struggle to breathe as soon as he or she is born, or difficulty may develop within a few hours. Breathing becomes rapid and shallow, the nostrils flare, and the infant grunts with each breath. Muscles around the ribs and structures in the neck strain inward with each breath, showing the extreme effort that is being exerted. Before long, the intercostal muscles that move the ribs and diaphragm to draw air into the lungs become fatigued, making the breaths even more shallow. This shallow breathing diminishes the oxygen level in the **blood** so severely that the infant becomes cyanotic (the skin turns bluish). Tiny, very premature infants may not even have signs of trouble breathing. Their lungs may be so filled with hyaline membrane that when they are born they cannot even start breathing without assistance.

There are two major complications of RDS. One is **pneumothorax**, which means "air in the chest." When the infant itself or a ventilator breathing for the infant forces air into the lungs in an attempt to expand them, a lung may rupture, causing air to leak into the chest cavity. This air puts pressure on the lung, collapsing it and making breathing even more labored. Because pneumothorax interferes with blood flow in the pulmonary arteries, the infant's **blood pressure** may drop suddenly, diminishing blood supply to the **brain**. The other complication is intraventricular hemorrhage (bleeding into the ventricles of the brain), which can be fatal.

Diagnosis

When a premature infant has obvious trouble breathing at birth or within a few hours of birth, RDS

KEY TERMS

Alveoli—The small air sacs located at the ends of the breathing tubes of the lung, where oxygen normally passes from inhaled air through the membranes into the capillaries and the bloodstream.

Amniocentesis—Analysis of amniotic fluid, extracted surgically by a hollow needle from the uterus of a pregnant woman, to determine the health or other characteristics of a fetus.

Amniotic fluid—The fluid cushioning the fetus inside the uterus, which may be sampled to determine whether the fetus is making enough surfactant to breathe independently.

Endotracheal tube—A metal or plastic tube inserted in the windpipe, which may be attached to a ventilator. It may also be used to deliver medications such as surfactant.

Hyaline membranes—A fibrous layer that develops in the alveoli of many premature infants, which prevents oxygen from passing through the alveolar sac into the capillaries.

Pneumothorax—Air in the chest outside the lung, which compresses the lung. It occurs as a result of the lung rupture, often caused by oxygen delivered under too high a pressure.

Steroids—Also known as corticosteroids or glucocorticoids, these naturally occurring substances are often given to women before they deliver a very premature infant to stimulate the fetal lungs to produce surfactant; this treatment is intended to prevent or minimize RDS.

Surfactant—A substance normally produced in fetal lungs after the 34th week of pregnancy that helps the air sacs to open up at the time of birth so that the infant can breathe independently.

Toxemia—A disease of pregnancy in which the mother's blood pressure is elevated; it is associated with both maternal and fetal complications, and sometimes with fetal death.

Ventilator—A machine that breathes for an infant with RDS until its lungs are producing enough surfactant and are able to function normally.

is a possible diagnosis. If premature birth is expected, or there is some condition that calls for delivery prior to term, the amount of surfactant in the amniotic fluid indicates the extent to which the lungs have matured. If little surfactant is found in an amniotic fluid sample obtained via **amniocentesis**, then there is a definite risk of RDS. In some cases where delivery is essential to maternal or fetal survival, amniocentesis is performed at regular intervals so that the infant may be delivered as soon as the lungs are sufficiently mature. If the amniotic sac has ruptured, surfactant levels may be easily measured using a sample of vaginal fluid.

RDS can also be diagnosed by **chest x ray**. The syndrome has a recognizable radiologic image, and an x ray will also reveal pneumothorax (if this has occurred). This test may be ordered if the infant suddenly becomes worse while on ventilation.

Treatment

If only a mild degree of RDS is present at birth, then placing the infant in an oxygen hood may be sufficient to sustain them until they can breathe independently. Nurses must closely monitor infants receiving oxygen, however, to prevent excessive oxygen saturation, which can damage the retina. This condition, called retinitis of

prematurity, causes blindness. The oxygen level in the blood may be tested by analyzing the levels of arterial gases present, or more easily, by using a device called a **pulse oximeter**, which is clipped to an earlobe. A laboratory technologist usually performs all necessary blood work.

In more severe cases, a drug that mimics the action of natural surfactant (Exosurf Neonatal or Survanta), may be dripped into the lungs through an endotracheal tube. Typically, the infant will be able to breathe more easily within a few days, and complications such as lung rupture are less likely to occur. The drug is continued until the infant starts producing its own surfactant. There is a risk of bleeding into the lungs from surfactant treatment; this affects about 10% of the smallest infants.

Infants with severe RDS may also be placed on a ventilator, a machine that delivers air under pressure through a tracheal tube to the lungs. This is performed as an emergency procedure for infants who do not breathe when born. Assisted ventilation must be closely supervised, as too much pressure can cause further lung damage, injure vocal cords, and increase the baby's risk of pulmonary **infection**. A gentler way to assist breathing is continuous positive airway pressure (CPAP), which delivers an oxygen mixture through nasal prongs or a tube placed through the nose rather than an endotracheal tube. CPAP may be tried before resorting to a ventilator, or after an infant placed on a ventilator begins to improve. Drugs that stimulate breathing may speed the recovery process.

Pneumothorax, which is a possible complication of assisted ventilation, is a medical emergency requiring immediate intervention. Air may be removed from the chest using a needle and syringe. A tube is then inserted into the lung cavity, and suction applied.

Prognosis

If an infant born with RDS is not treated promptly, lack of an adequate oxygen supply will damage the body's organs. They will eventually stop functioning, after which death follows. The **central nervous system** in particular—made up of the brain and spinal cord—is very dependent on a steady oxygen supply and is one of the first organ systems to feel the effects of RDS. On the other hand, if the infant's breathing is supported immediately after birth until the lungs mature and make their own surfactant, complete recovery within a few day to a week is the rule.

Health care team roles

Premature infants with respiratory disorders are usually cared for in a neonatal intensive care unit by a neonatologist, certified neonatal intensive care nurse specialist, anesthesia provider (to maintain the airway), and respiratory therapist. Once the infant has recovered, a pediatrician, family practice physician, and a pediatric nurse practitioner may provide continuing medical care. Parents and siblings of critically ill newborns may require additional support from social workers, pastoral counselors, self-help support groups, or other mental health professionals.

Prevention

The best way to prevent RDS is to delay delivery until fetal lungs have matured and are producing enough surfactant—generally at about 37 weeks of pregnancy. If delivery cannot be delayed, the mother may be given a steroid hormone, similar to a natural substance produced in the body, which crosses the placental barrier and helps the fetal lungs produce surfactant. The steroid should be given at least 24 hours before the expected delivery. If the infant does develop RDS, this treatment sharply reduces the risk of cerebral hemorrhage.

If a very premature infant is born without symptoms of RDS, the decision may be made to deliver surfactant to its lungs anyway. This treatment may prevent RDS, or

QUESTIONS TO ASK YOUR DOCTOR

1. Since it seems likely that I will deliver prematurely, can you test for the level of surfactant in my amniotic fluid?
2. What factors determine the type of treatment you follow if my baby is born with RDS?
3. Are there ways my pregnancy can be prolonged in order to decrease the chance my baby will develop RDS?
4. What long-term health problems may develop in my child if he/she has RDS?

make it less severe if it does develop. An alternative is to wait until the first symptoms of RDS appear and then give surfactant immediately. Pneumothorax may be prevented by frequently monitoring blood oxygen content, and limiting oxygen treatment under pressure to the minimum.

Resources

BOOKS
Linden, Dana W. *Preemies: The Essential Guide for Parents of Premature Babies,* 2nd ed. New York: Gallery Books, 2010.

Walsh, Brian K., Michael P. Czervinske, and Robert M. DiBlasi. *Perinatal and Pediatric Respiratory Care,* 3rd ed. Philadelphia: Saunders, 2009.

OTHER
Pramanik, Arun K. Respiratory Distress Syndrome. Medscape Reference March 9, 2012 [accessed April 13, 2012]. http://emedicine.medscape.com/article/976034-overview

Respiratory Distress Syndrome (RDS). American Lung Association 2010 accessed [April 13, 2012]. http://www.lung.org/assets/documents/publications/solddc-chapters/rds.pdf

Tidy, Colin. Infant Respiratory Distress Syndrome. Patient.co.uk 2009 [accessed April 13, 2012]. http://www.patient.co.uk/doctor/Infant-Respiratory-Distress-Syndrome-%28RDS%29.htm.

What is Respiratory Distress Syndrome? National Heart Lung and Blood Institute. January 24, 2012 [accessed April 13, 2012] http://www.nhlbi.nih.gov/health/health-topics/topics/rds

ORGANIZATIONS
American Academy of Pediatrics, 141 Northwest Point Boulevard, Elk Grove Village, IL 60007-1098, (847) 434-4000, Fax: (847) 434-8000, http://www.aap.org

American Lung Association, 1301 Pennsylvania Ave., NW Suite 800, Washington, DC 20004, (212) 315-8700, (800) LUNG-USA (548-8252), http://www.lungusa.org

Association of Women's Health, Obstetric, and Neonatal Nurses, 2000 L St., NW, Suite. 740, Washington, DC 20036, (202) 261-2400, (800) 673-8499. Toll free in Canada (800) 245-0231, Fax: (202) 728-0575, customer-service@awhonn.org, http://www.awhonn.org

National Heart Lung and Blood Institute Health Information Center, P.O. Box 30105, Bethesda, MD 20824-0105, (301) 592-8573; TTY: (240) 629-3255, Fax: (240) 629-3246, :nhlbiinfo@nhlbi.nih.gov, http://www. nhlbi.nih.gov.

Barbara Wexler
Tish Davidson, AM

Respiratory failure

Definition

Respiratory failure occurs when the lungs' ability to either add oxygen to the bloodstream or remove carbon dioxide from it is impaired. Respiratory failure is a syndrome rather than a single disease. It can have any one of several causes, such as lung disease or **infection**, electrolyte imbalance, interruption of the nerve signals that regulate breathing or nervous system damage, structural (rib cage) collapse, or airway obstruction.

Description

During respiration, the **lungs** extract oxygen from inhaled air, oxygenate the bloodstream, and eliminate carbon dioxide (CO_2) from the **blood** into exhaled air. In respiratory failure, the level of oxygen in the blood becomes dangerously low, and/or the level of CO_2 becomes dangerously high. This can happen if the gas-exchange process breaks down or if ventilation is inhibited.

There are two main types of respiratory failure. Hypoxemic failure occurs when normal **gas exchange** is interrupted, causing a condition called hypoxemia. When this happens, there is too little oxygen in the blood, and all of the body's organs and tissues suffer as a result. One common type of hypoxemic respiratory failure, which occurs in both adults and **premature infants**, is **respiratory distress syndrome**, a condition in which fluid or tissue changes or physical immaturity prevent oxygen from passing out of the lungs' air sacs and into the circulating blood. Hypoxemia is also caused by exposure to high altitudes, where there is less oxygen in

the air, lung diseases that impair the transfer of oxygen into the blood through the alveolar capillaries, severe anemia (i.e., not enough red blood cells to carry the oxygen throughout the body), and blood vessel disorders that shunt blood away from the lungs, thus preventing the lungs from picking up oxygen.

Ventilatory failure occurs when the body cannot exhale CO_2 properly. The resulting buildup in the blood is called hypercapnia. Ventilatory failure can result when the respiratory center in the brainstem fails to drive breathing, when muscle disease prevents the chest wall from expanding during inhalation, or when a patient has **chronic obstructive pulmonary disease** that impairs exhalation. Many of the diseases and conditions that produce respiratory failure can cause both hypoxemia and hypercapnia simultaneously.

Causes and symptoms

Respiratory failure can have a variety of causes; all of them inhibit breathing in some way.

• Airway obstructions: Chronic bronchitis with heavy secretions, emphysema, cystic fibrosis, asthma, and obstructive sleep apnea, in which patients stop breathing for short periods during sleep.

• Depressed respiration: Weakened breathing that is caused by drug abuse (especially narcotics or opiates) and/or alcohol intoxication, both of which depress the respiratory center. Extreme obesity can also be a factor, because it restricts chest wall expansion during inhalation, diminishing the body's ability to acquire enough oxygen.

• Muscle weakness: This can be caused by neuromuscular diseases such as myasthenia gravis, muscular dystrophy, multiple sclerosis, polio, and amyotrophic lateral sclerosis (ALS or Lou Gehrig's disease), as well as strokes that paralyze respiratory muscles and spinal cord injuries.

• Lung diseases and disorders: Severe pneumonia, respiratory distress syndrome, pulmonary fibrosis and other scarring diseases of the lung, radiation exposure, burn injury from smoke inhalation, and widespread lung cancer. Pulmonary edema, often a result of heart disease, can also cause respiratory failure.

• Chest wall abnormalities: These can be caused by scoliosis or severe thoracic injuries, including trauma to the phrenic nerve, which supplies the lungs and diaphragm.

• Cellular disorders: Any interruption of the Krebs cycle can impede respiration, as can electrolyte disorders such as hypokalemia.

Arrhythmia—Abnormal heart rhythm.

Chest percussion—A method of loosening deep lung secretions by rhythmically beating the chest with a cupped hand or mechanical vibrator directly over the affected lung areas.

Chronic obstructive pulmonary disease (COPD)—Lung diseases, such as emphysema and chronic bronchitis, in which airflow is obstructed, causing labored breathing and impairing gas exchange.

Cyanosis—A bluish tinge to the skin caused by low oxygen levels in the blood.

Gas exchange—The process by which oxygen is extracted from inhaled air into the bloodstream, and at the same time, carbon dioxide is eliminated from the blood and exhaled.

Hypokalemia—Potassium deficiency in the blood.

Hypoxemia—An abnormally low amount of oxygen in the blood, one of the major consequences of respiratory failure.

Krebs cycle—One of a series of chemical reactions in which the body's cells metabolize glucose for energy.

Pulmonary edema—Fluid accumulation in the lungs; it is frequently a complication of heart disease and other medical disorders.

Pulmonary fibrosis—The conversion of inflamed lung tissue to scarred, fibrotic tissue that cannot carry out gas exchange. Pulmonary fibrosis is caused by occupational toxins such as asbestos and silica, connective tissue diseases like rheumatoid arthritis and lupus, and exposure to some types of medications, including bleomycin and methotrexate.

Pulmonary hypertension—Potentially life-threatening condition in which blood pressure in the pulmonary artery increases to abnormal levels. Primary pulmonary hypertension, which is rare, occurs without any known cause. Secondary pulmonary hypertension is often a complication of lung diseases like emphysema and bronchitis.

Ventilation—The movement of air in and out of the lungs.

Patients with respiratory failure often have a rapid, weak, or shallow pulse. They also are usually short of breath, restless, and may become confused and disoriented when normal blood gas levels are altered. High blood CO_2 levels can cause headaches and, in time, a semi-conscious state, or even **coma**. Low blood oxygen causes **cyanosis** and can produce cardiac **arrhythmias**. Lung disease may cause abnormal breath sounds that are audible through a **stethoscope**: **wheezing** in **asthma**, rales in **pneumonia**, or distant breath sounds in obstructive lung disease. A patient with ventilatory failure is prone to gasp for breath, and may use the neck and shoulder muscles to help expand the chest.

Diagnosis

The signs and symptoms of respiratory failure depend on the underlying condition causing it. The key to diagnosis and treatment is measuring the levels of oxygen, carbon dioxide, and acid in the blood at regular intervals. Generally, laboratory technologists and respiratory therapists perform all needed blood work and lung-function testing.

Treatment

Nearly all patients are given oxygen as the first treatment. Then the underlying cause of respiratory failure must be addressed. **Antibiotics** are used to fight a lung infection; bronchodilators, like albuterol, and steroid therapy are commonly prescribed for patients with asthma.

Nurses and respiratory therapists have a number of methods to help patients overcome respiratory failure. These include:

- Suctioning the lungs through a small plastic tube passed through the nose. This removes secretions from the airway that the patient is unable to cough up.

- Postural drainage therapy, in which the patient's position is adjusted frequently to help secretions drain into the central airways. Chest percussion and mechanical vibrators are also applied to help loosen deep secretions. The patient is then encouraged to cough up the secretions. If the patient is not strong enough to do this, they are suctioned out.

- Deep-breathing exercises, which are often prescribed after the patient recovers, help strengthen the muscles that aid breathing. One technique has the patient breathe out against pursed lips to increase pressure in the airways, preventing them from collapsing. A device called a volumetric incentive spirometer is also used to encourage deep breathing while giving visual feedback. The patient inhales slowly through a plastic tube attached to a clear plastic cylinder. The cylinder contains a piston and a ball that rests on top of it. Inhalation raises the ball; the patient has to inhale deeply enough to move it to a predetermined mark.

Patients whose breathing remains very poor may require a ventilator until the lungs can resume their function. Although ventilation is a life-saving treatment, it is very important to use no more pressure than necessary to provide sufficient oxygen; otherwise ventilation may cause further lung damage. Drugs are administered to keep the patient calm, and the amount of fluid in the body is carefully monitored so that the **heart** and lungs can function as normally as possible. Steroids, which combat inflammation, may sometimes be helpful but can cause complications, including weakening of the muscles of respiration.

Prognosis

The outlook for patients with respiratory failure depends chiefly on the underlying cause. If it can be effectively treated and the patient's breathing supported during treatment, the outlook is usually promising. Good general health and some degree of lung function improve the prognosis considerably.

When respiratory failure develops slowly, secondary pulmonary **hypertension** may develop. This condition may damage the **blood vessels**, worsen hypoxemia, and eventually cause the heart to fail. If it is not possible to provide enough oxygen to the body, complications involving either the **brain** or the heart may prove fatal.

If the **kidneys** fail or the patient's lungs become infected, the prognosis worsens. In some cases, the primary disease causing the lungs to fail is irreversible. The patient, family, and physician must then decide whether to prolong life by ventilator support.

Health care team roles

Patients with respiratory failure are often cared for in the intensive care unit by critical care or intensive care physicians and nurses. Depending on the underlying cause of respiratory failure, patients may be treated by pulmonologists, cardiologists, internists, surgeons, or oncologists. The treatment team also may include respiratory therapists, laboratory technologists, **radiology** technologists, and physical therapists. Patients and families facing decisions about end-of-life or **hospice** care may benefit from counseling from social workers, religious counselors, or mental health professionals.

Prevention

Because respiratory failure is not a disease itself, but the result of another disorder, the best prevention is to treat any lung disease promptly and effectively, and to ensure that patients whose blood electrolyte chemistry is out of balance receive supplemental therapy. Patients with lung problems should, to every extent possible, also avoid exposure to pollutants. Once respiratory failure is present, it is best for a patient to receive treatment in an intensive care unit, where specialized personnel and equipment are available. Close supervision of treatment, especially **mechanical ventilation**, help to minimize the risk of complications.

Resources

WEBSITES

Kaynar, Alta M. Respiratory Failure. Medscape Reference January 5, 2012 [accessed April 13, 2012]. http://emedicine.medscape.com/article/167981-overview.

Lung Diseases. MedlinePlus April 31, 2012 [accessed April 13, 2012]. http://www.nlm.nih.gov/medlineplus/lungdiseases.html.

Respiratory Failure. Merck Manual Home Health Handbook (Online) January 2008 [accessed April 13, 2012]. http://www.merckmanuals.com/home/lung_and_airway_disorders/respiratory_failure_and_acute_respiratory_distress_syndrome/respiratory_failure.html.

Springer, Shelley C. Pediatric Respiratory Failure. Medscape Reference January 25, 2012 [accessed April 13, 2012]. http://emedicine.medscape.com/article/908172-overview.

What Is Respiratory Failure? National Heart Lung and Blood Institute December 19, 2011 [accessed April 13, 2012]. http://www.nhlbi.nih.gov/health/health-topics/topics/rf.

ORGANIZATIONS

American Lung Association, 1301 Pennsylvania Ave., NW Suite 800, Washington, DC 20004, (212) 315-8700, (800) LUNG-USA (548-8252), http://www.lungusa.org

American Association for Respiratory Care, 9425 N. MacArthur Blvd, Ste 100, Irving, TX 75063-4706, (972) 243-2272, Fax: 972) 484-2720, info@www.aarc.org, http://www.aarc.org

Global Alliance Against Chronic Respiratory Diseases (GARD), World Health Organization, Department of Chronic Diseases and Health Promotion, 20, Avenue Appia, CH-1211 27, Geneva, Switzerland.http://www.who.int/gard/en/index.html

National Heart Lung and Blood Institute Health Information Center, P.O. Box 30105, Bethesda, MD 20824-0105, (301) 592-8573; TTY: (240) 629-3255, Fax: (240) 629-3246, :nhlbiinfo@nhlbi.nih.gov, http://www.nhlbi.nih.gov.

Barbara Wexler
Amy Loerch Strumolo
Tish Davidson, AM

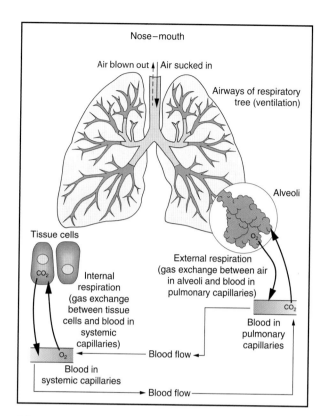

(The respiratory system and the gas-exchange process.)

Respiratory system

Definition

The respiratory system consists of organs that deliver oxygen to the circulatory system for transport to all the cells of the body. The respiratory system also assists in the removal of carbon dioxide (CO_2), thus preventing a deadly buildup of this waste product in the body.

Description

The respiratory system consists of the upper and lower respiratory tracts, extending from the nose to the **lungs**.

The upper respiratory tract encompasses the:

• nose

• pharynx, more commonly called the throat

The lower respiratory tract includes the:

• larynx, also called the voice box

• the trachea or windpipe, which splits into two main branches called bronchi

• tiny branches of the bronchi called bronchioles

• the lungs

These organs all work together to provide air to and from the lungs. The lungs then operate in conjunction with the circulatory system to deliver oxygen and remove carbon dioxide.

Nasal passages

The flow of air begins in the nose, which is divided into the left and right nasal passages and ends in the lungs. The nasal passages are lined with epithelial cells, a mucous membrane composed mostly of a layer of flat, closely packed cells. Each epithelial cell is fringed with thousands of tiny fingerlike extensions of the cells called cilia. Goblet cells are specialized cells that produce mucus, and are among the epithelial cells. Mucus is a thick, moist fluid that coats epithelial cells and cilia. Beneath the mucous membrane, near the surface of the nasal passages, are many tiny **blood vessels** called capillaries. The nasal passages play two critical roles in transporting air to the pharynx. First, the nasal passages filter air to remove potentially disease-causing particles. Secondly, they moisten and warm the air to protect the respiratory system.

Filtering air through the nasal passage prevents airborne **bacteria**, **viruses**, smog, dust particles, and other potentially disease-causing substances from entering the lungs or the bronchioles. Just inside the nostrils are coarse hairs that assist in trapping airborne particles as they are inhaled. The particles then drop down onto

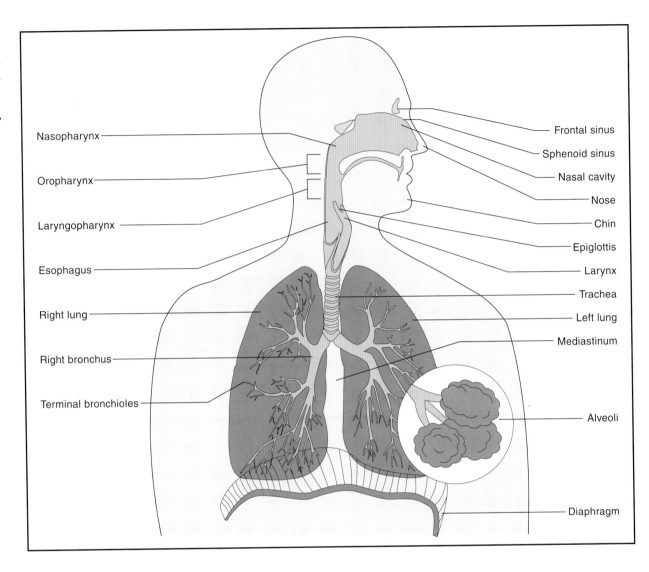

Nasopharynx

Oropharynx

Laryngopharynx

Esophagus

Right lung

Right bronchus

Terminal bronchioles

Frontal sinus

Sphenoid sinus

Nasal cavity

Nose

Chin

Epiglottis

Larynx

Trachea

Left lung

Mediastinum

Alveoli

Diaphragm

the mucous membranes in the lining of the nasal passages. The particles are then propelled out of the nose or downward to the pharynx by the wave of mucus created by the cilia in the mucous membranes. From the pharynx, mucus is swallowed and travels to the **stomach** where subsequently the particles are destroyed by stomach acid. If there are more particles in the nasal passages than the cilia can cope with, a reflex will be triggered producing a sneeze. The sneeze, designed to flush out the polluted air, is due to particles building up on the mucus and irritating the membrane below it.

Pharynx

As air leaves the nasal passages, it flows to the pharynx, which is a short, funnel-shaped tube about 13 cm (5 inches) long. The pharynx is also lined with a mucous membrane and ciliated cells that filter air from the nasal passages. The pharynx also includes the tonsils,

which are lymphatic tissues that contain white **blood** cells. If any impurities escape the hairs, cilia, and mucus of the nasal passages and pharynx, the white blood cells attack the disease-causing organisms. To prevent these organisms from moving further into the body, the tonsils are strategically located. One pair of growths of lymphoid tissue, referred to as the adenoids, is located high in the rear wall of the pharynx. Two tonsils called the palatine tonsils are positioned on either side of the tongue at the back of the pharynx. Another pair called the lingual tonsils is found deep in the pharynx at the base of the tongue. The tonsils may become swollen with **infection** during their fight against disease-causing organisms.

Larynx

Air passes from the pharynx to the larynx, which is approximately 2 inches (5 cm) long and situated near the middle of the neck. The larynx is comprised of several layers of cartilage, a tough and flexible tissue.

In addition to transporting air to the trachea, the larynx serves other functions such as:

- It prevents food and fluid from entering the air passage which would cause choking.
- Its mucous membranes and cilia-bearing cells help filter air.
- It plays a primary role in producing sound.
- The cilia in the larynx move airborne particles up toward the pharynx to be swallowed.

A thin, leaflike flap of tissue called the epiglottis prevents food and fluids from entering the larynx from the pharnyx. The epiglottis is held in a vertical position, like an open trap door when a person is breathing. When swallowing, a reflex forces the larynx and the epiglottis to move toward each other. This reflex diverts food and fluids to the esophagus. The swallowing reflex may not work if one eats or drinks too rapidly, or laughs while swallowing. Food or fluid enters the larynx and a coughing reflex is initiated to clear the obstruction. This situation may cause life-threatening **choking** if coughing does not clear the larynx of the obstruction.

Trachea, bronchi, and bronchioles

Air is passed from the larynx into the trachea, the largest airway in the respiratory system. The trachea is a tube located just below the larynx, approximately 5 to 6 inches (12 to 15 cm) long. Fifteen to 20 C-shaped rings of cartilage form the trachea. Air passes freely at all times because the trachea is held open by the rings of sturdy cartilage. The open part of the C-shaped cartilage rings is situated at the back of the trachea with the ends connected by muscle tissue. The trachea branches into two tubes at its base, located just below where the neck meets the trunk of the body. These two tubes are called the left and right bronchi and they deliver air to the left and right lungs, respectively. The bronchi branch into smaller tubes called bronchioles within the lungs. The trachea, bronchi, and the first few bronchioles are lined with mucous membranes and ciliated cells; thus they contribute to the cleansing action of the respiratory system by moving mucus upward to the pharynx.

Alveoli and lungs

The bronchioles divide many more times in the lungs into an upside-down tree-like structure with progressively smaller branches. Tiny air sacs called alveoli are at the end of the branches. Some of the bronchioles are no larger than 0.5 mm (0.02 inches) in diameter. The alveoli comprise most of the lung tissue, with about 150 million alveoli per lung, and resemble bunches of grapes. The alveoli send oxygen to the circulatory system while removing carbon dioxide. Alveoli have thin elastic walls, thus allowing air to flow into them when they expand; they collapse when the air is exhaled. Alveoli are arranged in clusters, and each cluster is surrounded by a dense network of capillaries. The walls of the capillaries are very thin; thus the air in the wall of the alveoli is very near to the blood in the capillaries (only about 0.1 to 0.2 microns). Carbon dioxide is a waste product that is dumped into the bloodstream from the cells. It flows throughout the body in the bloodstream to the **heart**, and then to the alveolar capillaries. The oxygen diffuses from the alveoli to the capillaries since the concentration of oxygen is much higher in the alveoli than in the capillaries. From the capillaries, the oxygen flows into larger vessels and is then carried to the heart where it is pumped to the rest of the body. The forces of exhalation cause the carbon dioxide to go back up through the respiratory passages and out of the body. Numerous macrophages are interspersed among the alveoli. Macrophages are large white blood cells that remove foreign substances from the alveoli that have not been previously filtered out. The presence of the macrophages ensures that the alveoli are protected from infection; they are the last line of defense of the respiratory system.

The lungs are the largest organ in the respiratory system and resemble large pink sponges. The left lung is slightly smaller than the right lung since it shares space with the heart, which is also located in the left side of the chest. Each lung is divided into lobes, with two in the left lung and three in the right. A slippery membrane called the pleura covers the lungs and lines the inside of the chest wall. It helps the lungs move smoothly during each breath. Normally, the two lubricated layers of the pleura have very little space between them. They glide smoothly over each other when the lungs expand and contract.

The diaphragm is the most important muscle involved in respiration. It lies just under the lungs and is a muscle shaped like a large dome. The sternum (or breastbone), ribs, and spine protect the lungs and the other organs in the chest. Twelve pairs of ribs curve around the chest and are joined to the vertebrae of the spine. The intercostal muscles are also important for respiration. They lie between the ribs and assist in breathing by helping to move the rib cage.

Function

The main function of the respiratory system is the delivery of oxygen and removal of carbon dioxide. To achieve this purpose, the nervous system controls the flow of air in and out of the lungs while maintaining a regular rate and pattern of breathing. Regulation is controlled by the respiratory center, a cluster of nerve cells in the **brain** stem. These cells simultaneously send signals to the muscles involved in inhalation: the diaphragm and rib muscles. The diaphragm flattens out when stimulated by a nervous impulse. The thoracic or chest cavity contains the lungs. The volume of the cavity expands with the downward movement of the diaphragm, thus expanding the lungs. The rib muscles also contract when stimulated, which pulls the rib cage up and out, at the same time expanding the thoracic cavity. This movement reduces pressure in the chest. When the volume is increased in the thoracic cavity, air rushes into the lungs to equalize the pressure. This nervous stimulation is quick, and when it is over, the diaphragm and rib muscles relax and a person exhales.

Working in conjunction with the circulatory system, the oxygen-rich blood travels from the lungs through the pulmonary veins into the left side of the heart. From there, blood is pumped to the rest of the body. Blood that is oxygen-depleted, but carbon dioxide-rich, returns to the right side of the heart through two large veins called the superior and inferior venae cavae. This blood is then pumped through the pulmonary artery to the lungs, where oxygen is picked up and carbon dioxide is released. This process is repeated continually under normal circumstances.

Other functions the respiratory system assist in just by normal respiration are the regulation of acid–base balance in the body, a critical process for normal cellular function. It also protects the body against toxic substances inhaled as well as against disease–causing organisms in the air. The respiratory system also assists in detecting **smell** using the olfactory receptors located in the nasal passages. Furthermore, it aids in producing sounds for speech.

Role in human health

Breathing is an unconscious process carried out on a constant basis and is necessary for survival. Under normal conditions, a person takes 12–20 breaths per minute, although newborns breathe at a faster rate, at approximately 30–50 breaths per minute. The breathing rate set by the respiratory center can be altered by conscious control, for example, by holding the breath. This alteration occurs when the part of the brain involved in thinking, the cerebral cortex, sends signals to the diaphragm and rib muscles to momentarily ignore the signals from the respiratory center. If a person holds his or her breath too long, carbon dioxide accumulates in the blood, which then causes the blood to become more acidic. The increased acidity interferes with the action of enzymes, which are specialized **proteins** that coordinate all biochemical reactions in the body. To prevent too much acid from building up in the blood, special receptors located in the brainstem and in the blood vessels of the neck called chemoreceptors monitor the acid level in the blood. These chemoreceptors send nervous signals to the respiratory center when acid levels are too high, which overrides the signals from the cerebral cortex, forcing a person to exhale and then resume breathing. The blood acid level is brought back to normal levels by exhalation, which expels the carbon dioxide. Irreversible damage to tissues occurs, followed by the failure of all body systems, and ultimately, death if the respiratory system's tasks are interrupted for more than a few minutes.

Common diseases and disorders

The diseases and disorders of the respiratory system can affect any part of the respiratory tract and may range from mild to life-threatening conditions such as:

- Colds—A virus that targets the nasal passages and pharynx. Symptoms include a stuffy and runny nose.
- Hay fever and asthma—Allergic reactions that may occur when the immune system is stimulated by pollen, dust, or other irritants. A runny nose, watery eyes, and sneezing characterizes hay fever. In asthma, because the bronchi and bronchioles are temporarily constricted and inflamed, a person has difficulty breathing.
- Bronchitis—Characterized by inflamed bronchi or bronchiole membranes, resulting from viral or bacterial infection or from chemical irritants.
- Emphysema—A non-contagious disease that results from multiple factors including: smog, cigarette smoke, infection, and a genetic predisposition to the condition. Emphysema partially destroys the alveolar tissue and leaves the remaining alveoli weakened and enlarged. When a person exhales, the bronchioles collapse, trapping air in the alveoli. This process eventually impedes the ability to exchange oxygen and carbon dioxide, leading to breathing difficulties.
- Pneumonia—Infections caused by bacteria or viruses can lead to this potentially serious condition. The alveoli become inflamed and fill with fluid, impairing the flow of oxygen and carbon dioxide between the capillaries and the alveoli.
- Tuberculosis—A condition caused by a bacterium that attacks the lungs and occasionally other body tissues. Left untreated, the disease destroys lung tissue.
- Laryngitis—An inflammation of the larynx caused by irritants such as cigarette smoke, overuse of the voice, or a viral infection. People with laryngitis may become

KEY TERMS

Acidosis—A dangerous condition in which the blood and body tissues are less alkaline (or more acidic) than normal.

Alkalosis—Excessive alkalinity of the blood and body tissue.

Bronchi—The trachea branches into two tubes at the base of the trachea called the left and right bronchi, which extend from the trachea to deliver air to the left and right lungs, respectively. The bronchi branch into smaller tubes called bronchioles within the lungs.

Bronchioles—The bronchioles are no larger than 0.5mm (0.02 inches) in diameter and divide many times in the lungs to form a tree-like structure; they have progressively smaller branches and tiny air sacs called alveoli at the end.

Capillaries—Tiny blood vessels that lie beneath the mucous membrane, near the surface of the nasal passages.

Carbon dioxide (CO_2)—A gaseous waste product that is dumped into the bloodstream from the cells; a byproduct of respiration, it is released upon exhalation of air from the body.

Cilia—Each epithelial cell is fringed with thousands of these tiny fingerlike extensions of the cells.

Diaphragm—The diaphragm is involved in inhalation. It lies just under the lungs and is a muscle shaped like a large dome.

Epiglottis—A thin, leaflike flap of tissue that prevents food and fluids from entering the larynx from the pharynx.

Mucus—A thick, moist fluid that coats epithelial cells and cilia.

pH—the negative logarithm of H+ (hydrogen) concentration. Acid-base balance can be defined as homeostatis (equilibrium) of the body fluids at a normal arterial blood pH ranging between 7.37 and 7.43.

Thoracic cavity—Also called the chest cavity, it is the portion of the ventral body cavity located between the neck and the diaphragm. It is enclosed by the ribs, the vertebral column, and the sternum. It is separated from the abdominal cavity by the diaphragm.

---

hoarse, or they may only be able to whisper until the inflammation is reduced.

• Lung cancer—Occurs in those individuals who are exposed to cancer-causing agents, such as tobacco smoke, asbestos, or uranium; or who have a genetic predisposition to the disease. Treatments are very effective if the cancer is detected before the cancer has spread to other parts of the body. About 85% of cases are diagnosed after the cancer has spread; thus the prognosis is very poor.

• Respiratory distress syndrome (RDS)—Refers to a group of symptoms that indicate severe malfunctioning of the lungs affecting adults and infants. Adult respiratory distress syndrome (ARDS) is a life-threatening condition that results when the lungs are severely injured, for example, by poisonous gases, in an automobile accident, or as a response to inflammation in the lungs.

• Wheezing—A high-pitched whistling sound produced due to air flowing through narrowed breathing tubes. It may have many causes such as asthma, emphysema, pneumonia, bronchitis, etc.

• Shortness of breath or dyspnea—This condition may have multiple causes such as asthma, emphysema, hyperventilation, obesity, cigarette smoking, lung disease, excessive exercise, etc.

• Chronic respiratory insufficiency (or chronic obstructive pulmonary disease; COPD)—A prolonged or persistent condition characterized by breathing or respiratory dysfunction resulting in reduced rates of oxygenation or the ability to eliminate carbon dioxide. These rates are insufficient to meet the requirements of the body and may be severe enough to impair or threaten the function of vital organs (respiratory failure).

Some of the most common symptoms of respiratory disorders are a **cough**, shortness of breath, chest **pain**, **wheezing**, **cyanosis** (bluish discoloration), finger clubbing, stridor (a crowing sound when breathing), hemoptysis (coughing up of blood), and **respiratory failure**. These symptoms do not necessarily signify a respiratory problem, but can be a sign of another problem. For example, chest pain may be due to a heart or a gastrointestinal problem.

Cystic fibrosis is a genetic disease that causes excessive mucus production and clogs the airways.

Acidosis is a condition resulting from higher than normal acid levels in the body fluids. It is not a disease but may be an indicator of disease. Respiratory acidosis is due to a failure by the lungs to remove carbon dioxide, therefore reducing the pH in the body. Several conditions such as chest injury, blockage of the upper air passages, and severe lung disease may result in respiratory acidosis. Blockage of the air passages may be due to **bronchitis**, **asthma**, or airway obstruction resulting in mild or severe acidosis. Regular, consistent retention of carbon dioxide in the lungs is referred to as chronic respiratory acidosis. This disorder results in only mild acidosis because of an increased bicarbonate (alkali) production by the **kidneys**.

Alkalosis is a condition resulting from a higher than normal level of base or alkali in the body fluids. Respiratory alkalosis results from decreased carbon dioxide levels caused by conditions such as hyperventilation (a faster breathing rate), **anxiety**, and **fever**. The pH becomes elevated in the body. Hyperventilation causes the body to lose excess carbon dioxide in expired air and can be triggered by altitude or a disease that reduces the amount of oxygen in the blood. Symptoms of respiratory alkalosis may include **dizziness**, lightheadedness, and numbing of the hands and feet. Treatments include breathing into a paper bag or a mask that induces rebreathing of carbon dioxide.

Resources

BOOKS

Ganong, William F. *Review of Medical Physiology,* 20th ed. New York: McGraw-Hill Professional Publishing, 2001.

Hlastala, Michael P., and Albert J. Berger. *Physiology of Respiration,* 2nd ed. Oxford, UK: Oxford University Press, 2001.

Murray, John F., and Jay A. Nadel. *Textbook of Respiratory Medicine (Two-Volume Set),* 3rd ed. Philadelphia: WB Saunders Co, 2000.

West, John B. *Respiratory Physiology: The Essentials,* 6th ed. Philadelphia: Lippincott, Williams and Wilkins, 2000.

PERIODICAL

Napoli, Maryann. "Alleviating cold symptoms: what works, what doesn't." *Healthfacts* (January 2001). *http://www. findarticles.com/cf_0/m0815/2001_Jan/68277444/p1/ article.jhtml.*

ORGANIZATIONS

The American Lung Association. 1740 Broadway, NY, NY, 10019. (212) 315–8700. http://www.lungusa.org.

National Center for Complementary and Alternative Medicine (NCCAM). 31 Center Dr., Room #5B-58, Bethesda, MD 20892-2182. (800) NIH-NCAM Fax: (301) 495-4957. http://nccam.nih.gov.

National Heart, Lung and Blood Institute. Building 31, Room 4A21, Bethesda, MD 20892. (301) 496-4236. http://www. nhlbi.nih.gov.

Crystal Heather Kaczkowski, MSc.

▌ Respiratory therapy

Definition

Respiratory therapy is a therapeutic treatment for respiratory diseases and conditions. A respiratory therapist (RT) is a healthcare professional who usually provides these treatments and evaluates the patient's response to the treatments.

Purpose

The purpose of respiratory therapy is to maintain an open airway for trauma, intensive care, and surgical patients, assist in **cardiopulmonary resuscitation** and support, provide **life support** for patients who cannot breathe on their own, provide assistance to the anesthesiologist in the operating room, provide inhaled drugs and **medical gases**, provide results from the testing of measuring lung function, and assist with **patient education**.

Description

Respiratory therapy is performed in hospitals, in neonatal, emergency, intensive care, surgical and cardiac units, and various other health care facilities. Respiratory therapy treats many kinds of patients, and provides temporary relief to patients suffering from respiratory ailments. The therapies most commonly administered are oxygen and aerosol medications, and ventilator support after intubation. RTs are assigned to patients during their shift and continuously monitor those patients and respiratory equipment.

It is essential to assess a patient's respiratory function if he/she has a known or suspected pulmonary condition. Therapists perform procedures that are both diagnostic and therapeutic.

Diagnostic therapy includes:

• Obtaining and analyzing sputum and breath specimens. Blood specimens are also obtained and analyzed for levels of oxygen, carbon dioxide, and other gases.

- Interpreting data obtained from these specimens.
- Measuring the capacity of a patient's lungs to determine if there is impaired function.
- Performing other studies of the cardiopulmonary system.
- Studying disorders of people with disruptive sleep patterns.

Treatment therapy includes:

- Operating and maintaining various types of highly sophisticated equipment to administer oxygen or assist with breathing.
- Employing mechanical ventilation for treating patients who cannot breathe adequately on their own.
- Monitoring and managing therapy that will help a patient recover lung function.
- Administering medications in aerosol form to help alleviate breathing problems and to help prevent respiratory infections.
- Monitoring equipment and patient response to therapy.
- Maintaining the patient's artificial airway.

The following are the most commonly performed procedures in respiratory therapy:

- Oxygen therapy—Oxygen therapy involves the administration of oxygen at concentrations greater than that in ambient air with the intent of treating or preventing the symptoms and manifestations of hypoxia. Indications include documented hypoxemia, severe trauma, acute myocardial infarction, and short-term therapy as in post-anesthesia recovery. The need for oxygen therapy is determined by measurement of inadequate oxygen saturations, by invasive or noninvasive means or the presence of clinical indicators. Low-flow oxygen therapy systems deliver 100% oxygen at flows lower than the patient's inspiratory flow rate. The concentration inhaled may be low or high, depending on the specific device and the patient's inspiratory flow rate. Nasal cannulas can provide 24–40% oxygen with flow rates up to 6 L/min in adults. In infants and newborns, flow should be limited to a maximum of 2 L/min. If the oxygen supplied to adults via nasal cannula is at a flow rate lower than or equal to 4 L/min, it does not have to be humidified. Simple oxygen masks can provide 35–50% oxygen at flow rates of 5-10 L/min. Rates should be maintained at 5 L/min or more to avoid rebreathing exhaled CO_2 that may be retained in the mask. Masks with reservoir bags (partial and non-rebreathers) provide FIO_2 (fraction-inspired oxygen, or the concentration of oxygen as delivered to the patient) of 0.5 or greater. High-flow systems deliver a prescribed gas mixture—either high or low FDO_2—at flow rates that exceed patient demand. Aerosol masks, tracheostomy collars, T-tube adaptors and face tents can be used with high-flow supplemental oxygen systems. O_2 therapy should be administered continuously unless needed only in specific situations, as with exercise or sleep.

- Pulse oximetry—Indications for pulse oximetry include the need to monitor the adequacy of arterial oxyhemoglobin saturation, gauge the response of O_2 saturation to therapeutic interventions, and complying with regulations. SpO_2 (a measure of oxygen saturation) is used for continuous and prolonged monitoring as in during sleep, exercise or surgical procedures. Results of SpO_2 tests validate the basis for ordering the test by reflecting the patient's clinical condition. Documentation of results should be noted in the patient's chart.

- Incentive spirometry—I.S. encourages patients to take long, slow, deep breaths. It is a device that provides patients with positive feedback during inhalation at a predetermined flow rate or volume and sustains the inflations for a minimum of three seconds. I.S. is used to increase transpulmonary pressure and inspiratory volumes, improve inspiratory muscle performance, and reestablish or simulate the normal pattern of pulmonary hyperinflation. Airway patency is maintained and atelectasis prevented and/or reversed if the procedure is performed on a repeat basis. It is not effective unless performed as ordered, so proper teaching is mandatory. I.S. is used in post-surgical procedures, especially those involving the thorax or upper abdomen; or conditions that portend atelectasis, as in immobility, abdominal binders, and less than optimal pain control.

- Selection of aerosol delivery devices—for delivery of aerosol to the lower airways. Devices include metered dose inhalers (MDIs), dry powder inhalers, and nebulizers. Drugs used in delivery include beta-adrenergic agents, anticholinergics, anti-inflammatory agents, and mucokinetics. For maximum success, the technique is important—for instance, coordination, breathing pattern, and inspiratory hold. Patient compliance may be a limiting factor in the procedure.

- Arterial blood gases (ABGs)—for arterial blood gas analysis. Blood is drawn from a peripheral artery (radial, brachial, femoral) via a single percutaneous needle puncture or from an indwelling arterial cannula, for a direct measurement of partial pressures of carbon dioxide ($PaCO_2$) and oxygen (PaO_2), hydrogen ion activity (pH), total hemoglobin (Hbtotal), and oxyhemoglobin saturation (HbO_2). The procedure is performed by trained health care personnel (usually the RT). ABGs are utilized to quantify the patient's response to therapeutic interventions and/or diagnostic evaluation and to monitor disease severity or progression. The sampling of arterial blood must be done

KEY TERMS

Artificial airway—A passage for respiration that is created and maintained by a device, such as tubing. Artificial airways are usually established for patients who are at risk of having their own natural airways collapse because of trauma or another medical condition.

Mechanical ventilation—The process of maintaining respiration in a patient who cannot breathe naturally by means of a respiratory device.

according to protocol or test results may be rendered invalid.

• Nasotracheal suctioning (NTS)—to remove secretions, blood or vomitus from the trachea, especially if the patient is unable to cough spontaneously, to maintain a patent airway. To accomplish NTS, a suction catheter is inserted through the nasal passage and pharynx into the trachea to aspiration secretions or foreign material.

• Patient-ventilator system checks—documented evaluation of a mechanical ventilator and of the patient's response to ventilatory support. Objectives of ventilator checks include: evaluating the patient's response to mechanical ventilation; assuring proper operation of the ventilator, that it is functioning properly and alarms are activated; and verifying that inspired oxygen concentration is measured with every change in FIO_2 and that ventilator settings comply with physician orders. All of the above are documented in the patient's chart. Clinical observations of the patient's response to ventilation are also charted in narrative form.

In order for respiratory therapy to be effective, RTs have to evaluate, document, and report all of the above procedures so that appropriate action can be taken by other members of the health care team.

Aftercare

Another important part of respiratory therapy is planning and implementing safe and effective care after discharge from the medical institution. The patient must be successfully transferred from the health care facility to another care site. Patient evaluation involves assessing the patient's current medical condition and ascertaining the type of respiratory care and support needed. The patient's physical, functional, and psychological ability is assessed, as well as the family's psychosocial

condition. The goals of care for the patient and family are also evaluated.

Complications

• Pulse oximetry is usually considered a safe procedure. Device limitations and false-negative results for hypoxemia, though, may lead to inappropriate treatment of the patient. At times, tissue injury at the monitoring site may occur due to misuse of the probe.

• Incentive spirometry. Unless closely supervised, pulse oximetry may be ineffective. It is also inappropriate as a sole treatment for major lung collapse. There may be discomfort secondary to inadequate pain control. Hyperventilation and fatigue may also occur.

• Aerosol delivery devices. Malfunction of the device or improper technique may result in underdosing or overdosing. There may be complications of specific pharmacologic agents and repeated aerosol exposure may produce asthmatic symptoms in caregivers.

• Arterial blood gases. Dangers encountered during this procedure include air or clotted-blood emboli, introduction of contagion at sampling site and infection, hemorrhage, trauma to the vessel, arterial occlusion, and pain.

• Nasotracheal suctioning. Mechanical trauma (laceration of nasal turbinates, perforation of pharynx, nasal irritation, mucosal hemorrhage) are hazards of this procedure. Other complications of NTS include hypoxia, cardiac dysrhythmias, hyper- or hypotension, respiratory arrest, coughing, gagging or vomiting, bronchoconstriction, atelectasis, misdirection of catheter, and increased intracranial pressure.

• Patient-ventilator system checks. Disconnecting the patient from the ventilator during system checks may result in hypoventilation, hypoxemia, bradycardia, and hypotension.

Health care team roles

Physicians, registered nurses, respiratory therapists, and pulmonologists all work to maintain respiratory health in the patient. Physicians diagnose respiratory illnesses and determine which kinds of therapy will be most effective in alleviating them. Registered nurses monitor the effects of the therapy on the patient, administer tests, and make recommendations for any needed changes to the therapy program. Respiratory therapists are trained in the use of therapy equipment and are responsible for maintaining the welfare of patients while they are undergoing therapy. Pulmonologists specialize in the study of the heart-lung system and may also recommend or adjust therapy.

Resources

PERIODICAL

Myers, C. "Facility Profile: Expanding the Reach of Respiratory Therapists." *RT Magazine* (December 2000).

OTHER

Bureau of Labor Statistics, United States Department of Labor Occupational Outlook Handbook (December 2000). http://stats.bis.gov/oco/ocos/084.htm.

ORGANIZATIONS

American Association for Respiratory Care. 11030 Ables Lane, Dallas, TX 75229-4593. (972) 243-2272. http://www.rcjournal.com/online_resources/cpgs/pcgtcpg.html.

Canadian Society of Respiratory Therapy. 1785 Alta Vista Drive, Suite 102, Ottawa, Ontario K1G3Y6. (800) 267-3422. http://www.csrt.com.

René A. Jackson, RN

Respiratory therapy apparatus

Definition

Respiratory therapy apparatus refers to a group of different inhalation devices and equipment used to treat a variety of respiratory ailments.

Purpose

Respiratory therapy apparatus is used to aid a patient's breathing or heal damage to a patient's **lungs** and bronchial tubes due to **infection** and disease.

Description

Simply put, respiratory therapists help patients breathe more effectively. Patients may have mechanical difficulties within the lungs and trachea that make it difficult to get enough oxygen. Often these instances are life threatening and must be treated immediately. Obstructions (e.g., When a child swallows an object) and injury (automobile accidents, **sports injuries**, natural disasters, etc.) are common situations in which breathing assistance is necessary. In these cases, intubation (the insertion of a tube into the trachea) is necessary to open the airway so that oxygen can be administered. **Ventilators** regulate the amount of oxygen that the patient receives and even how often the patient breathes. Disease and atrophy of the lungs may require the use of a ventilator to help a patient breathe.

Premature infants and some other newborns may not have lungs that are mature enough to allow them to breathe on their own. Oxygen is often administered as a life-support measure. In some cases, oxygen is given to ease the burden on the lungs until the baby is strong enough to breathe on its own.

Some patients may be suffering from **chronic obstructive pulmonary disease** (COPD), a group of diseases that affect the lungs, and which includes **emphysema**, **bronchitis**, and **asthma**. Other patients may have **cystic fibrosis**, **lung cancer**, **pneumonia**, or **AIDS**. In these cases, the respiratory therapist may administer medications through an inhaler or a hand-held nebulizer.

Other patients may have **heart** disease. The therapist may administer oxygen and also provide **rehabilitation** devices and techniques to increase lung capacity.

Nebulizers and inhalers

Nebulizers and inhalers provide medications in a fine mist that the patient breathes. Inhalers provide metered doses of medication and come prepackaged. They are portable and can be tucked into a pocket or handbag. So-called "rescue" inhalers are often carried by people with asthma and used when they have an episode. Special dry powder inhalers provide medications that do not work well in liquid form. These inhalers deliver the medication in fine, dry particles that are inhaled.

Metered-dose inhalers dispense specific medications and can be grouped according to type of medication. They are usually bronchodilators, inhaled steroids, cromolyn, nedrocromil, and ipratropium bromide.

Nebulizers are hand-held machines with an airflow meter that measures oxygen flow. These machines administer a variety of medications. The respiratory therapist must prepare a mixture of medication and saline solution according to the physician's written order. Nebulizers vaporize this mixture and deliver it as a fine mist or steam. Nebulizers are usually used in the hospital or nursing home setting. Disposable nebulizers are often sent home with a patient and are cleaned and reused for a limited time. There are three types of nebulizers: large volume, small volume, and ultrasonic.

Intubation catheters and ventilators

Intubation catheters are inserted into the airway and fill the lungs with oxygen at a specific respiratory rate. Ventilators provide mechanical breathing though the catheters and are said to "breathe" for the patient. The amount of oxygen can be varied as well as the breathing rate.

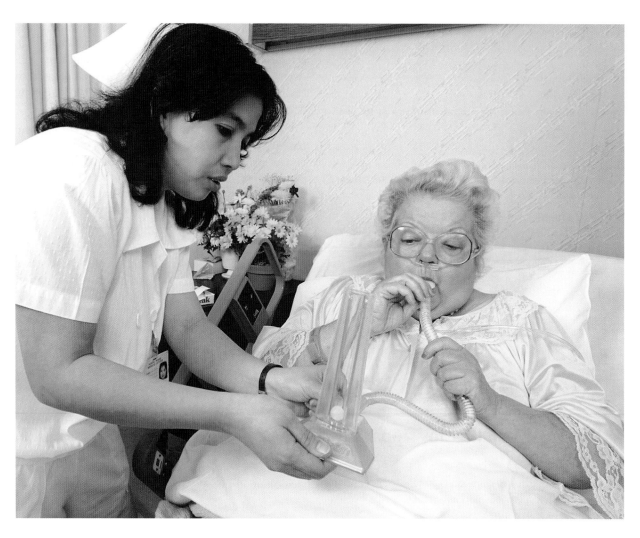

(A female nurse assists an elderly female patient (in a hospital bed) with a breathing apparatus, photograph. © Royalty-Free/Corbis)

Oxygen masks, nasal cannulas, and oxygen tanks

Oxygen masks, nasal cannulas, and oxygen tanks provide **oxygen therapy** and assistance in maintaining specific oxygen levels within the lungs. Oxygen masks fit over the mouth and nose, whereas cannulas are thin tubes inserted into the nasal openings. Tubing connects the mask or cannula to the oxygen tank from which oxygen is delivered.

Oxygen masks come in a variety of sizes. There are very small ones used to fit premature infants' faces. Adult-size masks come in small, medium, and large. Masks usually provide high flow and a high concentration of oxygen within a range to the patient. Ventilator masks come with a series of different adaptors that allow a specific percentage of oxygen flow. These adaptors are preset and can be installed on the mask to provide oxygen at a specific rate (e.g., 50% oxygen).

Nasal cannulas provide low flow and a lower concentration of oxygen. Cannulas deliver oxygen within a range. These are usually used in home health situations because of their ease of use.

Operation

The respiratory therapist will need to make sure that the equipment is running efficiently and that the medication formula is properly mixed. Masks must be of the correct size and must fit the patient snugly. Since therapy often involves patient cooperation, the therapist should instruct conscious patients clearly about the procedure and what is expected of them during treatment. For example, when using inhalers, the patient should be instructed in creating a tight seal around the inhaler nozzle with the lips and to hold the inhalation for a few seconds.

For unconscious patients, the therapist will need to make sure that oxygen masks fit properly or that intubation and ventilation is done correctly.

KEY TERMS

Bronchodilators—Medications that expand the bronchial tubes so that patients can breathe better.

Intubation—The insertion of a tube into the trachea.

Nasal cannula—A tube placed inside the nostrils to bring oxygen to the patient's lungs.

Nebulizer—A hand-held device that distributes medication to the lungs via a steam or mist derived from a mixture of medication and saline solution. The respiratory therapist prepares the mix per the physician's written order.

Trachea—Windpipe; the airway by which oxygen passes to the lungs and carbon dioxide is expelled from the body.

Maintenance

Most respiratory therapy devices are one-use only and disposable. Only in the case of pocket inhalers and take-home nebulizers does the therapist need to instruct the patient in proper cleaning of the devices. Inhalers often just need rinsing with soap and water and drying after use. Nebulizers will need to be cleaned with distilled water and vinegar, or other approved disinfectant solution. Even in hospital settings, nebulizers are changed every day, though they may be reused several times during that day. Some nebulizers may be cleaned by running them through a cycle in a dishwasher, but the therapist should check with the manufacturer first.

Intubation catheters need to be as sterile as possible in order to prevent infection or **sepsis**. Therefore, they are one-use disposable products.

Nebulizers will need to be inspected for wear to insure their proper working. Machines with an air compressor or motor often have air filters; these filters will need to be replaced regularly.

Health care team roles

The respiratory therapist is a member of a large medical team that treats a patient's specific diseases and injuries and can work in hospitals, **nursing homes**, outpatient clinics, physicians' offices, and in homes. Since respiratory therapy requires trust and cooperation from the patient, the therapist will need to be able to instruct patients clearly and in a friendly manner. The therapist will also need to be adaptable and able to deal with a variety of people across a wide age range.

The respiratory therapist is responsible for maintaining the respiratory therapy equipment, cleaning it if necessary, and requisitioning parts and apparatus (masks, catheters, etc.). The therapist also administers treatment via this equipment and monitors patient performance and response.

Training

Formal training and licensure by the state in which the therapist works is necessary for these professionals. Training programs graduate registered or certified respiratory therapists. According to the Commission on accreditation of Allied Health Education, 329 advanced respiratory therapy programs and 51 entry-level programs were accredited in the United States and Puerto Rico in 2005. Registered respiratory therapists usually study for two years and earn an associate degree, though some receive a bachelor's degree after four years of coursework. Respiratory therapists take courses in **physiology** and **anatomy**, chemistry, **microbiology**, physics, and mathematics. They are also trained in the use and maintenance of respiratory therapy apparatus. Apart from formal education, many therapists are receiving additional on-the-job training to administer stress tests and electrocardiograms, or draw **blood**.

Resources

BOOK

Kacmarek, Robert M., and James K. Stoller, A. H. Heuer. *Egan's Fundamentals of Respiratory Care*, 10th edition. Mosby, 2012.

WEBSITE

"Respiratory Therapists." Bureau of Labor Statistics, U.S. Department of Labor. *Occupational Outlook Handbook, 2012-13 Edition*. April 6, 2012. http://www.bls.gov/ooh/healthcare/respiratory-therapists.htm (accessed November 2, 2012).

ORGANIZATIONS

American Association for Respiratory Care. 11030 Ables Lane, Dallas, TX 75229. (972) 243-2272.

National Board for Respiratory Care. 8310 Nieman Road, Lenexa, KS 66214- 1579. (913) 599-4200.

Janie F. Franz

Restorative dental materials

Definition

Restorative dental materials are substances that are used to repair, replace, or enhance a patient's teeth. These materials include metals, porcelains, and composite resins (often made from plastics).

Purpose

Restorative dental materials are used to create fillings, bridges, crowns, and inlays in order to restore a tooth's appearance, structure, or function.

Description

The end of the twentieth century witnessed a dramatic decline in **dental caries** and an increased interest in dental health and enhancement. Smaller cavities are being discovered in the general population and in children, with more than half of those aged five to 17 having no tooth decay at all. At the other end of the spectrum, older Americans are retaining more and more of their natural teeth and are beginning to seek out dentists for restorative work.

Visits to prosthodontists (dentists who specialize in mouth reconstructions, such as crowns, fixed bridges, dentures, and implants) and cosmetic or esthetic dentists (those who repair and enhance teeth through whitening, veneer application, or attachment of permanent restorations) increased from the 1990s into the twenty-first century. An American Dental Association (ADA) survey in 2000 indicated that 84% of responding dentists reported offering some form of cosmetic services to their patients.

Dentists now have more tools with which to diagnose a patient's unique problems, and they are able to find more creative, conservative solutions for them. The dentistry of the 1970s provided limited options. A patient had a tooth filled or extracted, had teeth straightened with braces, or had a crown or bridge installed. Often, the crown cracked and had to be replaced, or the bridge that was fitted was a plastic tooth set in a maze of wires.

Thirty years later, dentists can whiten teeth, alter their shape, fill gaps between them, or build up a tooth that is cracked. Dentists can fill a cavity with a tooth-colored filling that appears invisible to the naked eye. They can replace a missing tooth with a porcelain bridge or a resin implant. Even crooked teeth can be greatly improved with veneers and bonding or invisible plastic braces.

Cosmetic dentists and prosthodontists create restorations in order to repair, replace, or enhance a patient's tooth or teeth.

Restoration types

All restorations perform one of three main functions. They repair, replace, or enhance. Among the types of restorations that repair are fillings. These are used to restore tooth damage that occurs as a result of dental caries (tooth decay). Metal amalgams or composite resins are used to fill cavities and restore the function and esthetics of a tooth. Inlays and crowns, used to repair damage to the teeth, replace tooth structure lost to decay or injury, protect what remains, and restore the tooth's shape and function. Inlays are more durable than amalgam fillings.

Crowns may be necessary when a tooth cracks, has its entire structure weakened by decay, or becomes brittle after a root canal. Crowns can also cover dental implants or abutment (adjacent) teeth when fitting a bridge.

Bonding and contouring

Bonding is a low-cost alternative to crowns or veneers. A tooth-colored composite resin is molded over the tooth, exposed to a special light, and then polished. It is used to restore chipped or slightly ill-shaped teeth. It is less durable and subject to chipping. Bonding is also limited to areas of the mouth that do not experience strong chewing forces, such as the front teeth.

Contouring is done to correct the shape of a tooth. This is mainly an extractive procedure because small amounts of tooth enamel are removed. This technique can be combined with bonding or veneer application.

Restorations that replace

BRIDGES. Bridges fill in a gap left by missing teeth, preventing the remaining teeth from shifting and providing a more stable surface for chewing. Bridges consist of a metal framework and one or more artificial teeth anchored to adjacent teeth (abutment teeth). Sometimes, a two-implant bridge is required. It is then cemented into place.

IMPLANTS, DENTURES, AND PARTIAL DENTURES. Implants, dentures, and partial dentures also replace missing teeth. Individual artificial teeth may be implanted or inserted into the patient's jaw. Partial dentures are dental appliances that have more than one artificial tooth inserted into a metal framework. They are usually removable and can be designed for one or both sides of the mouth.

Restorations that enhance

Crowns are used less frequently to enhance stained or damaged teeth. Newer techniques, such as bleaching or veneer application, are less invasive, save more original tooth structure, and cost less than crowns.

Veneers are ultra-thin coatings used to close gaps between teeth or cover discolored teeth. They are also used to fill in spaces between teeth, repair broken or chipped teeth, and straighten out misshapen or crooked teeth.

Materials used in fillings

The dentist cleans out the decayed part of the tooth and fills the opening with an artificial material (a filling) to protect the tooth's structure and restore the beauty and utility of the tooth.

METALS. The most common and strongest filling material is amalgam. It is a silver filling that is usually placed on the rear molars, which endure more **stress** during chewing. Amalgam fillings are strong and very resistant to wear, and are used for large, deep fillings. Amalgam has been in use since 1833. It is a mixture (an amalgam) of several metals, including liquid mercury (35% silver, 15% tin or tin and **copper**, 50% mercury, and a trace of **zinc**). When it is prepared, it has a malleable consistency that can easily be shaped to fit the prepared tooth. It hardens to a durable metal.

Despite its durability, many dentists and patients avoid using amalgam fillings. They have found that amalgam has a tendency to expand with time. As a result, teeth become fractured from the inside and often split. Patients are not choosing amalgam, but this is strictly for aesthetic reasons. They darken over time and make teeth appear decayed. There has also been a question about the safety of amalgam since it contains mercury; the ADA has maintained that it is safe to use as a restorative material.

Gold fillings or inlays are created outside of the mouth by a dental technician, then cemented into place. They are also used to fill the back molars and are very durable. Like amalgam, however, they are not as aesthetically pleasing as tooth-colored fillings. Still, gold has been a good source for foundation materials for porcelain over metal crowns.

Alloys of palladium, nickel, or chromium are frequently used for inlays and overlays, as well as for some base material for porcelain over metal crowns. Palladium is the metal of choice for porcelain-to-metal reconstructions. It is strong and generates fewer allergic reactions. Low-fusing porcelain allows lab technicians to add onto existing restorations.

PORCELAINS. Implants, partial dentures, dentures, crowns, and veneers are usually made from porcelain. Thin veneers made from porcelain are quite durable. All-porcelain products in the twenty-first century tend to fracture less often than those of the past. Some crowns and implants are made with porcelain-covered metals. They are extremely durable, but sometimes recede from the gums, exposing the metals. Porcelain-over-gold crowns often have a golden glow that is caused by the metal beneath. This glow creates a more aesthetically pleasing crown, but it is more expensive than a crown made of other materials.

When inlays are required for teeth exposed by a smile, tooth-colored composites and porcelains are used. Reinforced porcelain and lucite porcelain are durable, but still may not be suitable for patients who grind their teeth because metal fillings withstand the stress of grinding better.

COMPOSITE RESIN. Composite fillings, often called white fillings, are made of a plastic resin and finely ground glass. They must be applied to the tooth surface in thin layers. Dentists try to match the color of composites with neighboring teeth for a more natural look, making the fillings appear invisible. Composite resin fillings are often made smaller than amalgam fillings and require less tooth preparation, thereby saving more natural tooth surface.

The composite filling is bonded to the tooth so that the tooth becomes stronger than it was before. A composite filling is also less sensitive to temperature changes in the mouth, which can damage the tooth. Thus, there is less chance that the tooth will shatter because of the filling.

The major drawback of the composite resin filling is cost. The average cost is 1.5 to 2 times greater than the price of an amalgam filling. The composite resin filling can be stained by coffee and tea. Further, the large composite filling tends to wear out sooner than the large amalgam filling. However, the composite combined with porcelain is an excellent material for thin veneers. Finally, the light-cured composite's flexibility allows restorations to be repaired directly in the mouth. They are not abrasive and feel much like a natural tooth.

Operation

Crowns

The dentist first removes the decayed portion of the tooth. The tooth is then prepared for a crown. It may be tapered on the outside edges to a peg, reinforced with a cast metal core, or rebuilt with both a cast metal core and a post. An impression is made of the prepared tooth and its adjacent teeth. A retraction cord is placed around the tooth to get the impression medium under the gum, where the crown will be fitted.

A new crown will be created by the dental technician, who will use a cast made from this impression. The technique the technician uses is called lost-wax casting. A wax model is made of the crown. Another mold is made around the wax model and both are fired in a kiln. The wax melts, leaving an opening into which a restorative material can be poured. The crown may be made of gold or stainless steel alone, metal with a veneer of tooth-colored porcelain or resin, or of porcelain or resin alone. The finished crown is then placed over the prepared tooth, adjusted, and cemented into place.

When a tooth has had a root canal procedure and the root has been filled, the tooth may not be strong. In these cases, post crowns are used. The tooth is leveled at the gum line and a stainless steel or gold post is fitted into the root canal. This post can then receive the new crown and hold it in place.

For other patients, it may be necessary to implant the crown. In this case, a steel post is embedded in the patient's jawbone. It is left in place until the **bone** adheres to the post. The post is exposed and the crown is made and fitted.

Inlays

After the decay is removed and the cavity walls are shaped, the dentist makes a wax pattern of the space. A mold is cast from the wax pattern. An inlay is made from this mold and sealed into the tooth with dental cement.

When a restoration is cemented in place, the dentist and the dental assistant clean off all uncured restorative materials left on the tooth. Pumice or another mild abrasive is more effective in removing leftover materials than air or water spray, or even a roll of cotton.

Partial dentures, dentures, and implants

Partial dentures, dentures, implants, and veneers are created in much the same way as crowns and inlays. Teeth may already be absent, or they may need to be extracted. Impressions of the patient's mouth are taken and restorations are created from a variety of materials in a dental laboratory. The final product is fitted and/or cemented into place at the dentist's office. For a veneer, the tooth is etched and a strong bonding agent is applied. The veneer is then cemented to the tooth.

Bonding

For bonding, thin layers of enamel are removed. The bonding material is laid over the tooth and shaped. It is cured with a special light and then polished.

Maintenance

Restoration materials are durable. Composite and amalgam fillings can last seven to 10 years. They should

---

KEY TERMS

Abutment tooth—A crowned tooth that stabilizes a bridge or partial denture.

Amalgam—A mixture of metals, primarily mercury and silver, used to make large, durable fillings. Also called silver fillings.

Composite filling—A resin material that is tooth colored and used to fill a tooth after decay has been removed. It is used most often in front teeth, but may be used in any tooth for aesthetic reasons.

Crown—A protective shell that fits over the tooth.

Denture—A dental prosthetic device consisting of a full set of teeth to fill the upper or lower jaw or both jaws. Also called false teeth.

Enamel—The hard outermost surface of a tooth.

Impression—An exact copy of the teeth and mouth using materials that will set sufficiently so that a more durable cast of the mouth can be made from plaster, dental stone, or other casting materials.

Inlay—A filling that is made outside the tooth and then cemented into place.

Onlay—A restoration like an inlay that wraps over the crown and sides of a tooth.

Partial dentures—A dental prosthetic of two or more teeth used to replace missing teeth.

Porcelain—A strong, translucent ceramic material.

Prosthodontist—A dentist who specializes in mouth reconstructions such as crowns, fixed bridges, dentures, and implants.

Restoration—Any prosthetic device or process used to replace or improve the structure or appearance of a tooth or teeth.

---

be maintained with good **oral hygiene** and replaced as necessary. Some of the composite resins are sensitive to staining from coffee and tea. Amalgam fillings have a tendency to expand over time. As a result, teeth become fractured from the inside, and they often split. When a fracture occurs, a crown is needed. Unfortunately, amalgam fillings also darken over time and make teeth look as if they are decayed.

Cracks can occur in materials used for dentures and partial dentures, but far less frequently in older porcelain materials.

Composite resins are used to bond teeth, but they may not stand up to the patient who eats hard candy, popcorn kernels, or ice. They may require repair or touch-ups. Porcelain—a strong, translucent ceramic material—is used to make veneers, which can change the shape of teeth and fill in unsightly gaps. Porcelain veneers can become chipped or otherwise damaged, and may need to be replaced every five to 12 years.

Health care team roles

Dentists are assisted by dental assistants, who prepare patients for prosthodontic procedures. These usually involve taking x rays, making impressions of patients' teeth, making casts from the impressions, preparing restorative materials, and assisting the dentist in installing dental **prosthetics** or applying restorative materials. Cleaning and disinfecting of instruments and the treatment area are also the responsibility of the dental assistant. They take an active role in educating patients about the care and maintenance of their restorations, and instruct patients in proper aftercare, especially if there has been some invasive procedure (such as extraction or surgery). Dental assistants must be well trained in the preparation of dental materials and their applications, and must also have good communication skills, as they need to instruct patients and have the ability to reassure those who may be uncomfortable in a dentist's office.

In the laboratory, dental technicians are responsible for the creation of dental prosthetics. They must possess excellent manual dexterity and some creative skill. With recent advances in digital dentistry, the technician will require computer skills as well as manual ones.

Resources

BOOK

Shillingburg, Jr., Herbert T., Sumiya Hobo, and Lowell D. Whitsett. *Fundamentals of Fixed Prosthodontics.* Chicago: Quintessence Publishing Co., 1997.

PERIODICALS

Duff, Kerry. "New Technology Creates Cosmetic Dentistry Revolution." *Business Journal* 20, no. 32 (May 12, 2000): 49.

Sherman, Jenny. "All Smiles." *MPLS-St. Paul Magazine* 29, no. 2 (February 2001): 88.

OTHER

Porcelain Laminate Veneers. April 2001. http://www.newsmile. com/personal/solutions/veneers.html/.

Veneers. 2004 (April 24, 2006). http://www.qualitydentistry. com/dental/restorative/veneers.html/.

ORGANIZATIONS

Academy of General Dentistry. Suite 1200, 211 East Chicago Avenue, Chicago, IL 60611. (312) 440-4300. http://www. agd.org.

American College of Prosthodontists. 211 East Chicago Avenue, Suite 1000, Chicago, IL 60611. (312) 573-1260. http://222.prosthodontics.org.

American Dental Association. 211 East Chicago Avenue, Chicago, IL 60611. (312) 440-2500. http://www.ada.org.

American Prosthodontic Society. 3703 West Lake Avenue, Suite 100, Glenview, IL 60025. (877) 499-3500. http:// www.prostho.com.

National Association of Dental Laboratories. 1530 Metropolitan Blvd., Tallahassee, FL 32308. (800) 950-1150.

Janie F. Franz

Restraint use

Definition

A restraint, or physical restraint, is a piece of equipment or device that restricts a patient's ability to move. Restraints may keep a patient from getting out of bed or moving arms and legs excessively.

Purpose

Restraints are used to control a patient who is in danger of harming him/herself or others. It is sometimes necessary to restrain children, who may not be capable of remaining still when they are frightened or in **pain** during some procedures. The use of physical restraints in the health care arena should be used as a last-resort option.

Precautions

Many safety measures should be considered before applying restraints. According to federal law, first and foremost is the need to try other methods to promote safety and avoid the use of physical restraints. Some examples of alternative methods are patient reorientation to physical surroundings, discussion with family and friends about staying with patient, moving the patient's room nearer to staff members, teaching **relaxation** techniques in order to decrease **anxiety** and fear, and decreasing overstimulation. Documentation of these methods is extremely important.

Description

Several types of medical manufacturers have different names for the same types of physical restraints. The most common names and types of physical restraints are:

- soft wrist and ankle restraints
- strap fastening vest (posey jacket)

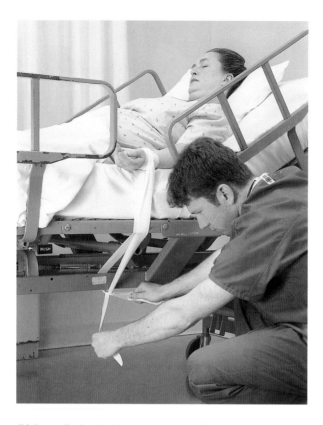

(Male medical technician or nurse squatting on the floor, fastening wrist restraints to the bottom bed rail, female patient lying in bed, photograph. From Fundamentals of Nursing, Standards and Practices 2nd edition by Delaune/Ladner. © 2002. Reprinted with permission of Delmar Learning: www.thomsonrights.com Fax 800-730-2215.)

- seat belt with buckle (restraint belt)
- mittens (restraint mitts)
- leather wrist and ankle restraints

The most common reasons for the use of physical restraints are:

- When a confused patient roams through the health care facility endangering him/herself.

- When a confused patient tries to remove medically necessary tubes, intravenous lines, or protective dressings.

- When a patient has an unsteady gait (walk) and is at risk for falls.

- When a patient needs to be kept from inflicting self-harm or injury (suicidal).

- When a patient needs to be kept from inflicting harm on health care workers, other patients, and/or visitors (homicidal).

- When a professional is performing minor surgical procedures on a child who is not able to remain still.

Preparation

Before restraint application, the health care provider should be familiar with the restraint device that will be used. Also, if a patient is violent, a five-person team is optimal for the restraining process. Each person will be responsible for one extremity, with the fifth person supervising and positioning the patient's head.

Each restraint device will have different directions for application. However, there are some universal standards for proper application. When using any type of restraining device, it is extremely important to tie or lock the restraint to the bed frame and not the bed rails, thus allowing for proper movement. With soft restraints, posey jackets, and restraint belts, a quick-release slipknot should be used to allow immediate release if needed. When leather restraints are used and applied to both arms and legs, one arm should be positioned above the patient's head while the other is positioned by the patient's side. This will decrease the possibility of the patient's rocking or tipping over the bed.

Aftercare

The nurse has to reassess restraints at least every 30 minutes. Neurovascular assessment (circulation to hands, fingers, feet, toes); skin assessment (bruising of restrained area); and meeting a patient's activities of daily living such as toileting, eating, and drinking are all aspects of restraint reassessment and care. Documentation of these interventions must be clearly identified on the patient's chart.

Complications

Most common restraint complications include:

- accidental or intentional removal of restraints by patient, family, or staff, resulting in possible removal of tubes, intravenous lines, or injury to patient or others

- injury to restrained extremity (arm or leg)

- fracture or muscle strains during application with violent patient

- dislocation or contusion of extremity

- exposure to blood or body fluid while restraining violent patient (biting, spitting, urinating, etc.)

- numbness and/or tingling in restrained extremity

Results

The end results of using physical restraints are the maintenance of safety to the patient and others and the administration of medically necessary interventions.

KEY TERMS

Extremity—A term referring to an arm or leg.

Gait—A characteristic pace of a person's walk.

Neurovascular—Referring to the combined status of the neurological and circulatory systems.

Physical restraint—A piece of equipment or device that restricts a patient's ability to move.

Health care team roles

The **registered nurse** (RN) or **licensed practical nurse** (LPN) has a tremendous responsibility when caring for a patient in physical restraints. Many times restraints are needed immediately and violent attacks on health care workers can happen. The emphasis on proper documentation of alternative methods is an absolute must. Obtaining a physician's order for physical restraints is a top priority as well. Rationale for the application of restraints must be discussed with the patient and family. Adequate explanation of the interference with medical treatment or the diversion of suicidal or homicidal acts is important. Reassessment of proper restraint positioning and re-evaluation of the patient's continued need for physical restraints are also aspects of complete nursing care.

Paramedics and emergency medical technicians (EMTs) are confronted with the need to use physical restraints in the field (outside the hospital). In these cases, they are allowed to use a "reasonable amount of force" in order to manage a combative patient during transport to the health care facility. Physical restraints utilized by paramedics and EMTs are plastic bound straps (zip straps), vests, and blankets. When physical restraints are necessary, law enforcement is usually involved.

Resources

BOOKS

Bledsoe, Bryan E., Robert S. Porter, and Richard S. Cherry. "Medical/Legal Aspects of Advanced Prehospital Care." In *Paramedic Care: Principles & Practice: Introduction to Advanced Prehospital Care.* Upper Saddle River, NJ: Prentice-Hall, 2000, pp. 108–137.

Mulryan, Kathleen. "Applying Restraints." In *Clinical Nursing Skills & Techniques*, 4th ed. Edited by Susan R. Epstein. St. Louis: Mosby-Year Book, 1998, pp. 78–84.

Mulryan, Kathleen. "Designing a Restraint-Free Environment." In *Clinical Nursing Skills & Techniques*, 4th ed. Edited by Susan R. Epstein. St. Louis: Mosby-Year Book, 1998, pp. 74–78.

OTHER

Wigder, Herbert N. "Restraints from Emergency Medicine/Legal Aspects of Emergency Medicine." emedicine.com January 2001. http://www.emedicine.com/emerg/topic776.htm.

ORGANIZATION

National Association of Psychiatric Health Systems. 325 Seventh Street, N.W., Suite 625, Washington, D.C. 20004-2802. (202) 393-6700. http://www.haphs.org/News/guidingprinc.html.

Lori Beck, RN, MSN, FNP-C

Retainers *see* **Orthodontic appliances**

Reticulocyte Count

Definition

A reticulocyte count is a test that measures the rate at which new (immature) red **blood** cells (called reticulocytes) are manufactured by **bone** marrow and released into the bloodstream already containing mature red blood cells. The test is usually performed when medical professionals suspect a patient has anemia or during treatment for anemia, but is also used for other conditions relating to blood disorders.

Purpose

The reticulocyte count test will determine if immature red blood cells are being produced at an increased rate, a normal rate, or at a decreased rate. The test is also used to monitor and evaluate the response of the bone marrow during treatment for anemia.

On the first day that bone marrow makes a red blood cell, it is a large bluish-colored cell filled with ribonucleic acid (RNA). Over the next two days, the cell diminishes in size and changes to a pinkish color as the amount of RNA decreases and the amount of hemoglobin increases. The cell's nucleus then clusters together. The cell is now considered a reticulocyte, an immature red blood cell. After about three days inside the bone marrow, the reticulocyte is ejected into the bloodstream. The reticulocyte circulates for about two days until it becomes a mature red blood cell—after about a total of five days of maturation. Normally, at any given time, about 1–2% of all red blood cells in the bloodstream are reticulocytes.

Precautions

The reticulocyte count may be adversely affected by:

- pregnancy
- medications such as azathioprine (Imuran), chloramphericol (Chloromycetin), corticotrophin (ACTH),

levodopa (L-dopa), and dactinomycin (Cosmegen), along with medications to treat fever, cancer, or malaria

• radiation therapy

• sulfonamide antibiotics (such as Bactrim or Septra)

• recent transfusion of blood

Description

The first step in measuring the reticulocyte count is to perform a blood draw. Blood is drawn by a medical professional using a needle inserted in a vein usually located on the arm or hand. The area is cleaned with antiseptic or alcohol. An elastic band is placed around the upper arm to apply pressure to the vein. The needle is inserted into a vein and approximately 17 ounces (5 mL) of blood is collected in an airtight vial or syringe. After the approximate 5–10 minute procedure, the band is removed to reinstate circulation. After the collection is complete, the needle is removed and the site is covered with a gauze pad or a cotton ball to stop any bleeding. Pressure is applied for a few minutes with the arm slightly elevated. A small bandage is placed over the gauze pad or cotton ball.

The blood sample is then delivered to a laboratory for analysis. A technician places the sample in a test tube with methylene blue, a dye that identifies RNA, a protein found in immature red blood cells but not in mature ones. Drops of the mixture are smeared on slides and viewed under a **microscope**. The reticulocytes are seen as deep dark blue granules or a blue mesh network. A technician will count one thousand red blood cells manually, determining which ones are reticulocytes and which ones are not, or let a flow cytometer automatically count between (usually) 10,000 and 50,000 red blood cells. In either case, the final reticulocyte count is stated as a percentage of reticulocytes to the total number of red blood cells. The number of reticulocytes in the blood indicates how quickly or slowly they are being produced and released by the bone marrow.

Preparation

The medical professional should be aware of any prescription medications that the patient is taking before performing the blood draw. The health care professional should observe **universal precautions** when drawing blood.

Aftercare

The bandage placed over the puncture area should be removed by the patient later in the day and the area cleaned with soap and water.

Complications

When the needle is inserted to draw blood, some people feel some **pain**, while others feel a tiny prick of the skin. Some people feel minor pain or discomfort while the needle is in the vein. Other people feel no pain. The amount of pain is usually determined by the skill of the medical professional, the condition of the patient's veins, and the patient's sensitivity to pain. Afterwards, there may be some minor throbbing of the arm or bruising at the blood draw site.

The main complication is a slight chance of mild **dizziness** or fainting immediately after the blood draw. Other small risks include excessive bleeding, hematoma, **infection**, inflammation, multiple punctures, or localized bruises or swelling. People with **bleeding disorders** may bleed more than usual.

Results

A reticulocyte count is usually given as the percentage of immature red blood cells to the total number of red blood cells in the bloodstream. A normal range, which varies among laboratories, is from 0.5–2.0%. Generally, women and children have higher reticulocyte counts than men.

A lower-than-normal percentage of reticulocytes usually indicates decreased production of red blood cells, which may be caused by a nutritional deficiency. It may also indicate a need for a **bone marrow biopsy** and further testing, to determine whether there is a problem with the production of new reticulocytes by the bone marrow. Conditions that may indicate a lower-than-normal count include:

- bone marrow failure from such conditions as toxicity, tumor, fibrosis, or infection
- cirrhosis of the liver
- folate (folic acid), iron (Fe), or vitamin B_{12} deficiencies
- radiation therapy
- kidney disease with decreased erythropoietin production

A higher-than-normal percentage indicates an increased production of red blood cells. This reading shows an indication that there has been blood loss (excess bleeding) or red blood cell breakdown or destruction (hemolysis). It may also indicate a need for further tests. These conditions may be present:

- erythroblastosis fetalis
- h anemia
- post-hemorrhage (bleeding)
- kidney disease with increased erythropoietin production

Health care team roles

The medical team is responsible for administering the blood draw, analyzing the blood sample, providing results to the patient, and determining a course of action based on the results of the reticulocyte count.

Resources

BOOKS

Corbett, Jane V., and Angela Banks. *Laboratory Tests and Diagnostic Procedures with Nursing Diagnoses*, 8th edition. Prentice Hall, 2012.

Malarkey, Louise M., and Mary Ellen McMorrow. *Saunders Nurse's Guide to Laboratory and Diagnostic Tests*. Philadelphia: W.B. Saunders Co., 2005.

OTHER

Health A to Z, Medical Network Inc. "Reticulocyte Count," 2002. http://www.healthatoz.com/healthatoz/ Atoz/ency/reticulocyte_count.jsphtml (December 9, 2005).

WebMD, Healthwise, Inc. "Reticulocyte Count," October 28, 2004. http://www.webmd.com/hw/health_guide_atoz/ hw203366.asp?printing=true (December 9, 2005).

William Arthur Atkins

Retinal detachment

Definition

Retinal detachment is movement of the transparent sensory part of the retina away from the outer pigmented layer of the retina. In other words, the moving away of the retina from the outer wall of the eyeball.

Description

There are three layers of the eyeball. The outer, tough, white sclera. Lining the sclera is the choroid, a thin membrane that supplies nutrients to part of the retina. The innermost layer is the retina.

The retina is the light-sensitive membrane that receives images and transmits them to the **brain**. It is made up of several layers. One layer contains the photoreceptors. The photoreceptors, the rods and cones, send the visual message to the brain. Between the photoreceptor layer (also called the sensory layer) and the choroid is the pigmented epithelium.

The vitreous is a clear gel-like substance that fills up most of the inner space of the eyeball. It lies behind the lens and is in contact with the retina.

A retinal detachment occurs between the two outermost layers of the retina—the photoreceptor layer and the outermost pigmented epithelium. Because the choroid supplies the photoreceptors with nutrients, a detachment can basically starve the photoreceptors. If a detachment is not repaired within 24-72 hours, permanent damage may occur.

Causes and symptoms

Several conditions may cause retinal detachment:

- Scarring or shrinkage of the vitreous can pull the retina inward.
- Small tears in the retina allow liquid to seep behind the retina and push it forward.
- Injury to the eye can simply knock the retina loose.
- Bleeding behind the retina, most often due to diabetic retinopathy or injury, can push it forward.
- Retinal detachment may be spontaneous. This occurs more often in the elderly or in very nearsighted (myopic) eyes.
- Cataract surgery causes retinal detachment 2% of the time.
- Tumors can cause the retina to detach.

Retinal detachment will cause a sudden defect in **vision**. It may look as if a curtain or shadow has just

KEY TERMS

Cauterize—To damage with heat or cold so that tissues shrink. It is an effective way to stop bleeding.

Diabetic retinopathy—Disease that damages the blood vessels in the back of the eye caused by diabetes.

Saline—A salt solution equivalent to that in the body–0.9% salt in water.

descended before the eye. If most of the retina is detached, there may be only a small hole of vision remaining. If just a part of the retina is involved, there will be a blind spot that may not even be noticed. It is often associated with *floaters*–little dark spots that float across the eye and can be mistaken for flies in the room. There may also be *flashes* of light. Anyone experiencing a sudden onset of flashes and/or floaters should contact their eye doctor immediately, as this may signal a detachment.

Diagnosis

If the eye is clear–that is, if there is no clouding of the liquids inside the eye–the detachment can be seen by looking into the eye with a hand-held instrument called an ophthalmoscope. To evaluate the **blood vessels** in the retina, a fluorescent dye (fluorescein) may be injected into a vein and photographed with ultraviolet light as it passes through the retina. Further studies may include computed tomography scan (CT scan), **magnetic resonance imaging** (MRI), or ultrasound study. Other lenses may be used to examine the back of the eyes. One example is binocular indirect ophthalmoscopy. The doctor dilates the patient's eyes with eyedrops and then examines the back of the eyes with a handheld lens.

Treatment

Reattaching the retina to the inner surface of the eye requires making a scar that will hold it in place and then bringing the retina close to the scarred area. The scar can be made from the outside, through the sclera, using either a laser or a freezing cold probe (cryopexy). Bringing the retina close to the scar can be done in two ways. A tiny belt tightened around the eyeball will bring the sclera in until it reaches the retina. This procedure is called scleral buckling and may be done under **general anesthesia**. Using this procedure

permits the repair of retinal detachments without entering the eyeball. Sometimes, the eye must be entered to pump in air or gas, forcing the retina outward against the sclera and its scar. This is called pneumatic retinopexy and can generally be done under **local anesthesia**.

If all else fails, and especially if there is disease in the vitreous, the vitreous may have to be removed in a procedure called vitrectomy. This can be done through tiny holes in the eye, through which equally tiny instruments are placed to suck out the vitreous and replace it with saline, a salt solution. The procedure must maintain pressure inside the eye so that the eye does not collapse.

Prognosis

Retinal reattachment has an 80-90% success rate.

Prevention

In diseases such as diabetes, with a high incidence of retinal disease, routine eye examinations can detect early changes. Early treatment can prevent both progressing to detachment and blindness from other events like hemorrhage. The most common problem is weakness of **blood** vessels that causes them to break down and bleed. When enough vessels have been damaged, new vessels grow to replace them. These new vessels may grow into the vitreous, producing blind spots and scarring. The scarring can in turn pull the retina loose. Other diseases can cause the tiny holes and tears in the retina through which fluid can leak. Preventive treatment uses a laser to cauterize the blood vessels, so that they do not bleed and the holes, so they do not leak.

Good control of diabetes can help prevent diabetic eye disease. **Blood pressure** control can prevent **hypertension** from damaging the retinal blood vessels. Eye protection can prevent direct injury to the eyes. Regular eye exams can also detect changes that the patient may not be aware of. This is important for patients with high **myopia** who may be more prone to detachment.

Resources

ORGANIZATIONS

American Academy of Ophthalmology (AAO), P. O. Box 7424, San Francisco, CA 94120-7424, ((415)) 561-8500, Fax: (415) 561-8500, http://www.aao.org

American Optometric Association, 243 North Lindbergh Blvd., St. Louis, MO 63141, (314) 991-4100, Fax: ((314)) 991-4101, (800) 365-2219, http://www.aoa.org/

J. Ricker Polsdorfer, MD

Retinol *see* **Vitamin A**

Retinopathy

Definition

Retinopathy is not a single disease but a condition in which the retina of the eye degenerates as a result of acute or persistent damage associated with such systemic diseases as **hypertension** or diabetes, or with premature birth. Retinopathy may also result from exposure to radiation or staring at the sun without proper protection (solar retinopathy).

Description

To understand retinopathy, it is helpful to begin with a review of the **anatomy** of the human eye. The retina is an outward extension of the **central nervous system** that lines the inside of the eye. It has 10 layers and is comprised of the photoreceptor rods and cones and such support cells as Mueller cells. The retinal pigment epithelium (RPE) is a single cell layer located behind the retina, which services the photo-receptors. Bruch's membrane is a basement membrane found between the RPE and the choroid, a highly vascular layer that includes the choriocapillaris, which supplies nutrients to the RPE and to the photorecep-tors. The central retinal artery and its branches supply **blood** to the rest of the retina. The cilio-retinal artery that emerges from the optic nerve supplies the macula.

The macula is located temporal to the optic nerve and is the part of the retina that contains the highest concentration of photoreceptors, especially cones. The part of the macula with the highest concentration of cones is the fovea. The vitreous humor is a gelatinous body that is located between the retina and the lens of the eye. The optic nerve is a large nerve in the posterior part of the eye through which the central artery and vein pass. It is actually formed from the axons of cells in the retina. It is through the optic nerve that visual stimuli leave the eye for the occipital lobe of the **brain**, where **vision** is processed. Hemoglobin is a molecule in red blood cells responsible for the transport of oxygen.

The presentation and pathogenesis of each of these retinal diseases are unique; and the signs can be seen by an ophthalmologist or an optometrist on dilation of the eye. All retinopathies can lead to blindness.

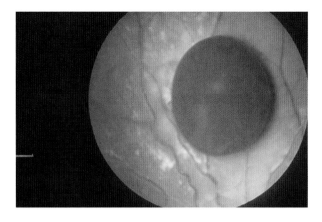

(Retinopathies (retinal hermorrhage), photograph. Custom Medical Stock Photo. Reproduced by permission.)

Demographics

Retinopathy affects millions of people in the United States and Canada as of 2012. The National Eye Institute (NEI) estimated in 2009 that 40% to 45% of all persons diagnosed with diabetes have some form of diabetic retinopathy, while the number of diabetics with diabetic retinopathy is projected to increase from 5.5 million in 2005 to 16 million in 2050. Approximately 700,000 persons in the United States have proliferative diabetic retinopathy, with an annual incidence of 65,000. Diabetic retinopathy is the single most common cause of new blindness in adults between the ages of 25 and 74. African Americans and Hispanics are at greater risk of diabetic retinopathy than members of other ethnic groups; Mexican Americans in particular have twice the rate of diabetic retinopathy as Caucasians.

Retinopathy of prematurity (ROP), a form of retinopathy that affects babies born before 25 to 28 weeks' gestation, affects between 20% and 29% of preterm infants worldwide. Risk factors include birth before 25 to 28 weeks' gestation and a birth weight below 2.75 pounds (1250 grams). Boys are more likely than girls to develop ROP. African American infants have a lower risk of this form of retinopathy; the reason for this ethnic difference is not known as of 2012. About 1200 infants in the United States each year develop a stage of ROP that is severe enough to require treatment; between 400 and 500 will become legally blind.

Hypertensive retinopathy (retinopathy associated with high **blood pressure**) may affect as many as 50 million adults in the United States. It is more common in African Americans than in any other racial or ethnic group; men are affected more often than women. People whose hypertension is untreated or poorly controlled are at increased risk of hypertensive retinopathy.

Solar retinopathy is relatively uncommon because most people blink reflexively when looking at the sun. This form of retinopathy has been reported, however, in people who stare at the sun under the influence of mind-altering drugs as well as those who are viewing a solar eclipse without adequate eye protection.

Causes and symptoms

Diabetic retinopathy

Risk factors for diabetic retinopathy include hypertension, elevated HgA1C (a **hemoglobin test**), a history of **smoking**, and the number of years as a diabetic. Within 10 years of diagnosis, over 70% of type I diabetics will have some retinopathy, and within 16 years of diagnosis, 60% of type II diabetics will have retinopathy. A diabetic person may have normal vision, yet still have severe retinopathy.

The underlying pathogenesis of diabetic retinopathy is hypoxia, a decreased oxygen supply that is caused by elevated blood sugar or hyperglycemia. Glucose is needed in the cells of the body for energy, and oxygen and insulin are required for entry of the glucose molecules. The diabetic, because of insufficient insulin or because of cellular resistance to insulin, cannot absorb glucose into the cell effectively. The pathologic response of the retina to a decreased oxygen supply is first a thickening of, and then a breakdown of the retinal capillary basement membrane. Pericytes, which are cells that surround the capillaries and produce an inhibitor for angiogenesis, also degenerate. In the absence of this inhibitor, retinal neovascularization, or new vessel formation, is stimulated by vascular endothelial growth factor (VEGF). The newly formed vessels are very fragile and can easily rupture, causing bleeding in the vitreous and subsequently leading to vitreous traction. Degeneration of retinal neural cells precedes the vascular changes of diabetic retinopathy.

Diabetic retinopathy is a condition that initially affects only the posterior pole of the retina. The peripheral retina is affected only in the extreme cases. Diabetic retinopathy is divided into two phases: nonproliferative and proliferative. In the nonproliferative phase the retina has microaneurysms, dot and blot hemorrhages, hard lipid exudates, a beading pattern of some of the venules, areas of local **ischemia** where there is little or no oxygen perfusion (called cotton-wool spots), or macular **edema**. The macular edema is called clinically significant macula (CSME) when there are hard exudates and macular thickening or edema, close to the fovea. In the proliferative phase of diabetic retinopathy, neovascularization of the retina and of the optic nerve can be observed. A fibrous substance that materializes when the new retinal vessels form adheres to the vitreous humor, causing retinal traction and retinal detachments. The newly formed **blood vessels** can invade the anterior part of the eye, causing neovascular **glaucoma**. Vitreous hemorrhaging occurs when the blood vessels attach to the vitreous. Venous and arterial occlusions are also seen in diabetic retinopathy.

Arteriosclerotic retinopathy

Arteriosclerotic retinopathy is the ocular manifestation of arteriosclerosis, a systemic condition in which the arterial walls thicken and harden. The risk factors for arteriosclerotic retinopathy include **heart** disease and elevated blood serum **cholesterol** levels. Arteriosclerotic retinopathy can be involved in hypertensive retinopathy. One of the first ophthalmoscopic signs of arteriosclerotic retinopathy is an increased arterial reflex due to thickening of the retinal arterial walls. As the arteriosclerosis progresses, the vessels undergo color changes to a copper-wire and then to a silver-wire appearance. Arteriovenous or A-V crossing defects are also synonymous with arteriosclerotic retinopathy. In advanced arteriosclerosis, banking—a type of A-V crossing that completely cuts off distal venous circulation, forming a large dilated vein—often occurs.

Arterial occlusion can occur as a result of arteriosclerotic retinopathy. An embolus from the carotid artery or from the aortic arch of the heart can travel to the retina, occluding either the central retinal artery (CRAO) or one of its branches (BRAO). An embolus from the carotid artery usually is a cholesterol plaque; and that from the heart is usually fibrotic in appearance. Immediately after a CRAO, the retina becomes ischemic and then edematous. Due to the surrounding ischemia, the fovea takes on a characteristic cherry-red appearance. A pupil abnormality, called an afferent pupillary defect (APD), may be noted. The vision loss in a CRAO is severe, sudden, and painless, although the patient may have a history of amaurosis fugax. After resolution of the CRAO the retina takes on a normal appearance, but the retinal blood vessels are narrowed and the optic nerve shows pallor. Macular function will be intact if there is cilioretinal circulation. Patients with a BRAO may be asymptomatic if there is no macular involvement, but usually there is field loss in the affected quadrant as well as decreased visual acuity.

Hypertensive retinopathy

Hypertensive retinopathy is an ocular presentation of the effects of systemic hypertension, defined as systolic pressure over 140 mm/Hg and diastolic pressure over 90 mm/Hg. This type of retinopathy is usually bilateral. There is narrowing of retinal arterioles in systemic hypertension. Constriction of vessels in older hypertensive patients may not be observed because of involutional sclerosis of the arteries, which occurs during **aging**. When the integrity of the retinal vessels is compromised because of long-term hypertension, leakage of blood occurs, and flame-shaped hemorrhages that are characteristic of hypertensive retinopathy can be observed in the retina. Also, a star-shaped pattern of exudation appears in the macula. In the advanced stages of hypertensive retinopathy there will be cotton wool spots close to the optic nerve. In malignant hypertension the optic nerve will become swollen and the patient will often experience blurred vision, and, if the blood pressure is extremely elevated, **encephalopathy** can develop.

Retinal vein occlusions

Retinal vein occlusions block the drainage of the retina. They can be either central (CRVO) or branched (BRVO). They are usually seen in older patients who have arteriosclerosis, hypertension or diabetes. Vein occlusions can also strike patients with sickle-cell anemia. Papillophlebitis is a form of retinal vein occlusion that is inflammatory in nature and seen in younger patients. A hemi-central vein occlusion is similar to a CRVO, but affects only one-half of the retina. A CRVO occurs when the central retinal artery compresses the central vein as it leaves the lamina cribosa. A BRVO occurs when there is constriction of a venule by a sclerotic artery that affects only one quadrant, usually the superior temporal one.

A CRVO can be either ischemic (characterized by decreased blood flow) or nonischemic. Approximately 80% of CRVO events are nonischemic. In the nonischemic CRVO, hemorrhages are evident throughout the retina, but usually there are no cotton-wool spots. The optic nerve swelling is usually mild and macular edema is not always present. The visual acuity may be only mildly reduced. Months after such an occlusion, collateral blood vessels may appear on the optic nerve. Up to 20% of individuals with a nonischemic CRVO may progress to an ischemic event. The hallmark of ischemic CRVO is extensive capillary nonperfusion. Ophthalmoscopic examination following an ischemic event reveals extensive venous tortuosity (twisting) and enlargement of the retinal veins. Edema (swelling) of the macula and optic nerve are always present and cotton wool spots are common. Visual acuity is usually less than 20/200. Neovascularization of the iris and neovascular glaucoma are common complications of CRVO. There can be optic nerve neovascularization, bleeding into the vitreous, and vitreal traction, which increases the risk of a

retinal detachment. The signs of a BRAO are similar, but present in just one quadrant.

Sickle-cell retinopathy

The underlying cause of sickle-cell retinopathy is different from that of the other retinopathies. Sickle-cell anemia is a genetically inherited condition seen primarily in persons of African descent. Close to 10% of African Americans carry one of the sickle-cell traits. Sickle-cell anemia is caused by mutant hemoglobin molecules that form either because of an amino acid substitution of valine for glutamic acid, causing a structural defect in the hemoglobin molecule, or because of a deficiency in the synthesis of one of the hemoglobin peptide chains. A normal red blood cell has a biconcave appearance and can easily pass through the capillary bed. A sickled cell does not have this biconcave shape, is less pliable than a normal red blood cell, and thus does not move well through the capillaries, thus triggering retinal microvascular occlusions and then ischemia.

Sickle-cell retinopathy can be nonproliferative or proliferative and affects primarily the peripheral retina. In the nonproliferative stage, the retinal vessel walls begin to deteriorate. The ophthalmoscopic signs of nonproliferative sickle-cell retinopathy include: venous tortuosity; intraretinal "salmon patch" hemorrhages, found near a vessel occlusion; "black sunburst" lesions, that develop when a vascular occlusion damages the RPE; silver-wired arterioles; and breaks in Bruch's membrane called angioid streaks. Sickle-cell retinopathy becomes proliferative when neovascularization, in the form of arteriovenous anastomoses or connections between veins and arteries, appears in a sea-shaped formation. These vessels can adhere to the vitreous, but usually regress, forming a characteristic white tuft. Vitreous traction and retinal detachments are not common in sickle-cell retinopathy.

Retinopathy of prematurity

Retinopathy of prematurity is a type of retinopathy that was first diagnosed in 1942. It develops in extremely preterm infants. In some cases it heals, but it can also lead to permanent low vision or blindness. The infants at greatest risk are those with very low birth weight, a young gestational age, and other illnesses associated with prematurity, such as **respiratory distress syndrome** or **sepsis**. The disorder is caused by the abnormal proliferation of blood vessels in the retina following premature birth. In normal prenatal development, the retinal blood vessels begin to develop around 16 weeks after conception. The vascularization of the nasal portion of the retina is completed by 32 weeks and the larger temporal area by 40 weeks (full term). If the baby is born before the retinal blood vessels are mature, normal development of the capillaries on the periphery of the retina shuts down temporarily. New capillaries develop in an irregular pattern, forming a ridge between the vascularized central portion of the retina and the unvascularized peripheral portion. The abnormal new blood vessels are fragile and may leak, scarring the retina and pulling it out of position, eventually causing partial or complete retinal detachment.

ROP is classified in five stages, from mild to severe. Most infants with ROP are at Stages I and II:

- Stage I: Mildly abnormal growth of new blood vessels. In most cases this stage resolves by itself and the child develops normal vision.

- Stage II: Moderately abnormal blood vessel growth. The new blood vessels typically form an elevated ridge of tissue in this stage. In many cases these children also develop normal vision and do not require treatment.

- Stage III: Severely abnormal blood vessel growth. The abnormal blood vessels grow toward the center of the eye outside the retina instead of following their normal growth pattern along the surface of the retina. Treatment is considered at this stage if the infant develops what is called "plus disease," marked by the dilation and twisting of the blood vessels in the posterior retina. Plus disease reflects an increase of blood flow through the retina and a worsening of the disease.

- Stage IV: Partial detachment of the retina.

- Stage V: Complete detachment of the retina. If Stage V ROP is not treated, the child will have severe visual impairment or blindness.

Solar and radiation retinopathy

Solar and radiation retinopathy are forms of retinopathy related to exposure to sunlight or radiation. In solar retinopathy, damage to the retina is caused by photochemical reactions rather than thermal injury. The symptoms of solar retinopathy are reduced visual acuity and scotomas (blank spots in the visual field). In most cases vision loss due to solar retinopathy is reversible, usually within a month in mild cases to over a year in more severe cases.

Radiation retinopathy can be caused by exposure to radiation during **radiotherapy**, accidental exposure, or a nuclear incident. Risk factors for retinal damage from radiation include type 2 diabetes, hypertension, and male sex.

Diagnosis

The diagnosis of retinopathy can be made by an ophthalmologist or an optometrist. The diagnosis of ROP in infants is usually made in the course of screening in the neonatal intensive care unit (NICU) by an ophthalmologist with special training in examining newborns. In adult patients, careful history-taking is important because hypertensive and diabetic retinopathy can develop slowly over years without any noticeable symptoms. In patients with a history of diabetes or hypertension, the ophthalmologist performs an examination with an ophthalmoscope, an instrument that allows visual examination of the retina and the vitreous humor. Ophthalmoscopy (also called fundoscopy) may also be performed by a primary care physician as part of a routine physical checkup.

The ophthalmologist or optometrist uses fluorescein **angiography** to determine the extent of vessel leakage and perfusion in the retinopathies. The fluorescein dye is injected into the body through a vein in the hand. Rarely does a patient have a reaction to the dye, but a localized redness at the injection site is occasionally observed. The fluorescein molecule binds to **proteins** in the blood and it excited by light of 490 nanometers (blue light). A retinal camera filters the light, such that only blue light enters the eye. Photos taken in rapid succession reveal the extent of perfusion, leakage, and ischemia in the retina. The results of this angiography help the doctor to determine if laser photocoagulation can benefit the patient.

Optical coherence tomography (OCT) may also be used to assess the severity of damage in diabetic retinopathy and to evaluate the patient's response to treatment. OCT is a new technique for obtaining images of translucent or opaque materials below the surface of tissue at a resolution equivalent to a low-power **microscope**. OCT is sometimes described as "optical ultrasound."

Treatment

In laser treatment of retinopathy, the light energy of the laser is absorbed by certain cells in the retina, destroying them and thus reducing the oxygen demand of the area, while leaving the surrounding tissue intact. Pan-retinal photocoagulation (PRP) treats neovascularization following a BRAO or hemi-retinal arterial occlusion and the neovascularization of the optic nerve in diabetic retinopathy. The macular edema of arterial occlusions and diabetic retinopathy is treated by focal argon photocoagulation. **Laser surgery** is not performed close to the fovea. Often the edema that develops during an arterial occlusion will dissipate

KEY TERMS

Acuity—The ability to see clearly at a distance.

Choroid—The vascular layer of the eye, containing connective tissue and lying between the retina and the sclera.

Fovea—A tiny pit in the macula that is responsible for sharp vision.

Fundus—The interior surface of the eye opposite the lens. It includes the retina, macula, fovea, and the optic disc. Examination of the fundus with an ophthalmoscope is sometimes referred to as fundoscopy.

Neovascularization—Growth of new capillaries.

Ophthalmologist—A physician who specializes in disorders and diseases of the eye, and is qualified to perform surgery as well as administer drugs. Ophthalmologists hold the M.D. degree.

Optometrist—A licensed medical professional trained to prescribe and fit lenses to improve vision, and to diagnose and treat various eye diseases with medications. Optometrists hold the degree of Doctor of Optometry.

Proliferative retinopathy—Retinopathy with neovascularization.

Retina—The innermost layer of the eye containing light-sensitive nerve cells and fibers. The retina is connected to the brain via the optic nerve.

Retinal pigment epithelium (RPE)—A single layer of hexagonal cells in the retina that are closely packed with pigment. The RPE shields the retina from excessive amounts of incoming light and is closely attached to the choroid beneath it. One form of wet ARMD is characterized by a buildup of fluid between the choroid and the RPE.

Scotoma—An area of visual loss in one's field of vision surrounded by a field of normal (or better-preserved) vision. A scotoma may involve any part of the visual field and may be any shape or size.

Vitrectomy—The surgical removal of the vitreous humor. The gel is replaced with saline or another clear fluid.

Vitreous humor—The clear gel that fills the space between the lens and the retina of the eye.

without treatment. Laser treatment is not usually beneficial in CRAO. Peripheral scatter photocoagulation treats the neovascularization of sickle-cell retinopathy.

The vitreous hemorrhaging of diabetic and sickle-cell retinopathy may require either a vitrectomy, which is a surgical removal of part or all of the vitreous, or cryopexy, the use of low-temperature probes to kill the blood vessels. Vitrectomy has been especially beneficial in restoring vision in diabetic patients in whom retinopathy has already affected visual acuity.

There is little that can be done to treat a CRAO. Massage of the globe to dislodge the embolus, the use of carbogen to increase blood carbon dioxide levels, and anterior chamber **paracentesis** have all been employed with limited success. **Hyperbaric oxygen therapy** has been successful in treatment of CRAO in one study.

In treatment of the patient with malignant hypertension it is important to slowly lower the blood pressure in order to reduce the risk of ischemic optic neuropathy. Patients with hypertensive retinopathy may also be treated with injections of **corticosteroids** or anti-vascular endothelial growth factor (VEGF)

drugs into the vitreous to lower retinal edema. The intraocular pressure must be lowered in the patient with a CRAO. Nonmedical treatments of hypertensive retinopathy may include changes in diet and **exercise** regimens.

The most effective treatments for ROP are cryotherapy and laser therapy. Laser therapy **burns** away the periphery of the retina, where there are no normal blood vessels. Cryotherapy uses extreme cold to destroy the abnormal blood vessels. These treatments are usually used only on babies with Stage III ROP with "plus disease." Stages IV and V can be treated by vitrectomy or by inserting a scleral buckle, a silicone band around the eye. The buckle prevents the vitreous from pulling on the scar tissue, allowing the retina to move back down onto the wall of the eye. The buckle is removed at a later time as the child's eye continues to grow. Newer treatments include the use of anti-VEGF medications and preventive dietary supplementation with omega-3 polyunsaturated fatty acid.

Solar retinopathy does not usually need treatment in mild cases. Intravitreous injections of bevacizumab (Avastin), an anti-VEGF medication, have been found useful in treating radiation retinopathy.

Prognosis

Except when vitrectomy is performed (when indicated), and once the retinopathies have had an effect on vision, there is little that can be done to restore it. The goal of many of the treatments is to prevent further damage. If the proliferative phases of these retinopathies are treated early enough, normal vision is possible. The prognosis for patients with nonproliferative retinopathy is better than for patients with proliferative disease. When diagnosed early, the progress of diabetic retinopathy from the nonproliferative to the proliferative form can be slowed significantly by tight control of blood sugar levels. In proliferative diabetic neuropathy, 95 percent of patients will keep their sight for at least 5 years if treated promptly. If they are treated late, only 50 percent will keep their sight for 5 years.

The prognosis for infants with Stage I or II ROP is good. The prognosis for infants in the later stages depends on the presence of "plus disease" and the initiation of treatment for the disorder.

Health care team roles

The role of the allied health professional in diagnosis and treatment of retinopathy is to assist the ophthalmologist or optometrist in diagnosis. Ophthalmic technicians or nurses may instill the drops for dilation of the eye, inject the fluorescein dye used in angiography. The ophthalmic technician or a retinal photographer takes the photos needed for analysis of retinopathy. Dietitians assist diabetics, hypertensives, and those with heart disease.

Infants diagnosed with ROP may be cared for by pediatric ophthalmologists and neonatologists (doctors with specialized training in care of newborns). Nurses may assist in the care of these infants.

Prevention

The first line in prevention of the retinopathies is an annual dilated eye exam performed by an ophthalmologist or an optometrist. Patients with systemic disease that can lead to retinopathy must understand the ocular complications of their disease and the consequences if medical therapy is not followed as recommended by a physician.

Depending on the type of retinopathy, other preventive measures need to be taken. All patients with retinal emboli need a cardiac workup, including analysis of blood lipid levels. This is the case even in the absence of an occlusion. Older patients need testing for temporal arteritis once CRAO is detected. Over 65% of patients with temporal arteritis will have a

---

QUESTIONS TO ASK YOUR DOCTOR

- Am I at risk for diabetic or hypertensive retinopathy?
- What can I do to lower my risk?
- What diagnostic techniques will you use to check my eyes?
- How often should I have an eye exam?
- What is your opinion of the current therapies for hypertensive and diabetic retinopathy?
- I am having radiotherapy for cancer. What is my risk of radiation retinopathy?

CRAO in the fellow eye within days of the initial event. Since 70% of patients with BRAO have hypertension, all patients with such occlusions need to be evaluated for hypertension. Since sickle-cell anemia can cause a BRVO, African Americans need a Sickledex test. In the event of unilateral hypertensive retinopathy, a carotid artery obstruction should be suspected and a carotid workup is imperative. Finally, the best prevention of the retinopathies is management of the underlying systemic diseases.

Retinopathy of prematurity can be prevented in some cases by taking measures to reduce the risk of premature birth. Solar retinopathy can be prevented by taking proper precautions to protect the eyes before looking at the sun.

Resources

BOOKS

Anderson, Robert E., et al., eds.*Retinal Degenerative Diseases: Laboratory and Therapeutic Investigations*. New York: Springer, 2010.

Cunha-Vaz, José, ed. *Diabetic Retinopathy*. Hackensack, NJ: World Scientific, 2010.

Joussen, A.M., ed. *Retinal Vascular Disease*. New York: Springer, 2007.

Wahler, Connie, and Lauren Wilkinson, eds.*Retinopathy: New Research*. Hauppauge, NY: Nova Science Publishers, 2011.

PERIODICALS

Antonetti, D.A., et al. "Diabetic Retinopathy." *New England Journal of Medicine* 366 (March 29, 2012): 1227–1239.

Elagouz, M., et al. "Sickle Cell Disease and the Eye: Old and New Concepts." *Survey of Ophthalmology* 55 (July-August 2010): 359–377.

Grosso, A., et al. "Similarities and Differences in Early Retinal Phenotypes in Hypertension and Diabetes." *Journal of Hypertension* 29 (September 2011): 1667–1675.

Gupta, A., et al. "Radiation Retinopathy: Case Report and Review." *BMJ Ophthalmology* 7 (April 5, 2007): 6.

Henderson, A.D., et al. "Hypertension-related Eye Abnormalities and the Risk of Stroke." *Reviews in Neurological Diseases* 8 (2011): 1–9.

Myung, J.S., et al. "Evaluation of Vascular Disease Progression in Retinopathy of Prematurity Using Static and Dynamic Retinal Images." *American Journal of Ophthalmology* 153 (March 2012): 544–551.

Rivera, J.C., et al. "Understanding Retinopathy of Prematurity: Update on Pathogenesis." *Neonatology* 100 (April 2011): 343–353.

Stewart, M.W. "The Expanding Role of Vascular Endothelial Growth Factor Inhibitors in Ophthalmology." *Mayo Clinic Proceedings* 87 (January 2012): 77–88.

Suhr, C.L., et al. "The Use of Optical Coherence Tomography to Aid in Diagnosing Solar Retinopathy." *Optometry* 82 August 2011): 481–484.

Wu, W.C., et al. "Modified 23-gauge Vitrectomy System for Stage 4 Retinopathy of Prematurity." *Archives of Ophthalmology* 129 (October 2011): 1326–1331.

WEBSITES

Canada.com. "The Facts on Retinopathy." http://bodyand-health.canada.com/channel_condition_info_details.asp?disease_id=196&channel_id=2022&relation_id=16665 (accessed May 5, 2012).

Lighthouse International. "Diabetic Retinopathy Overview." http://lighthouse.org/about-low-vision-blindness/vision-disorders/diabetic-retinopathy/diabetic-retinopathy-overview/ (accessed May 5, 2012).

Lighthouse International. "Retinopathy of Prematurity." http://www.lighthouse.org/about-low-vision-blindness/childrens-vision/pediatric-eye-disorders/retinopathy-prematurity/ (accessed May 5, 2012).

Medscape. "Diabetic Retinopathy." http://emedicine.medscape.com/article/1225122-overview (accessed May 5, 2012).

Medscape. "Ophthalmologic Manifestations of Hypertension." http://emedicine.medscape.com/article/1201779-overview (accessed May 5, 2012).

Medscape. "Retinopathy of Prematurity." http://emedicine.medscape.com/article/1225022-overview (accessed May 5, 2012).

Merck Manual for Health Care Professionals. "Hypertensive Retinopathy." http://www.merckmanuals.com/professional/eye_disorders/retinal_disorders/hypertensive_retinopathy.html (accessed May 5, 2012).

Midwest Eye Care. "Solar Retinopathy." http://www.midwes-teyecare.com/SubSection/index.php?SectionID=7&SubSectionID=183&ParentID=60 (accessed May 5, 2012).

National Eye Institute (NEI). "Facts about Diabetic Retinopathy." http://www.nei.nih.gov/health/diabetic/retinopathy.asp (accessed May 5, 2012).

National Eye Institute (NEI). "Facts about Retinopathy of Prematurity." http://www.nei.nih.gov/health/rop/rop.asp (accessed May 5, 2012).

ORGANIZATIONS

American Academy of Ophthalmology (AAO), P.O. Box 7424, San Francisco, CA United States 94120-7424, (415) 561-8500, Fax: (415) 561-8533, http://www.aao.org/

American Optometric Association (AOA), 243 N. Lindbergh Blvd., St. Louis, MO United States 63141, (800) 365-2219, http://www.aoa.org/x4674.xml, http://www.aoa.org/

Lighthouse International, 111 East 59th Street, New York, NY United States 10022-1202, (212) 821-9200, Fax: (212) 821-9707, (800) 829-0500, info@lighthouse.org, http://www.lighthouse.org/

National Eye Institute (NEI), 31 Center Drive, MSC 2510, Bethesda, MD United States 20892-2510, (301) 496-5248, 2020@nei.nih.gov, http://www.nei.nih.gov/index.asp.

Martha S. Reilly, O.D.
Rebecca J. Frey, Ph.D.

Retrograde cystography

Definition

A retrograde cystogram is a radiographic study of the bladder, made after a direct injection of a radiopaque contrast material by means of a urethral catheter.

Purpose

A retrograde cystogram is performed to evaluate the structure of the bladder and identify such bladder disorders as cystitis, polyps, stones, and tumors. It may also be used to diagnose recurrent urinary tract infections due to urine reflux (backward flow) into the ureters. This examination is commonly performed as an emergency procedure on patients with gross hematuria (**blood** in urine) due to a pelvic fracture or severe trauma to the **abdomen**, in order to detect rupture of the bladder. Retrograde cystography is frequently done on children being evaluated for a congenital abnormality, obstruction, or urethral stricture. When the urethra is also being evaluated, the study is called a cystourethrogram. If the bladder or urethra is evaluated while the patient is voiding (urinating), the study is called a voiding cystourethrogram or VCUG. A voiding cystourethrogram is often performed when the bladder is full to check for any reflux or other problems during urination.

Complications

The physician should be alerted to any previous history of an allergic reaction to an iodine-based contrast material. Since the contrast medium is injected directly

KEY TERMS

Bladder—A balloon-like organ located in the lower pelvis that stores urine.

Catheter—A thin tube used to inject fluids into or withdraw fluids from the body.

Fluoroscope—An under-table x-ray tube used in conjunction with a television monitor that allows immediate visualization of the x-ray image.

Hematuria—The presence of blood in the urine.

Stones—Also known as calculi, stones result from an excessive build-up of mineral crystals in the kidney. Symptoms of stones include intense pain in the lower back or abdomen, urinary tract infection, fever, burning sensation on urination, and/or blood in the urine.

Ureter—The tube that carries urine from the kidney to the bladder.

Urethra—The tube that empties urine from the bladder to the outside of the body.

into the bladder instead of the venous circulation, allergic reactions are extremely rare. A retrograde cystogram should not be performed, however, on patients who have had recent bladder surgery or an obstruction that interferes with the placement of a urinary catheter. Patients with an active urinary tract **infection** or who may be pregnant should not be given a retrograde cystogram.

Description

To administer a retrograde cystogram, a doctor or nurse will insert a thin tube-like instrument called a Foley catheter through the patient's urethra and into the bladder. The contrast medium is then injected through the catheter into the bladder. The catheter can be inserted in an outpatient clinic before the patient is taken to the **radiology** department. It may also be inserted by an emergency physician when a retrograde cystogram is ordered on a severe trauma patient. The cystogram can be performed in the emergency department using a portable x-ray machine.

After the Foley catheter is inserted, 250–300 mL of a water-soluble contrast medium is injected into the bladder and the catheter is clamped. A diluted contrast agent (usually 30% sodium iodide) is used since the contrast medium is not injected intravenously. An AP (anteroposterior) view of the full bladder is taken with the tube angled 10–15 degrees caudal (in the direction of the patient's feet) to project the pubic symphysis away from the base of the

bladder. The patient is turned 45 degrees onto each side for two oblique views of the bladder and completely sideways for a true lateral view. The films are reviewed by the radiologist. If no other films are needed the catheter will be removed and a post-void film is taken. If the patient is unable to urinate, the clamp will be removed, the contrast medium will then empty from the bladder through the tube, and a post-drainage film will be taken. During a voiding cystogram, films are taken by the radiologist under fluoroscopy while the patient is voiding in order to image any urethral abnormalities or urinary reflux.

A retrograde cystogram usually takes from 30 minutes to one hour, depending on how many films are requested by the radiologist.

This examination can also be performed with a radioactive tracer (isotope) in the nuclear medicine department. A cystogram performed with a tracer is known as a radionuclide retrograde cystogram.

A CT scan of the bladder may also be ordered after the injection of a radiopaque contrast material.

Preparation

Laxatives or enemas are sometimes given before the procedure to eliminate gas and fecal material that may prevent proper visualization of the bladder. The patient will be given a hospital gown. The x-ray technologist will explain the procedure and take a detailed patient history concerning **allergies**, the possibility of **pregnancy**, and current medical problems. The patient is usually requested to sign a consent form.

Aftercare

The patient may have some burning on urination for a few hours after the test, due to the irritation of the urethra from the catheter. The discomfort can be reduced by a liberal fluid intake, which will dilute the urine.

Results

A normal result reveals no anatomical or functional abnormalities of the bladder.

Abnormal results may indicate:

• calculi (stones)

• inflammation (cystitis)

• blood clots

• polyps

• injury (bladder tear)

• diverticula

• cystocele (prolapse of the bladder into the vaginal cavity, common after childbith)

- ruptures (imaged as flame-like leakages of the contrast material superior or lateral to the bladder)

- tumors (visualized in the bladder or in an adjacent structure such as the vagina or prostate)

- reflux (urine passing backward from the bladder into the ureters, causing infection)

Health care team roles

The procedure is ordered by the physician. The patient may be catheterized by a physician or nurse. The x-ray technologist prepares the contrast medium for injection and takes all the overhead views of the bladder. If the portable x-ray machine is used to perform the cystogram, all staff members remaining in the room must be shielded. The x-ray technologist works closely with the doctors and nurses to make sure the patients are catheterized before arriving in the radiology department and that an **enema** or laxative has been administered.

Patient education

The x-ray technologist must explain to the patient that it is necessary to fill the bladder completely to see a detailed image of the bladder outline. The patient may experience some discomfort with a full bladder; however, the films are taken at once and the catheter is removed or unclamped. If a film must be taken while the patient is voiding, the lights can be dimmed and the water tap turned on to help the patient relax. The radiology technologist must be certified and registered with the American Society of Radiologic Technologists.

Resources

BOOKS

Clinical Evaluation of Genitourinary Disorders. *The Merck Manual of Diagnosis and Therapy*, 17th edition, ed. Mark H. Beers, MD, and Robert Berkow, MD. Whitehouse Station, NJ: Merck Research Laboratories, 1999.

Eisenberg, Ronald. *Clinical Imaging: Atlas of Differential Diagnosis*, 3rd ed. New York: Thieme Publishing, 1997.

Malarkey, Louise M., and Mary Ellen McMorrow. *Nurse's Manual of Laboratory Tests and Diagnostic Procedures*. Philadelphia: W. B. Saunders Company, 1996.

ORGANIZATIONS

American Kidney Fund. 6110 Executive Blvd., #1010, Rockville, MD 20852. 800-638-8299.

National Kidney and Urologic Diseases Information Clearinghouse. 3 Information Way, Bethesda, MD 20892-3580. (301) 654-4415.

National Kidney Foundation. 30 East 33rd St., New York, NY 10016. (800) 622-9010 or (212) 889-2210.

Lorraine K. Ehresman

Rh factor

Definition

Rh (Rhesus) factor is a **blood** protein that plays a critical role in some pregnancies. People without Rh factor are known as Rh negative, while people with the Rh factor are Rh positive. If a woman who is Rh negative is pregnant with a fetus who is Rh positive, her body may make **antibodies** against the fetus's blood. This can cause Rh disease in the baby, also known as hemolytic disease of the newborn, or erythroblastosis fetalis. In severe cases, Rh disease leads to **brain** damage and even death. Since 1968 a vaccine has existed to prevent the mother's body from making antibodies against the fetus's blood.

Description

Rh factor is an antigen found on the red blood cells of most people. Rh factor, like the blood types A, B, and O, is inherited from one's parents. A simple blood test can determine blood type, including the presence of the Rh factor. About 85% of white Americans and 95% of African-Americans are Rh positive. A person's own health is not affected by the presence or absence of Rh factor.

Rh factor is important only during a **pregnancy** in which an Rh negative woman is carrying a fetus who might be Rh positive. This can occur when an Rh negative woman conceives a baby with an Rh positive man. The gene for Rh positive blood is dominant over the gene for Rh negative blood, so their baby will be Rh positive. If the Rh positive father also carries the gene for Rh negative blood, his babies have a 50% chance of inheriting Rh negative blood and a 50% chance of inheriting Rh positive blood. If both parents are Rh negative, their babies will always be Rh negative. In order to protect their future babies from Rh disease, all women of childbearing age should know their Rh status before becoming pregnant.

Role in human health

Rh factor in pregnancy

The danger of Rh disease begins when the mother's Rh negative blood is exposed to the baby's Rh positive blood. This mixing of blood can occur at the time of birth, and after an **abortion** or **miscarriage**. It may also happen during prenatal tests such as **amniocentesis** and **chorionic villus sampling**. More rarely, blood from the mother and fetus may mingle during pregnancy, before birth. When this contact

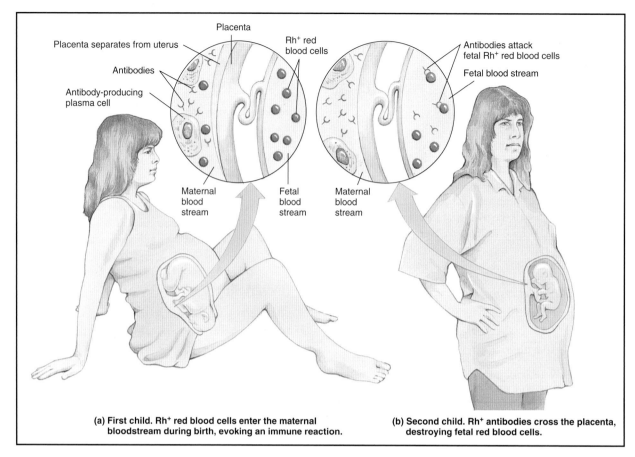

Placenta separates from uterus

Placenta

Rh⁺ red blood cells

Antibodies attack fetal Rh⁺ red blood cells

Antibodies

Fetal blood stream

Antibody-producing plasma cell

Maternal blood stream

Fetal blood stream

Maternal blood stream

(a) First child. Rh⁺ red blood cells enter the maternal bloodstream during birth, evoking an immune reaction.

(b) Second child. Rh⁺ antibodies cross the placenta, destroying fetal red blood cells.

(From Delmar's Medical Terminology Image Library 1st edition by DELMAR. © 1999. Reprinted with permission of Delmar Learning, a division of Thomson Learning: www.thomsonrights.com. Fax 800-730-2215.)

occurs, the mother's body responds by building antibodies to fight the foreign Rh blood protein. The mother's blood is now said to be "sensitized" against Rh factor blood.

Common diseases and disorders

Rh incompatibility

Once a mother's blood has become sensitized, her antibodies will attack the blood of any Rh positive fetus that she carries. The antibodies will destroy the fetus's red blood cells. If this happens, the infant will suffer from Rh factor incompatibility. It will become anemic, a condition caused by a reduction in red blood cells and marked by **weakness** and fatigue. Severe anemia can lead to **heart failure** and death. The breakdown of red blood cells will also cause the formation of a reddish-yellow substance known as bilirubin. An infant with high levels of bilirubin will look yellowish. This is known as **jaundice**. Brain damage can occur if the bilirubin level gets high enough. However, Rh incompatibility occurs in varying degrees of severity, with brain damage at the far end of a spectrum.

Rh disease is usually not a problem during a first pregnancy. This is because the Rh negative mother probably will not become sensitized until her blood mixes with the baby's blood during birth. Her baby will be born before her blood can produce antibodies against the baby's Rh positive blood. Once a mother is sensitized, however, any future babies with Rh positive blood will be at risk for Rh disease.

PREVENTION AND TREATMENT. Since 1968 a vaccine has existed to prevent sensitization from occurring. This is the best way to eliminate Rh disease. Available as an injection, the vaccine is called Rh immune globulin (brand name RhoGAM). It blocks the action of the antibodies and prevents the mother's blood from attacking the baby's blood. To be effective, the vaccine must be given any time fetal blood mixes with maternal blood: after birth, abortion, miscarriage, or prenatal tests like amniocentesis and chorionic villus sampling. The vaccine is typically given within 72 hours of any of these events. Since mixing of the blood may also occur during the last three months of pregnancy, the vaccine is also administered at 28 weeks of pregnancy.

A pregnant woman who has already been sensitized from a previous pregnancy will want her doctor to carefully monitor the level of antibodies in her blood throughout her pregnancy. As long as the antibody levels remain relatively low, no problem exists. But if those levels rise, the fetus will need special attention. High antibody levels mean that the fetus's red blood cells are being attacked and destroyed.

A fetus whose red blood cells are being destroyed will need a blood transfusion while it is still in the uterus. Two or three transfusions may be necessary before the baby is born. If the fetus shows signs of illness close to its anticipated birth, the physician may elect to deliver the baby early, either by inducing birth or by **cesarean section**. The baby will then receive a transfusion after birth.

Eliminating Rh disease

Until the introduction of the Rh immune globulin vaccine, Rh disease could not be prevented. About 45 babies per 10,000 births developed the disease each year before widespread use of the vaccine in the early 1970s. Use of the Rh immune globulin vaccine has reduced the chances of the mother becoming sensitized from approximately 12–13% to 1–2%.

Nevertheless, the disease is not completely eradicated. Further steps must be taken, since this is a preventable disease. The majority of cases of Rh disease are the result of women not receiving the vaccine at the appropriate time. Poor women without health insurance, who are likely to lack adequate **prenatal care**, are especially vulnerable to this oversight. Older women may have become sensitized before the vaccine was available; foreign-born women may not have had access to the vaccine.

Resources

WEBSITES

"Rh factor." MayoClinic.com. June 16, 2012. http://www.mayoclinic.com/health/rh-factor/MY01163 (accessed November 2, 2012).

Salem, Leon. "Rh Incompatibility." Medscape Reference. March 12, 2012. http://emedicine.medscape.com/article/797150-overview (accessed November 2, 2012).

"What Is Rh Incompatibility?" National Heart, Lung, and Blood Institute (NHLBI), National Institutes of Health. January 1, 2011. http://www.nhlbi.nih.gov/health/health-topics/topics/rh/ (accessed November 2, 2012).

Liz Marshall

Rh sensitivity *see* **Rh factor**

Rh typing *see* **Type and screen**

Rheumatic fever

Definition

Rheumatic **fever** (RF) is an illness which arises as a complication of untreated or inadequately treated **strep throat infection**. Rheumatic fever can seriously damage the valves of the **heart**.

Description

Throat infection with a member of the Group A streptococcus (strep) **bacteria** is a common problem among school-aged children. It is easily treated with a 10-day course of **antibiotics** by mouth. However, when such a throat infection occurs without symptoms, or when a course of medication is not taken for the full 10 days, there is a 3% chance of that person developing rheumatic fever. Other types of strep infections (such as of the skin) do not put the patient at risk for RF.

Children between the ages of 5 and 15 are most susceptible to strep throat, and therefore most susceptible to rheumatic fever. Other risk factors include poverty, overcrowding (as in military camps), and lack of access to good medical care. Just as strep throat occurs most frequently in fall, winter, and early spring, so does rheumatic fever.

Causes and symptoms

Two different theories exist as to how a bacterial throat infection can develop into the disease called rheumatic fever. One theory, less supported by research evidence, suggests that the bacteria produce some kind of poisonous chemical (toxin). This toxin is sent into circulation throughout the bloodstream, thus affecting other systems of the body.

Research seems to point to a different theory, however. This theory suggests that the disease is caused by the body's **immune system** acting inappropriately. The body produces immune cells (called **antibodies**), which are specifically designed to recognize and destroy invading agents; in this case, streptococcal bacteria. The antibodies are able to recognize the bacteria because the bacteria contain special markers called antigens. Due to a resemblance between Group A streptococcus bacteria's antigens and antigens present on the body's own cells, the antibodies mistakenly attack the body itself.

It is interesting to note that members of certain families seem to have a greater tendency to develop rheumatic fever than do others. This could be related to the above theory, in that these families may have cell antigens which more closely resemble streptococcal antigens than do members of other families.

In addition to fever, in about 75% of all cases of RF one of the first symptoms is arthritis. The joints (especially those of the ankles, knees, elbows, and wrists) become red, hot, swollen, shiny, and extraordinarily painful. Unlike many other forms of arthritis, the arthritis may not occur symmetrically (affecting a particular joint on both the right and left sides, simultaneously). The arthritis of RF rarely strikes the fingers, toes, or spine. The joints become so tender that even the touch of bedsheets or clothing is terribly painful.

A peculiar type of involuntary movement, coupled with emotional instability, occurs in about 10% of all RF patients (the figure used to be about 50%). The patient begins experiencing a change in coordination, often first noted by changes in handwriting. The arms or legs may flail or jerk uncontrollably. The patient seems to develop a low threshold for anger and sadness. This feature of RF is called Sydenham's chorea or St. Vitus' Dance.

A number of skin changes are common to RF. A **rash** called erythema marginatum develops (especially in those patients who will develop heart problems from their illness), composed of pink splotches, which may eventually spread into each other. It does not itch. Bumps the size of peas may occur under the skin. These are called subcutaneous nodules; they are hard to the touch, but not painful. These nodules most commonly occur over the knee and elbow joint, as well as over the spine.

The most serious problem occurring in RF is called pancarditis ("pan" means total; "carditis" refers to inflammation of the heart). Pancarditis is an inflammation that affects all aspects of the heart, including the lining of the heart (endocardium), the sac containing the heart (pericardium), and the heart muscle itself (myocardium). About 40–80% of all RF patients develop pancarditis. This RF complication has the most serious, long-term effects. The valves within the heart (structures which allow the **blood** to flow only in the correct direction, and only at the correct time in the heart's pumping cycle) are frequently damaged during the course of pancarditis. This may result in blood which either leaks back in the wrong direction, or has a difficult time passing a stiff, poorly moving valve. Either way, damage to a valve can result in the heart having to work very hard in order to move the blood properly. The heart may not be able to "work around" the damaged valve, which may result in a consistently inadequate amount of blood entering the circulation.

Diagnosis

Diagnosis of RF is done by carefully examining the patient. A list of diagnostic criteria has been created. These "Jones Criteria" are divided into major and minor criteria. A patient can be diagnosed with RF if he or she has either two major criteria (conditions), or one major and two minor criteria. In either case, it must also be proved that the individual has had a previous infection with streptococcus.

The major criteria include:

• carditis
• arthritis
• chorea
• subcutaneous nodules
• erythema marginatum

The minor criteria include:

• fever
• joint pain (without actual arthritis)
• evidence of electrical changes in the heart (determined by measuring electrical characteristics of the heart's functioning during a test called an electrocardiogram, or EKG)
• evidence (through a blood test) of the presence in the blood of certain proteins, which are produced early in an inflammatory/infectious disease.

Antibodies—Specialized cells of the immune system which can recognize organisms that invade the body (such as bacteria, viruses, and fungi). The antibodies are then able to set off a complex chain of events designed to kill these foreign invaders.

Antigen—A special, identifying marker on the outside of cells.

Arthritis—Inflammation of the joints.

Autoimmune disorder—A disorder in which the body's antibodies mistake the body's own tissues for foreign invaders. The immune system therefore attacks and causes damage to these tissues.

Chorea—Involuntary movements in which the arms or legs may jerk or flail uncontrollably.

Immune system—The system of specialized organs, lymph nodes, and blood cells throughout the body, which work together to prevent foreign invaders (bacteria, viruses, fungi, etc.) from taking hold and growing.

Inflammation—The body's response to tissue damage. Includes hotness, swelling, redness, and pain in the affected part.

Pancarditis—Inflammation of the lining of the heart, the sac around the heart, and the muscle of the heart.

Tests are also performed to provide evidence of recent infection with group A streptococcal bacteria. A swab of the throat can be taken, and smeared on a substance in a petri dish, to see if bacteria will multiply and grow over 24–72 hours. These bacteria can then be specially processed, and examined under a **microscope**, to identify streptococcal bacteria. Other tests can be performed to see if the patient is producing specific antibodies; that are only made in response to a recent strep infection.

Treatment

A 10-day course of penicillin by mouth, or a single injection of penicillin G is the first line of treatment for RF. Patients will need to remain on some regular dose of penicillin to prevent recurrence of RF. This can mean a small daily dose of penicillin by mouth, or an injection every three weeks. Some practitioners keep patients on this regimen for five years, or until they reach 18 years of age (whichever comes first). Other practitioners prefer to continue treating those patients who will be regularly exposed to streptococcal bacteria (teachers, medical workers), as well as those patients with known RF heart disease.

Arthritis quickly improves when the patient is given a preparation containing aspirin, or some other anti-inflammatory agent (ibuprofen). Mild carditis will also improve with such anti-inflammatory agents, although more severe cases of carditis will require steroid medications. A number of medications are available to treat the involuntary movements of chorea, including diazepam for mild cases, and haloperidol for more severe cases.

Prognosis

The long-term prognosis of an RF patient depends primarily on whether he or she develops carditis. This is the only manifestation of RF which can have permanent effects. Those patients with no or mild carditis have an excellent prognosis. Those with more severe carditis have a risk of **heart failure**, as well as a risk of future heart problems, which may lead to the need for valve replacement surgery.

Prevention

Prevention of the development of RF involves proper diagnosis of initial strep throat infections, and adequate treatment within 10 days with an appropriate antibiotic. Prevention of RF recurrence requires continued antibiotic treatment, perhaps for life. Prevention of complications of already-existing RF heart disease requires that the patient always take a special course of antibiotics when he or she undergoes any kind of procedure (even dental cleanings) that might allow bacteria to gain access to the bloodstream.

Resources

ORGANIZATION

Centers for Disease Control and Prevention (CDC), 1600 Clifton Road, Atlanta, GA 30333, (800) 232-4636, cdcinfo@cdc.gov, http://www.cdc.gov

Rosalyn Carson-DeWitt, MD

Rheumatoid arthritis

Definition

Rheumatoid arthritis is a chronic inflammatory autoimmune joint disease that causes **pain**, stiffness, swelling, and decreased movement in joints. Unchecked, it can lead to joint destruction.

Description

Rheumatoid arthritis is a painful disease that causes joints to swell and become stiff and restricts their range of motion. People of any age, including children, can get rheumatoid arthritis, but it most commonly appears between the ages of 35 and 50 years. About three times more women than men develop rheumatoid arthritis. Between .03% and 1.5% of the population in the United States, have rheumatoid arthritis. Worldwide incidence is about 3 cases per 100,000 population. The disease occurs in all ethnic groups worldwide; however it is more common among some Native American groups and less common among people of Afro-Caribbean origin.

Causes and symptoms

Although researchers are not sure of the exact cause of rheumatoid arthritis, they do know that it is an autoimmune disease in which **immune system** cells function incorrectly, leading them to attack the ligaments and joints of the body. Both genetic and environmental factors appear to be involved in developing the disease. People with first-degree relatives (parents, siblings) who have rheumatoid arthritis are two to three times more likely to develop the disease than people without affected relatives. On the other hand, genetics alone do not determine who develops rheumatoid, as only 15–20% of monozygotic (identical) twins both develop the disease.

Symptoms vary from person to person and can mimic other **bone** and joint diseases such as **osteoarthritis**. For most people, the symptoms of rheumatoid arthritis appear gradually, although about one-third of individuals develop serious symptoms within a few months. In many people, symptoms tend to change from day to day, with periods of improvement followed by periods of worsening symptoms. In more serious cases, symptoms simply worsen progressively without periods of improvement. The wrists and hand joints are affected in more than 85% of individuals with rheumatoid arthritis. Usually if a joint on one side of the body is inflamed, the same joint on the other side will also be affected.

Signs and symptoms of rheumatoid arthritis include:

- sore, stiff, swollen, and warm joints
- involvement of multiple joints
- prolonged stiffness of over an hour in the morning
- general feelings of illness and fatigue, especially when joint pain has worsened
- chronic low fever
- appetite loss and weight loss
- anemia
- formation of rheumatoid nodules or bumps under the skin often around the elbow, spine, and fingers
- inflammation of the tear and salivary glands, causing dry eyes and mouth.

Diagnosis

Although a family physician can diagnose rheumatoid arthritis, a rheumatologist who specializes in bone and joint diseases usually is consulted. Rheumatoid arthritis is difficult to diagnose because symptoms are common to many other diseases. Diagnosis is made based on medical history supplemented with x rays and **blood** tests that look for inflammatory disease factors (e.g., C-reactive protein) and autoantibodies to rheumatoid factor. Diagnosis often involves tests to rule out other causes of joint distress.

The American Rheumatology Association designates that at least four of the following seven criteria must be present for at least six weeks to diagnose rheumatoid arthritis.

- morning joint stiffness lasting more than one hour
- pain simultaneously in three or more joint areas
- arthritis in the wrist or hand
- joint pain in symmetrical joint areas (e.g., both wrists, both knees)
- presence of rheumatoid nodules
- presence of serum rheumatoid factor, a protein found in blood
- x rays that show typical rheumatoid arthritis changes in the affected joints

X rays often appear normal until rheumatoid arthritis is quite advanced and serious joint damage has already occurred. Rheumatoid factor is an antibody or immune system protein. It is found in 80–90% of people with rheumatoid arthritis, but it is also found in about 30% of people who have no symptoms of the disease, so its presence is not a definitive diagnosis.

Treatment

There is no cure for rheumatoid arthritis. Treatment is divided into two categories: treatment of symptoms and treatment to stop or slow joint damage. Treatment to improve symptoms includes the use of various pain medications including **nonsteroidal anti-inflammatory drugs** (e.g., aspirin, ibuprophen, naproxen sodium) and **analgesics** (acetaminophen, tramadol), either alone or in combination with narcotic pain medications. **Corticosteroids** such as prednisone and cortisone are also used in the lowest effective dose to control pain and stiffness. **Exercise** and **physical therapy** to increase strength and flexibility are also beneficial.

Drugs to stop or slow joint damage are collectively called disease-modifying antirheumatic drugs (DMARDs). These drugs, especially when given early in the course of the disease, interfere with the disease process in ways that slow or stop joint damage. DMARDs are often given in combination with drugs to improve symptoms. Some common DMARDs include methotrexate (Rheumatrex, Trexall), hydroxychloroquinine (Plaquenil), sulfasalazine (Azulfidine), leflunomide (Arava), D-pencillamine (Dpen, Cuprimine), azathioprine (Imuran), cyclosporine (Neoral, Sandimmune) and minocycline (Minocin, Dynacin). All these drugs have potentially serious side effects and may require regular blood or other tests.

Rheumatoid arthritis can also be treated with biologic response modifiers (BMRs). BMRs target specific **proteins** of the immune system that are involved in rheumatoid arthritis. Many BMRs are approved for use in adults only. The exception is etanercept (Enbrel), which is approved for individuals over age four. Other BMRs used to treat rheumatoid arthritis include infliximab (Remicade), anakinra (Kineret), and adalimumab (Humira). BMRs interfere with and may weaken the immune system. Individuals should not receive live-virus vaccinations while taking BMRs. Other side effects are also possible.

Many complementary and alternative cures are heavily advertised for rheumatoid arthritis. The National Center for Complementary and Alternative Medicine has investigated many of these alternative cures. Most do not provide any benefit to individuals with rheumatoid arthritis. Those complementary and alternative treatments that may have possible benefit include thunder god vine (*Tripteryguim wilfordii*, gamma-linolenic acid (GLA), fish oil, mind-body **stress** reduction techniques, and **acupuncture**. Individuals should not replace conventional treatment with alternative therapies, and before adding any herbal or other complementary treatments should consult their physician, as some complementary therapies may interfere with the conventional treatment and/or have serious side effects.

When treatment fails to control pain and joint damage, joint replacement surgery followed by guided **rehabilitation** may be necessary. Knee and hip replacement surgery are the most common types of surgery done on individuals with rheumatoid arthritis.

Prognosis

There is no cure for rheumatoid arthritis. The course of the disease is variable. Some people have the disease for only a year or two, and then for unknown reasons it goes away on its own without joint damage. Most people have periods when the disease is quiet and symptoms disappear, only to flare up again for unknown reasons. For some people the disease is continuous, chronic, and progressively worsens. It is estimated that rheumatoid arthritis reduces the lifespan of men by 7.5 years and of women by 3.5 years.

Health care team roles

A rheumatologist normally oversees the health care team treating an individual with rheumatoid arthritis. Nurses play an important role in **patient education** by teaching individuals with rheumatoid arthritis how to balance activity and rest. Physical therapists evaluate an individual's range of motion and teach appropriate exercises to promote joint mobility and muscle fitness and the appropriate use of heat and cold treatments. Physical therapists also have special equipment that can provide electrical stimulation to reduce pain and improve joint movement. Occupational therapists teach individuals how to move in ways that protect their joints and how to perform tasks of daily living in ways that reduce pain and stress on the joints. Both PT and OT are essential after surgery, but may also be helpful to individuals with advanced rheumatoid arthritis undergoing non-surgical treatments.

KEY TERMS

Autoimmune disease—A disease in which the immune system of the body inappropriately attacks the body's own tissues.

Osteoarthritis—A noninflammatory wearing away of bone and cartilage most often associated with aging.

Prevention

Rheumatoid arthritis cannot be prevented. Early detection and treatment can help slow the disease. Clinical trials of new medications and complementary and alternative therapies for rheumatoid arthritis are ongoing. A list of clinical trials currently enrolling patients is available at www.clinicaltrials.gov.

Resources

BOOKS

Ebringer, Alan. *Rheumatoid Arthritis and Proteus.* New York: Springer, 2012.

Haskell, Gretchen. *Arthritis Foundation's Guide to Good Living with Rheumatoid Arthritis*, 2nd ed. Atlanta, GA: Arthritis Foundation, 2005.

Weisman, Michael H. *Rheumatoid Arthritis.* New York: Oxford University Press, 2011

PERIODICALS

Ernst, E. and P. Posadzki "Complementary and Alternative Medicine for Rheumatoid Arthritis and Osteoarthritis: An Overview of Systematic Reviews." *Current Pain and Headache Reports.* (December 2011) 15(6):431–7. PMID: 2197910.

Mandema,J. W. et al. "A Dose-Response Meta-Analysis for Quantifying Relative Efficacy of Biologics in Rheumatoid Arthritis." *Clinical Pharmacology and Therapeutics.* (December 2011) 90(6): 828–35. PMID: 22048227.

OTHER

Juvenile Rheumatoid Arthritis. MedlinePlus April 12, 2012 [accessed April 14, 2012]. http://www.nlm.nih.gov/medlineplus/juvenilerheumatoidarthritis.html

Rheumatoid Arthritis. MedlinePlus April 12, 2012 [accessed April 14, 2012]. http://www.nlm.nih.gov/medlineplus/rheumatoidarthritis.html

Temprano, Kathrerine. Rheumatoid Arthritis Medscape Reference December 29, 2011 [accessed April 14, 2012]. http://emedicine.medscape.com/article/331715-overview

What is Rheumatoid Arthritis? Arthritis Foundation 2012 [accessed April 14, 2012]. http://www.arthritis.org/types-what-is-rheumatoid-arthritis.php

ORGANIZATIONS

American College of Rheumatology, 2200 Lake Blvd NE, Atlanta, GA 30319, (404) 633-3777, Fax: (404) 366-1870, arc@rhemuatology.org, http://www.rheumatology.org

Arthritis Foundation, PO Box 7669, Atlanta, GA 30357-0669, (800) 283-7800, http://www.arthritis.org

National Institute of Arthritis and Musculoskeletal and Skin Diseases (NIAMS)Information Clearinghouse, 1 AMS Circle, Bethesda, MD 20892-3675, (301) 495-4484, 877) 22-NIAMS (226-4267); TTY: (301) 565–2966, Fax: (301) 718-6366, NIAMSinfo@mail.nih.gov, http://www.niams.nih.gov.

Tish Davidson, AM

Rheumatoid factor test *see* **Autoimmune disease tests**

Rhinovirus infection *see* **Common cold**

Riboflavin

Description

Riboflavin, also known as Vitamin B_2, has many functions in common with the other members of the B complex family. These include support of the immune and nervous systems, and formation of healthy red **blood** cells. Riboflavin provides essential factors for the production of cellular enzymes that turn **proteins**, fats, and **carbohydrates** into energy. It also participates in cell reproduction, and keeps skin, hair, nails, eyes, and mucous membranes healthy. **Folic acid** (vitamin B_9) and pyridoxine (vitamin B_6) are activated by riboflavin.

General use

The RDA of riboflavin for infants under six months is 0.4 milligrams (mg). It goes up incrementally with age and caloric intake. Babies from six months to one year of age require 0.5 mg. Children need 0.8 mg at one to three years of age, 1.1 mg at four to six years, and 1.2 mg at seven to 10 years. Women need 1.3 mg from 11-50 years, and 1.2 mg thereafter. Slightly more is required during **pregnancy** (1.6 mg) and **lactation** (1.7-1.8 mg). Men require 1.5 mg from 11-14 years of age, 1.8 mg from 15-18 years, 1.7 mg from 19-50 years, and 1.4 mg at

51 years and older. Riboflavin is water-soluble, and is not stored in significant quantities in the body.

High doses of riboflavin, as much as 400 mg per day, have been shown to reduce the frequency of migraine headaches by half in susceptible people. The severity of the events was also reportedly decreased. This may be an effect of improved use of cellular energy in the **brain**. It is theorized that riboflavin may help decrease the odds of getting **cataracts**, but the evidence for this protection is not definitive. One large study had a group taking both **niacin** (vitamin B_3) and riboflavin, and while the group had a significantly lower total incidence of cataracts, they had a somewhat higher than average incidence of a specific cataract subtype. **Memory** may be improved by these supplements, according to some research done on older people. Riboflavin and **vitamin C** both help boost the body's level of glutathione, which is an antioxidant with many beneficial effects. There is not enough evidence to support the effectiveness of riboflavin for sickle-cell anemia, **canker sores**, or as an athletic performance aid.

Preparations

Natural sources

Beef **liver** is a very rich source of riboflavin, but dairy products also supply ample amounts. Higher-fat sources contain less than those with low fat. Many processed grain products are fortified with riboflavin, as well as other B **vitamins**. Good vegetable choices include avocados, mushrooms, spinach, and other dark green, leafy vegetables. Nuts, legumes, nutritional yeast, and brewer's yeast contain riboflavin as well. Cooked foods provide as much of this vitamin as raw ones do, since the substance is heat stable. Light, however, does break down riboflavin. To preserve it, be sure to either store dairy and grain products in something opaque or keep them away from light.

Supplemental sources

Riboflavin is available as an oral single vitamin product. Consider taking a balanced B complex supplement rather than high doses of an individual vitamin unless there is a specific indication to do so. Store supplements in a cool, dry place, away from light, and out of the reach of children.

Deficiency

Ariboflavinosis is the term for the condition of vitamin B_2 deficiency. Since small amounts can be stored in the liver and **kidneys**, a dietary inadequacy

may not become apparent for several months. Insufficient levels of riboflavin have noticeable effects on several areas of the skin. Commonly the corners of the mouth are cracked. Facial skin and scalp tend to itch and scale, as does the scrotal skin. The eyes fatigue easily and are sensitive to light, and may also become watery, sore, or bloodshot. Trembling, neuropathy, **dizziness**, insomnia, poor digestion, slow growth, and **sore throat** and tongue have also been reported. Anemia may develop if the deficiency is severe. People who are deficient in riboflavin are likely to be lacking in other B vitamins, and possibly additional nutrients as well.

Risk factors for deficiency

Riboflavin deficiency is uncommon, but some populations may need more than the RDA in order to maintain good health. Vegans and others who do not use dairy products would do well to take a balanced B vitamin supplement. Those with increased need for riboflavin and other B vitamins may include people under high **stress**, including those experiencing surgery, chronic illnesses, liver disease, or poor nutritional status. Diabetics may have a tendency to be low on riboflavin as a result of increased urinary excretion. Athletes and anyone else with a high-energy output will need additional vitamin B_2. This includes anyone who exercises with some regularity. The elderly are more likely to suffer from nutritional inadequacy as well as problems with absorption. Smokers and alcoholics are at higher risk for deficiency, as tobacco and alcohol suppress absorption. Birth control pills may possibly reduce riboflavin levels, as can phenothiazine tranquilizers, tricyclic antidepressants, and probenecid. Consult a health care professional to determine if supplementation is appropriate.

Precautions

Riboflavin should not be taken by anyone with a B vitamin allergy or chronic renal disease. Other populations are unlikely to experience any difficulty from taking supplemental B$_2$.

Side effects

Taking supplemental riboflavin causes a harmless intense orange or yellow discoloration of the urine.

Interactions

Probenecid (a drug treating **gout**) impairs riboflavin absorption, and propantheline bromide (a drug treating peptic ulcers) reportedly both delays and increases absorption. Phenothiazines (**antipsychotic drugs**) increase the excretion of riboflavin, thus lowering serum levels; and oral contraceptives may also decrease serum levels. Supplementation should be discussed with a health care provider if these medications are being used. Absorption of riboflavin is improved when taken together with other B vitamins and vitamin C.

Resources

BOOKS

Bratman, Steven, and David Kroll. *Natural Health Bible.* Prima Publishing, 1999.

Feinstein, Alice. *Prevention's Healing with Vitamins.* Emmaus, PA: Rodale Press, 1996.

Griffith, H. Winter. *Vitamins, Herbs, Minerals & Supplements: The Complete Guide.* Arizona: Fisher Books, 1998.

Jellin, Jeff, Forrest Batz, and Kathy Hitchens. *Pharmacist's Letter/Prescriber's Letter Natural Medicines Comprehensive Database.* California: Therapeutic Research Faculty, 1999.

Pressman, Alan H., and Sheila Buff. *The Complete Idiot's Guide to Vitamins and Minerals.* New York: Alpha Books, 1997.

Judith Turner

Ribs *see* **Thorax**

Rinne and Weber tests

Definition

Both the Rinne and the Weber tests employ the use of metal tuning forks to provide a rough assessment of a patient's **hearing** level at various frequencies. A tuning fork is a metal instrument with a handle and two prongs,

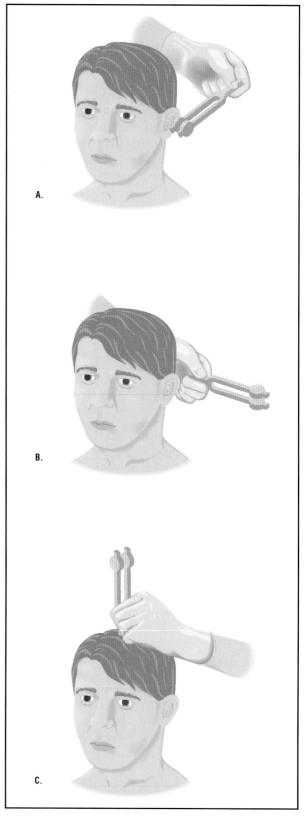

(Three hearing tests using a tuning fork in different positions on or near the head. Illustration by GGS Information Services, Inc. The Gale Group.)

or tines. Tuning forks, made of steel, aluminum, or **magnesium** alloy, will vibrate at a set frequency to produce a musical tone when struck. The vibrations produced can be used to assess a person's ability to hear different sound frequencies.

Purpose

A vibrating tuning fork held next to the ear or placed against the **skull** will stimulate the inner ear to vibrate, and can help determine if there is **hearing loss**. The Rinne tuning fork test helps evaluate a patient's hearing ability by air conduction compared to that of **bone** conduction. The Weber tuning fork test helps determine a patient's hearing ability by bone conduction only, and is useful when hearing loss is asymmetrical.

Precautions

No special patient precautions are necessary when tuning forks are used to conduct hearing tests.

Description

Two types of hearing tests using tuning forks are typically conducted. In the Rinne test, the vibrating tuning fork is held against the skull, usually on the bone behind the ear (mastoid process) to cause vibrations through the bones of the skull and inner ear. It is also held next to, but not touching, the ear, to cause vibrations in the air next to the ear. The patient is asked to determine which sound is louder, the sound heard through the bone or through the air. For the Weber test, the stem or handle of the vibrating tuning fork is placed at various points along the midline of the skull and face. The patient is then asked to identify which ear hears the sound created by the vibrations. Tuning forks of different sizes produce different frequencies of vibrations and can be used to establish the range of hearing for an individual patient.

Preparation

No special patient preparation is required for either of these hearing tests.

Aftercare

No special patient aftercare is required following the hearing tests. If hearing loss is detected using either tuning-fork test, the patient may require further testing to determine the cause and extent of hearing loss.

Complications

There are no known complications associated with the use of tuning forks to screen for hearing loss.

Results

With the Rinne test, a patient with normal hearing will hear the tone of the vibration longer and louder when the tuning fork is held next to the ear, as opposed to when it is held against the mastoid bone. Conversely, the test detects a hearing loss when a patient hears a louder and longer tone when the vibrating tuning fork is held against the mastoid bone, than when it is held next to the ear. This result is often referred to as "reversed Rinne."

For the Weber test, the patient is considered to have normal hearing if the tone produced when the tuning fork is placed along the center of the skull or face sounds about the same volume in each ear. The volume of sound vibrations conducted through parts of the skull and face during the Weber test can indicate which ear may have a hearing loss, if the patient hears louder sound vibrations in one ear compared to sounds picked up by the opposite ear.

If either method of testing reveals abnormal results, the patient will require further evaluation.

Health care team roles

Nurses should explain the procedure to patients and answer any questions.

Patient education

Patients should be instructed to listen carefully to directions for either test and be reassured that there are no **pain** or complications associated with either test.

Training

No special training is required.

Resources

BOOK

The Merck Manual, edited by Robert S. Porter. 19th ed. Whitehouse Station, NJ: Merck Research Laboratories, 2011.

OTHER

Carr, M.M., D.D.S., M.D, M.Ed. "How to Perform and Interpret Weber and Rinne Tests." 1998. http://icarus.med. utoronto.ca/carr/manual/tuningfork.html (March 15, 2001).

Susan Joanne Cadwallader

RK surgery *see* **Radial keratotomy**

RN *see* **Registered nurse**

Robot-assisted surgery

Definition

Robot-assisted surgery involves the use of a robot under the direction and guidance of a surgeon.

Purpose

Robot-assisted surgery provides many benefits in the surgical care of patients. Computer-assisted robots provide exact motion and trajectories to minimize the side effects of surgical intervention. Robot-assisted surgeries can use three-dimensional imaging and smaller surgical tools to operate in a closed environment through smaller incisions. For example, traditional methods of cardiac surgery usually required a six-to-eight inch incision in the sternum and the use of a heart-lung machine to maintain the functions of the **heart** and **lungs** while they are stopped for the surgery. Robot-assisted surgery has furthered the use of the keyhole approach, in which multiple small incisions are made between the ribs. With robot-assisted surgery, the surgeon is also able to make more precise movements using motion scaling. In this practice, an image is enlarged and the movements of the surgeon's hands are translated by the computer into smaller movements. This allows surgeons to perform more precisely, which can be especially important when the surgery is to be performed on particularly small parts of the body.

Demographics

Patients undergoing surgical procedures classified as **neurosurgery**, orthopedic surgery, radio surgery and **radiotherapy**, prostatectomy, endoscopy, **laparoscopy**, cardiac surgery and craniofacial surgery may experience robot-assisted surgical techniques.

Description

Neurosurgery

A high level of accuracy is required when operating on the **brain** to avoid damage to the sensitive brain tissue. Biopsies and minor interventions are best assisted by the robotic device. Interventions include drilling into the **skull** and making an incision through the dura mater to gain brain tissue samples, empty cysts, or eliminate hemorrhages.

Orthopedic surgery

Applications such as cementless hip-replacement, total knee arthroplasties, and pedicle screw placement can benefit from the more accurate cutting and drilling provided by a robot. Femur bone-cutting devices provide improved drilling to carve a cavity in the **bone** for prosthesis implant. Pins inserted into the bone before surgery are used as landmarks for computerized tomography (CT) imaging. The CT image provides the surgeon with the necessary information for choosing an implant. The surgeon removes the head from the femur bone, eliminating the joint. The leg is secured in position and the robot is brought into position. A high speed cutter is then applied to create the cavity, and then followed by a smoothing tool. The surgeon manually inserts the implant into the femur and completes the cap implant into the pelvic bone.

Radiosurgery and radiotherapy

Radiation treatment is provided by a robot. The CT image or magnetic resonance image (MRI) is used to determine where the radiation treatment should be delivered. The robot aligns with patient **anatomy**, delivering specific doses of radiation to the intended location.

Prostatectomy

Removal of all or part of the prostate is another robot-assisted procedure. The robot controls instruments inserted through the urethra to the prostate gland. A diathermic hot wire cutting loop is guided to remove tissue in an appropriate pattern around the urethra. Fastening the guiding frame to the upper legs of the patient secures the device for accurate guidance.

Endoscopy

Endoscopy is used to examine patient cavities for the presence of polyps, tumors, and other diseases. The **endoscope** can be better passed through cavities such as

KEY TERMS

Arthoplastic—Manufactured replacement joint.

Cardiac surgery—Surgery performed on the heart.

Craniofacial surgery—Surgery of the facial tissue and skull.

Endoscopy—Used to visualize internal structures of the body, such as the trachea, esophagus or intestines.

Laparoscopy—Surgery on internal structures through small incisions and visualized with the laparoscope.

Neurosurgery—Surgery performed on the brain.

Orthopedic surgery—Surgery performed on the bones. May include joint replacements and surgery of the vertebrae.

Prostatectomy—Performed for the treatment of prostate disease including prostate cancer.

Radio surgery and radiotherapy—Used in the treatment of cancerous growths or kidney stones.

the colon or trachea. Three-dimensional images of the cavity are obtained and used to dictate the path taken by the endoscope. Sedation and heavy analgesia can be avoided.

Laparoscopy

In laparoscopic surgeries, three to four small incisions are made in the abdominal or thoracic cavity to insert the instruments and video equipment. The surgeon performs the operation from a remote console that provides the human-machine interface. The console provides video monitoring images that are three-dimensional. Joysticks are used to manipulate the tools within the chest cavity to complete the surgical procedure.

Cardiac surgery

Robots can be used in the coronary artery bypass grafting surgeries and cardiac valve replacement and repair surgeries. The harvesting of artery and vein grafts can also be accomplished with the aid of laparoscopic techniques.

Craniofacial surgery

Difficult bone cuts and bone tumor removals are accomplished successfully using robotic instruments. Pre-planned trajectories are programmed into the machine. Precision cuts are made in the manner desired to achieve an aesthetically satisfactory result. As the

QUESTIONS TO ASK THE DOCTOR

- Is there an institution in the vicinity which uses robot-assisted surgery?
- How experienced is the surgeon with robot-assisted surgical techniques?
- What benefits would the robot-assisted surgery provide?
- What complications can be avoided and which may be encountered with robot-assisted surgery?

surgeon manipulates the saw, he or she is guided along the path by a predetermined trajectory determined during an initial run on a model of the surgical site.

Aftercare

The patient should expect a faster recovery then that achieved by traditional surgery procedures.

Risks

With some of these procedures, a longer surgical time is required to achieve the same desired outcome as the traditional surgical approach. There is an increased risk of anesthesia related complications as surgical times increase. Additionally, if the robotic procedure is not completed successfully, the surgeon may need to complete the procedure with a traditional technique.

Normal results

Results for each procedure are comparable to or better than the standard surgical procedure.

Morbidity and mortality rates

Complications should be comparable to the standard surgical procedure, and even reduced. Some complications may only be associated with the robot-assisted procedure.

Alternatives

The alternative to using robot-assisted surgery is for the surgeon to employ a traditional surgical approach.

Resources

BOOKS

DiGioia, Anthony et al, eds. *Computer and Robotic Assisted Hip and Knee Surgery.* New York: Oxford University Press, 2004.

Faust, Russel A., ed. *Robotics in Surgery: History, Current and Future Applications.* New York: Nova Science Publishers, 2007.

Stiehl, James B., Werner H. Konermann and Rolf G. Haaker, eds. *Navigation and Robotics in Total Joint and Spine Surgery.* New York: Springer, 2004.

PERIODICALS

Bates, Betsy. "Robots Can Assist in Improving Care." *Internal Medicine News* 39.17 (Sept. 1, 2006): 1-3.

Diks, J., D. Nio, V. Jongkind, M. A. Cuesta, J. A. Rauwerda and W. Wisselink. "Robot-Assisted Laparoscopic Surgery of the Infrarenal Aorta; The Early Learning Curve." *Surgical Endoscopy* 21.11 (Nov 2007): 2118-2120.

Allison Joan Spiwak, MSBME
Robert Bockstiegel

Root canal therapy

Definition

Root canal therapy, also known as endodontic treatment, is a dental procedure in which the diseased or damaged pulp (nerve) of a tooth is removed and the inside areas of the nerve chambers or root canals are filled and sealed.

Purpose

Root canal therapy has become a common dental procedure. More than 14 million are performed each year, with a success rate of 95%, according to the American Association of Endodontists. Inflamed or infected pulp (pulpitis), often causing a toothache, is removed to relieve the **pain** and prevent further complications for the patient.

Precautions

Once root canal therapy is finished and the nerve is removed, the tooth becomes brittle over time and can fracture and break easily. Therefore the tooth requires extra protection and will need a crown.

Description

Root canal therapy may be performed by a general dentist or by an endodontist, a dentist who specializes in endodontic procedures. The pulp of the tooth consists of soft tissue containing the **blood** supply from which the tooth gets its nutrients and by which the tooth senses hot and cold. This tissue is vulnerable to damage from deep dental decay, accidental injury, tooth fracture, or trauma from repeated dental procedures (such as multiple fillings over time). **Infection** may produce pain that is severe, constant, or throbbing, as well as prolonged sensitivity to heat or cold. Swelling in and around the surrounding gums along

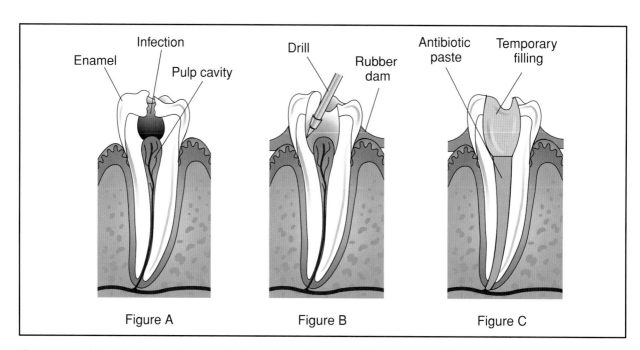

(Root canal treatment, illustration. Electronic Illustrators Group. Reproduced by permission of The Gale Group.)

KEY TERMS

Abscess—Gum tissue filled with pus as the result of infection. This swelling exerts pressure on the surrounding tissues, causing pain.

Apicoectomy—Also called root resectioning. The root tip of a tooth is accessed in the bone and a small amount is taken off away. A small filling is placed to reseal the canal.

Crown—The natural crown of a tooth is that part of the tooth covered by enamel. Also, a restorative crown is a protective shell that fits over a tooth.

Endodontic—Pertaining to the inside structures of the tooth, including the dental pulp and tooth root, and the periapical tissue surrounding the root.

Endodontist—A dentist who specializes in the diagnosis and treatment of disorders affecting the inside structures of the tooth.

Extraction—The surgical removal of a tooth from its socket in the bone.

Gutta-percha—An inert latex-like substance used for filling root canals.

Pulp—The soft innermost layer of a tooth, containing blood vessels and nerves.

Pulp chamber—The area within the natural crown of the tooth occupied by dental pulp.

Pulpitis—Inflammation of the pulp of a tooth involving the blood vessels and nerves.

Root canal—The space within a tooth that runs from the pulp chamber to the tip of the root.

Root canal treatment—The process of removing diseased or damaged pulp from a tooth, then filling and sealing the pulp chamber and root canals.

with facial swelling may be seen. However, in some cases, the pulp may die so gradually that there is little noticeable pain or swelling.

Root canal therapy is performed under **local anesthesia**. A thin sheet of rubber, called a rubber dam, is placed in the mouth to isolate the tooth. The endodontist makes an opening through the natural crown of the tooth into the pulp chamber. He will then determine the length of the root canal, usually with a series of x rays. Small wire-like files, called broaches, are used to clean the entire canal space of diseased pulp tissue and **bacteria**. The debris is flushed out (irrigated) with sterile water. The canals are also slightly enlarged and shaped to receive an inert (non-reactive) filling material called gutta-percha. However, the tooth is not filled and permanently sealed until it is completely free of the active infection and/or bacteria. The endodontist will place a temporary seal, or leave the tooth open to drain, and prescribe an antibiotic to counter any spread of infection from the tooth. The patient may need a number of return visits to the dental office while the root canal is being treated, and the infection brought under control.

Preparation

There is no typical preparation for root canal therapy, as the treatment is done on an emergency basis due to sudden injury or pain. The reasons why root canals are thought to be so painful are due to the sudden injury and buildup of infection in the tooth. Normal doses of local anesthetic used by the dentist are not always effective against the degree of pain the patient is already feeling. Occasionally, even high amounts of anesthesia aren't effective until the infection can be drained and brought under control.

Aftercare

The tooth may be sore for several days after filling. Pain relievers, such as ibuprofen (Advil, Motrin) may be taken to ease the soreness. Ibuprofen is an effective anti-inflammatory drug and can help reduce the inflammation caused by the infection. The tissues surrounding the tooth may also be irritated due to the infection, but also due to the rubber dam used to isolate the tooth during the root canal treatment. Rinsing the mouth with warm salt-water rinses several times a day is helpful. The patient should avoid chewing on the treated tooth for several days. A follow-up appointment should be scheduled with the dentist for six months after treatment to make sure the tooth and surrounding structures are healthy.

Risks

There is the possibility that the root canal treatment will not be successful the first time. If infection and inflammation recur and an x ray indicates retreatment is feasible, the old filling material is removed and the canals are thoroughly cleaned out. The dentist will try to identify and correct problems with the first root canal treatment before filling and sealing the tooth a second time.

In cases in which an x ray indicates that retreatment cannot correct the problem, endodontic surgery may be performed. An apicoectomy, or root resectioning, is the procedure by which the root portion of the tooth is accessed through the gum tissue above or below the tooth in the **bone**. A small portion of the root tip is taken off and a small filling is placed to reseal the canal.

In some cases, root canal treatment, retreatment, and apicoectomy surgery are not effective and the tooth must be extracted.

Results

With successful root canal treatment, the restored tooth can last a lifetime.

Resources

OTHER

Dentistry on the Web. 497 Main Street, Ansonia, CT 06401. (203) 735-4701 http://www.smilekeepers.com/Dental_Links/dental_links.htm.

Root Canal—Saving Precious Teeth (television clip). ADA Dental Minutes, August 17, 2000.

"Root Canal Therapy." Tooth Talk and Your Health with Dr. Frank Gober. Radio Talk Show, Fort Lauderdale, Florida. http://www.toothtalk.com/.

ORGANIZATIONS

American Association of Endodontists. 211 East Chicago Avenue, Suite 1100, Chicago, IL 60611-2691. (800) 872-3636. http://www.aae.org.

American Dental Association. 211 East Chicago Avenue, Chicago, IL 60611. (312) 440-2500. http://www.ada.org.

Cindy F. Ovard, RDA

Root planing *see* **Nonsurgical periodontal therapy**

Rotator cuff injury

Definition

A rotator cuff injury is a tear or inflammation of the rotator cuff muscles and tendons that surround the shoulder.

Description

Rotator cuff injury is known by several names, including pitcher's shoulder, swimmer's shoulder, and tennis shoulder. As these names imply, the injury often occurs in athletes practicing sports that require the arm to be moved over the head repeatedly, such as pitching, swimming, tennis, and weight lifting. Rotator cuff tendonitis is an inflammation of the shoulder tendons while a rotator cuff tear is a ripping of one or more of the tendons.

The four muscles make up the rotator cuff are the supraspinatus, infraspinatus, teres minor, and subscapularis. Via their tendons, the muscles of the rotator cuff attach the humerus (upper arm **bone**) to the scapula (shoulder blade). These muscles are used to make rotational movements at the glenohumeral joint. The rotator cuff tendons can also degenerate due to age, usually starting around age 40. Rotator cuff injury may also be caused by falling on the outstretched arm or joint of the elbow. Either of these may produce enough force to drive the humerus into the shoulder socket.

Causes and symptoms

Some areas of the rotator cuff tendons have poor **blood** supply. Thus, the tissue is very slow to heal and maintain itself during normal use. Tearing and inflammation in athletes is usually due to hard and repetitive use, especially in baseball pitchers. In non-athletes over age 40, the injuries usually occur as a result of lifting heavy objects. The two primary symptoms are **pain** and **weakness** in the shoulder or arm, especially with arm movement or at night. A partial tear may cause pain but still allow normal arm movement. A complete tear usually leaves the injured person unable to raise the arm away from the side.

Diagnosis

Diagnosis is usually made after a **physical examination**, often by a sports medicine physician. X rays are also sometimes used in diagnosis as well as an arthrogram, an x ray of the inside of a damaged joint made after a substance that shows up on a x ray has been injected into the joint. However, the arthrogram is an invasive procedure and may be painful afterwards. For this reason, **magnetic resonance imaging** (MRI) is preferred to determine tendon tears as it also show greater detail than the arthrogram. MRI is an imaging technique that uses electromagnetic radiation to obtain images of the body's soft tissues, for example, in this case the rotator cuff tendons.

Treatment

The primary treatment is resting the shoulder and, for minor tears and inflammation, applying ice packs. Anti-inflammatory medications may also be prescribed. As soon as pain decreases, **physical therapy** is usually started to help regain normal motion. If pain persists after

KEY TERMS

Arthrogram—A test done by injecting dye into the shoulder joint and then taking x rays. Areas where the dye leaks out indicate a tear in the tendons.

Arthroscope—An instrument for the visual examination of the interior of a joint.

Arthroscopy—Examination of a joint with an arthroscope or joint surgery using an arthroscope.

Cortisone—A hormone produced naturally by the adrenal glands or made synthetically.

Magnetic resonance imaging (MRI) scan—A special radiological test used diagnostically that uses electromagnetic waves to create pictures of an area, including bones, muscles, and tendons.

Spur—Any projection from a bone.

several weeks, the physician may inject cortisone into the affected area.

Serious tears to the rotator cuff tendons may require surgery to repair. An instrument called an arthroscope is used to view the shoulder joint and confirm the presence of a tear. The arthroscope can also be used to remove any bone spurs that may be present in the shoulder area. Current arthroscopic procedures usually involve a two-inch (5.1 centimeter) incision in the outer shoulder. Through this incision the torn rotator edge may be reattached to the humerus with stitches.

Prognosis

The prognosis for recovery from minor rotator cuff injuries is excellent. For serious injuries, the prognosis is usually good, some six weeks of physical therapy being required following surgery. Full recovery may take several more months. In some cases, the injury is so severe that it requires tendon grafts and muscle transfers. In rare cases, a severe injury is not repairable, usually because the tendon has been torn for too long a time.

Health care team roles

Besides an orthopedic surgeon, the primary health care professional involved with rotator cuff injury is a

physical therapist who assists in non-surgical treatment and **rehabilitation**. Physical therapy (PT) can teach patients specific exercises, stretches, and techniques, and use specialized equipment to address problems. A physical therapy program usually may include range-of-motion and resistive exercises, then incorporates power, aerobic and muscular endurance, flexibility, and coordination drills. Depending on the severity of the injury, physical therapy may take from three weeks to several months.

Prevention

The best prevention is to avoid repetitive overhead arm movements and to develop shoulder strength. It is also helpful to do stretching and warm-up exercises before engaging in extensive use of the rotator cuff, such as before pitching in a baseball game.

Resources

BOOKS

Donatelli, Robert. *Physical Therapy of the Shoulder.* London: Churchill Livingstone, 2003.

Icon Health Publications. *The Official Patient's Sourcebook on Rotator Cuff Injury: A Revised and Updated Directory for the Internet Age.* San Diego: Icon Health Publications, 2002.

PERIODICALS

Ebell, Mark H. "Diagnosing Rotator Cuff Tears."*American Family Physician* (April 15, 2005): 1587-1589.

Marx, Robert. "Rotator-Cuff Tendonitis of the Shoulder." *Muscle & Fitness* (December 2004): 190.

Quillen, David M, et al. "Acute Shoulder Injuries." *American Family Physician* (November 15, 2004): 1947–1958.

ORGANIZATIONS

American Academy of Orthopaedic Surgeons. 6300 North River Road, Rosemont, IL 60018-4262; (847) 823-7186; Fax: ((847) 823-8125; www.aaos.org.

The American Orthopaedic Society for Sports Medicine. 6300 North River Road, Suite 500, Rosemont, IL 60018; (847) 292-4900; Fax (847) 292-4905; www.sportsmed.org.

Ken R. Wells

Routine urinalysis *see* **Urinalysis**

Rubella test *see* **TORCH test**

Ruptured disk *see* **Herniated disk**

S

Salivary gland scan

Definition

A salivary gland scan is a nuclear medicine test that establishes the function of the salivary glands. The salivary glands include the parotid glands and submandibular glands, which are located on both sides of the neck below the ears and jaw. Salivary gland function is determined by the pattern of uptake and secretion of a radioactive tracer, usually Tc99m (Technium 99). The scan also demonstrates the relative size and shape of the salivary glands.

Purpose

A salivary gland scan is indicated when a patient has recurring salivary gland swelling due to either **infection**, inflammation, or obstruction. Salivary gland scans can detect salivary gland tumors, and can help evaluate the glands of patients with persistent dry mouth.

Precautions

Salivary gland scans are a safe, effective way to diagnose salivary gland pathology. The level of radioactivity used to obtain the images is low, however, pregnant patients are cautioned not to have this test unless necessary. Women who are breastfeeding are advised to stop breast feeding for a specific period of time, depending on the dose administered. Other recent nuclear medicine tests may affect the results of this scan, and it may be necessary to wait until previously administered radiopharmaceuticals have been cleared from the body before undergoing this test.

Description

A salivary gland scan, also called a parotid gland scan, is a non-invasive test. It is typically performed in a hospital **radiology** or nuclear medicine department or

out patient radiology facility. The patient is injected with a low-level radioactive marker and is positioned in front of or under a gamma scintillation camera, which detects the radiation and produces an image. In some facilities, imaging begins immediately after the injection to observe the progressive accumulation of the radioactive tracer in the glands. If indicated, an additional procedure can be done after the initial images are obtained. The patient is given a sour substance, known as a sialogogue, such as a lemon drop or some lemon juice, to stimulate the emptying of the salivary glands. Another set of images is then made for comparison purposes. The entire process takes about 30 to 45 minutes.

Preparation

No special preparations are needed for this test. It is not necessary to fast or to restrict medications before testing. Any **blood** to be drawn for other tests may need to be taken before the radiopharmaceutical is injected. Patients must remove any metal objects from the face and neck and may be asked to remove dentures.

Images of the **thyroid gland** is typically included when imaging the salivary glands. Therefore, it should be

Sarcomas

noted if the patient is taking any medication that inhibits the uptake of the radiopharmaceutical in the thyroid gland.

Aftercare

Patients can return to normal activities immediately.

Complications

A salivary gland scan is a safe test, and there are generally no complications associated with it.

Results

A normal study reflects a normal position, size, and shape of the salivary glands, and will also demonstrate proper emptying of the glands after the oral administration of the sialogogue. Abnormally functioning salivary glands, due to conditions such as Sjögren's syndrome, fail to exhibit a normal uptake and secretion pattern. Some tumors, such as a Warthin's tumor, prevent the emptying of the salivary gland and are seen as areas of increased concentration of radionuclide. Metastatic lesions, cysts, and abscesses are seen as areas of decreased concentration of radionuclide. This test does not differentiate between benign and malignant lesions. This requires other diagnostic imaging tests such as CT, MRI, or ultrasound.

Health care team roles

The radionuclide is administered by a nuclear medicine technologist, who is specially trained to handle radioactive materials and operate the equipment in a nuclear medicine department. The technologist may obtain pertinent patient medical history and describe the testing procedure to the patient. All data collected is interpreted by a radiologist or nuclear medicine specialist. Results of the test are sent to the referring physician.

Resources

BOOK

Klingensmith III, M.D., Wm. C., Dennis Eshima, Ph.D., John Goddard, Ph.D. *Nuclear Medicine Procedure Manual.* 2000.

OTHER

Payne, Kattie. "Salivary Gland Scan." WebMD. January 9, 2004 (April 7, 2006). http://www.webmd.com/hw/lab_tests/hw234444.asp.

Christine Miner Minderovic, B.S., R.T., R.D.M.S.

Salmonella food poisoning *see* **Foodborne illness**

Sarcomas

Definition

A sarcoma is a malignant tumor (neoplasm), or **cancer**. Certain sarcomas characteristically spread throughout the body. The word "sarcoma" has its origin in a Greek word whose definition is "fleshy." Tumors come from the mesenchymal tissue, from which connective tissues, **blood**, lymphatics, **bone**, and cartilage come. The blood carries sarcomas throughout the body into neighboring tissue, or via the bloodstream. Frequent sites of extension of the tumors are the lung, the **liver**, and the **brain**.

Description

When the original site of the cancer is the bone, there is a primary bone cancer. The tumor originates in or near a bone. Most primary bone tumors are benign, and the cells that compose them do not metastasize (spread) to nearby tissue or to other parts of the body.

Sarcomas account for fewer than 1% of all cancers diagnosed in the United States. They can infiltrate nearby tissues, enter the bloodstream, and metastasize to other bones, tissues, and organs far from the site of the original malignancy. Malignant primary bone tumors are characterized as either:

- cancers that originate in the hard material of the bone
- soft-tissue sarcomas that begin in blood vessels, nerves, or tissues containing muscles, fat, or fiber

Types of bone tumors

Osteogenic sarcoma, or osteosarcoma, is the most common form of primary bone cancer, accounting for about 5% of all cancers in children. Every year, 900 new cases of osteosarcoma are diagnosed in the United States. The disease usually affects teenagers and young adults, and is almost twice as common in males as in females.

Osteosarcomas grow very rapidly. Although they can develop in any bone, but they are most often seen along the edge or on the end of one of the fast-growing long bones that support the arms and legs. Approximately 80% of all osteosarcomas develop in the distal femur or in the proximal tibia (parts of the upper and lower leg nearest the knee). The next likely location for

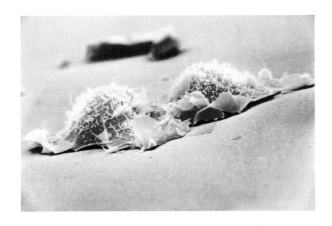

(Color enhanced scanning electron micrograph (SEM) of sarcoma cells, photograph. Keith R. Porter / Photo Researchers, Inc.)

an osteosarcoma is the proximal humerus (the bone of the upper arm closest to the shoulder).

Ewing's sarcoma is the second most common form of childhood bone cancer. Accounting for less than 5% of bone tumors in children, Ewing's sarcoma usually begins in the soft tissue or nerves. It rapidly metastasizes to the **lungs**, and may metastasize to bones in other parts of the body.

Ewing's sarcoma occurs most frequently in children aged 11 to 15. It is more often diagnosed in taller teens. Slightly more males than females develop common bone cancer—but this type is the most frequently found carcinoma in children. The disease is rarely diagnosed in children younger than five and adults older than 30. It primarily affects Caucasians, and rarely occurs in African Americans and native Chinese persons.

Chondrosarcomas are cancerous bone tumors that most often appear in middle age. Usually originating in cartilage in ribs, leg, or hip bones, chondrosarcomas grow slowly. They rarely metastasize to the lungs. It takes years for a chondrosarcoma to metastasize to other parts of the body, and some of these tumors never spread.

Parosteal osteogenic sarcomas, fibrosarcomas, and chordomas are rare. Parosteal osteosarcomas generally involve both the bone and the periosteum, the membrane that covers bones. Fibrosarcomas originate in the ends of the bones in the arm or leg, and then spread to soft tissue. Chordomas develop on the **skull** or **spinal cord**.

Osteochondromas, which usually develop between persons aged 10–20 years, are the most common noncancerous primary bone tumors. Giant cell tumors generally develop in a section of the femur near the knee. Giant cell tumors are originally benign, but sometimes become malignant.

Causes and symptoms

The cause of bone cancer is unknown, but the tendency to develop it may be inherited. Children who develop bone tumors are often tall for their age, and the disease seems to be associated with growth spurts during childhood and adolescence. Injuries can make the presence of tumors more apparent, but do not cause them.

A bone that has been broken or exposed to high doses of radiation that has been used to treat other cancers is more likely than other bones to develop osteosarcoma. It should be noted, however, that the amount of radiation in diagnostic x rays poses little or no danger of bone cancer development. A history of noncancerous bone disease also increases bone cancer risk.

Cancer of the eye (retinoblastoma) is a rare tumor of the eye that develops in the cells of the retina, and occurs mostly in patients under five years of age. It is known to be hereditary—the condition is an autosomal-dominant trait.

Both benign and malignant bone tumors can distort and weaken bone, causing **pain**, but benign tumors are generally painless and asymptomatic.

Patients may feel a lump or mass, but pain in the affected area is the most common early symptom of bone cancer. Pain is not constant in the initial stages of the disease; it is aggravated by activity and may be worst at night. If the tumor is located on a leg bone, the patient may limp. Swelling and **weakness** of the limb may not be noticed until weeks after the pain began.

Other symptoms of bone cancer include:

- a bone that breaks with minimal trauma, also known as a pathologic fracture
- difficulty moving the affected part of the body
- fatigue
- fever
- a lump or swelling on the trunk, an arm or leg, or another bone
- persistent, unexplained back pain
- weight loss

Diagnosis

Physical examination and routine x rays may provide enough evidence to diagnose benign bone tumors, but biopsy (removal of tumor tissue for microscopic analysis) is the only definitive way to determine the nature of the tumor.

A needle biopsy involves using a fine, thin needle to remove small bits of tumor, or a thick needle to extract tissue samples from the innermost part (the core) of the growth. An excisional biopsy is the surgical removal of a small, accessible tumor and a margin of surrounding normal tissue. An incisional biopsy is performed on tumors too large or inaccessible to be completely removed. A portion of the tumor is removed by the surgeon performing an incisional biopsy. Performed under local or **general anesthesia**, biopsy reveals whether a tumor is benign or malignant, and ideally identifies the type of cancer cells the malignant tumor contains.

Primary bone cancer is usually diagnosed about three months after symptoms first appear. Twenty percent of these malignant tumors will have already metastasized to the lungs or to other parts of the body.

Imaging techniques

The following procedures are used, in conjunction with biopsy, to diagnose bone cancer:

- Plain x rays. These x rays usually provide a clear image of osteosarcomas.

- The computerized tomography (CAT) scan, or computed tomographic scanning (CT), is a specialized x ray that uses a rotating beam to obtain detailed information about an abnormality and its physical relationship to other parts of the body.

- A CAT scan can show differentiation between osteosarcomas and other types of bone tumors, reveal if tumor cells have spread to other tissues, and help surgeons decide which portion of a growth is best to biopsy. Since malignant bone tumors frequently metastasize to the lungs, a CAT scan of the chest should also be performed. The CAT scan can provide information about other organs that may have been affected. Chest and abdominal CAT scans are used to determine whether Ewing's sarcoma has spread to the lungs, liver, or lymph nodes.

- Magnetic resonance imaging (MRI) is a specialized scan that relies on radio waves and powerful magnets to reflect energy patterns created by tissue abnormalities and specific diseases. MRI provides more detailed information than a CAT scan about tumors and marrow cavities of the bone, and can sometimes detect clusters of cancerous cells that have separated from the original tumor. This valuable information helps physicians select the best approach for treatment.

- Radionuclide bone scans involve the injection of a small amount of radioactive material into a vein. Primary tumors, or cells that have metastasized, absorb the radioactive material and present as dark spots on the scan.

Cytogenic and molecular genetic studies, which assess the structure and composition of chromosomes and genes, may also be used to diagnose osteosarcoma. These tests sometimes help to determine the most appropriate form of treatment.

Laboratory studies

A **complete blood count** (CBC) reveals abnormalities in the blood, and may indicate whether bone marrow has been affected. A blood test that measures levels of the enzyme lactate dehydrogenase (LDH), can be used determine the prognosis for the survival of a given patient.

Immunohistochemistry involves adding special **antibodies** and chemicals, or stains, to tumor samples. This technique effectively helps the pathologist to identify cells that are found in Ewing's sarcoma, but that are not present in other malignant tumors.

Reverse transcription polymerase chain reaction (RTPCR) relies on chemical analysis of RNA (the substance in the body that transmits genetic information) to:

- Evaluate the effectiveness of cancer therapies.

- Identify mutations consistent with the presence of Ewing's sarcoma.

- Reveal cancer that recurs after treatment has been completed.

Staging

Once bone cancer has been diagnosed, the tumor is staged. This process indicates how far the tumor has spread from its original location. The stage of a tumor helps the oncologist decide which form of treatment is indicated, and to predict how the condition will probably respond to therapy.

An osteosarcoma may be localized or metastatic. A localized osteosarcoma has not spread beyond the bone where it, originated, or beyond nearby muscles, tendons, and other tissues. Metastatic osteosarcoma has spread to the lungs, to bones not directly connected to the bone, or to other tissues or organs.

Treatment

Since the 1960s, when amputation was the only treatment for bone cancer, **chemotherapy** and innovative surgical techniques have improved survival with intact limbs. Because osteosarcoma is rare, treatment is most often sought at a cancer center staffed by specialists familiar with the disease. A treatment plan for bone cancer, which is devised after the tumor has been diagnosed and staged, may include:

- Radiation therapy. Radiation therapy is used often to treat Ewing's sarcoma.

- Surgery. Surgery, coordinated with diagnostic biopsy, enhances the probability that limb-salvage surgery can be used to remove the cancer, while preserving nearby blood vessels and bones. A metal rod or bone graft is used to replace the area of bone removed. Subsequent surgery may be needed to repair or replace rods that have become loose or broken. Patients who have undergone limb salvage surgery require intensive rehabilitation. It may take as long as one year for a patient to regain full use of a leg following limb salvage surgery. Some patients who undergo this procedure eventually require amputation.

- Chemotherapy. In addition to surgery, chemotherapy is usually administered to kill cancer cells that have separated from the original tumor and spread to other parts of the body. Although chemotherapy can increase the likelihood of future development of another form of cancer, the American Cancer Society maintains that the benefit of chemotherapeutic bone cancer treatment is much greater than its potential risk.

- Amputation. Amputation may be the only therapeutic option for large tumors involving nerves or blood vessels that have not responded to chemotherapy. MRI scans demonstrate the extent of disease in the limb, providing information about how much of it must be removed. The treatment, surgery, is designed to create a cuff (formed of muscles and skin) around the amputated bone. Following surgery, a prosthetic (artificial) leg is fitted over the cuff. Patients who actively participate in the rehabilitation may be walking independently as soon as three months after the amputation.

- Rotationoplasty. Rotationoplasty, sometimes performed after a leg amputation, involves attaching the lower leg and foot to the femur, so that the ankle replaces the knee. A prosthetic is later added to make the leg as long as it is normally. Prosthetic devices are not used to lengthen limbs that remain functional after amputation to remove osteosarcomas located on the upper arm. When an osteosarcoma develops in the jaw bone, the entire lower jaw is removed. Bones from other parts of the body are later grafted onto remaining bone to create a new jaw.

Follow-up treatments

After a patient completes the final course of chemotherapy, a number of tests—CAT or **CT scans**, bone scans, x rays, and other diagnostic tests—may be repeated to determine if any traces of tumor remain. If none are found, treatment is discontinued, but patients are advised to see their oncologists and orthopedic surgeons every two or three months for the subsequent year. X rays of the chest and affected bone are taken every four months. An annual echocardiogram is recommended to determine whether there have been any adverse cardiovascular effects of chemotherapy, and CT scans are performed every six months.

Patients who have received treatment for Ewing's sarcoma are examined regularly—at gradually lengthening intervals—after completing therapy. Accurate growth measurements are taken at each visit and blood is drawn to test for side effects of treatment. X rays, CAT or CT scans, bone scans, and/or other imaging studies are generally performed every three months during the first year. If no evidence of tumor growth or recurrence is revealed, these tests are performed less frequently in the following years.

Some benign bone tumors shrink or disappear without treatment. However, regular examinations are recommended to determine whether these tumors have changed in any way.

Alternative treatment

Alternative treatments should never be substituted for conventional anticancer treatments or used without the approval of a physician. Some alternative treatments may be used as adjunctive and supportive therapies during and following conventional treatments.

Many patients find that alternative and complementary therapies help to reduce the **stress** associated with illness, improve immune function and feel better. While there is no evidence that these therapies specifically combat disease, activities such as biofeedback, **relaxation**, **therapeutic touch**, **massage therapy**, and guided imagery have been reported to enhance well-being.

Some cancer patients find that **acupuncture** alleviates pain, nausea, and **vomiting**. It may also be effective in helping to maintain energy and relative wellness during surgery, chemotherapy, and radiation. Massage, reflexology, and relaxation techniques are reported to relieve pain, tension, **anxiety**, and depression.

Claims of effectiveness in fighting cancer have been made for a variety of herbal medicines. These botanical remedies should only be used when prescribed by a practitioner familiar with cancer treatment.

Prognosis

Benign bone tumors rarely recur, but sarcomas can reappear, even after treatment considered effective in eliminating all the cancerous cells.

KEY TERMS

Biofeedback—The technique of making unconscious or involuntary bodily processes (as heartbeat or brain waves) perceptible to the senses in order to manipulate them by conscious mental control.

CAT scan (CT scan)—Computerized axial tomography, or computed tomography, tomographic scanning; a specialized x ray that uses a rotating beam to obtain detailed information about an abnormality and its physical relationship to other parts of the body.

Chondrosarcoma—A malignant tumor derived from cartilage cells or their precursors.

Chordoma—Malignant tumor composed of remnants of the embryonic notochord—a flexible rod of cells that in the embryos of higher vertebrates forms the supporting axis of the body—and is found along the spine, attacking especially the bones at the base of the skull, or near the coccyx.

Echocardiogram (ECHO)—The use of beeps of ultrasonic waves directed through the chest wall to record the position and motion of the heart walls or internal structures of the heart.

Ewing's sarcoma—A tumor that invades the shaft of a long bone and that tends to recur, but metastasizes infrequently.

Fibrosarcoma—A sarcoma of relatively low malignancy, consisting mostly of spindle-shaped cells that generally form collagenous fibers of connective tissue.

Magnetic resonance imaging (MRI)—A specialized scan that uses radio waves and powerful magnets to reflect energy created by abnormal tissue and specific diseases.

Metastasis—Transfer of disease from one organ of the body to another not directly connected with it, as a result of transfer of pathogenic microorganisms or to transfer of cells.

Likelihood of long-term survival depends on:

• the type and location of the tumor

• how much the tumor has metastasized, and the organs, bones, or tissues affected

More than 85% of patients survive for more than five years after complete surgical removal of low-grade osteosarcomas (tumors that arise in mature tissue and contain a small number of cancerous cells). About 25–30% of patients diagnosed with high-grade osteosarcomas (tumors that develop in immature tissue and contain a large number of cancer cells) will die of the disease.

Two-thirds of all children diagnosed with Ewing's sarcoma live for more than five years after the disease is detected. The outlook is most favorable for children under age 10, and least favorable in patients whose cancer is not diagnosed until after it has metastasized: fewer than three of every 10 of these patients remain alive five years later. More than 80% of patients whose Ewing's sarcoma is confined to a small area, and surgically removed live for at least five years. Postsurgical radiation and chemotherapy add years to their lives. More than 70% of patients live five years or more with a small Ewing's sarcoma that cannot be removed, but only three out of five patients with large, unremovable tumors survive that long. Patients with tumors that do not respond to treatment and those who suffer recurrences have poor outlooks for long-term survival.

Health care team roles

Like other cancer patients, patients with sarcoma are usually cared for by a multidisciplinary team of health professionals. The patient's family physician or primary care provider collaborates with other physician specialists, such as surgeons and oncologists. Radiologic technicians perform x-ray, CT, and MRI scans; nurses and laboratory technicians may obtain samples of blood, urine and other laboratory tests.

Before and after any surgical procedures, including biopsies, the procedures may be explained by nurses or physicians, who are also called upon to help prepare patients and families. Depending on the tumor location and treatment plan, patients may also benefit from **rehabilitation** therapy with physical therapists, nutritional counseling from dietitians, and counseling from social workers or other mental health professionals.

Prevention

Since the causes of most sarcomas are not known, there are no formal recommendations about how to prevent their development. Among families with an inherited tendency to develop soft tissue sarcomas, careful monitoring may help to ensure early diagnosis and treatment of the disease.

In 1999 and 2000, there were a number of studies that reported both genetic and biologic factors in sarcomas. The reports generated by these studies provide evidence that more and more sarcomas possess the same chromosome abnormalities. The reports also point to the high complexity of these genetic changes; which further complicate identifying any single abnormality associated with sarcomas. Despite their limitations, continuing studies can yield new, therapeutic treatment modalities. These approaches will be experimental, yet they will facilitate advancement in this arena toward even better disease management.

Resources

BOOK

Campanacci, M. *Bone and Soft Tissue Tumors: Clinical Features, Imaging, Pathology, and Treatment.* Springer Verlag, 1999.

PERIODICAL

Merimsky, Ofer, Yehuda Kollender, Josephine Issakov, et al. "Multiple Primary Malignancies in Association with Soft Tissue Sarcomas." *Cancer* 91, no. 7 (April 1, 2001): 1363-69.

OTHER

Bone Tumors. http://housecall.orbisnews.com/databases/ami/convert/001230.html. (April 11, 1998).

Ewing's Family of Tumors Cancer Information. http://www.cancer.org/cidSpecificCancers/ewing's. (April 6, 1998).

Osteosarcoma Cancer Information. http://www.cancer.org/cidSpecificCancers/osteo/index/html. (April 11, 1998).

ORGANIZATIONS

American Cancer Society. 1599 Clifton Road NE, Atlanta, GA 30329. (800) ACS-2345. http://www.cancer.org/main.html.

Cancer Care, Inc. 1180 Avenue of the Americas, New York, NY 10036. (800) 813-HOPE. http://www.cancercare.org.

National Institutes of Health. National Cancer Institute. 9000 Rockville Pike, Bethesda, MD 20892. (800) 4-CANCER. http://www.cancenet.nci.nih.gov/.

Barbara Wexler

Scaling *see* **Nonsurgical periodontal therapy**

Schizophrenia

Definition

Schizophrenia is a psychotic disorder (or a group of disorders) marked by severely impaired thinking, emotions, and behaviors. Schizophrenic persons are typically unable to filter sensory stimuli and may have enhanced perceptions of sounds, colors, and other features of their environment. Most schizophrenics, if untreated, gradually withdraw from interactions with other people, and lose their ability to take care of personal needs and grooming.

Description

The course of schizophrenia in adults can be divided into three phases or stages. In the acute phase, a person has an overt loss of contact with reality (psychotic episode) that requires intervention and treatment. In the second or stabilization phase, the initial psychotic symptoms have been brought under control but the person is at risk for relapse if treatment is interrupted. In the third or maintenance phase, an individual is relatively stable and can be kept indefinitely on antipsychotic medications. Even in the maintenance phase, however, relapses are not unusual, and people do not always return to full functioning.

The term schizophrenia comes from two Greek words that mean split mind. It was first used by a Swiss doctor named Eugen Bleuler in 1908 to describe the splitting apart of mental functions that he regarded as the central characteristic of schizophrenia.

Recently, some psychotherapists have begun to use a classification of schizophrenia based on two main types. People with Type I, or positive schizophrenia, have a rapid (acute) onset of symptoms and tend to respond well to drugs. They also tend to suffer more from so-called positive symptoms, such as delusions and hallucinations. People with Type II, or negative schizophrenia, are usually described as poorly adjusted before their schizophrenia slowly overtakes them. They have predominantly negative symptoms, such as withdrawal from others and a slowing of mental and physical reactions (psychomotor retardation).

The latest (2000) edition of the *Diagnostic and Statistical Manual of Mental Disorders* (*DSM-IV-TR*) specifies five subtypes of schizophrenia.

PARANOID. The key feature of this subtype of schizophrenia is the combination of false beliefs (delusions) and **hearing** voices (auditory hallucinations), with more nearly normal emotions and cognitive functioning (cognitive functions include reasoning, judgment, and **memory**). The delusions of paranoid schizophrenics usually involve thoughts of being persecuted or harmed by others or exaggerated opinions of their own importance, but may also reflect feelings of jealousy or excessive religiosity. The delusions are typically organized into a coherent framework. Paranoid schizophrenics function at a higher level than other subtypes, but are at risk for suicidal or violent behavior under the influence of their delusions.

DISORGANIZED. Disorganized schizophrenia (formerly called hebephrenic schizophrenia) is marked by disorganized speech, thinking, and behavior by an affected person, coupled with flat or inappropriate emotional responses to a situation (affect). An individual may act silly or withdraw socially to an extreme extent. Most people in this category have weak personality structures prior to their initial acute psychotic episode.

CATATONIC. Catatonic schizophrenia is characterized by disturbances of movement that may include rigidity, stupor, agitation, bizarre posturing, and repetitive imitations of the movements or speech of other people. These people are at risk for malnutrition, exhaustion, or self-injury. This subtype is presently uncommon in Europe and the United States. Catatonia as a symptom is most commonly associated with mood disorders.

UNDIFFERENTIATED. Persons in this category have the characteristic positive and negative symptoms of schizophrenia but do not meet the specific criteria for the paranoid, disorganized, or catatonic subtypes.

RESIDUAL. This category is used for persons who have had at least one acute schizophrenic episode but do not presently have strong positive psychotic symptoms, such as delusions and hallucinations. They may have negative symptoms, such as withdrawal from others, or mild forms of positive symptoms, which indicate that the disorder has not completely resolved.

Genetic profile

The risk of schizophrenia among first-degree biological relatives is 10 times greater than that observed in the general population. Furthermore the presence of the same disorder is higher in monozygotic (identical) twins than in dizygotic (non-identical) twins. Research concerning adoption studies and identical twins also supports the notion that environmental factors are important, because not all relatives have the disorder or express it. There are several chromosomes and loci (specific areas on chromosomes that contain mutated genes) that have been identified. Research is ongoing to elucidate the causes, types and variations of these mutations.

Demographics

A number of studies indicate that about 1% of the world's population is affected by schizophrenia, without regard to race, social class, level of education, or cultural influences. The outcome may vary from culture to culture, depending on the familial support of an affected person. Most people are diagnosed in their late teens or early twenties, but the symptoms of schizophrenia can emerge at any age in the life cycle. The male-female ratio in adults is about 1.2:1. Males typically have their first acute episode in their early 20s, while females are usually closer to age 30 when they are recognized with active symptoms.

Schizophrenia is rarely diagnosed in preadolescent children, although individuals as young as five or six have been reported. Childhood schizophrenia is at the upper end of the spectrum of severity and shows a greater gender disparity. It affects one or two children in every 10,000; the male to female ratio is 2:1.

Causes and symptoms

Theories of causality

One of the reasons for the ongoing difficulty in classifying schizophrenic disorders is incomplete understanding of their causes. It is thought that these disorders are the end result of a combination of genetic, neurobiological, and environmental causes. A leading neurobiological hypothesis emphasizes the connection between the disease and excessive levels of dopamine, a chemical that transmits signals in the **brain** (neurotransmitter). The genetic factor in schizophrenia has been underscored by recent findings that first-degree biological relatives of schizophrenics are 10 times more likely to develop the disorder than are members of the general population.

Prior to recent findings of abnormalities in the brain structure of schizophrenic persons, several generations of psychotherapists advanced a number of psychoanalytic and sociological theories about the origins of schizophrenia. These theories ranged from hypotheses about a person's problems with **anxiety** or aggression to theories about **stress** reactions or interactions with disturbed parents. Psychosocial factors are now thought to influence the expression or severity of schizophrenia, rather than directly cause it.

Another hypothesis suggests that schizophrenia may be caused by a virus that attacks the hippocampus, a part of the brain that processes sense perceptions. Damage to the hippocampus would account for a schizophrenic person's vulnerability to sensory overload.

Symptoms of schizophrenia

People with a possible diagnosis of schizophrenia are evaluated on the basis of a set or constellation of symptoms. There is no single symptom that is unique to schizophrenia. In 1959, the German psychiatrist Kurt Schneider proposed a list of so-called first-rank symptoms, which he regarded as diagnostic of the disorder.

These symptoms include:

- delusions
- somatic hallucinations
- hallucinations
- hearing voices commenting on a person's behavior
- thought insertion or thought withdrawal

Somatic hallucinations refer to sensations or perceptions concerning body organs that have no known medical cause or reason, such as the notion that one's brain is radioactive. Thought insertion and/or withdrawal refer to delusions that an outside force (for example, the FBI, the CIA, Martians) has the power to put thoughts into one's mind or remove them.

POSITIVE SYMPTOMS. The positive symptoms of schizophrenia are those that represent an excessive or distorted version of normal functions. Positive symptoms include Schneider's first-rank symptoms as well as disorganized thought processes (reflected mainly in speech) and disorganized or catatonic behavior. Disorganized thought processes are marked by such characteristics as looseness of association, in which a person rambles from topic to topic in a disconnected way; tangentiality, which means that an individual gives unrelated answers to questions; and flights of ideas or "word salad," in which a person's speech is so incoherent that it makes no grammatical or linguistic sense. Disorganized behavior means that a person has difficulty with any type of purposeful or goal-oriented behavior, including personal self-care or preparing meals. Other forms of disorganized behavior may include dressing in odd or inappropriate ways, sexual self-stimulation in public, or agitated shouting or cursing.

NEGATIVE SYMPTOMS. The *DSM-IV-TR* definition of schizophrenia includes three so-called negative symptoms. They are called negative because they represent the lack or absence of behaviors. The negative symptoms that are considered diagnostic of schizophrenia are a lack of emotional response (affective flattening), poverty of speech, and absence of volition or will. In general, the negative symptoms are more difficult for doctors to evaluate than the positive symptoms.

Diagnosis

A doctor must make a diagnosis of schizophrenia on the basis of a standardized list of outwardly observable symptoms, not on the basis of internal psychological processes. There are no specific laboratory tests that can be used to diagnose schizophrenia. Researchers have, however, discovered that persons with schizophrenia have certain abnormalities in the structure and functioning of the brain compared to normal test subjects. These discoveries

have been made with the help of imaging techniques such as **computed tomography scans (CT scans)**.

When a psychiatrist assesses an individual for schizophrenia, the doctor will begin by excluding physical conditions that can cause abnormal thinking and some other behaviors associated with schizophrenia. These conditions include organic brain disorders (including traumatic injuries of the brain), temporal lobe epilepsy, Wilson's disease, Huntington's chorea, and **encephalitis**. The doctor will also need to rule out **substance abuse** disorders, especially amphetamine use.

After ruling out organic disorders, a clinician will consider other psychiatric conditions that may include psychotic symptoms or symptoms resembling **psychosis**. These disorders include mood disorders with psychotic features; delusional disorder; dissociative disorder not otherwise specified (DDNOS) or **multiple personality disorder**; schizotypal, schizoid, or paranoid **personality disorders**; and atypical reactive disorders. In the past, many individuals were incorrectly diagnosed as being schizophrenic. Some people who were diagnosed prior to the changes in categorization introduced by *DSM-IV-TR* should have their diagnoses, and treatment, reevaluated. In children, a doctor must distinguish between psychotic symptoms and a vivid fantasy life, and also identify learning problems or disorders. After other conditions have been ruled out, a person must meet a set of criteria specified by *DSM-IV-TR*:

- Characteristic symptoms. To make a diagnosis of schizophrenia, a person must exhibit two (or more) of the following symptoms during a one-month period: delusions; hallucinations; disorganized speech; disorganized or catatonic behavior; negative symptoms.

- Decline in social, interpersonal, or occupational functioning, including self-care.

- Duration. The disturbed behavior must last for at least six months.

- Diagnostic exclusions. Mood disorders, substance abuse disorders, medical conditions, and developmental disorders have been ruled out.

Treatment

The treatment of schizophrenia depends in part on an individual's stage or phase. People in the acute phase are hospitalized in most cases, to prevent harm to themselves or to others and to begin treatment with antipsychotic medications. A person having a first psychotic episode should be given a CT (computed tomography) or MRI (**magnetic resonance imaging**) scan to rule out structural brain abnormalities or disease.

KEY TERMS

Affective flattening—A loss or lack of emotional expressiveness. It is sometimes called blunted or restricted affect.

Akathisia—Agitated or restless movement, usually affecting the legs and accompanied by a sense of discomfort. It is a common side effect of neuroleptic medications.

Catatonic behavior—Behavior characterized by muscular tightness or rigidity and lack of response to the environment. In some persons, rigidity alternates with excited or hyperactive behavior.

Delusion—A fixed, false belief that is resistant to reason or factual disproof.

Depot dosage—A form of medication that can be stored in a person's body tissues for several days or weeks, thus minimizing the risk of forgetting daily doses. Haloperidol and fluphenazine can be given in depot form.

Dopamine receptor antagonists (DAs)—The older class of antipsychotic medications, also called neuroleptics. These primarily block the site on nerve

cells that normally receives the brain chemical dopamine.

Dystonia—Painful involuntary muscle cramps or spasms. Dystonia is one of the extrapyramidal side effects associated with some antipsychotic medications.

Extrapyramidal symptoms (EPS)—A group of side effects associated with antipsychotic medications. EPS include parkinsonism, akathisia, dystonia, and tardive dyskinesia.

First-rank symptoms—A set of symptoms designated by Kurt Schneider in 1959 as the most important diagnostic indicators of schizophrenia. These symptoms include delusions, hallucinations, thought insertion or removal, and thought broadcasting. First-rank symptoms are sometimes referred to as Schneiderian symptoms.

Hallucination—A sensory experience of something that does not exist outside the mind. A person can experience a hallucination in any of the five senses. Auditory hallucinations are a common symptom of schizophrenia.

Antipsychotic medications

The primary form of treatment of schizophrenia is antipsychotic medication. **Antipsychotic drugs** help to control almost all the positive symptoms of the disorder. They have minimal effect on disorganized behavior and negative symptoms. Between 60–70% of schizophrenics will respond to antipsychotics. In the acute phase of the illness, people are usually given medications by mouth or by **intramuscular injection**. After an affected person has been stabilized, the antipsychotic drug may be given in a long-acting form called a depot dose. Depot medications last for two to four weeks and have the advantage of protecting a person against the consequences of forgetting or skipping daily doses. In addition, some people who do not respond to oral neuroleptic medications have better results with depot form. Persons whose long-term treatment includes depot medications are introduced to the depot form gradually during their stabilization period. Most people with schizophrenia are kept on antipsychotic medications indefinitely during the maintenance phase of their disorder to minimize the possibility of relapse.

The most frequently used antipsychotics fell into two classes: the older dopamine receptor antagonists, or

DAs; and the newer serotonin dopamine antagonists, or SDAs. Antagonists block the action of some other substance. For example, dopamine antagonists counteract the action of dopamine. The exact mechanisms of action of these medications are not known, but it is thought that they lower a person's sensitivity to sensory stimuli and so indirectly improve the person's ability to interact with others.

DOPAMINE RECEPTOR ANTAGONIST. The dopamine antagonists include the older antipsychotic (also called neuroleptic) drugs, such as haloperidol (Haldol), chlorpromazine (Thorazine), and fluphenazine (Prolixin). These drugs have two major drawbacks. It is often difficult to find the best dosage level for a given individual, and a dosage level high enough to control psychotic symptoms frequently produces extrapyramidal side effects, or EPS. EPSs include parkinsonism, in which a person cannot walk normally and usually develops a tremor; dystonia, or painful muscle spasms of the head, tongue, or neck; and akathisia, or restlessness. A type of long-term EPS is called tardive dyskinesia, which features slow, rhythmic, automatic movements. Schizophrenics with **AIDS** are especially vulnerable to developing EPS.

Huntington's chorea—A hereditary disease that typically appears in midlife, marked by gradual loss of brain function and involuntary movements. Some of its symptoms resemble those of schizophrenia.

Negative symptoms—Symptoms of schizophrenia that are characterized by the absence or elimination of certain behaviors. DSM-IV-TR specifies three negative symptoms: affective flattening, poverty of speech, and loss of will or initiative.

Neuroleptic—Another name for the older type of antipsychotic medications given to schizophrenic persons.

Parkinsonism—A set of symptoms originally associated with Parkinson's disease that can occur as side effects of neuroleptic medications. The symptoms include trembling of the fingers or hands, a shuffling gait, and tight or rigid muscles.

Positive symptoms—Symptoms of schizophrenia that are characterized by the production or presence of behaviors that are grossly abnormal or excessive, including hallucinations and thought-process

disorder. DSM-IV-TR subdivides positive symptoms into psychotic and disorganized.

Poverty of speech—A negative symptom of schizophrenia, characterized by brief and empty replies to questions. It should not be confused with shyness or reluctance to talk.

Psychotic disorder—A mental disorder characterized by delusions, hallucinations, or other symptoms of lack of contact with reality. The schizophrenias are psychotic disorders.

Serotonin dopamine antagonists (SDAs)—The newer second-generation antipsychotic drugs, also called atypical antipsychotics. SDAs include clozapine (Clozaril), risperidone (Risperdal), and olanzapine (Zyprexa).

Wilson's disease—A rare hereditary disease marked by high levels of copper deposits in the brain, eyes and liver. It can cause psychiatric symptoms resembling schizophrenia.

Word salad—Speech that is so disorganized that it makes no linguistic or grammatical sense.

SERATONIN DOPAMINE ANTAGONISTS. The serotonin dopamine antagonists, also called atypical antipsychotics, are newer medications that include clozapine (Clozaril), risperidone (Risperdal), and olanzapine (Zyprexa). The SDAs have a better effect on the negative symptoms of schizophrenia than do the older drugs and are less likely to produce EPS than the older compounds. The newer drugs are significantly more expensive in the short term, although the SDAs may reduce long-term costs by reducing the need for hospitalization. They are also presently unavailable in injectable forms. The SDAs are commonly used to treat persons who respond poorly to the DAs. However, many psychotherapists now regard the use of these atypical antipsychotics as the treatment of first choice.

Psychotherapy

Most schizophrenics can benefit from **psychotherapy** once their acute symptoms have been brought under control by antipsychotic medication. Psychoanalytic approaches are not recommended. Behavior therapy, however, is often helpful in assisting people to acquire skills for daily living and social interaction. It can be

combined with **occupational therapy** to prepare individuals for eventual employment.

Family therapy

Family therapy is often recommended for the families of schizophrenic patients, to relieve the feelings of guilt that they often have as well as to help them understand a schizophrenic's disorder. The family's attitude and behaviors toward the schizophrenic are key factors in minimizing relapses (for example, by reducing stress in an individual's life), and family therapy can often strengthen the family's ability to cope with the stresses caused by the schizophrenic's illness. Family therapy that focuses on communication skills and problem-solving strategies is particularly helpful. In addition to formal treatment, many families benefit from support groups and similar mutual help organizations for relatives of schizophrenics.

Prognosis

One important prognostic sign is a person's age at onset of psychotic symptoms. People with early onset of schizophrenia are more often male, have a lower level of

QUESTIONS TO ASK YOUR DOCTOR

- How will you determine the type of schizophrenia experienced by my parent?
- How does your diagnosis of the type of schizophrenia involved affect the type of treatment to be used?
- What treatment do you think is most likely to be successful in this case?
- What prognosis can you make for the course of this disorder?

functioning prior to onset, a higher rate of brain abnormalities, more noticeable negative symptoms, and worse outcomes. Persons with later onset are more likely to be female, with fewer brain abnormalities and thought impairment, and more hopeful prognoses.

The average course and outcome for schizophrenics are less favorable than those for most other mental disorders, although as many as 30% of people diagnosed with schizophrenia recover completely and the majority experience some improvement. Two factors that influence outcomes are stressful life events and a hostile or emotionally intense family environment. Schizophrenics with a high number of stressful changes in their lives, or who have frequent contacts with critical or emotionally over-involved family members, are more likely to relapse. Overall, the most important component of long-term care for schizophrenic individuals is complying with their regimen of antipsychotic medications.

Health care team roles

Physicians such as a family doctor or internist often make an initial diagnosis of schizophrenia. Psychiatrists, psychologists, or other therapists may also provide an initial diagnosis. Psychiatrists, clinical psychologists, or other trained professionals provide intervention treatment and therapy. Counselors may provide support during and after treatment. Nurses often administer medications.

Prevention

With present levels of understanding about schizophrenia, there does not appear to be any way to prevent the disease. Better understanding holds the promise of prevention if specific causal factors are environmental, chemical or viral.

Resources

BOOKS

American Psychiatric Association. *Diagnostic and Statistical Manual of Mental Disorders*, 4th ed. Washington, DC: American Psychiatric Association Press, Inc., 2000.

Haycock, Dean A., and Elias K. Shaya. *The Everything Health Guide to Schizophrenia: The Latest Information on Treatment, Medication, and Coping Strategies.* Avon, MA: Adams Media, 2009.

Mueser, Kim Tornvall, and Dilip V. Jeste. *Clinical Handbook of Schizophrenia.* New York: Guilford Press, 2011.

Weinberger, Daniel R., and P.J. Harrison. *Schizophrenia*, 3rd ed. Chichester, West Sussex, UK; Hoboken, NJ: Wiley-Blackwell, 2011.

PERIODICALS

Calkins, Monica E., and Karin E. Borgmann-Winter. "Evaluation and Treatment of Children and Adolescents With Psychotic Symptoms." *Current Psychiatry Reports* 14, 2 (2012): 101–110.

Doherty, J.L., M.C. O'Donovan, and M.J. Owen. "Recent Genomic Advances in Schizophrenia." *Clinical Genetics* 81, 2 (2012): 103–109.

Holttum, Sue. "Condition Management and the Causes of Psychosis." *Mental Health and Social Inclusion* 16, 1 (2012): 8–13.

Schaub, Daniela, and Martin Brune. "Comparison of Self- and Clinician's Ratings of Personal and Social Performance in Patients with Schizophrenia: The Role of Insight." *Psychopathology* 45, 2 (2012): 109–116.

OTHER

Bengston, Michael. *Schizophrenia and Psychosis.* PsychCentral. http://psychcentral.com/disorders/schizophrenia/ (accessed May 10, 2012).

Schizophrenia. MedicineNet.com. http://www.medicinenet.com/schizophrenia/article.htm (accessed May 10, 2012).

Schizophrenia. PubMed Health. http://www.ncbi.nlm.nih.gov/pubmedhealth/PMH0001925/ (accessed May 10, 2012).

Schizophrenia.com. http://www.schizophrenia.com/ (accessed May 10, 2012).

ORGANIZATIONS

American Psychological Association. 750 First St. NE, Washington, DC 20002-4242. (202) 336-5500. http://www.apa.org. http://www.apa.org/about/contact/contact.aspx.

Brain and Behavior Research Foundation. 60 Cutter Mill Rd., Suite 404, Great Neck, NY 11021. (516) 829-0091. Fax: (516) 487-6930. http://www.mhsource.com/narsad/. info@bbrfoundation.org.

National Alliance for the Mentally Ill. 3803 N. Fairfax Dr., Suite 100, Arlington, VA 22203. (703) 524-7600. http://www.nami.org/.

National Institute of Mental Health. Science Writing, Press, and Dissemination Branch, 6001 Executive Blvd., Room 8184, MSC 9663, Bethesda, MD 20892-9663. (866) 615-6464. http://www.nimh.nih.gov/index.shtml. nimhinfo@nih.gov.

L. Fleming Fallon, Jr., M.D., Dr.P.H.

Sciatica

Definition

Sciatica describes **pain** or discomfort in the distribution of the sciatic nerve or its components. This nerve runs from the lower part of the **spinal cord**, down the back of the leg, to the foot. Injury to, or pressure on, the sciatic nerve can cause the characteristic pain of sciatica—a sharp or burning pain that radiates from the lower back or hip, following the path of the sciatic nerve to the foot.

Description

The sciatic nerve is the largest and longest nerve in the body. It supplies sensation from the lower back to the foot. The nerve originates in the lumbar region of the spinal cord. As it branches off from the spinal cord, it passes between the bony vertebrae (the component bones of the spine) and runs through the pelvic girdle (hipbones). The nerve passes near the hip joint and continues down the back of the leg to the foot.

Sciatica is a fairly common disorder. Approximately 40% of the population suffers from it at some point in their lives; however, only about 1% experience any sensory or motor deficits. Sciatic pain has several root causes, and its treatment is directed to the underlying problem.

Of the identifiable causes of sciatic pain, lumbosacral (LS) radiculopathy and back strain are the most frequently suspected. The LS area is the lower part of the spine, and radiculopathy describes pain radiating from pressure on a spinal nerve roots. This area between the vertebrae (hard bones) is cushioned with a disk of shock-absorbing tissue. The spinal canal, comprising the spinal cord and other nerve roots, is hollow and lies in the middle of the spinal column. It is the disks between the vertebrae that enable the back to bend or flex.

A "ring" of cartilage, gristle-like in character, is found on the outer edge of the disk (the annulus). The disk's center (nucleus) is a substance like gel. When a disk ruptures, or herniates, it does so because of wear-and-tear, excessive weight, poor posture, injury (perhaps due to improper lifting), or disease. The center nucleus pushes the outer edge of the disk into the spinal canal, putting pressure on the nerves. The spinal nerve root may become compressed by the shifted tissue or the vertebrae. This compression of the nerve root sends a pain signal to the **brain**. Although the injury is actually suffered by the nerve roots, the pain may be perceived as originating anywhere along the sciatic nerve. Further, if fragments of the disk lodge in the spinal canal, the nerves that control bowel and urinary functions may be damaged. Incontinence may result.

Sciatica is largely a symptom of a **herniated disk**. However, compression of the sciatic nerve can also present as muscle spasms in the lower back (back strain). In this case, pressure is placed on the sciatic nerve. In rare cases, **infection**, **cancer**, **bone** inflammation, or other diseases may cause pressure. Another possible cause of sciatica is piriformis syndrome.

As the sciatic nerve passes behind the hip joint, it shares the space with several muscles. One of these muscles, the piriformis muscle, is closely associated with the sciatic nerve. In some people, the nerve actually runs through the muscle. If this muscle is injured or has a spasm, it places pressure on the sciatic nerve, in effect, compressing it.

In many sciatica cases, the specific cause is never identified. About half of affected individuals recover from an episode within a month. Some cases persist and may require aggressive treatment. In other cases, the pain returns or becomes chronic.

Demographics

Sciatica is generally reported in about 1% to 10% of the U.S. population. It is most frequently found in people from the ages of 25 to 45 years. Pain involving the sciatic nerve usually disappears within six to 12 weeks; however, if serious underlying conditions are present the pain may last longer—for weeks, months or even years. In addition, depending on the cause of the sciatica pain, symptoms may not be constant, but appear and disappear on a frequent basis. Generally, about 90% of all sciatica cases will resolve themselves with traditional treatments such as a short-period of rest followed with moderate **exercise** that will not aggravate the condition (such as swimming or walking) and medications such as **nonsteroidal anti-inflammatory drugs** (NSAIDs, such as ibuprofen or naproxen) and **analgesics** (such as paracetamol).

Causes and symptoms

Patients with sciatica may experience low **back pain**, but the most common symptom is pain that radiates through one buttock and down the back of the leg. The most frequently identified cause of pain is compression or pressure on the sciatic nerve. The extent of the pain varies. Some patients describe pain that centers in the

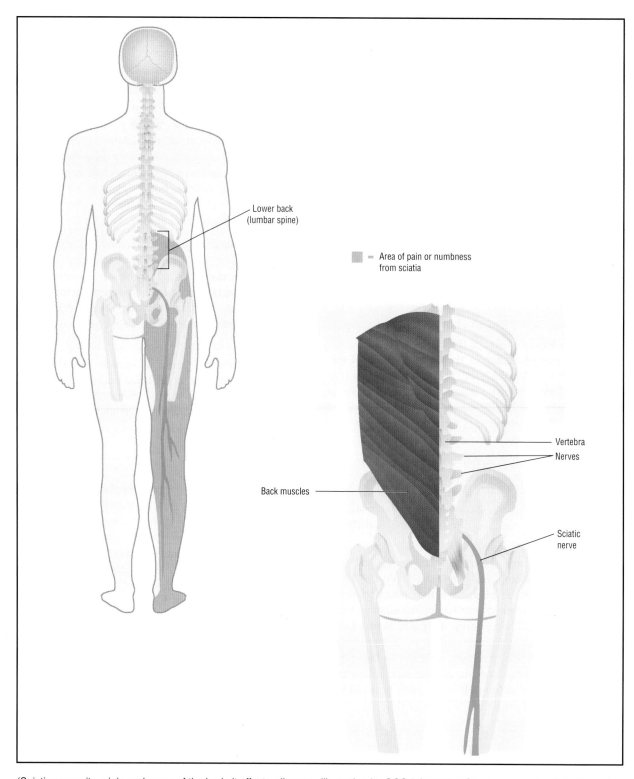

Lower back
(lumbar spine)

▦ = Area of pain or numbness
from sciatia

Vertebra

Nerves

Back muscles

Sciatic
nerve

(Sciatic nerve, its origin and areas of the body it affects, diagram. Illustration by GGS Information Services, Inc. The Gale Group.)

area of the hip; others feel discomfort all the way to the foot. The quality of the pain also varies; it may be described as tingling, burning, prickly, aching, or stabbing.

Onset of sciatica may be sudden, but it might also develop gradually. The pain may be intermittent or continuous. Certain activities (such as bending, coughing, sneezing, or sitting) can worsen the pain.

Sudden loss of bowel or bladder control, **weakness** in the legs, buttocks, or torso, as well as numbness that goes upwards from the toes or the feet, may indicate a sciatic condition.

Chronic pain may arise from more than simple compression of the nerve root. Discogenic pain, the result of injury to the innervated portions of the annulus fibrosus, is a common cause of sciatica. Pain is generally felt in the buttocks and in the posterior thigh.

According to some pain researchers, physical damage to a nerve is only half of the equation. A theory developed in 2001 proposes that some nerve injuries result when certain neurotransmitters and **immune system** chemicals that exacerbate and sustain a pain message. Even after the injury has healed or the damage has been repaired, the pain lingers. Effective management of this type of pain is difficult. Another theory that has been put forward is that back problems may be inherited. This theory presupposes that a genetic abnormality is responsible for a number of cases of spinal disk disease cases. This defect makes people susceptible to rupture when the back is strained. The investigators claimed that 25% of all cases of sciatica, lower back problems, and discomfort higher in the spine, might be attributable to this gene defect. When classic symptoms are absent, identification of the defect could enable diagnosis of disease, thereby facilitating the therapeutic process. In the 2010s, these theories and others continue to be investigated by medical researchers.

Diagnosis

Establishing the diagnosis requires taking a thorough medical history and performing a focused **physical examination**. The patient is asked about the location, nature, and duration of the pain, and the details of any accidents, injuries or unusual activities that may have occurred prior to the onset of sciatica. This information provides clues that may point to back strain or injury to a specific location.

Back pain from disk disease, piriformis syndrome, and back strain must be differentiated from more serious conditions, such as cancer or infection. For instance, hidden infections in patients who suffered from persistent pain originating in the sciatic nerve have been thought to result from minor trauma. When patients suffered such trauma, studies have shown that an organism may have entered the body, which then causes inflammation in and around the sciatic nerve.

More investigations need to be done, however, evaluating the success of **antibiotics** (used to fight infections) in treating sciatica. Lumbar spine stenosis, an overgrowth of the covering layers of the vertebrae that narrows the spinal canal, must also be considered.

A straight leg-raising test is often performed. The patient lies supine, and the health care provider raises the affected leg to various heights. This test pinpoints the location of the pain and may reveal whether it is caused by a disk problem. Other tests, such as observing the patient rotate the hip joint, may provide information about involvement of the piriformis muscle if the patient experience pain. Piriformis weakness is tested with additional leg-strength maneuvers.

Further tests may be conducted depending on the patient's history, results of the physical examination, and response to initial treatment. Diagnostic tests may include traditional x rays, **magnetic resonance imaging** (MRI) scans, and **computed tomography (CT) scans**. Other tests include **electromyography** (studies of the electrical activity generated as muscles contract), nerve conduction velocity testing, and evoked potential testing. **Myelography**, a more invasive test, involves injecting a contrast medium into the spinal subarachnoid space between the vertebrae and taking x-ray images of the spinal cord. Myelography is usually ordered when surgical treatment is considered. Since the advent of MRI, however, myelography is very rarely used. The MRI does not use ionizing radiation. Noninvasive, it produces excellent computerized images of soft tissues, such as seen in herniated discs and tumors. The MRI is based on nuclear magnetic resonance of atoms within the body; the atoms are generated by the use of radio waves. All these tests can reveal problems with the vertebrae, the disk, or the nerve itself.

Treatment

Pharmacological therapy—initial treatment for sciatica—focuses on pain relief. Regardless of the cause of the pain, analgesics (such as acetaminophen) may help relieve pain. **Muscle relaxants** are also used, but it has not been medically proved whether they really work. Such medicines include carisoprodol (Soma), cyclobenzaprine (Flexeril), diazepam (Valium), and methocarbamol (Robaxin). Furthermore, the side effects of muscle relaxants may be greater than their benefits, particularly in the elderly. Generally, pain relief is accomplished with over-the-counter (OTC) nonsteroidal anti-inflammatory drugs (NSAIDs) such as aspirin, ibuprofen (Advil, Motrin IB, Nuprin, Rufen), naproxen (Aleve), and ketoprofen (Actron, Orudis KT). Prescription NSAIDs include dexibuprofen (Seractil), diclofenac (Voltaren), flurbiprofen (Ansaid), ibuprofen (Motrin), ketoprofen (Orudis, Oruvail), naproxen (Naprosyn, Anaprox), and tolmetin (Tolectin). It should be noted, however, that anti-inflammatory medications should be administered generally for only two to four weeks, and only if medical contraindications are not present.

In 2001, the Food and Drug Administration (FDA) approved labeling two drugs for the relief of pain; they were an NSAID with selective cyclo-oxygenase 2 inhibition (COX-2)—rofecoxib (Vioxx)—and the COX-2 drug celecoxib (Celebrex). In 2004, Vioxx was withdrawn from the market by its manufacturer, Merck, because it was shown to double patients' risks of **heart** attack and **stroke**. It also caused skin rashes and other negative effects. Valdecoxib (Bextra) was also taken off the U.S. market. As of April 2012, celecoxib (Celebrex) is still available in the United States; however, patients should discuss with their doctor if it is safe for them to take for sciatica.

If the pain is unremitting, opioids may be prescribed for short-term use or a local anesthetic may be injected directly into the lower back. Opioids include hydrocodone (Vicodin), oxycodone (Percodan, Percocet, OxyContin), and oxymorphone (Numorphan). Massage and heat application may be suggested as adjunct therapies.

If the pain is chronic, different pain relief medications are used to avoid long-term dosing of NSAIDs, muscle relaxants, and opioids. **Antidepressant drugs**, which have been shown to be effective in treating pain, may be prescribed in conjunction with a short-term course of a muscle relaxants or a NSAID. Local anesthetic injections, or epidural steroids, are used in selected cases.

Tramadol (Ultram) is a synthetic analgesic (pain reliever) that is used to treat moderate to moderately-severe pain. It is often prescribed as an alternative to opioids. It possesses opioid-like properties but is not nearly as addictive as opioids. A drug containing both tramadol and acetaminophen, called Ultracet, is now available in the United States for the treatment of sciatica. Rather than oral opioids, a skin patch called transdermal fentanyl (Duragesic) is also used to relieve chronic pain from sciatic. Because it is applied directly onto the pain site, it often is more effective than oral dosages.

Corticosteroid injections are also sometimes used to treat sciatica. The injection site should be close to the affected location in order to maximize the benefit. However, medical studies on such corticosteroid injections for sciatica are not consistent. Although short-term benefit (over a one- to two-month period) has been shown for many patients in such studies, longer term benefits have not been proven.

The botulinum toxin (produced by the bacterium *Clostridium botulinum*), commonly called Botox, has been studied for the treatment of sciatica. Such injections temporarily paralyze muscle tissue, and some preliminary studies indicate that it may also help to relieve sciatica. However, a definitive answer is yet to be proven.

As pain permits, **physical therapy** is introduced into the treatment regime. Stretching exercises that focus on the lower back, buttocks, and hamstring muscles are suggested. The exercises may also include identifying and practicing comfortable, pain-reducing positions. Corsets and braces may be useful in some cases, but there is no clinical evidence for their general effectiveness. However, they may be helpful in the prevention of exacerbation of sciatica as related to certain activities.

With less pain and the success of early therapy, the patient is encouraged to follow a long-term exercise program to maintain a healthy back and prevent re-injury. A physical therapist may suggest exercises and regular activity, such as water exercise or walking. Patients are instructed in proper posture and body mechanics as means of minimizing symptoms during light lifting, prolonged sitting or standing, and other activities.

If the pain is chronic and conservative treatment fails—suggesting that a disk fragment has lodged in the spinal canal and is pressing on the nerve (and perhaps causing a loss of function—surgery may be required. A procedure to repair a herniated disk or excise part, or all of the piriformis muscle, may be suggested, particularly if there is neurologic evidence of nerve or nerve-root damage (radiculopathy). It should be noted, however, that newer and minimally invasive procedures are available to relieve the pain of sciatica. A local anesthetic is used, and surgery is performed on an ambulatory basis. The recovery period is two to six weeks.

Massage is a recommended form of therapy, especially when the sciatic pain arises from muscle spasm. Patients may be able to relieve symptoms by icing the painful area as soon as pain occurs. The physical therapist or nurse may instruct the patient to place ice on the affected area for 20 minutes, several times a day. After two to three days, a hot water bottle or heating pad can replace the ice. **Chiropractic** or osteopathic therapy may offer solutions for relieving pressure on the sciatic nerve and the accompanying pain. **Acupuncture** and biofeedback may also be useful as pain control methods.

KEY TERMS

Acupuncture—The Chinese practice of piercing specific areas of the body along peripheral nerves with fine needles to relieve pain, to induce surgical anesthesia, and for therapeutic purposes.

Biofeedback—The process of furnishing an individual with information on the state of one or more physiologic variables, such as heart rate, blood pressure, or skin temperature. The goal is to enable the patient to gain some voluntary control over them.

Disk—Dense tissue between the vertebrae that acts as a shock absorber and prevents damage to nerves and blood vessels along the spine.

Electromyography—A diagnostic test in which a nerve's ability to conduct an impulse is measured.

Lumbosacral (LS)—Referring to the lower part of the backbone or spine.

Myelography—A medical test in which a special dye—a contrast medium—is injected the spinal subarachnoid space (through which cerebrospinal fluid [CSF] circulates, and across which extend delicate connective tissue pass) to make it visible on radiographic visualization.

NSAID—Nonsteroidal anti-inflammatory drugs are medications that produce analgesic and anti-inflammatory effects.

Opioid—A synthetic narcotic that has opiate-like qualities, but is not derived from opium.

Orthotics—Serving to protect or to restore or improve function; relating to the use or application of an orthosis.

Piriformis—A muscle in the pelvic girdle that is closely associated with the sciatic nerve.

Radiculopathy—A condition in which the nerve root of a nerve has been injured or damaged.

Spasm—Involuntary contraction of a muscle.

Spinal subarachnoid space—Space through which cerebrospinal fluid circulates, and across which extend delicate connective tissue pass.

Vertebrae—The component bones of the spine.

Prognosis

Most cases of sciatica are treatable with pain medication and physical therapy. After four to six weeks of treatment, most patients should be able to resume normal activities.

Prevention

Some sources of sciatica are not preventable, such as disk degeneration, back strain resulting from **pregnancy**, or accidental injuries from **falls**. Other sources of back strain, such as poor posture, overexertion, **obesity**, or wearing high heels, may be corrected or avoided. **Smoking** may also predispose patients to pain, as it the supply of **blood** to invertebral discs, and interferes with healing. An orthopedist with the Gwinnett Health System in Lawrenceville, Georgia, Dr. Walker states that "Smoking leads to drying and stiffness of the discs, making them more susceptible to injury, including herniation, and prolonged recovery time."

General suggestions for avoiding sciatica or preventing future episodes include sleeping on a firm mattress, using chairs with firm back supports, and sitting with both feet flat on the floor. Habitually crossing the legs while sitting may place excess pressure on the sciatic nerve. Sitting for prolonged periods of time also places pressure on the sciatic nerves, so patients are advised to take short breaks and move around during the workday, when on long trips, or in other situations that require sitting for extended lengths of time. When sitting for long periods, the patient should put his or her feet up on a low stool. If it is required that something be lifted without another person, the back should be kept straight and the legs should provide the lift. The knees should be bent, and the individual should get as close to the object as possible. This will reduce the load on the lower back. To give one a wider base of support and to distribute the weight of the object being lifted, the feet should be kept apart.

Regular exercise, such as swimming and walking, can build stamina, strengthen back muscles, improve flexibility, and improve posture. Exercise also helps to maintain proper body weight and lessens the likelihood of back strain.

Health care team roles

The diagnosis of sciatica is usually made by a primary care physician (PCP) or a mid-level practitioner (physician assistant [PA] or nurse practitioner [NP]). Other physician specialists, such as neurologists, orthopedists, and physiatrists (specialists in physical medicine) also may provide consultative services. Radiologic technologists generally perform diagnostic imaging studies.

QUESTIONS TO ASK YOUR DOCTOR

- What is causing my sciatica?
- Based on my lifestyle, medical history, and family background, am I at increased risk for further sciatica?
- How can I prevent sciatica?
- Will I need surgery for sciatica?
- What medications, if any, do you prescribe for sciatica?
- What are the side effects of medications used to treat sciatica?
- Are there any alternative or complementary therapies that could help me with sciatica?
- Should I exercise? If so, what types of exercise are best for me? How often should I exercise? And, at what intensity?
- Will losing weight help me with my sciatica problems?

The treatment plan may involve physical therapists (PTs) and physical therapist assistants (PTAs), who instruct and supervise prescribed exercise programs. Patients also may be referred to specialists in orthotics, who prescribe appliances/apparatuses to support, align, prevent, or correct deformities, improve posture, or ease the function of movable body parts. Sometimes specialists work with ergonomics. The patient may be taught proper body mechanics at home and in the workplace.

Patient education

Patient education focuses on adhering to prescribed treatment, including exercise and body mechanics (above), and preventing future injuries. Nurses, PTs, PTAs, occupational therapists, and exercise physiologists may be involved in helping patients learn how to perform the activities of daily living (ADL) without exacerbating existing injuries.

Resources

BOOKS

Cooper, J. Allen D., and Peter G. Pappas. *Cecil Review of General Internal Medicine.* Philadelphia: Elsevier Saunders, 2004.

Fishman, Loren, and Carol Ardman. *Sciatica Solutions: Diagnosis, Treatment, and Cure for Spinal and Piriformis Problems.* New York: W.W. Norton, 2006.

Habermann, Thomas M., and Amit K. Ghosh, editors. *Mayo Clinic Internal Medicine: Concise Textbook.* Rochester, MN: Mayo Clinic Scientific Press, 2008.

Longo, Dan L, and Tinsley Randolph Harrison. *Harrison's Principles of Internal Medicine.* New York: McGraw-Hill, 2012.

WEBSITES

Sciatica. Mayo Clinic. (April 22, 2010). http://www.mayoclinic.com/health/sciatica/DS00516 (April 25, 2012).

Sciatica. MedicineNet. http://www.medicinenet.com/sciatica/article.htm (April 25, 2012).

Sciatica. Medline Plus. (April 17, 2012). http://www.nlm.nih.gov/medlineplus/sciatica.html (April 25, 2012).

Sciatica. The New York Times. (April 22, 2010). http://health.nytimes.com/health/guides/disease/sciatica/medications.html (April 25, 2012).

ORGANIZATIONS

American Chronic Pain Organization, P.O. Box 850, Rocklin, CA 95677, Fax: (916) 632-3208, (800) 533-3231, acpa@pacbell.net, http://theacpa.org/default.aspx.

ORGANIZATIONS

American Pain Foundation, 201 N. Charles St., Ste. 710, Baltimore, MD 21201-4111, (888) 615-7246, http://www.painfoundation.org/.

ORGANIZATIONS

National Institute of Arthritis and Musculoskeletal and Skin Diseases, 1 AMS Circle, Bethesda, MD 20892-3675, Fax: (301) 495-4484, (877) 226-4267, NIAMSinfo@mail.nih.gov, http://www.niams.nih.gov/.

Barbara Wexler
William A. Atkins, BB, BS, MBA

Scoliosis

Definition

Scoliosis is a side-to-side (lateral) curvature of the spine of 10 degrees or greater.

Description

When viewed from the rear, the spine usually appears to form a straight vertical line. Scoliosis is a lateral (side-to-side) curve in the spine, usually combined with a rotation of the vertebrae. The lateral curvature of scoliosis should not be confused with the normal set of front-to-back spinal curves visible from the side. While a small degree of lateral curvature does not cause any medical problems, larger curves can cause postural imbalance and lead to muscle fatigue and **pain**. More

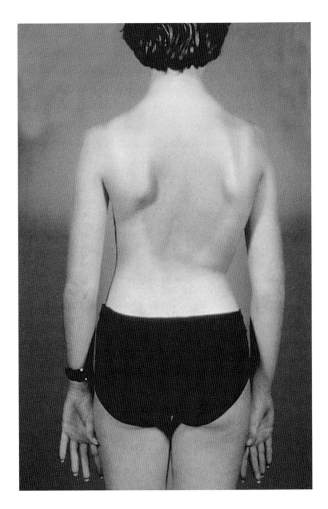

(Idiopathic scoliosis, photograph. Custom Medical Stock Photo. Reproduced by permission.)

severe scoliosis can interfere with breathing and lead to arthritis of the spine (spondylosis).

Four out of five cases of scoliosis are idiopathic, meaning their cause is unknown. Children with idiopathic scoliosis appear to be otherwise entirely healthy, and have not had any **bone** or joint disease early in life. Scoliosis is not caused by poor posture, diet, or carrying a heavy bookbag exclusively on one shoulder.

Idiopathic scoliosis is further classified according to age of onset:

- Infantile. Curvature appears before age three. This type is quite rare in the United States, but is more common in Europe.

- Juvenile. Curvature appears between ages three and 10. This type may be equivalent to the adolescent type, except for the age of onset.

- Adolescent. Curvature appears between ages of 10 and 13, near the beginning of puberty. This is the most common type of idiopathic scoliosis.

- Adult. Curvature begins after physical maturation is completed.

Causes are known for three other types of scoliosis:

- Congenital scoliosis is due to congenital birth defects in the spine, often associated with other structural defects.

- Neuromuscular scoliosis is due to loss of control of the nerves or muscles which support the spine. The most common causes of this type of scoliosis are cerebral palsy and muscular dystrophy.

- Degenerative scoliosis may be caused by degeneration of the discs which separate the vertebrae or arthritis in the joints that link them.

Genetic profile

Idiopathic scoliosis has long been observed to run in families. Twin and family studies have consistently indicated a genetic contribution to the condition. However, no consistent pattern of transmission has been observed in familial cases. No genes have been identified which specifically cause or predispose individuals to the idiopathic form of scoliosis.

There are several genetic syndromes which involve a predisposition to scoliosis. Several studies have investigated whether or not the genes which cause these syndromes may also be responsible for idiopathic scoliosis. Using this candidate gene approach, the genes responsible for Marfan syndrome (fibrillin), Stickler syndrome, and some forms of osteogenesis imperfecta (collagen types I and II) have been shown not to correlate with idiopathic scoliosis.

Attempts to map a gene or genes for scoliosis have not shown consistent linkages to any particular chromosome region.

Most researchers have concluded that scoliosis is a complex trait. As such, there are likely to be multiple genetic, environmental, and potentially additional factors that contribute to the etiology of the condition. Complex traits are difficult to study due to the difficulty in identifying and isolating multiple factors.

Demographics

The incidence of scoliosis in the general population is approximately 2–3%. Among adolescents, however, 10% have some degree of scoliosis, though fewer than 1% have curves that require treatment.

Scoliosis is found in both males and females, but a female's spinal curve is much more likely to progress than a male's. Females require scoliosis treatment about five times as often as males. The reason for these differences is not known with certainty but they may relate to increased levels of estrogen and other hormones in females.

Causes and symptoms

Scoliosis causes a noticeable asymmetry in the torso when viewed from the front or back. The first sign of scoliosis is often seen when a child is wearing a bathing suit or underwear. A child may appear to be standing with one shoulder higher than the other, or to have a tilt in the waistline. One shoulder blade may appear more prominent than the other due to rotation. In girls, one breast may appear higher than the other, or larger if rotation pushes that side forward.

Curve progression is greatest near the adolescent growth spurt. Scoliosis that begins early in life is more likely to progress significantly than scoliosis that begins later in **puberty**.

More than 30 states have screening programs in schools for adolescent scoliosis. These are usually conducted by physicians, school nurses or trained physical education teachers.

Diagnosis

Scoliosis is initially noticed during a screening program or during a routine **physical examination** conducted by a pediatrician or family physician. Confirmatory diagnosis of scoliosis is often conducted by an orthopedic surgeon. A complete medical history is taken, including questions about family history of scoliosis. The physical examination includes determination of pubertal development in adolescents, a neurological exam (which may reveal a neuromuscular cause), and measurements of trunk asymmetry. Examination of the trunk is done while the person is standing, bending over, and lying down, and involves both visual inspection and use of a simple mechanical device called a scoliometer.

If a curve is detected, one or more x rays will usually be taken to define more precisely the curve or curves. An x ray is used to document spinal maturity, any pelvic tilt or hip asymmetry, and the location, extent, and degree of curvature. The curve is defined in terms of where it begins and ends, in which direction it bends, and by an angular measure known as the Cobb angle. The Cobb angle is found by projecting lines parallel to the vertebrae tops at the extremes of the curve; projecting perpendiculars from these lines; and measuring their angle of intersection. To properly track the progress of scoliosis, it is important to project from the same points of the spine each time.

Occasionally, **magnetic resonance imaging** (MRI) is used, primarily to look more closely at the condition of the **spinal cord** and nerve roots extending from it if neurological problems are suspected.

Treatment

Treatment decisions for scoliosis are based on the degree of curvature, the likelihood of significant progression, and the presence of pain, if any.

Curves less than 20 degrees are not usually treated, except by regular follow-up for children who are still growing. Watchful waiting is usually all that is required in adolescents with curves of 20–25 degrees, or adults with curves up to 40 degrees or slightly more, as long as there is no pain.

For children or adolescents whose curves progress to 25 degrees, and who have a year or more of growth left, bracing may be required. Bracing cannot correct curvature, but may be effective in halting or slowing its progression. Bracing is rarely used in adults, except where pain is significant and surgery is not an option, as in some elderly patients.

There are two different categories of braces, those designed for nearly 24-hour daily use and those designed for night use. The full-time brace styles are designed to hold the spine in a vertical position, while the night use braces are designed to bend the spine in the direction opposite the curve.

The Milwaukee brace is a full-time brace which consists of metal uprights attached to pads at the hips, rib cage, and neck. Other types of full-time braces, such as the Boston brace, involve underarm rigid plastic molding to encircle the lower rib cage, **abdomen**, and hips. Because they can be worn out of sight beneath clothing, underarm braces are better tolerated and often lead to better compliance. The Boston brace is currently the most commonly used. Full-time braces are often prescribed to be worn for 22–23 hours per day, though some clinicians believe that recommending brace use of 16 hours leads to better compliance and results.

Night-use braces bend an individual's scoliosis into a correct angle, and are prescribed for eight hours of use during sleep. Some investigators have found that night-use braces are not as effective as the day-use types.

Bracing may be appropriate for scoliosis due to some types of neuromuscular disease, including spinal muscular atrophy, before growth is finished. Duchenne **muscular dystrophy** is not treated by bracing, since surgery is likely to be required, and since later surgery is complicated by loss of respiratory capacity.

KEY TERMS

Cobb angle—A measure of the curvature of scoliosis, determined by measurements made on x rays.

Scoliometer—A tool for measuring trunk asymmetry; it includes a bubble level and angle measure.

Spondylosis—Arthritis of the spine.

Surgery for idiopathic scoliosis is usually recommended if:

• The curve has progressed despite bracing.

• The curve is greater than 40–50 degrees before growth has stopped in an adolescent.

• The curve is greater than 50 degrees and continues to increase in an adult.

• There is significant pain.

Orthopedic surgery for neuromuscular scoliosis is often done early in life. The goals of surgery are to correct the deformity as much as possible, to prevent further deformity, and to eliminate pain as much as possible. Surgery can usually correct 40–50% of the curve, and sometimes as much as 80%. Surgery cannot always completely remove pain.

The surgical procedure for scoliosis is called spinal fusion, because the goal is to straighten the spine as much as possible, and then to fuse the vertebrae together to prevent further curvature. To achieve fusion, the involved vertebra are first exposed, and then scraped to promote re-growth. Bone chips are usually used to splint together the vertebrae to increase the likelihood of fusion. To maintain the proper spinal posture before fusion occurs, metal rods are inserted alongside the spine, and are attached to the vertebrae by hooks, screws, or wires. Fusion of the spine makes it rigid and resistant to further curvature. The metal rods are no longer needed once fusion is complete, but are rarely removed unless their presence leads to complications.

Spinal fusion leaves the involved portion of the spine permanently stiff and inflexible. While this leads to some loss of normal motion, most functional activities are not strongly affected, unless the very lowest portion of the spine (the lumbar region) is fused. Normal mobility, **exercise**, and even contact sports are usually all possible after spinal fusion. Full recovery takes approximately six months.

Prognosis

The prognosis for a person with scoliosis depends on many factors, including the age at which scoliosis begins and the treatment received. Most cases of mild adolescent idiopathic scoliosis need no treatment, do not progress, and do not cause pain or functional limitations. Untreated severe scoliosis often leads to spondylosis, and may impair breathing.

Health care team roles

A pediatrician or family physician usually makes an initial diagnosis of scoliosis. Orthopedic surgeons may provide surgical treatment. Physical therapists may provide therapeutic exercises for a person with scoliosis.

Prevention

There is no known way to prevent any of the forms of scoliosis.

Resources

BOOKS

Canale, S. Terry, Kay Daugherty, and Linda Jones. *Campbell's Operative Orthopaedics,* 9th ed. St. Louis: Mosby, 1998.

Eisenpreis, B. *Coping with Scoliosis.* New York: Rosen Publishing Group, 1999.

Neuwirth, Michael and Kevin Osborn. *Scoliosis Sourcebook,* 2nd ed. Lincolnwood, IL: NTC/Contemporary Publishing, 2001.

Thompson, George H. and Peter V. Scoles "Congenital scoliosis." In *Nelson Textbook of Pediatrics,* 16th ed. Ed. by Richard E. Behrman et al., Philadelphia: Saunders, 2000, 2084–2085.

Thompson, George H. and Peter V. Scoles. "Idiopathic scoliosis." In *Nelson Textbook of Pediatrics,* 16th ed. Ed. by Richard E. Behrman et al., Philadelphia: Saunders, 2000, 2083–2084.

Thompson, George H. and Peter V. Scoles. "Kyphosis." In *Nelson Textbook of Pediatrics,* 16th ed., Ed. by Richard E. Behrman et al., Philadelphia: Saunders, 2000, 2086–2087.

Thompson, George H. and Peter V. Scoles. "Neuromuscular scoliosis, syndromes, and compensatory scoliosis." In *Nelson Textbook of Pediatrics,* 16th ed. Ed. by Richard E. Behrman et al., Philadelphia: Saunders, 2000, 2085–2086.

PERIODICALS

Gross, G.W., and W.G. Mackenzie. "Scoliosis in Children: Surgical Management and Postoperative Radiographic Appearances." *Seminars in Musculoskeletal Radiology* 3, no. 3 (1999): 267–288.

Jason Lowry, K, J. Tobias, D. Kittle, T. Burd, and R.W. Gaines. "Postoperative pain control using epidural catheters after anterior spinal fusion for adolescent scoliosis." *Spine* 26, no. 11 (2001): 1290–1293.

Padua, R., S. Padua, L. Aulisa, E. Ceccarelli, L. Padua, E. Romanini, G. Zanoli, and A. Campi. "Patient outcomes after Harrington instrumentation for idiopathic scoliosis: a 15- to 28-year evaluation." *Spine* 26, no. 11 (2001): 1268–1273.

Redla, S., T. Sikdar, and A. Saifuddin. "Magnetic resonance imaging of scoliosis." *Clinical Radiology* 56, no. 5 (2001): 360–371.

Trivedi, J.M., and J.D. Thomson. "Results of Charleston bracing in skeletally immature patients with idiopathic scoliosis." *Journal of Pediatric Orthopedics* 21, no. 3 (2001): 277–280.

ORGANIZATIONS

American Academy of Orthopedic Surgeons. 6300 North River Road, Rosemont, IL 60018-4262. (847) 823-7186 or (800) 346-2267. Fax: (847) 823-8125. http://www.aaos.org/.

American Academy of Physical Medicine and Rehabilitation. One IBM Plaza, Suite 2500, Chicago, IL 60611-3604. (312) 464-9700. Fax: (312) 464-0227. http://www.aapmr.org/consumers/public/amputations.htm. info@aapmr.org.

American Thoracic Society. 1740 Broadway, New York, NY 10019. (212) 315-8700. Fax: (212) 315-6498. http://www.thoracic.org/.

National Scoliosis Foundation. 5 Cabot Place, Stoughton, MA 02072. (800) 673-6922, or (781) 341-6333. Fax: (781) 341-8333. http://www.scoliosis.org/. nsf@scoliosis.org.

OTHER

American Academy of Family Physicians. http://familydoctor.org/handouts/107.html.

American Academy of Orthopedic Surgeons. http://orthoinfo.aaos.org/brochure/thr_report.cfm?Thread_ID=14&topcategory=Spine.

National Institute of Arthritis and Musculoskeletal and Skin Diseases. http://www.nih.gov/niams/healthinfo/scochild.htm.

Nemours Foundation. http://kidshealth.org/teen/health_problems/diseases/scoliosis.html.

Scoliosis Association, Inc. http://www.scoliosis-assoc.org

Scoliosis Research Society. http://www.srs.org.

University of Iowa Hospitals. http://www.vh.org/Providers/Textbooks/AIS/AIS.html.

L. Fleming Fallon, Jr., M.D., Dr.P.H.

Scrotal nuclear medicine scan

Definition

Scrotal nuclear medicine scan is a study of the tissues in the scrotum, using a radioactive contrast agent to identify masses, **blood** flow, and areas of **infection**.

Purpose

The scrotal nuclear medicine scan is used to assess blood flow within the testicles and damage caused by injury. It is also used to ascertain the cause of swollen testes (testicles) which may be due to infection or the twisting of the entire tissues of the testicle. This is done in an emergency setting if the testicle swells suddenly and painfully.

This scan can be used to diagnose tumors and cysts (pockets of fluid), but testicular ultrasound has become the diagnostic tool of choice for these growths.

Precautions

There are no precautions with a scrotal nuclear medicine scan, except that the patient must remain still during the procedure.

Description

A radioisotope, technetium-99, combined with a chemical (pertechnate) is injected intravenously while the patient is under a gamma camera that detects radiation. This special camera scans the scrotum at one minute intervals for about five minutes, then less often for another 10 or 15 minutes. It then creates pictures (either x ray or Polaroid) that reveal where the isotope is in the scrotum. Because both sides of the scrotum are scanned, even greater accuracy is obtained by comparison.

Some areas accumulate the tracer in greater than normal amounts. These are called hot spots and may indicate tumors or other masses. Areas that have less than normal amounts of the tracer or none at all are called cold spots and may indicated cysts or infection.

It is important to differentiate infection from twisting torsion and infection. A common infection called **epididymitis** involves a collection of tubules on top of the testicle called the epididymis that carry sperm. Twisting of the spermatic cord inside the scrotum, outside the testicle often shuts off the testes' blood supply and is called **testicular torsion**. Both conditions cause a very painful, swollen testicle on one side of the scrotum. Epididymitis and testicular torsion occur most often in young men, although infection usually occurs at a slightly older age. Infection increases the blood supply, showing up as a "hot" spot on the scan, whereas testicular torsion cuts off the blood supply, appearing as a "cold" spot. The distinction is critically important, because testicular torsion must be untwisted immediately by surgery or the testicle will die. On the other hand, epididymitis responds to **antibiotics**, and surgery might further injure it.

KEY TERMS

Epididymitis—A common infection involving a collection of tubules on top of the testicle called the epididymis that carry sperm.

Radioisotope—An unstable form of an element that gives off radiation to become stable.

Scrotum—The bag of skin below the penis that contains the testes.

Testicular torsion—A condition involving the twisting of the spermatic cord inside the testicle that shuts off its blood supply and can seriously damage the testicle.

After the patient has changed into gown, he will lie on a scanning table. The penis will be taped to the **abdomen** to prevent it from shadowing the scan. A towel may be used to support the testicles during the test. The tracer will be injected into a vein on the inside of the elbow, and the camera will begin taking pictures of the testicles. It is important that the patient remain still during the scans.

Two complete passes are made about 15 minutes apart. The total scrotal scan takes about 45 minutes.

Preparation

There is no preparation prior to a scrotal nuclear medicine scan. The day of the test, the patient will need to remove any jewelry, watches, and metal (e.g., belts, hairpins) and change into a gown.

Aftercare

The patient should be able to go about normal activities after the scan. However, if surgery is performed immediately after the scan, normal post-surgical precautions should be undertaken.

Complications

The risk of complications is minimal due to the small amount of radiation to which the body is exposed. Even sensitive testicular tissue is at minimum risk. The tracer is eliminated from the body within 24 hours, and allergic reactions to the tracer are rare.

Results

Results are usually available in two days. In an emergency, results are made available in one hour.

Normal results show unobstructed blood flow with no "hot" or "cold" spots. Abnormal results are shown in the scan images as:

- "Hot" spots, where the tracer accumulates in greater amounts than normal, can indicate epididymitis or a tumor.

- "Cold" spots have no accumulation of the tracer or very little. These may point to cysts, abscesses, or blood clots.

- Blood flow is uneven throughout the testicles. This indicates a narrowing or blockage of the blood vessels, including from torsion, or possibly direct damage from injury. Sometimes the blood flow pattern appears in a "doughnut" shape, which suggests that testicular torsion has occurred but that it has resolved itself within the last few days.

Abnormal results may require further investigation through other tests, such as testicular biopsy or ultrasound.

Health care team roles

The nuclear medicine technologist will need to educate the patient about the procedure (for example, how the scan is done, what happens during it, what kinds of information the scan can produce for the doctor). This is very necessary to keep the patient informed and to ensure cooperation during the procedure. It is crucial that the patient remain still during the scan.

The nuclear medicine technologist who performs the scrotal scan will need to reassure the patient before and during the scan in order to keep the patient relaxed and still during the scan.

Resources

BOOKS

Rajfer, Jacob. "Congenital Anomalies of the Testes and Scrotum." In *Campbell's Urology*, edited by Patrick C. Walsh, et al. Philadelphia: W.B. Saunders, 1998, pp. 2184–2186.

Rozauski, Thomas, et al. "Surgery of the Scrotum and Testis in Children." In *Campbell's Urology*, edited by Patrick C. Walsh, et al. Philadelphia: W.B. Saunders, 1998, pp. 2200–2202.

OTHER

Nissl, Jan. "Testicular Scan." Health Library. Altru Health Systems. April 18, 2005 (April 18, 2006). http://www.altru.org/library/healthguide/en-us/Medicaltests/topic.asp?hwid=hw234999&.

Janie F. Franz

Scrotal ultrasound

Definition

Scrotal ultrasound is an imaging technique used for the diagnosis of suspected abnormalities of the scrotum and testes. It uses harmless, high-frequency sound waves to form an image. The sound waves are reflected by scrotal tissue to form a picture of internal structures. It is not invasive and involves no radiation.

Purpose

Ultrasound of the scrotum is the primary imaging method used to evaluate disorders of the testicles and surrounding tissues. It is used when a man has acute **pain** in the scrotum. Some of the medical problems for which the use of scrotal ultrasound is valuable include an absent or undescended testicle, inflammation of the testicle or associated structures, **testicular torsion**, a fluid collection (hydrocele), abnormal **blood vessels** (varicocele), or a mass (lump or tumor).

A sudden onset of pain in the scrotum is considered a serious problem. Delay in diagnosis and treatment can lead to loss of function. **Epididymitis** is the most common cause of this type of pain. Epididymitis is an inflammation of the epididymis, a tubular structure that transports sperm from the testes. It is most often caused by bacterial **infection**, but may occur after injury, or arise from an unknown cause. Epididymitis is treatable with **antibiotics**, which usually resolves pain quickly and ice to reduce swelling. Left untreated, this condition can lead to **abscess** formation or loss of **blood** supply to the testicle. The latter condition can cause testicular loss.

Testicular torsion is the twisting of the spermatic cord that containing the blood vessels that supply the testicles. It is caused by abnormally loose attachments of tissues that are formed during **fetal development**. Torsion can be complete, incomplete, or intermittent. Spontaneous detorsion, or untwisting, can occur, making diagnosis difficult. Testicular torsion arises most commonly during adolescence, and is acutely painful. Scrotal ultrasound is used to distinguish this condition from inflammatory problems, such as epididymitis. Testicular torsion is a surgical emergency; it should be operated on as soon as possible to avoid permanent damage to the testes.

A scrotal sac with an absent testicle may be the result of a congenital anomaly (an abnormality present at birth), where a testicle fails to develop. More often, it is due to an undescended testicle. In the fetus, the testicles normally develop just outside the **abdomen** and descend into the scrotum during the seventh month. Approximately 3% of full term baby boys have undescended testicles. It is important to distinguish between an undescended testicle and an absent testicle, as an undescended testicle has a very high probability of developing **cancer** if left untreated.

Ultrasound can be used to locate and evaluate masses in the scrotum. Most masses within the testicle are malignant or cancerous, and most outside the testicle are benign. Primary cancer of the testicles is the most common malignancy in men between the ages of 20 and 35. Fluid collections and abnormalities of the blood vessels in the scrotum may appear to the physician as masses and need evaluation by ultrasound. A hydrocele, the most common cause of painless scrotal swelling, is a collection of fluid between two layers of tissue surrounding the testicle. An abnormal enlargement of the veins which drain the testicles is called a varicocele. It can cause discomfort and swelling, which can be examined by touch (palpated). Varicocele is a common cause of male **infertility**, and is more common on the left testicle.

Precautions

Clear scrotal ultrasound images are difficult to obtain if a person is unable to remain still. Other than cleaning the surface of the skin upon which a transducer will be placed, there are no special precautions that are associated with **ultrasonography**.

Description

A transducer (an electronic imaging device) is used to both generate and receive acoustic images. It is placed against the skin over the structure to be examined. The transducer is moved over the area creating images from reflected sound waves, which appear on a monitor screen. There is no discomfort from the study itself. However, if the scrotum is very tender, even the slight pressure involved may be painful.

Preparation

The patient lies on his back on an examining table. The technologist will usually take a history of the problem, then gently palpate the scrotum. A rolled towel is placed between the patient's legs to support the scrotum. The penis is lifted up onto the abdomen and covered. A gel that enhances sound transmission is applied directly on the scrotum. The technologist then gently places a transducer (an electronic imaging device) against the skin.

KEY TERMS

Epididymis—A tubular structure that transports sperm from the testes to the vas defens, which transports it to the prostate gland.

Hydrocele—A collection of fluid between two layers of tissue surrounding the testicle; the most common cause of painless scrotal swelling.

Scrotum—The structure of skin that surrounds and protects the testicles.

Testicular torsion—A twisting of the spermatic cord that containing the blood vessels supplying the testicles.

Varicocele—An abnormal enlargement of the veins which drain the testicles.

Aftercare

The transducing gel is removed with soap and water. Any underlying medical condition is treated. There is no aftercare for the scrotal ultrasound examination.

Complications

There are no complications associated with ultrasonography.

Results

A normal study reveals testicles of normal size and shape, with no masses or abnormalities.

An abnormal result of an ultrasound of the scrotum may reveal an absent or undescended testicle, an inflammation problem, testicular torsion, a fluid collection, abnormal blood vessels, or a mass.

Health care team roles

A family physician, pediatrician, urologist, or emergency room doctor usually orders a scrotal ultrasound examination. An ultrasonographer or radiologist performs the examination. A radiologist interprets the images obtained.

Resources

BOOKS

Allan, Paul L. et al. *Clinical Doppler Ultrasound, 2nd edition* London: Churchill Livingstone, 2006.

Evans, David H., and W. N. McDicken. *Doppler Ultrasound: Physics, Instrumental, and Clinical Applications,* 2nd ed. New York: Wiley, 2000.

Gill, Katheryn A. *Abdominal Ultrasound: A Practitioner's Guide.* Philadelphia: Saunders, 2001.

Hofer, Matthias, and Stanley Platypus. *Teaching Manual of Color Duplex Sonography.* New York: Thieme Medical Publishers, 2001.

Kurjak, Asim, and Sanja Jupesic. *Clinical Application of 3D Sonography.* Pearl River, NY: Parthenon Publishing Group, 2000.

Papadakis, Emmanuel. *Ultrasonic Instruments and Devices: Reference for Modern Instrumentation, Techniques, and Technology.* New York: Academic Press, 2000.

PERIODICALS

Frauscher F., A. Klauser, A. Stenzl, G. Helweg, B. Amort, and D. zur Nedden. "Ultrasound findings in the scrotum of extreme mountain bikers." *Radiology* 219, no. 2 (2001): 427–431.

Gordon, S.J., U. Otite, P. Maheshkumar, P. Cannon, and V. H. Nargund. "The use of scrotal ultrasonography in male infertility." *British Journal of Ultrasonography International* 87, no. 4 (2001): 417–418.

Simon, S.D., R.D. Lee, and J.P. Mulhall. "Should all infertile males undergo urologic evaluation before assisted reproductive technologies? Two cases of testicular cancer presenting with infertility." *Fertility and Sterility* 75, no. 6 (2001): 1226–1227.

OTHER

Medical College of Georgia. http://www.mcghealthcare. org/radiology/ultra/ultra.htm.

Scrotal Ultrasound pictures. http://www.gemedical systems. com/rad/us/products/log_700pro/msu302.html and http://www.gemedicalsystems. com/rad/us/products/log_700pro/ msu301.html and http://ultrasound.ucsf.edu/scrotal.html and http://www.drgdiaz.com/pat/scrotal_hernia.shtml.

University of Iowa. http://www.vh.org/Providers/Lectures/ IROCH/ScrotalUS/Captions/UStwo34.html.

University of Maryland College of Medicine. http://www.umm. edu/radiology/ultra.htm.

University of Michigan College of Medicine. http://www.med. umich.edu/1libr/tests/testu08.htm.

ORGANIZATIONS

American College of Radiology. 1891 Preston White Drive, Reston, VA 20191. (703) 648-8900. Fax: (703) 262-9319. http://www.acr.org. info@acr.org.

American Foundation for Urologic Disease. 1128 North Charles Street, Baltimore, MD 21201. (800) 242-2383 or (410) 468-1800. http://www.afud.org. admin@afud.org.

American Infertility Association. 666 Fifth Avenue, Suite 278, New York, NY 10103. (718) 621-5083. http://www. americaninfertility.org/. info@americaninfertility.org.

American Institute of Ultrasound In Medicine. 14750 Sweitzer Lane, Suite 100, Laurel, Maryland 20707-5906. (301) 498-4100 or (800) 638-5352. Fax: (301) 498-4450. http://www.aium.org/.

American Osteopathic College of Radiology. 119 East Second St, Milan, MO 63556. (660) 265-4011. Fax: (660) 265-3494. http://www.aocr.org/. aocr@nemr.net.

American Registry of Diagnostic Medical Sonographers. 600 Jefferson Plaza, Suite 360, Rockville, Maryland 20852-1150. (301) 738-8401 or (800) 541-9754. Fax: (301) 738-0312/0313. http://www.ardms.org.

American Urological Association. 1120 North Charles Street, Baltimore, MD 21201. (410) 727-1100. Fax: (410) 223-4370. http://www.auanet.org/index_hi.cfm. aua@auanet.org.

Society of Radiologists in Ultrasound. 44211 Slatestone Court, Leesburg, VA 20176-5109. (703) 858-9210. Fax: (703) 729-4839. http://www.sru.org/. info@sru.org.

L. Fleming Fallon, Jr., M.D., Dr.P.H.

Sedimentation rate test

Definition

The sedimentation rate test, also called the erythrocyte sedimentation rate (ESR) or sed rate test, measures the speed at which the red **blood** cells (erythrocytes or RBCs) separate from the liquid part of the blood (plasma) and settle to the bottom in a tube of anticoagulated blood.

Purpose

The sedimentation rate is a non-specific indicator of the presence of inflammation or **infection**. Although newer methods for diagnosing specific diseases have decreased the test's usefulness, it is still an important tool for the diagnosis and monitoring of two diseases: polymyalgia rheumatica and temporal arteritis. Sedimentation rate testing at regular intervals can also be helpful in predicting relapse in patients with chronic diseases such as Hodgkin's disease and other cancers.

Precautions

Patients who have **bleeding disorders** or are taking blood thinners might have trouble with bleeding following a venipuncture. Before having a blood sample drawn, such patients should tell the phlebotomist about their condition.

Description

The sedimentation rate test dates back to the early 1900s. In 1921, Westergren introduced a new method for performing the test that has become the time-honored classic. It is the recommended method of the International Committee for Standardization in Haematology and the National Committee for Clinical Laboratory Science. While automated methods can perform the sed rate in less time and with smaller samples of blood, many labs continue to use the Westergren method because it is simple and inexpensive.

For accurate results, the blood sample should be fresh (within two hours of collection is best). The sample might be rejected because it is too old or because the collection tube is underfilled, not labeled correctly, or contains blood that is hemolyzed or clotted.

The standard Westergren method includes the following steps:

- Diluting whole blood, or blood anticoagulated with EDTA, in citrate (1 volume of citrate to 4 volumes of blood).
- Aspirating the diluted blood to the 200 mm mark of a Westergren tube (30 cm in length and 2.55 mm in diameter with a uniform bore diameter) by means of a mechanical device or teat.
- Placing the tube in a vertical position in a Westergren rack in a location that is free of vibration and that is not exposed to direct sunlight.
- After exactly one hour, reading the distance the erythrocytes have fallen, and recording this value as the sedimentation rate.

Preparation

This test requires no special preparation.

Aftercare

To prevent bruising, pressure should be applied to the site of the venipuncture as soon as the needle is withdrawn. Pressure should be maintained until the bleeding stops.

Complications

No complications are associated with this test other than the possibility of having a slight bruise from having blood drawn from a vein. In very rare cases, vein inflammation or continued bleeding at the puncture site might be a problem.

Results

The sedimentation rate is measured in millimeters per hour (mm/hr). Normal values vary with age and sex, and can vary from lab to lab. A normal result does not rule out a diagnosis of inflammatory disease. An abnormal result does not diagnose any specific disease,

KEY TERMS

Arteritis—The inflammation of an artery.

Aspirate (verb)—To draw or move by suction.

Phlebotomist—A person who draws blood from a vein.

Phlebotomy—A procedure in which a vein is punctured to obtain a blood sample.

Polymyalgia rheumatica—A disease that causes aching and stiffness in the neck, shoulder, or pelvis.

Temporal (giant cell) arteritis—A disease caused by arterial inflammation that usually results in headaches and facial pain. The production of giant cells is characteristic of this type of arteritis. If the ophthalmic artery and its branches become involved, it can also cause blindness.

Venipuncture—The puncture of a vein to withdraw a blood sample.

and should be evaluated in conjunction with the patient's physical exam, medical history, and other more specific blood tests. In general, an abnormal result correlates with active inflammatory disease, and the sedimentation rate test is a useful way of monitoring disease progression or treatment. If the result is abnormal, the test should be repeated to verify its accuracy. A number of factors (such as medications, hormones, **obesity**, and improper collection or handling of the blood sample) can affect the outcome of this test.

Normal values

• Males under 50: 0 to 15 mm/hr.

• Males 50 and older: 0 to 20 mm/hr.

• Females under 50: 0 to 20 mm/hr.

• Females 50 and older: 0 to 30 mm/hr.

• Children: 3 to 13 mm/hr.

• Newborns: 0 to 2 mm/hr.

Greater than normal values

A greater than normal value can indicate inflammation due to infection, autoimmune disease (such as **rheumatoid arthritis**), or certain types of **cancer** (such as **multiple myeloma** and Hodgkin's disease). An elevated sed rate usually occurs when the level of plasma **proteins** in the blood is higher than normal. These plasma proteins (primarily fibrinogen) bind to the red blood cells, reducing the negative surface charge which normally causes the cells to repel each other. The red blood cells stack and settle to bottom of the tube faster than single red blood cells.

Lower than normal values

A lower than normal value can indicate diseases such as congestive **heart failure**, sickle cell anemia, and polycythemia (abnormally high numbers of circulating red blood cells).

Health care team roles

A phlebotomist usually draws and labels the blood sample for the sedimentation rate. However, any health care professionals trained in **phlebotomy** (such as doctors, nurses, clinical laboratory scientists, or medical technologists) can perform this task.

When the blood sample arrives at the lab, a clinical laboratory scientist (CLS [NCA]), medical technologist (MT [ASCP]), clinical laboratory technician (CLT [NCA]), or medical laboratory technician (MLT [ASCP]) will set up the test and record the sedimentation rate after the specified period of time, usually one hour.

Resources

BOOKS

University of Texas Medical Branch Department of Pathology. *Laboratory Survival Guide.* December 2001.

Zaret, Barry L, Peter I. Jatlow, and Lee D. Katz, eds. *The Yale University School of Medicine Patient's Guide to Medical Tests.* Boston, MA: Houghton Mifflin. 1997.

PERIODICAL

Bridgen, Malcolm L. "Clinical Utility of the Erythrocyte Sedimentation Rate." *American Family Physician* 60, no. 5 (October 1999): 1443.

OTHER

Cornett, Patricia. "Sedimentation Rate." Reader's Digest Health. 2000. http://www.rdhealth.com/kbase/topic/medtest/hw43353/descrip.htm (January 23, 1998).

"Guideline: Laboratory Medicine: Number 1403 Erythrocyte Sedimentation Rate." The College of Physicians and Surgeons of Manitoba College On the Web. (1999). http://www.umanitoba.ca/cgi-bin/colleges/cps/college.cgi/1403.html (May 1999).

Kramer, Robert J. "Sedimentation Rate." MyHeartDr: Heart Health Encyclopedia 2001. http://www.heartcenteronline.com/ (October 11, 2000).

MedTech1-Information on Medical Technology Solutions. 125 Cambridge Park Drive, Cambridge, MA 02140. http://medtech1.com.

Yale Medical Test Guide. 2001. http://webmd.com.

ORGANIZATION

Yale University School of Medicine. 367 Cedar Street, New Haven, CT 06510. (203) 785-2643. http://www.info. med. yale.edu/ysm/ysminfo/index.html.

Beverly G. Miller, MT(ASCP)

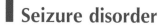

Seizure disorder

Definition

Seizure disorders are a group of neurological disorders characterized by sudden disruption of the brain's normal electrical activity, accompanied by an alteration in consciousness or other neurological and behavioral manifestations. Instead of the normal pattern of signal transmission in the **brain**, the nerve cells misfire as many as 500 times a second, which is much faster than their usual rate. The affected person's symptoms may range from a few seconds of blank staring to several minutes of convulsions (repetitive jerking or twitching of the body), loss of consciousness, or muscle spasms. Epilepsy is a condition characterized by recurrent seizures that may include convulsions.

It is important to keep in mind that seizure disorder is not caused by a psychiatric disorder or by mental retardation. While some mentally retarded people do have seizures, having seizures does not mean that the affected person is or will become mentally retarded.

Description

Demographics

Doctors estimate that about 1 person in every 100 around the world, or about 50 million people in all, has a seizure disorder. In the United States, there are about 3 million people with seizure disorder as of 2012; about 200,000 people are diagnosed with seizure disorder each year, 45,000 of them children below the age of 15. There is no apparent cause of the seizures in over half of newly diagnosed cases. About half of newly diagnosed patients have generalized seizures. Generalized seizures are more common in children under the age of 10 than in adults. In some developing countries, parasitic infections account for an increased incidence of seizures and epilepsy.

Historical background

Seizure disorder has been known to doctors for thousands of years. The loss of control, strange

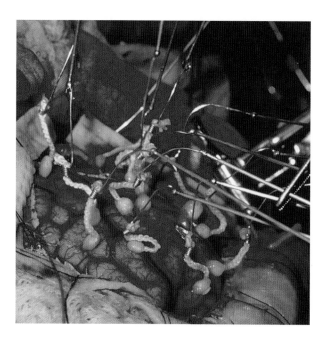

(Seizure disorder, surgery-resection of mass, photograph. Custom Medical Stock Photo. Reproduced by permission.)

movements, and unpredictable behaviors of people having seizures caused some ancient Babylonian writers to wonder whether these patients were possessed by gods or demons. An ancient Egyptian medical papyrus reported the case of a man who developed seizures after a **head injury**. Hippocrates in the fifth century BC attributed seizures to a problem within the brain. His insight proved to be correct. It was not until the 1870s, however, that medical researchers in Europe were able to demonstrate from animal studies that seizures result from abnormal electrical activity in the brain. The first measurement of electrical signals in the human brain by attaching electrodes to the scalp was made in 1929; this was the first electroencephalogram or EEG. **Electroencephalography** allowed doctors to make a systematic classification of seizure disorders.

In 1964, the Commission on Classification and Terminology of the International League against Epilepsy (ILAE) devised the first official classification of seizures, which was revised in 1981, 1989, and 2005–2009. The commission has proposed to use a diagnostic scheme of five diagnostic levels or axes rather than a classification scheme for characterizing seizures. These axes are (1) the events that occur during the seizure; (2) the type of seizure, chosen from a list that can include where the seizure localizes in the brain and what stimulates it; (3) the type of epileptic syndrome most closely associated with the seizure; (4) the underlying medical or other causes of the syndrome; and (5) the level of impairment the seizure causes. These are proposed recommendations that are still under discussion.

Types of seizures

The older ILAE classification, meanwhile, is accepted worldwide and is based on electroencephalographic (EEG) studies. This system classifies seizures as either focal or generalized. Each of these categories can be further subdivided.

Focal seizures

The human brain has two cerebral hemispheres, a right and a left hemisphere. A focal or partial seizure develops when a small number of nerve cells fire their impulses abnormally within one hemisphere of the brain. Focal seizures are divided into simple or complex based on the level of consciousness (wakefulness) during an attack. Simple partial seizures occur in patients who are conscious, whereas complex partial seizures demonstrate impaired **levels of consciousness**. About 60 percent of people with epilepsy have focal seizures.

Generalized seizures

A generalized seizure results from initial abnormal firing of brain nerve cells throughout both the left and right hemispheres. Generalized seizures can be classified as follows:

- Tonic-clonic seizures: This is the most common type among all age groups and is categorized into several phases beginning with vague symptoms that appear hours or days before an attack. These seizures are sometimes called grand mal seizures.
- Tonic seizures: These are typically characterized by a sustained nonvibratory contraction of muscles in the legs and arms. Consciousness is also impaired during these episodes.
- Atonic seizures (also called drop attacks): These are characterized by sudden, limp posture and a brief period of unconsciousness; they last for one to two seconds.
- Clonic seizures: These are characterized by a rapid loss of consciousness with loss of muscle tone, tonic spasms, and jerks. The muscles become rigid for about 30 seconds during the tonic phase of the seizure and alternately contract and relax during the clonic phase, which lasts 30–60 seconds.
- Absence seizures: These are subdivided into typical and atypical forms based on duration of attack and level of consciousness. Absence (petit mal) seizures generally begin at about the age of four and stop by the time the child becomes an adolescent. They usually begin with a brief loss of consciousness and last 1 to 10 seconds.

People having petit mal seizures become very quiet and may blink, stare blankly, roll their eyes, or move their lips. A petit mal seizure lasts 15 to 20 seconds. When it ends, individuals resume whatever they were doing before the seizure began, will not remember the seizure, and may not realize that anything unusual happened. Untreated, petit mal seizures can recur as many as 100 times a day and may progress to grand mal seizures.

- Myoclonic seizures: These are characterized by rapid muscular contractions accompanied with jerking movements in the facial and pelvic muscles.

Subcategories are commonly diagnosed based on electroencephalographic (EEG) results. Terminology for the classification of seizures in infants and newborns is still controversial.

It is possible for a person with seizure disorder to have more than one type of seizure.

Some people with seizure disorder find that their seizures are triggered by certain conditions or activities while others do not have recognizable triggers. The most common trigger for a seizure is failure to take prescribed antiseizure medication. Other triggers include heavy drinking, lack of sleep, emotional **stress**, or (in women) hormonal changes associated with the menstrual cycle. Seizure triggers do not cause seizures in the strict sense, they simply set them off.

Most seizures are benign, but a seizure that lasts a long time can lead to status epilepticus, a life-threatening condition characterized by continuous seizures, sustained loss of consciousness, and respiratory distress. Nonconvulsive epilepsy can impair physical coordination, **vision**, and other senses. Undiagnosed seizures can lead to conditions that are more serious and more difficult to manage.

Causes and symptoms

Causes

Seizure disorder can have a number of different possible causes. Genetic factors have long been suspected; researchers at the National Institute of Neurological Disorders and **Stroke** (NINDS) estimate that as many as 500 different genes may be involved in some way in seizure disorders, but it is clear as of 2012 that genes play only a partial role. Genetic factors do, however, appear to affect a person's susceptibility to seizures, or seizure threshold. A few rare types of epilepsy have been traced to specific genes; a few other types are known to run in families even though they have not been linked to specific genes.

In some cases, people develop seizures as a result of Alzheimer disease, alcohol abuse, brain tumors, **AIDS**, and other infectious diseases that affect the brain, including measles, mumps, and diphtheria. Other possible causes include head injuries, **cerebral palsy**, and **autism**. In about 50 to 70 percent of cases, however, doctors cannot identify a specific cause of the patient's seizure disorder.

Less common causes of epilepsy include:

• A brain abscess or inflammation of the meninges (membranes covering the brain or spinal cord)

• Phenylketonuria (PKU). A disease that is present at birth, PKU is often characterized by seizures, and can result in mental retardation and other inherited disorders.

• Lead poisoning, mercury poisoning, carbon monoxide poisoning, or ingestion of some other poisonous substance

Simple partial seizures can be caused by congenital abnormalities (abnormalities present at birth), tumor growths, head trauma, stroke, and infections of the brain or nearby structures. Generalized tonic-clonic seizures are associated with drug and alcohol abuse, and low levels of **blood** glucose (blood sugar) and sodium. Certain psychiatric medications, **antihistamines**, and even **antibiotics** can precipitate tonic-clonic seizures. Absence seizures are implicated with an imbalance of certain chemicals in the brain that modulate nerve cell activity (one of these neurotransmitters is called gamma-aminobutyric acid or GABA, which functions as an inhibitor). Myoclonic seizures are commonly diagnosed in newborns and children.

Status epilepticus, a life-threatening condition in which a person suffers from continuous seizures and may have trouble breathing, can be caused by:

• Sudden discontinuance of antiseizure medication

• Hypoxic or metabolic encephalopathy (brain disease resulting from lack of oxygen or malfunctioning of other physical or chemical processes)

• Acute head injury

• Blood infection caused by inflammation of the brain or the membranes that cover it.

Risk factors

Risk factors for seizure disorder include:

• Age: Children younger than 2 years and adults over 65 are more likely to develop the condition.

• Sex: Males are slightly more likely to develop seizure disorder than females.

• Race: African Americans are more likely to develop seizure disorder than members of other racial groups.

• Personal history of head injury.

The rate of seizure disorder is higher in people with other disorders that affect the nervous system:

• 10 percent of patients with Alzheimer's disease

• 22 percent of patients with stroke

• 10 percent of children with cerebral palsy

• 10 percent of children with mental retardation

• 8.7 percent of children whose mothers have seizure disorder

• 2.4 percent of children whose fathers have seizure disorder

Symptoms

Symptoms for the different types of seizures are specific.

PARTIAL SEIZURES. Simple partial seizures: Multiple signs and symptoms may be present during a single simple partial seizure. These symptoms include specific muscles tensing and then alternately contracting and relaxing, speech arrest, vocalizations, and involuntary turning of the eyes or head. There could be changes in vision, **hearing**, balance, **taste**, and **smell**. In addition, patients with simple partial seizures may have a cramping sensation in the **abdomen**, sweating, paleness, flushing, hair follicles standing up (piloerection), and dilated pupils (the dark center in the eye enlarges). Seizures with psychological symptoms include thinking disturbances and hallucinations, or illusions of **memory**, sound, sight, time, and self-image.

Complex partial seizures. Complex partial seizures often begin with a motionless stare or arrest of activity; this is followed by a series of involuntary movements, speech disturbances, and eye movements.

GENERALIZED SEIZURES. Generalized seizures have a more complex set of signs and symptoms.

Tonic-clonic seizures. Tonic-clonic seizures usually have vague prodromal (warning) symptoms that can start hours or days before a seizure. These symptoms include **anxiety**, mood changes, irritability, **weakness**, **dizziness**, lightheadedness, and changes in appetite. The tonic phases may be preceded by brief muscle contractions on both sides of affected muscle groups. The tonic phase typically begins with a brief flexing of trunk muscles, upward movement of the eyes, and pupil dilation. Patients usually emit a characteristic outcry. This sound is caused by contraction of trunk muscles that forces air from the **lungs** across abnormally tensed throat muscles. This sound is followed by a very short period (10–15 seconds) of general muscle **relaxation**. The clonic phase consists of muscular contractions with alternating periods of no movements (muscle atonia) that gradually increase in length until the abnormal muscular contractions stop. Tonic-clonic seizures end in a final generalized spasm. The affected person can lose consciousness during the tonic and clonic phases of the seizure.

Tonic-clonic seizures can also produce chemical changes in the body. Patients commonly experience lowered levels of carbon dioxide (hypocarbia) due to breathing alterations; increased levels of blood glucose (blood sugar); and an elevated level of a hormone called prolactin. Once affected people regain consciousness, they are usually weak, and have a **headache** and muscle **pain**. Tonic-clonic seizures can cause such serious medical problems as trauma to the head and mouth, **fractures** in the spinal column, pulmonary **edema** (water in the lungs), aspiration **pneumonia** (a pneumonia caused by a foreign body being lodged in the lungs), and sudden death. Attacks are generally one minute in duration.

Tonic seizures. Tonic and atonic seizures have distinct differences but are often present in the same patient. Tonic seizures are characterized by nonvibratory muscle contractions, usually involving flexing of the arms and relaxing or flexing of the legs. The seizure usually lasts less than 10 seconds but may be as long as one minute. Tonic seizures are usually abrupt and patients lose consciousness. Tonic seizures commonly occur during nonrapid eye movement (non-REM) sleep and drowsiness. Tonic seizures that occur during wakeful states commonly produce physical injuries due to abrupt and unexpected **falls**.

Atonic seizures. Atonic seizures, also called drop attacks, are abrupt, with loss of muscle tone lasting one to two seconds, but with rapid recovery. Consciousness is usually impaired. The rapid loss of muscular tone may be limited to head and neck muscles, resulting in the head drooping, or it may be more extensive, involving the muscles needed for balance, causing unexpected falls with physical injury.

Clonic seizures. Generalized clonic seizures are rare and seen typically in children with elevated **fever**. These seizures are characterized by a rapid loss of consciousness, decreased muscle tone, and a generalized spasm that is followed by jerky movements.

Absence seizures. Absence seizures are classified as either typical or atypical. The typical absence seizure is characterized by unresponsiveness, behavioral arrest, and abnormal muscular movements of the face and eyelids. It lasts less than 10 seconds. In atypical absence seizures, the affected person is generally more conscious, the seizures begin and end more gradually, and do not exceed 10 seconds in duration.

Myoclonic seizures. People with myoclonic seizures commonly exhibit rapid muscular contractions. Myoclonic seizures are seen in newborns and children who have either symptomatic or idiopathic (unknown cause) epilepsy.

Diagnosis

The diagnosis of seizure disorder can be difficult because the doctor will first of all need to find out whether the patient's seizure is their first or whether they have had others in the recent past. A first seizure can be caused by **meningitis**, **encephalitis**, or a stroke, and needs emergency attention. In other cases the person having the seizure may not remember what happened when they return to normal consciousness and the doctor will have to ask a family member or bystander to describe the patient's symptoms and whether they have had previous seizures.

If the patient does not need emergency medical treatment for a head injury or acute **infection**, the next step in diagnosis is a neurological examination. The doctor will test the patient's **reflexes**, sight, hearing, muscle tone, gait, posture, balance, coordination, and ability to talk normally and answer simple questions.

The specific laboratory tests and imaging studies that may be ordered depend on the specific symptoms associated with the seizure:

- Blood and urine tests. These are done to look for evidence of infection, diabetes, or anemia. A complete blood count (CBC) can be helpful in determining whether a seizure is caused by a neurological infection, which is typically accompanied by high fever. If drugs or toxins in the blood are suspected to be the cause of the seizure(s), blood and urine screening tests for these compounds may be necessary.

- Lumbar puncture. In some cases a lumbar puncture, also known as a spinal tap, will be performed to rule out meningitis or another infectious disease.

- Electroencephalogram (EEG). This test is the main test used to diagnose epilepsy. EEGs are performed with electrodes placed on or within the skull to record the brain's electrical activity and pinpoint the exact location of abnormal discharges. A person may be asked to remain motionless during a short-term EEG or to go about normal activities during extended monitoring. Some people are deprived of sleep or exposed to such seizure triggers as rapid deep breathing (hyperventilation) or flashing lights (photic stimulation). In some cases, people may be hospitalized for EEG monitoring that can last as long as two weeks. Video EEGs also document what an individual was doing when the seizure occurred and how the seizure altered the patient's behavior. In some types of seizure disorder, the patient's brain waves will be abnormal even when they are not having a seizure.

- Computed tomography (CT) scan, magnetic resonance imaging (MRI), positron emission tomography (PET), or single photon emission tomography (SPECT) scans of the head. These studies can identify brain tumors, evidence of a stroke, or other structural abnormalities of the brain. PET and SPECT can also be used to identify the parts of the brain responsible for focal seizures.

The last step in diagnosis is using the test results to determine which type of seizure disorder the patient has and if possible, the likely cause of the seizures. Identifying the type of seizure involved helps to guide treatment decisions.

Treatment

The goal of epilepsy treatment is to eliminate seizures or make the symptoms less frequent and less severe. Long-term anticonvulsant drug therapy is the most common form of epilepsy treatment.

Drugs

Anticonvulsants (antiseizure medications) are the first line of treatment for seizure disorder. Most patients need only one medication, but some may need a combination of two or more. It may take several trials of different drugs for the doctor to find which one works best for the patient and what dosage is most effective.

There are a number of different drugs used to treat seizure disorder. Simple and complex partial seizures respond to such drugs as carbamazepine, valproic acid (valproate), phenytoin, gabapentin, tiagabine, lamotrigine, and topiramate. Tonic-clonic seizures tend to respond to valproate, carbamazepine, phenytoin, and lamotrigine. Absence seizures seem to be sensitive to ethosuximide, valproate, and lamotrigine. Myoclonic seizures can be treated with valproate and clonazepam. Tonic seizures seem to respond favorably to valproate, felbamate, and clonazepam.

People treated with a class of medications called barbiturates (Mysoline, Mebral, phenobarbital) sometimes have adverse effects on their cognition (thinking). These cognitive effects can include decreased general intelligence, attention, memory, problem solving, motor speed, and visual motor functions. The drug phenytoin (Dilantin) can adversely affect the speed of response, memory, and attention. Other medications used for treatment of seizures do not appear to impair cognition.

Even a person whose seizures are well controlled should have regular blood tests to measure levels of antiseizure medication in the blood stream and to check to see whether the medication is causing any changes in the blood or **liver**. A doctor should be notified if any signs of drug toxicity appear, including uncontrolled eye movements; sluggishness, dizziness, or hyperactivity; inability to see clearly or speak distinctly; nausea or **vomiting**; or sleep problems.

Status epilepticus requires emergency treatment, usually with Ativan (Valium), phenytoin, or phenobarbital. An intravenous dextrose (sugar) solution is given to persons whose condition is due to low blood sugar, and a vitamin B_1 preparation is administered intravenously when status epilepticus results from chronic alcohol withdrawal. Because dextrose and **thiamine** are essentially harmless and because delay in treatment can be disastrous, these medications are given routinely, as it is usually difficult to obtain an adequate history from a person suffering from status epilepticus.

Surgery

Intractable seizures are seizures that cannot be controlled with medication or without sedation or other unacceptable side effects. Surgery may be used to eliminate or control intractable seizures. Some other patients whose seizures are caused by a small portion of the brain may also benefit from surgery. Surgical treatment is an option, however, only if the affected part of the brain does not control sight, hearing, or other vital functions.

Each year, as many as 5,000 new people may become suitable candidates for surgery, which is most often performed at a comprehensive epilepsy center. Potential surgical candidates include people with:

- Partial seizures and secondarily generalized seizures (attacks that begin in one area and spread to both sides of the brain)
- Seizures and childhood paralysis on one side of the body (hemiplegia)
- Complex partial seizures originating in the temporal lobe (the part of the brain associated with speech, hearing, and smell) or other focal seizures (However, the risk of surgery involving the speech centers is that a person will lose speech function.)
- Generalized myoclonic seizures or generalized seizures featuring temporary paralysis (akinetic) or loss of muscle tone (atonal)

A **physical examination** is conducted to verify that a person's seizures are caused by epilepsy. Surgery is not used to treat people with severe psychiatric disturbances or medical problems that raise risk factors to unacceptable levels.

Surgery is never indicated unless:

- The best available antiseizure medications have failed to control the person's symptoms satisfactorily.
- The origin of a person's seizures has been precisely located.
- There is good reason to believe that surgery will significantly improve the person's health and quality of life.

Every person considering epilepsy surgery is carefully evaluated by one or more neurologists, neurosurgeons, neuropsychologists, and/or social workers. A psychiatrist, chaplain, or other spiritual advisor may help an affected individual and family members family cope with the stresses that occur during and after the selection process.

Patients who are treated surgically for epilepsy are usually asked to continue taking antiseizure medications for two years after the procedure even if the surgery is successful. Continuing the medication for that period of time reduces the risk of new seizures.

TYPES OF SURGERY. Surgical techniques used to treat intractable epilepsy include:

- Lesionectomy. Removing the lesion (diseased brain tissue) and some surrounding brain tissue is very effective in controlling seizures. Lesionectomy is generally more successful than surgery performed on persons whose seizures are not caused by clearly defined lesions, but removing only part of the lesion lessens the effectiveness of the procedure.
- Temporal resections. Removing part of the temporal lobe and the part of the brain associated with feelings, memory, and emotions (the hippocampus) provides good or excellent seizure control in 75% to 80% of properly selected individuals with appropriate types of temporal lobe epilepsy. Some people experience post-operative speech and memory problems.
- Extratemporal resection. This procedure involves removing some or all of the frontal lobe, the part of the brain directly behind the forehead. The frontal lobe helps regulate movement, planning, judgment, and personality, and special care must be taken to prevent post-operative problems with movement and speech. Extra-temporal resection is most successful in people whose seizures are not widespread.
- Hemispherectomy. This method of removing brain tissue is restricted to persons with severe epilepsy and abnormal discharges that often extend from one side of the brain to the other. Hemispherectomies are most often performed on infants or young children who have had an extensive brain disease or disorder since birth or from a very young age.

- Corpus callosotomy. This procedure, an alternative to hemispherectomy in persons with congenital hemiplegia, removes some or all of the white matter that connects the two halves of the brain. Corpus callosotomy is performed almost exclusively on children who are frequently injured during falls caused by seizures. If removing two-thirds of the corpus callosum doesn't produce lasting improvement in a person's condition, the remaining one-third will be removed during another operation.
- Multiple subpial transection. This procedure is used to control the spread of seizures that originate in or affect the so-called eloquent cortex, the area of the brain responsible for complex thought and reasoning.

Other treatments

VAGUS NERVE STIMULATION. The United States Food and Drug Administration (FDA) has approved the use of vagus nerve stimulation (VNS) in persons over the age of 16 who have intractable partial seizures. This nonsurgical procedure uses a pacemaker-like device implanted under the skin in the upper left chest, to provide intermittent stimulation to the vagus nerve. Stretching from the side of the neck into the brain, the vagus nerve affects swallowing, speech, breathing, and many other functions, and VNS may prevent or shorten some seizures. It is not clear as of 2012 why stimulation of this particular nerve helps to control seizures, but it is reported to lower the number of seizures by 20–40 percent in most patients who try it.

KETOGENIC DIET. Another treatment approach that has been found to reduce seizures in some children is the ketogenic diet. This diet reduces the amount of available glucose (sugar) in the body, forcing the child's body to turn to fat stores for energy. It is a high-fat diet that results in the person getting about 80 percent of their calories from fat. No one is exactly sure why this diet, which mimics the effects of starvation on the body, works to prevent seizures. It also does not work for every child, and the reasons for that also are unclear.

The goal of this controversial approach is to maintain or improve seizure control while reducing medication. The ketogenic diet works best with children between the ages of one and 10. It is introduced over a period of several days, and most children are hospitalized during the early stages of treatment.

If a child following this diet remains seizure-free for at least six months, increased amounts of **carbohydrates** and protein are gradually added. If the child shows no improvement after three months, the diet is gradually discontinued.

Introduced in the 1920s, the ketogenic diet has had limited short-term success in controlling seizure activity. Its use also exposes people to such potentially harmful side effects as:

- staphylococcal infections
- stunted or delayed growth
- low blood sugar (hypoglycemia)
- excess fat in the blood (hyperlipidemia)
- disease resulting from calcium deposits in the urinary tract (urolithiasis)
- disease of the optic nerve (optic neuropathy)

Alternative

Stress increases seizure activity in 30% of people who have epilepsy. Relaxation techniques can provide some sense of control over the disorder, but they should never be used instead of anti-seizure medication or used without the approval of a person's doctor. **Yoga**, **meditation**, and favorite pastimes help some people relax and more successfully manage stress. Biofeedback can teach adults and older adolescents how to recognize an aura and what to do to stop its spread. Children under 14 are not usually able to understand and apply principles of biofeedback. **Acupuncture** treatments (acupuncture needles inserted for a few minutes or left in place for as long as half an hour) make some people feel pleasantly relaxed. **Acupressure** can have the same relaxing effect on children or on adults who dislike needles.

Aromatherapy involves mixing aromatic plant oils into water or other oils and massaging them into the skin or using a special burner to waft their fragrance throughout the room. Aromatherapy oils affect the body and the brain, and undiluted oils should never be applied directly to the skin. Ylang ylang, chamomile, or lavender can create a soothing mood. People who have epilepsy should not use rosemary, hyssop, sage, or sweet fennel, which seem to make the brain more alert.

Dietary changes that emphasize whole foods and eliminate processed foods may be helpful. Homeopathic therapy also can work for people with seizures, especially constitutional homeopathic treatment that acts at the deepest levels to address the needs of an individual.

First aid for seizures

It is helpful for family members or bystanders to know the essentials of **first aid** for people with seizure disorders. A person having a seizure should not be restrained; however, sharp or dangerous objects should be moved out of reach. Anyone having a complex partial seizure can be warned away from danger by someone calling out his or her name in a clear, calm voice. The relative or bystander should time the length of the seizure with a watch if possible.

A person having a grand mal seizure should be helped to lie down. Tight clothing should be loosened. A soft, flat object like a towel or the palm of a hand should be placed under the person's head. Forcing a hard object into the mouth of someone having a grand mal seizure could cause injuries or breathing problems. If the person's mouth is open, placing a folded cloth or other soft object between the teeth will protect the tongue. Turning the head to the side will help breathing. After a grand mal seizure has ended, the person who had the seizure should be told what has happened and reminded of their present location. Those nearby should offer to call a taxi, friend, or relative to help the person get home if he or she seems confused or unable to get home by him- or herself.

Prognosis

The prognosis of seizure disorder varies according to the patient's age at the time of the first seizure as well as the type of seizure. Usually the prognosis is better if seizures can be controlled by one medication; if the frequency of seizures decreases; and if there is a normal EEG and neurological examination prior to taking the patient off medication.

About 80 percent of people with seizure disorder can be successfully treated with medications; the remaining 20 percent are said to have intractable (difficult-to-treat) epilepsy. About 75 percent of people who are seizure-free on medication for 2 to 5 years can be successfully withdrawn from medication. Seizure disorder does carry with it, however, an increased risk of sudden unexplained death or of status epilepticus. The factors that cause SUDEP (sudden unexplained death from epilepsy) are poorly understood as of 2012; it is not yet known whether SUDEP results from not taking prescribed doses of antiseizure medications; from having a more severe form of epilepsy; or from genetic factors that affect the patient's cardiac and respiratory function. About 42,000 people die each year in the United States from status epilepticus. There is also an increased chance of dying due to accidents, primarily drowning. Other causes of seizure-associated death include abnormal **heart** rhythms, water in the lungs, or heart attack.

In addition to a somewhat shortened life expectancy, people with seizure disorder have difficulty with finishing school and with employment in adult life. One reason is social misunderstanding; another is the effect of antiseizure drugs on a person's ability to

KEY TERMS

Acupuncture—An ancient Chinese method of relieving pain or treating illness by piercing specific areas of the body with fine needles.

Akinetic seizure—Seizure characterized by limp posture and a brief period of unconsciousness; also called a drop attack.

Anticonvulsant—A drug given to treat seizures.

Aura—A distinctive smell, taste, or other unusual sensation that precedes the onset of a seizure.

Biofeedback—A learning technique that helps individuals influence automatic body functions.

Clonic—Referring to clonus, a series of muscle contractions and partial relaxations that alternate in some nervous diseases in the form of convulsive spasms.

Electroencephalograph (EEG)—An instrument that measures the electrical activity of the brain. The EEG traces the electrical activity in the form of wave patterns onto recording paper. Wave patterns with sudden spikes or sharp waves strongly suggest seizures. An EEG with a seizure-type wave pattern is called an epileptiform EEG.

Hallucination—False sensory perceptions. A person experiencing a hallucination may hear sounds or see people or objects that are not really present. Hallucinations can also affect the senses of smell, touch, and taste.

Idiopathic—Arising spontaneously or from an obscure or unknown cause.

Ketogenic diet—A special high-fat low-carbohydrate diet used since the 1920s to reduce seizures in children and some adult patients diagnosed with epilepsy.

Lumbar puncture (LP)—A medical test in which a very narrow needle is inserted into a specific space between the vertebrae of the lower back in order to obtain a sample of CSF for examination. It is also known as a spinal tap.

Myoclonic seizures—Brief, involuntary spasms of the tongue or muscles of the face, arms, or legs.

Petit mal seizure—An older term for absence seizure.

Post-ictal state—A period of disorientation usually followed by sleep that occurs after a seizure.

Seizure threshold—A term that refers to a person's susceptibility to seizures.

Status epilepticus—A potentially life-threatening condition in which a person either has an abnormally prolonged seizure or does not fully regain consciousness between seizures.

Tonic—Characterized by tonus, a state of partial contraction that is maintained at least in part by a continuous bombardment of motor impulses.

---

concentrate. Employment difficulties in adult life are usually related to the restrictions that most states place on driving. Most states require a person with a history of seizure disorder to show that they have been seizure-free for a specified period of time before they can apply for a driver's license.

Health care team roles

First aid may be provided by trained individuals when someone has a seizure nearby. Physicians make the initial diagnosis of seizure disorders. Endocrinologists and radiologists may assist in refining a diagnosis. Neurologists, neurosurgeons, neuropsychologists, and social workers may assess persons prior to receiving surgery for a seizure disorder. Neurosurgeons may perform surgery to remove structures in the brain that are known to cause seizures. Psychiatrists, chaplains, or other spiritual advisors may help an affected individual

and relations cope with the stresses that occur during and after surgery. Nurses also teach family and friends about emergency care of patient when having a seizure, as well as **home care** following a seizure and hospitalization.

Prevention

Seizure disorder is difficult to prevent, given that it has so many different forms and the fact that doctors cannot identify a cause in about half of all cases. In terms of preventing seizures in persons already diagnosed with seizure disorder, eating properly, getting sufficient sleep, and controlling stress and fevers can help prevent some seizures.

A person who has epilepsy should be careful not to hyperventilate. A person who experiences an aura should find a safe place to lie down and stay there until the seizure passes. Anticonvulsant medications should not be

QUESTIONS TO ASK YOUR DOCTOR

- What type of seizure disorder do I have?
- What is the cause?
- What is the prognosis?
- What treatments will you recommend? Will I need surgery?
- Will I have to give up driving?
- What is your opinion of vagus nerve stimulation as a treatment for seizure disorder?
- What are my risks of SUDEP?

stopped suddenly; and, if other medications are prescribed or discontinued, the doctor treating the seizures should be notified. In some conditions, such as severe head injury, brain surgery, or subarachnoid hemorrhage, anticonvulsant medications may be given to a person to prevent seizures. Seizures that are caused by ingesting such substances as alcohol or drugs can be prevented by discontinuing use of the offending substance.

Resources

BOOKS

Cascino, Gregory D., and Joseph I. Sirven. *Adult Epilepsy.* Chichester, UK: Wiley-Blackwell, 2011.

Committee on the Public Health Dimensions of the Epilepsies, Board on Health Sciences Policy, Institute of Medicine of the National Academies. *Epilepsy across the Spectrum: Promoting Health and Understanding.* Washington, DC: National Academies Press, 2012.

Engel, Jerome Jr. *Seizures and Epilepsy,* 2nd ed. New York: Oxford University Press, 2013.

Yudofsky, Stuart C., and Robert E. Hales. *Clinical Manual of Neuropsychiatry.* Washington, DC: American Psychiatric Publishing, 2012.

PERIODICALS

Alavi, A., et al. "Positron Emission Tomography in Seizure Disorders." *Annals of the New York Academy of Sciences* 1228 (June 2011): E1–E12.

Berg, Anne T., et al. "Revised Terminology and Concepts for Organization of Seizures and Epilepsies: Report of the ILAE Commission on Classification and Terminology, 2005–2009." *Epilepsia* 51 (April 2010): 676–685. Available online at http://www.ilae.org/Visitors/Centre/ctf/documents/ClassificationReport_2010_000.pdf.

Brodie, M.J., and P. Kwan. "Newer Drugs for Focal Epilepsy in Adults." *BMJ* (January 26, 2012): 344–345.

Fisher, R.S. "Therapeutic Devices for Epilepsy." *Annals of Neurology* 71 (February 2012): 157–168.

Fridley, J., et al. "Brain Stimulation for the Treatment of Epilepsy." *Neurosurgical Focus* 32 (March 2012): E13.

Galanopoulou, A.S., et al. "Identification of New Epilepsy Treatments: Issues in Preclinical Methodology." *Epilepsia* 53 (March 2012): 571–582.

Lambrechts, D.A., et al. "The Ketogenic Diet as a Treatment Option in Adults with Chronic Refractory Epilepsy: Efficacy and Tolerability in Clinical Practice." *Epilepsy and Behavior* 23 (March 2012): 310–314,

Lüders, H.O., et al. "Modern Technology Calls for a Modern Approach to Classification of Epileptic Seizures and the Epilepsies." *Epilepsia* 53 (March 2012): 405–411.

Shorvon, S., and T. Tomson. "Sudden Unexplained Death in Epilepsy." *Lancet* 378 (December 10, 2011): 2028–2038.

WEBSITES

Epilepsy Foundation. About Epilepsy Home Page. http://www.epilepsyfoundation.org/aboutepilepsy/ (accessed May 3, 2012).

Epilepsy Foundation. "Ketogenic Diet." http://www.epilepsyfoundation.org/aboutepilepsy/treatment/ketogenicdiet/index.cfm (accessed May 3, 2012).

Epilepsy Foundation. "SUDEP (Sudden Unexplained Death in Epilepsy)." http://www.epilepsyfoundation.org/aboutepilepsy/healthrisks/sudep/index.cfm (accessed May 3, 2012).

Epilepsy Therapy Project (ETP). All about Epilepsy and Seizures Home Page. http://www.epilepsy.com/EPILEPSY/main_epilepsy (accessed May 3, 2012).

Mayo Clinic. "Epilepsy." http://www.mayoclinic.com/health/epilepsy/DS00342 (accessed May 3, 2012).

Medscape. "Epilepsy and Seizures." http://emedicine.medscape.com/article/1184846-overview (accessed May 3, 2012).

Merck Manual for Health Care Professionals. "Seizure Disorders." http://www.merckmanuals.com/professional/neurologic_disorders/seizure_disorders/seizure_disorders.html (accessed May 3, 2012).

National Institute of Neurological Disorders and Stroke (NINDS). "Epilepsy: Hope through Research." http://www.ninds.nih.gov/disorders/epilepsy/detail_epilepsy.htm (accessed May 2, 2012).

ORGANIZATIONS

American Academy of Neurology (AAN), 1080 Montreal Avenue, Saint Paul, MN United States 55116, (651) 695-2717, Fax: (651) 695-2791, (800) 879-1960, http://www.aan.com/go/home

Epilepsy Foundation, 8301 Professional Place, Landover, MD United States 20785-7223, Fax: (301) 577-2684, (800) 332-1000, ContactUs@efa.org, http://www.epilepsyfoundation.org/

Epilepsy Therapy Project (ETP), P.O. Box 742, 10 N. Pendleton Street, Middleburg, VA United States 20118, (540) 687-8077, Fax: (540) 687-8066, info@epilepsytherapyproject.org, http://www.epilepsy.com/epilepsy_therapy_project

International League Against Epilepsy (ILAE), 342 North Main Street, West Hartford, CT United States 06117-2507, (860) 586-7547, Fax: (860) 586-7550, http://www.ilae.org/

National Institute of Neurological Disorders and Stroke (NINDS), P.O. Box 5801, Bethesda, MD United States 20824, (301) 496-5751, (800) 352-9424, http://www.ninds.nih.gov/index.htm

L. Fleming Fallon, M.D., Dr.P.H.
Rebecca J. Frey, Ph.D.

Selective polishing *see* **Tooth polishing**
Selenium deficiency *see* **Mineral deficiency**

Semen analysis

Definition

A semen analysis is the examination of freshly ejaculated seminal fluid. Seminal fluid is a viscous, turbid fluid produced mainly from secretions of the seminal vesicles (45–80% of volume) and prostate gland (15–30% of the volume). About 1% of the total volume is spermatozoa and testicular fluid produced by the testes. A routine analysis of seminal fluid includes the measurement of fluid volume, viscosity, pH, and fructose; and measurement of sperm concentration, count, motility, viability, and morphology. Additional tests are performed as indicated. These are usually performed by andrology laboratories and include testing for sperm autoantibodies, zona free hamster oocyte penetration, cervical mucus penetration, the acrosomal reaction test, and computer-assisted sperm analysis (CASA).

Purpose

In the United States, the **infertility** rate for married couples is approximately 15%. A semen analysis is the examination of a male's ejaculate, performed to determine if the cause of a couple's infertility is attributed to the male's inability to fertilize the ovum. It is also used to confirm the absence of sperm following vasectomy. In addition, a microscopic exam for sperm is performed on vaginal swabs and clothing taken in suspected rape cases as part of the crime scene investigation. This is used along with tests for acid phosphatase and prostate specific antigen to determine the presence of seminal fluid.

Precautions

The patient should abstain from intercourse for three days prior sample collection and refrain from drinking alcoholic beverages for at least 24 hours before testing. Antineoplastic agents and estrogen may lower test results. Additionally, several herbal supplements have been found to affect sperm counts and/or characteristics.

A semen specimen to investigate infertility must kept at room temperature. It should be collected by masturbation into a disposable sterile, wide-mouth container. A room close to the testing site is preferred for collection, since specimen quality deteriorates rapidly. If possible, examinations for motility and viability should be performed and smears prepared within one hour of collection. Timing is not as critical for postvasectomy testing. Physiological and environmental factors can increase the variability of semen analysis, and the World Health Organization (WHO) recommends the evaluation of two ejaculates collected at least seven days but not more than three months apart.

Description

Male infertility may be caused by many conditions that affect the production of functional sperm. The most common cause is varicocele (hardening of the veins that drain the testes) which accounts for about 40% of cases and is treated surgically. Testicular failure accounts for approximately 10% of cases and may result from numerous causes including malignancy, mumps, Klinefelter's syndrome, injury, and radio- or **chemotherapy**. Hyperspermia, increased seminal fluid volume, also accounts for about 10% of cases. Endocrine diseases affecting spermatogenesis account for approximately 9% of cases and usually involve pituitary or adrenal hypoplasia or hyperthyroidism. Obstruction of the ejaculatory duct accounts for about 5% of cases and sperm autoantibodies for 1–2%.

Physical characteristics of the semen sample that are evaluated include volume, gross appearance (color, turbidity), viscosity, and liquifaction. Seminal fluid will coagulate within five minutes of collection due to coagulating protein secreted by seminal vesicles. The seminal fluid should liquefy within one hour at room temperature, due to the action of prostatic secretions. Failure to do so inhibits motility. After liquifaction, viscosity may be measured by observing the fluid as it drains from the tip of a 5 mL serological pipet. The fluid should flow from the tip in discrete droplets. Formation of a thread of two or more centimeters at the tip indicates abnormally high viscosity. Volume is determined by determining the amount of fluid that can be drawn into a 10 mL serological pipet.

Sperm counting methods

The sperm concentration is usually performed using a 1:20 dilution of seminal fluid in a diluent containing formalin which immobilizes the sperm. Usually five of the 0.2×0.2 mm squares of a hemacytometer grid are counted. The number of cells counted is equal to the sperm concentration in millions per mL. All 25 squares are counted if there are less than 10 sperm (spermatozoons) per square. A Mackler chamber, a grid consisting of 1 square millimeter divided into 100 equal squares, (0.1×0.1 mm, 0.01 mm deep) can be used in place of a hemacytometer. Undiluted seminal fluid is heated to 50–60°C to immobilize the sperm. Heads are counted in 10 of the squares and the total is equal to the sperm concentration in millions per milliliter. A sperm concentration less than 20 million per milliliter is termed oligozoospermia, and often results from ductal obstruction, regurgitation of sperm into bladder, or testicular failure. The total sperm count is determined by multiplying the sperm concentration per mL by the seminal fluid volume.

Motility and viability evaluation

Sperm motility should be performed within one hour of ejaculation. During this portion of the analysis, 10 microliters of semen are placed on a standard microscopic slide, and a coverglass is applied. Ten random fields are then examined at 250× to 400× magnification using phase contrast or brightfield microscopy. Two hundred sperm are graded for motility using a scale ranging from zero to four, with zero signifying no motility, and four describing sperm that exhibit rapid, progressive movement. A more detailed analysis of sperm motility is obtained using CASA. This procedure produces a computer analysis of video camera generated microscopic images of sperm movements. Various aspects of sperm movement such as curvilinear and straight-line velocity are measured and analyzed statistically.

Sperm viability is measured when the motility test is abnormal. The test is based upon the fact that living sperm exclude the dye eosin Y, but dead sperm do not. A slide is prepared by mixing a sample of the seminal fluid and the dye, and 200 sperm are counted under the **microscope**. The percentage of living sperm (unstained sperm) is recorded.

Morphology evaluation

The morphology of sperm is also assessed from a stained smear. To prepare a stained specimen, a drop of semen is placed on a glass slide and a second slide is used to spread the drop over the slide surface. The smear is air dried and fixed using ethanol-ether. The slide is stained with Papanicolaou or other suitable stain. (Wright stain is not recommended.) Two hundred mature sperm are evaluated for head, neck, and tail

defects. Any white **blood** cells (WBCs) or immature sperm cells (round cells) are also counted per 200 mature sperm. WBCs and rounds cells are estimated from the average number seen per 400× field. When more than one WBC or five round cells are seen on average per field, the respective cell count should be performed. Each cell per field equates to approximately one million cells per mL of seminal fluid. There are two alternative ways of classifying sperm that give very different results. The majority of clinical labs use nonstrict criteria. This process identifies only gross abnormalities of the sperm. The alternative method, strict criteria, is used by andrology and some clinical labs. For example, the WHO criteria for the normal sperm head is as follows: length 4.0–4.5 microns, width 2.5–3.5 microns, length:width ratio 1.5–1.75, acrosomal area 40–70%, vacuolization less than 20% of head area. Studies have shown that the probability of successful fertilization via assisted reproductive technology diminishes significantly when less than 15% of the sperm are normal by strict criteria. There are several strict criteria in use, including those developed by WHO.

Other tests

Chemical tests routinely performed on seminal fluid include pH and fructose. pH is measured with pH paper, and fructose may be measured quantitatively using an enzymatic assay.

Antibodies to sperm have the potential to impair fertility. While sperm agglutinins (antibodies) may be detected in the male or female partner of up to 10% of infertile couples, they are not always responsible for infertility. There are several tests for sperm agglutinins including direct microscopic observation, the mixed antiglobulin test, and the immunobead test.

Preparation

Sterile, wide-mouth containers should be used for specimen collection. The best quality sperm are obtained when the specimen is collected after three days of sexual abstinence, but not more than five to seven days. Because the initial portion of the ejaculate contains the majority of the sperm cells, and the volume of ejaculate may provide clues regarding infertility, *coitus interruptus* should not be used as the method of collection.

The specimen should be examined in the laboratory within one hour of collection. Typically, two to three specimens are examined over a period of several weeks. When results from two testing days are different, additional specimens collected over a two- to three-month period should be analyzed.

KEY TERMS

Autoantibody—An antibody formed in response to, and reacting against, an antigenic constituent of the individual's own tissues.

Infertility—The diminution of absence of ability to produce offspring.

Morphology—The biological study of the form and function of living organisms.

Motility—The the ability to move spontaneously.

Semen—Fluid discharged at ejaculation in the male, consisting of secretion of glands associated with the urogenital tract and containing spermatozoa.

Sperm—Vernacular term for spermatozoon, which is a mature male germ cell, the specific output of the testes, which impregnates the ovum in sexual reproduction.

Vasectomy—An operation done to sterilize a man by stopping the release of sperm into semen.

Aftercare

There are no aftercare requirements.

Complications

There are no complications associated this test.

Results

Each laboratory defines its own set of normal values. Many follow the recommendation of WHO. The values below are representative for the procedures described above.

- Volume: 2.0 to 5.0 mL
- pH: 7.2-8.0
- Sperm concentration: Greater than or equal to 20 million per mL
- Sperm count: Greater than or equal to 40 million per ejaculate
- Motility: Greater than or equal to 50% demonstrating forward progressive movement or 25% or more demonstrating rapid progressive movement. Prolonged abstinence may depress sperm motility. Frequent sperm agglutination suggests the presence of antisperm antibodies
- Morphology: Nonstrict criteria: greater than 60% normal sperm. Strict criteria: 15–40% normal sperm

- White blood cells: Less than 1 million per mL
- Round cells: Less than 5 million per mL
- Viability: Equal to or greater than 75%
- Viscosity: Droplets to threads less than 2 cm

Post-vasectomy

Semen analysis to confirm the success of a vasectomy is concerned only with the absence or presence of sperm. Semen is collected six weeks after surgery, or after at least 20 ejaculations. Sperm should not be seen. If sperm are seen, another specimen is collected two to four weeks later. The test should be repeated several months later to ensure that the vas deferens have not reattached.

Health care team roles

Physicians, nurses, or laboratory scientists provide collection and delivery instructions. Laboratory tests are performed by clinical laboratory scientists CLS(NCA)/ medical technologists MT(ASCP), or pathologists.

Resources

BOOKS

Chernecky, Cynthia C, and Barbara J. Berger. *Laboratory Tests and Diagnostic Procedures,* 3rd ed. Philadelphia, PA: W.B. Saunders Company, 2001.

Kee, Joyce LeFever. *Handbook of Laboratory and Diagnostic Tests,* 4th ed. Upper Saddle River, NJ: Prentice Hall, 2001.

Walsh, P. *Campbell's Urology,* 7th ed. Philadelphia, PA: W.B. Saunders Company, 1998.

OTHER

Laboratory Corporation of America. "Semen Analysis, Basic." Copyright 2001. http://www.labcorp.com

Walsh, P. Campbell's Urology, 7th ed. W.B. Saunders Company, 1998. http://www.vasectomy-information.com/journal/sanalyse.htm.

Victoria E. DeMoranville

Senna *see* **Laxatives**

Sensory reeducation

Definition

Sensory reeducation is a therapeutic program using sensory stimulation to help sensory-impaired patients recover functional sensibility in the damaged area and learn adaptive functioning.

Purpose

Following disease, such as **stroke**, or accident, sensory reeducation helps patients with various forms of sensory loss and impairment retrain their sensory pathways, adapt to changed abilities, and regain function.

Precautions

There may be contraindications related to particular modalities used in sensory reeducation or related to coexisting conditions. For example, some coexisting conditions that may contraindicate electrical stimulation include thrombophlebitis, cardiac demand pacemaker, disturbances in cardiac rhythm, local inflammation or **infection**, or **cancer**. Extreme caution should be used when applying heat, cold, or electrical stimulation to sensory impaired areas to avoid possible damage due to the patient's inability to feel symptoms that may indicate dangerous temperature or stimulation levels.

A thorough medical history and examination should be conducted and any coexisting conditions noted and taken into consideration during treatment design and implementation. The patient should be educated and monitored to help prevent further damage to the sensory-impaired area.

Description

Sensory reeducation uses a variety of therapeutic, **rehabilitation**, and educational techniques to help sensory-impaired patients recover sensibility, fine discrimination abilities, and the ability to perform other tasks involved in daily living and work activities. In addition to actual loss of sensibility and related functional ability, paresthesias (abnormal sensations), such as numbness, tingling, or burning sensations, may be present. Some of the many possible causes of sensory impairment may include nerve damage, nerve repair surgery, stroke, **aneurysm**, other forms of **central nervous system** damage, and diabetes-related nerve impairment.

Many techniques of sensory stimulation are used to provide input to sensory receptors and pathways. Some forms of stimulation used include electrical stimulation; stroking the skin with textured, friction-producing items such as Velcro; and the use of specially modified tools and instruments (Dannenbaum). Other procedures and modalities that may be used include massage, vibration, pressure, biofeedback, various forms of movement and tactile stimulation, or other activities that require use of and attention to the senses. Sensory reeducation may be delivered in indirect ways as part of a larger therapeutic program, rather than being an independent, distinct therapy.

In addition to loss of tactile sensibility and related inability to distinguish heat, cold, textures, shapes, and other types of stimulation on the skin, losses related to other senses may also be addressed. One example is visual field impairment that may be caused by a stroke. Patients with visual field impairments might be taught to attend to the neglected side, or helped to use other senses to compensate for sensory impairment and loss.

Another form of impairment that may be treated with sensory reeducation is hypersensitivity, a condition in which a patient overreacts to mild forms of stimulation. One such condition is called regional **pain** syndrome. When treating such conditions tactile stimulation, weight bearing activities, and other forms of sensory reeducation are used to desensitize the patient's sensory responses and reduce perceived discomfort.

Among the goals of sensory reeducation is the retraining of neural pathways and responses to stimuli in order to restore the patient's sensory perception. Increased sensory input and activity may help to stimulate nerve regeneration and growth. In addition, previously unused neural connections may be trained to take over for damaged pathways. This neural plasticity can be used to the advantage of the patient with nerve damage or impairment.

Some scientists believe it may be possible for a remapping to occur in the **brain** so that connections between areas of the brain and certain parts of the body, as represented on Penfield maps, can adapt and change after nerve injury or amputation, causing new connections that relay sensation.

In general, in addition to actually retraining the senses and nervous system activities, much of sensory reeducation may focus on teaching the patient functional adaptation—new ways of using the abilities they have to compensate for sensory impairments and other disabilities. Adaptation may be used to help the patient function until full rehabilitation is achieved, but it may also be a permanent adaptation when full rehabilitation is not possible.

Preparation

The patient will be interviewed and examined by the therapist to determine the types and extent of sensory impairment. An individualized rehabilitation

KEY TERMS

Functional sensibility—The ability to make fine sensory discriminations in order to carry out specific somatosensory tasks.

Paresthesia—The presence of unusual sensations, such as numbness, tingling, or burning.

Penfield maps—Graphical depictions of the connections between areas in the brain and body parts with which they communicate; created by Wilder Penfield.

Reeducation—Rehabilitation by special training, such as physical therapy, that helps to restimulate nerve connections associated with sensory perception and related functional ability.

and sensory reeducation program will be designed in accord with the patient's needs, abilities, and goals.

Aftercare

Patients may continue to see their physician and therapist for follow-up exams and treatment after completion of initial sensory reeducation to record and maintain progress made.

Complications

The therapist should be alert to any possible complications related to the primary and coexisting conditions and associated with any of the modalities used. With careful diagnosis, treatment planning, and monitoring, complications should be minimal. Special caution and supervision should be used when working with sensory-impaired patients.

Results

The patient should be helped to regain sensibility and related functions such as two-point discrimination and object recognition, and minimize discomfort. To the degree that full recover of sensibility is not possible, the patient should learn adaptive behaviors that will aid in function.

Health care team roles

The surgeon, neurologist, or primary physician may prescribe and monitor the therapy. Physical or occupational therapists and their assistants may perform sensory reeducation. Nurses and other hospital personnel may also be involved in the general rehabilitation and sensory reeducation of the patient, along with social workers, speech therapists, cognitive therapists, and other allied health care providers.

Resources

BOOKS

APTA Guide to Physical Therapist Practice, Revised 2nd ed. American Physical Therapy Association, 2003.

Callahan, A.D. "Methods of Compensation and Reeducation for Sensory Dysfunction." In *Rehabilitation of the Hand: Surgery and Therapy,* 4th ed. James M. Hunter, Evelyn J. Mackin, and Anne D. Callahan, editors. St. Louis: Mosby, 1995, 701-714.

Ramachandran V.S., and Sandra Blakeslee. "Knowing Where to Scratch." *Phantoms in the Brain.* New York: William Morrow and Company, Inc., 1998, pp. 21–38.

Yekutiel, M. *Sensory Re-Education of the Hand After Stroke.* London: Whurr Publishers, 2000.

ORGANIZATION

American Physical Therapy Association (APTA). 1111 North Fairfax Street. Alexandria, VA 22314. (703) 684-2782. (800) 999-2782. http://www.apta.org.

Diane Fanucchi, C.M.T., C.C.R.A.

Sensory testing

Definition

Sensory testing involves the evaluation of a patient's perception in an effort to assess the integrity of the peripheral nervous system. There are many sensory receptors in the human body that provide information to the **brain** concerning an individual's surroundings. The information from sensory receptors helps the human being move and interact within the environment. For example, information from various sensory organs such as the eyes, vestibular (inner ear), and light touch are all integrated and organized by the brain to help the body complete safe and efficient movement. If sensory impairment is present, the patient's movement will likely be affected, making common tasks cumbersome and even dangerous. Therefore, individuals with possible sensory impairment need to have a full sensory evaluation to assess the integrity of sensation.

Purpose

There are many pathologies that can cause impairments in sensation. Injury or disease can compromise the integrity of a nerve and thus impair sensory function. **Peripheral neuropathy** is a broad classification that describes disease or dysfunction of a peripheral nerve. A peripheral neuropathy can be acquired or inherited.

Acquired peripheral neuropathy

A common acquired peripheral neuropathy is Guillain-Barre syndrome. This syndrome is usually considered an autoimmune disorder, but the etiology (cause) is unknown. Guillain-Barre syndrome is classified as a myelinopathy where the myelin sheath (an insulating wrapping which surrounds the axons of many nerves) disintegrates. In this disorder there is marked **weakness** and sensory impairment on both sides of the body. Two other types of acquired peripheral neuropathy are alcoholic and diabetic neuropathies. Alcoholic neuropathy is due to **alcoholism** and diabetic neuropathy is due to diabetes, a metabolic disease. In alcoholic neuropathy, sensory and motor losses are typical, especially in the feet and lower legs. The actual cause is unknown, but may be due to the toxic effects of alcohol on the nervous system. In diabetic neuropathy sensory loss also is prominent, especially in the lower limbs. Other acquired neuropathies can be caused by laceration (e.g., knife injury), crushing injuries to the nerve, or **ischemia** (a condition characterized by a decreased supply of oxygenated **blood**). All can lead to sensory and/or motor impairment by compromising the integrity of the nerve.

Inherited peripheral neuropathy

The most common inherited peripheral neuropathy is Charcot-Marie-Tooth disease. It is a genetic disorder that is categorized by weakness or atrophy of the lower limbs, especially the lower leg and foot.

There are many sensory receptors corresponding to various sensations within the human body. The purpose of sensory receptors is to gather pertinent information on the surrounding environment. Sensory receptors respond to stimuli in the environment, and thus provide valuable information on a person's surroundings. Therefore, the disorders categorized as peripheral neuropathies can impair the gathering and transmission of information. The purpose of sensory testing is to evaluate the proficiency and integration of information from sensory receptors in individuals who have known disease or injury.

Precautions

Sensory testing gives valuable information to the clinician on an individual's sensation and perception. Care must be taken when performing sensory tests if sensory loss is suspected. Applying increased pressure or heat on an individual who has a sensory deficit may injure the patient. For example, if a patient cannot sense the application of heat, there is a risk that the patient will be burned.

Description

Sensory testing should be done on both sides of the body so that comparisons can be made between sides, that is, affected side versus non-affected side. If there is a deficit noted, it is usually termed absent, diminished, or exaggerated. If there is no deficit, sensation is termed intact.

There are seven common tests used to evaluate sensation and perception. They are: stereognosis, touch and pressure, kinesthesia, proprioception, touch localization, two-point discrimination, and recognition of textures.

Stereognosis

Stereognosis refers to the ability of an individual to identify objects placed in his/her hand, while his/her eyes are closed. The individual should be able to identify objects based on size, shape, and texture.

Touch and pressure

Touch can be assessed by gently rubbing a ball of cotton on the surface of the skin to be tested. The clinician's finger can be used to apply pressure to various locations in order to assess pressure sensation. While touch and pressure are being assessed, the subject's eyes should be closed.

Proprioception

This test evaluates the individual's perception of movement specifically related to the limbs. In this test the individual's eyes are closed while the examiner moves the unaffected limb into a position and holds the position. The examiner then asks the individual to move the affected side into the same position.

Kinesthesia

This test assesses the individual's perception of joint movement rather than position (proprioception). In this test, the examiner moves the unaffected limb and, as the limb is moved, the individual being tested must copy the movement and follow the path with the affected or involved side. This test also is done with the individual's eyes are closed.

Touch localization

While the subject's eyes are closed, the examiner touches different areas on the skin and asks the subject, "Where am I touching?" The subject must verbally identify the location of the examiner's touch.

Two-point discrimination

This test evaluates an individual's ability to discern two points at the same time. While the subject's eyes are closed, the examiner applies point pressure in two spots separated by one to two inches. The examiner asks the subject, "Can you feel two points?" If the subject can discern two points, the examiner moves the points closer together and the test is repeated. This continues until two points cannot be discerned. These results are compared with results from the opposite side.

Recognition of textures

Various textures are placed in the individual's hand, while his/her eyes are closed. The individual must verbally identify the texture. Cotton and sandpaper are examples of items used in this test.

Another testing device, the Weinstein Enhanced Sensory Test (WEST), is primarily used to assess touch sensation. It is a precision instrument that uses hair-like filaments to record pressure or force. The instrument is a safe, valid, and reliable way of recording sensory loss.

Results

Results or outcomes of treatment are variable. Usually the initial severity of the deficit reflects the possible outcome. The greater the deficit, the greater the likelihood of long-term or total impairment.

Health care team roles

Nurses and other allied health team members need to be aware of potential sensory and perceptive disorders and their relationship to function. Early identification of sensory or perceptive impairments may minimize further complications. Physicians, nurses, and allied health professionals, such as occupational and physical therapists, usually perform sensation testing. Nurses are now becoming more familiar with the WEST device and this technology is now available for assessing the feet. This is especially useful for patients with diabetic neuropathy.

KEY TERMS

Kinesthesia—The ability to perceive where a limb or the body is moving in space. Information about the surrounding environment is processed in the brain and received from muscles, tendons, and joints.

Proprioception—The ability to perceive where a limb or the body is in space. Usually refers to a static situation.

Sensation—Awareness (as of heat or pain) due to stimulation of a sense organ.

Resources

BOOKS

Bennett, S. E., and J. L. Karnes. *Neurological Disabilities, Assessment and Treatment.* Philadelphia: Lippincott, 1998.

Fredericks, C. M., and L.K. Saladin. *Pathophysiology of the Motor Systems.* Philadelphia: F.A. Davis Co., 1996.

Magee, D. J. *Orthopedic Physical Assessment.* Philadelphia: W.B. Saunders Co., 1997.

ORGANIZATIONS

American Diabetes Association. 1701 North Beauregard St., Alexandria, VA 22311. (800) 342-2383. http://www.diabetes.org.

American Physical Therapy Association. 1111 North Fairfax St., Alexandria, VA 22314-1488. (703) 684-APTA or (800) 999-APTA. TDD: (703) 683-6748. Fax: (703) 684-7343. http://www.apta.org.

Mark Damian Rossi, Ph.D., P.T., C.S.C.S.

Sepsis

Definition

Sepsis refers to a bacterial **infection** in the bloodstream or body tissues. This very broad term covers the presence of many types of microscopic disease-causing organisms.

Demographics

In the general population, the incidence of sepsis is two people in 10,000. The number of deaths from sepsis each year has almost doubled in the United States since

---

1980 because more patients are developing the condition. There are three major factors responsible for this increase: a rise in the number of organ transplants and other surgical procedures that require suppressing the patient's **immune system**; the greater number of elderly people in the population; and the overuse of **antibiotics** to treat infectious illnesses, resulting in the development of drug-resistant **bacteria**.

Description

Sepsis is also called bacteremia. Closely related terms include septicemia and septic syndrome. In sepsis, there is active multiplication of bacteria in the bloodstream which may or may not result in organ dysfunction. If sepsis is not promptly recognized and treated, pulmonary, hepatic, and renal function may be impaired.

Causes and symptoms

Sepsis can originate anywhere bacteria can gain entry to the body. Common sites include the genitourinary tract, the **liver** and its bile ducts, the gastrointestinal tract, and the **lungs**. Broken or ulcerated skin can also provide access to bacteria commonly present in the environment. Invasive medical procedures, including dental work, can introduce bacteria or permit them to accumulate in the body. Entry points and equipment left in place for any length of time present a particular risk. **Heart** valve replacement, catheters, ostomy sites, intravenous (IV) or arterial lines, surgical **wounds**, or surgical drains are examples. IV drug users are at high risk as well.

People with inefficient immune systems, such as those with HIV infection; **spinal cord** injuries; or **blood** disorders are at particular risk for sepsis and have a higher death rate (up to 60%). In people who have no underlying chronic disease, the death rate is far lower (about five percent). The growing problem of antibiotic resistance has increased the incidence of sepsis, partly because ordinary preventive measures (such as prophylactic antibiotics) are less effective.

Cancer patients are at an increased risk of developing sepsis because **chemotherapy** and other forms of treatment for cancer weaken their immune systems.

The most common symptom of sepsis is **fever**, often accompanied by chills or shaking, or other flu-like symptoms. A history of any recent invasive procedure or dental work should raise the suspicion of sepsis and medical help should be sought promptly.

KEY TERMS

Bacteremia—The medical term for sepsis.

Prophylactic—Referring to medications or other treatments given to prevent disease.

Diagnosis

An accurate and detailed patient history is helpful in determining the source of the sepsis and in designing an appropriate course of treatment.

The presence of sepsis is indicated by blood tests showing particularly high or low white blood cell counts. The causative agent is determined by **blood culture**.

In some cases the doctor may order imaging studies to rule out **pneumonia**, or to determine whether the sepsis has developed from a ruptured appendix or other leakage from the digestive tract into the **abdomen**.

Treatment

Identifying the specific causative agent ultimately determines how sepsis is treated. However, time is of the essence, so a broad-spectrum antibiotic or multiple antibiotics will be administered until blood cultures reveal the culprit and treatment can be designed specific to the organism. Intravenous antibiotic therapy is usually necessary and is administered in a hospital setting.

Prognosis

The prognosis associated with sepsis is dependent on several factors such as the general condition of the patient, including the patient's immune status, and early recognition and initiation of prompt, appropriate treatment of the cause of the sepsis.

In severe cases, the patient's chances of survival are enhanced by rapid admission to an intensive care unit followed by aggressive treatment with antibiotics and by careful monitoring of response to treatment.

Prevention

Prompt recognition and appropriate treatment of bacterial infections can often prevent the progression of bacteremia to sepsis.

Resources

BOOK

Cunha, Burke A. "Sepsis and Its Mimics in the Critical Care Unit." In Cunha, Burke A. *Infectious Diseases in Critical*

Care Medicine, 2nd ed. New York: Informa Healthcare, Inc., 2007.

PERIODICALS

Girard, T.D., and E.W. Ely. "Bacteremia and Sepsis in Older Adults." *Clinics in Geriatric Medicine.* 23(3) (August 2007): 633–47.

Mackenzie, I. and A. Lever. "Management of Sepsis." *BMJ.* 335(7626) (November 3, 2007): 929–32.

Winters, B.D., et al. "Long-term Mortality and Quality of Life in Sepsis: A Systematic Review." *Critical Care Medicine.* 38(5) (May 2010): 1276–83.

OTHER

Cunha, B.A. "Sepsis, Bacterial." eMedicine (July 15, 2010) 2010]. http://www.emedicine.medscape.com (accessed September 14, 2010).

ORGANIZATIONS

American College of Epidemiology (ACE), 1500 Sunday Dr., Suite 102, Raleigh, NC 27607, (919) 861-5573, http:// www.acepidemiology.org

American Public Health Association (APHA), 800 I St. NW, Washington, DC 20001-3710, (202) 777-APHA, http:// www.apha.org

Centers for Disease Control and Prevention (CDC), 1600 Clifton Rd., Atlanta, GA 30333, (800) 232-4636, http:// www.cdc.gov.

Jill S. Lasker
Rebecca J. Frey, Ph.D.
Melinda G. Oberleitner, RN, DNS, APRN, CNS

Sepsis syndrome *see* **Septic shock**

Septic shock

Definition

Septic **shock** is a syndrome in which a potentially lethal drop in **blood pressure** occurs as a result of an overwhelming bacterial **infection**.

Description

Septic shock is a possible consequence of bacteremia, which is also called **sepsis**. Bacterial toxins, and the immune system's hyperactive response to them, can cause a dramatic drop in circulating **blood** volume and blood pressure and may result in underperfusion to various organs. Septic shock can lead to multiple organ failure, including **respiratory failure**, and may cause rapid death. Toxic shock syndrome is one type of septic shock.

The rate of septic shock in the United States has been increasing. Researchers suggest that this is because more people are taking immunosuppressive drugs following organ transplant or as **cancer** treatment, and more people are living with weakened **immune system** as the treatment of HIV/AIDS improves. One study in the late 2000s estimated that there were 200,000 cases of septic shock annually in the United States. The mortality rate in these cases was about 50% More black Americans develop and die from septic shock than white Americans. Researchers suggest this occurs because black Americans have a higher rate of diabetes and renal disease which generally weaken the body's resistance to infection.

Causes and symptoms

During an infection, certain **bacteria** release complex molecules called endotoxins that may provoke a dramatic response by the body's immune system. Endotoxins are particularly dangerous; as they become widely dispersed, they cause arteries and the smaller arterioles to dilate. At the same time, the walls of the **blood vessels** become leaky, allowing fluid to seep into the tissues, lowering intravascular volume (the amount of fluid left in circulation). This combination, of arterial dilation and decreased intravascular volume, causes a dramatic decrease in blood pressure and impaired blood flow to multiple organs. Other changes seen in septic shock are disseminated intravascular coagulation (DIC), which can further impair organ perfusion (blood flow).

Septic shock is seen most often in patients with impaired host defenses (i.e., patients who are immunosuppressed), and is often due to nosocomial (hospital-acquired) infections. The immune system is suppressed by drugs used to treat cancer, **autoimmune disorders**, organ transplants, and diseases of immune deficiency such as **AIDS**. Malnutrition, chronic drug abuse, and long-term illness also increase the likelihood of succumbing to bacterial infection. Bacteremia is more likely with preexisting infections such as urinary or gastrointestinal tract infections, or skin ulcers. Bacteria may be introduced to the blood stream by surgical procedures, catheters, or intravenous equipment.

Toxic shock syndrome (TSS) is a potentially fatal disorder resulting from infection with Staphylococcus aureus, a toxin-producing strain of bacteria. When it was first reported in 1978, toxic shock syndrome was associated with menstruation and linked to super-absorbent tampon use. Today, it is recognized that use of super-absorbent tampons does increase the risk of TSS, as does use of a contraceptive sponge or diaphragm.

Postpartum patients (women who have just given birth) and patients with wound infections, or recovering from nasal surgery also are at risk for TSS. The illness appears suddenly, with **fever**, **rash**, low blood pressure, and episodes of fainting. Mortality rate for women with menstrual-related toxic shock is about, 1.8%. Patients recovering from TSS face increased risk of recurrence. To prevent TSS, menstruating women are advised to avoid use of super-absorbent tampons.

Symptoms

Septic shock usually is preceded by bacteremia, which causes fever, malaise, chills, and nausea. The first sign of shock is often confusion and decreased consciousness. In this beginning stage, the extremities are usually warm. Later, as the blood pressure drops, they may become cool, pale, and cyanotic (bluish). Fever may subside to normal temperatures later on in sepsis.

Other symptoms include:

- rapid heartbeat
- shallow, rapid breathing
- decreased urination
- reddish patches in the skin

Septic shock may progress to cause "adult respiratory distress syndrome," (also called non-cardiogenic pulmonary **edema**) in which the pulmonary capillaries become leaky and the **lungs** fill with fluid. This can lead to respiratory failure. When this occurs, the patient can no longer breathe without **mechanical ventilation** and supplemental oxygen.

Diagnosis

Diagnosis of septic shock is made when a patient with a severe infection has **hypotension** (low blood pressure) for which other causes such as major bleeding, **dehydration**, or massive **myocardial infarction** have been excluded. Pulmonary artery pressure may be monitored with a Swan-Ganz catheter, a catheter inserted into the pulmonary artery. Blood, urine, sputum, and cultures from other possible sites of infection determine the type of bacteria responsible for the infection. Arterial **blood gases** are also monitored to assess changes in respiratory function.

Treatment

Septic shock is treated initially with a combination of **antibiotics** and fluid replacement. The antibiotic is chosen based on the bacteria known or suspected to be present. Usually, two or more types of antibiotics are started until the organism is identified. Intravenous fluids replenish the intravascular fluid lost by leakage. Impaired coagulation and hemorrhage may be treated with transfusions of plasma, platelets, or red blood cells. Dopamine may be given to increase blood pressure further if necessary.

Respiratory distress is treated with mechanical ventilation and supplemental oxygen, either using a nosepiece or a tube into the trachea through the throat. The mainstay of therapy is to treat the underlying infection that caused the septic shock.

Prognosis

Septic shock is most likely to develop in the hospital, since it frequently results from hospital-acquired infection. Close monitoring and early, aggressive therapy can minimize the likelihood of progression. Nonetheless, death occurs in 25–50% of all cases.

The likelihood of recovery from septic shock depends on many factors, including the degree of immunosuppression of the patient, underlying disease, timeliness of treatment, and type of bacteria responsible. Mortality is highest in the very young, the elderly, those with persistent or recurrent infection, and those with compromised immune systems.

Health care team roles

Generally, care for the septic patient is delivered by hospital-based health care professionals in the hospital ICU (intensive care unit). Physicians, intensive care nurses, and other nursing personnel closely monitor patients' **vital signs** and administer antibiotics and fluids. Laboratory technologists perform necessary blood tests, and respiratory therapists may provide oxygen to patients in respiratory distress.

Prevention

The risk of developing septic shock can be minimized through treatment of underlying bacterial infections and prompt attention to signs of bacteremia. In the hospital, scrupulous **aseptic technique** on the part of medical professionals reduces the risk of introducing bacteria into the bloodstream.

Resources

PERIODICAL

Rivers, E.P., et al. "Early Interventions in Severe Sepsis and Septic Shock: A Review of the Evidence One Decade Later." *Minerva Anestesiologica.* 23 March 2012 (ePub) PMID: 22447123.

OTHER

Pinsky, Michael R. Septic Shock. Medscape Reference October 25, 2011 [accessed April 10, 2012]. http://emedicine. medscape.com/article/168402-overview

Sepsis. MedlinePlus April 6, 2012. [accessed April 9, 2012]. http://www.nlm.nih.gov/medlineplus/sepsis.html

Septic Shock. PubMed Health January 14, 2012 [accessed April 9, 2012]. http://www.ncbi.nlm.nih.gov/ pubmedhealth/PMH0001689

Venkataraman, Ramesh. Toxic Shock Syndrome. Medscape Reference July 16, 2010 [accessed April 9, 2012]. http:// emedicine.medscape.com/article/169177-overview

ORGANIZATIONS

Infectious Diseases Society of America (IDSA), 1300 Wilson Boulevard, Suite 300, Arlington, VA 22209, (703) 299-0200, Fax: (703) 299-0204, info@idsociety.org, http:// www.idsociety.org

National Institute of Allergy and Infectious Diseases Office of Communications and Government Relations, 6610 Rockledge Drive, MSC 6612, Bethesda, MD 20892-6612, (301) 496-5717, (866) 284-4107 or TDD: (800)877-8339 (for hearing impaired), Fax: (301) 402-3573, http://www3. niaid.nih.gov.

Barbara Wexler
Tish Davidson, AM

Serum electrolyte tests *see* **Electrolyte tests**

Serum iron test *see* **Iron tests**

Serum protein electrophoresis test *see* **Protein electrophoresis test**

Sex hormones tests

Definition

Sex hormones tests include tests that measure levels of estrogen (estradiol and estriol), progesterone, and testosterone (total and free).

Purpose

In non-pregnant women, a test of estradiol (E2) levels is ordered to evaluate delayed sexual maturity, precocious **puberty**, menstrual problems, and **infertility**, and ovarian failure. It is also used to test for tumors in both males and females that secrete estrogen. The test is also used to measure estrogen secretion in males who present with gynecomastia and feminization in male children.

Estriol (E3), another estrogen, is only ordered for pregnant women (typically at 15–18 weeks gestation). The test is used as part of the triple marker screen (in association with alpha fetoprotein and chorionic gonadotropin) for **Down syndrome**.

A progesterone test is ordered to evaluate women for anovulation, and to investigate precocious puberty. Progesterone may be measured in those persons with ovarian or adrenal **cancer** that secrete progesterone.

The testosterone test (free testosterone and/or total testosterone) is used to evaluate delayed sexual development, male sexual precocity, testicular failure, virilism in females, infertility, and tumors that secrete testosterone.

Precautions

Both the estrogen and testosterone test are most often measured by radioimmunosasay and results can be affected by radioactive scans. When RIA is used the estradiol or estriol tests should not be performed on a patient who has received radioactive dye within 48 hours prior to the test. For RIA testosterone tests, the period between the scan and the test should be at least seven days. Oral contraceptives may interfere with progesterone and estradiol results. Tetracycline, some phenothiazines, diazepam, clomiphene, and some **vitamins** may interfere with estradiol results.

Estradiol and progesterone results vary with the phase of the menstrual cycle, and this must be taken into account when interpreting the results of these tests.

Sex hormone tests are performed on **blood** collected by venipuncture. The nurse or phlebotomist performing the procedure should observe **universal precautions** for the prevention of transmission of bloodborne pathogens.

Description

The sex hormones control the development of primary and secondary sexual characteristics and regulate the sex-related functions of the body, such as the menstrual cycle, and the production of eggs or sperm. Because of their normally low concentration in plasma the sex hormones are typically measured by radioimmunoassay (RIA), chemiluminescence immunoassay, or fluorescent immunoassay.

Estradiol

While there have been more than 30 of these hormones identified, only estradiol (E2) is necessary to evaluate ovarian function. Estradiol is the most potent of the estrogens, but it accounts for only one-third of the total estrogen in premenopausal females. In the nonpregnant female the ovaries are responsible for almost all estradiol production. In **pregnancy**, some estradiol is also produced by the placenta. Estradiol is produced from **cholesterol**, androstenedione, and testosterone. In males, estradiol is mainly produced from testosterone by the testes, but a small amount is also made by the adrenal cortex.

In **menopause**, the ovaries stop producing estradiol and estrone (E1) becomes the principal estrogen. A small amount of estradiol is formed from adrenal conversion of androstenedione, but this accounts for only about 15% of total estrogens. Plasma estradiol will be low in menopause, and FSH and LH will usually be increased. The measurement of estrone is seldom needed, but may be used to investigate vaginal bleeding after menopause or when estrone secreting ectopic hormone production is suspected.

Prior to menopause, estradiol is most often measured to evaluate amenorrhea and ovarian failure. In primary ovarian failure the ovaries may either fail to develop (as in Turner syndrome) or fail to produce estrogens as a result of autoimmune, metabolic, or endocrine disease. The plasma estradiol will be low, but the plasma levels of both LH and FSH are elevated. If secondary sexual characteristics are undeveloped, and the person is of short stature, chromosomal studies may reveal Turner syndrome as the cause. Primary amenorrhea results in failure to have a menses by age 16. In addition to ovarian failure, primary amenorrhea may be caused by endometriosis, polycystic ovary syndrome, anatomic defects in the vagina or uterus, and other disorders. In secondary ovarian failure, amenorrhea may be caused by pituitary failure or prolactinoma. In the former, both plasma and urinary LH and FSH will be low. In prolactinoma, LH and FSH are low because their release is suppressed by excessive secretion of prolactin which inhibits corticotropin releasing hormone.

An increased plasma level of estrogen indicates ovarian hyperfunction which may occur as a result of an ovarian tumor such as a granulosa-thecal cell tumor or signals the presence of an ectopic estradiol-producing tumor.

Estradiol is also measured to evaluate the response of patients to progesterone challenge and to determine responsiveness to clomiphene. In a person with amenorrhea, estradiol greater than 40 pg/mL following progestin administration excludes estrogen deficiency as a cause of amenorrhea. Clomiphene blocks the hypothalamic response to estrogen and is a treatment for patients with anovulation who have adequate estrogen and normal pituitary function. Use of the drug requires demonstration that the ovaries can produce estradiol.

Estriol (E3)

Estriol (E3) is the principal estrogen produced during pregnancy. Estriol is produced by the placenta from dehydroepiandosterone sulfate derived from the fetal **liver** and adrenals. Estriol levels are low by approximately 25% in Down syndrome and other trisomies. Tests on maternal plasma for alpha-fetoprotein, chorionic gonadotropin, and unconjugated estriol are perfomed at 15–18 weeks gestation. Measurement of unconjugated estriol (uE3) is a better reflection of fetal-derived estriol than is total estriol, and is measured by RIA. Estriol levels are also low for the gestational age in spontaneous abortions and in threatened pregnancy, but are no longer needed for the diagnosis of these conditions.

Progesterone

Progesterone in the nonpregnant female is produced mainly by the ovaries with a small fraction also made by the adrenals. Progesterone levels in plasma are very low prior to ovulation. At ovulation, the level begins to rise due to secretion by the corpus luteum. The progesterone level peaks in the middle of the luteal phase (about one week prior to the next menses). Progesterone causes thickening of the endometrium in order to prepare the ovum for implantation should it be fertilized. In the absence of fertilization, negative feedback of progesterone on the hypothalamus results in suppression of luteinizing hormone and the corpus luteum involutes causing the wall of the uterus to breakdown. If fertilization occurs, the corpus luteum and placenta produce large amounts of progesterone. The most common use of plasma progesterone measurement is to evaluate ovulation. Progesterone is often measured on days 21 and 22 of the menstrual cycle. At this point the progesterone should represent the midluteal peak and levels above 5 ng/L are considered evidence of ovulation. Lower levels indicate a disruption of the normal luteal phase of progesterone production.

Testosterone

In males testosterone is produced by the testes under the control of luteinizing hormone. It is responsible for development of the testes, secondary sexual characteristics, and spermatogenesis. Testosterone is subject to diurnal variation in response to LH and highest plasma levels occur at six to nine AM. Approximately 60% of plasma testosterone is bound to sex hormone binding globulin (SHBG) and almost 40% is bound to albumin. Only about 2% of the hormone is in the free form and is physiologically active. Measurement of free hormone levels is more sensitive than total hormone because small changes in SHBG concentration can increase free hormone levels. A reduction in binding of testosterone to SHBG can be caused by drugs or other steroid hormones, and will increase free hormone levels. In males, plasma testosterone is low in hypogonadism and is measured in male children with delayed or absent sexual maturation. Primary testicular failure may result from Klinefelter syndrome, testicular **infection**, injury, and other causes. In these cases the plasma testosterone is low, but the LH and FSH are increased. In secondary testicular failure, plasma testosterone, FSH, and LH are decreased. Testosterone levels are also useful for the differential diagnosis of gynecomastia. In addition to low testosterone, gynecomastia can be caused by drugs that interfere with testosterone action, or ectopic tumors that secrete estrogen or chorionic gonadotropin.

Testosterone levels may be measured in both males and females to identify tumors that secrete the hormone. Testosterone is produced by some testicular and ovarian tumors as well as some others. Overproduction of testosterone caused by testicular, adrenal, or pituitary tumors in the young male may result in precocious puberty. Overproduction in females caused by an ovarian tumor or adrenal adenoma causes virilization and hursitism (excessive hair growth). In cases of ambiguous sex or virilization in female children, testosterone and adrenal androgens such as androstenedione may be measured. Most cases of congenital adrenal hyperplasia are caused by 21-hydroxylase deficiency which is associated with excessive androgen production. The enzyme deficiency blocks cortisol synthesis and causes intermediate steroids to accumulate that are converted to testosterone and other androgens. Androgens are most often measured by RIA or gas chromatography-mass spectroscopy (GC-MS).

Preparation

Progesterone and testosterone tests require a blood sample; it is not necessary for the patient to restrict food or fluids before the test. However, testosterone specimens should be drawn in the morning, because testosterone levels are highest in the early morning hours. For progesterone tests, the date of the patient's last menstrual cycle or week of gestation should be noted on the test request slip.

The estrogen test can be performed on blood and/or urine. It is not necessary for the patient to restrict food or fluids for either test. If a 24-hour urine test has been requested, the patient should be instructed to discard the first morning specimen, then save all urine voided during the next 24 hours. The blood sample should be placed on ice immediately after it is drawn. It is also important to note the patient's sex, age, and menstrual cycle phase on the test request slip.

Aftercare

Discomfort or bruising may occur at the puncture site. Applying pressure to the puncture site until the bleeding stops helps to reduce bruising; warm packs relieve discomfort. Some people feel dizzy or faint after blood has been drawn and should be treated accordingly.

Complications

Other than potential bruising at the puncture site, and/or **dizziness**, there are no complications associated with these tests.

Results

Normal values for sex hormone tests are highly dependent upon age and sex and in females the time of the collection relative to the menstrual cycle. Ranges vary from laboratory to laboratory depending upon the method used. Representative values for some patient groups are shown below.

Estradiol: For adult women, estradiol levels range from 20–150 pg/mL during the follicular phase, 100–500 pg/mL during the mid-cycle phase, and 50–150 pg/mL during the luteal phase. Menopausal women have estradiol levels of less than 18 pg/mL. The normal range for adult males is approximately 18–75 pg/mL.

Increased levels of estrogen are found in the following conditions:

- ovarian tumor
- adrenocortical tumor
- some testicular tumors
- pregnancy

KEY TERMS

Amenorrhea—Cessation of the menstrual cycle.

Gynecomastia—Excessive development of the male mammary glands, even to the functional state.

Hirsutism—Excessive bodily and facial hair, especially in women.

Hypogonadism—Underactivity of the testes.

Orchiectomy—Removal of one or both testes.

Spermatogenesis—The production of sperm.

Virilism—The presence of male characteristics in women.

Decreased levels of estrogen are found in the following conditions:

• ovarian dysfunction

• interuterine death in pregnancy

• anorexia nervosa

• primary and secondary hypogonadism

• turner syndrome

• infantilism

• menopausal and post-menopausal symptoms

• pituitary insufficiency

• psychogenic stress

Progesterone levels for women during the follicular phase normally range from 0.1–1.5 ng/mL and 2–24 ng/mL during the luteal phase. The normal range for the mid-luteal peak is 4.5–25.5 ng/mL. For post meanopausal women, results fall below 1.0 ng/mL. Results for pregnant women are as follows:

• first trimester: 9–50 ng/mL

• second trimester: 18–150 ng/mL

• third trimester: 60–260 ng/mL

For men, the normal progesterone value is 0.1–0.3 ng/mL. For children, normal values run from 7–51 ng/mL.

Increased levels of progesterone are seen:

• during ovulation and pregnancy

• with certain types of ovarian cysts

• with a tumor of the ovary known as a choriocarcinoma

Decreased levels of progesterone are seen:

• in toxemia of pregnancy

• with a threatened abortion

• during placental failure

• after fetal death

• with amenorrhea

• due to gonadal dysfunction

Normal ranges for testosterone are generally 300–1,200 ng/dL for men, and 30-95 ng/dL for women. Boys between the ages of six and nine have normal values in the range of 3–30 ng/dL, while for girls of the same age the range is 2–20 ng/dL.

In men, increased levels are found in:

• sexual precocity

• adrenal hyperplasia

• testicular tumor

• hyperthyroidism

• testicular feminization

In men, decreased levels are found in:

• Klinefelter syndrome

• primary and secondary hypogonadism

• Down syndrome

• orchiectomy

• impotence

• gynecomastia

In women, increased levels of testosterone are most commonly associated with ovarian and adrenal tumors and hirsutism.

Health care team roles

Physicians order sex hormone tests and interpret the results often with the assistance of endocrinologists. A nurse or phlebotomist collect the blood samples. Testing is performed by clinical laboratory scientists/medical technologists.

Resources

BOOKS

Chernecky, Cynthia C., and Barbara J. Berger. *Laboratory Tests and Diagnostic Procedures,* 3rd ed. Philadelphia, PA: W.B. Saunders Company, 2001.

Kee, Joyce LeFever. *Handbook of Laboratory and Diagnostic Tests,* 4th ed. Upper Saddle River, NJ: Prentice Hall, 2001.

Pagana, Kathleen Deska. *Mosby's Manual of Diagnostic and Laboratory Tests.* St. Louis, MO: Mosby, Inc., 1998.

Victoria E. DeMoranville

Sexual arousal disorders *see* **Sexual dysfunction**

Sexual desire disorders *see* **Sexual dysfunction**

Sexual dysfunction

Definition

Sexual dysfunction is broadly defined as the inability to fully enjoy sexual intercourse. Specifically, sexual dysfunctions are disorders that interfere with a full sexual response cycle. These disorders make it difficult for a person to enjoy or to have sexual intercourse. While sexual dysfunction rarely threatens physical health, it can take a heavy psychological toll, bringing depression, **anxiety**, and debilitating feelings of inadequacy.

Description

Sexual dysfunction takes different forms in men and women. A dysfunction can be life-long and always present; acquired; situational; or generalized, occurring despite the situation. A man may have a sexual problem if he:

- Ejaculates before he or his partner desires
- Does not ejaculate, or experiences delayed ejaculation
- Is unable to have an erection sufficient for pleasurable intercourse
- Feels pain during intercourse
- Lacks or loses sexual desire

A woman may have a sexual problem if she:

- Lacks or loses sexual desire
- Has difficulty achieving orgasm
- Feels anxiety during intercourse
- Feels pain during intercourse
- Feels vaginal or other muscles contract involuntarily before or during sex
- Has inadequate lubrication

The most common sexual dysfunctions in men include:

- Erectile dysfunction: an impairment of the erectile reflex. The man is unable to have or maintain an erection that is firm enough for coitus or intercourse.
- Premature ejaculation, or rapid ejaculation with minimal sexual stimulation before, on, or shortly after penetration and before the person wishes it.

- Ejaculatory incompetence: the inability to ejaculate within the vagina despite a firm erection and relatively high levels of sexual arousal.
- Retrograde ejaculation: a condition in which the bladder neck does not close off properly during orgasm so that the semen spurts backward into the bladder.

Until recently, it was presumed that women were less sexual than men. In the past two decades, traditional views of female sexuality were all but demolished, and women's sexual needs became accepted as legitimate in their own right.

Female sexual dysfunctions include:

- Sexual arousal disorder: the inhibition of the general arousal aspect of sexual response. A woman with this disorder does not lubricate, her vagina does not swell, and the muscle that surrounds the outer third of the vagina does not tighten—a series of changes that normally prepare the body for orgasm ("the orgasmic platform"). Also, in this disorder, the woman typically does not feel erotic sensations.
- Orgasmic disorder: the impairment of the orgasmic component of the female sexual response. The woman may be sexually aroused but never reach orgasm. Orgasmic capacity is less than would be reasonable for her age, sexual experience, and the adequacy of sexual stimulation she receives.
- Vaginismus: a condition in which the muscles around the outer third of the vagina have involuntary spasms in response to attempts at vaginal penetration.
- Painful intercourse: a condition that can occur at any age. Pain can appear at the start of intercourse, midway through coital activities, at the time of orgasm, or after intercourse is completed. The pain can be felt as burning, sharp searing, or cramping; it can be external, within the vagina, or deep in the pelvic region or abdomen.

Causes and symptoms

Many factors, of both physical and psychological natures, can affect sexual response and performance. Injuries, ailments, and drugs are among the physical influences; in addition, there is increasing evidence that chemicals and other environmental pollutants depress sexual function. As for psychological factors, sexual dysfunction may have roots in traumatic events such as rape or incest, feelings of guilt, a poor self-image, depression, chronic fatigue, certain religious beliefs, or marital problems. Dysfunction is often associated with anxiety. If a man operates under the misconception that all sexual activity must lead to intercourse and to orgasm by his partner, and if the expectation is not met, he may consider the act a failure.

Men

With premature ejaculation, physical causes are rare, although the problem is sometimes linked to a neurological disorder, prostate **infection**, or urethritis. Possible psychological causes include anxiety (mainly performance anxiety), guilty feelings about sex, and ambivalence toward women. However, research has failed to show a direct link between premature ejaculation and anxiety. Rather, premature ejaculation seems more related to sexual inexperience in learning to modulate arousal.

When men experience painful intercourse, the cause is usually physical; an infection of the prostate, urethra, or testes, or an allergic reaction to spermicide or condoms. Painful erections may be caused by Peyronie's disease, fibrous plaques on the upper side of the penis that often produce a bend during erection. **Cancer** of the penis or testis and arthritis of the lower back can also cause **pain**.

Retrograde ejaculation occurs in men who have had prostate or urethral surgery, take medication that keeps the bladder open, or suffer from diabetes, a disease that can injure the nerves that normally close the bladder during ejaculation.

Erectile dysfunction is more likely than other dysfunctions to have a physical cause. Drugs, diabetes (the most common physical cause), **Parkinson's disease**, **multiple sclerosis**, and **spinal cord** lesions can all be causes of erectile dysfunction. When physical causes are ruled out, anxiety is the most likely psychological cause of erectile dysfunction.

Female

Dysfunctions of arousal and orgasm in women also may be physical or psychological in origin. Among the most common causes are day-to-day discord with one's partner and inadequate stimulation by the partner. Finally, sexual desire can wane as one ages, although this varies greatly from person to person.

Pain during intercourse can occur for any number of reasons, and location is sometimes a clue to the cause. Pain in the vaginal area may be due to infection, such as urethritis; also, vaginal tissues may become thinner and more sensitive during breastfeeding and after **menopause**. Deeper pain may have a pelvic source, such as endometriosis, pelvic adhesions, or uterine abnormalities. Pain can also have a psychological cause, such as fear of injury, guilt feelings about sex, fear of **pregnancy** or injury to the fetus during pregnancy, or recollection of a previous painful experience.

Vaginismus may be provoked by these psychological causes as well, or it may begin as a response to pain, and continue after the pain is gone. Both partners should understand that the vaginal contraction is an involuntary response, outside the woman's control.

Similarly, insufficient lubrication is involuntary, and may be part of a complex cycle. Low sexual response may lead to inadequate lubrication, which may lead to discomfort, and so on.

Diagnosis

In deciding when a sexual dysfunction is present, it is necessary to remember that while some people may be interested in sex at almost any time, others have low or seemingly nonexistent levels of sexual interest. Only when it is a source of personal or relationship distress, instead of voluntary choice, is it classified as a sexual dysfunction.

The first step in diagnosing a sexual dysfunction is usually discussing the problem with a health care professional, who will need to ask further questions in an attempt to differentiate among the types of sexual dysfunction. A physical exam of the genitals may be performed, and further medical tests may be ordered, including measurement of hormone levels in the **blood**. Men may be referred to a specialist in diseases of the urinary and genital organs (urologist), and primary care physicians may refer women to a gynecologist.

In general, causes of sexual dysfunction are either physical or psychological. Physical causes often have an underlying condition that effect sexual function including:

- diabetes
- heart disease
- neurological disorders
- pelvic surgery or trauma
- alcoholism and drug abuse
- chronic disease such as kidney or liver failure
- side effects of medicines
- hormone imbalance
- heavy smoking

Psychological factors including the following:

- stress or anxiety
- insecurity about sexual performance
- relationship discord
- confusion regarding sexual orientation
- depression
- trauma in previous sexual experiences

The following agents have been associated with sexual dysfunction, so patients should speak to their doctors if they have concerns regarding: Tamoxifen, Luminal, Dilantin, Mysloine, Tegretol, Tricyclic, Anafranil, Prozac, Paxil, Inderal, Lopressor, Corgard, Blocadren, Tenormin, Cimetidine, Tagament, Thorazine, Haldol, Zyprexa, Xanax, Valium, and some progestin-dominant birth control pills. It is important to note that there may be alternate medications available that do not affect sexual function. Other agents may also be available to counteract any sexual dysfunctions experienced with these medications. Prescribed medication should not be discontinued without first speaking with a physician.

Treatment

Treatments break down into two main kinds, physical and behavioral **psychotherapy**.

In many cases, doctors or advance practice nurses may prescribe medications to treat an underlying physical cause or sexual dysfunction. Possible medical treatments include:

- Viagra (Sildenafil) is a treatment for erectile dysfunction in men.

- Papaverine and prostaglandin are used for erectile difficulties.

- MUSE (Medical Urethral System for Erection), a prostaglandin E-1 pellet which can be inserted into the urethra. In addition, Caverject and Edex are prostaglandin E-1 injection medications for erectile dysfunction.

- Surgically implanted inflatable penile prosthesis for erectile dysfunction.

- Androgel, a topical gel for testosterone/androgen replacement in men. Testosterone injections and patches may also be used in men and women to stimulate sexual desire.

- Clomipramine, fluoxetine, as well as serotonin re-uptake inhibitors such as Prozac, Zoloft, and Anafranil for premature ejaculation.

- Hormone replacement therapy for female dysfunctions.

- EROS-CTD, a clitoral therapy device approved by the FDA in May 2000 is designed to enhance lubrication and sensation in women who have arousal disorders. With a gentle suction, it increases blood flow to the clitoris and surrounding area.

Other agents include:

- ICOS is an agent for treatment of erectile dysfunction.

- Uprima (apomorphine) claims to induce erection in men and arousal in women.

- Vasomax, an oral tablet, is said to facilitate an erection within 10–15 minutes. It is anticipated that Vasomax may aid women as well as men.

- Viagra for women.

- SS Cream is a topical agent with natural plant extracts which appears to desensitize the penis and is used to treat premature ejaculation.

In some cases, a specific technique may be used during intercourse to correct a dysfunction. One of the most common is the "squeeze technique" to prevent premature ejaculation. When a man feels that an orgasm is imminent, he withdraws from his partner. Then, the man or his partner gently squeezes the head of the penis to halt the orgasm. After 20–30 seconds, the couple may resume intercourse. The couple may do this several times before the man proceeds to ejaculation.

In cases where significant sexual dysfunction is linked to a broader emotional problem, such as depression or **substance abuse**, intensive psychotherapy and/or pharmaceutical intervention may be appropriate.

A variety of alternative therapies can be useful in the treatment of sexual dysfunction. Counseling or psychotherapy is highly recommended to address any emotional or mental components of the disorder. Botanical medicine, either western, Chinese, or ayurvedic, as well as nutritional supplementation, can help resolve biochemical causes of sexual dysfunction. **Acupuncture** and homeopathic treatment can be helpful by focusing on the energetic aspects of the disorder.

Some problems with sexual function are normal. For example, women starting a new or first relationship may feel sore or bruised after intercourse and find that an over-the-counter lubricant makes sex more pleasurable. Simple techniques, such as soaking in a warm bath, may relax a person before intercourse and improve the experience. **Yoga** and **meditation** provide needed mental and physical **relaxation** for several conditions, such as vaginismus. Relaxation therapy eases and relieves anxiety about dysfunction. Massage is extremely effective at reducing **stress**, especially if performed by the partner.

Prognosis

There is no single cure for sexual dysfunction, but almost all can be controlled. Most people who have a level of sexual dysfunction fare well once they get into a treatment program. For example, a high percentage of men with premature ejaculation can be successfully treated in two to three months. Furthermore, the gains made in sex therapy tend to be long-lasting rather than

KEY TERMS

Ejaculatory incompetence—The inability to ejaculate within the vagina.

Erectile dysfunction—Difficulty achieving or maintaining an erect penis.

Impotence—The inability to achieve and sustain an erection suitable for intercourse.

Orgasmic disorder—The impairment of the ability to reach sexual climax.

Painful intercourse (dyspareunia)—Generally thought of as a female dysfunction but it also affects males. Pain can occur anywhere.

Premature ejaculation—Rapid ejaculation before the person wishes it, usually in less than one to two minutes after beginning intercourse.

Retrograde ejaculation—A condition in which the semen spurts backward into the bladder.

Sexual arousal disorder—The inhibition of the general arousal aspect of sexual response.

Vaginismus—Muscles around the outer third of the vagina have involuntary spasms in response to attempts at vaginal penetration, not allowing for penetration.

short-lived. Viagra produces an erection in 75% of men with erectile dysfunction. For men who are not responsive to drug treatment, studies with surgically implanted inflatable penile prosthesis claim a success rate at approximately 98%.

Health care team roles

Nursing and allied health professionals play a critical part in the diagnosis and treatment of sexual dysfunction. Sex therapy, which is ideally provided by a member of the American Association of Sexual Educators, Counselors, and Therapists (AASECT), universally emphasizes correcting sexual misinformation, the importance of improved partner communication and honesty, anxiety reduction, sensual experience and pleasure, and interpersonal tolerance and acceptance. Sex therapists believe that many sexual disorders are rooted in learned patterns and values. These are termed psychogenic. An underlying assumption of sex therapy is that relatively short-term outpatient therapy can alleviate learned patterns, restrict symptoms, and allow a greater satisfaction with sexual experiences.

Registered dietitians and nutritionists can be instrumental in giving dietary guidance and **nutrition** supplementation that may improve overall health and energy levels. Health improvements may impact general well-being and sexual function.

Resources

BOOKS

Berman, Jennifer, M.D., Laura Berman, Ph.D., and Elisabeth Bumiller. *For Women Only: A Revolutionary Guide to Overcoming Sexual Dysfunction and Reclaiming Your Sex Life.* New York: Henry Holt, 2001.

Masters, William H., Virginia E. Johnson, and Robert C. Kolodny. *Human Sexuality.* New York: HarperCollins Publishers, 1992.

Weiner D. N., and R. C. Rosen. "Medications and Their Impact." Chap. 6 in *Sexual Function in People with Disability and Chronic Illness: A Health Professionals Guide.* Gaithersburg: Aspen Publications, 1997, p. 437.

PERIODICAL

Phillips, N., M.D. "Female sexual dysfunction: evaluation and treatment." *American Family Physician* 62 (2000): 127–36. *http://www.aafp.org/afp/20000701/127.html.*

ORGANIZATIONS

American Academy of Clinical Sexologists. 1929 18th Street NW, Suite 1166, Washington, DC 20009. (202) 462-2122.

American Association for Marriage and Family Therapy. 1100 17th Street NW, 10th Floor, Washington, DC 20036-4601. (202) 452-0109.

American Association of Sex Educators, Counselors & Therapists. P.O. Box 238, Mt. Vernon, IA 52314.

American Foundation for Urologic Disease, Sexual Function Health Council. 1126 N. Charles Street, Baltimore, MD 21201. (410) 468-1800. http://www.impotence.org.

National Kidney and Urologic Diseases, Information Clearinghouse. 3 Information Way, Bethesda, MD 20892-3580. http://www.niddk.nih.gov.

Network for Excellence in Women's Sexual Health (NEWSHE). Female Sexual Medicine Center, UCLA Medical Center, 924 Westwood Blvd., Suite 520, Los Angeles, California 90095. (310) 825-0025. Fax: (310) 794-0211. http://www.newshe.com.

Crystal Heather Kaczkowski, M.Sc.

Sexual pain disorders *see* **Sexual dysfunction**

Sexuality and disability

Definition

Sexuality is a wide term that encompasses more than just the sexual organs or secondary sexual characteristics of a human being. It includes body image, self image, gender identity, beliefs and feelings about sex, capacities for love and friendship, and social behavior as well as overt physical expression of love or sexual desire. A person's sexuality is influenced by ethical, spiritual, cultural, and moral concerns. It can also be greatly impacted by mental, emotional, or physical disabilities.

Description

Simply put, sexuality is a natural part of life, and it should be addressed with sensitivity, but as any other occupation or activity would be by a **rehabilitation** therapist or other health professional treating a patient. While the sexual activity of persons with disabilities has been studied by medical and mental health researchers for the last thirty years, however, the subject rarely arises in ordinary conversations between persons with disabilites and their health care providers. This silence reflects both the embarrassment that people feel in discussing sexual problems, as well as the social attitude that persons with disabilities are not fully human, that is, they do not have sexual desires.

Sexual activity is a complex set of behaviors that involves most of the systems of the body as well as the mind and emotions. Consequently, a physical or mental disability that interferes with cognition, motor skills, coordination, and/or sensory skills can affect one's sexuality and/or sexual activity. Such physical impairments as **brain** and **spinal cord injury**, **multiple sclerosis**, arthritis, or seizures produce muscle **weakness**, loss of endurance, a decreased range of motion, and **back pain**. Such developmental and cognitive disabilities as attention span deficit, **dementia**, mental retardation, and depression affect a person's ability to form healthy relationships with trustworthy sexual partners. Lastly, the damaged self-image that can result from such surgical procedures as mastectomy or amputation can affect a person's desire to resume or maintain sexual activity.

Health professionals should note that sexuality is a concern of most people in contemporary society, not just of those with some form of disability. The widespread use of sex in advertising to sell consumer goods, the saturation of the mass media with images of physically perfect men and women, and the increased availability of pornography leave many adults confused about "normal" sexual behaviors, "normal" aspects of attractiveness to others, and "normal" levels of sexual desire. It is often helpful to reassure persons with disabilities that "normal" covers a wide range of degrees of interest in sexual relationships or sexual behaviors.

Human sexuality is not a "one-size-fits-all" entity in either men or women.

Patients of occupational therapists, physical therapists, social workers, and other health professionals should understand that they can discuss sexual concerns. Patients should be reminded throughout the process of rehabilitation that the return of sexual feelings is a sign of healing and recovery. It is equally important, however, for practitioners to keep in mind that a patient with a chronic stressful health problem may not consider sexual activity a high priority. That decision, too, should be respected.

Physical disabilities

SPINAL CORD INJURIES. Sexual function or dysfunction following **spinal cord** injury (SCI) depends on the severity of injury. Sensation can be affected throughout the limbs and body, affecting erectile function in men and lubrication in women. Just below half of studied men have reported they could have erections and achieve orgasm. Most women report that they still can achieve lubrication and orgasm, but sometimes in an altered manner. Males with spinal cord injuries often use their mouths more frequently to arouse and give pleasure to their partners.

STROKE AND TRAUMATIC BRAIN INJURY. Survivors of **stroke** are often concerned about the impact of changes in their physical appearance on their partner, since strokes often produce such symptoms as drooling or a droop on one side of the mouth. In addition, many persons who have had a stroke worry about having another stroke during sexual activity. Lastly, either emotional depression or medications can cause stroke patients to lose interest in sex. Frank discussion with the partner as well as experimentation with different positions for intercourse are often helpful. In no case, however, should a stroke patient stop taking a prescribed medication without consulting his or her physician.

Not much research exists on the sexual function following traumatic brain injury (TBI). However, sexual activity has been found to decrease following TBI. Existing studies report conflicting evidence regarding men and **erectile dysfunction**. While many men report no erectile dysfunction, other studies have shown that a majority of men are impotent following TBI. It is also possible, depending on the portion of the brain affected by TBI, for a person to exhibit inappropriate sexual behavior, which is also known as hypersexuality.

NEUROMUSCULAR DISORDERS. Neuromuscular disorders, such as **muscular dystrophy**, can result in underdeveloped genitalia, which in turn, can affect sexual function. Although few studies exist, most experts believe that given the **physiology** of neuromuscular disorders, people with these disorders still are able to become aroused, have erections, and experience orgasms.

The age at onset of the disorder determines how sexually active a person can be. A patient who experiences neuromuscular disorders at an early age may never gain full physical dependence, and that subsequently could hinder sexual function. Physical disability leads to lessened socialization, which also can hinder sexual expression. It is also common for the parents of children with disabilities to never fully acknowledge sexual maturation or the possibility of normal sexual function in their children.

ARTHRITIS. Arthritis causes stiffness in the joints, fatigue, and **pain**. A decreased desire for sex may directly result from the tiredness and discomfort, but it may also be a side effect of arthritis medications. Arthritis patients should be assessed for joint range of motion, inflammation, deformity, and muscle strength and flexibility. Because arthritis affects the use of the hands, masturbation can be difficult. Positioning during sex can be difficult because of the body's loss of flexibility. Low back pain is common in patients with **osteoarthritis**, and sexual activity may result in muscle spasms.

Rheumatoid arthritis causes **bone** erosion and may cause problems with erection. Some persons with rheumatoid arthritis have reported that the symptoms of the disorder become temporarily worse following sexual activity.

DIABETES. Many studies exist examining the effects of diabetes on sexual function and sex drive. Most experts believe that sexual desire in men is virtually unaffected by diabetes. Women, however, are reported to experience a decrease in sexual desire. Diabetic women also experience a higher rate of occurrence of vaginal infections, which results in a decrease in lubrication, discharge, odor, **itching**, and tenderness, all which affect sexual desire and function.

Diabetes greatly impacts **contraception**, fertility, successful gestation, and the long-term health of women. Diabetic women are less likely than nondiabetic to carry a child full term and have a live birth. There is a risk of **miscarriage**, **birth defects**, and complications during **childbirth**.

Mental disabilities

Cognitive or mental impairment does not preclude a person's engaging in sexual activity. For a patient with mental retardation, information should be presented in simple, short terms. The Association for Retarded Citizens believes that persons with mental retardation have a fundamental right to learn about sexual functions and relationships as well as safe sex, and that they should be able to make informed decisions regarding their sexuality. The Arc, a national organization for people with mental retardation maintains that the retarded should not be involuntarily sterilized nor denied sterilization if they choose it for themselves.

Having a developmental disability does not preclude a person from ever having an appropriate sexual relationship. Although some individuals may be too impaired to have a safe and appropriate sexual relationship, there are many individuals with moderate developmental impairments who can engage in self-stimulation.

The Arc also urges that people with mental retardation be given education and support to protect them from abuse and exploitation while respecting their human dignity.

Children with disabilities

Children with disabilities should not be treated as if they are asexual beings, without sexual feelings and drives. At the same time they, like people with mental retardation, require appropriate protections against exploitation and abuse by adults. These protections are all the more necessary because of the increased emphasis on sexual activity in the mass media and the general culture.

Because masturbation and certain other behaviors that may be related to children's self-discovery are clearly inappropriate if performed in public, it is important for practitioners to point out their inappropriateness to children. Practitioners should not, however, refer to these behaviors as "bad," but rather as improper at certain times.

The elderly

In general, older adults are often regarded as "over the hill" with regard to sexual attractiveness, interest or activity, purely apart from any physical or mental disabilities that may accompany the **aging** process. This prejudice is particularly strong in the case of postmenopausal women. The National **Women's Health** Information Center reports that many medical professionals are misinformed about the sexual potential of women of any age with disabilities and consequently do not encourage them to resume normal sexual activities. But many older women also reported to the agency that they do not receive adequate education on sexual function related to disability. It is important for health professionals to inform themselves about the effects of aging on sexuality in the elderly—particularly about the side effects of medications frequently prescribed for older adults—and convey an openness to discussing these matters with their patients.

Viewpoints

The Sexuality Information and Education Council of the United States (SIECUS), which takes stands on issues of sexuality believes that persons with disabilities have a right to sexuality education, sexual health care, and opportunities for sexual expression. It further states that public and private health agencies should ensure that persons with disabilities should be eligible for services dealing with sexuality and sexual function.

Professional implications

Rehabilitation should include advice about resuming sexual activity when such discussion is appropriate. It is important, however, for the practitioner to consider this issue prior to addressing it with a patient. The practitioner should first analyze his or her own attitudes about sexuality, and understand that the patient may want to discuss an aspect of sexuality or sexual function that the practitioner does not agree with or is uncomfortable discussing. If a practitioner plans to avoid discussion of a particular sexual issue with a patient, they should be prepared to refer the patient to appropriate counseling or therapy that will meet this need. The practitioner always should remain nonjudgmental with the patient when discussing any sexuality issue.

Much like any other activity of daily living, sexuality should be addressed by the practitioner during the normal course of treatment. The issue can easily be raised in the context of such other everyday activities as grooming, bathing, or dressing. Sexual issues can be addressed in the context of communication and intimacy among partners rather than focusing on physical abilities or limitations. Practitioners can bring up the subject with an open-ended question asking the patient if he/she has any questions regarding sexual activity. If the practitioner avoids discussion of sexuality, the patient may assume that the subject is inappropriate or that the practitioner is uncomfortable. Practitioners uneasy about the subject should at least put the issue on the table, leave it open for discussion, and give the patient the option of declining to address it. It is also appropriate to allow the patient to invite their spouse or partner to a treatment session dealing with sexuality.

Resources

BOOKS

Neistadt, Maureen E., and Elizabeth Blesedell Crepeau. *Willard and Spackman's Occupational Therapy*, 9th ed. Philadelphia: Lippincott-Raven Publishers, 1998.

Sipski, Marcia L., and Craig J. Alexander. *Sexual Function in People With Disability and Chronic Illness.* Gaithersburg, MD: Aspen Publishers, Inc, 1997.

Umphred, Darcy Ann, ed. *Neurological Rehabilitation*, 3rd ed. St. Louis, MO: Mosby-Year Book, Inc., 1995.

PERIODICALS

Couldrick, Lorna. "Sexual Issues: An Area of Concern for Occupational Therapists?" *British Journal of Occupational Therapy* 61 (November 1998): 493–49.

Holmes, Maria. "An Evaluation of Staff Attitudes towards the Sexual Activity of People with Learning Disabilities." *British Journal of Occupational Therapy* 61 (March 1998): 111–115.

Joe, Barbara E. "Coming to Terms with Sexuality."*OT Week* (19 September 1996): 214–216.

ORGANIZATIONS

The American Occupational Therapy Association, Inc. 4720 Montgomery Lane, Bethesda, MD 20824-1220. (301) 652-2682. http://www.aota.org.

The ARC of the United States. 1010 Wayne Ave., Suite 650, Silver Spring, MD 20910. (301) 565-3842. http://www.thearc.org.

Center for Research on Women with Disabilities, Department of Physical Medicine and Rehabilitation, Baylor College of Medicine. 3440 Richmond Ave., Suite B, Houston, TX 77046. (800) 442-7693. http://www.bcm.edu/crowd.

National Information Center for Children and Youth with Disabilities. P.O. Box 1492, Washington, DC, 20013. (800) 695-0285. http://www.nichcy.org.

National Institute on Aging (NIA) Age Page: Sexuality in Later Life. NIA Information Center, P.O. Box 8057, Gaithersburg, MD 20898. (800) 222-2225. TTY: (800) 222-4225.

The National Women's Health Information Center. 8550 Arlington Blvd., Suite 300, Fairfax, VA 22031. (800) 994-WOMAN. http://www.4woman.gov.

Sexuality Information and Education Council of the United States (SIECUS). 1638 R Street, Suite 220, Washington, DC 20009. (202) 265-2405. http://www.siecus.org.

Meghan M. Gourley

Sexually transmitted disease

Definition

Sexually transmitted disease (STD) is a term used to describe more than 20 different infections that are transmitted through exchange of semen, **blood**, and other body fluids, or by direct contact with the affected body areas of people with an STD. Sexually transmitted diseases are also called venereal diseases.

Demographics

The Centers for Disease Control and Prevention (CDC) has reported that 85% of the most prevalent infectious diseases in the United States are sexually transmitted. The rate of STDs in this country is 50 to 100 times higher than that of any other industrialized nation. One in four sexually active Americans will be affected by an STD at some time in his or her life.

The CDC estimates that about 19 million new STD infections occur in the United States each year. Almost half of these infections occurs in someone between the ages of 15 and 24. It is estimated that STDs have an economic cost of as much as $15.9billion dollars each year in the United States alone.

The two most commonly reported STDs are Chlamydia and gonorrhea, with more than 1.5 million new cases being reported annually. The most frequently affected group is girls between 15 and 19 years of age, and women between 20 and 24 years of age. Other STDs may occur more frequently than Chlamydia and gonorrhea, but because some STDs such as human papillomavirus (**HPV**) and **genital herpes** do not get reported to the CDC they tend to be undercounted.

Description

Types of STDs

Some of the most common and potentially serious STDs in the United States include:

• Chlamydia. This STD is caused by the bacterium *Chlamydia trachomatis*, a microscopic organism that lives as a parasite inside human cells. In 2008, there were 1,210,523 reported cases of Chlamydia. That means that Chlamydia affects more about 40 out of every 1,000 people. Chlamydia has been increasing in frequency in the United States in recent years, with a 9.2% increase in reported cases from 2007 to 2008. Approximately 40% of women will develop pelvic inflammatory disease (PID) as a result of Chlamydia infection, a leading cause of infertility.

• Human papillomavirus (HPV). HPV causes genital warts and is the single most important risk factor for cervical cancer in women. Over 100 types of HPV exist, but only about 30 of them can cause genital warts and are spread through sexual contact. In some instances, warts are passed from mother to child during childbirth, leading to a potentially life-threatening condition for newborns in which warts develop in the throat (laryngeal papillomatosis).

• Genital herpes. Herpes is an incurable viral infection thought to be one of the most common STDs in the United States. It is caused by one of two types of herpes simplex viruses: HSV-1 (commonly causing oral herpes) or HSV-2 (usually causing genital herpes). The CDC estimates that there were 292,000 new cases of genital herpes in 2008. It is believed to affect more than 45 million Americans (one out of every five individuals 12 years of age or older) are infected with HSV-2; this number has increased 30% since the 1970s. HSV-2 infection is more common in women (one out of every four women) than men (one out of every five men) and in African Americans than Caucasians.

• Gonorrhea. The bacterium *Neisseria gonorrhoeae* is the causative agent of gonorrhea and can be spread by vaginal, oral, or anal contact. The CDC reports that 336,742 new cases of gonorrhea were reported in 2008. This is about 111.6 cases per 100,000 people. This was a decrease of 5.4% from 2007. Since 1975 reported cases of gonorrhea have declined more than 70%.

• Syphilis. Syphilis is a potentially life-threatening infection that increases the likelihood of acquiring or transmitting HIV. In 2008, the CDC reported approximately 13,500 new cases of syphilis in the United States. This was the highest number of new cases reported since 1995. The rate of primary and secondary syphilis is about 4.5 cases per 100,000 people, and the rate of congenital syphilis is about 10.1 per 100,000 live births. Congenital syphilis causes irreversible health problems or death in as many as 40% of all live babies born to women with untreated syphilis.

• Human immunodeficiencyvirus (HIV) infection. The CDC estimates that there are approximately 1,106,400 people in the United States living with HIV/AIDS, and that about one fifth of them were not aware of the HIV infection. In 2007 there were 35,962 diagnosed cases of AIDS in the United States, with 28 of them occurring in children under the age of 13. As of 2010, the World Health Organization estimated that there were 33.4 million people living with HIV worldwide. There is no cure for this STD.

STDs can have very painful long-term consequences as well as immediate health problems. They can cause:

• birth defects

• blindness

• bone deformities

• brain damage

• cancer

• heart disease

KEY TERMS

Chlamydia—A microorganism that resembles certain types of bacteria and causes several sexually transmitted diseases in humans.

Condom—A thin sheath worn over the penis during sexual intercourse to prevent pregnancy or the transmission of STDs. There are also female condoms.

Diaphragm—A dome-shaped device used to cover the back of a woman's vagina during intercourse in order to prevent pregnancy.

Pelvic inflammatory disease (PID)—An inflammation of the tubes leading from a woman's ovaries to the uterus (the Fallopian tubes), caused by a bacterial infection. PID is a leading cause of fertility problems in women.

Venereal disease—Another term for sexually transmitted disease.

• infertility and other abnormalities of the reproductive system

• mental retardation

• death

Social groups and STDs

STDs affect certain population groups more severely than others. Women, young people, and members of minority groups are particularly affected. Women in any age bracket are more likely than men to develop medical complications related to STDs. Ethnic minorities are more likely to be affected by STDs than Caucasians, with African Americans especially at risk, although this may be changing. For example, in 2008, the incidence of **syphilis** among white women was 0.5 cases per 100,000, while the incidence among African American women was 7.6 cases per 100,000.

Causes and symptoms

The symptoms of STDs vary according to the disease agent (virus or bacterium), the sex of the patient, and the body systems affected. The symptoms of some STDs are easy to identify, others produce infections that may either go unnoticed for some time or are easy to confuse with other diseases. Syphilis in particular can be confused with disorders ranging from **infectious mononucleosis** to allergic reactions to prescription medications. In addition, the incubation periods of STDs varies. Some produce symptoms close enough to the time of sexual contact—often less than 48 hours later—for the individual to recognize the connection between the behavior and the symptoms. Others have a longer incubation period, so that the individual may not recognize the early symptoms as those of a sexually transmitted **infection**.

Some symptoms of STDs affect the genitals and reproductive organs:

• A woman who has an STD may bleed when she is not menstruating or have abnormal vaginal discharge. Vaginal burning, itching, and odor are common, and she may experience pain in her pelvic area while having sex.

• A discharge from the tip of the penis may be a sign that a man has an STD. Males may also have painful or burning sensations when they urinate.

• There may be swelling of the lymph nodes near the groin area.

• Both men and women may develop skin rashes, sores, bumps, or blisters near the mouth or genitals. Homosexual men frequently develop these symptoms in the area around the anus.

Other symptoms of STDs are systemic, which means that they affect the body as a whole. These symptoms may include:

• fever, chills, and similar flu-like symptoms

• skin rashes over large parts of the body

• arthritis-like pains or aching in the joints

• throat swelling and redness that lasts for three weeks or longer

Diagnosis

A sexually active person who has symptoms of an STD should be examined without delay by one of the following health care professionals:

• a specialist in women's health (gynecologist)

• a specialist in disorders of the urinary tract and the male sexual organs (urologist)

- a family physician

- a nurse practitioner

- a specialist in skin disorders (dermatologist).

The diagnostic process begins with a thorough **physical examination** and a detailed medical history that documents the patient's sexual history and assesses the risk of infection.

The doctor or other health care professional will:

- Describe the testing process. This includes all blood tests and other tests that may be relevant to the specific infection.

- Explain the meaning of the test results.

- Provide the patient with information regarding high-risk behaviors and any necessary treatments or procedures.

The doctor may suggest that a patient diagnosed with one STD be tested for others, as its possible to have more than one STD at a time. One infection may hide the symptoms of another or create a climate that fosters its growth. At present, it is particularly important that people who are HIV-positive be tested for syphilis as well.

Notification

The law in some parts of the United States requires **public health** officials to trace and contact the partners of people with some STDs. Minors, however, can get treatment without their parents' permission. Public health departments in most states can provide information about STD clinic locations, and Planned Parenthood facilities are available to provide testing and counseling. These agencies can also help with or assume the responsibility of notifying sexual partners who should be tested and may require treatment.

Treatment

Although self-care can relieve some of the **pain** of genital herpes or genital warts that has recurred after being diagnosed and treated by a physician, other STD symptoms require immediate medical attention.

Antibiotics are prescribed to treat gonorrhea, Chlamydia, syphilis, and other STDs caused by **bacteria**. Although prompt diagnosis and early treatment can almost always cure these STDs, new infections can develop if exposure continues or is renewed. Viral infections can be treated symptomatically and possibly with antiviral medications.

Prognosis

The prognosis for recovery from STDs varies among the different diseases. The prognosis for recovery from gonorrhea, syphilis, and other STDs caused by bacteria is generally good, provided that the disease is diagnosed early and treated promptly. Untreated syphilis in particular can lead to long-term complications and disability. Viral STDs (genital herpes, genital warts, HIV) cannot be cured but must be treated on a long-term basis to relieve symptoms and prevent life-threatening complications.

Prevention

Vaccines

Vaccines for the prevention of hepatitis A and hepatitis B are currently available, and are recommended, especially for gay and bisexual men, users of illegal drugs, health care workers, and others at risk of contracting these diseases. Vaccine for HPV also is available and is recommended for young women. Vaccines to prevent other STDs are being actively researched and tested.

Research into vaccinations to prevent HIV infection are underway. Although some have undergone clinical trials, as of 2010 there are no vaccines approved by the United States Food and Drug Administration (FDA) to prevent the disease.

Lifestyle choices

The risk of becoming infected with an STD can be reduced or eliminated by making certain choices. Abstaining from sexual contact, maintaining a mutually monogamous relationship, or being informed about a partner's medical status can all reduce the risk. The risk of contracting an STD can also be reduced by avoiding sexual contact with partners who are known to be infected with an STD, whose health status is unknown, who abuse drugs, or who are involved in the sex trade.

Use of condoms and other contraceptives

Condoms are the only known contraceptive method to reduce the risk of STD transmission. It is important to make sure a new condom is used every time there is genital, oral, or anal contact. Used correctly and consistently, male condoms provide good protection against HIV and other STDs such as gonorrhea, Chlamydia, and syphilis. Female condoms (lubricated sheaths inserted into the vagina) have also been shown to be effective in preventing HIV and other STDs.

Condoms also provide a measure of protection against genital herpes, genital warts, and hepatitis B.

There is some evidence that spermicides and diaphragms may provide a small amount of protection from some STDs, but that claim remains extremely controversial, and it recommended that people do not use these instead of other methods of STD protection. They do not protect women from contracting HIV. Birth-control pills, patches, or injections do not prevent STDs. Neither do surgical sterilization or hysterectomy.

Hygienic measures

Urinating and washing the genital area with soap and water immediately after having sex may eliminate some germs before they cause infection. Douching, however, can spread infection deeper. It may also increase a woman's risk of developing pelvic inflammatory disease (PID).

Resources

BOOKS

Egendorf, Laura, ed. *Sexually Transmitted Diseases.* Detroit, MI: Greenhaven Press, 2007.

Grimes, Jill.*Seductive Delusions: How Everyday People Catch STDs.* Baltimore: The Johns Hopkins University Press, 2008.

Marr, Lisa. *Sexually Transmitted Diseases: A Physician Tells You What You Need to Know* 2nd ed. Baltimore: The Johns Hopkins University Press, 2007.

Nack, Adina.*Damaged goods?: women living with incurable sexually transmitted diseases.* Philadelphia: Temple University Press, 2008.

OTHER

Medline Plus. Sexually Transmitted Diseases. February 3, 2010. http://www.nlm.nih.gov/medlineplus/sexuallytransmitteddiseases.html

National STD and AIDS Hotline. (800) 227-8922.

ORGANIZATIONS

AIDS Education and Training Centers (AETC) National Resource Center, 65 Bergen Street, 8th floor, Newark, NJ 07101.info@aidsetc.org, http://www.aidsetc.org

CDC National Prevention Information Network, P.O. Box 6003, Rockville, MD 20849-6003, (404) 639-3113, (888) CDC-INFO (888) 232-4636, a 24-hour information number., cdcinfo@cdc.gov, http://www.cdc.gov

Planned Parenthood Federation of America, 434 West 33rd St., New York, NY 10001, (212) 541-7800, (800) 230-PLAN, Fax: (212) 245-1845, http://www.plannedparenthood.org

United States Centers for Disease Control and Prevention (CDC), 1600 Clifton Road, Atlanta, GA 30333, (404) 639-3534, 800-CDC-INFO (800-232-4636). TTY: (888) 232-6348, inquiry@cdc.gov, http://www.cdc.gov.

Maureen Haggerty
Tish Davidson, AM

Sexually transmitted disease cultures

Definition

Sexually transmitted diseases are infections spread from person to person through sexual contact. A culture is a test in which a laboratory attempts to grow and identify the microorganism causing an **infection**. Laboratory culture is performed to isolate and identify the causes of several sexually transmitted infections.

Purpose

Sexually transmitted diseases (STDs) produce symptoms such as genital discharge, **pain** during urination, bleeding, pelvic pain, skin ulcers, or urethritis. Often, however, they produce no immediate symptoms. Therefore, the decision to test for these diseases must be based not only on the presence of symptoms, but on whether or not a person is at risk of having one or more of the diseases. Activities such as drug use and sex with more than one partner put a person at high risk for these diseases. STD cultures are necessary to diagnose certain types of STDs. Only after the infection is diagnosed can it be treated and further spread of the infection prevented. Left untreated, consequences of these diseases range from discomfort to **infertility** to death. In addition, these diseases in a pregnant woman can be passed from mother to fetus.

Precautions

Some infections, particularly gonorrhea, can be difficult to culture. It may be necessary to culture other sites that may be infected, such as the anus and mouth if the patient has corresponding sexual habits that may put him or her at risk. Also, health care workers should be aware that testing of anyone who mentions a sexual assault must be done very carefully, following a protocol which is usually best carried out in the emergency room. The physician, nurse, or physician assistant performing sample collection should observe **universal precautions** for the prevention of transmission of bloodborne pathogens.

Description

Gonorrhea, bacterial vaginosis, candidiasis, chancroid, chlamydiosis, herpes, and mycoplasma are common sexually transmitted diseases that can be cultured. The organisms that cause the first three conditions are cultured routinely while those that cause the last four are more difficult to grow and are more frequently identified immunologically or by DNA amplification. **Syphilis**, human **immunodeficiency** virus, and trichomoniasis are sexually transmitted diseases that usually are not cultured because they do not grow on artificial culture medium.

The female patient will be in the dorsal lithotomy position (lying on the back with legs raised and bent) typical for Pap testing. A speculum is moistened with warm water (no lubricant should be used) and inserted into the vagina to secure good visualization of the cervix. Any excess cervical mucous should be removed with a cotton ball (held by ring forceps). A sterile swab is inserted just inside the opening of the cervix (the os) and rotated gently for 30 seconds. Genital swabs are usually placed in a transport medium that contains charcoal to absorb toxins that inhibit the growth of gonococcus.

Care should be taken not to touch the vaginal surfaces with the swab in order to avoid the transfer of normal vaginal flora. For culture, the sample is placed in Stuart or Amies transport medium with charcoal added and delivered to the laboratory at room temperature. Since *Neisseria gonorrhoeae* are very sensitive to drying and temperature changes, plating is performed as soon as possible. For DNA probe or immunological testing (in which organisms are not cultured), the swab is broken off at the top of the sterile tube provided, and the tube is capped and sent to the laboratory. For immediate viewing, a swab sample may be placed in normal saline. One drop can then be placed between a slide and coverslip, and viewed beneath the **microscope**. This is called a "wet prep." A wet prep is useful for diagnosing yeast infection and trichomoniasis. Pelvic inflammatory disease samples and samples from genital lesions such as chancres are collected by aspiration. Plating for *H. ducreyi* should be done from the chancre aspirate and performed immediately because the organism is fastidious.

In the male patient, a smaller sterile swab is used to remove cells and any discharge from the last 0.75 inch (2 cm) of the urethra, and the swab is transported for culture (or DNA probe or immunological testing) as described for the female patient. If visible discharge is present on the surface of the penis, this should be swabbed, and it is unnecessary to enter the urethra. For anal specimens the physician inserts a sterile, cotton-tipped swab about 1 inch (2.5 cm) into the anus and rotates the swab for 30 seconds. Stool must not contaminate the swab. For oropharynx (throat) specimens the person's tongue is held down with a tongue depressor, as a health care worker moves a sterile, cotton-tipped swab across the back of the throat and tonsilar region.

Gonorrhea

Neisseria gonorrhoeae, also called gonococcus or GC, causes gonorrhea. It infects the mucosal surfaces of the genitourinary tract, primarily the urethra in males and the cervix in females. When seen on **Gram stain**, *Neisseria gonorrhoeae* are gram-negative diplococci (pairs of round or bean-shaped **bacteria**) often located inside white **blood** cells. The best specimen from which to culture *Neisseria gonorrhoeae* is a swab of the urethra in a male or the cervix in a female. Other possible specimens include the mouth, anus, or a swab of a genital lesion. All swabs are plated on modified Thayer-Martin (MTM) agar or New York City (NYC) agar. These media are selective for the growth of *N. gonorrhoeae*. MTM is chocolate agar (heated sheep blood agar) containing colistin to inhibit the growth of gram negative bacilli, nystatin or anisomycin to inhibit yeast, vancomycin to inhibit growth of gram-positive bacteria, and trimethoprim to inhibit *Proteus spp*. NYC agar contains amphotericin B instead of nystatin and consists of clear proteose-peptone supplemented agar. In addition, the sample is plated on either 5% sheep blood agar or Columbia agar with 5% sheep blood and colistin and nalidixic acid (CNA) to isolate *Candida albicans* which causes a yeast infection in the vagina and *Gardnerella vaginalis* which causes vaginosis as well. Plates are incubated at 96.8°F (36°C). in 5–10% carbon dioxide. MTM or NYC agar are examined for growth at 24 hours and if negative again at 48 hours. After 24 hours, any suspicious colonies are Gram-stained and tested for oxidase which provides presumptive identification of *Neisseria* if positive. The physician can be notified at this point by a preliminary report that gonococcus has been identified presumptively. Further biochemical testing may be performed to differentiate *N. gonorrhoeae* from *N. meningitides* which is sometimes isolated from homosexual males. Isolated colonies should also be tested for penicillin resistance. Plates may be discarded at 48 hours if no growth is seen. Rapid nonculture DNA amplification and enzyme **immunoassay tests** are available to test for *Neisseria gonorrhoeae* and provide results on the same day.

Microscopic analysis should always be included with **genital culture**. Wet preparations can identify yeast, *Trichomonas vaginalis*, and *G. vaginalis*. The latter can be seen as rods attached to large squamous epithelial cells called clue cells. A Gram stain of the swab material can identify gram-negative diplococci, which is presumptive evidence of gonococcal infection. In males, a positive finding on the Gram stain obviates the need for culture and the patient can begin antibiotic treatment. In females, the diplocicci must be located intracellularly in order to make a presumptive diagnosis of gonorrhea infection, and culture must be performed to confirm the diagnosis. The presence of clue cells, epithelial cells containing gram-negative or gram-variable coccobacilli, can signal the presence of *Gardnerella vaginalis*.

Chancroid

Chancroid is caused by *Haemophilus ducreyi*. It is characterized by genital ulcers with nearby swollen lymph nodes. The specimen is collected by swabbing one of these pus-filled ulcers. The Gram stain cannot differentiate *Haemophilus ducreyi* from other *Haemophilus* species. The physician must request a specific culture for a person who has symptoms of chancroid. Even using special culture, *Haemophilus ducreyi* is isolated from less than 80% of the ulcers it infects. If a culture is negative, the physician must diagnose chancroid based on the person's symptoms, and by ruling out other possible causes of these symptoms, such as syphilis (which is diagnosed by a blood test for **antibodies**).

H. ducreyi is fastidious and culture media should be inoculated within 10 minutes of sample collection. The swab should be spread over a chocolate (heated sheep blood agar) plate and incubated at 96.8°F (36°C) in 5–10% carbon dioxide. Isolated colonies are Gram-stained to identify the bacteria as small gram-negative bacilli, a colony is transferred to trypticase soy broth and a suspension is made. This is plated onto Mueller-Hinton or trypticase soy agar and strips of factor X (hemin) and factor V (NAD) are applied. *Haemophilus ducreyi* requires X factor but not V factor for growth. Like other *Haemophilus* species the organism is oxidase positive and reduces nitrate. Unlike most other *Haemophilus* species it does not produce catalase and does not ferment glucose, and these tests can be used for positive identification.

Mycoplasma *and* Ureaplasma

Three types of mycoplasmal organisms cause **sexually transmitted disease**: *Mycoplasma hominis*, *Mycoplasma gentialium*, and *Ureaplasma urealyticum*. *M. hominis* causes pelvic inflammatory disease (PID) and pyelonephritis in females but does not cause urethritis, vaginitis, or cervicitis. *Ureaplasma urealyticum* can cause urethritis in males and may cause PID in females but does not cause vaginitis or cervicitis. *M. gentialium* has been implicated as a cause of urethritis and PID. Samples are collected from the cervix in a female, and from the urethra (or urine) in a male. Swabs must be immediately placed in sucrose-phosphate or other acceptable transport medium and transported to the lab immediately. These organisms will grow on New York City agar and *M. hominis* will also grow on CNA plates, but swabs should be inoculated onto a selective agar or broth such as SP-4, which differentiates *Mycoplasma* from *Ureaplasma* based upon the ability of the latter to hydrolyze urea. Cultures are incubated aerobically at 96.8°F (36°C) and grow for two to four days. Colonies are very small and difficult to see with the unaided eye. When growth is seen, a portion of the agar is removed and stained with Dienes stain. The colonies are examined under a microscope for their characteristic fried egg appearance. They will have a dark blue center and light blue periphery. These organisms cannot be seen with the Gram stain.

Chlamydiosis

Chlamydiosis is caused by the gram-negative bacterium *Chlamydia trachomatis*. It is one of the most common STDs in the United States (approximately three million cases occur each year), and generally appears in sexually active adolescents and young adults. While chlamydiosis often does not have any initial symptoms, it can if left untreated lead to PID and sterility. Samples are collected from one or more of these infection sites: cervix in a female, urethra in a male, or the rectum. Swabs must be immediately placed in sucrose-phosphate or other acceptable transport medium and transported to the lab immediately. Culture is successful in recovering *Chlamydia trachomatis* about 80% of the time. The organism is inoculated onto monolayers of malignant tissue culture cells such as HeLa cells or McCoy cells in shell vials. The cultures are incubated for two to three days at 96.8°F (36°C) in 5–10% carbon dioxide. Following this they are stained with flourescent-labeled **monoclonal antibodies** to the major outer membrane protein (MOMP) to identify the characteristic chlamydial inclusions. This technique is expensive and requires a high level of tissue culture expertise. Consequently most labs use non-culture tests such as enzyme immunoassay or DNA amplication methods to diagnose chlamydial infections.

Genital herpes

Herpes is generally diagnosed based on the patient's symptoms and the physical exam. Approximately two-thirds of **genital herpes** is caused by herpes simplex 2 (HSV-2), and the remainder by herpes simplex 1 (HSV-1). Extremely painful blisters around the genital area are classic for initial herpes presentation. However, if questions remain, the herpes virus can be cultured from a vesicle (blister) which has been "unroofed" carefully with a scalpel blade. The base of the vesicle is swabbed with a sterile cotton applicator, and the virus taken to the laboratory in a tube of viral transport medium. Herpes can be cultured in several cell lines including human diploid fibroblasts (HDF), HEp2 cells (epithelial **cancer** cells from the larynx), primary monkey kidney cells (PMK), and rabbit kidney cells (RK). Cell cultures are inoculated and allowed to grow for one to three days at 96.8°F (36°C) in 5–10% carbon dioxide. Usually by the end of the first day of culture the cytopathic effect (CPE) can be seen by observing the cells under a microscope. Herpes induces the formation of giant cells.

Antibiotic susceptibility testing

Antibiotic susceptibility is not usually required for organisms isolated from a genital culture. Gonorrhea is treated with penicillin or related drugs. Chlamydiosis and mycoplasmal infections are treated with erythromycin. Herpes is treated with acyclovir or related antivirals. Candida is treated with clotrimazole or other antifungal. Bacterial vaginosis is treated with metronidazole, *Haemophilus ducryi* is treated with ceftriaxone or erythromycin.

For both male and female patients, urine tests for the DNA of *Chlamydia trachomatis* and *Neisseria gonorrhoeae* are available. In recent years, use of these nucleic acid amplification tests (NAATs) has increased, particularly for screening and where urethral and vervical culture samples are not possible because patients do not accept the procedure or because of logistics. These tests measure bacterial DNA that is amplified either by the ligase chain reaction (LCR) or the polymerase chain reaction (PCR). Both methods can detect the organisms within four hours, affording more rapid treatment. However, the tests do not detect any other genital tract pathogens that might be present in the patient.

Preparation

Cultures should always be collected before the person begins taking **antibiotics**. Men should not urinate within one hour before collection of a urethral specimen. Women should not douche or take a bath within 24 hours of collection of a cervical or vaginal culture.

Aftercare

Patients should be instructed to have no sexual contacts until test results are reported.

Complications

The minor discomforts of genital testing are short lived, and no significant complications are common.

Results

With the exception of *Mycoplasma* and *Ureaplasma*, these microorganisms are not found under normal conditions, so tests should be negative. *M. hominis* can be found in the male urethra, and *Ureaplasma urealyticum* can be found in the female genital tract in the absence of disease. Therefore, positive cultures for these organisms may indicate colonization without infection, and the physician must differentiate these conditions on the basis of the **physical examination** and symptoms. Therefore, these organisms are treated at the discretion of the physician. If a person has a positive culture for any other of these microorganisms, antibiotic treatment is started, and his or her sexual partners should be notified and tested. After treatment is completed, the physician may request a follow-up culture to confirm that the infection is cured.

Health care team roles

Genital cultures are ordered by a physician and collected by a physician, nurse, or physician assistant. Culture, microscopic analysis, immunoassay, and DNA testing are performed by clinical laboratory scientists or medical technologists. Wet preparations may also be performed by the physician or physician assistant or nurse practitioner with appropriate training. Nursing staff have a very important task in educating the patient in what to expect, assisting with obtaining samples, and helping to explain test results to patients. Many patients undergoing genital testing are in need of counseling regarding the risks of careless sexual behavior, and the opportunity should be used by staff for education to reduce risks in the future.

Resources

BOOKS

Fishbach, Frances Talaska. *A Manual of Laboratory and Diagnostic Tests,* 6th ed. Lippincott: 2000: 563–565.

Malarky, Louise M., and Mary Ellen McMorrow. *Nurses Manual of Laboratory Tests and Diagnostic Procedures.* WB Saunders Co., 2000: 177–179.

Tierney, Lawrence M., Stephen J. McPhee and Maxine A. Papadakis. *Current Medical Diagnosis and Treatment 2001.* Lange Medical Books/McGraw-Hill, 2001: 1309.

PERIODICAL

Campos-Outcalt, Doug. "Sexually Transmitted Disease: Easier Screening Tests, Single-Dose Therapies." *The Journal of Family Practice* (December 2003): 965–969.

ORGANIZATION

Centers for Disease Control and Prevention. National Center for HIV, STD, and TB Prevention. 1600 Clifton Road NE, Atlanta, GA 30333. (404) 639-8000. http://www.cdc.gov/nchstp/od/nchstp.html.

Erika J. Norris
Teresa G. Odle

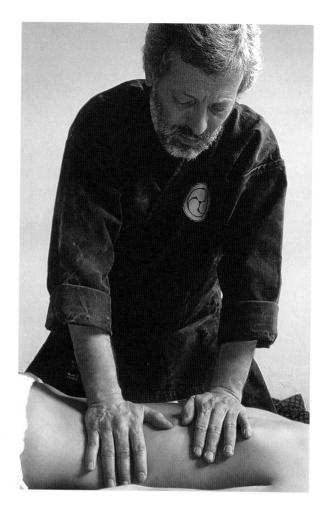

(A trained masseur administers shiatsu massage, photograph. Mauro Fermariello / Photo Researchers, Inc.)

Shiatsu

Definition

Shiatsu is a manipulative therapy developed in Japan and incorporating techniques of *anma* (Japanese traditional massage), **acupressure**, stretching, and Western massage. Shiatsu involves applying pressure to special points or areas on the body in order to maintain physical and mental well being, treat disease, or alleviate discomfort. This therapy is considered holistic because it attempts to treat the whole person instead of a specific medical complaint. All types of acupressure generally focus on the same pressure points and so-called energy pathways, but may differ in terms of massage technique. Shiatsu, which can be translated as finger pressure, has been described as needle-free **acupuncture**.

Origins

Shiatsu is an offshoot of anma that developed during the period after the Meiji Restoration in 1868. Traditional massage (anma) used during the age of shoguns was being criticized, and practitioners of *koho anma* (ancient way) displeased with it introduced new practices and new names for their therapies.

During the twentieth century, shiatsu distinguished itself from anma through the merging of Western knowledge of **anatomy**, koho anma, *ampuku* (abdominal massage), acupressure, *Do-In* (breathing practices), and Buddhism. Based on the work of Tamai Tempaku, shiatsu established itself in Japan and worldwide. The Shiatsu Therapists Association was found in 1925 and clinics and schools followed. Students of Tempaku began teaching their own brand of shiatsu, creating branch disciplines. By 1955, the Japanese Ministry of Health and Welfare acknowledged shiatsu as a beneficial treatment and licensing was established for practitioners.

Benefits

Shiatsu has a strong reputation for reducing **stress** and relieving nausea and **vomiting**. Shiatsu is also believed to improve circulation and boost the **immune system**. Some people use it to treat **diarrhea**, indigestion, constipation, and other disorders of the gastrointestinal tract; menstrual and menopausal problems; chronic **pain**; migraine; arthritis; toothache; **anxiety**; and depression. Shiatsu can be used to relieve muscular pain or tension, especially neck and **back pain**. It also appears to have sedative effects and may alleviate insomnia. In a broader sense, shiatsu is believed to enhance physical vitality and emotional well being.

Description

Shiatsu and other forms of Japanese acupressure are based on the concept of *ki*, the Japanese term for the all-pervading energy that flows through everything in the universe. (This notion is borrowed from the Chinese, who refer to the omnipresent energy as qi or chi.) Ki tends to flow through the body along special energy pathways called meridians, each of which is associated with a vital organ. In Asian systems of traditional medicine, diseases are often believed to occur due to disruptions in the flow this energy through the body. These disruptions may stem from emotional factors, climate, or a host of other causes including stress, the presence of impurities in the body, and physical trauma.

The aim of shiatsu is to restore the proper flow of bodily energy by massaging the surface of the skin along the meridian lines. Pressure may also be applied to any of the 600 or so acupoints. Acupoints, which are supposedly located just under the skin along the meridians, are tiny energy structures that affect the flow of ki through the body. When ki either stagnates and becomes deflected or accumulates in excess along one of these channels, stimulation to the acupoints, which are sensitive to pressure, can unblock and regulate the ki flow through toning or sedating treatment.

Western medicine hasn't proven the existence of meridians and acupoints. However, in one study, two French medical doctors conducted an experiment at Necher Hospital in Paris to test validity of theory that energy is being transported along acupuncture meridians. They injected and traced isotpes with gamma-camera imaging. The meridians may actually correspond to nerve transmission lines. In this view, shiatsu and other forms of healing massage may trigger the emission of naturally occurring chemicals called neurotransmitters. Release of these chemical messengers may be responsible for some of the therapeutic effects associated with shiatsu, such as pain relief.

Preparations

People usually receive shiatsu therapy while lying on a floor mat or massage table or sitting up. The massage is performed through the clothing—preferably a thin garment made from natural fibers—and disrobing is not required. Pressure is often applied using the thumbs, though various other parts of the body may be employed, including fingertips, palms, knuckles, elbows, and knees—some therapists even use their feet. Shiatsu typically consists of sustained pressure (lasting up to 10 seconds at a time), squeezing, and stretching exercises. It may also involve gentle holding as well as rocking motions. A treatment session lasts anywhere from 30 to 90 minutes.

Before shiatsu treatment begins, the therapist usually performs a general health assessment. This involves taking a family medical history and discussing the physical and emotional health of the person seeking therapy. Typically, the practitioner also conducts a diagnostic examination by palpating the **abdomen** or back for any energy imbalances present in other parts of the body.

Precautions

While shiatsu is generally considered safe, there are a few precautions to consider. Because it may increase **blood** flow, this type of therapy is not recommended in people with bleeding problems, **heart** disease, or **cancer**. **Massage therapy** should always be used with caution in those with **osteoporosis**, fresh **wounds** or scar tissue, **bone fractures**, or inflammation.

Applying pressure to areas of the head is not recommended in people with epilepsy or high **blood pressure**, according to some practitioners of shiatsu.

Shiatsu is not considered effective in the treatment of **fever**, **burns**, and infectious diseases.

Shiatsu should not be performed right after a meal.

Side effects

When performed properly, shiatsu is not associated with any significant side effects. Some people may experience mild discomfort, which usually disappears during the course of the treatment session.

Research and general acceptance

Like many forms of massage, shiatsu is widely believed to have a relaxing effect on the body. There is also a significant amount of research suggesting that acupressure techniques can relieve nausea and vomiting associated with a variety of causes, including **pregnancy** and anesthetics and other drugs. In one study, published in the *Journal of Nurse-Midwifery* in 1989, acupressure was shown to significantly reduce the effects of nausea in 12 of 16 women suffering from morning sickness. Five days of this therapy also appeared to reduce anxiety and improve mood. Another investigation, published in the *British Journal of Anaesthesia* in 1999, studied the effects of acupressure on nausea resulting from the use of anesthetics. Pressure applied to an acupoint on the inside of the wrist appeared to alleviate nausea in patients who received anesthetics during the course of laparoscopic surgery.

Shiatsu may also produce sedative and analgesic effects. The sedative powers of acupressure were investigated in a study published in the *Journals of Gerontology* in 1999, which involved over 80 elderly people who suffered from sleeping difficulties. Compared to the people in the control groups, the 28 participants who received acupressure were able to sleep better. They slept for longer periods of time and were less likely to wake up during the night. The researchers concluded that acupressure may improve the quality of sleep in older adults. The use of acupressure in postoperative pain was investigated in a study published in the *Clinical Journal of Pain* in 1996. In this study, which involved 40 knee surgery patients, one group received acupressure (15 acupoints were stimulated) while the control group received sham acupressure. Within an hour of treatment, members of the acupressure group reported less pain than those in the control group. The pain-relieving effects associated with acupressure lasted for 24 hours.

Shiatsu may benefit **stroke** victims. The results of at least one study (which did not include a control group) suggest that shiatsu may be useful during stroke **rehabilitation** when combined with other treatments.

Training and certification

A qualified shiatsu therapist must have completed courses in this form of therapy and should be nationally certified or licensed by the state (most are certified by the American Oriental Bodywork Therapy Association). Asking a medical doctor for a recommendation is a great place to start. It can also be helpful to consult friends and family members who have tried shiatsu. There are several massage-related organizations that offer information on locating a qualified therapist. These include the National Certification Board for Therapeutic Massage and Bodywork, the American Massage Therapy Association, the International School of Shiatsu, and the American Oriental Bodywork Therapy Association.

Resources

BOOK

Cook, Allan R. *Alternative Medicine Sourcebook.* Detroit: Omnigraphics, 1999.

PERIODICALS

Chen, M.L., L.C. Lin, S.C. Wu, et al. "The effectiveness of acupressure in improving the quality of sleep of institutionalized residents." *J Gerontol A Biol Sci Med Sci* (1999): M389-94.

Felhendler, D., and B. Lisander. "Pressure on acupoints decreases postoperative pain." *Clin J Pain* (1996): 326–329.

ORGANIZATIONS

Acupressure Institute. 1533 Shattuck Avenue, Berkeley, CA 94709.

American Massage Therapy Association. 820 Davis Street, Suite 100, Evanston, IL.

American Oriental Bodywork Therapy Association. 50 Maple Place, Manhassett, NY 11030.

International School of Shiatsu. 10 South Clinton Street, Doylestown, PA 18901.

National Certification Board for Therapeutic Massage and Bodywork. 8201 Greensboro Drive, Suite 300, McLean, VA 22102.

Greg Annussek

Shingles (herpes zoster)

Definition

Shingles, or herpes zoster, is a condition caused by the reactivation of the varicella zoster virus (VZV) that causes chickenpox (varicella). After a bout of chickenpox, the virus remains dormant in the sensory nerve ganglia that are adjacent to the **spinal cord** and **brain**. Years later the virus reemerges, traveling along the nerves to the skin where it causes red rashes that develop into blisters. In the process the virus can damage nerves, leading to a very painful inflammation called postherpetic neuralgia (PHN), which can persist long after the **rash** disappears.

Demographics

Anyone who has had chickenpox or been vaccinated against varicella can develop shingles. Virtually all American adults have had chickenpox, even if the disease was so mild as to pass unnoticed. Nearly one in three Americans eventually develops shingles, and there are at least one million cases in the United States each year.

Although shingles can occur at any age, even in children, the incidence increases steadily with age. About half of all cases occur in people aged 60 or older. About 20% of people with shingles develop PHN. It is more common in women than in men. In the United States, between 120,000 and 200,000 people suffer from PHN each year. It occurs more frequently among the elderly and is one of the most common causes of pain-related suicide in older adults. The incidence of PHN increases with age and tends to last longer in older patients:

• PHN is rare in those under age 30.

• By age 40 the risk of PHN lasting longer than one month is 33%.

• By age 70 the risk increases to 74%.

Some scientists believe that the incidence of shingles is likely to increase over the next 40–50 years due to the introduction of a childhood vaccine against chickenpox in 1995. With far fewer children contracting chickenpox, adults have far less exposure to the virus, which would otherwise boost the immunity they acquired during childhood and help prevent reactivation of latent virus in their bodies.

Description

Varicella zoster virus is a member of the herpes virus family. It causes chickenpox or varicella, which is highly contagious and spreads through the air. Following this initial or primary VZV **infection**, which usually occurs in childhood, the virus remains in an inactive or latent state in nerve tissue. Years later—usually after age 50—VZV can be reactivated to cause herpes zoster or shingles. The name "varicella" is derived from "variola," the Latin name for smallpox, a now-eradicated deadly disease, which can resemble chickenpox. "Zoster" is the Greek word for girdle, and "shingles" derives from "cingulum," the Latin word for belt or girdle, which refer to the shingles lesions or blisters that form on one side of the waist. Scientists suspected as early as 1909 that chickenpox and shingles were caused by the same virus; this was confirmed in 1958.

Shingles is an infection of the **central nervous system**, particularly the dorsal root ganglia of the spine. From there the virus migrates through sensory nerve fibers to the skin, usually on the trunk, where it causes painful, fluid-filled eruptions or vesicles. Because the sensory nerves serve sharply bounded, non-overlapping areas of the skin called dermatomes, the shingles lesions appear within these dermatomes and do not cross the midline of the body.

Unlike chickenpox, shingles is not contagious because the virus is not usually in the **lungs** from which it could spread through the air. However, the fluid-filled eruptions on the skin contain large amounts of virus, which can be transmitted through direct contact and infect a person, usually a child, who has not previously been exposed to VZV. The infected person will develop a case of primary chickenpox. A vaccine that prevents or ameliorates the symptoms of shingles became available in 2006. Immunization against chickenpox does not prevent shingles although it may reduce its incidence.

Risk factors

Anyone who has ever had chickenpox or been vaccinated against it is at risk for shingles. Overall, approximately 20% of those who had chickenpox as children eventually develop shingles. Susceptibility to shingles appears to be genetically determined and the condition runs in families. The risk of shingles increases with age and with any condition that weakens the **immune system**. Those at particular risk for shingles include:

• children who had chickenpox in infancy or whose mothers had chickenpox late in pregnancy

• bone marrow and other transplant recipients

• those with compromised immune systems from diseases such as HIV/AIDS

• those with suppressed immune systems from chemotherapy drugs or other medications

Causes and symptoms

It is not clear why VZV reactivates to cause shingles, but it appears to be related to a decreased **immune response** due to advancing age, emotional or physical **stress**, fatigue, certain medications, **chemotherapy**, or diseases such as **cancer** or HIV/AIDS. Shingles is sometimes an early sign of **immunodeficiency** in people infected with HIV. In some cases, the virus appears to be reactivated by mechanical irritation or minor surgical procedures.

Mild cases of shingles often go unnoticed. The earliest signs may be vague and can easily be mistaken for other illnesses. The condition may begin with **fever**, chills, gastrointestinal discomfort, and malaise (a vague feeling of **weakness** or discomfort). Lymph nodes may swell. Within two to four days, localized areas of intense **pain**, **itching**, and numbness/tingling (paresthesia) or extreme sensitivity to touch (hyperesthesia) can develop, usually on the trunk. The second most common place is

Acyclovir—An antiviral drug that is available in oral, intravenous, and topical forms and that blocks replication of the varicella zoster virus.

Antibody—A specific protein produced by the immune system in response to a specific foreign protein or particle called an antigen.

Capsaicin—An active ingredient from hot chili peppers that is used in topical ointments to relieve pain. It appears to work by reducing the levels of a chemical substance involved in transmitting pain signals from nerve endings to the brain.

Corticosteroids—A group of hormones produced by the adrenal glands or manufactured synthetically. They are often used to treat inflammation. Examples include cortisone and prednisone.

Famciclovir—An oral antiviral drug that blocks replication of the varicella zoster virus.

Ganglion—A mass of nerve tissue outside of the central nervous system.

Immunocompromised—A weakened or poorly functioning immune system due to disease.

Immunosuppressed—Suppression of the immune system by medications during the treatment of diseases such as cancer or following an organ transplantation.

Post-herpetic neuralgia (PHN)—Long-lasting nerve pain caused by herpes zoster.

Tzanck preparation—A procedure in which skin cells from a blister are stained and examined under the microscope.

Valacyclovir—An oral antiviral drug that blocks the replication of the varicella zoster virus.

Vesicle—A small, raised lesion filled with clear fluid.

on one side of the face around the eye (ophthalmic shingles) or on the forehead. However, shingles can occur on the arms or legs or elsewhere on the body. The pain may be continuous or intermittent, usually lasting from one to four weeks. The pain may accompany skin eruptions or precede the eruptions by days.

The red rash or oozing blisters appear along the course of the affected nerve. There is usually a vague streak or band from the spine along the path of the nerve on one side of the body. About five days after they appear, the vesicles begin to crust or scab, and the disease resolves within the next two to three weeks. There may be no visible after effects or a slight scarring from the vesicles.

Shingles can be more debilitating in the elderly or those in poor health. The eruptions may be more extensive and inflammatory; they may also include bleeding blisters, areas of skin death, secondary bacterial infection, or extensive and permanent scarring. Ophthalmic shingles can cause painful eye infections and **vision** loss. Shingles infections within or near the ear can cause **hearing** or **balance problems**. Sometimes shingles can cause temporary or permanent tremors or **paralysis**; rarely, the condition spreads to the brain or spinal cord and causes **stroke** or **meningitis**.

Shingles pain usually subsides when the rash disappears, but it may last much longer, especially in the elderly. PHN can persist for months or years. It is caused by damage to the dorsal root ganglia, with the nerves becoming either spontaneously active—which is perceived as chronic pain—or hypersensitive to slight stimuli such as light touch. In the most severe cases, PHN can cause insomnia, weight loss, depression, and disability.

Diagnosis

Examination

Diagnosis of shingles is based on a medical history and **physical examination**. A definite diagnosis is difficult before eruption of the characteristic vesicles or bumps on the skin. The vesicles have a clear dermatome-bounded distribution usually on the midsection of the body.

Tests

Tests for shingles are rarely necessary but may include:

• polymerase chain reaction (PCR) testing for viral DNA

• viral culture of skin lesions

• a Tzanck preparation—stained cells from a blister, which will appear under the microscope to have many very large dark nuclei if infected with VZV

• a complete blood count (CBC) to test for elevated white blood cells that are indicative of infection

• blood serum levels of antibodies against VZV

Treatment

Traditional

Shingles almost always resolves spontaneously within a few weeks. Unless complicated by conditions such as HIV/AIDS or cancer, a primary care physician can provide treatment for easing painful symptoms. Rarely, transcutaneous electrical nerve stimulation (TENS) or a permanent nerve block is used to relieve the pain of PHN.

Drugs

The **antiviral drugs** acyclovir, valacyclovir, and famciclovir are used to treat shingles. These drugs can shorten the course of the illness. If started within 72 hours of the onset of the rash, antiviral therapy can heal the blisters more rapidly and sometimes even halt the disease. If taken after the disease has progressed, these drugs are less effective but may still lessen the pain. Antiviral drug treatment reduces the incidence of PHN by about one half and may also shorten its duration. Severely immunocompromised individuals, such as those with HIV/AIDS, may require intravenous administration of antiviral drugs or taking the drugs on an ongoing basis.

Various other drugs may be prescribed for shingles and PHN:

- corticosteroids, such as prednisone, to reduce inflammation from shingles, especially if the eye or other facial nerves are involved, and to reduce severe pain

- anticonvulsants such as pregabalin (Lyrica) or gabapentin to relieve pain

- the tricylcic antidepressants (TCAs) desipramine and nortriptyline

- opioid painkillers such as oxycodone, morphine, tramadol, or methadone

- tranquilizers or sedatives

- topical local anesthetics for application to the painful skin area and for post-herpetic itch; especially lidocaine, available as a cream, gel, spray, or patch

- capsaicin cream, which is available without a prescription but usually causes burning pain during application

Alternative

Alternative remedies and therapies will not cure shingles but they may relieve pain, reduce inflammation, and speed recovery:

- The amino acid lysine has also been reported to ease the symptoms of shingles and other herpes infections. Foods that are high in lysine include soybeans, black bean sprouts, lentils, parsley, and peas.

- Vitamin B12 supplementation during the first two days of the illness and ongoing vitamin B complex, vitamin C with bioflavonoids, and calcium supplements may boost the immune system.

- Echinacea can boost the immune system and help fight viral infections.

- Red pepper (capsicum or cayenne) is an ingredient in commercial ointments including Zostrix and Capzasin-P. It should be applied only to healed blisters and is useful for treating painful PHN. Seasoning food with red pepper may also provide relief.

- Calendula or licorice (*Glycyrrhiza glabra*) ointment or lotion may help treat shingles.

- Topical applications of lemon balm (*Melissa officinalis*), licorice, or peppermint (*Mentha piperita*) may reduce pain and blistering. These can also be consumed as teas.

- Sedative herbs such as passionflower can be brewed for a tea to treat PHN.

- Vervain helps relieve pain and inflammation.

- St. John's wort, lavender, chamomile, and marjoram help relieve inflammation.

- Homeopathic remedies include *Rhus toxicodendron* for blisters, *Mezereum* and *Arsenicum album* for pain, and *Ranunculus* for itching.

- Several drops of "Rescue Remedy" placed under the tongue or taken in water throughout the day are prescribed for relieving stress.

- Ayurvedic treatments for shingles include the application of turmeric paste.

- Acupuncture and acupressure can alleviate pain and PHN.

- Biofeedback or spinal cord stimulators may help relieve PHN.

- Relaxation techniques such as hypnotherapy and yoga may help relieve pain.

- Reflexology may help balance the body.

Practitioners of traditional Chinese medicine (TCM) may recommend herbal remedies:

- Chinese gentian root is used to treat the liver.

- Skullcap root in water is a Chinese folk remedy for shingles.

- Long Dan Xie Gan Tang is used to quell the accumulation of damp, toxic heat in the liver.

- For damp, infected, painful eruptions on the torso, Huang Qin Gao can be applied to the surrounding area.

Home remedies

Home remedies for shingles include plenty of rest, a healthy diet, regular **exercise**, and minimizing stress. The skin should be kept clean and contaminated items should not be reused. Cool compresses may help reduce pain from blisters. Blisters or crusting can be treated with compresses made with one-quarter cup (60 mL) of white vinegar in two quarts (1.9 L) of lukewarm water and applied twice daily for 10 minutes. The compresses should be discontinued when the blisters have dried up. Soothing baths and lotions with colloidal oatmeal, starch, or calamine may help to relieve itching and discomfort. If the skin becomes dry, tight, and cracked as the crusts and scabs separate, a small amount of plain petroleum jelly can be applied three or four times daily. The pain of PHN may be relieved with hot and cold compresses.

Prognosis

Shingles is almost never life-threatening in otherwise healthy patients and usually resolves without treatment in a few weeks. Because shingles boosts the immune response to VZV, repeat episodes are rare, occurring in less than 4% of patients. Although PHN usually diminishes over time, it can be disabling and difficult to treat.

Shingles can be much more severe in immunocompromised patients. The condition can last for months, recur frequently, and spread to the lungs, **liver**, gastrointestinal tract, brain, or other vital organs. Complications of shingles in immunocompromised or immunosuppressed patients may resemble those of primary varicella infection in adults, including viral **pneumonia**, male sterility, acute liver failure, and **birth defects** in children born to infected mothers. Depletion of CD4+ T lymphocytes in HIV/AIDS patients is associated with severe and chronic or recurrent VZV infection.

Prevention

A lifestyle that promotes immune system function and overall health may help prevent shingles. Factors include a well-balanced diet rich in essential **vitamins** and **minerals**, adequate sleep, regular exercise, and reduced stress. Patients with shingles should avoid contact with anyone who has not had chickenpox or been vaccinated against the disease, particularly pregnant women, newborns, and those with weakened immune systems.

In the United States, it is now recommended that all children between 18 months and adolescence be immunized against chickenpox. Because a weakened (attenuated) form of the virus is used in this vaccine, it is thought that **vaccination** will reduce the likelihood of shingles later on in life. A single-dose vaccine against shingles (Zostavax) became available in 2006 and is recommended for most people aged 60 and older who have previously had chickenpox. It appears to prevent shingles in about 50% of vaccinated people and reduces the pain associated with shingles in others. It also can help prevent post-herpetic neuralgia.

Resources

BOOKS

Kirschmann, John D. *Nutrition Almanac,* 6th ed. New York: McGraw-Hill, 2007.

Shannon, Joyce Brennfleck. *Pain Sourcebook,* 3rd ed. Detroit: Omnigraphics, 2008.

Siegel, Mary-Ellen, and Gray Williams. *Shingles: New Hope for an Old Disease,* updated ed. Lanham M. Evans and Company, Inc., 2008.

PERIODICALS

Froelich, Janis D. "How Did a Gal Like Me Come Down with Shingles?" *Tampa Tribune* (June 21, 2008): 16.

Gutpa, Sanjay. "Rash Redux." *Time* 172, no. 4 (July 28, 2008): 53.

OTHER

"Herpes Zoster." *American Academy of Dermatology.* [Accessed December 3, 2010] http://www.aad.org/ public/ publications/pamphlets/viral_herpes_zoster.htm.

Office of Communications and Public Liaison, National Institute of Neurological Disorders and Stroke. "Shingles: Hope Through Research." *NIH Publication No. 06-307.* [Accessed December 3, 2010] http://www.ninds. nih.gov/ disorders/shingles/detail_shingles.htm.

"Shingles & After-Shingles Pain." *AfterShingles.com.* [Accessed December 3, 2010] http://www.aftershingles. com/after-shingles-pain.aspx.

"Shingles (Herpes Zoster) Vaccination." *Vaccines & Immunizations.* [Accessed December 3, 2010] http://www.cdc. gov/vaccines/vpd-vac/shingles/default.htm.

"Shingles." *National Institute of Allergy and Infectious Diseases.* [Accessed December 3, 2010] http://www3. niaid.nih.gov/topics/shingles/

ORGANIZATIONS

American Academy of Dermatology, P.O. Box 4014, Schaumburg, IL 60168, (847) 240-1280, (866) 503-SKIN (7546), Fax: (847) 240-1859, http://www.aad.org

American Botanical Council, 6200 Manor Rd., Austin, TX 78723, (512) 926-4900, Fax: (512) 926-2345, abc@ herbalgram.org, http://cms.herbalgram.org

National Institute of Allergy and Infectious Diseases (NIAID), Office of Communications and Public Liaison, 6610 Rockledge Drive, Bethesda, MD 20892-66123, (866) 284-4107, http://www3.niaid.nih.gov

National Institute of Neurological Disorders and Stroke (NINDS), NIH Neurological Institute, P.O. Box 5801,

Bethesda, MD 20824, (301) 496-5751, (800) 352-9424, http://www.ninds.nih.gov.

National Shingles Foundation, 590 Madison Ave., 21st Floor, New York 10022(212) 222-3390, Fax: (212) 222-8627, http://www.vzvfoundation.org.

U.S. Centers for Disease Control and Prevention (CDC), 1600 Clifton Road, Atlanta, GA 30333, (800)-CDC-INFO (232-4636), cdcinfo@cdc.gov, http://www.cdc.gov.

Rebecca J. Frey, Ph.D.
Larry Gilman, Ph.D.
Margaret Alic, Ph.D.

Shock

Definition

Shock occurs when the body's organs and tissues do not receive an adequate flow of **blood**. Inadequate blood flow deprives the organs and tissues of oxygen and allows the buildup of waste products. Shock is a medical emergency and can result in serious damage or even death.

Description

There are three stages of shock: Stage I (also called compensated, or nonprogressive), Stage II (also called decompensated or progressive), and Stage III (also called irreversible).

In Stage I of shock, when low blood flow (perfusion) is first detected, a number of systems are activated in order to maintain or restore perfusion. The result is that the **heart** beats faster, the **blood vessels** throughout the body become slightly smaller in diameter, and the kidney works to retain fluid in the circulatory system. All this serves to maximize blood flow to the most important organs and systems in the body. A person in this stage of shock has very few symptoms, and treatment can completely halt any progression.

In Stage II of shock, the body's standard methods of compensation begin to fail and are unable to improve perfusion any longer. Oxygen deprivation in the **brain** causes the person to become confused and disoriented, while oxygen deprivation in the heart may cause chest **pain**. With quick and appropriate treatment, this stage of shock can be reversed.

In Stage III of shock, the length of time that poor perfusion has existed begins to take a permanent toll on the body's organs and tissues. The heart's functioning continues to spiral downward, and the **kidneys** usually shut down completely. Cells in organs and tissues throughout the body are injured and dying. The endpoint of Stage III shock is death.

Causes and symptoms

Shock is caused by three major categories of problems: cardiogenic (problems associated with the heart's functioning); hypovolemic (total volume of blood available to circulate is low); and **septic shock** (overwhelming **infection**, usually by **bacteria**).

Cardiogenic shock can be caused by any disease or event which prevents the heart muscle from pumping strongly and consistently enough to circulate the blood in a normal fashion. Heart attack, conditions that cause inflammation of the heart muscle (**myocarditis**), disturbances of the electrical rhythm of the heart, and any kind of mass or fluid accumulation or blood clot that interferes with flow out of the heart can significantly affect the heart's ability to pump a normal quantity of blood.

Hypovolemic shock occurs when the total volume of blood in the body falls well below normal. This can occur when there is excess fluid loss, as in **dehydration** due to severe **vomiting** or **diarrhea**, diseases which cause excess urination (**diabetes insipidus**, **diabetes mellitus**, and kidney failure), extensive **burns**, blockage in the intestine, inflammation of the **pancreas (pancreatitis)**, or severe bleeding of any kind.

Septic shock can occur when an untreated or inadequately treated infection (usually bacterial) is allowed to progress. Bacteria often produce poisonous chemicals (toxins) that can cause injury throughout the body. When large quantities of these bacteria and their toxins begin circulating in the bloodstream, every organ and tissue is at risk of their damaging effects. The most damaging consequences include:

- poor functioning of the heart muscle
- widening of the diameter of the blood vessels
- a drop in blood pressure
- activation of the blood clotting system, causing blood clots, followed by a risk of uncontrollable bleeding
- damage to the lungs, causing acute respiratory distress syndrome
- liver failure
- kidney failure
- coma

Initial symptoms of shock include cold, clammy hands and feet, pale or blue-tinged skin tone, weak and fast pulse rate, fast rate of breathing, and low **blood**

KEY TERMS

Cardiogenic—Originating with the heart.

Deprivation—A condition of having too little of something.

Hypovolemic—Having a low volume.

Perfusion—Blood flow through an organ or tissue.

Sepsis—An overwhelming infection throughout the body, usually caused by bacteria in the bloodstream.

QUESTIONS TO ASK THE DOCTOR

1. What type and stage shock is my loved one experiencing?
2. Have you diagnosed the underlying condition that caused this shock?
3. Are there likely to be lasting or permanent effects from this episode of shock?
4. What should I tell my friends and family about my condition?

pressure. A variety of other symptoms may be present, but they are dependent on the underlying cause of shock.

Diagnosis

Diagnosis of shock is based on a person's symptoms, as well as criteria including a significant drop in blood pressure, extremely low urine output, and blood tests that reveal overly acidic blood with a low circulating concentration of carbon dioxide. Other tests are performed, as appropriate, to try to determine the underlying condition responsible for an individual's state of shock.

Treatment

The most important goals in treating shock include quickly diagnosing a person's state of shock; quickly intervening to halt the underlying condition (e.g., stopping bleeding, re-starting the heart, giving **antibiotics** to combat an infection,); treating the effects of shock (e.g., low oxygen, increased acid in the blood, activation of the blood clotting system); and supporting vital functions (e.g., blood pressure, urine flow, heart function).

Treatment includes keeping a person warm, with legs raised and head down to improve blood flow to the brain, putting a needle in a vein in order to give fluids or blood transfusions, as necessary; giving a person extra oxygen to breathe and medications to improve the heart's functioning; and treating the underlying condition which led to shock.

Prognosis

The prognosis of an individual in shock depends on the stage of shock when treatment was begun, the underlying condition causing shock, and the general medical state of the person.

Health care team roles

First aid is often given by appropriately trained individuals. Physicians supervise the treatment of shock in a hospital setting. Nurses provide bedside management and patient-family education.

Prevention

The most preventable type of shock is caused by dehydration during illnesses with severe vomiting or diarrhea. Shock can be avoided by recognizing that a person who is unable to drink in order to replace lost fluids and needs to be given fluids intravenously (through a needle in a vein). Other types of shock are only preventable insofar as one can prevent their underlying conditions or can monitor and manage those conditions well enough so that they never progress to the point of shock.

Resources

BOOK

Limmer, Daniel and Michael F. O'Keefe, *Emergency Care*, 12th ed. Boston: Brady, 2012.

OTHER

Cunha, John P. Medical Shock. MedicineNet.com October 20, 2011 [accessed April 10, 2012]. http://www.medicinenet.com/shock/article.htm

Pinsky, Michael R. Septic Shock. Medscape Reference October 25, 2011 [accessed April 10, 2012]. http://emedicine.medscape.com/article/168402-overview

Shock. MedlinePlus April 6, 2012 [accessed April 10, 2012]. http://www.nlm.nih.gov/medlineplus/shock.html

Wedrow, Benjamin. Shock. eMedicineHealth April 5, 2012 [accessed April 10, 2011]. http://www.emedicinehealth.com/shock/article_em.htm

ORGANIZATIONS

American Academy of Emergency Medicine, 555 East Wells Street, Suite 1100, Milwaukee, WI 53202-3823, (800) 884-2236, Fax: (414) 276-3349, http://www.aaem.org

American College of Emergency Physicians, P.O. Box 619911, Dallas, TX 75261-9911, (972) 550-0911, (800) 798-1822, Fax: (972) 580-2816, www.acep.org.

L. Fleming Fallon, Jr., M.D., Dr.P.H.
Tish Davidson, A.M.

Sickle cell disease

Definition

Sickle cell disease describes a group of inherited **blood** disorders characterized by chronic anemia, painful events, and various complications due to associated tissue and organ damage.

Description

The most common and well-known type of sickle cell disease is sickle cell anemia, also called SS disease. All types of sickle cell disease are caused by a genetic change in hemoglobin, the oxygen-carrying protein inside the red blood cells. The red blood cells of affected individuals contain a predominance of a structural variant of the usual adult hemoglobin. This variant hemoglobin, called sickle hemoglobin, has a tendency to polymerize into rod-like structures that alter the shape of the usually flexible red blood cells. The cells take on a shape that resembles the curved blade of a sickle, an agricultural tool. Sickle cells have a shorter life span than normally shaped red blood cells. This results in chronic anemia characterized by low levels of hemoglobin and decreased numbers of red blood cells. Sickle cells are also less flexible and more sticky than normal red blood cells and can become trapped in small **blood vessels**, preventing blood flow. This condition compromises the delivery of oxygen, which can result in **pain** and damage to associated tissues and organs. Sickle cell disease presents with marked variability, even within families.

Demographics

Carriers of the sickle cell gene are said to have sickle cell trait. Unlike sickle cell disease, sickle cell trait does not cause health problems. In fact, sickle cell trait is protective against **malaria**, a disease caused by blood-borne **parasites** transmitted through mosquito bites. According to a widely accepted theory, the genetic mutation associated with the sickle cell trait occurred thousands of years ago. Coincidentally, this mutation increased the likelihood that carriers would survive malaria **infection**. Survivors then passed the mutation

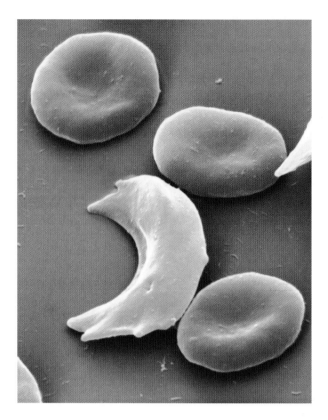

(Sickle cell disease, production of abnormal hemoglobin (Hbs) in red blood cells, photograph. Eye of Science / Photo Researchers, Inc.)

on to their offspring, and the trait became established throughout areas where malaria was common. As populations migrated, so did the sickle cell trait. Today, approximately one in 12 African Americans has sickle cell trait.

Worldwide, it has been estimated that one in every 250,000 babies is born with sickle cell disease. Sickle cell disease affects primarily people with African, Mediterranean, Middle Eastern, and Asian Indian ancestry. In the United States, sickle cell disease is most often seen in African Americans, in whom the disease occurs in one out of every 400 births. The disease has been described in individuals from several different ethnic backgrounds and is also seen with increased frequency in Latino Americans, particularly those of Caribbean, Central American, and South American ancestry. Approximately one in every 1,000–1,400 Latino births is affected.

Genetic profile

Humans normally make several types of the oxygen-carrying protein hemoglobin. An individual's stage in development determines whether primarily embryonic, fetal, or adult hemoglobins will be made. All types of hemoglobin are made of three components: heme, alpha (or alpha-like) globin, and beta (or beta-like) globin. Sickle hemoglobin is the result of a genetic change in the beta globin component of normal adult hemoglobin. The beta globin gene is located on chromosome 11. The sickle cell form of the beta globin gene results from the substitution of a single DNA nucleotide, or genetic building-block. The change from adenine to thymine at codon (position) 6 of the beta globin gene leads to insertion of the amino acid valine instead of glutamic acid at this same position in the beta globin protein. As a result of this change, sickle hemoglobin has unique properties in comparison to the usual type of adult hemoglobin.

Most individuals have two normal copies of the beta globin gene, which make normal beta globin that is incorporated into adult hemoglobin. Individuals who have sickle cell trait (called sickle cell carriers) have one normal beta globin gene and one sickle cell gene. These individuals make both the usual adult hemoglobin and sickle hemoglobin in roughly equal proportions, so they do not experience any health problems as a result of having the trait. Although traces of blood in the urine and difficulty in concentrating the urine can occur, neither represents a significant health problem due to sickle cell trait. Of the millions of people with sickle cell trait worldwide, a small handful of individuals have experienced acute symptoms. In these very rare cases, individuals were subject to very severe physical strain.

When both members of a couple are carriers of sickle cell trait, there is a 25% chance in each **pregnancy** for their baby to inherit two sickle cell genes and have sickle cell anemia, or SS disease. Correspondingly, there is a 50% chance their baby will have sickle cell trait and a 25% chance that the baby will have the usual type of hemoglobin. Other types of sickle cell disease include SC disease, SD disease, and S/beta thalassemia. These conditions are caused by the co-inheritance of the sickle cell gene and another altered beta globin gene. For example, one parent may have sickle cell trait, and the other parent may have hemoglobin C trait (another hemoglobin trait that does not cause health problems). For such a couple, there would be a 25% chance of SC disease in each pregnancy.

Causes and symptoms

Normal adult hemoglobin transports oxygen from the **lungs** to tissues throughout the body. Sickle hemoglobin can also transport oxygen. However, once the oxygen is released, sickle hemoglobin tends to polymerize (line-up) into rigid rods that alter the shape of the red blood cell. Sickling of the red blood cell can be triggered by low oxygen, such as occurs in organs with slow blood flow. It can also be triggered by cold temperatures and **dehydration**.

Sickle cells have a decreased life span in comparison to normal red blood cells. Normal red blood cells survive for approximately 120 days in the bloodstream; sickle cells last only 10–12 days. As a result, the bloodstream is chronically short of red blood cells and hemoglobin, and an affected individual develops anemia.

The sickle cells can create other complications. Due to their shape, they do not fit well through small blood vessels. As an aggravating factor, the outside surfaces of sickle cells may have altered chemical properties that increases their stickiness. These sticky sickle cells are more likely to adhere to the inside surfaces of small blood vessels, as well as to other blood cells. As a result of the sickle cells' shape and stickiness, blockages form in small blood vessels. Such blockages prevent oxygenated blood from reaching areas where it is needed, causing pain, as well as organ and tissue damage.

The severity of symptoms cannot be predicted based solely on the genetic inheritance. Some individuals with sickle cell disease may develop problems in infancy that affect their health and can be life-threatening. Others may experience only mild symptoms throughout their lives. Individuals may experience varying degrees of health at different stages in the life cycle. For the most part, this clinical variability is unpredictable, and the reasons for the observed variability can not usually be determined. However, certain types of sickle cell disease (i.e., SC disease) tend to result in fewer and less severe symptoms on average than other types of sickle cell disease (i.e., SS disease). Some additional modifying factors are known. For example, elevated levels of fetal hemoglobin in a child or adult can decrease the quantity and severity of some symptoms and complications. Fetal hemoglobin is a normally occurring hemoglobin that usually decreases from over 90% of the total hemoglobin to under 1% during the first year of life. This change is genetically determined, although some individuals may experience elevated levels of fetal hemoglobin due to variation in the genes that control fetal hemoglobin production. Such individuals often experience a reduction in their symptoms and complications due to the ability of fetal hemoglobin to prevent the polymerization of sickle hemoglobin, which leads to sickling of the red blood cell.

There are several symptoms that warrant immediate medical attention, including the following:

- signs of infection (fever above 101°F or 38.3°C, frequent coughing or breathing problems, unusual crankiness, feeding difficulties)
- signs of severe anemia (pale skin or lips, yellowing of the skin or eyes, very tired, very weak)

- signs indicating possible dehydration (vomiting, diarrhea, fewer wet diapers)
- other signs (pain or swelling in the abdomen, swollen hands or feet, screams when touched)

The following can be signs of various complications that occur in sickle cell disease.

Infections and effects on the spleen

Children with sickle cell disease who are under age three are particularly prone to life-threatening bacterial infections. *Streptococcus pneumoniae* is the most common offending bacterium, and invasive infection from this organism leads to death in 15% of cases. The spleen, an organ that helps to fight bacterial infections, is particularly vulnerable to the effects of sickling. Sickle cells can impede blood flow through the spleen, causing organ damage, which usually results in the loss of spleen function by late childhood. The spleen can also become enlarged due to blockages and/or increased activity of the spleen. Rapid enlargement of the spleen may be a sign of another complication called splenic sequestration, which occurs mostly in young children and can be life-threatening. Widespread sickling in the spleen prevents adequate blood flow from the organ, removing increasing volumes of blood from the circulation and leading to accompanying signs of severe anemia.

Painful events

Painful events, also known as vaso-occlusive events, are a hallmark symptom of sickle cell disease. The frequency and duration of the pain can vary tremendously from person to person and over an individual's life cycle. Painful events are the most common cause of hospitalizations in sickle cell disease. However, only a small proportion of individuals with sickle cell disease experience frequent and severe painful events. Most painful events can be managed at home. Pain results when small blood vessel blockages prevent oxygen from reaching tissues. Pain can affect any area of the body, although the extremities, chest, **abdomen**, and bones are frequently affected sites. There is some evidence that cold temperatures or infection can trigger a painful event, but most events occur for unknown reasons. The hand-foot syndrome, or dactylitis, is a particular type of painful event. Most common in toddlers, dactylitis results in pain and swelling in the hands and feet and is sometimes accompanied by a **fever**.

Anemia

Sickle cells have a high turnover rate, and there is a deficit of red blood cells in the bloodstream. Common symptoms of anemia include fatigue, paleness, and a shortness of breath. A particularly severe form of anemia called aplastic anemia may occur following infection with parvovirus. Parvovirus infection causes extensive destruction of the **bone** marrow, bringing production of new red blood cells to a halt. Bone marrow production resumes after seven to 10 days. However, given the short lives of sickle cells, even a brief shut-down in red blood cell production can cause a rapid decline in hemoglobin concentrations.

Delayed growth

The energy demands of the bone marrow for red blood cell production compete with the demands of a growing body. Children with sickle cell anemia may have delayed growth and reach **puberty** at a later age than normal. By early adulthood, they catch up on growth and attain normal height. However, their weight typically remains below average.

Stroke

Children with sickle cell disease have a significantly elevated risk of having a **stroke**, which can be one of the most serious complications of sickle cell disease. Approximately 11% of individuals with sickle cell disease will have a recognizable stroke by the age of 20. **Magnetic resonance imaging** (MRI) studies have found that 17% of children with sickle cell anemia have evidence of a previous stroke or clinically "silent" stroke-like events called transient ischemic attacks (TIAs). Stroke in sickle cell disease is usually caused by a blockage of a blood vessel. However, approximately one-fourth of the time they may be caused by a hemorrhage (or rupture) of a blood vessel.

Strokes result in compromised delivery of oxygen to an area of the **brain**. The consequences of stroke can range from life-threatening, to severe physical or cognitive impairments, to apparent or subtle learning disabilities, to undetectable effects. Common stroke symptoms include **weakness** or numbness that affects one side of the body, sudden behavioral changes, loss of **vision**, confusion, loss of speech or the ability to understand spoken words, **dizziness**, **headache**, seizures, **vomiting**, or even **coma**.

Approximately two-thirds of children who have a stroke will have at least one more. Transfusions have been shown to decrease the incidence of a second stroke. A recent study showed that children at highest risk of experiencing a first stroke were ten times more likely to stroke if untreated when compared to high-risk children treated with chronic blood **transfusion therapy**. High-risk children were identified using transcranial Doppler ultrasound technology to detect individuals with increased blood flow speeds due to constricted intracranial blood vessels.

Acute chest syndrome

Acute chest syndrome (ACS) is a leading cause of death for individuals with sickle cell disease, and recurrent attacks can lead to permanent lung damage. Therefore rapid diagnosis and treatment is of great importance. ACS can occur at any age and is similar to but distinct from **pneumonia**. Affected persons may experience fever, **cough**, chest pain, and shortness of breath. ACS seems to have multiple causes including infection, sickling in the small blood vessels of the lungs, fat embolisms to the lungs, or a combination of factors.

Priapism

Males with sickle cell anemia may experience priapism, a condition characterized by a persistent and painful erection of the penis. Due to blood vessel blockage by sickle cells, blood is trapped in the tissue of the penis. Priapism may be short in duration, or it may be prolonged. Priapism can be triggered by low oxygen (hypoxemia), alcohol consumption, or sexual intercourse. Since priapism can be extremely painful and can result in damage to this tissue (causing impotence), rapid treatment is essential.

Kidney disease

The internal environment of the kidney is particularly prone to damage from sickle cells. Signs of kidney damage can include blood in the urine, incontinence, and enlarged **kidneys**. Adults with sickle cell disease often experience insufficient functioning of the kidneys, which can progress to kidney failure in a small percentage of adults with sickle cell disease.

Jaundice and gallstones

Jaundice is indicated by a yellow tone in the skin and eyes, and alone it is not a health concern. Jaundice may occur if bilirubin levels increase, which can occur with high levels of red blood cell destruction. Bilirubin is the final product of hemoglobin degradation, and is typically removed from the bloodstream by the **liver**. Therefore, jaundice can also be a sign of a poorly functioning liver, which may also be evidenced by an enlarged liver (hepatomegaly). Increased bilirubin also leads to increased chance for gallstones in children with sickle cell disease. Treatment, which may include removal of the gall bladder, may be selected if the gallstones start causing symptoms.

Retinopathy

The blood vessels that supply oxygen to the retina, the tissue at the back of the eye, may be blocked by sickle cells, leading to a condition called **retinopathy**. This is one of the only complications that is actually more common in SC disease as compared to SS disease. Retinopathy can be identified through regular **ophthalmology** evaluations and effectively treated in order to avoid damage to vision.

Joint problems

Avascular necrosis of the hip and shoulder joints, in which bone damage occurs due to compromised blood flow due to sickling, can occur later in childhood. This complication can affect an individual's physical abilities and result in substantial pain.

Diagnosis

In the United States, African Americans and Latino Americans have the highest risk of having the disease or trait. Sickle cell is also common among individuals of Mediterranean, Middle Eastern, and Eastern Indian descent. Individuals from these ethnic groups should consider screening for sickle cell disease.

A **complete blood count** (CBC) will describe several aspects of an individual's blood cells. A person with sickle cell disease will have a lower-than-normal hemoglobin level, together with other characteristic red blood cell abnormalities. Hemoglobin electrophoresis is a test that can help identify the types and quantities of hemoglobin made by an individual. This test uses an electric field applied across a slab of gel-like material. Hemoglobins migrate through this gel at various rates and go to specific locations, depending on their size, shape, and electrical charge. Although sickle hemoglobin (Hb S) and regular adult hemoglobin (called Hb A) differ by only one amino acid, they can be clearly separated using hemoglobin electrophoresis. Isoelectric focusing and high-performance liquid chromatography (HPLC) use similar principles to separate hemoglobins and can be used instead of or in various combinations with hemoglobin electrophoresis to determine the types of hemoglobin present.

Another test, called the sickledex can help confirm the presence of sickle hemoglobin, although this test cannot provide accurate or reliable diagnosis when used alone. When Hb S is present, but there is an absence or only a trace of Hb A, sickle cell anemia is a likely diagnosis. Additional beta globin DNA test that directly assays the beta globin gene can be performed to help confirm the diagnosis and establish the exact genetic type of sickle cell disease. CBC and hemoglobin electrophoresis are also typically used to diagnosis sickle cell trait and various other types of beta globin traits.

Diagnosis of sickle cell disease can occur under various circumstances. If an individual has symptoms that are suggestive of this diagnosis, the above-described screening tests can be performed followed by DNA testing, if indicated. Screening at birth using HPLC or a related technique offers the opportunity for early intervention. More than 40 states include sickle cell screening as part of the usual battery of blood tests done for newborns. This allows for early identification and treatment. Hemoglobin trait screening is recommended for any individual of a high-risk ethnic background who may be considering having children. When both members of a couple are found to have sickle cell trait or other related hemoglobin traits, they can receive **genetic counseling** regarding the risk of sickle cell disease in their future children and various testing options.

Sickle cell disease can be identified before birth through the use of prenatal diagnosis. **Chorionic villus sampling** (CVS) can be offered as early as 10 weeks of pregnancy and involves removing a sample of the placenta made by the baby and testing the cells. CVS carries a risk of causing a **miscarriage** that is between 0.5 and 1%.

Amniocentesis is generally offered between 15 and 22 weeks of pregnancy, but can sometimes be offered earlier. Two to three tablespoons of the fluid surrounding a baby are removed. This fluid contains fetal cells that can be tested. Although both tests carry a risk of causing a miscarriage, the risk is not greater than 1%. Pregnant woman and couples may choose prenatal testing in order to prepare for the birth of a baby that may have sickle cell disease. Alternately, knowing the diagnosis during pregnancy allows for the option of pregnancy termination.

Preimplantation genetic diagnosis (PGD) is a relatively new technique that involves in-vitro fertilization followed by **genetic testing** of one cell from each developing embryo. Only the embryos unaffected by sickle cell disease are transferred back into the uterus. PGD is currently available on a research basis only and is relatively expensive.

Treatment

There are several practices that are intended to prevent some of the symptoms and complications of sickle cell disease. These include preventative **antibiotics**, good hydration, immunizations, and access to comprehensive care. Maintaining good health through adequate **nutrition**, avoiding stresses and infection, and getting proper rest is also important. Following these guidelines usually improves the health of individuals with sickle cell disease.

Penicillin

Infants are typically started on a course of penicillin that extends from infancy to age six. Use of this antibiotic is meant to ward off potentially fatal infections. Infections at any age are treated aggressively with antibiotics. Vaccines for common infections, such as *pneumococcal pneumonia*, are also recommended.

Pain management

Pain is one of the primary symptoms of sickle cell anemia, and controlling it is an important concern. The methods necessary for pain control are based on individual factors. Some people can gain adequate pain control through over-the-counter oral painkillers (**analgesics**). Others individuals or painful events may require stronger methods, which can include administration of narcotics. Alternative therapies may be useful in avoiding or controlling pain, including **relaxation**, hydration, avoiding extremes of temperature, and the application of local warmth.

Blood transfusions

Blood transfusions are not usually given on a regular basis but are used to treat individuals with frequent and severe painful events, severe anemia, and other emergencies. In some cases blood transfusions are given as preventive measures, for example, to treat spleen enlargement (splenomegaly) or prevent a second stroke (or a first stroke in an individual shown to be at high risk).

Regular blood transfusions have the potential to decrease formation of hemoglobin S, and reduce associated symptoms. However, there are limitations and risks associated with regular blood transfusions, including the risk of blood-borne infection and sensitization to **proteins** in the transfused blood that can make future transfusions very difficult. Most importantly, chronic blood transfusions can lead to **iron** overload. The body tends to store excess iron, such as that received through transfusions, in various organs. Over time, this iron storage can cause damage to various tissues and organs, such as the **heart** and endocrine organs.

Some of this damage can be prevented by the administration of a medication called desferrioxamine

Amino acid—A type of molecule used as a building block for protein construction.

Anemia—A condition in which the level of hemoglobin or the number of red blood cells falls below normal values. Common symptoms include paleness, fatigue, and shortness of breath.

Bilirubin—A yellow pigment that is the end result of hemoglobin breakdown. Bilirubin is cleared from the blood by action of liver enzymes and excreted from the body.

Bone marrow—A spongy tissue located in the hollow centers of certain bones, such as the skull and hip bones. Bone marrow is the site of blood cell generation.

Bone marrow transplantation—A medical procedure in which normal bone marrow is transferred from a healthy donor to an ailing recipient. An illness such as sickle cell anemia that prevents production of normal blood cells may be treated with a bone marrow transplant.

Globin—One of the component protein molecules found in hemoglobin. Normal adult hemoglobin has a pair each of alpha-globin and beta-globin molecules.

Heme—The iron-containing molecule in hemoglobin that serves as the site for oxygen binding.

Hemoglobin—The red pigment found within red blood cells that enables them to transport oxygen throughout the body. Hemoglobin is a large molecule composed of five components: a heme molecule and two pairs of globin molecules.

Hemoglobin A—Normal adult hemoglobin contains a heme molecule, two alpha-globin molecules, and two beta-globin molecules.

Hemoglobin electrophoresis—A laboratory test that separates molecules based on their size, shape, or electrical charge.

Hemoglobin S—Hemoglobin that is produced in association with the sickle cell trait. The beta-globin molecules of hemoglobin S are defective.

Hydroxyurea—A drug that has been shown to induce production of fetal hemoglobin. Fetal hemoglobin has a pair of gamma-globin molecules in place of the typical beta-globins of adult hemoglobin. Higher-than-normal levels of fetal hemoglobin can prevent sickling from occurring.

Impotence—The inability to have a penile erection, which can be due to tissue damage resulting from sickling within the penis (priapism).

Iron overload—A side effect of frequent transfusions in which the body accumulates abnormally high levels of iron. Iron deposits can form in organs, particularly the heart, and cause life-threatening damage.

Jaundice—A condition characterized by higher-than-normal levels of bilirubin in the bloodstream and an accompanying yellowing of the skin and eyes.

Magnetic resonance imaging—A type of imaging technique that allows the visualization of internal structures, such as the brain.

Mutation—A change in a gene's DNA. Whether a mutation is harmful is determined by the effect on the product for which the gene codes.

Narcotic—Strong, prescription medication that can be effective in treating sickle cell pain. Narcotics have the potential to be habit-forming if their use is not adequately supervised.

Ophthalmology—The medical specialty of vision and the eye.

Placenta—The organ responsible for oxygen and nutrition exchange between a pregnant mother and her developing baby.

Red blood cell—Hemoglobin-containing blood cells that transport oxygen from the lungs to tissues. In the tissues, the red blood cells exchange their oxygen for carbon dioxide, which is brought back to the lungs to be exhaled.

Screening—Process through which carriers of a trait may be identified within a population.

Sickle cell—A red blood cell that has assumed a elongated shape due to the presence of hemoglobin S.

that helps the body to eliminate excess iron through the urine. Alternately, some individuals receive a new, non-standard treatment called erythrocytophoresis. This procedure involves the automated removal of sickle cells and is used in conjunction with a reduced number of regular transfusions. This treatment also helps to reduce iron overload.

Hydroxyurea

Emphasis is being placed on developing drugs that treat sickle cell anemia directly. The most promising of these drugs is hydroxyurea, a drug that was originally designed for anticancer treatment. Hydroxyurea has been shown to reduce the frequency of painful crises and acute chest syndrome in adults, and to lessen the need for blood transfusions. Hydroxyurea, and other related medications, seem to work by inducing a higher production of fetal hemoglobin. The major side effects of the drug include decreased production of platelets, red blood cells, and certain white blood cells. The effects of long-term hydroxyurea treatment are unknown. The drug was approved for use against sickle cell disease by the U.S. Food and Drug Administration (FDA) in 1998.

Bone marrow transplantation

Bone marrow transplantation has been shown to cure sickle cell anemia in some cases. This treatment is reserved primarily for severely affected children with a healthy donor whose marrow proteins match those of the recipient, namely a brother or sister who has inherited the same tissue type. Indications for a bone marrow transplant are stroke, recurrent acute chest syndrome, and chronic unrelieved pain.

Bone marrow transplantations tend to be the most successful in children. Adults have a higher rate of transplant rejection and other complications. There is approximately a 10% fatality rate associated with bone marrow transplants performed for sickle cell disease. Survivors face potential long-term complications, such as chronic graft-versus-host disease (an immune-mediated attack by the donor marrow against the recipient's tissues), **infertility**, and development of some forms of **cancer**. A relatively recent advance in transplantation involves the use of donor stem cells obtained from cord blood, the blood from the placenta that is otherwise discarded following the birth of a new baby. Cord blood cells, as opposed to fully mature bone marrow cells, appear to be less likely to result in graft-versus-host disease in a recipient. This increases the safety and efficacy of the transplant procedure.

Surgery

Certain surgical interventions are utilized in the treatment of specific sickle cell-related complications. Removal of a dysfunctional **gallbladder** (cholecystectomy) or spleen (splenectomy) can often lead to improvements in health. Investigations are currently underway to establish the efficacy of hip coring surgery, in which a portion of affected bone is removed to treat avascular necrosis of the hip. The hope is that this procedure may provide an effective treatment to alleviate some pain and restore function in an affected hip.

PSYCHOSOCIAL SUPPORT. As in any life-long, chronic disease, comprehensive care is important. Assistance in coping with the emotional, social, family-planning, economic, vocational, and other consequences of sickle cell disease can enable affected individuals to better access and benefit from their medical care providers.

Prognosis

Sickle cell disease is characteristically variable between and within affected individuals. Predicting the course of the disorder based solely on genes is not possible. Several factors aside from genetic inheritance determine the prognosis for affected individuals, including the frequency, severity, and nature of specific complications in any given individual. The availability and access of comprehensive medical care also plays an important role in preventing and treating serious, acute complications that cause the majority of sickle cell-related deaths. For those individuals who do not experience such acute events, life-expectancy is probably substantially greater than the average for all people with sickle cell disease. The impact of recent medical advances supports the hypothesis that current life-expectancies may be significantly greater than those estimated in the early 1990s. At that time, individuals with SS disease lived, on average, to their early- to mid-40s, and those with SC disease lived into the upper 50s. With early detection and comprehensive medical care, most people with sickle cell disease enjoy fairly good health throughout most of their lives. Most individuals can be expected to live well into adulthood, enjoying an improved quality of life including the ability to choose a variety of education, career, and family-planning options for themselves.

Health care team roles

Sickle cell disease is often initially identified as a result of a screening test. Such tests may be ordered by a pediatrician, obstetrician or family physician. A phlebotomist or nurse often obtains a sample of blood. A laboratory technician processes the sample. A pathologist or hematologist analyzes the results of a test. A family doctor may return results to individuals who have been tested. A genetic counselor or other person with training in test interpretation and ethics must be available to assist tested persons to accurately assess their options in the future.

Prevention

Inheritance of sickle cell disease or trait cannot be prevented, but it may be predicted. Screening is recommended for individuals in high-risk populations.

QUESTIONS TO ASK YOUR DOCTOR

- Do you recommend that my partner and I have a screening test for sickle cell disease? On what do you base this recommendation?
- If such a test were positive, to whom can we speak about the significance of those results for our future offspring?
- What procedures do you recommend for the treatment of the pain associated with sickle cell disease?
- What are the risks and benefits of using blood transfusions to treat my sickle cell disease?
- What local resources are available for additional information and support on the subject of sickle cell disease?

Resources

BOOKS

Dick, Moira. *Sickle Cell Disease in Childhood: Standards and Guidelines for Clinical Care*, 2nd ed. London: NHS Sickle Cell and Thalassaemia Screening Programme: Sickle Cell Society, 2010.

Dyson, Simon, and Karl Atkin, eds. *Genetics and Global Public Health: Sickle Cell and Thalassaemia*. London; New York: Routledge, 2012.

Howard, Jo. *Sickle Cell Disease in Clinical Practice*. New York: Springer Verlag 2012.

Platt, Allan F., James Eckman, and Lewis Hsu. *Hope and Destiny: The Patient and Parent's Guide to Sickle Cell Disease and Sickle Cell Trait*, 3rd rev. ed. Indianapolis, IN: Hilton Publishing Company, 2011.

Rouse, Carolyn Moxley. *Uncertain Suffering: Racial Health Care Disparities and Sickle Cell Disease*. Berkeley: University of California Press, 2009.

PERIODICALS

Brown, M. "Managing the Acutely Ill Adult with Sickle Cell Disease." *British Journal of Nursing* 21, 2 (2012): 90–96.

Erskine, R. "Adolescent Boys with Sickle Cell Disease: A Qualitative Study." *Clinical Child Psychology and Psychiatry* 17, 1 (2012): 17–31.

Fisak, B., M.H. Belkin, A.C. von Lehe, and M. M. Bansal. "The Relation between Health-related Quality of Life, Treatment Adherence and Disease Severity in a Paediatric Sickle Cell Disease Sample." *Child: Care, Health and Development* 38, 2 (2012): 204–210.

Howard, Jo, and Eugene Oteng-Ntim. "The Obstetric Management of Sickle Cell Disease." *Best Practice & Research Clinical Obstetrics & Gynaecology* 26, 1 (2012): 25–36.

OTHER

Learning about Sickle Cell Disease. National Human Genome Research Institute. http://www.genome.gov/10001219 (accessed May 10, 2012).

Sickle Cell Disease. http://sickle.bwh.harvard.edu/menu_sickle. html (accessed May 10, 2012).

Sickle Cell Disease. Genetics Home Reference. http://ghr.nlm. nih.gov/condition/sickle-cell-disease (accessed May 10, 2012).

Sickle Cell Disease. Kids' Health. http://kidshealth.org/parent/medical/heart/sickle_cell_anemia.html (accessed May 10, 2012).

Sickle Cell Disease. Your Genes Your Health. http://www.yourgenesyourhealth.org/sickle/whatisit.htm (accessed May 10, 2012).

ORGANIZATIONS

American Academy of Pediatrics, 141 Northwest Point Blvd., Elk Grove Village, IL 60007-1098. (847) 434-4000. Fax: (847) 434-8000. http://www.aap.org/default.htm. http://www2.aap.org/visit/contact.htm.

American Society of Hematology. 2021 L St. NW, Suite 900, Washington, DC 20036. (202) 776-0544. Fax (202) 776-0545. http://www.hematology.org/. http://www.hematology.org/About-ASH/Contact-Us.aspx.

Sickle Cell Disease Association of America, Inc. 231 E. Baltimore St., Suite 800, Baltimore, MD 21202. (800) 421-8453. Fax: (410) 528-1495. http://www.sicklecelldisease.org/. scdaa@sicklecelldisease.org.

L. Fleming Fallon, Jr., M.D., Dr.P.H.

Sigmoidoscopy

Definition

Sigmoidoscopy is a diagnostic and screening procedure in which a rigid or flexible tube with a camera on the end (a sigmoidoscope) is inserted into the anus to examine the rectum and lower colon (bowel) for bowel disease, **cancer**, precancerous conditions, or causes of bleeding and **pain**.

Purpose

Sigmoidoscopy is used most often in screening for **colorectal cancer** or to determine the cause of rectal bleeding. It is also used in diagnosis of inflammatory bowel disease, microscopic and ulcerative **colitis**, and **Crohn's disease**.

Cancer of the rectum and colon is the second most common cancer in the United States. About 155,000

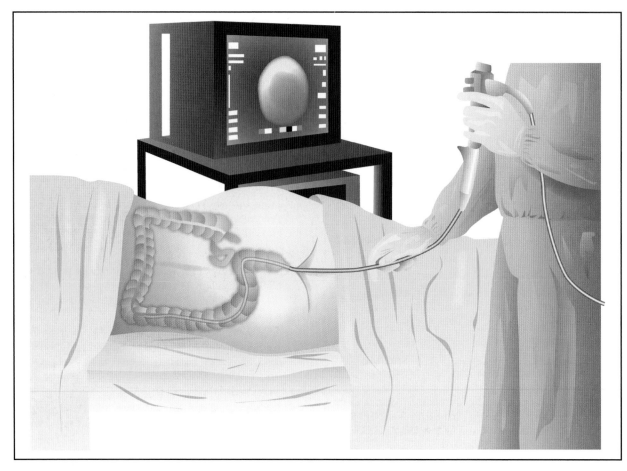

(Sigmoidoscope inserted into a patient's intestine through the rectum while patient reclines on left side, illustration by GGS Information Services, Inc. Reproduced by permission of Gale, a part of Cengage Learning.)

cases are diagnosed annually. About 55,000–60,000 Americans die each year of colorectal cancer.

A number of studies have suggested, and it is now recommended by cancer authorities that people over 50 be screened for colorectal cancer using endoscopy every three to five years. Individuals with inflammatory bowel disease, such as Crohn's disease or ulcerative colitis, who are at increased risk for colorectal cancer, may begin their screenings at a younger age, depending on when their disease was diagnosed. Many physicians screen such patients more often than every three to five years. Screening should also be done in patients who have a family history of colon or rectal cancer or small growths in the colon (polyps).

Some physicians do this screening with a colonoscope, which allows them to see the entire colon. However, most physicians prefer sigmoidoscopy, which is less time consuming, less uncomfortable, and less costly.

Studies have shown that one quarter to one-third of all precancerous or small cancerous growths can be seen with a sigmoidoscope. About one-half are found with a 1 ft (30 cm) scope, and two-thirds to three-quarters can be seen using a 2 ft (60 cm) scope.

In some cases, the sigmoidoscope can be used therapeutically in conjunction with other equipment, such as electrosurgical devices, to remove polyps and other lesions found during the sigmoidoscopy.

Precautions

Sigmoidoscopy can usually be conducted in a physician's office or an outpatient clinic. However, some individuals should have the procedure done in a hospital day-surgery facility. Those with rectal bleeding may need full **colonoscopy** in a hospital setting. Patients whose **blood** does not clot well (possibly as a result of blood thinning medications) may need the procedure performed in a hospital setting as well.

Individuals with renal insufficiency or congestive **heart failure** need to be prepared in an alternative way, and must be carefully monitored during the procedure.

Sigmoidoscopy may be contraindicated in patients with severe active colitis or toxic megacolon (an extremely dilated colon). In general, patients on continuous ambulatory **peritoneal dialysis** are not candidates due to a high risk of developing intraperitoneal bleeding.

Description

Sigmoidoscopy may be performed using either a rigid or flexible sigmoidoscope, a thin tube with fiberoptics, electronics, a light source, and camera. The physician inserts the sigmoidoscope into the anus to examine the rectum (the first 1 ft/30 cm of the colon) and its interior walls. If a 2 ft/60 cm scope is used, the next portion of the colon can also be examined for any irregularities. The sigmoidoscope's camera is connected to a viewing monitor (television screen), so the rectum and colon are enlarged and viewed on a monitor. Images can then be recorded as still pictures for hard copy or the entire procedure can be videotaped.

If polyps, lesions, or other suspicious areas are found, the physician biopsies them for analysis. During the sigmoidoscopy, the physician may also use forceps, graspers, snares, or electrosurgical devices to remove polyps, lesions, or tumors.

The sigmoidoscopy procedure takes five to 20 minutes. Preparation begins one day before the procedure. There is some discomfort when the scope is inserted and throughout the procedure, similar to that experienced when a physician performs a rectal exam using a finger to test for occult blood in the stool (another major colorectal cancer screening test). The patient may also feel some minor cramping pain. There is rarely severe pain, except for individuals with active inflammatory bowel disease.

Private insurance plans almost always cover the $150 to $200 cost of sigmoidoscopy for screening in healthy individuals over 50, or for diagnostic purposes. **Medicare** covers the cost for diagnostic exams, and may cover the costs for screening exams. **Medicaid** varies by state, but does not cover the procedure in most states. Some community health clinics offer the procedure at reduced cost, but this can only be done if a local gastroenterologist (a physician who specializes in treating **stomach** and intestinal disorders) is willing to donate his or her time.

Preparation

The purpose of preparation for sigmoidoscopy is to cleanse the lower bowel of stool so the physician can see the lining. Preparation begins 24 hours before the procedure, when the individual must begin a clear liquid diet. Preparation kits are available in drug stores. In normal preparation, about 20 hours before the exam, the patient begins taking a series of **laxatives**, which may be oral tablets or liquid. The individual must stop drinking four hours before the exam. An hour or two prior to the exam, the patient uses an **enema** or laxative suppository to finish cleansing the lower bowel.

Individuals need to be careful about medication before having sigmoidoscopy. They should not take aspirin, products containing aspirin, or ibuprofen products (Nuprin, Advil, or Motrin) for one week prior to the exam, because these medications can exacerbate bleeding during the procedure. They should not take any **iron** or **vitamins** with iron for one week prior to the exam, since iron can cause color changes in the bowel lining that interfere with the examination. They should take any routine prescription medication, but may need to stop certain medications; the physician should be consulted regarding routine prescriptions and their possible effect on sigmoidoscopy.

Aftercare

There is no specific aftercare necessary following sigmoidoscopy. If a biopsy was taken, a small amount of blood may appear in the next stool. Patients should be encouraged to pass gas following the procedure to relieve any bloating and cramping that may occur after the procedure. In addition, an **infection** may develop following sigmoidoscopy, and patients should be instructed to call their physician if a **fever** or pain in the **abdomen** develops over the few days after the procedure.

Complications

There is a slight risk of bleeding from the procedure. This risk is heightened in individuals whose blood does not clot well, either due to disease or medication, and in those with active inflammatory bowel disease. Rarely, trauma to the bowel or other organs can occur, resulting in an injury (perforation) that needs to be repaired or peritonitis, which must be treated with medication.

Results

A normal exam shows a smooth colon wall, with sufficient **blood vessels** for good blood flow.

For a cancer screening sigmoidoscopy, an abnormal result is one or more noncancerous or precancerous polyps, or clearly cancerous polyps. People with polyps have an increased risk of developing colorectal cancer in the future and may be required to undergo additional procedures, such as colonoscopy, or more frequent examinations.

KEY TERMS

Biopsy—The removal a small portion of tissue during sigmoidoscopy to perform laboratory tests to determine if the tissue is cancerous.

Colonoscopy—A diagnostic endoscopic procedure that uses a long flexible tube called a colonoscope to examine the inner lining of the entire colon; used for colorectal cancer screening and more thorough examination of the colon.

Colorectal cancer—Cancer of the large intestine, or colon, including the rectum (the last 16 in of the large intestine before the anus).

Congestive heart failure—Excess fluid accumulation in the lungs and surrounding tissues due to the weakness of the heart muscle and the inability to pump sufficiently.

Electrosurgical device—A medical device that uses electrical current to cauterize or coagulate tissue during surgical procedures, often used in conjunction with laparoscopy.

Inflammatory bowel disease—Ulcerative colitis or Crohn's disease; chronic conditions characterized by periods of diarrhea, bloating, abdominal cramps, and pain, sometimes accompanied by weight loss and malnutrition because of the inability to absorb nutrients.

Pathologist—A doctor who specializes in the diagnosis of disease by studying cells and tissues under a microscope.

Polyp—A small growth, usually not cancerous, but often precancerous when it appears in the colon.

Renal insufficiency—The inability of the kidneys to process fluid fast enough to flush the body of impurities.

Small polyps can be completely removed. Larger polyps may require the physician to remove a portion of the growth for laboratory biopsy. Depending on the laboratory results, the patient is then scheduled to have the polyp removed surgically, either as an "urgent" matter if it is cancerous or as an elective surgery within a few months if it is noncancerous.

In a diagnostic sigmoidoscopy, an abnormal result shows signs of active inflammatory bowel disease, either a thickening of the intestinal lining consistent with ulcerative colitis, or ulcerations or fissures consistent with Crohn's disease.

Health care team roles

Sigmoidoscopy is performed by an experienced family physician or gastroenterologist. Nurses or physician assistants may be present during the procedure to assist the physician and monitor the patient. Biopsy specimens taken during the sigmoidoscopy are analyzed in the clinical laboratory by a pathologist. Sigmoidoscopes and procedural accessories must be sterilized or disinfected by clinical staff trained in proper scope reprocessing techniques.

Resources

BOOKS

Beers, Mark H., and Robert Berkow, eds. *Merck Manual of Diagnosis and Therapy,* 17th ed. Merck Research Laboratories, 1999.

Fauci, Anthony S., et al., eds. *Harrison's Principles of Internal Medicine,* 14th ed. New York: McGraw-Hill, 1998.

PERIODICAL

Johnson, Brett Andrew. "Flexible Sigmoidoscopy: Screening for Colorectal Cancer." *American Family Physician* (January 15, 1999). *http://www.aafp.org/afp/990115ap/313.html.*

ORGANIZATIONS

Colorectal Cancer Network (CCNetwork). P.O. Box 182, Kensington, MD 20895-0182. (301) 879-1500. http://www.colorectal-cancer.net.

National Digestive Diseases Information Clearinghouse. 2 Information Way, Bethesda, MD 20892-3570. http://www.niddk.nih.gov.

Society of American Gastrointestinal Endoscopic Surgeons (SAGES). 2716 Ocean Park Boulevard, Suite 3000, Santa Monica, CA 90405. (310) 314-2404. http://www.sages.org.

Society of Gastroenterology Nurses and Associates Inc. 401 North Michigan Avenue, Chicago, IL 60611-4267. (800) 245-7462. http://www.sgna.org.

Jennifer E. Sisk, M.A.

Sinus endoscopy

Definition

Sinus endoscopy is a procedure used to examine, diagnose, and treat disorders of the nose, sinuses, or throat. During sinus endoscopy, an endoscope—a narrow, flexible tube fitted with a fiber-optic device such as a telescope or magnifying lens—is inserted into the nose, the interior of the nasal passages, sinuses, and throat.

Purpose

Sinus endoscopy is used diagnostically to evaluate structural defects, **infection** or damage to the sinuses, or structures in the nose and throat. It may be used to view polyps (growths) in the sinuses and to investigate causes of recurrent **sinusitis** (infection of the sinuses). During treatment, an **endoscope** may be used to view the affected area before, during, and after surgical procedures to correct anatomical malformations, sinus-drainage problems, or to remove polyps from the nose and throat.

Precautions

Insertion of the endoscope may cause a gag reflex and some discomfort, however, no special precautions are required to prepare for nasal endoscopy. Before the procedure begins, the nurse generally describes this and any other discomfort the patient may experience.

Description

This procedure is usually performed in a physician's office or other outpatient setting, such as a clinic or ambulatory surgical center. The endoscope is inserted into a nostril and threaded through the sinus passages to the throat. To visualize these areas more easily, and to record the areas being examined, the endoscope is fitted with a camera, monitor, or other viewing device.

Preparation

During the procedure, the patient is usually awake and seated upright in a chair. A local anesthetic spray or liquid may be applied to the throat to ease insertion of the endoscope and minimize discomfort.

Aftercare

Following sinus endoscopy procedures, most patients may immediately resume normal activities. If anesthetic was used, the patient may have to wait until the numbness wears off before eating or drinking.

Complications

The insertion and removal of the endoscope may trigger a gag reflex and can cause some discomfort. The procedure may also irritate the tissues of the nose and throat, causing a nosebleed or coughing.

KEY TERMS

Fiber-optic—Relating to the transmission of light through very fine, flexible glass or plastic fibers.

Polyp—A usually nonmalignant growth or tumor protruding from the mucous lining of an organ such as the nose, bladder, or intestine, often causing obstruction.

Results

Under normal conditions, no polyps are found in the sinuses. There should also be no evidence of infection, swelling, injury, or an anatomical or structural defect that would prevent normal draining of the sinuses.

Polyps, growths, infections, or structural defects of the nasal passages are considered abnormal.

Health care team roles

Sinus endoscopy is usually performed by an otolaryngologist (a physician specializing in disorders of the ear, nose and throat). Before the procedure, some patients may undergo **computed tomography (CT) scans** or other imaging studies performed by radiological technologists.

Patient education

Generally, the procedure is explained by the physician who will perform it. Since the procedure is generally performed in the physician's office or other outpatient setting, **patient education** also may be provided by nurses, nursing assistants, or certified medical assistants working in the medical office.

Resources

BOOKS

Gates, George A. *Current Therapy in Otolaryngology–Head and Neck Surgery.* St. Louis, MO: Mosby, 1998.

Nasal Endoscopy. In *The Patient's Guide to Medical Tests,* edited by Barry L. Zaret. Boston, MA: Houghton Mifflin Company, 1997.

ORGANIZATIONS

American Academy of Otolaryngology—Head and Neck Surgery. One Prince St, Alexandria, VA 22314. (703) 836-4444.

Ear Foundation. 2000 Church St., Box 111, Nashville, TN 37236. (615) 329-7807, (800) 545-HEAR.

Barbara Wexler

Sinusitis

Definition

Sinusitis refers to an inflammation of the tissues that line the sinuses, which are air spaces within the bones of the face close to the nose. Sinusitis is most often caused by an **infection** within these spaces.

Sinusitis is usually classified as either acute or chronic. Acute sinusitis usually has a rapid onset; it is often a complication of the **common cold** but can also be triggered by **allergies**, bacterial infections, or fungal infections. Sinusitis that lasts longer than eight weeks, or keeps recurring (four or more times per year), is called chronic sinusitis.

Demographics

Acute sinusitis is a very common condition in Canada and the United States with 31–37 million cases reported each year and 200,000 surgical procedures performed to treat the disorder. It is possible that the actual number of cases is much higher because the symptoms of bacterial sinusitis often mimic those of colds or allergies, and many patients never see a doctor for proper diagnosis and treatment. About half of all diagnosed cases of acute sinusitis are caused by **bacteria**. The cost to the U.S. economy of acute sinusitis is estimated at $3 billion per year.

About 90% of people will have an episode of sinusitis at some point in life. Most people diagnosed with sinusitis are young or middle-aged adults. Sinusitis is very rare in children younger than 18 months because the sinuses are not yet fully developed in infants.

Sinusitis is equally common in males and females and in all racial and ethnic groups.

Description

The sinuses are paired air pockets located within the bones of the face. They are:

- the frontal sinuses; located above the eyes, in the center region of each eyebrow
- the maxillary sinuses; located within the cheekbones, just to either side of the nose
- the ethmoid sinuses; located between the eyes, just behind the bridge of the nose
- the sphenoid sinuses; located just behind the ethmoid sinuses and behind the eyes

The sinuses are connected with the nose. They are lined with the same kind of skin found elsewhere within the respiratory tract. This skin has tiny little hairs projecting from it called cilia. The cilia beat constantly, to help move the mucus produced in the sinuses into the respiratory tract. The beating cilia sweeping the mucus along the respiratory tract help to clear the respiratory tract of any debris, or any organisms which may be present. When the lining of the sinuses is at all swollen, the swelling interferes with the normal flow of mucus. Trapped mucus can then fill the sinuses, causing an uncomfortable sensation of pressure and providing an excellent environment for the growth of infection-causing bacteria.

Risk factors

The risk factors for acute sinusitis and chronic sinusitis are similar. Risk factors for acute sinusitis include:

- A history of hay fever or other allergies affecting the nose.
- A structural abnormality in the nose, such as polyps or a deviated septum.
- Being a heavy smoker or being exposed to cigarette smoke in the home or at work.
- A history of cystic fibrosis, sarcoidosis, or gastroesophageal reflux disease (GERD).
- Having a disorder of the immune system or an antibody deficiency.
- Severe malnutrition, burns, liver disease, or cancer.
- Recent hospitalization, particularly in an intensive care unit.

In addition to these risk factors, there are two additional risk factors for chronic sinusitis:

- Asthma. About 20% of people with chronic sinusitis have asthma.
- Aspirin sensitivity that causes upper respiratory symptoms.

Causes and symptoms

Sinusitis is almost always due to an infection, although swelling from allergies can mimic the symptoms of pressure, **pain**, and congestion; and allergies can set the stage for a bacterial infection. Bacteria are the most common cause of sinus infection. *Streptococcus pneumoniae* causes about 33% of all cases, while *Haemophilus influenzae* causes about 25% of all cases. As of 2010, *Staphylococcus aureus* is seen more frequently as a cause of bacterial sinusitis in adults. About 2% of cases of viral sinusitis lead to secondary bacterial sinusitis. Some doctors think that nasal irritation from nose blowing leads to the secondary bacterial infection.

KEY TERMS

Cilia (singular, cilium)—Tiny hair-like projections from a cell. Within the respiratory tract, the cilia act to move mucus along, in an effort to continually flush out and clean the respiratory tract.

Polyp—An abnormal growth of tissue projecting from a mucous membrane. Nasal polyps are tissue growths arising from the mucous membranes lining the nasal passages. They are a risk factor for sinusitis.

Septum—A structure comprised of cartilage and bony plates that separates the nasal cavity into two nostrils. A septum that is not in line with the center line of the nose is called a deviated septum and is a risk factor for sinusitis.

Sinus—An air-filled body cavity.

In some cases, sinusitis may result from a dental infection, a foreign body in the nose, **cocaine** abuse, or occupational exposure to such chemical irritants as chlorine gas.

Sinusitis in children may be caused by *Moraxella catarrhalis* (20%). In people with weakened immune systems (including patients with diabetes; acquired **immunodeficiency** syndrome or **AIDS**; and patients who are taking medications which lower their immune resistance, such as **cancer** and transplant patients), sinusitis may be caused by **fungi** such as *Aspergillus*, *Candida*, or *Mucorales*.

Acute sinusitis usually follows some type of upper respiratory tract infection or cold. Viral sinusitis generally lasts from 7–10 days, while bacterial sinusitis tends to be more persistent. Instead of ending, the "cold" seems to linger on, with constant or even worsening congestion. Drainage from the nose often changes from a clear color to a thicker, yellowish-green discharge. There may be **fever**. **Headache** and pain over the affected sinuses may occur, as well as a feeling of pressure which may worsen when the patient bends over or lies down. There may be pain in the jaws or teeth. Some children, in particular, get upset stomachs from the infected drainage going down the back of their throats, and being swallowed into their stomachs. Some patients develop a **cough**.

Chronic sinusitis occurs when the problem has existed for at least eight weeks. There is rarely a fever with chronic sinusitis. Sinus pain and pressure is frequent, as is nasal congestion. Because of the nature of the swelling in the sinuses, they may not be able to drain out the nose. Drainage, therefore, drips constantly down the back of the throat, resulting in a continuously **sore throat** and bad breath.

Sinusitis in children is harder to distinguish from ordinary colds. Children younger than 6 years rarely develop headaches with sinusitis. However, swelling around the eyes or unusual irritability and fatigue are often associated with sinusitis in children, as are a discharge of yellowish or green mucus, sore throat, bad breath, fever above 100.4°F, and symptoms lasting longer than 10–14 days.

Diagnosis

Diagnosis of sinusitis can be made by a family doctor or by an otolaryngologist, a doctor who specializes in ear, nose, and throat disorders. In rare cases, the patient's dentist may be consulted to see whether a tooth infection is triggering the sinusitis.

Examination

Diagnosis of sinusitis is sometimes tricky because the symptoms so often resemble those of an uncomplicated cold. Sinusitis should be strongly suspected, however, when a cold lingers beyond a week's time. In some cases, the patient's history suggests the diagnosis, particularly a history of **asthma**, hay fever, **smoking**, or an occupational history of exposure to secondhand smoke or industrial chemicals. About 40% of cases of chronic sinusitis are associated with secondhand smoke.

Medical practitioners have differing levels of trust of certain basic examinations commonly conducted in the office. For example, tapping over the sinuses may cause pain in patients with sinusitis but it may not. A procedure called sinus transillumination may or may not also be helpful. Using a flashlight pressed up against the skin of the cheek, the practitioner will look in the patient's open mouth. When the sinuses are full of air (under normal conditions), the light will project through the sinus and will be visible on the roof of the mouth as a lit-up, reddened area. When the sinuses are full of mucus, the light will be blocked. While this simple test can be helpful, it is certainly not a perfect way to diagnose or rule out the diagnosis of sinusitis.

Tests

Imaging tests can be useful in diagnosing sinusitis. X-ray pictures and **CT scans** of the sinuses are helpful for both acute and chronic sinusitis. People with chronic sinusitis may require an examination with a nasal **endoscope** to see whether any kind of anatomic obstruction is causing their illness. For example, the septum (the cartilage which separates the two nasal cavities from each other) may be slightly displaced, which is called a deviated septum. This can result in chronic obstruction, setting the person up for the development of an infection.

Procedures

In some cases a sample of tissue from the patient's nasal passages can be taken for biopsy and culture. Tissue culture is particularly useful in detecting fungal sinusitis.

If the doctor suspects that a previously undiagnosed allergy is triggering chronic sinusitis, he or she may recommend an allergy skin test to identify the specific allergens responsible for the sinusitis.

Treatment

Traditional

Drugs

Antibiotic medications are used to treat acute sinusitis. Suitable **antibiotics** include sulfa drugs, amoxicillin, and a variety of cephalosporins. These medications are usually given for about two weeks but may be given for even longer periods of time. Decongestants, or the short-term use of decongestant nose sprays, can be useful. Acetaminophen and ibuprofen can decrease the pain and headache associated with sinusitis. Also, running a humidifier can prevent mucus within the nasal passages from drying out uncomfortably and can help soothe any accompanying sore throat or cough.

Surgery

Chronic sinusitis is often treated initially with antibiotics. Steroid nasal sprays may be used to decrease swelling in the nasal passages. If an anatomic reason is found for chronic sinusitis, it may need to be corrected with surgery. If a surgical procedure is necessary, samples are usually taken at the same time to allow identification of any organisms present that may be causing infection.

Fungal sinusitis will require surgery to clean out the sinuses. Then, a relatively long course of a very strong antifungal medication called amphotericin B is given through a needle in the vein (intravenously).

Alternative

Chronic sinusitis is often associated with **food allergies**. An elimination/challenge diet is recommended to identify and eliminate allergenic foods. Irrigating the sinuses with a salt water solution is often recommended for sinusitis and allergies, in order to clear the nasal passages of mucus. Another solution for nasal lavage (washing) utilizes powdered goldenseal (*Hydrastis canadensis*). Other herbal treatments, taken internally, include a mixture made of eyebright (*Euphrasia officinalis*), goldenseal, yarrow (*Achillea millefolium*), horseradish, and ephedra (*Ephedra sinica*), or, when infection is present, a mixture made of echinacea (*Echinacea* spp.), wild indigo, and poke root (*Phytolacca decandra-Americana*).

Homeopathic practitioners find a number of remedies useful for treating sinusitis. Among those they recommend are: *Arsenicum album*, *Kalium bichromium*, *Nux vomica*, *Mercurius iodatus*, and *Silica*.

Acupuncture has been used to treat sinusitis, as have a variety of dietary supplements, including **vitamins** A, C, and E, and the mineral **zinc**. Contrast **hydrotherapy** (hot and cold compresses, alternating 3 minutes hot, 30 seconds cold, repeated 3 times always ending with cold) applied directly over the sinuses can relieve pressure and enhance healing. A direct inhalation of essential oils (2 drops of oil to 2 cups of water) using thyme, rosemary, and lavender can help open the sinuses and kill bacteria that cause infection.

Prognosis

Prognosis for sinus infections is usually excellent, although some individuals may find that they are particularly prone to contracting such infections after a cold. The chief risk for serious illness resulting from sinusitis is the closeness of the nasal passages to the **central nervous system**, the lymph nodes in the neck, and the **blood vessels** in the neck and throat. Complications of sinusitis can include osteomyelitis, an infection of the **bone**; orbital cellulitis, inflammation of the tissues surrounding the eye; and **meningitis**, inflammation of the membranes covering the **brain** and **spinal cord**. Fungal sinusitis, however, has a relatively high death rate.

Prevention

Prevention of sinusitis involves the usual standards of good hygiene to cut down on the number of colds an individual catches. Quitting smoking or avoiding exposure to cigarette smoke, identifying and treating allergies, and avoiding deep dives in swimming pools may help prevent sinus infections. During the winter, it is a good idea to use a humidifier. Dry nasal passages may crack, allowing bacteria to enter. When allergies are diagnosed, a number of nasal sprays are available to try to prevent inflammation within the nasal passageways, thus allowing the normal flow of mucus.

The American Academy of Otolaryngology—Head and Neck Surgery adds the following suggestions for preventing sinusitis:

- Blowing the nose gently, blocking one nostril while blowing through the other.

- Avoiding air travel when other methods of transportation are available. Those who must travel by air should use a nasal spray decongestant before takeoff to prevent blockage of the sinuses.

- People with allergies should minimize their exposure to known allergens as well as using decongestants.

Resources

BOOKS

Bruce, Debra Fulghum, and Murray Grossan. *The Sinus Cure: Seven Simple Steps to Relieve Sinusitis and Other Ear, Nose, and Throat Conditions*, revised and updated. New York: Ballantine Books, 2007.

Goroll, Allan H., and Albert G. Mulley, Jr., eds. *Primary care medicine: office evaluation and management of the adult patient*, 6th ed. Philadelphia: Wolters Kluwer Health/ Lippincott Williams and Wilkins, 2009.

Wynn, Rhoda, and Winston C. Vaughn. *100 Questions and Answers about Sinusitis and Other Sinus Diseases*. Sudbury Jones and Bartlett, Publishers, 2008.

PERIODICALS

Anon, J.B. "Upper Respiratory Infections." *American Journal of Medicine* 123 (April 2010): s16–S25.

Bailey, J., and J. Change. "Antibiotics for Acute Maxillary Sinusitis." *American Family Physician* 79 (May 1, 2009): 757–58.

Brook, I. "Treatment Modalities for Bacterial Sinusitis." *Expert Opinion on Pharmacotherapy* 11 (April 2010): 755–69.

Cazzavillan, A., et al. "Treatment of Rhinosinusitis: The Role of Surgery." *International Journal of Immunopathology and Pharmacology* 23 (January-March 2010): 74–77.

Dykewicz, M.S., and D.L. Hamilos. "Rhinitis and Sinusitis." *Journal of Allergy and Clinical Immunology* 125 (February 2010): S103–S115.

Kelesidis, T., et al. "An Unusual Foreign Body as Cause of Chronic Sinusitis: A Case Report." *Journal of Medical Case Reports* 4 (May 26, 2010): 157.

Leibovitch, I., et al. "Severe Destructive Sinusitis and Orbital Apex Syndrome as a Complication of Intranasal Cocaine Abuse." *American Journal of Emergency Medicine* 24 (July 2006): 499–501.

Singh, N., et al. "Fine-Needle Aspiration Biopsy as an Initial Diagnostic Modality in a Clinically Unsuspected Case of Invasive Maxillary Fungal Sinusitis: A Case Report." *Diagnostic Cytopathology* 38 (April 2010): 290–93.

OTHER

American Academy of Otolaryngology—Head and Neck Surgery. *Sinusitis*. [Accessed December 6, 2010] http://www.entnet.org/HealthInformation/Sinusitis.cfm.

Centers for Disease Control and Prevention (CDC). *Sinus Infection (Sinusitis)*. http://www.cdc.gov/getsmart/antibiotic-use/URI/sinus-infection.html

Mayo Clinic. *Acute Sinusitis*. [Accessed December 6, 2010] http://www.mayoclinic.com/health/acute-sinusitis/DS00170.

Mayo Clinic. *Chronic Sinusitis*. [Accessed December 6, 2010] http://www.mayoclinic.com/health/chronic-sinusitis/DS00232.

National Institute of Allergy and Infectious Diseases (NIAID). *Sinus Infection (Sinusitis)*. [Accessed December 6, 2010] http://www.niaid.nih.gov/topics/sinusitis/Pages/index.aspx.

ORGANIZATIONS

American Academy of Family Physicians (AAFP), P.O. Box 11210, Shawnee Mission, KS 66207, (913) 906-6000, (800) 274-2237, Fax: (913) 906-6075, contactcenter @aafp. org, http://www.aafp.org/online/en/home.html

American Academy of Otolaryngology—Head and Neck Surgery, 1650 Diagonal Road, Alexandria, VA 22314, (703) 836-4444, http://www.entnet.org/

Centers for Disease Control and Prevention (CDC), 1600 Clifton Road, Atlanta, GA 30333, (800) 232-4636, cdcinfo@cdc.gov, http://www.cdc.gov.

National Institute of Allergy and Infectious Diseases (NIAID), 6610 Rockledge Drive, MSC 6612, Bethesda, MD 20892-6612, (301) 496-5717, (866) 284-4107, Fax: (301) 402-3573, http://www3.niaid.nih.gov.

Rosalyn Carson-DeWitt, M.D.
Rebecca J. Frey, Ph.D.

Skeletal muscles

Definition

Skeletal muscles have transverse striations and are under conscious or voluntary control by the **somatic nervous system**.

Description

Macroscopic

Skeletal muscles are often attached to **bone**, although this is not always the case. Tendons are a common means of attaching skeletal muscle to bone; they are composed of collagen, a structurally strong yet flexible substance. A muscle's origin is the end that moves least on contraction; the other end is referred to as the insertion. There is a large range of muscle sizes, types, and functions. Most human muscles have muscle fibers arranged parallel to a tendon. A unipinnate muscle, however, has all of its muscle fibers inserted at an angle into one side of a tendon.

Microscopic

Skeletal muscles are made up of bundles (called fascicles) of individual muscle fibers lined with connective tissue. Each muscle fiber is a giant multinucleated cell, formed by the fusion of myoblasts (muscle cell precursors) during development. Muscle fibers contain approximately one thousand myofibrils, tubular organelles that appear striated under a **microscope**; each myofibril is surrounded by a system of vesicles called the sarcoplasmic reticulum. The striations are due to alternating bands of light and dark regions called bands. The light regions are called I-bands, while the dark regions are called A-bands. A dividing line that runs through the A-band is called the Z-line, and the region between successive Z-lines is called the sarcomere.

The sarcomere is the functional unit of skeletal muscle and is associated with **muscle contraction**. It is composed primarily of two different contractile **proteins**: actin (or thin filaments) and myosin (or thick filaments). The filaments are arranged in an organized array so that their overlapping pattern produces the striations visible from under a microscope. The light I-bands are formed by actin filaments that are rooted at the Z-line, while the dark A-bands are composed of myosin filaments that overlap the actin filaments to varying degrees based on the extent of muscle contraction. The region in which there is no overlap (i.e., groups of actin filaments) in the center part of the A-band is called the H-band.

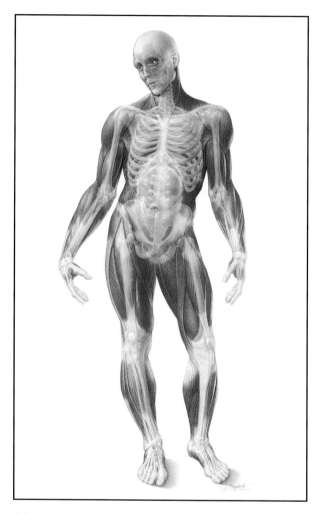

(Medical illustration showing placement and connection of skeletal muscle to bone, photograph. John M. Dougherty / Photo Researchers, Inc.)

Function

Contraction

In a resting muscle, opposing actin filaments overlap myosin filaments only partially, resulting in the characteristic H-band. When a muscle contracts, however, the opposing actin filaments slide along the myosin filaments and are pushed together so that the H-bands (and I-bands) become narrower, while the A-bands remain the same length. The result is that the Z-lines come closer together without the actual length of the filaments changing. This mode of action is called the sliding filament mechanism.

The sliding filament mechanism is regulated by the binding of adenoside triphosphate (ATP) to myosin. ATP is a molecule present in all living cells that acts as an energy source. When ATP is not bound to myosin, projections along the myosin filaments called heads remain tightly bound to actin and therefore no sliding

KEY TERMS

Actin—A contractile protein that forms thin filaments in myofibrils; forms the I-band of the sarcomere.

Adenosine triphosphate (ATP)—A molecule present in all living organisms that acts as an energy source.

Fascicle—Bundles of muscle fibers surrounded by connective tissue.

Muscle fibers—Tubular multinucleated cells containing approximately one thousand contracting myofibrils.

Myofibrils—Tubular organelles found in muscle fibers that appear striated under a microscope; they are surrounded by a system of vesicles called the sarcoplasmic retictulum, important in the regulation of muscle contraction.

Myosin—A contractile protein that forms thick filaments in myofibrils; forms the A-band of the sarcomere with some overlap with actin filaments.

Sarcomere—The functional unit of muscle contraction; composed of striated bands of contractile proteins (actin and myosin).

takes place (and subsequently, no muscle contraction). When ATP binds to myosin, however, a series of steps causes the myosin head to temporarily dissociate and change its conformation so that the actin and myosin filaments move relative to one another. This process, actively repeated in the many sarcomeres in a muscle fiber, results in muscle contraction.

Muscle contraction is also regulated by the **calcium** ion. A nerve impulse results in calcium being released from the sarcoplasmic reticulum. The calcium binds to various proteins that in turn cause conformational changes that expose the myosin-binding sites on the actin filaments so that contraction may occur.

Lactic acid fermentation

Glucose is a major fuel for most organisms; when energy is needed, glucose can be quickly released from the body's stores and processed metabolically to produce ATP. This metabolic process occurs optimally under high-oxygen (aerobic) conditions. When oxygen cannot be replenished to the muscles as fast as it is being used (as in short bursts of extreme activity), glucose can be broken down anaerobically (under no- or low-oxygen conditions). Use of this pathway, however, leads to a

buildup of the byproduct lactic acid in the muscles; this buildup causes muscle **pain** and cramps—uncontrollable shortening and hardening of muscle tissue—and limits the period of intense activity.

Role in human health

Neuromuscular disorders typically manifest themselves with one of four classes of symptoms (or any combination of the four):

- Weakness: Muscle weakness may be specific to a particular part of the body (e.g., neck, shoulder, arm, hand, leg, hip) or it may be generalized. Weakness may be caused by brain damage from a stroke or tumor, damage to the spinal cord, damage to a single nerve, or psychological problems.

- Fatigue: Individuals may suffer from chronic fatigue because of major depression, multiple sclerosis, stroke, neuromuscular transmission failure, or psychosomatic illness.

- Pain: Like muscle weakness, muscle pain may be specific (e.g., due to an muscle abscess) or general; it may also have a psychosomatic origin (e.g., associated with anxiety or depression).

- Cramps: Muscle pain caused by cramps is distinct from general muscle pain in that it often occurs in healthy individuals and causes intense pain.

Common diseases and disorders

- Spasmodic torticollis: This disease is characterized by painful spasms of the neck muscles that force the head to rotate and/or tilt. Its cause is usually unknown although occasionally conditions such as infections of the nervous system, tumors of the neck, or hyperthyroidism cause spasmodic torticollis.

- Fibromyalgia: Syndromes associated with fibromyalgia are characterized by localized or general pain or stiffness in muscles, tendons, and ligaments. There is no known cause for fibromyalgia but stress, inadequate sleep, injury, infections, and other conditions have been associated.

- Muscular dystrophy: The most common dystrophies (Duchenne's and Becker's) cause weakness in the muscles in or around the torso. In the case of Duchenne's muscular dystrophy (DMD), joint and muscle contractures develop in the form of cramps and amassment of fibrous tissue (including progressive destruction of muscle fibers).

- Tetanus: The bacillus *Clostridium tetani* produces a toxin called tetanospasmin that causes persistent spasms in the muscles of the jaw (hence the name lockjaw), the back, and/or the site of infection.

- Sports injuries: Muscle, ligament, and tendon injuries can be caused by inaccurate training advice, abnormalities in body structures, and overexertion. Common muscular injuries include ankle sprains, shin splints, hamstring injuries, and weightlifter's back. Such injuries can often be prevented by warming up before exercise, cooling down after exercise, performing strengthening and stretching exercises, and wearing protective gear.

Resources

BOOKS

Kakulas, B. A. "Pathologic Aspects of Muscle Contracture." In *Exercise Intolerance and Muscle Contracture*, edited by Georges Serratrice, Jean Pouget, and Jean-Philippe Azulay. France: Springer-Verlag, 1999.

McComas, Alan J. *Skeletal Muscle Form and Function.* Champaign, IL: Human Kinetics, 1996.

Schapira, Anthony H.V. and Robert C. Griggs, eds. *Muscle Diseases.* Woburn, MA: Butterworth-Heinemann, 1999.

OTHER

Berkow, Robert, Mark H. Beers, Andrew J. Fletcher, and Robert M. Bogin, eds. "Bone, Joint, and Muscle Disorders." The Merck Manual of Medical Information: Home Edition. 2001. http://www.merckhomeedition.com.

ORGANIZATION

Muscular Dystrophy Association. 3300 E. Sunrise Drive, Tucson, AZ 85718. (800) 572-1717. http://www.mdausa.org.

Stéphanie Islane Dionne

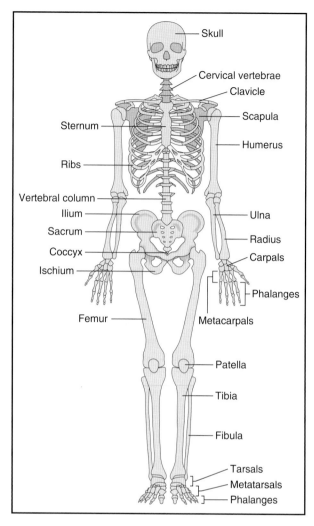

(From Delmar's Medical Terminology Image Library 1st edition by DELMAR. © 1999. Reprinted with permission of Delmar Learning, a division of Thomson Learning:www.thomsonrights. com. Fax: 800-730-2215.)

Skeletal system

Definition

The skeletal system is a living, dynamic, bony framework of the body, with networks of infiltrating **blood vessels**.

Description

Inside every person is a skeleton, a sturdy framework of about 206 bones that protects the body's organs, supports the body, provides attachment points for muscles to enable body movement, functions as a storage site for **minerals** such as **calcium** and **phosphorus**, and produces **blood** cells. Living mature **bone** is about 60% calcium compounds and about 40% collagen. Hence, bone is strong, hard, and slightly elastic. Humans are born with over 300 bones, but some of them, such as those in the **skull** and lower spine, fuse during growth, thereby reducing the number. Although mature bones consist largely of calcium—70% calcium salts and about 30% organic matrix, mostly collagen fibers—most bones in the skeleton of vertebrates, including humans, began as cartilage. Cartilage is a type of connective tissue, and contains collagen and elastin fibers. The hard outer part of bones are comprised mostly of a **proteins** such as collagen, in addition to a substance called hydroxyapatite. This substance is composed primarily of calcium and other minerals, and stores much of the body's calcium; it is primarily responsible for the strength of bones. At the center of each bone is the marrow, which is softer and less dense than the rest of the bone. The marrow contains specialized cells that produce blood cells that run through a bone, with nerves surrounding it.

Individual bones meet at areas called joints and are held in place by connective tissue. Most joints, such as the elbow, are called synovial joints, for the synovial membrane which envelopes the joint and secretes a lubricating fluid. Cartilage lines the surface of many joints and helps reduce friction between bones. The connective tissues linking the skeleton together at the joints are tendons and ligaments. Ligaments and tendons are both made up of collagen, but serve different functions. Ligaments link bones together and help prevent dislocated joints. Tendons link bone to muscle.

Because the bones making up the human skeleton are inside the body, the skeleton is called an endoskeleton. Some animals, such as the crab, have an external skeleton called an exoskeleton.

Types of bone

Bones may be classified according to their various traits, such as shape, origin, and texture. Four types are recognized based on shape. These are long bones, short bones, flat bones, and irregular bones. Long bones have a long central shaft, called the diaphysis, and two knobby ends, called the epiphysis. In growing long bones, the diaphysis and epiphysis are separated by a thin sheet of cartilage. Examples of long bones include bones of the arms and legs, the metacarpals of the hand, metatarsals of the foot, and the clavicle. Short bones are about as long as wide. The patella, carpels of the wrist, and tarsals of the ankle are short bones. Flat bones take several shapes, but are characterized by being relatively thin and flat. Examples include the sternum, ribs, hip bones, scapula, and cranial bones. Irregular bones are the odd-shaped bones of the skull, such as the sphenoid, the sacrum, and the vertebrae. The common characteristic of irregular bones is not that they are similar to each other in appearance, but that they cannot be placed in any of the other bone categories.

Bones may also be classified based on their origin. All bone (as well as muscles and connective tissue) originates from an embryonic connective tissue called mesenchyme, which makes mesoderm, also an embryonic tissue. Some mesoderm forms the cartilaginous skeleton of the fetus, the precursor for the bony skeleton. However, some bones, such as the clavicle and some of the facial and cranial bones of the skull, develop directly from mesenchyme, thereby bypassing the cartilaginous stage. These types of bone are called membrane bone (or dermal bone). Bone that originates from cartilage is called endochondral bone.

Finally, bones are classified based on texture. Smooth, hard bone called compact bone forms the outer layer of bones. Inside the outer compact bone is cancellous bone, sometimes called the bone marrow. Cancellous bone appears open and spongy, but is actually very strong, like compact bone. Together, the two types of bone produce a light, but strong, skeleton.

Structure

The human skeletal system is divided into two main groups: the axial skeleton and the appendicular skeleton. The axial skeleton includes bones associated with the body's main axis including:

• the skull
• the spine or vertebral column
• the ribs

The appendicular skeleton consists of the bones that anchor the body's appendages to the axial skeleton including:

• the pectoral girdle (shoulder area)
• the pelvic girdle (hip area)
• the upper extremities (arms)
• the lower extremities (legs)

AXIAL SKELETON. There are 28 bones in the skull. Of these, eight bones comprise the cranium and provide protection for the **brain**. In adults, these bones are flat and interlocking at their joints, making the cranium immobile. Fibrous joints, or sutures occur where the bony plates of the cranium meet and interlock. Cartilage-filled spaces between the cranial bones of infants, known as soft spots or fontanelles, allow their skull bones to move slightly during birth. This makes birth easier and helps prevent skull **fractures**, but may leave the infant with an odd-shaped head temporarily while the skull regains its shape. Eventually, the fontanelles in an infant's head are replaced by bone, and fibrous joints develop. In addition to protecting the brain, skull bones also support and protect the sensory organs responsible for sight, **hearing**, **smell** and **taste**.

The eight bones of the cranium are:

• frontal
• parietal (2)
• temporal (2)
• ethmoid
• sphenoid
• occipital

The frontal bone forms the forehead and eyebrows. Behind the frontal bone are the two parietal bones. Parietal bones form the roof of the cranium and curve down to form the sides of the cranium. Also forming the sides of the cranium are the two temporal bones, located behind the eyes. Each temporal bone encloses the cochlea and labyrinth of the inner ear, and the ossicles, three tiny bones of the middle ear which are not part of the cranium. The ossicles are the malleus (hammer), incus (anvil), and stapes (stirrups). The temporal bones also attach to the lower jaw, and this is the only moveable joint in the skull. Between the temporal bones is the irregular shaped sphenoid bone, which provides protection for the **pituitary gland**. The small ethmoid bone forms part of the eye socket next to the nose. Olfactory nerves, or sense of smell nerves, pass through the ethmoid bone on their way to the brain. Forming the base and rear of the cranium is the occipital bone. The occipital bone has a hole, called the foramen magnum, through which the **spinal cord** passes and connects to the brain.

Fourteen bones shape the cheeks, eyes, nose, and mouth. These include:

• the nasal (2)

• zygomatic (2)

• maxillae (2)

• mandible

The upper, bony bridge of the nose is formed by the nasal bones and provides an attachment site for the cartilage making up the softer part of the nose. The zygomatic bones form the cheeks and part of the eye sockets. Two bones fuse to form the maxillae, the upper jaw of the mouth. These bones also form the hard palate of the mouth. The mandible forms the lower jaw of the mouth and is moveable, enabling chewing of food and speech. The mandible is the bone which connects to the temporal bones.

Located behind these facial bones are other bones which shape the interior portions of the eyes, nose, and mouth. These include:

• lacrimal (2)

• palatine (2)

• conchae (2)

• vomer bones

In addition to these 28 skull bones is the hyoid bone, located at the base of the tongue. Technically, the hyoid bone is not part of the skull but it is often included with the skull bones. It provides an attachment site for the tongue and some neck muscles.

Several of the facial and cranial bones contain sinuses, or cavities, that connect to the nasal cavity and drain into it. These are the frontal, ethmoid, sphenoid, and maxillae bones, all located near the nose. Painful sinus headaches result from the build up of pressure in these cavities. Membranes that line these cavities may secrete mucus or become infected, causing additional aggravation for humans.

The skull rests atop of the spine, which encases and protects the spinal cord. The spine, also called the **vertebral column** or backbone, consists of 33 stacked vertebrae, the lower ones fused. Vertebra are flat with two main features. The main oval shaped, bony mass of the vertebra is called the centrum. From the centrum arises a bony ring called the neural arch which forms the neural canal (also called a vertebral foramen), a hole for the spinal cord to pass through. Short, bony projections (neural spines) arise from the neural arch and provide attachment points for muscles. Some of these projections (called transverse processes) also provide attachment points for the ribs. There are also small openings in the neural arch for the spinal nerves, which extend from the spinal cord throughout the body. Injury to the column of vertebrae may cause serious damage to the spinal cord and the spinal nerves, and could result in **paralysis** if the spinal cord or nerves are severed.

There are seven cervical, or neck, vertebrae. The first one, the atlas, supports the skull and allows the head to nod up and down. The atlas forms a condylar joint (a type of synovial joint) with the occipital bone of the skull. The second vertebra, the axis, allows the head to rotate from side to side. This rotating synovial joint is called a **pivot joint**. Together, these two vertebrae make possible a wide range of head motions.

Below the cervical vertebrae are the 12 thoracic, or upper back, vertebrae. The ribs are attached to these vertebrae. Thoracic vertebrae are followed by five lumbar, or lower back, vertebrae. Last is the sacrum, composed of five fused vertebrae, and the coccyx, or tail bone, composed of four fused bones.

The vertebral column helps to support the weight of the body and protects the spinal cord. Cartilaginous joints rather than synovial joints occur in the spine. Disks of cartilage lie between the bony vertebrae of the back and provide cushioning, like **shock** absorbers. The vertebrae of the spine are capable of only limited movement, such bending and some twisting.

A pair of ribs extends forward from each of the 12 thoracic vertebrae, for a total of 24 ribs. Occasionally, a person is born with an extra set of ribs. The joint between the ribs and vertebrae is a gliding (or plane) joint, a type of synovial joint, as ribs do move, expanding and contracting with breathing. Most of the ribs (the first seven pair) attach in the front of the body via cartilage to the long, flat breastbone, or sternum. These ribs are called true ribs. The next three pair of ribs are false ribs. False ribs attach to another rib in front instead of the sternum, and are connected by cartilage. The lower two pair of ribs which do not attach anteriorly are called floating ribs. Ribs give shape to the chest and support and protect the body's major organs, such as the **heart** and **lungs**. The rib cage also provides attachment points for connective tissue, to help hold organs in place. In adult humans, the sternum also produces red blood cells as well as providing an attachment site for ribs.

APPENDICULAR SKELETON. The appendicular skeleton joins with the axial skeleton at the shoulders and hips. Forming a loose attachment with the sternum is the pectoral girdle, or shoulder. Two bones, the clavicle (collar bone) and scapula (shoulder blade), form one shoulder. The scapula rests on top of the ribs in the back of the body. It connects to the clavicle, the bone that attaches the entire shoulder structure to the skeleton at the sternum. The clavicle is a slender bone that is easily broken. Because the scapula is so loosely attached, it is easily dislocated from the clavicle, hence the dislocated shoulder injuries commonly suffered by persons playing sports. The major advantage to the loose attachment of the pectoral girdle is that it allows for a wide range of shoulder motions and greater overall freedom of movement.

Unlike the pectoral girdle, the pelvic girdle, or hips, is strong and dense. Each hip, left and right, consists of three fused bones, the ilium, ischium, and pubic. Collectively, these three bones are known as the innominate bone.

The innominates fuse with the sacrum to form the pelvic girdle. Specifically, the iliums shape the hips and the two ischial bones support the body when a person sits. The two pubic bones meet anteriorly at a cartilaginous joint. The pelvic girdle is bowl-shaped, with an opening at the bottom. In a pregnant woman, this bony opening is a passageway through which her baby must pass during birth. To facilitate the baby's passage, the body secretes a hormone called relaxin which loosens the joint between the pubic bones. In addition, the pelvic girdle of women is generally wider than that of men. This also helps to facilitate birth, but is a slight impediment for walking and running. Hence, men, with their narrower hips, are better adapted for such activities. The pelvic girdle protects the lower abdominal organs, such as the intestines, and helps supports the weight of the body above it.

The arms and legs, the upper and lower appendages of the body, are very similar in form. Each attaches to the girdle, pectoral or pelvic, via a **ball and socket joint**, a special type of synovial joint. In the shoulder, the socket, called the glenoid cavity, is shallow. The shallowness of the glenoid cavity allows for great freedom of movement. The hip socket, or acetabulum, is larger and deeper. This deep socket, combined with the rigid and massive structure of the hips, give the legs much less mobility and flexibility than the arms.

The humerus, or upper arm bone, is the long bone between the elbow and the shoulder. It connects the arm to the pectoral girdle. In the leg the femur, or thigh bone, is the long bone between the knee and hip which connects the leg to the pelvic girdle. The humerus and femur are sturdy bones, especially the femur, which is a weight bearing bone. Since the arms and legs are jointed, the humerus and femur are connected to other bones at the end opposite the ball and socket joint. In the elbow, this second joint is a type of synovial joint called a **hinge joint**. Two types of synovial joints occur in the knee region, a condylar joint (like the condylar joint in the first vertebra) which connects the leg bones, and a plane, or **gliding joint**, between the patella (knee cap) and femur.

At the elbow the humerus attaches to a set of parallel bones, the ulna and radius, bones of the forearm. The radius is the bone below the thumb that rotates when the hand is turned over and back. The ulna and radius then attach to the carpel bones of the wrist. Eight small carpel bones make up the wrist and connect to the hand. The hand is made up of five long, slender metacarpal bones (the palms) and 14 phalanges of the hand (fingers and thumb). Some phalanges form joints with each other, giving the human hand great dexterity.

Similarly, in the leg, the femur forms a joint with the patella and with the fibula and tibia bones of the lower leg. The tibia, or shin bone, is larger than the fibula and forms the joint behind the patella with the femur. Like the femur, the tibia is also a weight bearing bone. At the ankle joint, the fibula and tibia connect to the tarsals of the upper foot. There are seven tarsals of the upper foot, forming the ankle and the heel. The tarsals in turn connect to five long, slender metatarsals of the lower foot. The metatarsals form the foot's arch and sole and connect to the phalanges of the feet (toes). The 14 foot phalanges are shorter and less agile than the hand phalanges. Several types of synovial joints occur in the hands and feet, including plane, ellipsoid and saddle. Plane joints occur between toe bones, allowing limited movement. Ellipsoid joints between the finger and palm bones give the fingers circular mobility, unlike the toes. The saddle joint at the base of the thumb helps make the hands the most important part of the body in terms of dexterity and manipulation. A saddle joint also occurs at the ankles.

Bone development and growth

Since most bone begins as cartilage, it must be converted to bone through a process called ossification. The key players in bone development are cartilage cells (chondrocytes), bone precursor cells (osteoprogenitor cells), bone deposition cells (osteoblasts), bone resorption cells (osteoclasts), and mature bone cells (osteocytes).

During ossification, blood vessels invade the cartilage and transport osteoprogenitor cells to a region called the center of ossification. At this site, the cartilage cells die, leaving behind small cavities. Osteoblast cells form from the progenitor cells and begin depositing bone tissue, spreading out from the center. Through this process, both the spongy textured cancellous bone and the smooth outer compact bone forms. Two types of bone marrow, red and yellow, occupy the spaces in cancellous bone. Red marrow produces red blood cells, while yellow marrow stores fat in addition to producing blood cells. Eventually, in compact bone, osteoblast cells become trapped in their bony cavities, called lacunae, and become osteocytes. Neighboring osteocytes form connections with each other and thus are able to transfer materials between cells. The osteocytes are part of a larger system called the Haversian system. These systems are like long tubes, squeezed tightly together in compact bone. Blood vessel, lymph vessels, and nerves run through the center of the tube, called the Haversian canal, and are surrounded by layers of bone, called lamellae, which house the osteocytes. Blood vessels are connected to each other by lateral canals called Volkmann's canals. Blood vessels are also found in spongy bone, without the Haversian system. A protective membrane called the periosteum surrounds all bones.

Bone development is a complex process, but it is only half the story. Bones must grow, and they do so via a process called remodeling. Remodeling involves resorption of existing bone inside the bone (enlarging the marrow cavities) and deposition of new bone on the exterior. The resorptive cells are the osteoclasts and osteoblast cells lay down the new bone material. As remodeling progresses in long bones, a new center of ossification develops, this one at the swollen ends of the bone, called the epiphysis. A thin layer of cartilage called the epiphyseal plate separates the epiphysis from the shaft and is the site of bone deposition. When growth is complete, this cartilage plate disappears, so that the only cartilage remaining is that which lines the joints, called hyaline cartilage. Remodeling does not end when growth ends. Osteocytes, responding to the body's need for calcium, resorb bone in adults to maintain a calcium balance.

Function

The skeletal system has several important functions:

• It provides shape and form to the body, while allowing for body movement.
• It supports and protects vital organs and muscles.

• It produces red blood cells for the body in the bone marrow. Each second, an average of 2.6 million red blood cells are to replace worn out blood cells and those destroyed by the liver.
• It stores minerals including calcium and phosphorus. When excess are present in the blood, the bones will store minerals. When the supply in the blood runs low, minerals will be withdrawn from the bones to replenish the blood supply.

Common diseases and disorders

Even though bones are very strong, they may be broken. Most fractures do heal. The healing process may be stymied if bones are not reset properly or if the injured person is the victim of malnutrition. Osteoprogenitor cells migrate to the site of the fracture and begin the process of making new bone (osteoblasts) and reabsorbing the injured bone (osteoclasts). With proper care, the fracture will fully heal, and in children, often without a trace.

The joint between the mandible and the temporal bones, called the temporomandibular joint, is the source of the painful condition known as temporomandibular joint dysfunction, or TMJ dysfunction. Sufferers of TMJ dysfunction experience a variety of symptoms including headaches, a sore jaw, and a snapping sensation when moving the jaw. There are several causes of the dysfunction. The cartilage disk between the bones may shift, or the connective tissue between the bones may be situated in a manner that causes misalignment of the jaw. Sometimes braces on the teeth can aggravate TMJ dysfunction. The condition may be corrected with **exercise**, or in severe cases, surgery. Another condition, cleft palate, is due to the failure of the maxillary bones in the jaw to completely fuse in the fetus.

Bones are affected by poor diet and are also subject to a number of diseases and disorders. Some examples include scurvy, rickets, **osteoporosis**, arthritis, and bone tumors. Scurvy results from the lack of **vitamin C**. In infants, scurvy causes poor bone development. It also causes membranes surrounding the bone to bleed, forming clots that are eventually ossified, and thin bones that break easy. In addition, adults are affected by bleeding gums and loss of teeth. Before modern times, sailors were often the victims of scurvy, due to extended periods of time at sea with limited food. They consequently tried to keep a good supply of citrus fruits, such as oranges and limes, on board because these fruits supply vitamin C. By the twenty-first century, scurvy had become extremely rare in Western societies.

Rickets is a children's disease resulting from a deficiency of **vitamin D**. This vitamin enables the body

KEY TERMS

Bone—Composed primarily of a non-living matrix of calcium salts and a living matrix of collagen fibers, bone is the major component that makes up the human skeleton. Bone produces blood cells and functions as a storage site for elements such as calcium and phosphorus.

Calcium—A naturally occurring element that primarily combines with phosphate to form the nonliving matrix of bones.

Cartilage—A type of connective tissue that takes three forms: elastic cartilage, fibrocartilage, and hyaline cartilage. Hyaline cartilage forms the embryonic skeleton and lines the joints of bones.

Haversian system—Tubular systems in compact bone with a central Haversian canal that houses blood and lymph vessels surrounded by circular layers of calcium salts and collagen, called lamellae, in which reside osteocytes.

Marrow—A type of connective tissue that fills the spaces of most cancellous bone. It produces blood cells and stores fat.

Ossification—The process of replacing connective tissue such as cartilage and mesenchyme with bone.

Osteoblast—The bone cell that deposits calcium salts and collagen during bone growth, bone remodeling, and bone repair.

Osteoclast—The bone cell responsible for re-absorbing bone tissue in bone remodeling and repair.

Osteocyte—Mature bone cell whose main function is to regulate the levels of calcium and phosphate in the body.

Skeleton—Consists of bones and cartilage that are linked together by ligaments. The skeleton protects vital organs of the body and enables body movement.

Synovial joint—One of three types of joints in the skeleton and by far the most common. Synovial joints are lined with a membrane that secretes a lubricating fluid. Includes ball and socket, pivot, plane, hinge, saddle, condylar, and ellipsoid joints.

Vertebrates—Includes all animals with a vertebral column protecting the spinal cord such as humans, dogs, birds, lizards, and fish.

to absorb calcium and phosphorus; without it, bones become soft and weak and actually bend, or bow out, under the body's weight. Vitamin D is found in milk, eggs and **liver**, and may also be produced by exposing the skin to sunlight. Pregnant women can also suffer from a vitamin D deficiency, osteomalacia, resulting in soft bones. The elderly, especially women who had several children in succession, sometimes suffer from osteoporosis, a condition in which a significant amount of calcium from bones is dissolved into the blood to maintain the body's calcium balance. Weak, brittle bones dotted with pits and pores are the result. Osteoporosis occurs most often in older people and in women after **menopause**. It affects nearly half of all those, men and women, over the age of 75. Women, however, are five times more likely than men to develop the disease. They have smaller, thinner bones than men to begin with, and they lose bone mass more rapidly after menopause (usually around age 50), when they stop producing a bone-protecting hormone called estrogen. In the five to seven years following menopause, women can lose about 20% of their bone mass. By age 65 or 70, though, men and women lose bone mass at the same rate. As an increasing number of men reach an older age, they are becoming more aware that osteoporosis is an important health issue for them as well.

Arthritis is another condition commonly afflicting the elderly. This is an often painful inflammation of the joints. Arthritis is not restricted to the elderly, and even young people can suffer from this condition. There are several types of arthritis, such as rheumatoid, rheumatic, and degenerative. Arthritis basically involves the inflammation and deterioration of cartilage and bone at the joint surface. In some cases, bony protuberances around the rim of the joint may develop. Most people will probably develop arthritis if they live to a significant older age. Degenerative arthritis is the type that commonly occurs with age. The knee, hip, shoulder, and elbow are the major targets of degenerative arthritis. A number of different types of tumors, some harmless and others more serious, may also affect bones.

Resources

BOOKS

Adams, John S., and Barbara P. Lukertet. *Osteoporosis: Genetics, Prevention and Treatment.* Boston, Kluwer Academic, 1999.

Browner, Bruce D. et al., ed. *Skeletal Trauma: Fractures, Dislocations, Ligamentous Injuries,* 2nd ed. Vols 1 and 2. Philadelphia, PA: W.B. Saunders Co, 1998.

Ganong, William F. *Review of Medical Physiology,* 20th ed. New York: McGraw-Hill Professional Publishing, 2001.

Kessler, George J. et al. *The Bone Density Diet: 6 Weeks to a Strong Body and Mind.* New York: Ballantine Books, 2000.

Praemer, A., et al., ed. *Musculoskeletal Conditions in the United States.* Rosemont, IL: American Academy of Orthopaedic Surgeons; 1999.

ORGANIZATIONS

Arthritis Foundation. 1330 W. Peachtree St., P.O. Box 7669, Atlanta, GA 30357-0669. (800) 283-7800. http://www.arthritis.org.

National Center for Complementary and Alternative Medicine (NCCAM), 31 Center Dr., Room #5B-58, Bethesda, MD 20892-2182. (800) NIH-NCAM, Fax (301) 495-4957. http://nccam.nih.gov.

National Osteoporosis Foundation. 1150 17th Street, Suite 500 NW, Washington, DC 20036-4603. (800) 223-9994. http://www.nof.org.

Osteoporosis and Related Bone Diseases-National Resource Center. 1150 17th St., NW, Ste. 500, Washington, DC 20036-4603. (800) 624-BONE. http://www.osteo.org.

Crystal Heather Kaczkowski, M.Sc.

Skin allergy tests *see* **Allergy tests**

Skin biopsy

Definition

A skin biopsy is a procedure in which a small piece of living skin is removed from the body for examination, usually under a **microscope**, to establish a precise diagnosis. Skin biopsies are usually brief, straightforward procedures performed by a skin specialist (dermatologist) or family physician.

Purpose

The word *biopsy* is taken from Greek words that mean "to view life." The term describes what a specialist in identifying diseases (pathologist) does with tissue obtained from a skin biopsy. The pathologist *visually* examines the tissue under a microscope.

A skin biopsy is used to make a diagnosis of many skin disorders. Information from the biopsy also helps the doctor choose the best treatment for the patient.

Doctors perform skin biopsies to:

• make a diagnosis

• confirm a diagnosis made from the patient's medical history and a physical examination

• check whether a treatment prescribed for a previously diagnosed condition is working

• check the edges of tissue removed with a tumor to make certain it contains all the diseased tissue.

Skin biopsies also can serve a therapeutic purpose. Many skin abnormalities (lesions) can be removed completely during the biopsy procedure.

Precautions

A patient taking aspirin or another **blood** thinner (anticoagulant) may be asked to stop taking them a week or more before the skin biopsy. This adjustment in medication will prevent excessive bleeding during the procedure and allow for normal blood clotting.

Some patients are allergic to lidocaine, the numbing agent most frequently used during a skin biopsy. The doctor can usually substitute another anesthetic agent.

Description

The first part of the skin biopsy test is obtaining a sample of tissue that best represents the lesion being evaluated. Many biopsy techniques are available. The choice of technique and precise location from which to take the biopsy material are determined by factors such as the type and shape of the lesion. Biopsies can be classified as excisional or incisional. In excisional biopsy, the lesion is completely removed; in incisional biopsy, a portion of the lesion is removed.

The most common biopsy techniques are:

• Shave biopsy. A scalpel or razor blade is used to shave off a thin layer of the lesion parallel to the skin.

• Punch biopsy. A small cylindrical punch is screwed into the lesion through the full thickness of the skin and a plug of tissue is removed. A stitch or two may be needed to close the wound.

• Scalpel biopsy. A scalpel is used to make a standard surgical incision or excision to remove tissue. This technique is most often used for large or deep lesions. The wound is closed with stitches.

• Scissors biopsy. Scissors are used to snip off surface (superficial) skin growths and lesions that grow from a stem or column of tissue. Such growths are sometimes seen on the eyelids or neck.

After the biopsy tissue is removed, bleeding may be controlled by applying pressure or by burning with

KEY TERMS

Benign—Noncancerous.

Dermatitis—A skin disorder that causes inflammation, that is, redness, swelling, heat, and pain.

Dermatologist—A doctor who specializes in skin care and treatment.

Dermatosis—A noninflammatory skin disorder.

Lesion—An area of abnormal or injured skin.

Malignant—Cancerous.

Pathologist—A person who specializes in studying diseases. In particular, this person examines the structural and functional changes in the tissues and organs of the body that are caused by disease or that cause disease themselves.

electricity or chemicals. **Antibiotics** often are applied to the wound to prevent **infection**. Stitches may be placed in the wound, or the wound may be bandaged and allowed to heal on its own.

The second part of the skin biopsy test is handling and examining the tissue sample. Drying and structural damage to the tissue sample must be prevented, so it should be placed immediately in an appropriate preservative, such as formaldehyde.

The pathologist can use a variety of laboratory techniques to process the biopsy tissue. Tissue stains and several different kinds of microscopes are used. Because there are many skin disorders (broadly called dermatosis and dermatitis), the pathologist has extensive training in their accurate identification. Cases of **melanoma**, the most malignant kind of skin **cancer**, have almost tripled in the past 30 years. Because melanoma grows very rapidly in the skin, quick and accurate diagnosis is important.

Preparation

The area of the biopsy is cleansed thoroughly with alcohol or a disinfectant containing iodine. Sterile cloths (drapes) may be positioned, and a local anesthetic, usually lidocaine, is injected into the skin near the lesion. Sometimes the anesthetic contains epinephrine, a drug that helps reduce bleeding during the biopsy. Sterile gloves and **surgical instruments** are always used to reduce the risk of infection.

Aftercare

If stitches have been placed, they should be kept clean and dry until removed. Stitches are usually removed five to 10 days after the biopsy. Sometimes the patient is instructed to put protective ointment on the stitches before showering. **Wounds** that have not been stitched should be cleaned with soap and water daily until

they heal. Adhesive strips should be left in place for two to three weeks. **Pain** medications usually are not necessary.

Risks

Infection and bleeding occur rarely after skin biopsy. If the skin biopsy may leave a scar, the patient usually is asked to give **informed consent** before the test.

Normal results

The biopsy reveals normal skin layers.

Abnormal results

The biopsy reveals a noncancerous (benign) or cancerous (malignant) lesion. Benign lesions may require treatment.

ORGANIZATION

American Academy of Dermatology, P.O. Box 4014, Schaumburg, IL 60168-4014, Fax: (847) 240-1859, (866) 503-SKIN (7546), http://www.aad.org.

Collette L. Placek

Skin cancer *see* **Melanoma**

Skin culture

Definition

A skin culture is a laboratory test used to isolate and identify the microorganism (bacterium, fungus, or virus) causing a skin **infection**, so the most effective antibiotic or other treatment for the infection can be determined.

Purpose

Skin infections are contagious and, if left untreated, can lead to serious complications. A skin culture helps the physician to diagnose and treat a skin infection.

Precautions

To avoid spreading pathogenic organisms to patients or other individuals, health care professionals should be cautious in the collection and handling of skin culture specimens.

Description

Skin infections may involve the superficial layer (epidermis) only or may involve the deeper dermis, including the sweat glands, oil glands, lymphatics and hair follicles within. Microorganisms can infect healthy skin, but more often they infect skin already damaged by an injury or an **abrasion**. The lesion produced by the infection is an early indication of which type of microorganism is causing the infection. For example, pustules are associated with impetigo (pyoderma) the most common bacterial skin infection. Pyoderma is most often caused by group A *Streptococcus*. Vesicular skin rashes are commonly caused by herpesviruses as in chickenpox. Scaly rashes are most commonly caused by dermatophytes, **fungi** that infect the keratinized skin (epidermis). Bacterial skin infections are the most common, and can result in ulcers, cellulitis, rashes, **boils**, abscesses, and other types of lesions.

The following types of microorganisms cause most skin infections and can be isolated by performing a skin culture:

• Bacteria: Aerobic gram positive cocci, *Streptococcus pyrogenes,* and *Staphylococcus aureus* are the most common isolates and are responsible for pyoderma. However many other bacteria cause skin infections less frequently. Usually, these are introduced through a wound in the skin caused by a bite, decubitus ulcer, burn, trauma, or puncture. Some notable genera are anaerobic bacteria such as *Bacteroides* and *Clostridium* from soils, gram negative rods such as *Aeromonas, Plesiomones,* and *Vibrio* from water. Organisms that live in the mouth of dogs and cats such as *Pasteurella multocida* can infect bite wounds.

• Fungi (molds and yeast): Three genera of fungi commonly cause ringworm of the skin, hair, and nails and are the most common fungi isolated from skin. These are *Trichophyton, Epidermophyton,* and *Microsporum.* Candida can colonize the epidermis as part of the normal flora but will infect burned skin and skin folds of newborns. Several other fungi may cause subcutaneous infection.

• Viruses: Rubella (German measles), rubeola (measles), roseola, and herpes varicella zoster (chickenpox) are common causes of viral rashes in children. Herpes simplex 1 and cytomegalovirus may cause more complex infections in immunosuppressed adults. In addition, skin infections can be caused by enteroviruses, poxviruses, and several others.

• Skin infections can also be caused by mycobacteria such as *Mycobacterium tuberculosis* and *M. leprae* the cause of leprosy, and skin lesions can be caused by some parasites when the larva enter the skin.

Based on the appearance of the lesion, the physician orders one or more types of skin cultures. Using **aseptic technique**, the physician, nurse, or other health care professional collects a specimen. For open epidermal infections a sample of the lesion such as skin cells, pus, or fluid can be collected using a swab. For crusted or closed lesions, the surface of the vesicle or pustule should be removed with a scalpel blade in order to expose the infected skin before swabbing. Ringworm should be scraped using a scalpel blade to collect the keratinized skin. Deeper infections should be sampled by aspiration. Swabs for bacterial culture are placed in a sterile container (often containing transport medium such as Stuart or Cary-Blair) before being sent to the laboratory for culture. If anaerobic culture is requested the specimen is immediately placed in prereduced oxygen-free transport medium.

Bacterial skin cultures

A **Gram stain** is prepared by rolling the smear across the center of a glass slide or dropping a liquid specimen onto the center and allowing it to air dry. Gram-positive cells retain the crystal violet stain and appear dark purple, while gram-negative cells do not. Gram-negative **bacteria** are counterstained by the safranin and appear pink. In addition to classifying the bacteria seen, the Gram stain can identifies yeast, hyphal elements, and organisms that require special culture media. For example, the presence of large gram-positive spore forming rods indicates the possible presence of *Clostridium spp.* and the need for anaerobic culture.

A routine bacterial skin culture involves inoculating (spreading a portion of the specimen on) several culture plates containing general-use enrichment media and selective media. Commonly used media include sheep **blood** agar plates, chocolate (heated blood) agar plates, MacConkey agar for isolation of gram-negative rods, and either phenylethyl alcohol (PEA) or colistin-naladixic acid (CNA) blood agar for isolation of gram positive cocci. Plates are incubated in air or 5–10% carbon dioxide and examined for growth daily for at least two days. Bacteria present in the specimen multiply and appear on the plates as visible colonies. These are Gram stained and subcultured (transferred) to other media in order to identify the organism. Complete identification usually requires one to two days following isolation of a pure culture. It is standard practice to perform an antibiotic sensitivity test on any bacterial pathogen isolated from a routine skin culture, except group A *Streptococcus*, which is susceptible to penicillin and related **antibiotics**. An antibiotic sensitivity test, also called an antibiotic susceptibility test, grows the bacteria in the presence of different antibiotics to determine which ones will effectively treat the infection by killing the bacteria.

Fungal skin cultures

Physicians request fungal skin cultures less frequently. A group of fungi called dermatophytes cause skin infections such as ringworm and athlete's foot. Yeast infections caused by *Candida* can thrive on moist skin, such as in diaper areas and in the folds of skin in the groin. Yeast infections can cause significant problems for newborns and patients with **AIDS** or depressed immune systems. Yeast infections are cultured on sheep blood agar and grow in one to two days. Dermatopohytes are usually identified by a **KOH test**. In this test, a sample of skin scraped with a scalpel blade and transferred to a slide. After adding KOH, the slide is allowed to stand for five minutes in order to dissolve skin cells, hair, and debris. Lactophenol cotton blue stain can be added to make the fungi easier to see, or if a fluorescent **microscope** is available, calcofluor white stain may be added to the KOH preparation. This will cause the fungi to become fluorescent making them easier to identify. Dermatophytes are easily recognized under the microscope by their long branch-like tubular structures called hyphae. Fungi causing ringworm infections produce septate (segmented) hyphae. Some show the presence of spores formed directly from the hyphae (arthroconidia). Yeast infections of the skin can also be identified by the KOH test. Yeast cells appear round or oval, and budding forms may be seen.

A culture is requested only when specific identification of the fungus is necessary. For a routine **fungal culture**, the specimen is spread on a culture plate or tube containing nutrient media designed to grow fungi, incubated for up to four weeks, and observed for growth at regular intervals. Stains and biochemical tests are usually used to identify yeast and other fungi. Dermatophytes may be cultured on a medium called dermatopohyte test medium (DTM). This is an agar slant containing phytone, dextrose, phenol red, cycloheximide, gentamicin, and chlortetracycline. The antibiotics inhibit the growth of normal skin flora. Skin scrapings, hair, or nail samples are added to the medium and allowed to grow at room temperature. Cultures are held for 14 days. Dermatophytes will turn the medium from yellow to red as they grow. Other fungi, called systemic fungi can enter the skin through puncture **wounds**, abrasions or cuts and cause subcutaneous infection. A common cause of systemic mycosis in the United States among gardeners and farmers is *Sporothrix schenckii*. Such fungi are cultured from skin aspirates on growth medium for fungi containing antibiotics to inhibit bacterial growth. Most commonly used are Sabouraud dextrose agar with antibiotics and mycosel agar with cycloheximide and chloramphenicol. Cultures are incubated at both 77° and 96.8°F (25° and 36°C). *Sporothrix schenckii* grows in about four days but other fungi grow more slowly, and plates should be held for 30 days before reporting as negative.

Viral skin cultures

Viruses, such as herpes, can also cause skin infections. A specimen for viral culture is mixed with commercially prepared animal cells usually grown on a coverslip in a shell vial. Characteristic changes to the animal cells caused by the growing virus help to identify the virus. For rapid diagnosis, some laboratories use an electron microscope to identify viruses on the basis of morphology. For example, the herpes virus can be cultured from a vesicle (blister) which has been removed carefully with a scalpel blade. The base of the vesicle is swabbed with a sterile cotton applicator, and the virus taken to the laboratory in a tube of viral transport medium. Herpes can be cultured in several cell lines including human diploid fibroblasts (HDF), HEp2 cells (epithelial **cancer** cells from the larynx), primary monkey kidney cells (PMK), and rabbit kidney cells (RK). Cell cultures are inoculated and allowed to grow for one to three days at 96.8°F (36°C) in 5–10% carbon dioxide. Usually by the end of the first day of culture the cytopathic effect (CPE), formation of giant cells, can be seen by observing the cells under a microscope.

Preparation

Before ordering a skin culture, the physician will ask the patient for a complete medical history and perform a **physical examination** to determine possible causes of the skin infection and whether a skin culture is appropriate. For acute skin infections, immediate treatment is sometimes necessary.

KEY TERMS

Antimicrobial—A substance or action that kills or inhibits the growth of microorganisms.

Aseptic technique—Practices performed before, during, and after a clinical procedure to prevent or reduce contamination and postprocedural infection.

Pathogen—An organism that causes disease.

Pyoderma—A pus-containing bacterial skin infection.

Selective media—Media designed to enhance the growth of one type of microorganism by inhibiting the growth of other types with antibiotics or other substances.

Sensitivity test—A laboratory test that shows which antibiotics will treat an infection by killing the bacteria.

All health care professionals who participate in collecting a skin culture specimen should be trained in aseptic technique. Before collecting the specimen, they should scrub their hands thoroughly with an antimicrobial soap and, in some cases, put on sterile gowns, masks, and gloves. Sterile instruments and containers should be assembled near the patient. If appropriate, a sterile drape can be placed around the site of the infection. After cleaning the infected area with alcohol and sterile saline, the physician, nurse, or other health care professional uses a sterile blade, swab, needle, syringe, or other instruments to collect a sample of skin cells, pus, or fluid from the lesion. It might be necessary to open the lesion before collecting the specimen.

Aftercare

Collection of the specimen could cause some slight bleeding at the infection site, which might require some attention. Otherwise, no special aftercare is necessary for the patient following a skin culture.

The health care professionals who collect the specimen should ensure that any drapes, gowns, gloves, or instruments used for the collection are placed in the proper containers for disposal or sterilization. Then they should again scrub their hands thoroughly with an antimicrobial soap before leaving the area.

Complications

If aseptic technique is not used to collect the specimen, the patient or the health care professionals could develop postprocedure infections. The infection could also be transmitted to other individuals by contaminated hands or objects.

Results

Results for bacterial cultures are usually available in one to three days. Cultures for fungi and viruses may take longer—up to three or more weeks.

Many microorganisms that are found on a person's skin are normally considered to be harmless. When these microorganisms grow on a skin culture, they are reported as "normal flora." One of the most common of these microorganisms is *Staphylococcus epidermidis*. Other bacteria that live in the high salt environment of the skin include *Propionibacterium acnes, Corynebacterium xerosis,* and some yeasts.

Besides normal flora, any microorganism that grows on a skin culture is considered to be the cause of the infection if it is the only microorganism or the predominant microorganism; if it grows in large numbers; or if it is known to produce infection. *Staphylococcus aureus* and group A *Streptococcus* cause most bacterial skin infections. *Candida albicans* causes most yeast skin infections, and *Herpes simplex* is the most frequent cause of viral skin infections.

Health care team roles

The physician determines whether a skin culture is needed to diagnose a skin infection, and orders the test when appropriate. Then the physician, nurse, or other health care professional trained in aseptic technique collects the specimen and sends it to the laboratory. The clinical laboratory scientist, CLS(NCA)/medical technologist, MT(ASCP) assumes responsibility for correct handling, culture, identification, and reporting of the results.

Resources

BOOKS

Fischbach, Francis. *A Manual of Laboratory and Diagnostic Tests.* 6th ed. Philadelphia: Lippincott Williams & Wilkins, 1999.

Fitzpatrick, Thomas B., et al. *Dermatology in General Medicine.* 5th ed. New York: McGraw-Hill, Inc., 1998.

Tierney, Lawrence M., Stephen J. McPhee, and Maxine A. Papadakis. *Current Medical Diagnosis and Treatment 2001 (Lange Series).* New York: McGraw-Hill Professional Book Group, 2000.

ORGANIZATIONS

American Society of Microbiology. 1752 N Street NW, Washington, DC 20036. (202) 737-3600. http://www.asmusa.org.

UTMB The University of Texas Medical Branch. 301 University Blvd., Galveston, TX 77555. (409) 772-1011. http://www.utmb.edu.

Yale University School of Medicine. 367 Cedar Street, New Haven, CT 06510. (203) 785-2643. http://www.info. med. yale.edu/ysm/ysminfo/index.html.

Beverly G. Miller, MT(ASCP)
Nancy J. Nordenson

Skull

Definition

The skull—or cranium—is the skeleton of the head It includes the **brain** case and the bones of the face and jaw.

Description

The skull is the bony part of the head. It rests on the first vertebra of the spine, called the atlas. It belongs to the axial skeleton, meaning the skeleton associated with the **central nervous system**. That includes the skull, all the bones of the spine, the ribs, and the breastbone.

At birth, the skull of a baby is large when compared to the rest of the body. It is fairly compressible, with soft spots (fontanelles) that eventually harden around the age of eighteen months. In the adult, some bones of the skull are paired, meaning that there is a left and a right, while others are unpaired. They are connected by sutures, which are saw-like bony edges that join bones. Bones of the skull are usually classified as cranial bones, facial bones (splanchocranium), or as bones that form the braincase (neurocranium). There are eight cranial bones and 14 facial bones. The facial **bone** assembly also includes air-filled spaces located all around the nose and called the paranasal sinuses.

Paired cranial bones

The paired cranial bones include parietal bones and the temporal bones.

The parietal bones are paired. Shaped like curved plates, they form the bulging sides and roof of the cranium. Fused in the middle along the sagittal suture, they meet the frontal bone along the coronal suture in the front of the skull. The point at which the two sutures meet is called the bregma. In the back of the skull, the parietals connect with the occipital bone along the lambdoid suture. The intersection of the lambdoid and sagittal sutures is called the lambda. The parietals meet the temporal bones in the lower portion of the skull along the squamosal and parieto-mastoid sutures. On the external surface near the center of the bone is the parietal eminence, or bulge. Slightly behind the bulge is found the parietal foramen (a foramen is an opening through bone that serves as a passageway for **blood vessels** and nerves). The parietals make contact with the following bones: occipital, frontal, temporal, sphenoid, and parietal.

The temporals form parts of the sides and base of the cranium. They are also paired left and right. Each temporal bone consists of two major sections, the squamous portion, or flat section, and a very thick and rugged part, the petrosal portion. The petrosal portion contains the cavity of the middle ear and the three smallest bones of the body. The smallest bones are the bones of the ear: the malleus, the incus and the stapes. Located near the lower edge is a gap, the external auditory meatus, that leads inward to the ear. At the lower end of the petrosal portion is the slender styloid process. A process is a bony extension or projection on a bone and the styloid is of variable length, it serves as a muscle attachment for various thin muscles to the tongue and other structures in the throat. Another projection, the mastoid process, provides an attachment for some of the muscles of the neck. The temporals also house the internal structures of the ear and have depressions, called mandibular fossae, that assist in forming the shallow socket of the jawbone joint. A zygomatic process projects from the front of the temporal bone where it joins the zygomatic bone to help form the prominence of the cheek. The temporals make contact with the following bones: the zygomatics, parietals, mandible, occipital, and sphenoid.

Unpaired cranial bones

The unpaired cranial bones include the frontal bone, occipital bone, sphenoid bone, and ethmoid bone.

The frontal bone consists of two major sections, a vertical squamous portion that connects with the paired parietals along the coronal suture and forms the forehead, and two orbital plates, which form the left and right eye sockets (orbits). On its external surface, the squamous portion very often displays a left and right frontal eminence, or bulge. Additionally, the frontal bone has two supra-orbital ridges, which are bumps above each of the eye sockets. The frontal and nasal bones connect along the fronto-nasal suture. The frontal bone makes contact with the following bones: lacrimals, nasals, zygomatics, sphenoid, maxillae, parietals, and ethmoid.

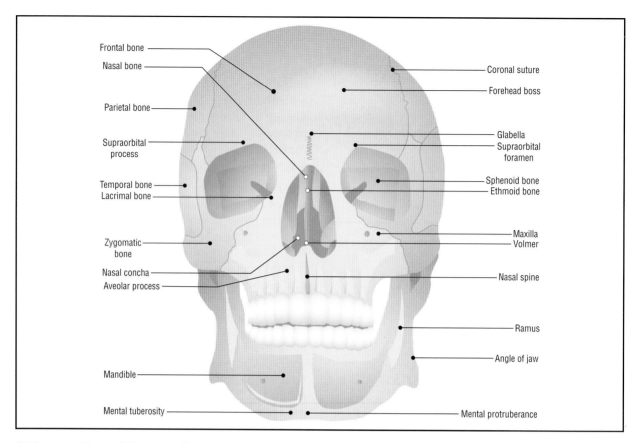

Frontal bone
Nasal bone
Parietal bone
Supraorbital process
Temporal bone
Lacrimal bone
Zygomatic bone
Nasal concha
Aveolar process
Mandible
Mental tuberosity

Coronal suture
Forehead boss
Glabella
Supraorbital foramen
Sphenoid bone
Ethmoid bone
Maxilla
Volmer
Nasal spine
Ramus
Angle of jaw
Mental protruberance

(Major parts of the skull, front view, illustration by GGS Information Services, Inc. Cengage Learning, Gale.)

The occipital bone forms the back of the skull and the base of the cranium. It consists of a large flattened section separated from a small thick portion by the foramen magnum—a large opening through which cranial nerves from the brain pass and enter the spine to become part of the **spinal cord**. On both sides of the foramen, there is a left and a right occipital condyle. A condyle is a rounded enlargement that has an articulating surface, or joint. The occipital condyles articulate with the first vertebra of the neck, the atlas (also known as the first cervical vertebra, or C1). The occipital makes contact with the following bones: parietals, temporals, sphenoid, and the atlas.

The sphenoid is a single bone that assists in connecting the cranial bones to the facial bones. It consists of a hollow part, which contains the sphenoidal sinus, and three pairs of bony projections. The first projections are called the lesser wings and they contain the optic foramen, through which the optic (or second) cranial nerve passes before reaching the eye. The second pair are called the greater wings, they assist in forming the orbital plates for each of the eye sockets. The third pair are the pterygoid processes that run along the back section of the nasal passages toward the palate and provide muscle attachments for the jawbones. The sphenoid makes contact with the following bones: vomer, ethmoid, frontal, occipital, parietals, temporals, zygomatics, and palatines.

Like the sphenoid, the ethmoid is a single bone that helps to connect the cranial bones to the facial bones. It consists of various plates and paired projections. The upper projections are the crista galli that assist in dividing the left and right frontal lobes of the brain. Side projections from the crista galli are the left and right cribriform plates which provide a seat for the olfactory nerves. The nerves go through these plates into the nasal cavity below. Directly under the crista galli is the perpendicular plate which connects with the vomer bone and helps to separate the left and right nasal passages. The ethmoid makes contact with the following bones: sphenoid, frontal, maxillae, palatines, vomer, and lacrimals.

Paired facial bones

Paired facial bones include the lacrimals, nasals, zygomatics, maxillae, palatines, and inferior nasal conchae.

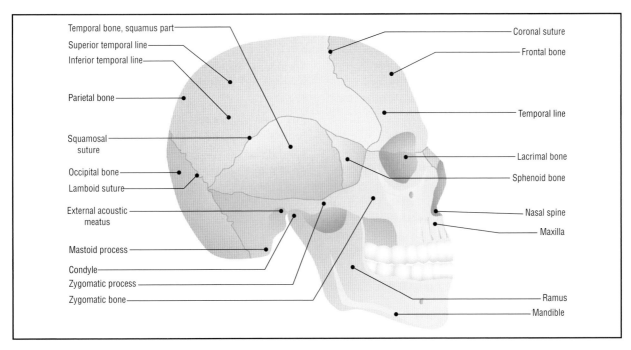

(Major parts of the skull, side view, illustration by GGS Information Services, Inc. Cengage Learning, Gale.)

The lacrimal bones are the smallest and most fragile of the facial bones and they are paired left and right. They help form the back portion of each eye socket, and are rectangular in shape with two surfaces and four borders. The lacrimals contain a feature, called the lacrimal sulcus, which helps to form the lacrimal fossa. The lacrimal fossa is an opening for the lacrimal ducts that connects the corner of the eye to the nasal passage, and allows the tears from the eye to be channeled into the nose. The lacrimals make contact with the following bones: frontal, ethmoid, and maxillae.

Each nasal bone is a small rectangular bone. Together they form the bridge of the nose above the nasal cavity. They join with each other along the internasal suture and with the frontal bone above along the fronto-nasal suture. The point of intersection of both sutures is called the nasion. Nasal bones make contact with the following bones: frontal, maxilla, and other nasals.

The zygomatics are the cheek bones. They have three major features that connect them with surrounding bones. The first is the frontal process. The frontal process forms the wall of the eye socket and connects above with the zygomatic process of the frontal bone. This section separates the eye orbit from the temporal fossa and has a projection called the marginal process. The third feature is the temporal process, and it connects with the zygomatic process of the temporal bone. Together these processes help to form the zygomatic arch which is the attachment for the masseter muscle, one of the major muscles used for chewing (mastication). The zygomatics make contact with the following bones: frontal, sphenoid, maxillae, and temporals.

The maxillae are also paired facial bones. They seat the upper teeth and form the upper jaw. In the upper part of the bone, the frontal process helps to form the nasal opening and ends by connecting with the frontal bone. A maxilla makes contact with the following bones: frontal, ethmoid, zygomatic, vomer, lacrimal, maxilla, nasal, palatine, mandible, and inferior nasal concha.

The palatines are paired left and right and connect with each other along the interpalatine suture. Both bones help form the back section of the hard palate as well as a portion of the nasal cavity. A palatine bone makes contact with the following bones: sphenoid, ethmoid, maxilla, vomer, and the other palatine bone.

The inferior nasal conchae are very thin and delicate paired bones that are elongated with curled-up ends. They are attached to the sides of the nasal cavity and connect to the maxilla and the bones that form the side wall of the nasal cavity. An inferior nasal concha makes contact with the following bones: ethmoid, lacrimal, maxilla, and palatines.

Unpaired facial bones

The unpaired facial bones include the vomer, mandible, and hyoid.

The vomer is a single flat bone. The upper part connects with the perpendicular plate of the ethmoid to

Atlas—The atlas is not part of the skull. It is the first of the seven vertebrae of the neck and the one upon which the base of the skull rests. It is also the bone around which the skull rotates.

Axial skeleton—The skeleton associated with the central nervous system—the cranium, all the bones of the vertebral column, the ribs, and the sternum.

Brain—One of the two components of the central nervous system (CNS), the brain is the center of higher thought and emotion. It is responsible for the coordination and control of all body activities and for the perception and the interpretation of sense information.

Bregma—The point where the coronal and sagittal sutures of the skull meet.

Calvaria—The skull cap, roof of the skull, or cranium without the facial bones attached.

Condyle—A rounded enlargement that has an articulating surface.

Coronal suture—The suture between the two parietal bones and the frontal bone in the skull.

Cranial bones—The eight bones of the skull that form the braincase, which encloses the brain. They are the parietals, the temporals, the frontal, the occipital, the sphenoid, and the ethmoid bones.

Cranial nerve—In humans, there are 12 cranial nerves. They are connected to the brain stem and basically 'run' the head as well as help regulate the organs of the thoracic and abdominal cavities.

Cranium—The bones of the head.

Ethmoid bone—Skull bone located behind the nose.

External auditory meatus—The passage or canal in the skull for the tissues involved in hearing.

Facial bones—The 14 bones of the skull that form the face and jaw. The paired facial bones are the lacrimals, nasals, zygomatics, maxillae, palatines, and inferior nasal conchae. The unpaired facial bones are the vomer, mandible and hyoid.

Foramen—A hole in a bone, usually for the passage of blood vessels and/or nerves.

Foramen magnum—The large opening at the base of the skull that allows passage of the spinal cord.

Fossa—A pit, depression, or concavity, on a bone or formed from several bones.

Lambda—The point where the sagittal and lamb-doid sutures of the skull meet.

Lambdoidal suture—The suture between the two parietal bones and the occipital bone in the skull.

Mandible—The lower jaw bone.

Maxillae—The upper jaw bones, connected to the orbit, hard palate and nasal cavity.

Neurocranium—The braincase of the skull.

Process—A general term describing any marked projection or prominence on a bone.

Sagittal suture—The suture between the two parietal bones in the top of the skull.

Sinuses—Air-filled cavities of the skull. The ethmoid sinus is in the ethmoid bone, the maxillary sinus in the maxilla, the frontal sinus in the frontal bones and the sphenoid sinus in the sphenoid bone.

Skull—All of the bones of the head.

Sphenoid bone—An irregularly shaped bone located in front of the occipital bone in the base of the skull.

Spinal cord—The elongated part of the central nervous system (CNS) that lies in the vertebral canal of the spine from which the spinal nerves emerge.

Squamosal suture—The suture between a temporal bone and a parietal bone in the skull.

Squamous—Adjective meaning scaly, flat, and plate-like.

Splanchocranium—The facial bones of the skull.

Suture—The saw-like edge of a cranial bone that serves as joint between bones of the skull.

Vertebrae—The flat bones that make up the spine or vertebral column. The spine has 33 vertebrae.

form the nasal septum, the dividing wall that runs down the middle of the nose. The vomer makes contact with the following bones: sphenoid, ethmoid, palatines, and maxillae.

The largest facial bone is the mandible. It is the only bone of the skull that contains a movable joint. It is a strong, curved-shaped bone that encases the lower teeth in the alveolar process. It has rounded projections, called mandibular condyles on each end. The condyles link it to the temporal bone by hinges called the temporomandibular joints. The mandible makes contact with the following bones: temporals and maxillae.

The hyoid is a single small U-shaped bone that does not join with any other bone. It hangs from the styloid process of each temporal bone by means of ligaments.

Function

The skull encloses and protects the brain, provides a base for the attachments of the muscles of the head and neck, and provides a structural element to form the first sections of the respiratory and digestive tracts. The bones of the skull are very hard, and protection of the brain is undoubtedly their most important function.

Common diseases and disorders

Disorders and conditions that affect the skull can be divided into two broad categories—craniofacial anomalies and trauma-related injuries. The most serious injury is a skull fracture, meaning a break or rupture in any of the skull bones. Cranofacial anomaly is a general term that includes malformations diagnosed at birth (congenital anomalies) and developmental anomalies that result from the abnormal growth of the skull and face after birth.

- Basal skull fractures: These are most commonly extensions of fractures of the roof of the skull. The usual locations are the temporal bone, the orbital surface of the frontal bone, and the occipital bone.

- Jaw fractures: These include mandibular fractures and maxillary fractures.

- Facial fractures: These can range from the fracture of one facial bone, for example a zygomatic fracture, to more severe trauma such as facial smash, which involves multiple fractures and extensive disruption of the bony architecture of the head.

- Hemifacial microsomia: Hemifacial microsomia is a condition that affects the growth of the face on one or both sides. The severity of this disorder can vary from mild to severe. Although different facial structures can be affected, the most common areas include the ear, the oral cavity, and the mandible.

- Goldenhar syndrome: This syndrome is a variant of hemifacial microsomia. The symptoms of this disorder match those of hemifacial microsomia with the addition of epibulbar dermoids, which are benign tumors located just inside the opening of the eye orbit.

- Treacher-Collins syndrome: Also known as mandibulofacial synostosis. The syndrome affects the size and shape of the ears, cheekbones, and upper and lower jaws.

Resources

BOOKS

Bryan, Glenda J. *Skeletal Anatomy*. Philadelphia: W.B. Saunders Co., 1996.

Simon, Seymour.*Bones: Our Skeletal System (Human Body)*. New York: Morrow (Harper Collins), 1998.

OTHER

Hohne, K. Voxel-Man Junior: Interactive 3d: Anatomy and Radiology in Virtual Reality. Scenes: Part 1: Brain & Skull, CD-ROM for Windows. New York: Springer Verlag, 1998.

South East Missouri Hospital Website. Craniofacial anomalies. http://www.southeastmissourihospital.com/health/kids/cranio~1/skullanat.htm.

ORGANIZATION

World Craniofacial Foundation. 7777 Forest Lane, Suite C-621, P.O. Box 515838, Dallas, TX, 75251-5838. (972) 566-6669. (800) 533-3315. http://www.worldcf.org/index.html.

Monique Laberge, Ph.D.

Skull x rays

Definition

Skull x rays are performed to examine the nose, sinuses, and facial bones. These studies may also be referred to as sinus or maxilofacial x rays. With advances in **computed tomography (CT) scans**, x rays of the skull have become increasingly rare.

X-ray studies produce films, also known as radiographs, by aiming x rays at bones and soft tissues of the body. X-ray beams are similar to light waves, except their shorter wavelength allows them to penetrate dense substances, producing images and shadows on film.

Purpose

Doctors may order skull x rays to aid in the diagnosis of a variety of diseases or injuries, such as:

Sinusitis

Sinus x rays may be ordered to confirm a diagnosis of **sinusitis**, or sinus **infection**.

Fractures

A skull x ray may detect **bone fractures**, resulting from injury or other disease. The skull x ray should

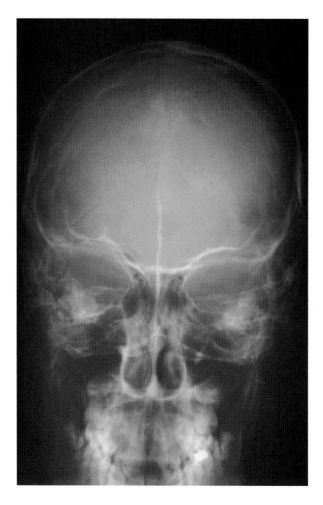

(K Beebe/CMSP)

clearly show the top of the skull, jaw bones (mandible), and facial bones. In larger facilities the computed tomography scan (CT) has begun to replace the skull x ray as a screening tool, since a CT scan can offer more information about craniofacial injuries.

Tumors

Skull radiographs may indicate tumors in facial bones, tissues, or the sinuses. Tumors may be benign (not cancerous) or malignant (cancerous). If a tumor is suspected the patient will then be referred to another imaging modality (MRI or CT) for a more thorough examination.

Other

Birth defects (referred to as congenital anomalies) may be detected on a skull x ray by changes in bone structure. Abnormal tissues or glands resulting from various conditions or diseases may also be shown on a skull radiograph.

Precautions

As with any x-ray procedure, women who may be pregnant are advised against having a skull x ray if it is not absolutely necessary. However, a lead apron may be worn across the **abdomen** during the procedure to protect the fetus. Children are also more sensitive to x-ray exposure. Children of both sexes should wear a protective covering (a lead apron) in the genital/reproductive area. In general, skull x-ray exposure is minimal and x-ray equipment and procedures are monitored to ensure radiation safety.

Description

In many instances, particularly for sinus views, the patient will sit upright in a chair, perhaps with the head held stable by a foam sponge. Sitting upright helps demonstrate air-fluid levels within the sinuses. (Air-fluid levels indicate acute disease, such as acute sinusitis or hemorrhage.) A film cassette is located behind the patient. The x-ray tube is in front of the patient and may be moved to allow for different positions and views. A patient may also be asked to move his or her head at various angles and positions.

In some cases, the technologist will ask the patient to lie on a table and will place the head and neck at various angles. In routine skull x rays, as many as five different views may be taken to allow a clear picture of various bones and tissues. The radiologist may request additional views to help better demonstrate pathology. The length of the test will vary depending on the number of views taken, but in general, it should last about 10 minutes. The technologist will usually ask a patient to wait while the films are being developed to ensure that they are clear before going to the radiologist.

Preparation

There is no preparation for the patient prior to arriving at the **radiology** facility. Patients will be asked to remove jewelry, dentures, or other metal objects that may produce artifacts on the film. The referring doctor or x-ray technologist can answer any questions regarding the procedure. Any woman who is, or may be, pregnant should inform the technologist.

Aftercare

There is no aftercare required following skull or sinus x-ray procedures.

Complications

There are no common side effects from skull or sinus x ray. The patient may feel some discomfort in the positioning of the head and neck, but will have no complications. Any x-ray procedure carries minimal radiation risk, and children and pregnant women should be protected from radiation exposure to the abdominal or genital areas.

Results

Normal results should indicate sinuses, bones, tissues, and other observed areas are of normal size, shape, and thickness for the patient's age and medical history. Results, whether normal or abnormal, will be provided to the referring physician in a written report.

Abnormal results may include:

Sinusitis

Air in sinuses will show up on a radiograph as black, but fluid will be cloudy or white (opaque). This helps the radiologist to identify fluid in the sinuses. In chronic sinusitis, the radiologist may also note thickening or hardening of the bony wall of an infected sinus.

Fractures

Radiologists may recognize facial bone fractures as a line of defect.

Tumors

Tumors may be visible if the bony sinus wall or other bones are distorted or destroyed. Abnormal findings may result in follow-up imaging studies, such as **magnetic resonance imaging** (MRI) and computed tomography (CT).

Other

Skull x rays may also detect disorders that show up as changes in bone structure, such as Paget's disease of the bone or acromegaly (a disorder associated with excess growth hormone from the **pituitary gland**). Areas of calcification (a gathering of **calcium** deposits), depending on their appearance and distribution, may indicate a condition such as an infection of bone or bone marrow (osteomyelitis).

Health care team roles

Skull or sinus x rays may be performed in a doctor's office that has x-ray equipment. A radiologic technologist performs the procedure, and a physician interprets the results. The exam may also be performed in an outpatient radiology facility or a hospital radiology department.

Resources

BOOK

Schull Patricia. *Illustrated Guide to Diagnostic Tests.* 2nd ed. Springhouse, PA: Springhouse Corporation, 1998.

ORGANIZATIONS

Cancer Information Clearinghouse, National Cancer Institute. Building 31, Room 10A24, 9000 Rockville Pike, Bethesda, MD 20892. (800) 4-Cancer. http://www.nci.nih.gov.
The National Head Injury Foundation, Inc. 1140 Connecticut Ave. NW, Suite 812, Washington, DC 20036. (800) 444-NHIF.
Radiological Society of North America. 2021 Spring Rd., Suite 600, Oak Brook, IL 60521-1860. (708) 571-2670. http://www.rsna.org.

J. Paul Dow, Jr.

Sleep and wakefulness

Definition

Sleep is a normal state of rest that is characterized by unconsciousness, reduced activity, and limited sensory responsiveness. Sleep differs from other states of reduced consciousness, such as drug intoxication or **coma**, because it is spontaneous, periodic, and readily reversible. Sleep is usually described by contrasting it with wakefulness, which is characterized by consciousness, sensory responsiveness, and purposeful activity.

Description

Sleep is one of the least understood aspects of human and animal behavior. It occurs in virtually every vertebrate species and seems to be necessary to healthy functioning, but science has been slow to discover how and why sleep occurs. The biological events that take

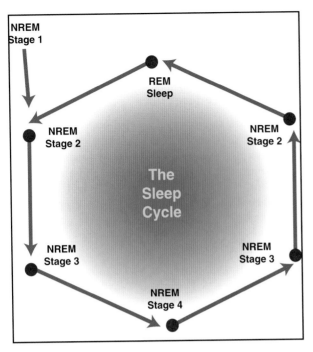

NREM
Stage 1

REM
Sleep

NREM
Stage 2

NREM
Stage 2

The
Sleep
Cycle

NREM
Stage 3

NREM
Stage 3

NREM
Stage 4

(Diagram showing the sleep cycle, hexagonal format, photograph. From Fundamentals of Nursing, Standards and Practices 2nd edition by Delaune/Ladner. © 2002. Reprinted with permission of Delmar Learning: www.thomsonrights.com Fax: 800-730-2215.)

place during sleep are subtle, and many seem to occur at a cellular level within the **brain**. These events are difficult to observe, and as a consequence our understanding of sleep has developed slowly.

Stages of sleep

Although the sleeping person seems inactive, the sleeping brain exhibits variations in activity throughout the sleep period. Recordings of brain activity, known as electroencephalograms (EEGs), show patterns that occur in a regular cycle lasting about 90 to 100 minutes. This cycle includes relatively brief periods of rapid-eye-movement (REM) sleep, characterized by back-and-forth movement of the eyes and changes in **autonomic nervous system** activity. REM is absent in the other phases of the sleep cycle, which are characterized as non-REM (NREM) sleep. Sleep can be divided into five distinct stages based on EEG and REM activity:

- Stage 1 NREM sleep: This lightest stage of sleep occurs as the person is just falling asleep. Stage 1 accounts for about 5% of a normal sleep period.

- Stage 2 NREM sleep: During this period the EEG exhibits characteristic patterns known as "sleep spindles" and K-complexes. This stage accounts for about 50% of a normal sleep period.

- Stage 3 NREM sleep: This stage is characterized by "slow wave" EEG activity, which is associated with deep sleep.

- Stage 4 NREM sleep This stage is very similar to Stage 3, the only difference being the amount of slow wave sleep that occurs. Together, Stages 3 and 4 account for about 20% of a normal sleep period.

- REM sleep. The EEG pattern of this stage is similar to that of Stage 1 NREM sleep. The sleeping person exhibits rapid eye movements and autonomic changes, as well as inactivity of the skeletal muscles. Most dreaming occurs during this stage of sleep. This stage accounts for about 20 to 25% of a normal sleep period.

The first 90-minute sleep cycle of the night begins with Stage 1 NREM sleep and progresses through Stages 2, 3, and 4, ending with a period of REM sleep. Subsequent cycles usually replace Stage 1 with the REM period. In a typical night of sleep, the earlier cycles tend to include more Stage 3 and 4 NREM sleep, with briefer REM periods. As the night progresses, the REM periods tend to get longer while the NREM periods get shorter.

Sleep and biological rhythms

Sleep is one of several biological processes that exhibit a pattern known as a circadian rhythm. A circadian rhythm recurs spontaneously on about a 24-hour cycle. Humans tend to sleep and wake up according to internal circadian rhythms, which seem to be part of our self-regulatory systems.

Circadian rhythms are regulated by a structure in the brain called the superchiasmatic nucleus, which is influenced by exposure to light. Damage to the superchiasmatic nucleus may result in loss of circadian rhythms, however, the individual still exhibits periodic tendencies to fall asleep. This is because a second, homeostatic process also regulates sleep. The individual seems to need sleep after periods of being awake, and the longer the period of wakefulness, the greater the likelihood that the person will fall asleep.

Sleep and the life cycle

The duration and patterning of sleep shows developmental changes throughout the life cycle. Newborns tend to sleep about 16 hours each day, with sleep occurring in relatively brief two to four-hour periods. As children grow, they sleep for longer periods at a time, with fewer sleep periods in a day, until they achieve the adult pattern of a single sleep period each day. The total amount of sleep also declines during childhood, until reaching the adult average of seven to nine hours per night.

In most adults, the amount of nightly sleep remains fairly stable until old age. Adults over 65 years of age tend to sleep less and report more frequent awakenings than younger adults. More than half of adults over 65 report some difficulty with sleep, although these sleep disturbances are often related to other problems, such as poor health or depression.

The patterns of REM and NREM sleep also show developmental changes. REM sleep tends to be much more prevalent in infants, with as much as 50% of their sleep time taken up by REM activity. This percentage declines throughout childhood and stabilizes at 20 to 25% in adolescence. In old age the percentage of sleep time devoted to REM declines to about 20%. Older adults also show a sharp decline in Stage 3 and Stage 4 NREM sleep.

Function

Experience suggests that sleep has some sort of restorative function. Humans feel refreshed and energized after a good night's sleep, or tired and ineffectual when we don't sleep well. But science has had difficulty going beyond this common-sense understanding of sleep. The physiological purpose of sleep continues to be something of a mystery.

The most common way to look for the purpose of sleep is to study people who have been deprived of sleep and measure the degree of impairment in their functioning. A large number of such studies have been done, with surprisingly slim results. Lack of sleep seems to have very little impact on functions such as motor coordination, sensory perception, or reflex activity, and most cognitive functions seem relatively unaffected as well. The biggest impact seems to be on short-term **memory** and sustained attention, both of which are impaired somewhat by sleep deprivation. This impairment may be due to the subjects' marked tendency to fall asleep for short periods as sleep deprivation is increased. By far, the most common outcome of sleep deprivation is increased sleepiness. As deprivation increases, the pressure to fall asleep intensifies to the point where it is almost impossible to keep subjects awake unless they are monitored constantly.

Role in human health

The quality and quantity of sleep are important indicators of overall health. Sleep is often affected by physical or emotional **stress**, and sleep disturbances are good indicators that something is amiss with a person. Although the majority of sleep complaints can be traced to psychosocial stress, sleep disturbance can be an important feature of many serious physical or psychological problems as well.

Sleep disturbance occurs in a wide variety of medical problems, including endocrine disturbances, gastrointestinal disorders, and **hypertension**. Chronic **pain** disorders such as arthritis and **fibromyalgia** also produce sleep disturbances, and sleep disruption is a common feature of a number of neurological disorders. Complaints about sleep are also very common with psychiatric illnesses, especially **anxiety** disorders and mood disorders, and they also occur in some forms of **psychosis**. Sleep disruption can be an important indicator of **substance abuse**. The most obvious case is the abuse of stimulants, such as **caffeine** or amphetamines, but alcohol abuse can also interfere with sleep, as can the abuse of sedatives.

Inadequate sleep is also a **public health** issue in its own right. A recent poll indicated that 63% of American adults fail to get the recommended amount of sleep at night, and 69% report frequent sleep problems. Chronic lack of sleep causes daytime sleepiness, which increases the risk of accidents of all types, especially automobile accidents. One estimate suggests that driver sleepiness plays a role in 10% of serious automobile accidents. Lack of sleep also impairs work performance and may contribute to industrial accidents.

Common diseases and disorders

Sleep disorders can be classified as primary or secondary, depending on the presumed cause of the disorder. Primary sleep disorders are those that arise in the absence of other medical or psychiatric conditions, while secondary sleep disorders are likely caused by some other condition.

Some of the more common primary sleep disturbances include the following:

• Primary insomnia: This disorder is defined as difficulty getting to sleep or staying asleep that lasts for over one month. Primary insomnia is often triggered by psychological stress, but it may persist long after a stressful event occurs. It is often related to anxiety about sleep, as well as poor sleep hygiene.

• Narcolepsy: Narcolepsy is characterized by periodic attacks of uncontrollable sleepiness, sometimes triggered by strong emotions. Patients with narcolepsy often experience cataplexy, a sudden loss of muscle tone, which can result in falling and injuries. Other symptoms of narcolepsy include hallucinations and

KEY TERMS

Cataplexy—An abrupt and reversible loss of muscle tone. Cataplexy is one of the key symptoms of narcolepsy.

Circadian rhythm—A body rhythm that occurs in a 24-hour cycle. Sleep, body temperature, and some endocrine functions exhibit circadian rhythms.

Electroencephalogram (EEG)—A recording of electrical activity in the brain.

Insomnia—Difficulty falling asleep or staying asleep.

Narcolepsy—A sleep disorder characterized by sudden attacks of sleep. Key symptoms include cataplexy, hallucinations, and sleep paralysis.

Nocturnal myoclonus—A sleep disorder in which sleep is disturbed by twitching or cramps in the leg muscles. Nocturnal myoclonus is also known as periodic limb movements in sleep (PMLS).

Non-rapid eye movement (NREM) sleep—Stages of sleep during which rapid eye movements do not occur. The majority of sleep consists of the four stages of NREM sleep.

Rapid eye movement (REM) sleep—A stage of sleep during which the sleeper's eyes move back and forth rapidly. Most dreams occur during REM sleep.

Restless leg syndrome (RLS)—A sleep disorder in which the person is awakened by uncomfortable "crawly" feelings in the legs.

Sleep apnea—Temporary cessation of breathing during sleep.

Sleep hygiene—A set of behaviors associated with the timing and conditions of sleep. Good sleep hygiene involves setting a regular sleep schedule, avoiding bedtime stress, and restricting activities so that the bed becomes a place for sleeping.

Sleep paralysis—A sudden inability to move that occurs at the point of falling asleep or awakening.

sleep paralysis. Narcolepsy occurs in around 04% of the general population.

- Breathing-related sleep disorders: This is a group of disorders that are all characterized by disturbed sleep due to periodic disruptions in breathing. The most common form is obstructive sleep apnea (OSA) syndrome, in which sleep is marked by periodic blockage of the upper airway. This disorder may affect 2 to 4% of the general population.

- Nocturnal myoclonus and restless leg syndrome: These are characterized by night-time discomfort and movement of the lower extremities. In nocturnal myoclonus, the person may be awakened by twitching or cramps in the legs. In restless leg syndrome, patients usually report a "crawly" feeling and the urge to move their legs. Both disorders interfere with sleep, and patients may complain of insomnia or daytime sleepiness.

- Circadian rhythm sleep disorders: In these disorders the timing of sleep is disturbed, so that the person's sleep schedule does not fit with external social demands. Shift work and long-distance travel can contribute to these disorders, but they are also common in elderly people. Often these disorders are treated by light exposure and other efforts to "reset" the patient's internal clock.

- Sleep terror disorder: This is a disorder in which the patient wakes up physically aroused and screaming or crying. Although these episodes resemble nightmares, they usually occur during NREM sleep rather than during the normal dreaming of REM sleep. The patient often cannot recall the episode the next morning. Sleepwalking disorder is a similar condition, involving complex movements and activities during sleep. It also occurs during NREM sleep. Both disorders are more common in children than adults.

Resources

BOOKS

Lashley, Felissa R., and M. de Menses. "Sleep Enhancement." In *Nursing Interventions: Effective Nursing Treatments.* ed. G.M. Bulechek and J.C. McCloskey. Philadelphia: W.B. Saunders, 1999.

Poceta, J. Steven, and Merrill M. Mitler, eds. *Sleep Disorders: Diagnosis and Treatment.* Totowa, NJ: Humana Press, 1998.

Shneerson, John M. *Handbook of Sleep Medicine.* Oxford: Blackwell Science, 2000.

PERIODICAL

Myslinski, Norbert R. "In the Arms of Morpheus." *World and I* 15 (December 2000): 130.

OTHER

"Less Fun, Less Sleep, More Work: An American Portrait." 2001 Sleep in America Poll results. National Sleep Foundation. 27 March 2001. http://www.sleepfoundation. org/PressArchives/lessfun_lesssleep.html.

ORGANIZATION

National Sleep Foundation. 1522 K Street NW. Suite 500, Washington, DC 20005. http://www.sleepfoundation.org.

Denise L. Schmutte, Ph.D.

Sleep apnea

Definition

Sleep apnea is a condition in which breathing stops for more than ten seconds during sleep. Sleep apnea is a major, though often unrecognized, cause of daytime sleepiness. It can have serious negative effects on a person's quality of life and is thought to be considerably underdiagnosed in the United States.

Demographics

Approximately 6–7% of the U.S. population, or 18 million Americans, are thought to have sleep apnea but only 10 million have symptoms, and only 0.6 million have yet been diagnosed. In Americans aged 30–60 years, obstructive sleep apnea affects nearly one in four men and one in ten women; men are twice as likely as women to have sleep apnea. As sleep apnea seldom occurs in premenopausal females, it is suggested that hormones may play some role in the disorder.

Other predisposing factors include age, as nearly 20–60% of the elderly may be affected; overweight status or **obesity**; or use of alcohol or sedatives. Some studies have demonstrated that elderly African-Americans are more than twice as likely as elderly whites to suffer from sleep apnea. Some families appear to have increased incidence of sleep apnea.

Description

A sleeping person normally breathes continuouusly and uninterruptedly throughout the night. A person with sleep apnea, however, has frequent episodes (up to 400–500 per night) in which he or she stops breathing. This interruption of breathing is called apnea. Breathing usually stops for about 30 seconds; then the person usually startles awake with a loud snort and begins to breathe again, gradually falling back to slep.

There are two forms of sleep apnea. In obstructive sleep apnea (OSA), breathing stops because tissue in the throat closes off the airway. In central sleep apnea, (CSA), the **brain** centers responsible for breathing fail to send messages to the breathing muscles. OSA is much more common than CSA. It is thought that about 1–10% of adults are affected by OSA; only about one tenth of that number have CSA. OSA can affect people of any age and of either sex, but it is most common in middle-aged, somewhat overweight men, especially those who use alcohol.

Causes and symptoms

Obstructive sleep apnea

Obstructive sleep apnea occurs when part of the airway is closed off (usually at the back of the throat) while a person is trying to inhale during sleep. People whose airways are slightly narrower than average are more likely to be affected by OSA. Obesity, especially obesity in the neck, can increase the risk of developing OSA because the fat tissue tends to narrow the airway. In some people, the airway is blocked by enlarged tonsils, an enlarged tongue, jaw deformities, or growths in the neck that compress the airway. Blocked nasal passages may also play a part in some people.

When a person begins to inhale, the expansion of the **lungs** lowers the air pressure inside the airway. If the muscles that keep the airway open are not working hard enough, the airway narrows and may collapse, shutting off the supply of air to the lungs. OSA occurs during sleep because the neck muscles that keep the airway open are not as active then. Congestion in the nose can make collapse more likely, since the extra effort needed to inhale will lower the pressure in the airway even more. Drinking alcohol or taking tranquilizers in the evening worsens this situation because these cause the neck muscles to relax. (These drugs also lower the "respiratory drive" in the nervous system, reducing breathing rate and strength.)

People with OSA almost always snore heavily because the same narrowing of the airway that causes **snoring** can also cause OSA. Snoring may actually help cause OSA as well because the vibration of the throat tissues can cause them to swell. However, most people who snore do not go on to develop OSA.

Other risk factors for developing OSA include male sex; **pregnancy**; a family history of the disorder; and **smoking**. With regard to gender, it has been found that male sex hormones sometimes cause changes in the size or structure of the upper airway. The weight gain that accompanies pregnancy can affect a woman's breathing patterns during sleep, particularly during the third trimester. With regard to family history, OSA is known to run in families even though no gene or genes associated with the disorder have been identified. Smoking increases the risk of developing OSA because it causes inflammation, swelling, and narrowing of the upper airway.

Some patients being treated for **head and neck cancer** develop OSA as a result of physical changes in the muscles and other tissues of the neck and throat. Doctors recommend prompt treatment of the OSA to improve the patient's quality of life.

Central sleep apnea

In central sleep apnea, the airway remains open but the nerve signals controlling the respiratory muscles are not regulated properly. This can cause wide fluctuations in the level of carbon dioxide (CO_2) in the **blood**. Normal activity in the body produces CO_2, which is brought by the blood to the lungs for exhalation. When the blood level of CO_2 rises, brain centers respond by increasing the rate of respiration, clearing the CO_2. As blood levels fall again, respiration slows down. Normally, this interaction of CO_2 and breathing rate maintains the CO_2 level within very narrow limits. CSA can occur when the regulation system becomes insensitive to CO_2 levels, allowing wide fluctuations in both CO_2 levels and breathing rates. High CO_2 levels cause very rapid breathing (hyperventilation), which then lowers CO_2 so much that breathing becomes very slow or even stops. CSA occurs during sleep because when a person is awake, breathing is usually stimulated by other signals, including conscious awareness of breathing rate.

A combination of the two forms is also possible and is called mixed sleep apnea. Mixed sleep apnea episodes usually begin with a reduced central respiratory drive, followed by obstruction.

OSA and CSA cause similar symptoms. The most common symptoms are:

• daytime sleepiness
• morning headaches
• a feeling that sleep is not restful
• disorientation upon waking
• poor judgment
• personality changes

Sleepiness is caused not only by the frequent interruption of sleep but by the inability to enter long periods of deep sleep, during which the body performs numerous restorative functions. OSA is one of the leading causes of daytime sleepiness and is a major risk factor for motor vehicle accidents. Headaches and disorientation are caused by low oxygen levels during sleep from the lack of regular breathing.

Other symptoms of sleep apnea may include **sexual dysfunction**, loss of concentration, **memory** loss, intellectual impairment, and behavioral changes including **anxiety** and depression.

Sleep apnea is also associated with night sweats and nocturia, or increased frequency of urination at night. Bedwetting in children is also linked to sleep apnea.

Sleep apnea can also cause serious changes in the **cardiovascular system**. Daytime **hypertension** (high **blood pressure**) is common. An increase in the number of red blood cells (polycythemia) is possible, as is an enlarged left ventricle of the **heart** (cor pulmonale), and left ventricular failure. In some people, sleep apnea causes life-threatening changes in the rhythm of the heart, including heartbeat slowing (bradycardia), racing (tachycardia), and other types of "arrhythmias." Sudden death may occur from such **arrhythmias**. Patients with the Pickwickian syndrome (named after a Charles Dickens character) are obese and sleepy, with right **heart failure**, pulmonary hypertension, and chronic daytime low blood oxygen (hypoxemia) and increased blood CO_2 (hypercapnia).

Diagnosis

Excessive daytime sleepiness is the complaint that usually brings a person to see the doctor. A careful medical history will include questions about alcohol or tranquilizer use, snoring (often reported by the person's partner), and morning headaches or disorientation. A physical exam will include examination of the throat to look for narrowing or obstruction. Blood pressure is also measured. Measuring heart rate or blood levels of oxygen and CO_2 during the daytime will not usually be done since these are abnormal only at night in most patients.

In some cases the person's dentist may suggest the diagnosis of OSA on the basis of a dental checkup or evaluation of the patient for oral surgery.

Confirmation of the diagnosis usually requires making measurements while the person sleeps. These tests are called a **polysomnography** study and are conducted during an overnight stay in a specialized sleep laboratory. Important parts of the polysomnography study include measurements of:

• heart rate
• airflow at the mouth and nose
• respiratory effort
• sleep stage (e.g., light sleep, deep sleep, dream sleep)
• oxygen level in the blood, using a noninvasive probe (ear oximetry)

Simplified studies done overnight at home are also possible, and may be appropriate for people whose profile strongly suggests the presence of obstructive sleep apnea; that is, middle-aged, somewhat overweight men, who snore and have high blood pressure. The home-based study usually includes ear oximetry and cardiac measurements. If these measurements support the diagnosis of OSA, initial treatment is usually suggested without polysomnography. Home-based measurements are not used to rule out OSA, however, and if the measurements do not support the OSA diagnosis,

KEY TERMS

Continuous positive airway pressure (CPAP)—A ventilation system that blows a gentle stream of air into the nose to keep the airway open.

Genioplasty—An operation performed to reshape the chin. Genioplasties are often done to treat OSA because the procedure changes the structure of the patient's upper airway.

Mandible—The medical term for the lower jaw. One type of oral appliance used to treat OSA pushes the mandible forward in order to ease breathing during sleep.

Nocturia—Excessive need to urinate at night. Nocturia is a symptom of OSA and often increases the patient's daytime sleepiness.

Polysomnography—A group of tests administered to analyze heart, blood, and breathing patterns during sleep.

Tracheotomy—A surgical procedure in which a small hole is cut into the trachea, or windpipe, below the level of the vocal cords.

Uvulopalatopharyngoplasty (UPPP)—An operation to remove excess tissue at the back of the throat to prevent it from closing off the airway during sleep.

---

polysomnography may be needed to define the problem further.

Treatment

Behavioral changes

Treatment of obstructive sleep apnea begins with reducing the use of alcohol or tranquilizers in the evening, if these have been contributing to the problem. Weight loss is also effective but if the weight returns, as it often does, so does the apnea. Changing sleeping position may be effective; snoring and sleep apnea are both most common when a person sleeps on his back. Turning to sleep on the side may be enough to clear up the symptoms. Raising the head of the bed may also help. Opening of the nasal passages can provide some relief. There are a variety of nasal devices such as clips, tapes, or holders which may help, though discomfort may limit their use. Nasal decongestants may be useful but should not be taken for sleep apnea without the consent of the treating physician.

Oxygen and drug therapy

Supplemental nighttime oxygen can be useful for some people with either central and obstructive sleep apnea. Tricyclic **antidepressant drugs** such as protriptyline (Vivactil) may help by increasing the muscle tone of the upper airway muscles but their side effects may severely limit their usefulness.

Mechanical ventilation

For moderate to severe sleep apnea, the most successful treatment is nighttime use of a ventilator, called a CPAP machine. CPAP (continuous positive airway pressure) blows air into the airway continuously, preventing its collapse. CPAP requires the use of a nasal mask. The appropriate pressure setting for the CPAP machine is determined by polysomnography in the sleep lab. Its effects are dramatic; daytime sleepiness usually disappears within one to two days after treatment begins. CPAP is used to treat both obstructive and central sleep apnea.

CPAP is tolerated well by about two-thirds of patients who try it. Bilevel positive airway pressure (BiPAP), is an alternative form of ventilation. With BiPAP, the ventilator reduces the air pressure when the person exhales. This is more comfortable for some.

Surgery

Surgery can be used to correct obstructions in the airways. The most common surgery is called UPPP, for uvulopalatopharngyoplasty. This surgery removes tissue from the rear of the mouth and top of the throat. The tissues removed include parts of the uvula (the flap of tissue that hangs down at the back of the mouth), the soft palate, and the pharynx. Tonsils and adenoids are usually removed in this operation. This operation significantly improves sleep apnea in slightly more than half of all cases.

Reconstructive surgery is possible for those whose OSA is due to constriction of the airway by lower jaw deformities. Genioplasty, which is a procedure that plastic surgeons usually perform to reshape a patient's chin to improve his or her appearance, is now being done to reshape the upper airway in patients with OSA.

When other forms of treatment are not successful, obstructive sleep apnea may be treated by a tracheostomy. In this procedure, an opening is made into the trachea (windpipe) below the obstruction, and a tube inserted to maintain an air passage. A tracheostomy requires a great deal of care to prevent **infection** of the tracheostomy site. In addition, since air is no longer being filtered and moistened by the nasal passages before entering the lungs, the lower airways can become dry and susceptible to infection as well. Tracheostomy is usually reserved for those whose apnea has led to life-threatening heart arrhythmias, and who have not been treated successfully with other treatments.

Oral appliances

Another approach to treating OSA involves the use of oral appliances intended to improve breathing either by holding the tongue in place or by pushing the lower jaw forward during sleep to increase the air volume in the upper airway. The first type of oral appliance is known as a tongue retaining device or TRD. The second type is variously called an oral protrusive device (OPD) or mandibular advancement splint (MAS), because it holds the mandible, or lower jaw, forward during sleep. These oral devices appear to work best for patients with mild-to-moderate OSA, and in some cases can postpone or prevent the need for surgery. Their rate of patient compliance is about 50%; most patients who stop using oral appliances do so because their teeth are in poor condition. TRDs and OPDs can be fitted by dentists; however, most dentists work together with the patient's physician following a polysomnogram rather than prescribing the device by themselves.

Prognosis

The combination of behavioral changes, **ventilation assistance**, drug therapy, and surgery allow most people with sleep apnea to be treated successfully, although it may take some time to determine the most effective and least intrusive treatment. Polysomnography testing is usually required after beginning a treatment to determine how effective it has been.

Prevention

For people who snore frequently, weight control, avoidance of evening alcohol or tranquilizers, and adjustment of sleeping position may help reduce the risk of developing obstructive sleep apnea.

Resources

BOOKS

Cummings, CW, et al. *Otolayrngology: Head and Neck Surgery.* 4th ed. St. Louis: Mosby, 2005.

Goetz, CG. *Goetz's Textbook of Clinical Neurology.* 3rd ed. Philadelphia: Saunders, 2007.

Goldman L, Ausiello D., eds. *Cecil Textbook of Internal Medicine.* 23rd ed. Philadelphia: Saunders, 2008.

Libby, P. et al. *Braunwald's Heart Disease.* 8th ed. Philadelphia: Saunders, 2007.

PERIODICALS

Chasens, E.R., and M.G. Umlauf. "Nocturia: A Problem That Disrupts Sleep and Predicts Obstructive Sleep Apnea" *Geriatric Nursing* 24 (March-April 2003): 76–81, 105.

Chung, S.A., S. Jairam, M.R. Hussain, and C.M. Shapiro. "How, What, and Why of Sleep Apnea. Perspectives for Primary Care Physicians." *Canadian Family Physician* 48 (June 2002): 1073–1080.

Edwards, N., P.G. Middleton, D.M. Blyton, and C.E. Sullivan. "Sleep Disordered Breathing and Pregnancy." *Thorax* 57 (June 2002): 555–558.

Hisanaga, A., T. Itoh, Y. Hasegawa, et al. "A Case of Sleep Choking Syndrome Improved by the Kampo Extract of Hange-Koboku-To." *Psychiatry and Clinical Neuroscience* 56 (June 2002): 325–327.

Koliha, C.A. "Obstructive Sleep Apnea in Head and Neck Cancer Patients Post Treatment ... Something to Consider?" *ORL—Head and Neck Nursing* 21 (Winter 2003): 10–14.

Neill, A., R. Whyman, S. Bannan, et al. "Mandibular Advancement Splint Improves Indices of Obstructive Sleep Apnoea and Snoring but Side Effects Are Common." *New Zealand Medical Journal* 115 (June 21, 2002): 289–292.

Rose, E., R. Staats, J. Schulte-Monting, et al. "Long-Term Compliance with an Oral Protrusive Appliance in Patients with Obstructive Sleep Apnoea." [in German] *Deutsche medizinische Wochenschrift* 127 (June 7, 2002): 1245–1249.

Shiomi, T., A.T. Arita, R. Sasanabe, et al. "Falling Asleep While Driving and Automobile Accidents Among Patients with Obstructive Sleep Apnea-Hypopnea Syndrome." *Psychiatry and Clinical Neuroscience* 56 (June 2002): 333–334.

Umlauf, M.G., and E.R. Chasens. "Bedwetting—Not Always What It Seems: A Sign of Sleep-Disordered Breathing in Children." *Journal for Specialists in Pediatric Nursing* 8 (January–March 2003): 22–30.

OTHER

American Sleep Apnea Association (ASAA). "Sleep Apnea Information." [Accessed December 15, 2010] http://www.sleepapnea.org/info/index.html.

National Heart, Lung, and Blood Institute (NHLBI). "Sleep Apnea." [Accessed December 15, 2010] http://www.nhlbi.nih.gov/health/dci/Diseases/SleepApnea/SleepApnea_WhatIs.html.

ORGANIZATIONS

American Academy of Otolaryngology, Head and Neck Surgery, Inc., One Prince Street, Alexandria, VA 22314-3357, (703) 836-4444, http://www.entnet.org

American Dental Association, 211 East Chicago Avenue, Chicago, IL 60611, (312) 440-2500, http://www.ada.org

American Sleep Apnea Association, 1424 K Street NW, Suite 302, Washington, DC 20005, (202) 293-3650, Fax: (202) 293-3656, http://www.sleepapnea.org

Canadian Coordinating Office for Health Technology Assessment, http://www.ccohta.ca/pubs/english/sleep/treatmnt

National Sleep Foundation, 1522 K Street, NW, Suite 500, Washington, DC 20005, http://www.sleepfoundation.org

Richard Robinson
Rebecca J. Frey, Ph.D.

Sleep disorders

Definition

Sleep disorders are a group of syndromes characterized by disturbance in a person's amount of sleep, quality or timing of sleep, or in behaviors or physiological conditions associated with sleep. There are about 70 different sleep disorders. To qualify for the diagnosis of sleep disorder, the condition must be a persistent problem, cause an individual significant emotional distress, and interfere with social or occupational functioning. The text revision of the fourth edition (2000) of the *Diagnostic and Statistical Manual of Mental Disorders (DSM-IV-TR)* specifically excludes temporary disruptions of sleeping patterns caused by travel or other short-term stresses.

Although sleep is a basic behavior in animals as well as humans, researchers still do not completely understand all of its functions in maintaining health. In the past 30 years, however, laboratory studies on human volunteers have yielded new information about the different types of sleep. Researchers have learned about the cyclical patterns of different types of sleep and their relationships to breathing, **heart** rate, **brain** waves, and other physical functions. These measurements are obtained by a technique called **polysomnography**.

There are five stages of human sleep. Four stages have non-rapid eye movement (NREM) sleep, with unique brain wave patterns and physical changes occurring. Dreaming occurs in the fifth stage, during rapid eye movement (REM) sleep.

- Stage 1 NREM sleep. This stage occurs while a person is falling asleep. It represents about 5% of a normal adult's sleep time.

- Stage 2 NREM sleep. In this stage, (the beginning of "true" sleep), the person's electroencephalogram (EEG)

will show distinctive wave forms called sleep spindles and K complexes. About 50% of sleep time is stage 2 NREM sleep.

- Stages 3 and 4 NREM sleep. Also called delta or slow wave sleep, these are the deepest levels of human sleep and represent 10-20% of sleep time. They usually occur during the first 30-50% of the sleeping period.

- REM sleep. REM sleep accounts for 20-25% of total sleep time. It usually begins about 90 minutes after a person falls asleep, an important measure called REM latency. It alternates with NREM sleep about every hour and a half throughout the night. REM periods increase in length over the course of the night.

Sleep cycles vary with a person's age. Children and adolescents have longer periods of stage 3 and stage 4 NREM sleep than do middle aged or elderly adults. Because of this difference, a doctor will need to take a person's age into account when evaluating a sleep disorder. Total REM sleep also declines with age.

The average length of nighttime sleep varies among people. Most individuals sleep between seven and nine hours a night. This population average appears to be constant throughout the world. In temperate climates, however, people often notice that sleep time varies with the seasons. It is not unusual for people in North America and Europe to sleep about 40 minutes longer per night during the winter.

Description

The *DSM-IV-TR* classifies sleep disorders based on their causes. Primary sleep disorders are distinguished from those that are not caused by other mental disorders, prescription medications, **substance abuse**, or medical conditions. The two major categories of primary sleep disorders are the dyssomnias and the parasomnias.

Dyssomnias

Dyssomnias are primary sleep disorders in which a person suffers from changes in the amount, restfulness, and timing of sleep. The most important dyssomnia is primary insomnia, which is defined as difficulty in falling asleep or remaining asleep that lasts for at least one month. It is estimated that 35% of adults in the United States experience insomnia during any given year, but the number of these adults who are experiencing true primary insomnia is unknown. Primary insomnia can be caused by a traumatic event related to sleep or bedtime, and it is often associated with increased physical or psychological arousal at night. People who experience primary insomnia are often anxious about not being able to sleep. Individuals may then associate all sleep-related things

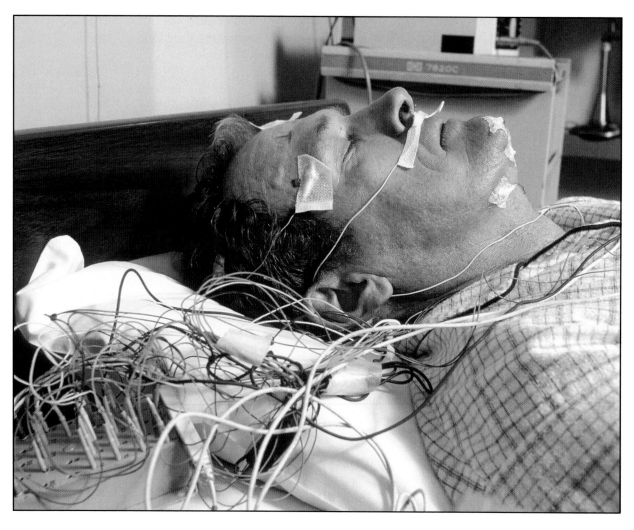

(Male patient with electrodes and wires attached to his face, photograph. Russ Curtis / Photo Researchers Inc.)

(e.g., their bed, bedtime) with frustration, making the problem worse. They then become more stressed about not sleeping. Primary insomnia often begins in young adulthood or in middle age.

Hypersomnia is a condition marked by excessive sleepiness during normal waking hours. Affected persons either have lengthy episodes of daytime sleep or episodes of daytime sleep on a daily basis even though they are sleeping normally at night. In some cases, persons with primary hypersomnia have difficulty waking in the morning and may appear confused or angry. This condition is sometimes called sleep drunkenness and is more common in males. The number of people with primary hypersomnia is unknown, although 5–10% of people in sleep disorder clinics have the disorder. Primary hypersomnia usually affects young adults between the ages of 15 and 30.

Nocturnal myoclonus and restless legs syndrome (RLS) can cause either insomnia or hypersomnia in

adults. Individuals with nocturnal myoclonus wake up because of cramps or twitches in the calves. These people feel sleepy the next day. Nocturnal myoclonus is sometimes called periodic limb movement disorder. RLS patients have a crawly or aching feeling in their calves that can be relieved by moving or rubbing the legs. RLS often prevents people from falling asleep until the early hours of the morning, when the condition is less intense.

Kleine-Levin syndrome is a recurrent form of hypersomnia that affects a person three or four times a year. Doctors do not know the cause of this syndrome. It is marked by two to three days of sleeping 18–20 hours per day, hypersexual behavior, compulsive eating, and irritability. Men are three times more likely than women to have the syndrome. There is no cure for this disorder.

Narcolepsy is a dyssomnia characterized by recurrent "sleep attacks" that a person cannot fight. The sleep attacks are about 10–20 minutes long. A person feels refreshed by the sleep, but typically feels sleepy again several hours later. Narcolepsy has three major symptoms in addition to sleep attacks: cataplexy, hallucinations, and sleep **paralysis**. Cataplexy is the sudden loss of muscle tone and stability ("drop attacks"). Hallucinations may occur just before falling asleep (hypnagogic) or right after waking up (hypnopompic) and are associated with an episode of REM sleep. Sleep paralysis occurs during the transition from being asleep to waking up. About 40% of patients with narcolepsy have or have had another mental disorder. Although narcolepsy is often regarded as an adult disorder, it has been reported in children as young as three years old. Almost 18% of people with narcolepsy are 10 years old or younger. It is estimated that 0.02–0.16% of the general population suffers from narcolepsy. Men and women are equally affected.

Breathing-related sleep disorders are syndromes in which a person's sleep is interrupted by problems with breathing. There are three types of breathing-related sleep disorders:

• Obstructive sleep apnea syndrome. This is the most common form of breathing-related sleep disorder, marked by episodes of blockage in the upper airway during sleep. It is found primarily in obese people. Persons with this disorder typically alternate between periods of snoring or gasping (when their airway is partly open) and periods of silence (when their airway is blocked). Very loud snoring is a clue to this disorder.

• Central sleep apnea syndrome. This disorder is primarily found in elderly people with heart or neurological conditions that affect their ability to breathe properly. It is not associated with airway blockage and may be related to brain disease.

• Central alveolar hypoventilation syndrome. This disorder is found most often in extremely obese people. Their airway is not blocked, but blood oxygen level is too low.

• Mixed-type sleep apnea syndrome. This disorder combines symptoms of both obstructive and central sleep apnea.

Circadian rhythm sleep disorders are dyssomnias resulting from a discrepancy between a person's daily sleep and wake patterns and demands of social activities, shift work, or travel. The term circadian comes from a Latin word meaning daily. There are three circadian rhythm sleep disorders. Delayed sleep phase type is characterized by going to bed and arising later than most people. Jet lag type is caused by travel to a new time zone. Shift work type is caused by the schedule of a person's job. People who are ordinarily early risers appear to be more vulnerable to jet lag and shift work-related circadian rhythm disorders than people who are "night owls." There are some individuals who do not fit the pattern of these three disorders and appear to be the opposite of the delayed sleep phase type. These people have an advanced sleep phase pattern and cannot stay awake in the evening, but wake up on their own in the early morning.

PARASOMNIAS. Parasomnias are primary sleep disorders in which a person's behavior is affected by specific sleep stages or transitions between sleeping and waking. They are sometimes described as disorders of physiological arousal during sleep.

Nightmare disorder is a parasomnia in which a person is repeatedly awakened from sleep by frightening dreams and is fully alert on awakening. The actual rate of occurrence of nightmare disorder is unknown. Approximately 10–50% of children between three and five years old experience nightmares. They occur during REM sleep, usually in the second half of the night. A child is usually able to remember the content of the nightmare and may be afraid to go back to sleep. More females than males have this disorder, but it is not known whether the gender difference reflects a difference in occurrence or a difference in reporting. Nightmare disorder is most likely to occur in children or adults under severe or traumatic **stress**.

Sleep terror disorder is a parasomnia in which a person awakens screaming or crying. The individual also has physical signs of arousal, like sweating or shaking. It is sometimes referred to as pavor nocturnus. Unlike nightmares, sleep terrors typically occur in stage 3 or stage 4 NREM sleep during the first third of the night. A person may be confused or disoriented for several minutes and cannot recall the content of the dream. There is usually a return to sleep without being able to remember the episode the next morning. Sleep terror disorder is most common in children four to 12 years old and is outgrown in adolescence. It affects about 3% of children. Fewer than 1% of adults have the disorder. In adults, it usually begins between the ages of 20 and 30. In children, more males than females have the disorder. In adults, men and women are equally affected.

Sleepwalking disorder, which is sometimes called somnambulism, occurs when a person is capable of complex movements during sleep, including walking. Like sleep terror disorder, sleepwalking occurs during stage 3 and stage 4 NREM sleep during the first part of the night. If individuals are awakened during a sleepwalking episode, they may be disoriented and have no **memory** of the behavior. In addition to walking around, persons with sleepwalking disorder have been reported to eat, use the bathroom, unlock doors, or talk to others. It is estimated that 10–30% of children have at least one episode of sleepwalking. However, only 1–5% meet the criteria for sleepwalking disorder. The disorder is most common in children eight to 12 years old. It is unusual for sleepwalking to occur for the first time in adults.

Unlike sleepwalking, REM sleep behavior disorder occurs later in the night and people can remember what they were dreaming. The physical activities of such persons are often violent.

Sleep disorders related to other conditions

In addition to the primary sleep disorders, the *DSM-IV-TR* specifies three categories of sleep disorders that are caused by or related to substance use or other physical or mental disorders.

Many mental disorders, especially depression or one of the **anxiety** disorders, can cause sleep disturbances. Psychiatric disorders are the most common cause of chronic insomnia.

Some people with chronic neurological conditions like **Parkinson's disease** or Huntington's disease may develop sleep disorders. Sleep disorders have also been associated with viral **encephalitis**, brain disease, and hypo- or hyperthyroidism.

The use of drugs, alcohol, and **caffeine** frequently produce disturbances in sleep patterns. Alcohol abuse is associated with insomnia. A person may initially feel sleepy after drinking, but wakes up or sleeps fitfully during the second half of the night. Alcohol can also increase the severity of breathing-related sleep disorders. With amphetamines or **cocaine**, a person typically suffers from insomnia during drug use and hypersomnia during drug withdrawal. Opioids usually make short-term users sleepy. However, long-term users develop tolerance and may suffer from insomnia.

In addition to alcohol and drugs that are abused, a variety of prescription medications can affect sleep patterns. These medications include **antihistamines**, **corticosteroids**, **asthma** medicines, and drugs that affect the **central nervous system**.

Sleep disorders in children and adolescents

Pediatricians estimate that 20–30% of children have difficulties with sleep that are serious enough to disturb their families. Although sleepwalking and night terror disorder occur more frequently in children than in adults, children can also suffer from narcolepsy and **sleep apnea** syndrome.

Causes and symptoms

The causes of sleep disorders have already been discussed with respect to the *DSM-IV-TR* classification of these disorders.

The most important symptoms of sleep disorders are insomnia and sleepiness during waking hours. Insomnia is by far the more common of the two symptoms. It covers a number of different patterns of sleep disturbance. These patterns include inability to fall asleep at bedtime, repeated awakening during the night, and/or inability to go back to sleep once awakened.

Diagnosis

Diagnosis of sleep disorders usually requires a psychological history as well as a medical history. With the exception of sleep apnea syndromes, physical examinations are not usually revealing. A person's gender and age are useful starting points in assessing the problem. A doctor may also talk to other family members to obtain information about a person's symptoms. A family's observations are particularly important to evaluate sleepwalking, kicking in bed, **snoring** loudly, or other behaviors that an individual cannot remember.

Sleep logs

Many doctors ask people to keep a sleep diary or sleep log for a minimum of one to two weeks in order to evaluate the severity and characteristics of the sleep disturbance. An individual records medications taken as well as the length of time spent in bed, the quality of the sleep, and similar information. Some sleep logs are designed to indicate circadian sleep patterns as well as simple duration or restfulness of sleep.

Psychological testing

A physician may use **psychological tests** or inventories to evaluate insomnia because it is frequently associated with mood or affective disorders. The Minnesota Multiphasic Personality Inventory (MMPI), the Millon Clinical Multiaxial Inventory (MCMI), the Beck Depression Inventory, and the Zung Depression Scale are the tests most commonly used in evaluating this symptom.

Self-report tests

The Epworth Sleepiness Scale, a self-rating form recently developed in Australia, consists of eight questions used to assess daytime sleepiness. Scores range from 0–24, with scores higher than 16 indicating severe daytime sleepiness.

Laboratory studies

If a doctor is considering breathing-related sleep disorders, myoclonus, or narcolepsy as possible diagnoses, an affected person may be tested in a sleep laboratory or at home with portable instruments.

POLYSOMNOGRAPHY. Polysomnography can be used to help diagnose sleep disorders as well as conduct research into sleep. In some cases a person is tested in a special sleep laboratory. The advantage of this testing is the availability and expertise of trained technologists, but it is expensive. Portable equipment is available for home recording of certain specific physiological functions.

MULTIPLE SLEEP LATENCY TEST. The multiple sleep latency test (MSLT) is frequently used to measure the severity of a person's daytime sleepiness. The test measures sleep latency (the speed with which an individual falls asleep) during a series of planned naps during the day. The test also measures the amount of REM sleep that occurs. Two or more episodes of REM sleep under these conditions indicates narcolepsy. This test can also be used to help diagnose primary hypersomnia.

REPEATED TEST OF SUSTAINED WAKEFULNESS. The repeated test of sustained wakefulness (RTSW) measures sleep latency by challenging a person's ability to stay awake. In the RTSW, a person is placed in a quiet room with dim lighting and is asked to stay awake. As with the MSLT, the testing pattern is repeated at intervals during the day.

Treatment

Treatment for a sleep disorder depends on what is causing the disorder. For example, if major depression is the cause of insomnia, then treatment of the depression with antidepressants should resolve the insomnia.

Medications

Sedative or hypnotic medications are generally recommended only for insomnia related to a temporary stress (such as surgery or grief) because of the potential for addiction or **overdose**. Trazodone, a sedating antidepressant, is often used for chronic insomnia that does not respond to other treatments. Sleep medications may also cause problems for elderly persons because of possible interactions with their other prescription medications. Among the safer hypnotic agents are lorazepam, temazepam, and zolpidem. Chloral hydrate is often preferred for short-term treatment in elderly people because of its mildness. Short-term treatment is recommended because this drug may be habit forming.

Narcolepsy is treated with stimulants such as dextroamphetamine sulfate or methylphenidate. Nocturnal myoclonus has been successfully treated with clonazepam.

Children with sleep terror disorder or sleepwalking are usually treated with benzodiazepines because this type of medication suppresses stage 3 and stage 4 NREM sleep.

Psychotherapy

Psychotherapy is recommended for persons with sleep disorders associated with other mental disorders. In many cases an individual's scores on the Beck or Zung inventories will suggest the appropriate direction of treatment.

Sleep education

"Sleep hygiene" or sleep education for sleep disorders often includes instructing a person in methods to enhance sleep. People are advised to:

- Wait until they feel sleepy before going to bed.
- Avoid using the bedroom for work, reading, or watching television.
- Get up at the same time every morning no matter how much or how little they have slept.
- Avoid smoking, and avoid drinking liquids with caffeine.
- Get some physical exercise on a daily basis, early in the day.
- Limit fluid intake after dinner; in particular, avoid alcohol because it frequently causes interrupted sleep.
- Learn to meditate or practice relaxation techniques.
- Avoid tossing and turning in bed; instead, people should get up and listen to relaxing music or read.

Lifestyle changes

People with sleep apnea or hypopnea are encouraged to stop **smoking**, avoid alcohol or drugs of abuse, and lose weight in order to improve the stability of the upper airway.

In some cases, individuals with sleep disorders related to jet lag or shift work may need to change employment or travel patterns. They may need to avoid rapid changes in shifts at work.

Children with nightmare disorder may benefit from limits on television or movies. Violent scenes or frightening science fiction stories appear to influence the frequency and intensity of children's nightmares.

Surgery

Although making a surgical opening into the windpipe (a tracheostomy) for sleep apnea or hypopnea in adults is a treatment of last resort, it is occasionally performed if a person's disorder is life threatening and cannot be treated by other methods. In children and adolescents, surgical removal of the tonsils and adenoids is a fairly common and successful treatment for sleep apnea. Most people with sleep apnea are treated with continuous positive airway pressure (CPAP). Sometimes an oral prosthesis is used for mild sleep apnea.

Alternative treatment

Some alternative approaches may be effective in treating insomnia caused by anxiety or emotional stress. **Meditation** practice, breathing exercises, and **yoga** can break the vicious cycle of sleeplessness, worry about inability to sleep, and further sleeplessness for some people. Yoga can help some people to relax muscular tension in a direct fashion. The breathing exercises and meditation can keep them from obsessing about sleep.

Homeopathic practitioners recommend that people with chronic insomnia see a professional homeopath. They do, however, prescribe specific remedies for at-home treatment of temporary insomnia: *Nux vomica* for alcohol or substance-related insomnia, *Ignatia* for insomnia caused by grief, *Arsenicum* for insomnia caused by fear or anxiety, and *Passiflora* for insomnia related to mental stress.

Melatonin has also been used as an alternative treatment for sleep disorders. Melatonin is produced in the body by the pineal gland at the base of the brain. This substance is thought to be related to the body's circadian rhythms.

Practitioners of Chinese medicine usually treat insomnia as a symptom of excess yang energy. Cinnabar is recommended for chronic nightmares. Either magnetic magnetite or "dragon bones" is recommended for insomnia associated with hysteria or fear. If the insomnia appears to be associated with excess yang energy arising from the **liver**, a practitioner will suggest oyster shells. **Acupuncture** treatments can help bring about balance and facilitate sleep.

Dietary changes such as eliminating stimulant foods (coffee, cola, chocolate) and late-night meals or snacks can be effective in treating some sleep disorders. Nutritional supplementation with **magnesium**, as well as botanical medicines that calm the nervous system, can

also be helpful. Among the botanical remedies that may be effective for sleep disorders are valerian (*Valeriana officinalis*), passionflower (*Passiflora incarnata*), and skullcap (*Scutellaria lateriflora*).

Prognosis

Prognosis depends on the specific disorder. Children usually outgrow sleep disorders. People with Kleine-Levin syndrome usually get better by age 40. Narcolepsy is a life-long disorder. The prognosis for sleep disorders related to other conditions depends on successful treatment of the substance abuse, medical condition, or other mental disorder. The prognosis for primary sleep disorders is affected by many things, including a person's age, gender, occupation, personality characteristics, family circumstances, neighborhood environment, and similar factors.

Health care team roles

Sleep experts are often trained in **physiology**, medicine or psychology. Such professionals often administer tests and make initial diagnoses. Physicians prescribe drugs for some forms of sleep disorders. Surgeons are occasionally called upon for surgical intervention. Nurses take part in any testing as well as providing pre-test **patient education**. Family members are often key members of a health care team when they provide information and help to make changes in the home. An affected person may become a member of the health care team when making dietary modifications, seeking alternative employment or deciding to undertake a course of therapy.

Prevention

Sleep disorders are difficult to prevent. Recognition of potential causes and avoidance of such situations or substances can prevent many forms of sleep disorders. Since many sleep disorders are relatively common and transitory, a good attitude about occasional problems with sleep is very helpful. This can prevent worrying.

Resources

BOOKS

Culebras, Antonio. *Sleep Disorders and Neurological Disease.* New York: Marcel Dekker, 1999.

Dement, William, and Christopher Vaughn. *The Promise of Sleep.* New York: Delacorte Press, 1999.

Diagnostic and Statistical Manual of Mental Disorders Revised IV. Washington, DC: American Psychiatric Press, 2000.

Jenkins, Renee R. "Sleep disorders." In *Nelson Textbook of Pediatrics, 16th ed.*, edited by Richard E. Behrman et al. Philadelphia: Saunders, 2000, 572.

Apnea—The temporary absence of breathing. Sleep apnea consists of repeated episodes of temporary suspension of breathing during sleep.

Cataplexy—Sudden loss of muscle tone (often causing a person to fall), usually triggered by intense emotion. It is regarded as a diagnostic sign of narcolepsy.

Circadian rhythm—Any body rhythm that recurs in 24-hour cycles. The sleep-wake cycle is an example of a circadian rhythm.

Dyssomnia—A primary sleep disorder in which the patient suffers from changes in the quantity, quality, or timing of sleep.

Electroencephalogram (EEG)—The record obtained by a device that measures electrical impulses in the brain.

Hypersomnia—An abnormal increase of 25% or more in time spent sleeping. Patients usually have excessive daytime sleepiness.

Hypnotic—A medication that makes a person sleep.

Hypopnea—Shallow or excessively slow breathing usually caused by partial closure of the upper airway during sleep, leading to disruption of sleep.

Insomnia—Difficulty in falling asleep or remaining asleep.

Jet lag—A temporary disruption of the body's sleep-wake rhythm following high-speed air travel across several time zones. Jet lag is most severe in people who have crossed eight or more time zones in 24 hours.

Kleine-Levin syndrome—A disorder that occurs primarily in young males, three or four times a year. The syndrome is marked by episodes of hypersomnia, hypersexual behavior, and excessive eating.

Narcolepsy—A life-long sleep disorder marked by four symptoms: sudden brief sleep attacks, cataplexy, temporary paralysis, and hallucinations. The hallucinations are associated with falling asleep or the transition from sleeping to waking.

Nocturnal myoclonus—A disorder in which the patient is awakened repeatedly during the night by cramps or twitches in the calf muscles. Nocturnal myoclonus is sometimes called periodic limb movement disorder (PLMD).

Non-rapid eye movement (NREM) sleep—A type of sleep that differs from rapid eye movement (REM) sleep. The four stages of NREM sleep account for 75–80% of total sleeping time.

Parasomnia—A primary sleep disorder in which a person's physiology or behaviors are affected by sleep, the sleep stage, or the transition from sleeping to waking.

Pavor nocturnus—Another term for sleep terror disorder.

Polysomnography—Laboratory measurement of a person's basic physiological processes during sleep. Polysomnography usually measures eye movement, brain waves, and muscular tension.

Primary sleep disorder—A sleep disorder that cannot be attributed to a medical condition, another mental disorder, or prescription medications or other substances.

Rapid eye movement (REM) sleep—A phase of sleep during which a person's eyes move rapidly beneath the lids. It accounts for 20–25% of sleep time. Dreaming occurs during REM sleep.

REM latency—After a person falls asleep, the amount of time it takes for the first onset of REM sleep.

Restless legs syndrome (RLS)—A disorder in which a person experiences crawling, aching, or other disagreeable sensations in the calves that can be relieved by movement. RLS is a frequent cause of difficulty falling asleep at night.

Sedative—A medication given to calm agitated individuals; sometimes used as a synonym for hypnotic.

Sleep latency—The amount of time that it takes to fall asleep. Sleep latency is measured in minutes and is important in diagnosing depression.

Somnambulism—Another term for sleepwalking.

Rosen, Carol L., and Gabriel G. Haddad. "Obstructive sleep apnea and hypoventilation in children." In *Nelson Textbook of Pediatrics*, 16th ed., edited by Richard E. Behrman et al. Philadelphia: Saunders, 2000, 1268-1271.

Shneerson, John. *Handbook of Sleep Medicine*. New York: Blackwell, 2000.

Simon, Roger, and Maria Sunseri. "Disorders of sleep and arousal." In *Cecil Textbook of Medicine*, 21st Ed., edited by Goldman, Lee Goldman and Bennett, J. Claude. Philadelphia: Saunders, 2000.

Thorpy, Michael, and Jan Yager. *The Encyclopedia of Sleep and Sleep Disorders, 2nd Ed.* New York: Facts on File, 2001.

PERIODICAL

Werra, R. "Restless legs syndrome." *American Family Physician* 63, no. 6 (2001): 1048.

ORGANIZATIONS

American Academy of Neurology. 1080 Montreal Avenue, St. Paul, Minnesota 55116, (651) 695-1940, http://www.aan.com/resources.html, web@aan.com

American Academy of Sleep Medicine. 6301 Bandel Road NW, Suite 101, Rochester, MN 55901. (507) 287-6006. Fax: (507) 287-6008, http://www.asda.org/, info@aasmnet.org

American Psychiatric Association. 1400 K Street NW, Washington, DC 20005. (888) 357-7924. Fax: (202) 682-6850. http://www.psych.org/, apa@psych.org.

L. Fleming Fallon, Jr., M.D., Dr.P.H.

Sleep study *see* **Polysomnography**

Sleepwalking *see* **Sleep disorders**

Slightly movable joint

Definition

A slightly movable joint (amphiarthrosis) is an articulation between bones in which the motion is limited due to either fibrous tissue or cartilage.

Description

Joints are classified as either fibrous or cartilaginous. Only one type of fibrous joint is slightly movable. It is known as a syndesmosis. In a syndesmosis, bones are separated by a substantial space and united by fibrous connective tissue.

In another classification of joints, cartilaginous also has only one type that is considered slightly movable. It is known as a symphysis. In a symphysis, bony surfaces are united by fibrocartilage.

Function

The function of a syndesmosis and symphysis is to bind two bones together, thus holding portions of the **skeletal system** intact. Also, the limited motion available

in either of these two types of joints allows certain movements to take place.

Role in human health

A syndesmosis connects two bones by connective tissue and is found throughout the human body. An example is the tibio-fibular syndesmosis, or the connective tissue that binds the distal ends of the fibula and tibia. A syndesmosis allows the fibula and tibia to work in unison as part of the lower leg. The limited motion available at this joint allows the tibia and fibula to move about each other yet still remain as a unit. This available movement is extremely important in the actions of the foot and ankle complex. This example describes how a syndesmosis provides stability as well as slight mobility.

A symphysis is a cartilaginous joint in which the uniting entity is fibrocartilage. Similar to the syndesmosis, the symphysis is stable but there is limited motion. In the syndesmosis, the bones are separated by a large space, unlike the symphysis, in which the articular surfaces are closer together. An example of a symphysis in the human body is the attachment of one vertebral body to another by way of an intervertebral disk. The intervertebral disk is a fibrocartilage ring that unites individual vertebral bodies. The sum attachment of many vertebrae gives rise to the **vertebral column**. The importance of this symphysis is that minimal motion occurs between vertebrae, thus maintaining stability. The combination of small movements between each successive vertebral attachment is what allows the vertebral column to move as a unit, that is, to flex and extend.

Common diseases and disorders

In the human body, a syndesmosis provides a stable environment between two bones and also allows for limited but important motion. In the example previously cited, the disorder that can affect a syndesmosis is primarily orthopedic. The tibio-fibular syndesmosis plays an integral role in stabilizing and allowing motion of the lower leg, foot, and ankle. Clearly, injury to this structure such as tearing would impair the stability and mobility of the lower leg, foot, and ankle. Thus, an injury to a syndesmosis described in this example could lead to impaired function such as walking.

A symphysis binds two bones by fibrocartilage. As cited previously, a good example of a symphysis in the human body is the attachment of one vertebra to another by a fibrocartilaginous disk. One of the most common and obvious disorders that can affect this joint is injury to the fibrocartilaginous disk. Injury to this fibrocartilage

Small intestine *see* **Intestine, small**

Small intestine radiography and fluoroscopy *see* **Upper GI exam**

KEY TERMS

Connective tissue—Tissue that has pliable fibers, which provide strength to the tissue and thus support to the structures it attaches to.

Fibrocartilage—Connective tissue made up of collagen fibers that unites two bones together as a joint.

Fibula—The outer or lateral bone of the lower leg.

Intervertebral disk—A fibrocartilaginous structure that attaches one vertebra to another. An intervertebral disk provides force attenuation in the spine and aids in the overall movement of the spine.

Tibia—The larger weight-bearing bone of the lower leg.

---

can be due to trauma, tumor, or **osteoarthritis**. Depending on which fibrocartilaginous disk is injured in the spine, associated problems could be **pain**, **weakness**, numbness, or tingling in the limbs, trunk, or both. Problems associated with an injured disk could affect overall human function and limit movement.

The syndesmosis and symphysis play important roles in human health. Moreover, injury to these joints could lead to reduced function and possible disability.

Resources

BOOKS

Hall, C.M., and L.T. Brody. *Therapeutic Exercise Moving Toward Function.* Philadelphia: Lippincott, Williams & Wilkins, 1998.

Lehmkuhl, L.D., and L.K. Smith. *Brunnstroms Clinical Kinesiology.* Philadelphia: F. A. Davis Co., 1996.

Magee, D.J. *Orthopedic Physical Assessment.* Philadelphia: W. B. Saunders Co., 1997.

Moore, K.L., and A.F. Dalley. *Clinically Oriented Anatomy.* Baltimore: Lippincott, Williams & Wilkins, 1999.

Rosse, C., P. Gaddum-Rosse, and W. Hollinshead. *Hollinshead's Textbook of Anatomy.* Baltimore: Lippincott, Williams & Wilkins, 1997.

Mark Damian Rossi, Ph.D., P.T.

Slipped disk *see* **Herniated disk**

Slit lamp examination *see* **Eye examination**

Small bowel follow-through (SBFT) *see* **Upper GI exam**

Smell

Definition

Smell is the ability of an organism to sense and identify a substance by detecting trace amounts of the substance that evaporate. Researchers have noted similarities in the sense of smell between widely differing species that reveal some of the details of how the chemical signal of an odor is detected and processed.

Description

The sense of smell has been a topic of debate from humankind's earliest days. The Greek philosopher Democritus of Abdera (460–360 B.C.), speculated that humans smell "atoms" of different size and shape that come from objects. His countryman Aristotle (384–322 B.C.), on the other hand, guessed that odors are detected when the "cold" sense of smell meets "hot" smoke or steam from the object being smelled. It was not until the late eighteenth century that most scientists and philosophers reached agreement that Democritus was basically right: the smell of an object is due to volatile, or easily evaporated, molecules that emanate from it.

In 1821, the French anatomist Hippolyte Cloquet (1787–1840) rightly noted the importance of smell for animal survival and reproduction; but his theorizing about the role of smell in human sex, as well as mental disorders, proved controversial. Many theories of the nineteenth century seem irrational or even malignant today. Many European scientists of that period fell into the trap of an essentially circular argument, that held that non-Europeans were more primitive, and therefore had a more developed sense of smell. The first half of the twentieth century saw progress in making the study of smell more rational. A Spanish neuroanatomist traced the architecture of the nerves leading from the nose to and through the **brain**. Other scientists carried out the first methodical investigations of how the nose detects scent molecules, the sensitivity of the human nose, and the differences between human and animal olfaction. But the most recent progress in studying the sense of smell and how it affects humans was made with the application of

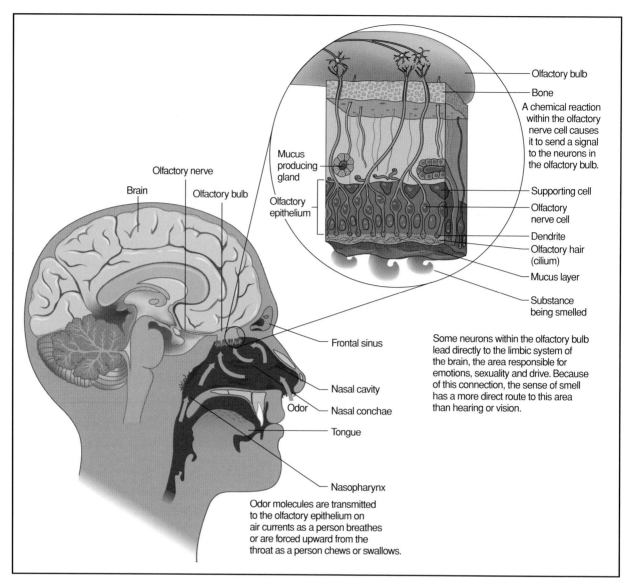

Olfactory bulb

Bone

A chemical reaction within the olfactory nerve cell causes it to send a signal to the neurons in the olfactory bulb.

Supporting cell

Olfactory nerve cell

Dendrite

Olfactory hair (cilium)

Mucus layer

Substance being smelled

Mucus producing gland

Olfactory epithelium

Olfactory nerve

Brain

Olfactory bulb

Frontal sinus

Nasal cavity

Odor

Nasal conchae

Tongue

Nasopharynx

Some neurons within the olfactory bulb lead directly to the limbic system of the brain, the area responsible for emotions, sexuality and drive. Because of this connection, the sense of smell has a more direct route to this area than hearing or vision.

Odor molecules are transmitted to the olfactory epithelium on air currents as a person breathes or are forced upward from the throat as a person chews or swallows.

(Sense of smell (human), illustration by Hans & Cassidy. Courtesy of Gale Research.)

molecular science to the odor-sensitive cells of the nasal cavity.

The sense of smell is the most important sense for most organisms. A wide variety of species use their sense of smell to locate prey, navigate, recognize and perhaps communicate with kin, and mark territory. In a broad sense, the workings of smell in animals as different as mammals, reptiles, fish, and even insects are remarkably similar.

The sense of smell differs from most other senses in its directness; humans and other mammals actually smell microscopic bits of a substance that have evaporated and made their way to the olfactory epithelium, a section of the mucus membrane in the roof of the olfactory cavity. The olfactory epithelium contains the smell-sensitive

ending of the olfactory nerve cells, also known as the olfactory epithelial cells. These cells detect odors through receptor **proteins** on the cell surface that bind to odor-carrying molecules. A specific odorant docks with an olfactory receptor protein in much the same way as a key fits in a lock; this in turn excites the nerve cell, causing it to send a signal to the brain. This is known as the stereospecific theory of smell.

Recently, molecular scientists have cloned the genes for the human olfactory receptor proteins. Although there are perhaps tens of thousands or more of odor-carrying molecules in the world, there are only hundreds, or at most about 1,000, kinds of specific receptors in any species of animal, including humans. Because of this, scientists do not believe that each receptor recognizes a unique odorant; rather, similar odorants can all bind to the same receptor. It appears that a few loose-fitting odorant "keys" of broadly similar shape can turn the same receptor "lock." Researchers do not yet know how many specific receptor proteins each olfactory nerve cell carries, but recent work suggests that the cells specialize just as the receptors do, and any one olfactory nerve cell has only one or a few receptors rather than many.

Function

It is the combined pattern of receptors that are tweaked by an odorant that allow the brain to identify it, much as yellow and red light together are interpreted by the brain as orange. (In fact, just as people can be color-blind to red or green, some can be "odor-blind" to certain simple molecules because they lack the receptor for that molecule.) In addition, real objects produce multiple odor-carrying molecules, so that the brain must analyze a complex mixture of odorants to recognize a smell.

Just as the sense of smell is direct in detecting fragments of the objects, it is also direct in the way the signals are transmitted to the brain. In most senses, such as **vision** this task is accomplished in several steps: a receptor cell detects light and passes the signal to a nerve cell, which passes it on to another nerve cell in the **central nervous system**, which then relays it to the visual center of the brain. But in olfaction, all these jobs are performed by the olfactory nerve cell. In a very real sense, the olfactory epithelium is a direct outgrowth of the brain.

Role in human health

In humans, the olfactory nerve cell takes the scent message directly to the nerve cells of the olfactory bulb of the brain. There multiple signals from different olfactory cells with different odor sensitivities are organized and processed. The signal then goes to the brain's olfactory cortex, where higher functions such as **memory** and emotion are coordinated with the sense of smell.

There is no doubt that many animals have a sense of smell far superior than humans. This is why, even today, humans use dogs to find lost persons, hidden drugs, and explosives although research on "artificial noses" that can detect scent even more reliably than dogs continues.

Because of their humble abilities of olfaction, humans are called microsmatic, rather than macrosmatic. Still, the human nose is capable of detecting over 10,000

KEY TERMS

Anosmia—A disorder in which one is able to detect no odors.

Olfactory bulb—The primitive part of the brain that first processes olfactory information.

Olfactory cortex—The cerebral cortex that makes use of information from the olfactory bulb.

Olfactory epithelium—The patch of mucus membrane at the top of the nasal cavity that is sensitive to odor.

Olfactory nerve cell—The cell in the olfactory epithelium that detects odor and transmits the information to the olfactory bulb of the brain.

Pheromones—Scent molecules made by the body that attract a mate and help initiate mating behaviors.

Receptor protein—A protein in a cell that sticks to a specific odorant or other signal molecule.

Stereospecific theory—The theory that the nose recognizes odorants when they bind to receptor proteins that recognize the odorants' molecular shape.

Volatile—Easily evaporated.

Vomeronasal—A pit on the roof of the mouth in most vertebrates that serves to detect odor molecules that are not as volatile as those detected by the nose.

---

different odors, some in the range of parts per trillion of air; and many researchers suspect that smell plays a greater role in human behavior and biology than has been previously thought. For instance, research has shown that human mothers can smell the difference between a vest worn by their baby and one worn by another baby only days after the child's birth.

Yet some olfactory abilities of animals are probably beyond humans. Most vertebrates have many more olfactory nerve cells in a proportionately larger olfactory epithelium than humans, which probably gives them much more sensitivity to odors. The olfactory bulb in these animals takes up a much larger portion of the brain than it does in humans, giving the animal more ability to process and analyze olfactory information. In addition, most land vertebrates have a specialized scent organ in the roof of the mouth called vomeronasal organ. This organ, believed to be vestigial in humans, is a pit lined by a layer of cells with a similar structure to the olfactory epithelium, which feeds into its own processing part of the brain, called accessory olfactory bulb, an area of the brain that is absent in humans.

Researchers have learned a lot about how the olfactory nerve cells detect odorants. However, they have not yet learned how this information is coded by the olfactory cell. Scientists are only beginning to understand the role that smell plays in animal and human behavior. The vomeronasal sense of animals is still largely not understood and some researchers have even suggested that the human vomeronasal organ might retain some function, and that humans may have pheromones that play a role in sexual attraction and mating. However, this hypothesis is still very controversial.

Detailed study of the biology of the olfactory system may yield gains in other fields. For instance, olfactory nerve cells are the only nerve cells that are derived from the central nervous system that can regenerate, possibly because the **stress** of their exposure to the outside world gives them a limited life span. Some researchers hope that studying regeneration in olfactory nerve cells or even transplanting them elsewhere in the body can lead to treatments for as yet irreversible damage to the spine and brain.

Common diseases and disorders

The most common complaint registered by patients is the loss of the sense of smell (anosmia). Smell disorders usually develop after an illness or an injury. Loss of the sense of smell is commonly caused by upper respiratory illnesses or a **head injury**. It can result from polyps in the nose or nasal cavity, sinus infections, hormonal fluctuations, or dental problems.

Resources

BOOKS

Schiffman, Harvey. *Sensation and Perception: An Integrated Approach.* New York: Wiley and Sons, 2001.

Watson, Lyall. *Jacobson's Organ: And the Remarkable Nature of Smell.* New York: W. W. Norton, 2000.

PERIODICALS

Dajer, Tony. "How the Nose Knows." *Discover*, January 1992.

Kreiter, Marcella S. "Brain Smells Out Signals." July 25, 2001. *http://www.nlm.nih.gov/medlineplus/news/fullstory_2928.html.*

OTHER

"Smell—Impaired." Medical Encyclopedia. Medline. 2001. http://www.nlm.nih.gov/medlineplus/ency/article/003052.htm).

Peggy Elaine Browning

Smoking

Definition

Smoking is the inhalation of the smoke of burning tobacco encased in cigarettes, pipes, and cigars. Casual smoking is the act of smoking only occasionally, usually in a social situation or to relieve **stress**. A smoking habit is a physical addiction to tobacco products. Many health experts now regard habitual smoking as a psychological addiction, too, and one with serious health consequences.

Description

The U.S. Food and Drug Administration has asserted that cigarettes and smokeless tobacco should be considered nicotine delivery devices. Nicotine, the active ingredient in tobacco, is inhaled into the **lungs**, where most of it stays. The rest passes into the bloodstream, reaching the **brain** in about 10 seconds and dispersing throughout the body in about 20 seconds.

Depending on the circumstances and the amount consumed, nicotine can act as either a stimulant or tranquilizer. This can explain why some people report that smoking gives them energy and stimulates their mental activity, while others note that smoking relieves **anxiety** and relaxes them. The initial "kick" results in part from the drug's stimulation of the **adrenal glands** and resulting release of epinephrine into the **blood**. Epinephrine causes several physiological changes—it temporarily narrows the arteries, raises the **blood pressure**, raises the levels of fat in the blood, and increases the **heart** rate and flow of blood from the heart. Some researchers think epinephrine contributes to smokers' increased risk of high blood pressure.

Nicotine, by itself, increases the risk of heart disease. However, when a person smokes, he or she is ingesting a lot more than nicotine. Smoke from a cigarette, pipe, or cigar is made up of many additional toxic chemicals, including tar and carbon monoxide. Tar is a sticky substance that forms into deposits in the lungs, causing **lung cancer** and respiratory distress. Carbon monoxide limits the amount of oxygen that the red blood cells can convey throughout your body. Also, it may damage the inner walls of the arteries, which allows fat to build up in them.

Besides tar, nicotine, and carbon monoxide, tobacco smoke contains 4,000 different chemicals. More than 200 of these chemicals are known be toxic. Nonsmokers who are exposed to tobacco smoke also take in these toxic chemicals. They inhale the smoke exhaled by the smoker as well as the more toxic *sidestream smoke*—the smoke from the end of the burning cigarette, cigar, or pipe.

Here's why sidestream smoke is more toxic than exhaled smoke: When a person smokes, the smoke he or she inhales and then breathes out leaves harmful deposits inside the body. But because lungs partially cleanse the smoke, exhaled smoke contains fewer poisonous chemicals. This is why exposure to tobacco smoke is dangerous even for a nonsmoker.

Causes and symptoms

No one starts smoking to become addicted to nicotine. It is not known how much nicotine may be consumed before the body becomes addicted. However, once smoking becomes a habit, the smoker faces a lifetime of health risks associated with one of the strongest addictions known to man.

About 70% of smokers in the United States would like to quit; in any given year, however, only about 3.6% of the country's 47 million smokers quit successfully. In 2008, the Centers for Disease Control and Prevention (CDC) reported that the prevalence of smoking in the United States fell in 2007 to 19.8%, almost a full percentage point decline from 20.8% in 2006.

Researchers conjecture that genetic factors contribute substantially to developing a smoking habit. Several twin studies have led to estimates of 46–84% heritability for smoking. It is thought that some genetic variations affect the speed of nicotine **metabolism** in the body and the activity level of nicotinic receptors in the brain.

Smoking risks

Smoking is recognized as the leading preventable cause of death, causing or contributing to the deaths of approximately 440,000 Americans each year. Anyone with a smoking habit has an increased chance of lung, cervical, and other types of **cancer**; respiratory diseases such as **emphysema**, **asthma**, and chronic **bronchitis**; and cardiovascular disease, such as heart attack, high blood pressure, **stroke**, and **atherosclerosis** (narrowing and hardening of the arteries). The risk of stroke is especially high in women who take birth control pills.

Smoking can damage fertility, making it harder to conceive, and it can interfere with the growth of the fetus during **pregnancy**. It accounts for an estimated 14% of premature births and 10% of infant deaths. There is some evidence that smoking may cause impotence in some men.

Because smoking affects so many of the body's systems, smokers often have vitamin deficiencies and suffer oxidative damage caused by free radicals. Free radicals are molecules that steal electrons from other molecules, turning the other molecules into free radicals and destabilizing the molecules in the body's cells.

Smoking is recognized as one of several factors that might be related to a higher risk of hip **fractures** in older adults.

Studies reveal that the more a person smokes, the more likely he is to sustain illnesses such as cancer, chronic bronchitis, and emphysema. But even smokers who indulge in the habit only occasionally are more prone to these diseases.

Some brands of cigarettes are advertised as "low tar" but no cigarette is truly safe. If a smoker switches to a low-tar cigarette, he or she is likely to inhale longer and more deeply to get the chemicals his body craves. A smoker has to quit the habit entirely in order to improve his health and decrease the chance of disease.

Though some people believe chewing tobacco is safer, it also carries health risks. People who chew tobacco have an increased risk of heart disease and mouth and throat cancer. Pipe and cigar smokers have increased health risks as well, even though these smokers generally do not inhale as deeply as cigarette smokers do. These groups haven't been studied as extensively as cigarette smokers but there is evidence that they may be at a slightly lower risk of cardiovascular problems but a higher risk of cancer and various types of circulatory conditions.

Recent research reveals that passive smokers, or those who unavoidably breathe in second-hand tobacco smoke, have an increased chance of many health problems such as lung cancer and asthma, and in children, sudden infant death syndrome.

Smokers' symptoms

Smokers are likely to exhibit a variety of symptoms that reveal the damage caused by smoking. A nagging morning **cough** may be one sign of a tobacco habit. Other symptoms include shortness of breath, **wheezing**, and frequent occurrences of respiratory illness, such as bronchitis. Smoking also increases fatigue and decreases the smoker's sense of **smell** and **taste**. Smokers are more likely to develop poor circulation, with cold hands and feet and premature wrinkles.

Sometimes the illnesses that result from smoking come on silently with little warning. For instance, **coronary artery disease** may exhibit few or no symptoms. At other times, there will be warning signs, such as bloody discharge from a woman's vagina, a sign of cancer of the cervix. Another warning sign is a hacking cough, worse than the usual smoker's cough, that brings up phlegm or blood—a sign of lung cancer.

Withdrawal symptoms

A smoker who tries to quit may expect one or more of these withdrawal symptoms: nausea, constipation or **diarrhea**, drowsiness, loss of concentration, insomnia, **headache**, nausea, and irritability.

Diagnosis

It is not easy to quit smoking, which is why it may be wise for a smoker to turn to his physician for help. For the greatest success in quitting and to help with the withdrawal symptoms, the smoker should talk over a treatment plan with his doctor or alternative practitioner. He should have a general **physical examination** to gauge his general health and uncover any deficiencies. He should also have a thorough evaluation for some of the serious diseases that smoking can cause.

Treatment

Research shows that most smokers who want to quit benefit from the support of other people. It helps to quit with a friend or to join a group such as those organized by the American Cancer Society. These groups provide support and teach behavior modification methods that can help the smoker quit. The smoker's physician can often refer him to such groups.

Other alternatives to help with the withdrawal symptoms of kicking the habit include nicotine replacement therapy in the form of gum, patches, nasal sprays, and oral inhalers. These are available by prescription or over the counter. A physician can provide advice on how to use them. They slowly release a small amount of nicotine into the bloodstream, satisfying the smoker's physical craving. Over time, the amount of gum the smoker chews is decreased and the amount of time between applying the patches is increased. This helps wean the smoker from nicotine slowly, eventually beating his addiction to the drug. But there's one important caution: If the smoker lights up while taking a nicotine replacement, a nicotine **overdose** may cause serious health problems.

The prescription drug Zyban (bupropion hydrochloride) has shown some success in helping smokers quit. This drug contains no nicotine and was originally developed as an antidepressant. It isn't known exactly how bupropion works to suppress the desire for nicotine. A five-year study of bupropion reported that the drug has a very good record for safety and effectiveness in treating tobacco dependence. Its most common side effect is insomnia, which can also result from nicotine withdrawal.

Researchers are investigating two new types of drugs as possible treatments for tobacco dependence. The first is an alkaloid known as 18-methoxycoronaridine (18-MC), which selectively blocks the nicotinic receptors in brain tissue. Another approach involves developing drugs that inhibit the activity of cytochrome P450 2A6 (CYP2A6), which controls the metabolism of nicotine.

Expected results

Research on smoking shows that most smokers desire to quit. But smoking is so addictive that fewer than 20% of the people who try ever successfully kick the habit. Still, many people attempt to quit smoking over and over again, despite the difficulties—the cravings and withdrawal symptoms, such as irritability and restlessness.

For those who do quit, the benefits to health are well worth the effort. The good news is that once a smoker quits the health effects are immediate and dramatic. After the first day, oxygen and carbon monoxide levels in the blood return to normal. At two days, nerve endings begin to grow back and the senses of taste and smell revive. Within two weeks to three months, circulation and breathing improve. After one year of not smoking, the risk of heart disease is reduced by 50%. After 15 years of abstinence, the risks of health problems from smoking virtually vanish. A smoker who quits for good often feels a lot better too, with less fatigue and fewer respiratory illnesses.

Alternative treatment

There are a wide range of alternative treatments that can help a smoker quit the habit, including hypnotherapy, herbs, **acupuncture**, and **meditation**. For example, a controlled trial demonstrated that self-massage can help smokers crave less intensely, smoke fewer cigarettes, and in some cases completely give them up.

Hypnotherapy

Hypnotherapy helps the smoker achieve a trance-like state, during which the deepest levels of the mind are accessed. A session with a hypnotherapist may begin with a discussion of whether the smoker really wants to and truly has the motivation to stop smoking. The therapist will explain how hypnosis can reduce the stress-related symptoms that sometimes come with kicking the habit.

Often the therapist will discuss the dangers of smoking with the patient and begin to "reframe" the patient's thinking about smoking. Many smokers are convinced they can't quit, and the therapist can help

KEY TERMS

Antioxidant—Any substance that reduces the damage caused by oxidation, such as the harm caused by free radicals.

Chronic bronchitis—A smoking-related respiratory illness in which the membranes that line the bronchi, or the lung's air passages, narrow over time. Symptoms include a morning cough that brings up phlegm, breathlessness, and wheezing.

Cytochrome—A substance that contains iron and acts as a hydrogen carrier for the eventual release of energy in aerobic respiration.

Emphysema—An incurable, smoking-related disease, in which the air sacs at the end of the lung's bronchi become weak and inefficient. People with emphysema often first notice shortness of breath, repeated wheezing and coughing that brings up phlegm.

Epinephrine—A nervous system hormone stimulated by the nicotine in tobacco. It increases heart rate and may raise smokers' blood pressure.

Flavonoid—A food chemical that helps to limit oxidative damage to the body's cells, and protects against heart disease and cancer.

Free radical—An unstable molecule that causes oxidative damage by stealing electrons from surrounding molecules, thereby disrupting activity in the body's cells.

Nicotine—The addictive ingredient of tobacco, it acts on the nervous system and is both stimulating and calming.

Nicotine replacement therapy—A method of weaning a smoker away from both nicotine and the oral fixation that accompanies a smoking habit by giving the smoker smaller and smaller doses of nicotine in the form of a patch or gum.

Sidestream smoke—The smoke that is emitted from the burning end of a cigarette or cigar, or that comes from the end of a pipe. Along with exhaled smoke, it is a constituent of second-hand smoke.

persuade them that they can change this behavior. These suggestions are then repeated while the smoker is under hypnosis. The therapist may also suggest while the smoker is under hypnosis that his feelings of worry, anxiety, and irritability will decrease.

In a review of 17 studies of the effectiveness of hypnotherapy, the percentage of people treated by hypnosis who still were not smoking after six months ranged from 4–8%. In programs that included several hours of treatment, intense interpersonal interaction, individualized suggestions, and follow-up treatment, success rates were above 50%.

Aromatherapy

One study demonstrated that inhaling the vapor from black pepper extract can reduce symptoms associated with smoking withdrawal. Other essential oils can be used for relieving the anxiety a smoker often experiences while quitting.

Herbs

A variety of herbs can help smokers reduce their cravings for nicotine, calm their irritability, and even reverse the oxidative cellular damage done by smoking. Lobelia, sometimes called Indian tobacco, has

historically been used as a substitute for tobacco. It contains a substance called lobeline, which decreases the craving for nicotine by bolstering the nervous system and calming the smoker. In high doses, lobelia can cause **vomiting** but the average dose—about 10 drops per day—should pose no problems.

Herbs that can help relax a smoker during withdrawal include wild oats and kava kava.

To reduce the oral fixation supplied by a nicotine habit, a smoker can chew on licorice root—the plant, not the candy. Licorice is good for the **liver**, which is a major player in the body's detoxification process. Licorice also acts as a tonic for the adrenal system, which helps reduce stress. And there's an added benefit: If a smoker tries to light up after chewing on licorice root, the cigarette tastes like burned cardboard.

Other botanicals that can help repair free-radical damage to the lungs and **cardiovascular system** are those high in flavonoids, such as hawthorn, gingko biloba, and bilberry, as well as antioxidants such as **vitamin A**, **vitamin C**, **zinc**, and selenium.

Acupuncture

This ancient Chinese method of healing is used commonly to help beat addictions, including smoking.

The acupuncturist will use hair-thin needles to stimulate the body's *qi*, or healthy energy. Acupuncture is a sophisticated treatment system based on revitalizing qi, which supposedly flows through the body in defined pathways called meridians. During an addiction like smoking, qi isn't flowing smoothly or gets stuck, the theory goes.

Points in the ear and feet are stimulated to help the smoker overcome his addiction. Often the acupuncturist will recommend keeping the needles in for five to seven days to calm the smoker and keep him balanced.

Vitamins

Smoking seriously depletes vitamin C in the body and leaves it more susceptible to infections. Vitamin C can prevent or reduce free-radical damage by acting as an antioxidant in the lungs. Smokers need additional C, in higher dosage than nonsmokers. Fish in the diet supplies Omega-3 fatty acids, which are associated with a reduced risk of **chronic obstructive pulmonary disease** (emphysema or chronic bronchitis) in smokers. Omega-3 fats also provide cardiovascular benefits as well as an anti-depressive effect. Vitamin therapy doesn't reduce craving but it can help beat some of the damage created by smoking. **Vitamin B$_{12}$** and **folic acid** may help protect against smoking-induced cancer.

Prevention

How do you give up your cigarettes for good and never go back to them again?

Here are a few tips from the experts:

- Have a plan and set a definite quit date.
- Get rid of all the cigarettes and ashtrays at home or in your desk at work.
- Don't allow others to smoke in your house.
- Tell your friends and neighbors that you're quitting. Doing so helps make quitting a matter of pride.
- Chew sugarless gum or eat sugar-free hard candy to redirect the oral fixation that comes with smoking. This will prevent weight gain, too.
- Eat as much as you want but only low-calorie foods and drinks. Drink plenty of water. This may help with the feelings of tension and restlessness that quitting can bring. After eight weeks, you'll lose your craving for tobacco so it's safe then to return to your usual eating habits.
- Stay away from social situations that prompt you to smoke. Dine in the nonsmoking section of restaurants.
- Spend the money you save not smoking on an occasional treat for yourself.

Resources

BOOK

Bevins, Rick A., and Anthony R. Caggiula. *The Motivational Impact of Nicotine and Its Role in Tobacco Use.* Nebraska Symposium on Motivation. New York: Springer, 2008.

PERIODICALS

Ferry, L., and J.A. Johnston. "Efficacy and Safety of Bupropion SR for Smoking Cessation: Data from Clinical Trials and Five Years of Postmarketing Experience." *International Journal of Clinical Practice* 57 (April 2003): 224–230.

Janson, Christer, Susan Chinn, Deborah Jarvis, et al. "Effect of Passive Smoking on Respiratory Symptoms, Bronchial Responsiveness, Lung Function, and Total Serum IgE in the European Community Respiratory Health Survey: A Cross-Sectional Study." *Lancet* 358 (December 22, 2001): 2103.

Maisonneuve, I.M., and S.D. Glick. "Anti-Addictive Actions of an Iboga Alkaloid Congener: A Novel Mechanism for a Novel Treatment." *Pharmacology, Biochemistry, and Behavior* 75 (June 2003): 607–618.

Sellers, E.M., R.F. Tyndale, and L.C. Fernandes. "Decreasing Smoking Behaviour and Risk through CYP2A6 Inhibition." *Drug Discovery Today* 8 (June 1, 2003): 487–493.

OTHER

Centers for Disease Control and Prevention (CDC). "Smokeless Tobacco" May 29, 2009. [Accessed December 15, 2010] http://www.cdc.gov/tobacco/basic_information/smokeless/.

Centers for Disease Control and Prevention (CDC). "Smoking and Tobacco Use." [Accessed December 15, 2010] http://www.cdc.gov/tobacco.

National Institutes of Health (NIH). "Smoking." [Accessed December 15, 2010] http://health.nih.gov/topic/Smoking .

United States Environmental Protection Agency (EPA). "Air: Indoor Air Pollution: Environmental Tobacco Smoke." [Accessed December 15, 2010] http://www.epa.gov/ebtpages/airindoorenvironmentaltobaccosmoke.html.

Virtual Office of the Surgeon General: Tobacco Cessation Guideline. [Accessed December 15, 2010] http://www.surgeongeneral.gov/tobacco.

World Health Organization (WHO). "Tobacco Free Initiative (TFI)." WHO Programs and Projects. [Accessed December 15, 2010] http://www.who.int/entity/tobacco/en.

World Health Organization (WHO). "WHO Framework Convention on Tobacco Control." WHO Programs and Projects. [Accessed December 15, 2010] http://www.who.int/entity/fctc/en.

ORGANIZATIONS

American Association of Oriental Medicine. 5530 Wisconsin Avenue, Suite 1210, Chevy Chase MD, 20815, (301) 941-1064, (888) 500-7999, http://www.aaom.org.

American Cancer Society. Contact the local organization or call (800) 227-2345, http://www.cancer.org.

American Lung Association. 1740 Broadway, New York NY, 10019, (800) 586-4872, (212) 315-8700, http://www.lungusa.org.

Herb Research Foundation. 1007 Pearl St., Suite 200, Boulder CO, 80302, (303) 449-2265, http://www.herbs.org.

National Heart, Lung, and Blood Institute (NHLBI). Building 31, Room 5A52, 31 Center Drive, MSC 2486, Bethesda MD, 20892, (301) 592-8573, http://www.nhlbi.nih.gov.

Smoking, Tobacco, and Health Information Line. Centers for Disease Control and Prevention. Mailstop K-50, 4770 Buford Highway NE, Atlanta GA, 30341-3724, (800) 232-1311, http://www.cdc.gov/tobacco.

Barbara Boughton

Smoking cessation

Definition

Smoking cessation means "quitting smoking," or "withdrawal from nicotine." Tobacco is highly addictive, therefore, quitting the habit often involves irritability, **headache**, mood swings, and cravings associated with the sudden cessation or reduction of tobacco use by a nicotine-dependent individual.

Purpose

There are many good reasons to stop smoking; one of them is that smoking cessation may speed post-surgery recovery. Smoking cessation helps a person heal and recover faster, especially in the incision area, or if the surgery involved any bones. Research shows that patients who underwent hip and knee replacements, or surgery on other **bone** joints, healed better and recovered more quickly if they had quit or cut down their tobacco intake several weeks before the operation. Smoking weakens the bone mineral that keeps the skeleton strong and undermines tissue and vessel health. One study suggested that even quitting tobacco for a few days could improve tissue **blood** flow and oxygenation, and might have a positive effect on wound healing. If a patient has had a history of **heart** problems, his chances of having a second heart attack will be lowered. Quitting may also reduce wound complications, and lower the risk of cardiovascular trouble after surgery. If surgery was performed to remove cancerous tumors, quitting will reduce the risk of a second tumor, especially if **cancer** in the lung, head, or neck has been successfully treated.

Description

Quitting smoking is one of the best things a person can do to increase their life expectancy. On average, male smokers who quit at 35 years old can be expected to live to be 76 years old instead of 69 years if they were still smoking. Women who quit would live to be 80 years old instead of 74 years.

Effects of smoking on the body

Nicotine acts as both a stimulant and a depressant on the body. Saliva and bronchial secretions increase along with bowel tone. Some inexperienced smokers may experience tremors or even convulsions with high doses of nicotine because of the stimulation of the **central nervous system**. The respiratory muscles are then depressed following stimulation.

Nicotine causes arousal as well as **relaxation** from stressful situations. Tobacco use increases the heart rate about 10–20 beats per minute; and because it constricts the **blood vessels**, it increases the **blood pressure** reading by 5–10 mm Hg.

Sweating, nausea, and **diarrhea** may also increase because of the effects of nicotine upon the central nervous system. Hormonal activities of the body are also affected. Nicotine elevates the blood glucose levels and increases insulin production; it can also lead to blood clots. Smoking does have some positive effects on the body by stimulating **memory** and alertness, and enhancing cognitive skills that require speed, reaction time, vigilance, and work performance. Smoking tends to alleviate boredom and reduce **stress** as well as reduce aggressive responses to stressful events because of its mood-altering ability. It also acts as an appetite suppressant, specifically decreasing the appetite for simple **carbohydrates** (sweets) and inhibiting the efficiency with which food is metabolized. The fear of weight gain prevents some people from quitting smoking. The addictive effects of tobacco have been well documented. It is considered mood- and behavior-altering, psychoactive, and prone to abuse. Tobacco's addictive potential is believed to be comparable to the addictive potentials of alcohol, **cocaine**, and morphine.

Health problems associated with smoking

In general, chronic use of nicotine may cause an acceleration of **coronary artery disease**, **hypertension**, reproductive disturbances, esophageal reflux, peptic ulcer disease, fetal illnesses and death, and delayed wound healing. The smoker is at greater risk of developing cancer (especially in the lung, mouth, larynx, esophagus, bladder, kidney, **pancreas**, and cervix); heart attacks and strokes; and chronic lung disease. Using tobacco during **pregnancy** increases the risk of **miscarriage**, intrauterine growth retardation (resulting in the birth of an infant

KEY TERMS

Addiction—Compulsive, overwhelming involvement with a specific activity. The activity may be smoking, gambling, alcohol, or may involve the use of almost any substance, such as a drug.

Appetite suppressant—To decrease the appetite.

Constrict—To squeeze tightly, compress, draw together.

Convulsion—To shake or effect with spasms; to agitate or disturb violently.

Depressant—A drug or other substance that soothes or lessens tension of the muscles or nerves.

Detoxification—To remove a poison or toxin or the effect of such a harmful substance; to free from an intoxicating or addictive substance in the body or from dependence on or addiction to a harmful substance.

Endorphins—Any of a group of proteins with analgesic properties that occur naturally in the brain.

Gestational age—The length of time of growth and development of the young in the mother's womb.

Metabolism—The sum of all the chemical processes that occur in living organisms; the rate at which the body consumes energy.

Nicotine—A poisonous, oily alkaloid in tobacco.

Oxygenation—To supply with oxygen.

Paraphernalia—Articles of equipment or accessory items.

Premature—Happening early or occurring before the usual time.

Psychoactive—Affecting the mind or behavior.

Respiratory infections—Infections that relate to or affect respiration or breathing.

Smoking cessation—The act of quitting smoking or withdrawal from nicotine.

Stimulant—A drug or other substance that increases the rate of activity of a body system.

Tremor—A trembling, quivering, or shaking.

Withdrawal—Stopping of administration or use of a drug; the syndrome of sometimes painful physical and psychological symptoms that follow the discontinuance.

small for gestational age), and the infant's risk for sudden infant death syndrome.

The specific health risks of tobacco use include: nicotine addiction, lung disease, **lung cancer**, **emphysema**, chronic **bronchitis**, coronary artery disease and **angina**, heart attack, atherosclerotic and **peripheral vascular disease**, aneurysms, hypertension, blood clots, strokes, oral/tooth/gum diseases including **oral cancer**, and cancer in the kidney, bladder, and pancreas. Nicotine is also associated with decreased senses of **taste** and **smell**. During pregnancy, nicotine may cause increased fetal death, premature labor, low birth weight infants, and sudden infant death syndrome.

Smoking is also increasingly harmful to a person's social acceptability. According to the National Institute on Drug Abuse (NIDA), students at the high school and college levels in the early twenty-first century are increasingly disapproving of smoking. In just one year, disapproval of smoking among high school seniors increased from 76.2% in 2004 to 79.8% in 2005. For young adults, smoking complicates finding housing, as many landlords will not rent to smokers and many potential roommates do not want to share their apartment with a smoker.

Nonsmokers who are regularly exposed to second-hand smoke also may experience specific health risks including:

- Increased risk of lung cancer.

- An increased frequency of respiratory infections in infants and children (e.g., bronchitis and pneumonia), asthma, and decreases in lung function as the lungs mature.

- Acute, sudden, and occasionally severe reactions including eye, nose, throat, and lower respiratory tract symptoms.

The specific health risks for smokeless tobacco users include many of the diseases of smokers, as well as a 50-fold greater risk for oral cancer with long-term or regular use.

In diabetics taking medication for high blood pressure, it has been reported that smoking may increase the risk of kidney disease and/or kidney failure.

Making a plan to quit

Long lead times for elective procedures like joint operations offer a good opportunity for doctors to encourage their patients to quit smoking, but only the smoker has the power to stop smoking. Before a smoker decides to quit, he should make sure he wants to quit smoking for himself, and not for other people. The following are some suggestions the smoker may want to consider:

- The first step is to set a quit date. Women should set their quit date to begin at the end of their period for best results.
- Make a written list of why you want to quit smoking.
- Consider using an aid to help you quit, which can be the patch, nicotine gum, Zyban, nicotine spray, soft laser therapy, nasal inhaler, or some other method. If you plan to use Zyban, set your quit date for one week after you begin to use it.
- Smoke only in certain places, preferably outdoors.
- Switch to a brand of cigarettes that you don't like.
- Buy a piggy bank or an attractive box or jar and put the money in it that you would ordinarily spend on cigarettes. With a pack of cigarettes costing over $10 in some states, the money in your savings bank will quickly add up.
- Do not buy cigarettes by the carton.
- Cut coffee consumption in half. You will not need to give it up.
- Practice putting off lighting up when the urge strikes.
- Go for a walk every day or begin an exercise program.
- Stock up on non-fattening safe snacks to help with weight control after quitting.
- Enlist the support of family and friends.
- Clean and put away all ashtrays the day before quitting.

Smokers who are trying to quit should remind themselves that they are doing the smartest thing they have ever done. Because of the preparation for smoking cessation, the smoker won't be surprised by or fearful of quitting. The quitter will be willing to do what's necessary, even though it won't be easy. Remember, this will likely add years to the lifespan. The quitting smoker should be prepared to spend more time with nonsmoking friends, if other smokers don't support the attempt to quit.

Since hospitals are smoke-free environments, if a smoking patient is in the hospital for elective surgery, it may be a good opportunity to quit smoking. It might be best to set the quit date around the time of the surgery and let the attending doctor know. As the smoker takes the first step, professional hospital staff will be there to give the support and help needed. Medical staff can start the patient on nicotine replacement therapy to help control the cravings and increase the chances of quitting permanently.

Methods of quitting

Cold turkey, or an abrupt cessation of nicotine, is one way to stop smoking. Cold turkey can provide cost savings because paraphernalia and smoking cessation aids are not required; however, not everyone can stop this way as tremendous willpower is needed.

Laser therapy is an entirely safe and **pain** free form of **acupuncture** that has been in use since the 1980s. Using a painless soft laser beam instead of needles the laser beam is applied to specific energy points on the body, stimulating production of endorphins. These natural body chemicals produce a calming, relaxing effect. It is the sudden drop in endorphin levels that leads to withdrawal symptoms and physical cravings when a person stops smoking. Laser treatment not only helps relieve these cravings, but helps with stress reduction and lung detoxification. Some studies indicate that laser therapy is the most effective method of smoking cessation, with an extraordinarily high success rate.

Acupuncture—small needles or springs are inserted into the skin—is another aid in smoking cessation. The needles or springs are sometimes left in the ears and touched lightly by the patient between visits.

Some smokers find hypnosis particularly useful, especially if there is any kind of mental conflict, such as phobias, panic attacks, or weight control. As a smoker struggles to stop smoking, the conscious mind, deciding to quit, battles the inner mind, which is governed by habit and body chemistry. Hypnosis, by talking directly to the inner mind, can help to resolve that inner battle.

Some people are helped to quit smoking by **psychotherapy**. As of 2007, cognitive behavioral therapy, or CBT, is considered the most effective form of psychotherapy for smoking cessation. A research team at Yale University reported in the fall of 2007 that CBT was more effective than brief behavioral interventions in helping adolescent smokers stay in a smoking cessation program as well as actually quitting smoking.

Aversion techniques attempt to make smoking seem unpleasant. This technique reminds the person of the distasteful aspects of smoking, such as the smell, dirty ashtrays, coughing, the high cost, and health issues. The most common technique prescribed by psychologists for "thought stopping"—stopping unwanted thoughts—is to wear a rubber band around the wrist. Every time there is an unwanted thought (a craving to smoke) the band is supposed to be pulled so that it hurts. The thought then becomes associated with pain and gradually neutralized.

Rapid smoking is a technique in which smoking times are strictly scheduled once a day for the first three days after quitting. Phrases are repeated such as "smoking irritates my throat" or "smoking **burns** my lips and tongue." This technique causes over-smoking in a way that makes the taste and sensations associated with smoking very unpleasant.

There are special mouthwashes available, which, when used before smoking, alter the taste, giving cigarettes a very unpleasant taste. The intention is to create a link in the smoker's mind between cigarettes and a bad taste in the mouth.

Smoking cessation aids wean a person off nicotine slowly, and the nicotine can be delivered where it does the least bodily harm. Unlike cigarettes, these aids do not introduce other harmful poisons to the body. They can be used for a short period of time; however, nicotine from any source (smoking, nicotine gum, or the nicotine patch) can make some health problems worse. These include heart or circulation problems, irregular heartbeat, chest pain, high blood pressure, overactive thyroid, **stomach** ulcers, or diabetes.

The four main brands of the patch are Nicotrol, Nicoderm, Prostep, and Habitrol. All four transmit low doses of nicotine to the body throughout the day. The patch comes in varying strengths ranging from 7 mg to 21 mg. The patch must be prescribed and used under a physician's care. Package instructions must be followed carefully. Other smoking cessation programs or materials should be used while using the patch.

Nicorette gum allows the nicotine to be absorbed through the membrane of the mouth between the cheek and gums. Past smoking habits determine the right strength to choose. The gum should be chewed slowly.

The nicotine nasal spray reduces cravings and withdrawal symptoms, allowing smokers to cut back slowly. The nasal spray acts quickly to stop the cravings, as it is rapidly absorbed through the nasal membranes. One of the drawbacks is a risk of addiction to the spray.

The nicotine inhaler uses a plastic mouthpiece with a nicotine plug, delivering nicotine to the mucous membranes of the mouth. It provides nicotine at about one-third the nicotine level of cigarettes.

Bupropion hydrochloride, sold under the trade name Zyban, is an oral medication that is making an impact in the fight to help smokers quit. It is a treatment for nicotine dependence. Another new medication, approved by the Food and Drug Administration (FDA) in 2006, is varenicline tartrate, sold under the trade name Chantix. Chantix is thought to work by affecting parts of the **brain** affected by nicotine in two ways: by providing some nicotine effects to ease withdrawal symptoms and by blocking the effects of nicotine from cigarettes if the patient resumes smoking. In November 2007, however, the FDA issued a warning regarding mood changes reported in persons taking Chantix. The drug is still considered safe, but anyone taking it in order to stop smoking should contact their doctor at once if they feel depressed or notice other sudden mood changes.

The nicotine lozenge is another smoking cessation aid recently added to the growing list of tools to combat nicotine withdrawal.

As of 2007, scientists are researching the possibility of developing medications that inhibit the function of CYP2A6, an enzyme that makes people more susceptible to nicotine addiction. Some people have a genetic variant that decreases the amount of CYP2A6 in the body, which is thought to protect these individuals against nicotine addiction. Thus medications that lower the amount of this enzyme might offer a new approach to smoking cessation.

Withdrawal symptoms

Generally, the longer one has smoked and the greater the number of cigarettes (and nicotine) consumed, the more likely it is that withdrawal symptoms will occur and the more severe they are likely to be. When a smoker switches from regular to low-nicotine cigarettes or significantly cuts back smoking, a milder form of nicotine withdrawal involving some or all of these symptoms can occur.

These are some of the withdrawal symptoms that most former smokers experience in the beginning of their new smoke-free life:

• dry mouth
• mood swings
• irritability
• feelings of depression
• gas in the digestive tract
• tension
• sleeplessness or sleeping too much
• difficulty in concentration
• intense cravings for a cigarette
• increased appetite and weight gain
• headaches.

These side effects are all temporary conditions that will probably subside in a short time for most people. These symptoms can last from one to three weeks and are strongest during the first week after quitting. Drinking plenty of water during the first week can help detoxify the body and shorten the duration of the withdrawal symptoms. A positive attitude, drive, commitment, and a willingness to get help from health care professionals and support groups will help a smoker kick the habit.

Researchers from the University of California San Diego strongly suggest that any of the above cessation aids should be used in combination with other types of smoking cessation help, such as counseling and/or support programs. These products are not designed to help with the behavioral aspects of smoking, but only the cravings associated with them. Counseling and support groups can offer tips on coping with difficult situations that can trigger the urge to smoke.

Even a new heart can't break a bad habit

Why do some people who have heart transplants continue to smoke? In a three-year study at the University of Pittsburgh of 202 heart transplant recipients, 71% of the recipients were smokers before surgery. The overall rate of post-transplant smoking was 27%. All but one of the smokers resumed the smoking habit they had before the transplant. The biggest reason for resuming smoking was addiction to nicotine. Smoking is a complex behavior, involving social interactions, visual cues, and other factors. Those who smoked until less than six months before the transplant were much more likely to resume smoking early and to smoke more. One of the major causes of early relapse was because of depression and **anxiety** within two months after the transplant. Another strong predictor of relapse was having a caretaker who smoked. The knowledge of these risk factors could help develop strategies for identifying those in greatest need of early intervention. According to European studies, the five-year survival rate for post-transplant smokers is 37%, compared to 80% for nonsmoking recipients. Smokers can develop inoperable lung cancers within five years after a transplant, thus resulting in a shorter survival rate. There is an alarming incidence of head and neck cancers in transplant recipients who resume smoking.

Overall, there is a 90% relapse rate in the general population; however, the more times a smoker tries to quit, the greater the chance of success with each new try.

Resources

BOOKS

Abrams, David B., et al. The Tobacco Dependence Treatment Handbook: A Guide to Best Practices. New York: Guilford Press, 2003.

American Cancer Society. Kicking Butts: Quit Smoking and Take Charge of Your Health. Atlanta, GA: American Cancer Society, 2002.

Britton, John, ed. ABC of Smoking Cessation. Malden, MA: BMJ Books, 2004.

Dodds, Bill. 1440 Reasons to Quit Smoking: 1 For Every Minute of the Day. Minnetonka, MN: Meadowbrook Press, 2000.

Mannoia, Richard J. NBAC Program: Never Buy Another Cigarette: A Cigarette Smoking Cessation Program. Paradise Publications, 2003.

National Institutes of Health. Clearing the Air: Quit Smoking Today. Bethesda, MD: National Institutes of Health, 2003.

Shipley, Robert H. Quit Smart: Stop Smoking Guide With the Quitsmart System, It's Easier Than You Think! Quitsmart, 2002.

PERIODICALS

Cavallo, D.A., J.L. Cooney, A.M. Duhig, et al. "Combining Cognitive Behavioral Therapy with Contingency Management for Smoking Cessation in Adolescent Smokers: A Preliminary Comparison of Two Different CBT Formats." American Journal on Addictions 16, no. 6 (November 2007): 468–474.

Lancaster, T., L. Stead, and K. Cahill. "An Update on Therapeutics for Tobacco Dependence." Expert Opinion on Pharmacotherapy 9, no. 1 (January 2008): 15–22.

Landman, Anne, Pamela M. Ling, and Stanton A. Glantz. "Tobacco Industry Youth Smoking Prevention Programs: Protecting the Industry and Hurting Tobacco Control." American Journal of Public Health 92, no. 6 (June 2002): 917–30.

Le Foll, B., and T.P. George. "Treatment of Tobacco Dependence: Integrating Recent Progress into Practice." Canadian Medical Association Journal 177, no. 11 (November 20, 2007): 1373–1380.

Mwenifumbo, J.C., and R.F. Tyndale. "Genetic Variability in CYP2A6 and the Pharmacokinetics of Nicotine." Pharmacogenomics 8, no. 10 (October 2007): 1385–1402.

OTHER

Illig, David. Stop Smoking. Audio CD. Seattle, WA: Successworld, 2001.

Mesmer. Stop Smoking With America's Foremost Hypnotist. Audio CD. Victoria, BC: Ace Mirage Entertainment, 2000.

"NIDA InfoFacts: Cigarettes and Other Tobacco Products." National Institute on Drug Abuse. July 2007. http://www.nida.nih.gov/infofacts/tobacco.html (April 7, 2008).

"Prevention and Cessation of Cigarette Smoking: Control of Tobacco Use," patient version. National Cancer Institute. 2008. http://www.cancer.gov/cancertopics/pdq/prevention/control-of-tobacco-use/Patient (April 7, 2008).

ORGANIZATIONS

Action on Smoking and Health, 2013 H Street, NW, Washington, DC 20006, (202) 659-4310, http://ash.org

American Cancer Society, 1875 Connecticut Avenue, NW, Suite 730, Washington, DC 20009, (800) ACS-2345, http://www.cancer.org

Centers for Disease Control and Prevention, Mail Stop K-50, 4770 Buford Highway, NE, Atlanta, GA 30341, (800) 232-4636, http://www.cdc.gov/tobacco/osh/index.htm.

Crystal H. Kaczkowski, M.Sc.
Rebecca Frey, Ph.D.

Smoking-cessation drugs

Definition

Smoking cessation drugs are medicines that help people stop **smoking** cigarettes or using other forms of tobacco.

Purpose

The known major health risks associated with smoking have led to efforts to dramatically reduce the number of people who do smoke and to encourage individuals, particularly young people, to not begin smoking. These efforts include restricting access to tobacco products to minors, substantially raising the costs of tobacco products, and using taxes which smokers pay on tobacco products to fund community-based tobacco reduction and cessation education and intervention programs. In addition, more and more communities and states have adopted smoke-free laws and regulations.

Although most smokers state they would like to quit smoking, people who smoke cigarettes or use other forms of tobacco often have a difficult time when they try to stop smoking. The difficulty is partly psychological; individuals get in the habit of using tobacco at certain times of day or while they are doing certain things, such as having a cup of coffee or reading the newspaper. But the habit is also hard to break for physical reasons. Tobacco contains nicotine, a drug that is as addictive as **cocaine** or heroin. Of those who have ever tried even a single cigarette, about a third become nicotine-dependent. A person who is addicted to nicotine has withdrawal symptoms, such as irritability, **anxiety**, difficulty concentrating, and craving for tobacco when he or she stops using the product.

Some people can stop smoking through willpower alone but most do better if they have support from friends, family, a physician or pharmacist, or a formal stop-smoking program. Heavy tobacco users may find that smoking cessation products also help by easing their withdrawal symptoms. Most smoking cessation products contain nicotine but the nicotine is delivered in small, steady doses spread out over many hours. In contrast, when a person inhales a cigarette, nicotine enters the **lungs** and then travels to the **brain** within seconds, delivering the "rush" that smokers crave. Another difference is that smoking cessation products do not contain the tar, carbon monoxide, and other toxins that make cigarettes so harmful to people's health.

Description

U.S. brand names

The brand names of nicotine replacement products which are sold either as over-the-counter (OTC) or non-prescription products or by prescription only in the United States are as follows:

- Nicotine patches: Habitrol (prescription), Nicoderm CQ (OTC), Nicotrol (OTC), ProStep (prescription)
- Nicotine Polacrilex Gums: Nicorette (OTC) and Nicorette DS (OTC)
- Nicotine Lozenges: Commit (OTC)
- Nicotine Inhaler: Nicotrol Inhaler (prescription)
- Nicotine Nasal Spray: Nicotrol NS (prescription)

Nicotine replacement products

Smoking cessation drugs that contain nicotine are also called nicotine substitution products or nicotine replacement therapy (NRT). Five forms are approved by the Food and Drug Administration (FDA) as of 2010—gum, skin patch, nasal spray, inhaler, and lozenges. Results of numerous research studies conducted in the United States and other countries have validated that nicotine replacement therapy (NRT) is an effective and safe approach when used as a first-line pharmacological treatment for tobacco reduction and/or cessation.

The nasal spray and inhaler are available only with a prescription, but gum, lozenges and some brands of the patch can be bought over-the-counter (without a prescription). People who buy the nonprescription products should check with a physician before starting to use them.

Other medications

Another type of smoking cessation drug, bupropion (Zyban), also reduces craving and withdrawal symptoms, although it is not a nicotine replacement product. Bupropion is an antidepressant medication that is thought to help people stop smoking by mimicking some of the effects of tobacco on brain tissue. Bupropion can be used together with nicotine replacement products. Several studies indicate that the combination helps more smokers quit than either method by itself. Bupropion is the only antidepressant currently approved by the FDA for use as a smoking cessation product.

Another non-nicotine product is the drug varenicline (Chantix). Varenicline is available only by prescription and is classified as a nicotinic receptor partial agonist. This drug works by targeting nicotine receptors in the brain. The drug attaches itself to the nicotine receptors

KEY TERMS

Acupuncture—A Chinese medical practice that treats illness or addictions by the insertion of very thin steel needles at specified points along the body's energy channels.

Bupropion—An antidepressant medication given to smokers for nicotine withdrawal symptoms. It is sold under the trade name Zyban.

Buspirone—An antianxiety medication that is also given for withdrawal symptoms. It is sold under the trade name BuSpar.

Nicotine—A colorless, oily chemical found in tobacco that makes people physically dependent on smoking. It is poisonous in large doses.

Withdrawal symptoms—A group of physical or mental symptoms that may occur when a person suddenly stops using a drug on which he or she has become dependent.

and blocks nicotine from reaching the receptors. This action blocks the pleasurable sensation smokers derive from smoking.

Alternative approaches

Other approaches that have been used to help smokers quit include hypnosis and **acupuncture**. The evidence for the usefulness of hypnosis is largely anecdotal. It appears to be most helpful when used in combination with nicotine replacement products or bupropion. Although acupuncture has been used in Western countries since the 1970s to help people quit smoking, it does not appear to be particularly effective in this regard.

Recommended dosage

The recommended dosage of nicotine replacement products depends on the method of administration. Each form of this medicine comes with detailed instructions for its use. Following directions exactly is very important. For example, nicotine gum should not be chewed like regular chewing gum. It must be chewed very slowly until it has a slight **taste** or causes a slight tingling sensation in the mouth; then "parked" between the cheek and gum until the taste and tingling goes away; then chewed and parked in the same way for about 30 minutes. Nicotine patches and other products also must be used correctly to be effective. Some patches are meant to be worn only during the day and removed at night; others are worn 24 hours a day.

Smokers who are heavily dependent on nicotine may want to ask their doctors about using a combination of nicotine replacement products. Some study results indicate that combining the transdermal patch with either the gum or the nasal spray helps more smokers quit than any of the three products by itself. Authorities believe

that the higher success rate is due to the different rates of speed at which these products deliver nicotine to the body. The nasal spray delivers nicotine very rapidly, and can be used to relieve intense cravings at times of the day when the smoker is accustomed to having a cigarette, while the patch delivers a smaller dosage of nicotine to the body at a steadier rate.

Precautions

Seeing a physician regularly while using smoking cessation drugs is important. The physician will check to make sure the medicine is working as it should and will watch for unwanted side effects.

Some side effects of smoking cessation drugs include:

- nausea
- vomiting
- severe pain in the stomach or abdomen
- severe diarrhea
- severe dizziness
- fainting
- convulsions (seizures)
- low blood pressure
- fast, weak, or irregular heartbeat
- hearing or vision problems
- severe breathing problems
- severe watering of the mouth or drooling
- cold sweat
- severe headache
- confusion
- severe weakness

Keep these drugs, including thrown-away patches and gum, out of the reach of children and pets. Even a small amount of nicotine can seriously harm a child or animal.

Nicotine in any form should not be used during **pregnancy**, as it may harm the fetus or cause **miscarriage**. Women who may become pregnant should use effective birth control while taking smoking cessation drugs. Women who become pregnant while taking this medicine should stop taking it immediately and check with their physicians.

Nicotine passes into breast milk and may cause problems for nursing babies. Women who are breastfeeding and want to use smoking cessation drugs may need to stop breastfeeding during treatment.

Anyone who has had unusual reactions to nicotine in the past should let his or her physician know before using a smoking cessation drug. The physician should also be told about any **allergies** to foods, dyes, preservatives, or other substances. People who have had a **rash** or irritation from adhesive bandages should check with a physician before using a nicotine patch.

Smoking cessation patches, gum, and other products may make certain medical problems worse. Before using a smoking cessation drug, people with any of these medical problems should make sure their physicians are aware of their conditions:

• heart or blood vessel disease

• high blood pressure

• diabetes

• overactive thyroid

• skin rash or irritation

• stomach ulcer

• pheochromocytoma (pcc) (a tumor of the adrenal medulla)

• dental problems or mouth sores

• sore throat

• jaw pain or temporomandibular joint disorder (TMJ)

There are also precautions to take with bupropion and buspirone. Bupropion should not be taken by patients with a history of seizures, high **blood pressure**, anorexia, or **bulimia nervosa**. People taking buspirone should be careful about driving or operating heavy machinery until they can tell whether the drug makes them drowsy as a side effect. Although buspirone does not interact with alcohol as intensely as most tranquilizers do, patients should still use alcohol cautiously if they are taking buspirone.

In 2009, the FDA directed the makers of the drugs varenicline (Chantix) and bupropion (Zyban) to include new warnings on the drug labels of their products related to the potential for the development of serious mental health side effects in individuals taking these drugs. Individuals with known psychiatric or mental health problems are at particularly high risk for the development of these mental health side effects, which include depression, agitation, and increased risk of suicide. Individuals without pre-existing mental health problems may also experience these serious side-effects

Side effects

Each type of smoking cessation product may cause minor side effects that usually go away as the body adjusts to the drug. These side effects usually do not need medical attention unless they continue or they interfere with normal activities. For example, nicotine gum may cause belching, jaw aches, or sore mouth or throat. Nicotine patches may cause redness, **itching**, or burning where the patch is applied. The nasal spray may irritate the nose and sinuses, while the inhaler may cause throat irritation or coughing.

If nicotine gum injures the mouth, teeth, or dental work, check with a dentist or physician as soon as possible. Other side effects are possible. Anyone who has unusual symptoms while using smoking cessation drugs should get in touch with his or her physician.

The side effects of bupropion include dry mouth and difficulty sleeping. The possible side effects of buspirone include headaches and drowsiness.

Bupropion and varenicline are associated with serious mental health side-effects including depression, agitation, thoughts of suicide, hostility, and attempted suicide. These side effects tend to occur shortly after the patient begins to take the medication and typically stop once the patient stops taking the drug. Patients experiencing these symptoms hould be closely monitored by a physician until the side-effects stop.

Interactions

People taking certain drugs may need to change their doses when they stop smoking. Anyone who uses a smoking cessation drug should let the physician know all other medicines he or she is taking and should ask whether the doses need to be changed. Examples of drugs that may be affected when a person stops smoking are:

• insulin

• airway opening drugs (bronchodilators) such as aminophylline (Somophyllin), oxtriphylline (Choledyl) and theophylline (Somophyllin-T)

• opioid (narcotic) pain relievers such as propoxyphene (Darvon)

• the beta blocker propranolol (Inderal)

Other drugs may also interact with smoking cessation drugs. Be sure to check with a physician or pharmacist before combining smoking cessation drugs with any other prescription or nonprescription (over-the-counter) medicine.

Bupropion should not be used by patients who are also taking monoamine oxidase inhibitor (MAOI) medications. These include such drugs as furazolidone, isocarboxazid, and phenelzine. Bupropion may also interact with phenytoin, carbamazepine, and levodopa. Buspirone also interacts with MAOIs, as well as with trazadone and haloperidol.

Resources

PERIODICALS

Aubin, H.J., et al. "Varenicline Versus Transdermal Nicotine Patch for Smoking Cessation: Results from a Randomized Open–Label Trial." *Thorax.* 63(8) (2008): 717–24.

Etter, J.F. and E. Laszlo. "Postintervention Effect of Nicotine Replacement Therapy for Smoking Reduction: A Randomized Trial with a 5–year Follow–up." *Journal of Clinical Psychopharmacology.* 27(2) (2007): 151–5.

Kralikova, E., et al. "Smoking Cessation or Reduction with Nicotine Replacement Therapy: A Placebo–controlled Double Blind Trial with Nicotine Gum and Inhaler." *BMC Public Health.* 9 (2009): 433.

Lemmens, V., et al. "Effectiveness of Smoking Cessation Interventions Among Adults: A Systematic Review." *European Journal of Cancer Prevention.* 17(6) (2008): 535–44.

Ray, R., R.A. Schnoll, and C. Lerman. "Pharmacogenetics and Smoking Cessation Replacement Therapy." *CNS Drugs.* 21(7) (2007): 525–33.

Schnoll, R.A., et al. "Effectiveness of Extended–Duration Transdermal Nicotine Therapy: A Randomized Trial." *Annals of Internal Medicine.* 152 (February 2, 2010): 144–151.

OTHER

"Prevention and Cessation of Cigarette Smoking: Control of Tobacco Use (PDQ)." National Cancer Institute. October 23, 2009. http://www.cancer.gov [Accessed September 15, 2010].

Stead, L.F., et al. "Nicotine Replacement Therapy for Smoking Cessation (Review). Cochrane Database for Systematic Reviews." 1:CD000146. [Accessed September 15, 2010] http://www2.cochrane.org/reviews/en/ab000146.html.

ORGANIZATIONS

American Association for Respiratory Care (AARC), 9425 N. MacArthur Blvd., Suite 100, Irving, TX 75063-4706, (972) 243-2272, http://www.aarc.org

American Cancer Society (ACS),(800) ACS-2345, Fax: (404) 329-7530, http://www.cancer.org

American Lung Association (ALA), 1301 Pennsylvania Ave. NW, Suite 800, Washington, DC 20004, (202) 785-3355, Fax: (201) 452-1805, http://www.lungusa.org

Office on Smoking and Health. Centers for Disease Control and Prevention (CDC-OSH), 4770 Buford Hwy, NE. MS K-50, Atlanta, GA 30341-3717, (800) CDC-INFO (232-4636), http://www.cdc.gov/tobacco.

Rebecca J. Frey, PhD
Melinda Granger Oberleitner, RN, DNS, APRN, CNS

Snoring

Definition

Snoring is a sound generated during sleep by vibration of loose tissue in the upper airway.

Description

Snoring is one symptom of a group of disorders known as sleep disordered breathing. It occurs when the soft palate, uvula, tongue, tonsils, and/or muscles in the back of the throat rub against each other and generate a vibrating sound during sleep. 20% of all adults are chronic snorers and 45% of normal adults snore occasionally. As people grow older, their chance of snoring increases. Approximately half of all individuals over 60 snore regularly.

In some cases, snoring is a symptom of a more serious disorder called obstructed **sleep apnea** (OSA). OSA occurs when part of the airway is closed off (usually at the back of the throat) while a person is trying to inhale during sleep, and breathing stops for more than 10 seconds before resuming again. These breathless episodes can occur as many as several hundred times a night.

People with OSA almost always snore heavily because the same narrowing of the airway that causes snoring can also cause OSA. Snoring may actually attribute to OSA as well, because the vibration of the throat tissues which occurs in snoring can cause the tissue to swell.

Snoring is associated with physical problems as well as social **stress**. People who do not suffer from OSA may be diagnosed with socially unacceptable snoring (SUS), which refers to snoring that is loud enough to prevent the sleeper's bed partner or roommate from sleeping. SUS is a factor in the breakup of some marriages and other long-term relationships. Moreover, a study published in 2002 indicates that people who snore are at increased risk of developing type 2 diabetes. Snoring appears to be a risk factor that is independent of body weight or a family history of diabetes.

Causes and symptoms

There are several major causes of snoring, including:

• Excessively relaxed throat muscles. Alcohol, drugs, and sedatives can cause the throat muscles to become lax, and/or the tongue to pull back into the airway.

• Large uvula. The piece of tissue that hangs from the back of the throat is called the uvula. Individuals with a large or longer than average uvula can suffer from snoring when the uvula vibrates in the airway.

• Large tonsils and/or adenoids. The tonsils (tissue at the back of either side of the throat) can also vibrate if they are larger than normal, as can the adenoids.

• Excessive weight. Overweight people are more likely to snore. This is frequently caused by the extra throat and neck tissue they are carrying around.

• Nasal congestion. Colds and allergies can plug the nose, creating a vacuum in the throat that results in snoring as airflow increases.

• Cysts and tumors. Cysts and/or tumors of the throat can trigger snoring.

• Structural problems of the nose. A deviated septum or other nasal problems can also cause snoring.

Diagnosis

A patient interview, and possibly an interview with the patient's spouse or anyone else in the household who has witnessed the snoring, is usually enough for a diagnosis of snoring. A medical history that includes questions about alcohol or tranquilizer use; past ear, nose, and throat problems; and the pattern and degree of snoring will be completed, and a physical exam will be performed to determine the cause of the problem. This will typically include examination of the throat to look for narrowing, obstruction, or malformations. If the snoring is suspected to be a symptom of a more serious disorder such as obstructive sleep apnea, the patient will require further testing. This testing is called a **polysomnography** study, and is conducted during an overnight stay in a specialized sleep laboratory. The polysomnography study include measurements of **heart** rate, airflow at the mouth and nose, respiratory effort, sleep stage (e.g., light sleep, deep sleep, dream sleep), and oxygen level in the **blood**.

In some cases the patient may be referred to a dentist or orthodontist for evaluation of the jaw structure and dentition.

In addition, the patient may be examined by sleep endoscopy. In this procedure, the patient is given a medication (midazolam) to induce sleep. His or her throat and nasal passages are then examined with a flexible laryngoscope. In many cases, sleep endoscopy reveals obstructions that are not apparent during a standard **physical examination** of the throat. Many patients are found to have obstructions at more than one level in their breathing passages.

Treatment

Several surgical procedures are available for treating chronic snoring, including

• Uvulopalathopharyngoplasty (UPPP), a surgical procedure which involves removing excess throat tissues (e.g., tonsils, parts of the soft palate) to expand the airway.

• Laser-assisted uvulopalatoplasty (LAUP) uses a surgical laser to remove part of the uvula and palate.

• Palatal stiffening is a minimally invasive surgical technique where a laser or a cauterizer is used to produce scar tissue in the soft palate in order to stop the vibrations that produce snoring.

• Radiofrequency ablation is another technique which uses scarring to shrink the uvula and/or soft palate. A needle electrode is used to shrink and scar the mouth and throat tissues.

Alternative treatment

There are a number of remedies for snoring, but few are proven clinically effective. Popular treatments include:

• Mechanical devices. Many splints, braces, and other devices are available which reposition the nose, jaw, and/or mouth in order to clear the airways. Other devices are designed to wake an individual when snoring occurs. Patients should consult a dentist or orthodontist about these devices, as most require custom fitting. In addition, persons with certain types of gum disease or dental problems should not be fitted with oral appliances to stop snoring.

• Nasal strips. Nasal strips that attach like an adhesive bandage to the bridge of the nose are available at most drugstores and can help stop snoring in some individuals by opening the nasal passages.

• Continuous positive airway pressure (CPAP). Some chronic snorers find relief by sleeping with a nasal mask which provides air pressure to the throat.

• Decongestants. Snoring caused by nasal congestion may be successfully treated with decongestants. Some

KEY TERMS

Ablation—The removal of abnormal tissue growths by surgery.

Cauterize—To seal tissue or blood vessels using a heat or electrical source.

Continuous positive airway pressure (CPAP)—A ventilation device that blows a gentle stream of air into the nose during sleep to keep the airway open.

Deviated septum—A hole or perforation in the septum, the wall that divides the two nasal cavities.

Endoscope—A slender optical instrument that allows a doctor to examine the inside of the throat or other hollow organ. Sleep endoscopy is a technique that allows the doctor to detect previously

unsuspected obstructions in the patient's nose and throat.

Obstructive sleep apnea (OSA)—A potentially life-threatening condition characterized by episodes of breathing cessation during sleep alternating with snoring or disordered breathing. The low levels of oxygen in the blood of patients with OSA may eventually cause heart problems or stroke.

Polysomnography—A technique for diagnosing sleep disorders with the use of a machine that records the pulse, breathing rate and other variables while the patient sleeps.

Soft palate—The structure at the roof of the mouth that separates the mouth and the pharynx.

---

effective herbal remedies that clear the nasal passages include golden rod (*Solidago virgauria*) and golden seal (*Hydrastis canadensis*). Steam inhalation of essential oils of eucalyptus blue gum (*Eucalyptus globulus*) or peppermint (*Mentha x piperata*) can also relieve congestion.

- Weight loss. Snoring thought to be caused by excessive weight may be curtailed by a sensible weight loss and exercise program.

- Sleep position. Snoring usually worsens when an individual sleeps on his or her back, so sleeping on one's side may alleviate the problem. Those who have difficulty staying in a side sleeping position may find sleeping with pillows behind them helps them maintain the position longer. Other devices include a new vest designed to prevent the sleeper from lying on his or her back.

- Bed adjustments. For some people, raising the head of the bed solves their snoring problem. A slight incline can prevent the tongue from retracting into the back of the throat. Bricks, wooden blocks, or specially designed wedges can be used to elevate the head of the bed approximately 4–l6 in (10–41 cm).

Alternative treatments that have been reported to be effective for patients whose snoring is caused by colds or **allergies** include **acupuncture**, **homeopathy**, and aromatherapy treatments. Aromatherapy treatments for snoring typically make use of marjoram oil, which is thought to be particularly effective in clearing the nasal passages.

Prevention

Adults with a history of snoring may be able to prevent snoring episodes with the following measures:

- avoid alcohol and sedatives before bedtime

- remove allergens from the bedroom

- use a decongestant before bed

- sleep on the side, not the back

Resources

BOOKS

Beers, Mark H., Robert S. Porter, and Thomas V. Jones, eds. *The Merck Manual of Diagnosis and Therapy*. 18th ed. Whitehouse Station, NJ: Merck Research Laboratories, 2006.

Pascualy, Ralph A. *Snoring and Sleep Apnea: Sleep Well, Feel Better*. New York: Demos Health, 2008.

PERIODICALS

Ellis, S.G., et al. "Dental Appliances for Snoring and Obstructive Sleep Apnoea: Construction Aspects for General Dental Practitioners." *Dental Update* 30 (January-February 2003): 16–22, 24–26.

Hassid, S., et al. "UPPP for Snoring: Long-Term Results and Patient Satisfaction." *Acta Otorhinolaryngologica Belgica* 56 (2002): 157–162.

Maurer, J.T., B.A. Stuck, G. Hein, et al. "Treatment of Obstructive Sleep Apnea with a New Vest Preventing the Supine Position." [in German] *Deutsche medizinische Wochenschrift* 128 (January 17, 2003): 71–75.

Nakano, H., T. Ikeda, M. Hayashi, et al. "Effects of Body Position on Snoring in Apneic and Nonapneic Snorers." *Sleep* 26 (March 15, 2003): 169–172.

Remacle, M., et al. "Laser-Assisted Surgery Addressing Snoring Long-Term Outcome Comparing CO_2 Laser vs. CO_2 Laser Combined with Diode Laser." *Acta Otorhinolaryngologica Belgica* 56 (2002): 177–182.

Trotter, M.I., A.R. D'Souza, and D.W. Morgan. "Medium-Term Outcome of Palatal Surgery for Snoring Using the Somnus Unit." *Journal of Laryngology and Otology* 116 (February 2002): 116–118.

OTHER

American Sleep Apnea Association (ASAA). Considering Surgery for Snoring? (Accessed December 15, 2010) http://www.sleepapnea.org/resources/pubs/snoring.html.

National Heart, Lung, and Blood Institute (NHLBI). Facts About Sleep Apnea. NIH Publication No. 95-3798. [cited April 13, 2003]. http://www.nhlbi.nih.gov/health/public/sleep/insomnia.txt.

ORGANIZATIONS

American Academy of Otolaryngology—Head and Neck Surgery, 1650 Diagonal Road, Alexandria, VA 22314-2857, (703) 836-4444, http://www.entnet.org

American Academy of Sleep Medicine (AASM), 2510 N. Frontage Road, Darien, IL 60561, (630) 737-9700, Fax: (630) 737-9790, inquiries@aasmnet.org, http://www.aasmnet.org

American Dental Association, 211 E. Chicago Ave., Chicago, IL 60611-2678, (312) 440-2500, http://www.ada.org

American Sleep Apnea Association, 6856 Eastern Avenue, NW, Suite 203, Washington, DC 20012, (202) 293-3650, Fax: (202) 293-3656, http://www.sleepapnea.org/

National Sleep Foundation, 1522 K St. NW, Suite 500, Washington, DC 20005, (202) 347-3471, Fax: (202) 347-2472, http://www.sleepfoundation.org

Paula Anne Ford-Martin
Rebecca J. Frey, Ph.D.

Social work in health care

Definition

Social work in health care helps people who are dealing with a medical problem to function within their situation. The social worker who specializes in health care works with clients and their families to provide services necessary to make their lives easier for the duration of the client's illness, and to help them deal with the consequences directly related to that illness.

Description

According to the code of ethics of the National Association of Social Workers (NASW), the profession of social work is dedicated to a set of core values. These values include social justice, service, dignity and worth of the person, importance of human relationships, integrity, and competence, and they form the foundation of social work. Social workers in the medical field provide a wide variety of services to clients who are going through a short-term medical crisis, suffering from chronic illnesses, facing a life-threatening disease, or in need of long-term care or **rehabilitation**.

The main concern of the social worker is to assist the client and the client's family in coping with their health care situation. Clients are faced with many problems when they have an accident, contract a sudden and debilitating illness, or are diagnosed with a chronic or life-threatening disease. Social workers help them assess these problems, identify their immediate and long term needs, and find resources to supply the needs.

Within the health care setting, the social worker has many responsibilities. The services provided by the social worker depend on the needs of the client. The worker acts as an advocate to secure the client's rights, directly counsels the client and the client's family, and refers the client to other social agencies, community resources, or facilities that can meet the client's immediate and long-term needs. The services provided by the social worker always depend upon the client's needs and the health care setting.

If the social worker is working in a hospital, these duties may include setting up home health care services after the client's discharge, arranging for meals to be delivered to the client's home, and setting appointments for follow-up care. The worker may also make arrangements for transportation to doctor's appointments and community social service agencies, and for long-term care within another facility.

Work settings

Duties of the social worker vary with the health care setting. Medical social workers may work in a hospital, **hospice**, assisted living center, nursing home, physical rehabilitation center, clinic, home health care agency, or drug rehabilitation or mental health center. Social workers may work in the health care facility or make home visits to work with their clients. They often work with other agencies and have to travel short distances for meetings with the agency members. Social workers confer with other agency workers or with health care team members to assess client needs and to make plans for the client's care.

Hours of work vary for the social worker, depending upon the facility or agency within which he is employed.

Usually the work hours are between 8 AM and 5 PM Monday through Friday, but the worker may be required to work hours as needed for emergencies. In larger urban areas or rural areas, the social worker may also be required to work during evening hours and on weekends to better serve the clients.

Education and training

Education, training, and licensing requirements may vary from state to state, but the NASW states that the minimum educational requirement for social workers is a baccalaureate degree in social work (BSW). However, people who hold a bachelor's degree in another discipline such as psychology, sociology, or urban studies may also qualify for entrance level jobs.

BSW programs prepare students for direct care of clients. Students who choose to major in social work must complete courses in social work practice, social work policies, human behavior and social environment, research methods, social work values and ethics, study of populations at risk, and the promotion of social justice. They must also complete 400 hours of supervised field work.

An advanced degree is the standard for many positions in social work including positions within the field of health care. A master's degree in social work (MSW) allows the social worker to be certified for clinical and supervisory work.

Advanced education and training

A master's degree in social work qualifies the social worker to make clinical assessments, choose an area of specialization, manage large caseloads, and supervise social workers with lesser degrees. In addition to courses of specialization and assessment, the MSW candidate must complete 900 hours of supervised field work, or an internship.

Social workers may also acquire a Ph.D. or D.W. in social work. This is required if they want to teach in an accredited program at a university or to work in a supervisory position as the head of a social service program.

The National Association of Social Workers requires social workers to complete 90 hours of continuing education classes every three years to continue their certification in the profession. Licensed professionals with advanced degrees may be required to complete more than 90 hours of continuing education classes.

KEY TERMS

BSW—Baccalaureate degree in social work.

Long-term care—Placement of client in a facility that provides nursing and basic needs care when client is no longer able to provide that care at home.

MSW—Master's degree in social work.

NASW—National Association of Social Workers.

Needs assessment—Social worker conducts an interview with client and family, reviews charts, interviews other health workers to determine what specific services are required by client.

Urban studies—Course work in the sociology of urban areas.

Future outlook

Social work is a growing profession. The occupational outlook is optimistic. The national Bureau of Labor Statistics predicts that growth will continue at a rate exceeding that of other occupations until at least 2008. There are several reasons why the field of social work in health care continues to grow:

- the aging population of "baby boomers"

- advanced medical treatment

- longer life expectancy

- growth of home health care due to growing trend of early release of patients from hospitals

- replacement of workers seeking career change

- stress and burnout among social workers causing them to leave profession

- increase in population of people living with AIDS

Resources

BOOK

Occupational Outlook Handbook, 2011-2012 Ed. Washington, DC: U.S. Department of Labor, 2011.

ORGANIZATION

National Association of Social Workers. 750 First Street NE, Suite 700, Washington, DC 20002-4241. http//www.naswdc.org.

Peggy Elaine Browning

Social work law

Definition

Social work law is a general term that refers to the legal aspects of social work practice, such as understanding the general relationship between the justice system and social work, having a working knowledge of the laws and regulatory agencies that affect one's particular area of social work, and being prepared to serve as a witness in courtroom cases.

Description

Since many social workers are employed by state or local government agencies, they need to know the extent of their powers and duties. In addition, the rapid rise in **malpractice** suits against social workers since the 1980s means that social workers need to inform themselves about their legal risks. Furthermore, social workers are subject to several sets of regulations or codes of ethics that may conflict at various points with civil or criminal law in their specific jurisdiction. These other sets of standards may include:

• professional licensing and disciplinary requirements

• codes of ethics such as the code revised by the National Association of Social Workers (NASW) in 1999

• regulations and policies established by the agency that employs the social worker

• local cultural or community standards of care

• the social worker's own sense of professionalism

The term "social work law" is also applied to the legal standards governing the training and certification of social workers. In the United Kingdom, for example, the title of "social worker" was defined by law in April 2005. It can be used only by persons who have met certain educational requirements and are registered either with the General Social Care Council (in England) or with its counterparts in Scotland, Wales, or Northern Ireland.

In the United States, the legal regulation of social work (like medicine, dentistry, and other health care professions) is delegated by the Constitution to the individual states. In most states, the legislature establishes a board of social work and gives it the necessary powers to define the practice of social work, determine the necessary qualifications, and license practitioners. In a few states, a department overseeing various advisory boards administers the practice act and other relevant law. Even a brief reading of the definitions of social work obtained from the 50 states and 10 Canadian provinces by the Association of Social Work Boards (ASWB), however, indicates considerable variety in length,

specificity, and areas of emphasis. In addition, the increasing division of social work into such specialties as **psychotherapy** and counseling, family crisis intervention, issues related to **aging**, employee assistance programs, policy planning and research, advocacy and community organizing, school and educational programs, refugee assistance, and many others, complicates any discussion of social work law.

History

Social work has been involved with the legal system of the United States for almost a century and a half. Unlike medicine, however, social work is a relatively new profession; it was not recognized as a separate vocation until the early twentieth century. Social work began around the time of the Civil War as a form of urban missionary outreach by the mainline Protestant churches. As the large cities of the United States grew at the expense of rural areas, and as millions of new immigrants from Europe and Asia entered the country, there was a great need for practical assistance in helping these new Americans find work, educate their children, and obtain satisfactory housing. Much of this early relief work was done by volunteers. The Sanitation Commission and the Freedmen's Bureau, government bodies that were established during the Civil War to provide **public health** measures and assist former slaves, were also precursors of modern social work. In addition, the 1860s saw the establishment of the first state-run institutions for orphans, the poor, and the mentally ill.

By the 1890s, it was obvious that the various forms of relief and social welfare work needed to be carried out on a systematic and "scientific" basis. Volunteer "friendly visitors," as they had been called, were gradually replaced by salaried case workers who saw themselves as detached and objective professionals. The term "social worker" itself was first used in the 1890s. The early professional social workers—most of whom were college-educated women who had few other opportunities to use their degrees—attended training programs to improve their casework skills. By 1900 social work began to expand into the fields of child welfare and the juvenile justice system. Social workers also were involved with the legal system through their involvement with local politics in order to improve the lives of their clients. These experiences convinced many that it was as important to change the structures of society as to help individuals.

After World War I (1914–1918), social workers began to specialize, creating such new fields as medical social work, psychiatric social work, and school social work. Psychiatry in particular became a large area of specialization; as of 2005 there are more social workers licensed as mental health care providers in the United States than psychiatrists, psychologists, and psychiatric nurses combined; and 40% of social workers presently list mental health care as their primary field of practice. The first professional organizations of social workers were formed during this period; the National Conference of Social Workers came into being in 1917. Colleges and universities began offering courses to prepare students as social workers; the first graduate school of social work was founded at the University of Chicago in 1920.

The Great Depression of the 1930s and the New Deal finally brought social work into the sphere of public policy. The first woman Cabinet member, Frances Perkins, had been a social worker before she became Secretary of Labor in 1933. As the scope of government involvement with health, education, and social issues continued to expand after World War II, social workers participated in public policy research as well as working with the criminal justice system through youth services, child protection services, domestic violence and **substance abuse** programs, and programs for prison inmates. In 1955, seven professional social work groups merged to form the National Association of Social Workers (NASW), which presently provides continuing education and credentialing for 150,000 social workers in the United States. The association states that it "is proud to be actively involved in state and national legislation." It also informs members on a regular basis of legal changes or decisions that may affect their work.

Professional liability

For most of the history of social work as a profession, lawsuits against social workers were uncommon. The number has risen sharply since the mid-1980s for several reasons:

- Social work has become more specialized. This trend means that clients expect higher standards of education, general competence, and specific skills from social workers.

- State legislatures and courts are abolishing the immunity from liability that formerly protected social workers in public agencies. In addition, courts and legislatures are continually revising and expanding such concepts as "protect and warn," which extends the range of duties that a social worker is required to fulfill. The *Tarasoff* case of 1976 was a particularly important ruling because it established warning potential victims of a client's intent to harm them, as a social worker's legal duty.

- Clients are more knowledgeable now than in the past about ways to pursue malpractice litigation or file ethics complaints against a social worker. Many people are aware, for example, that they can contact the state licensure board or professional organizations such as the NASW as well as file civil or criminal charges against a social worker.

- More and more social workers are employed on a fee-for-service basis. This change has detracted from the ideal of "pure service" that tended to discourage lawsuits against social workers in the past.

- Shrinking resources and cost-containment measures often result in premature termination of a social worker's services, which may lead to resentment on the client's part and a lawsuit for damages.

- Social work has a much higher profile as a profession in the early 2000s than it did even in the recent past. Greater visibility and higher status lead to increased demands for accountability.

Social workers in certain settings are at increased risk for lawsuits. These higher-risk types of practice include group practices, managed care settings, and child protection services. In group practices, all the members of the group may be held liable for the actions of one member. Managed care contexts are high-risk because cost-containment guidelines and the reimbursement system may put pressure on a social worker to terminate services to a client, who may then sue if he or she thinks their best interests have not been served. Lastly, child welfare settings carry special risks for liability, ranging from charges of inadequate investigation or wrongful removal of a child to overly intrusive investigation and returning a child to dangerous parents. Social workers who specialize in child welfare work frequently find themselves in "no-win" situations, caught between agency rules and regulations, the child's best interests, and the parents' wishes or demands.

There are several different classes of professional liability for social workers in the United States:

- Malpractice or negligence. Malpractice in law refers to "any professional misconduct, unreasonable lack of skill or fidelity in professional or fiduciary duties, evil practices, or immoral or illegal conduct." Negligence refers to carelessness or failure to take reasonable and prudent measures to ensure that others are not harmed by one's actions. It may include performing an action incorrectly (commission) as well as failing to take appropriate action (omission). Malpractice and negligence are classified as torts, which are civil cases involving wrongful acts that result in harm to another person or to property. Tort law covers intentional as well as unintentional acts. It is decided by common (court) law rather than statutory law; that is, a civil court rather than the legislature determines whether a wrongful act involves tort liability. Most malpractice actions against social workers involve negligence or failure to meet professional standards of care. According to the NASW, between 1969 and 1995, 53% of all malpractice suits against social workers were filed for incorrect treatment, sexual misconduct, breach of privacy, or a client's attempted suicide.

- Other civil violations. This category includes legal actions related to civil rights violations, violations of privacy, breaches of confidentiality, improper supervision, and breaches of contract. Improper supervision covers cases in which a field placement supervisor allows an intern or trainee to offer counseling to clients or perform other services above the trainee's level of competence and licensing. An example of a breach-of-contract case is a lawsuit brought by an insurance company against a social worker who had agreed to require co-payment from a client and then failed to bill the client.

- Criminal liability. In some states, sexual misconduct is a criminal rather than a civil offense; others allow criminal charges to be filed as well as a malpractice suit. Criminal cases differ from civil suits in two important respects. The first is that a higher standard of proof is required in criminal cases. In a malpractice or other civil suit, the case is decided on the basis of "preponderance of the evidence," which means that the evidence presented by one party in the case is considered more believable than that that produced by the other. In criminal cases, however, the defendant's guilt must be shown "beyond a reasonable doubt," which is a much more stringent criterion. The second major difference is that professional liability insurance cannot be used to cover the costs of defending oneself against a criminal charge.

- Infractions of professional licensing standards or regulations. These regulations may include title protection laws, which cover the use of such professional titles as "certified social worker" or "clinical social worker," practice regulation acts, which define the boundaries of a profession's services and activities, and registration laws, which define who is entitled to practice in each state. In the United States, a license to practice social work in one state is not transferable to another unless the two states in question have a reciprocity agreement to recognize each other's licensure procedures. In most cases, the social worker must apply for a new license if he or she moves to another state. The ASWB maintains a social work registry to facilitate the transfer of licensure documentation when a social worker moves. The ASWB also maintains a database of social workers who have been disciplined, known as the Disciplinary Action Reporting System or

DARS. As of the early 2000s, 42 of the 50 states send reports of disciplinary actions to DARS.

- Ethical violations. Ethical violations refer to breaking rules that reflect the values or goals of the profession. In the case of social work, these values include such ideals as respect for all persons, service to others, concern for social justice, maintaining high standards of competence, and the like. In most cases, state regulations simply incorporate the profession's recognized code of ethics and there are no conflicts between state law and professional standards. In instances of an actual or potential ethical dilemma, however, the social worker is advised to seek the advice of an attorney. Common examples of such ethical dilemmas include giving a client access to his or her clinical records, deciding whether to terminate or retain a client who is noncompliant or defaults on paying fees, or withholding potentially damaging information from some members of a family at the request of others.

Reducing the risk of litigation

Social workers in the early 2000s can lower the risk of a lawsuit by taking the following precautions:

- Maintain a high level of professional competence.

- Document *all* professional decisions and interventions clearly and completely.

- Obtain personal professional liability coverage rather than assuming that one will be covered by an employer's insurance.

- Become familiar with state and local licensing regulations.

- Find an attorney who is knowledgeable about malpractice, professional regulation, mental health law, and social welfare law, and have an initial consultation with him or her.

- Reread the NASW code of ethics periodically and abide by its recommendations.

Another aspect of risk reduction is dealing effectively with personal **stress** and avoiding substance abuse. According to several groups of researchers, marital or emotional stress is the most common cause of professional impairment among social workers. Social workers, however, also have a higher-than-average rate of alcohol and drug (AOD) problems compared to the general population. One study of 751 social workers, all of whom were members of NASW, reported that 21% had used illegal drugs since becoming social workers, 28% had had episodes of binge drinking in the previous year, 34% reported at least one incident in their practice that had occurred when they were impaired by substance use, and 39% reported that they had worked when they were too

KEY TERMS

Civil law—The branch of law that deals with matters between two individuals or between an individual and the government that do not concern criminal acts.

Common law—The system of law that originated in England between 1300 and 1500 and is based on custom or court decisions rather than laws enacted by a ruler or legislature. Common law is also known as case law.

Forensic—Referring to legal or courtroom matters.

Liability—The state or condition of being legally responsible for an act or event.

Negligence—Failure to perform one's professional duties according to an accepted standard of care.

Pro bono—Performed or donated without charge. The Latin phrase literally means "for the good."

Statutory law—Written law enacted by a legislature, as distinguished from unwritten law or common law.

Tarasoff case—A 1976 case in which the Supreme Court of California ruled that therapists or counselors have an "affirmative duty" to directly warn a potential victim of harm intended by the therapist's client; notifying the police is not considered sufficient to fulfill this duty. Tatiana Tarasoff was a university student who had been stalked and eventually killed by another student who was upset because she had rejected him.

Tort—A wrongful act against another person or property that results in harm. Torts are considered civil cases and are settled by common law (court decisions) rather than by statutory law.

upset to carry out their duties effectively. All of these are risk factors for making an error of judgment that may lead to a civil or criminal lawsuit.

Education and training

In the present legal climate, it is critical for social workers to understand the areas of social work practice regulated by their specific jurisdiction. Most states regulate four areas of practice based on academic degrees with or without additional qualifications. They are: bachelor's degree in social work (BSW) upon graduation; master's degree in social work (MSW) upon graduation; MSW plus two years of postgraduate supervised experience; and MSW with two years of

postgraduate direct clinical work experience. Some states, however, regulate only one or two of these areas. Only a few states license social workers with an associate's degree. The ASWB offers five competency examinations for different categories of state licensure: Associate, Bachelors, Masters, Advanced Generalist, and Clinical. The NASW has a Credentialing Center that certifies eligible candidates as Qualified Clinical Social Workers (QCSW; for entry-level clinicians) or as Diplomates in Clinical Social Work (DCSW; for private practitioners and advanced clinicians).

Advanced education and training

A growing number of social workers in the United States and Canada are earning advanced degrees in social work itself or in a closely related field. The United States Department of Labor noted in early 2005 that "while a bachelor's degree [in social work] is the minimum requirement, a master's degree ... has become the standard for many positions."

Certified specialties

In addition to credentialing clinical social workers, the NASW offers two specialty certifications for holders of the BSW and five for holders of the MSW. Social workers with a bachelor's degree may be certified as a Children, Youth, and Family Social Worker (C-CYFSW) or a Social Work Case Manager (C-SWCM). Those with an MSW may be certified as a School Social Work Specialist (C-SSWS), an Advanced Social Case Work Manager (C-ASWCM), a Clinical Alcohol, Tobacco, and Other Drugs Social Worker (C-CATODSW), a Social Worker in Healthcare (C-SWHC), or an Advanced Children, Youth, and Family Social Worker (C-ACYFSW).

Forensic social work

Some social workers choose to specialize in working with civil courts or the criminal justice system. Forensic social work developed within the profession around the turn of the twentieth century when the National Conference of Charities and Corrections (NCCC; one of the groups that preceded the NASW) was formed. As of 2005, forensic social work has become a credentialed specialty for social workers who meet regularly with judges, lawyers, corrections officers, and other personnel in the legal system. The National Organization of Forensic Social Work (NOFSW) defines the specialty as follows: "[Forensic social work] includes social work practice which in any way is related to legal issues and litigation, both criminal and civil. Child custody issues involving separation, divorce, **neglect**, termination of parental rights; the implications of child and spouse abuse; juvenile and adult justice services; corrections and mandated treatment; all fall under this definition." The organization provides professional certification at the diplomate level for members who meet its standards.

The emergence of forensic social work as a specialty, together with the expansion of interest in programs for social change and other fields requiring knowledge of the law, has led to the creation of joint degree programs in social work and law at a number of universities. Most of these programs allow a student to earn both a JD (Juris Doctor; the professional degree in law) and a master's degree in social work at the end of four years of courses. From the side of the legal profession, most law schools in the United States now offer students the option of working for a semester or longer in various public interest and pro bono (free of charge) programs that overlap with social work, such as clinics in tenants' rights, domestic violence, health law, and family law.

Future outlook

In spite of increasing concern about vulnerability to litigation, social work is an expanding field as of the early 2000s. The demand for social workers in hospitals is slowing because of limits on the length of patient stays. However, the aging of the baby boomer generation will generate an increased need for social workers trained in gerontology. Another area of increasing need is social work with substance abusers, as the legal system is placing more persons in treatment programs than in prison. Still another area of growth is social work in rural areas, which are often underserved in comparison to cities.

Resources

BOOKS

Houston-Vega, Mary Kay, and Elane M. Nuehring, with Elisabeth R. Daguio. *Prudent Practice: A Guide for Managing Malpractice Risk*. Washington, DC: NASW Press, 1997.

Johns, Robert. *Using the Law in Social Work*. Exeter, UK: Learning Matters, 2003.

Neighbors, Ira A., et al., eds. *Social Work and the Law: Proceedings of the National Organization of Forensic Social Work, 2000*. New York: The Haworth Press, 2002.

PERIODICALS

Herbert, P. B. "Psychotherapy as Law Enforcement." *Journal of the American Academy of Psychiatry and the Law* 32 (2004): 91–95.

Katsavdakis, K.A., G.O. Gabbard, and G.I. Athey, Jr. "Profiles of Impaired Health Professionals." *Bulletin of the Menninger Clinic* 68 (Winter 2004): 60–72.

Lynch, Joseph G., and Gregory R. Versen. "Social Work Supervisor Liability: Risk Factors and Strategies for Risk

Reduction." *Administration in Social Work* 27 (Summer 2003): 57–73.

Surface, David. "Malpractice Minefield—Eluding the Long Arm of the Law." *Social Work Today* 5 (March 2005): 28–33.

OTHER

Addictions Committee, New York City Chapter of the National Association of Social Workers. Helping Social Workers with Alcohol and Other Drug Problems: Options for Intervening with Colleagues. New York: NYCC-NASW, 1994.

National Association of Social Workers (NASW). Code of Ethics of the National Association of Social Workers. Approved by the 1996 NASW Delegate Assembly and revised by the 1999 NASW Delegate Assembly. http://www.socialworkers.org/pubs/code/code.asp.

National Association of Social Workers (NASW). The Power of Social Work. Washington, DC: NASW, 2004.

U.S. Department of Labor, Bureau of Labor Statistics. Occupational Outlook Handbook, 2004–05. http://www.bls.gov/oco/ocos060.htm.

ORGANIZATIONS

American Bar Association (ABA). 321 North Clark Street, Chicago, IL 60610. (312) 988-5000. http://www.abanet.org

Association of Social Work Boards (ASWB). 400 South Ridge Parkway, Suite B, Culpeper, VA 22701. (540) 829-6880 or (800) 225-6880. Fax: (540) 829-0142. http://www.aswb.org.

National Association of Social Workers (NASW). 750 First Street, NE, Suite 700, Washington, DC 20002. http://www.socialworkers.org.

National Organization of Forensic Social Work (NOFSW). 2600 Dixwell Avenue, Suite 7, Hamden, CT 06514. (203) 230-8289. Fax: (203) 248-8932. http://www.nofsw.org.

Rebecca J. Frey, Ph.D.

Sodium bicarbonate *see* **Antacids**

Sodium test *see* **Electrolyte tests**

Soft tissue mobilization *see* **Massage therapy**

Somatization disorder *see* **Somatoform disorders**

Somatoform disorders

Definition

Somatoform disorders is the umbrella term developed by the *Diagnostic and Statistical Manual of Mental Disorders (DSM-IV)* in 1980 to describe a group of conditions characterized by the presence of physical symptoms without evidence of a physiologic cause.

DSM-IV divides these conditions into six separate psychiatric disorders.

- somatization disorder
- undifferentiated somatoform disorder
- conversion disorder
- pain disorder
- hypochondriasis
- body dysmorphic disorder

Description

It is helpful to understand that the present classification of these disorders reflects recent historical changes in the practice of medicine and psychiatry. When psychiatry first became a separate branch of medicine at the end of the nineteenth century, the term hysteria was commonly used to describe mental disorders characterized by altered states of consciousness (for example, sleepwalking or trance states) or physical symptoms (for example, a "paralyzed" arm or leg with no neurologic cause) that could not be fully explained by a medical disease. The term dissociation was used for the psychological mechanism that allows the mind to split off uncomfortable feelings, memories, or ideas so that they are lost to conscious recall. Sigmund Freud and other pioneering psychoanalysts thought that the hysterical patient's symptoms resulted from dissociated thoughts or memories reemerging through bodily functions or trance states. Prior to the fourth edition of *DSM* in 1980, all mental disorders that were considered to be forms of hysteria were grouped together on the basis of this theory about their cause. Since 1980, however, the somatoform disorders and the so-called dissociative disorders have been placed in separate categories on the basis of their chief symptoms. In general, the somatoform disorders are characterized by disturbances in the patient's physical sensations or ability to move the limbs or walk, while the dissociative disorders are marked by disturbances in the patient's sense of identity or **memory**.

Somatization disorder

Somatization disorder was formerly called Briquet's syndrome, after the French physician who first recognized it. Z.J. Lipowski defined somatization in the *American Journal of Psychiatry* as "the tendency to experience and communicate somatic distress and symptoms not accounted for by pathologic findings, to attribute them to physical illness and to seek medical help for them."

Somatization disorder typically begins before the age of 30. It is estimated that worldwide, between 0.2%

and 2% of the population will develop this disorder in their lifetime. In the United States, it is nearly twice as common in women, but in other cultures, it is believed to be more widespread in men. Some psychiatrists think that the high female-to-male ratio in this disorder in North America reflects the cultural pressures on women and the social expectation that women are generally physically weak or sickly. It is also likely to run in families. As many as 20% of the mothers, sisters, or daughters of somatization disorder patients have the same illness. Their male first-degree relatives are more apt to have anti-social personality disorder or addiction problems. When asked to self-assess health, somatization disorder patients usually rate their well-being as worse than people suffering from actual long-term illness do. Physical complaints normally develop or increase during times of **stress**, and though these people look for help frequently, it is highly unusual for them to find relief.

Undifferentiated somatoform disorder

Undifferentiated somatoform disorder is generally less specific than somatization disorder, and requires only the presence of one symptom to be consistently present. But patients suffering from undifferentiated somatoform disorder often complain of fatigue, loss of appetite, or difficulty swallowing. Symptoms commonly develop when the person is under stress or is depressed, and to meet *DSM-IV* criteria, must have no physical basis and remain for more than six months.

Conversion disorder

In conversion disorders, people typically report a loss or change in the function of some part of their body that does not correlate with what medical science knows today of **anatomy** or **physiology**. Symptoms are often neurological in nature, such as seizures that are not seen on EEG, or an inability to move an arm or leg, or walk. The disorder gets its name from the notion that the patient is converting a psychological conflict or problem into an inability to move specific parts of the body or to use the senses normally. An example of a conversion reaction would be a patient who loses his or her voice in a situation in which he or she is afraid to speak. The symptom simultaneously contains the **anxiety** and serves to get the patient out of the threatening situation. The resolution of the emotion that underlies the physical symptom is called the patient's primary gain, and the change in the patient's social, occupational, or family situation that results from the symptom is called a secondary gain. Doctors sometimes use these terms when they discuss the aftereffects of conversion disorder or of other somatoform disorders on the patient's emotional adjustment and lifestyle.

Unlike somatization disorder, the symptoms of conversion disorder typically occur in adolescence or early adulthood, when the person is under extreme stress. It does not appear to run in families. It is estimated that as many as one in four people admitted to a general hospital have experienced conversion symptoms, but that the disorder is more likely to occur among less educated or sophisticated people. Females are at least twice as likely to develop conversion disorder symptoms, and men are more likely to develop such symptoms in occupational settings or military service.

Pain disorder

Pain disorder is marked by the experience of severe pain in the absence of physical cause for the pain, or markedly unwarranted complaint of pain from an actual illness. *DSM-IV* requirements include duration of a minimum of six months, a curtailing of normal activities such as work or school, and relationship problems. Prescription drug dependency often accompanies somatoform pain disorder, but drug-seeking does not cause it. Somatoform pain disorder is not deliberately put on. This category of somatoform disorder covers a range of patients with a variety of ailments, including chronic headaches, back problems, arthritis, muscle aches and cramps, or pelvic pain. In some cases the patient's pain appears to be largely due to psychological factors, but in other cases the pain is derived from a medical condition as well.

Pain disorder is frequently accompanied by what are termed the "Five Ds." These are:

• depressed mood

• disturbed sleep pattern

• dysfunction in social situations

• decreased activity level

• decreased physical activity

Because pain is such an individual experience, the incidence of somatoform pain disorder is unclear. It is known that between 10 and 15% percent of all of the population that suffer from **back pain** eventually become work-disabled. What percent of these people suffer from somatoform pain disorder is unclear.

Hypochondriasis

Hypochondriasis is a somatoform disorder marked by excessive fear of or preoccupation with having a serious illness that persists in spite of medical testing and reassurance. It was formerly called hypochondriacal **neurosis**.

Although hypochondriasis is usually considered a disorder of young adults, it is now increasingly recognized in children and adolescents. It may also develop in elderly people without previous histories of health-related fears. The disorder accounts for about 5% of psychiatric patients, and is equally common in men and women. Patients typically are abnormally attentive to normal bodily functions such as heartbeat or perspiring. *DSM-IV* criteria include the presence of unrealistic fears or beliefs for at least six months. During any six month period, between 4 and 6% of the population suffers from hypochondria. Episodes can last anywhere from months to years, and it is a persistent, relapsing condition. Chronic stress is believed to play a large role in its occurrence.

Body dysmorphic disorder

Body dysmorphic disorder is a new category in *DSM-IV*. It is defined as a preoccupation with an imagined or exaggerated defect in appearance. Most cases involve features on the patient's face or head, but other body parts—especially those associated with sexual attractiveness, such as the breasts or genitals—may also be the focus of concern. Patients with this disorder are often found in **plastic surgery** clinics. They frequently have histories of seeking or obtaining plastic surgery or other procedures to repair or treat supposed defects, but it seldom if ever provides them with long-term relief.

Though the average age of body dysmorphic disorder patients is thirty, it is regarded as a chronic condition that usually begins in the patient's late teens and fluctuates over the course of time. It was initially considered to be a relatively unusual disorder, but it is now estimated that two percent of those seeking plastic surgery may be dysmorphic disorder patients. It appears to affect men and women with equal frequency. Some may even meet the criteria for a delusional disorder of the somatic type.

Somatoform disorders in children and adolescents

In children and adolescents, the most common somatoform disorder is conversion disorder, though body dysmorphic disorders are being reported more frequently. Conversion reactions in this age group usually reflect stress in the family or problems with school, rather than long-term psychiatric disturbances. Some psychiatrists speculate that adolescents with conversion disorders frequently have overprotective or over-involved parents with a subconscious need to see their child as sick. In many cases the son or daughter's symptoms become the center of family attention. The rise in incidence of body dysmorphic disorder in adolescents is thought to reflect the increased influence of media preoccupation with physical perfection.

Causes and symptoms

In somatoform disorders, the patient's reported symptoms are considered to be the unconscious manifestation of very real emotional suffering. In classic psychoanalytic theories, unconscious conflicts are the result of painful early-life events that are re-awakened in adult life by similar stressors. Because the person is unable to express the re-awakened emotion because of fear or guilt, their emotions are repressed and changed into physical symptoms.

Because *DSM-IV* groups the somatoform disorders into their present category on the basis of symptom patterns, their causes as presently understood include several different factors.

Family stress

Family stress is believed to be one of the most common causes of somatoform disorders in children and adolescents. Conversion disorders in this age group may also be connected with physical or sexual abuse within the family of origin.

Parental modeling

Somatization disorder and hypochondriasis may result in part from the patient's unconscious reflection or imitation of parental behaviors. This "copycat" behavior is particularly likely if the patient's parent derived considerable secondary gain from his or her symptoms.

Cultural influences

Cultural influences appear to affect the gender ratios and body locations of somatoform disorders, as well as their frequency in a specific population. Some cultures (for example, Greek and Puerto Rican) report higher rates of somatization disorder among men than is the case for the United States. In addition, researchers found lower levels of somatization disorder among people with higher levels of education. People in Asia and Africa are more likely to report certain types of physical sensations (for example, burning hands or feet, or the feeling of ants crawling under the skin) than are Westerners.

Biological factors

Genetic or biological factors may also play a role. For example, people who suffer from somatization disorder may also differ in how they perceive and process pain.

Diagnosis

Accurate diagnosis of somatoform disorders is important to prevent unnecessary surgery, laboratory tests, or other treatments or procedures. But it is equally important for physicians and all health care staff to carefully evaluate the person to assure that an actual physical cause for the somatoform-appearing symptom is not being missed. Diagnosis of somatoform disorders requires a thorough physical workup. Pain disorder patients have, on occasion, later been discovered to actually have **cancer**, and a detailed examination is especially necessary when conversion disorder is a possible diagnosis, because some neurological conditions, including **multiple sclerosis** and myasthenia gravis, have been misdiagnosed as conversion disorder. Some patients who receive a diagnosis of somatoform disorder ultimately go on to develop neurologic disorders.

In addition to ruling out medical causes for the patient's symptoms, a doctor who is evaluating a patient for a somatization disorder will consider the possibility of other psychiatric diagnoses or of overlapping psychiatric disorders. Somatoform disorders often coexist with **personality disorders** because of the chicken-and-egg relationship between physical illness and certain types of character structure or personality traits. At one time, the influence of Freud's theory of hysteria led doctors to assume that the patient's hidden emotional needs cause the illness. But in many instances, the patient's personality may have changed over time due to the stresses of adjusting to a chronic disease. This gradual transformation is particularly likely in patients with pain disorder. Patients with somatization disorder often develop panic attacks or agoraphobia together with their physical symptoms. In addition to anxiety or personality disorders, the doctor will usually consider major depression as a possible diagnosis when evaluating a patient with symptoms of a somatoform disorder. Pain disorders may be associated with depression, and body dysmorphic disorder may be associated with obsessive-compulsive disorder.

Treatment

Psychiatric therapies

Patients with somatoform disorders are not considered good candidates for psychoanalysis or other forms of insight-oriented **psychotherapy**. They can benefit, however, from supportive approaches aimed at symptom reduction and stabilization of the patient's personality. Some patients with pain disorder benefit from group therapy or support groups, particularly if their social network has been limited by their pain symptoms. Cognitive-behavioral therapy is also used sometimes to treat pain disorder.

Family therapy is usually recommended for children or adolescents with somatoform disorders, particularly if the parents seem to be using the child as a focus to divert attention from other difficulties. Working with families of chronic pain patients also helps avoid reinforcing dependency within the family setting.

Medications

Patients with somatoform disorders are sometimes given anti-anxiety drugs or **antidepressant drugs** if they have been diagnosed with a coexisting mood or anxiety disorder. In general, though, it is considered better practice to avoid prescribing medications for these patients since they run the risk of becoming psychologically dependent on them.

Hypnosis is a time-honored technique used since Freud's time as part of a general psychotherapeutic approach to conversion disorder. It may allow patients to recover memories or thoughts connected with the onset of the physical symptoms.

Alternative treatment

Patients with somatization or pain disorders may be helped by a variety of alternative therapies including **acupuncture**, **hydrotherapy**, therapeutic massage, **yoga**, **meditation**, botanical medicine, and homeopathic treatment. These are often available through both pain and stress reduction clinics that many general hospitals now have.

Prognosis

Somatization disorder is considered to be a chronic disturbance that tends to persist throughout the patient's life, but a recent three year follow-up study reported in *Caring for the Mind: The Comprehensive Guide to Mental Health* showed that a consistent approach using education and reassurance resulted in noticeable improvement.

The prognosis for conversion disorder is considered to be good. Ninety percent of patients recover within a month, and only one in five will ever have a recurrence.

People suffering from hypochondriasis have a more optimistic outlook if treatment is initiated early, before they have gotten themselves into a cycle of medical tests and procedures. There has been very little research regarding the effectiveness of treatment in body dysmorphic disorder.

Health care team roles

In many cases a somatoform disorder diagnosis is made in a general medical clinic by a primary care practitioner, rather than by a psychiatrist. Children and adolescents with somatoform disorders are most likely to be diagnosed by their primary care physician, or pediatrician.

Primary care practitioner (PCP)

A PCP is typically a licensed medical doctor. Because somatoform disorders are associated with physical symptoms, patients are much more apt to be seen by primary care physicians. Their lengthy medical histories make a long-term relationship with a trusted PCP a safeguard against unnecessary treatments as well as being a comfort to the patient. Many PCPs prefer to schedule brief appointments on a regular basis with the patient and keep referrals to specialists to a minimum. This practice also allows them to monitor the patient for any new physical symptoms or diseases. However, some PCPs work with a psychiatric consultant.

Psychiatrist

Psychiatrists are licensed medical doctors that have undergone a three year psychiatric residency. They are often the providers of both education and support for patients with somatoform disorders.

Registered nurse (RN), psychiatric nurse, or licensed practical nurse (LPN)

Both RNs and LPNs must complete a prescribed course in nursing and pass a state examination. RNs typically have a degree in nursing, and psychiatric nurses have additional training specific to psychiatry. Both RNs and LPNs are often the people who deal the most with patients with somatoform disorders in general hospitals, clinics and on psychiatric units. An open mind and non-judgmental attitude toward the patient and careful, detailed observation of symptoms can be highly useful. The provision of education about the nature of these illnesses will typically come from both physicians and nurses.

Clinical laboratory scientist

Clinical laboratory scientists have specialized training and must pass a state examination. They draw **blood** samples or test urine or other specimens that are ordered by the physician to help in making a correct diagnosis.

Radiologic technologist

Radiologic technologists have specialized training and must pass a state examination. They take x rays or

Briquet's syndrome—Another name for somatization disorder.

Conversion disorder—A somatoform disorder characterized by the transformation of a psychological feeling or impulse into a physical symptom. Conversion disorder was previously called hysterical neurosis, conversion type.

CT scan—Computerized tomography scanning. A diagnostic technique in which the combined use of a computer and x rays passed through the body at different angles produces clear, cross-sectional images.

Dissociation—A psychological mechanism in which the mind splits off certain aspects of a traumatic event from conscious awareness. Dissociation can affect the patient's memory, sense of reality, and sense of identity.

Hysteria—The earliest term for a psychoneurotic disturbance marked by emotional outbursts and/or disturbances of movement and sense perception. Some forms of hysteria are now classified as somatoform disorders and others are grouped with the dissociative disorders.

Hysterical neurosis—An older term for conversion disorder or dissociative disorder.

MRI—Magnetic resonance imaging. A diagnostic technique that provides very clear cross-sectional images of organs and structures in the human body without x rays or other radiation.

Primary gain—The immediate relief from guilt, anxiety, or other unpleasant feelings that a patient derives from a symptom.

Repression—An unconscious psychological mechanism in which painful or unacceptable ideas, memories, or feelings are removed from conscious awareness or recall.

Secondary gain—The social, occupational, or interpersonal advantages that a patient derives from symptoms. A patient's being relieved of his or her share of household chores by other family members would be an example of secondary gain.

Somatoform disorder—A category of psychiatric disorder characterized by physical complaints that appear to be medical in origin but that cannot be explained in terms of a physical disease, the results of substance abuse, or by another mental disorder.

Stressor—Any interference that disturbs a person's healthy mental and physical well-being.

---

other imaging such as MRIs or **CT scans** that are ordered by the physician to help in making a correct diagnosis.

Social workers

Social workers are usually either certified (CSW) or licensed clinical social workers (LCSW). A two-year graduate program degree and specialized training including supervised clinical work in working with the mentally ill, and state licensure are typical requirements. Social workers often conduct supportive groups or programs that help people vent feelings or work on ways to be able to cope better.

Specialized therapists

Stress reduction therapists are a good example of this category. They are not necessarily licensed in all states, but typically have a degree in one of the human service fields such as social work, psychology, or nursing. They are often certified in a specific stress reduction program such as the now-nationwide one that was developed at University of Massachusetts Medical Center by Dr. Jon Kabat-Zinn. Most of these stress reduction programs incorporate standard supportive group therapy techniques with **alternative medicine** areas such as yoga and meditation.

Prevention

Generalizations regarding prevention of somatoform disorders are difficult because these syndromes affect different age groups, vary in their symptom patterns and persistence, and result from different problems of adjustment to the surrounding culture. In theory, allowing expression of emotional pain in children, rather than regarding it as a weakness, might reduce the secondary gain of physical symptoms that draw the care or attention of parents.

Resources

BOOKS

Clark, R. Barkley. "Psychosocial Aspects of Pediatrics and Psychiatric Disorders." In *Current Pediatric Diagnosis and Treatment,* edited by William W. Hay Jr., et al. Stamford, CT: Appleton & Lange, 1997.

Eisendrath, Stuart J. "Psychiatric Disorders." In *Current Medical Diagnosis & Treatment 1998,* edited by Lawrence M. Tierney Jr., et al. Stamford, CT: Appleton & Lange, 1997.

Hales, Dianne, and Robert E. Hales, M. D. *Caring for the Mind, The Comprehensive Guide to Mental Health* New York: Bantam Books, 1996.

Kaplan, David W., and Kathleen A. Mammel. "Adolescence." In *Current Pediatric Diagnosis & Treatment,* edited by William W. Hay Jr., et al. Stamford, CT: Appleton & Lange, 1997.

Stone, Timothy E., and Romaine Hain. "Somatoform Disorders." In *Current Diagnosis 9,* edited by Rex B. Conn, et al. Philadelphia: W. B. Saunders Company, 1997.

Joan M. Schonbeck

Somatosensory evoked potential study *see* **Evoked potential studies**

Sonogram unit *see* **Ultrasound unit**

Sore throat

Definition

Sore throat is an upper respiratory **infection** that may be caused by inflammation of the pharynx, larynx, or tonsils. Thus, it is a symptom of many conditions, but most often is associated with **common cold** or **influenza**. Sore throat may be caused by either a virus or **bacteria** in addition to certain environmental conditions. Most sore throats heal without complications, but they should not be ignored because some develop into serious illnesses.

Description

Almost everyone gets a sore throat at one time or another. Sore throat and cold are more prevalent among children in daycare centers or schools and seem to be related to their lack of resistance as compared to the adolescents and adults. It is interesting to note that women in the age of 20 to 30 are affected by more cold attacks than men, which may be attributed to their more frequent contacts with children. Sore throats are most common during the winter months when upper respiratory infections (colds) are more frequent. The National Center for Health Statistics has estimated that common cold symptoms (which include sore throat) amounted to 62 million cases, in 1996, that needed medical attention.

Sore throats can be either acute or chronic. Acute sore throats are more common. They last from three to seven days. A chronic sore throat lasts much longer and is a symptom of an unresolved underlying condition or disease, such as a sinus infection.

Causes and symptoms

Sore throats have many different causes, and may or may not be accompanied by cold symptoms, **fever**, or swollen lymph glands. Proper treatment depends on understanding the cause of the sore throat.

Viral sore throat

Viruses cause 90-95% of all sore throats. Cold and flu viruses are the main culprits although about 200 different viruses are known to cause the symptoms of sore throat. Rhinoviruses cause 30-35% of all adult colds in fall, spring, and summer. Coronaviruses cause the infections in winter and spring. These viruses cause an inflammation in the throat and occasionally the tonsils (**tonsillitis**). The causative agents of viral tonsillitis are Epstein-Barr virus, influenza virus, enterovirus, or adenoviruses. Cold symptoms almost always accompany a viral sore throat. These can include a runny nose, **cough**, congestion, hoarseness, conjunctivitis, and fever. The level of throat **pain** varies from uncomfortable to excruciating, when it is painful for the patient to eat, breathe, swallow, or speak.

Another group of viruses that cause sore throat are the adenoviruses. These may also cause infections of the **lungs** and ears. In addition to a sore throat, symptoms that accompany an adenovirus infection include cough, runny nose, white bumps on the tonsils and throat, mild **diarrhea**, **vomiting**, and a **rash**. The sore throat lasts about one week.

A third type of virus that can cause severe sore throat is the coxsackie virus. It can cause a disease called herpangina. Although anyone can get herpangina, it is most common in children up to age ten and is more prevalent in the summer or early autumn. Herpangina is sometimes called summer sore throat.

Three to six days after being exposed to the virus, an infected person develops a sudden sore throat that is accompanied by a substantial fever usually between 102–104°F (38.9–40°C). Tiny grayish-white blisters form on the throat that turn into ulcerative lesions. Throat pain is often severe, interfering with swallowing. Children may become dehydrated if they are reluctant to eat or drink because of the pain. In addition, people with herpangina may vomit, have **abdominal pain**, and generally feel ill and miserable.

One other common cause of a viral sore throat is mononucleosis. An estimated 90% of mononucleosis cases are caused by the Epstein-Barr virus (EBV), while the remaining cases may be attributed to the cytomegalovirus. EBV is known to infect B lymphocytes (a subset of white **blood** cells). The infection spreads to the **lymphatic system**, **respiratory system**, **liver**, spleen, throat and salivary glands. Symptoms appear 30–50 days after exposure.

Mononucleosis, sometimes called the "kissing disease," is extremely common. It is estimated that by the age of 35–40, 80–95% of Americans will have had mononucleosis. Often, symptoms are mild, especially in young children, and are diagnosed as a cold. Since symptoms are more severe in adolescents and adults, more cases are diagnosed as mononucleosis in this age group. One of the main symptoms of mononucleosis is severe sore throat.

Although a runny nose and cough are much more likely to accompany a sore throat caused by a virus than one caused by a bacteria, there is no absolute way to tell what is causing the sore throat without a laboratory test. Viral sore throats are contagious and are passed directly from person to person by coughing and sneezing.

Bacterial sore throat

About 5-10% of sore throats are caused by bacteria. The most common bacterial sore throat results from an infection by group A *Streptococcus*. This type of infection is commonly called **strep throat**. Anyone can get strep throat, This organism may also cause laryngitis, which is predominantly marked by hoarseness of voice, sore throat, dry and persistent cough, and fever. Yet another ailment caused by Streptococcus is pharyngitis, which is inflammation of pharynx leading to fever, tenderness in the neck glands, sore throat, abdominal pain, **headache**, cough, hoarseness, and skin rash. Other bacteria that are known to cause pharyngitis are groups C and G *Streptococcus*, *Yersinia enterocolitica*, and rarely *Corynebacterium diphtheriae*. Untreated streptococcal pharyngitis may lead to peritonsillar **abscess** that is accompanied by severe sore throat and hoarseness of voice. In these cases, immediate intervention by otolaryngologists is required to aspirate the abscess.

Pharyngeal gonorrhea, a sexually transmitted bacterial disease, causes severe sore throat. Gonorrhea in the throat is transmitted by having oral sex with an infected person.

Noninfectious sore throat

Not all sore throats are caused by infection. Postnasal drip can irritate the throat and make it sore. It can be caused by hay fever and other **allergies** that are irritating to the sinuses. Environmental and other conditions, such as heavy **smoking** or breathing secondhand smoke, heavy alcohol consumption, breathing polluted air or chemical fumes, or swallowing substances that burn or scratch the throat can also cause pharyngitis. Dry air, like that in airplanes or from forced hot air furnaces, can make the throat sore. People who breathe through their mouths at night because of nasal congestion often get sore throats that improve as the day progresses. Sore throat caused by environmental conditions is not contagious.

Diagnosis

It is easy for people to tell if they have a sore throat, but difficult to know what has caused it without laboratory tests. Most sore throats are minor and heal without any complications. A small number of bacterial sore throats do develop into serious diseases. Because of this, it is advisable to see a doctor if a sore throat lasts more than a few days or is accompanied by fever, nausea, or abdominal pain.

Diagnosis of a sore throat begins with a **physical examination** of the throat and chest. The examiner will also look for signs of other illness, such as a sinus infection or **bronchitis**. Since both bacterial and viral sore throat are contagious and pass easily from person to person, the health care provider will seek information about whether the patient has been around other people with flu, sore throat, colds, or strep throat. If it appears that the patient may have strep throat, laboratory tests will be performed.

If mononucleosis is suspected, the doctor may do a mono spot test to look for **antibodies** indicating the presence of the Epstein-Barr virus. The test is inexpensive, takes only a few minutes, and can be done in a physician's office. An inexpensive blood test can also determine increased lymphocytes and the presence of specific antibodies to the mononucleosis virus.

Treatment

Effective treatment varies depending on the cause of the sore throat. As frustrating as it may be to the patient, viral sore throat is best left to run its course without drug treatment. **Antibiotics** are ineffective against viruses. They do not shorten the length of the illness, nor do they lessen the symptoms.

Sore throat caused by a streptococci or another bacteria must be treated with antibiotics. Penicillin is the preferred medication. Oral penicillin must be taken for ten days. Patients need to take the entire course of antibiotic prescribed, even after symptoms of the sore throat improve. Incomplete treatment may lead to the relapse of the symptoms. Occasionally a single intramuscular injection of long-acting penicillin G is administered instead of ten days of oral treatment. In cases of penicillin allergy, cephalexin, cefuroxime, or cefprozil are the preferred alternative antibiotics that are recommended. These medications generally cost under fifteen dollars.

Mononucleosis, being a viral infection, is self-limiting with no means of therapeutic control. Rest, a healthy diet, plenty of fluids, avoiding strenuous exercises and competitive sports are recommended. The acute phase of infection is treated with acetaminophen (Datril, Tylenol, Panadol) or ibuprofen (Advil, Nuprin, Motrin, Medipren). Nearly 90% of mononucleosis infections are mild. The infected person does not normally get the disease again.

In the case of chronic sore throat, it is necessary to treat the underlying disease to heal the sore throat. If sore throat is caused by environmental factors, the aggravating stimulus should be eliminated from the sufferer's environment.

Home care for sore throat

Regardless of the cause of a sore throat, there are some **home care** steps that can be taken to ease discomfort. These include:

- Taking acetaminophen or ibuprofen for pain. Aspirin should not be given to children because of its association with increased risk for Reye's syndrome, a serious disease.
- Gargling with warm double strength tea or warm salt water made by adding one teaspoon of salt to eight ounces of water.
- Drinking plenty of fluids, but avoiding acid juices like orange juice, which can irritate the throat. Sucking on popsicles is a good way to get fluids into children.
- Eating soft, nutritious foods like noodle soup and avoiding spicy foods.
- Refraining from smoking.
- Resting until the fever is gone, then resuming strenuous activities gradually.
- Often minimizing the dryness by using room humidifier may improve the symptoms of sore throat, especially in pediatric population.
- Antiseptic lozenges and sprays may aggravate the sore throat rather than improve it.

Alternative treatment

Alternative treatment focuses on easing the symptoms of sore throat using herbs and botanical medicines.

- Aromatherapists recommend inhaling the fragrances of essential oils of lavender (*Lavandula officinalis*), thyme (*Thymus vulgaris*), eucalyptus (*Eucalyptus globulus*), sage (*Salvia officinalis*), and sandalwood.
- Ayurvedic practitioners suggest gargling with a mixture of water, salt, and turmeric (*Curcuma longa*) powder, or astringents such as alum, sumac, sage, and bayberry (*Myrica* spp.).
- Herbalists recommend taking osha root (*Ligusticum porteri*) internally for infection or drinking ginger (*Zingiber officinale*), slippery elm (*Ulmus fulva*), sage or marshmallow tea for pain. Also fresh juice of *Echinacea* along with the root of goldenseal may have a soothing effect on the throat. The tannins found in blueberries, blackberries, and red raspberries have also been shown to be effective for sore throats
- Homeopaths may treat sore throats with superdilute solutions of *Lachesis*, *Belladonna*, *Phytolacca*, or yellow jasmine (*Gelsemium*).
- Nutritional recommendations include zinc lozenges every two hours along with vitamin C with bioflavonoids, vitamin A, and beta-carotene supplements.

Prognosis

Sore throat caused by a viral infection generally clears up on its own within one week with no complications. The exception is mononucleosis. Ninety percent of cases of mononucleosis clear up without medical intervention or complications, so long as **dehydration** does not occur. In young children the symptoms may last only a week, but in adolescents the symptoms last longer. Adults over age 30 have the most severe and long-lasting symptoms. Adults may take up to six months to recover. In all age groups, fatigue and **weakness** may continue for up to six weeks after other symptoms disappear.

In rare cases of mononucleosis, breathing may be obstructed because of swollen tonsils, adenoids, and lymph glands. If this happens, the patient should immediately seek emergency medical care.

Patients with bacterial sore throat begin feeling better about 24 hours after starting antibiotics. If left untreated, strep throat may lead to scarlet fever, **rheumatic fever** resulting in rheumatic **heart** disease, or glomerulonephritis. Scarlet fever is a combination of sore throat with rash of sand paper consistency that may appear in the lower **abdomen** and gradually spread to the trunk. Rheumatic fever is marked by inflammation and pain in the joints. In severe cases, inflammation of the heart valves can lead to **heart failure**. Glomerulonephritis is inflammation of glomeruli, which serve as filters in the kidney. The damaged filters result in red urine due to the release of red blood cells. The treatment for this disorder is aimed at controlling the symptoms. Taking antibiotics within the first week of a strep infection will prevent these complications. People with strep throat remain contagious until after they have been taking antibiotics for 24 hours.

Health care team roles

Sore throat may not always need medical intervention, but persistent sore throats and accompanying symptoms should not be ignored. A general physician helps in determining whether the sore throat is a result of a viral or bacterial infection. A thorough physical examination followed by laboratory tests in cases of a doubtful bacterial infection is performed. If a bacterial sore throat is diagnosed by the physician, antibiotics are prescribed. Health care professionals, including the pharmacists, play a key role in cautioning the patient regarding the potential allergic reactions associated with the intake of antibiotics. Some of these reactions may be serious and need immediate medical intervention.

There may be lingering symptoms or changes in the symptoms after visiting the doctor. Some of the concerns will be:

• persistent fever

• continuing and severe sore throat

• discomfort in opening the mouth wide

• dizziness

In such cases, a doctor's advice is highly recommended. In addition, health care professionals will provide the best resources for **nutrition**, suggestions for pain relievers, and effective home remedies for viral sore throats.

Prevention

There is no way to prevent a sore throat; however, the risk of getting one or passing one on to another person can be minimized by:

• Washing hands well and frequently.

• Avoiding close contact with someone who has a sore throat.

• Not sharing food and eating utensils with anyone.

• Cleaning the environmental surfaces with a disinfectant.

• Not smoking.

• Avoiding polluted air.

• Using a room humidifier at home during the winter months when the dryness is maximum.

• Avoiding exposures to sudden and frequent changes in temperatures (in winter, being exposed to severe cold outside and heated room within the home).

KEY TERMS

Antigen—A foreign protein to which the body reacts by making antibodies.

Conjunctivitis—An inflammation of the membrane surrounding the eye; also known as pinkeye.

Lymphocyte—A type of white blood cell. Lymphocytes play an important role in fighting disease.

Pharynx—The pharynx is the part of the throat that lies between the mouth and the larynx or voice box.

Tonsils—Fleshy tissues located on either side of the back of the throat.

Toxin—A poison. In the case of scarlet fever, the toxin is secreted as a byproduct of the growth of the streptococcus bacteria and causes a rash.

Resources

BOOKS

Cummings, Stephen, and Dana Ullman. "Sore Throats." *Everybody's Guide to Homeopathic Medicine.* Health World Online, *http://www.healthy.net.*

Harrison's Principles of Internal Medicine, 18th ed. New York: McGraw-Hill, 2011.

PERIODICALS

National Institute of Allergy and Infectious Diseases. *The Common Cold Fact Sheet. http://www.niaid.nih.gov/factsheets/cold.htm* (March 26, 2001).

OTHER

"Laryngitis." Virtual health fair. March 19, 2001. http://www.vfair.com/conditions/laryngitis.htm.

"Mononucleosis." Virtual health fair. March 19, 2001. http://www.vfair.com/conditions/mononucleosis.htm.

"When you have a sore throat." American Family Physician http://www.aafp.org/afp/970100ap/970100a.htm.

Tish Davidson
Kausalya Santhanam

Speech disorders

Definition

A speech disorder is a communication disorder characterized by an impaired ability to produce speech sounds or normal voice, or to speak fluently.

Description

Speech disorders belong to a broad category of disorders called communication disorders that also include language and **hearing** disorders. Communication disorders affect one person out of every ten in the United States. Speech disorders refer to difficulties producing speech sounds or problems with voice quality. They may be characterized by an interruption in the flow or rhythm of speech such as **stuttering**, or by problems with the way sounds are formed, also called articulation or phonological disorders, or they may involve voice problems such as pitch, intensity, or quality. Often, there is a combination of several different problems.

Speech disorders can either be present at birth or acquired as a result of **stroke**, **head injury**, or illness. The production of intelligible speech is the result of very complex interactions originating in the **brain**. When the brain sends a series of speech signals to the speech muscles, the muscles need to produce the series of sounds that will convey the intended message. Major speech disorders that can impair this process include:

- Articulation disorders: Articulation is the production of speech sounds, and persons affected by articulation disorders experience difficulty in being understood because they produce incorrect speech sounds. As a result, their speech is not intelligible. They may substitute one sound for another or may distort the sound with the result that it sounds incorrect, even though still recognizable, or omit one or more sounds in a word.

- Phonological disorders: Phonology is the science of speech sounds and sound patterns and of the language rules that dictate how sounds may be combined to produce language. Persons affected by phonological disorders do not use the conventional rules for their native language but substitute their own variants. This affects classes of sounds, as opposed to single sounds. Sounds are characterized by where in the mouth they are produced, how they are produced, and by how the larynx (voice box) is used. Any unusual deviation in these features is called a phonological process. Fronting and backing are examples of phonological processes, characterized by the production of sounds at the front or at the back of the mouth when they should be produced the other way around. For example, the word "go," produced at the back of the mouth, might be used instead of "doe," which is produced in the front.

- Stuttering: Normal speech is fluent, in that it is spoken effortlessly and without hesitation. A break in fluent speech is called a dysfluency. Although some degree of dysfluency occurs in normal speech from time to time, stuttering has more dysfluencies than is considered average. Normally developing preschool children often demonstrate dysfluencies that are effortless and last for brief periods of time. However, changes in the types of dysfluency behavior and the frequency of occurrence may signal the development of a problem. Normal dysfluencies consist of word or sentence repetitions, fillers (um, ah), or interjections. Stuttering behavior includes sound or syllable repetition, prolongations (the unnatural stretching out of sounds), and blocks, which refers to an inability to produce the sound, as if it gets stuck and cannot come out. Stuttering dysfluencies are also often accompanied by tension and anxiety.

- Voice disorders: There are two types of voice disorders: organic voice and functional voice disorders. Organic voice disorders are associated with disease and require medical intervention. Functional voice disorders are the result of abuse or misuse of the larynx. Sounds are produced when the vocal cords of the throat come close together and vibrate with air coming from the lungs. These vibrations produce a series of pulses that then cause the air to resonate and produce voice sounds. People have unique voice characteristics and it is therefore difficult to define a normal voice. Generally speaking, a normal voice is pleasant sounding and has appropriate pitch and loudness for the age and gender of the speaker. A voice disorder is therefore present when the voice is not pleasant sounding, or when it is too loud or too soft or too high-pitched or low-pitched for the speaker's gender.

- Apraxia: This is a speech disorder in which voluntary muscle movement is impaired without muscle weakness. There are two main types of apraxias: buccofacial apraxia and verbal apraxia. Buccofacial apraxia impairs the ability to move the muscles of the mouth for non-speech purposes such as coughing, swallowing, and wiggling of the tongue. Verbal apraxia impairs the proper sequencing of speech sounds. Apraxias can either be acquired or developmental and have different degrees of severity, ranging from the inability to initiate speech to mild difficulties with the pronunciation of multi-syllabic words.

- Dysarthria: This is a speech disorder that affects the muscles involved in the production of speech. As a result, speech is slow, weak, inaccurate, and hesitant. The production of clear speech requires that several muscle systems work together. First, the lungs must provide the air required to activate speech. Then, the larynx must allow the air to vibrate. The soft palate that separates the oral and nasal cavities must also direct the air to one or both cavities to produce the different sounds. Finally, the lips, tongue, teeth, and jaw then must all move in a concerted way to shape the sounds into the various vowels, consonants, and syllables that make up the sounds of language. Dysarthria results from a weakness in any one of these elements or in the absence of proper coordination between them. If, for example, the lungs are weak, then speech will be too quiet or produced one word at a time. Childhood dysarthria can be present at birth or acquired as a result of disease or accident, as is the case for adult dysarthria.

Causes and symptoms

The causes of articulation and phonological disorders are unclear, although it has been observed that they tend to develop in children before age four and run in families. The symptoms vary, depending on whether other disorders are present, but typically involve difficulty in making specific speech sounds. Articulation is considered a disorder when it is unintelligible or draws negative attention to the speaker. For example, the word "super" is pronounced as "thuper."

The causes of stuttering are not very well understood. There is some evidence that stuttering has a genetic cause since it has been observed to run in some families. According to the National Stuttering Association (NSA), current research suggests a connection between stuttering and the brain's ability to coordinate speech. The major symptom of stuttering, found in preschoolers but not adults, is persistent dysfluency of language that exceeds 10%.

The main causes of organic **voice disorders** include neuromuscular disorder, **cancer**, vocal cord **paralysis**, endocrine changes, various benign tumors such as inflammatory growths (granulomas), or consisting of a mass of **blood vessels** (hemangiomas) or occurring on mucous membranes (papillomas). Functional voice disorders are caused by abuse or misuse of the larynx. Misuse of the voice includes talking for excessively long periods of time or yelling. Abuse occurs as a result of excessive throat clearing, laughing, crying, coughing, or **smoking**. Both abuse and misuse of the voice can damage the vocal cords, or may result in nodules, polyps, contact ulcers, or **edema**.

Acquired apraxias occur as a result of brain damage and can often be linked to specific lesion sites on the brain. They can result from stroke, head injury, brain tumors, toxins, or infections. In the case of developmental **apraxia** of speech (DAS), it is usually present at birth. There are no specific lesion sites in the brain associated with DAS, and no direct cause has been identified. However, since young children only use a few words, it has been proposed that delays in language expression can impair a child's ability to gain control over the speech muscles.

Childhood **dysarthria** can be present at birth or acquired with diseases such as **cerebral palsy**, Duchenne **muscular dystrophy**, or myotonic dystrophy. Adult dysarthria may be caused by stroke, degenerative diseases such as Parkinson's or Huntington's disease, amyotrophic lateral sclerosis, **multiple sclerosis**, myasthenia gravis, **meningitis**, brain tumors, toxins, drug or alcohol abuse, or lead **poisoning**.

Diagnosis

Speech disorders are usually identified using a combination of hearing tests and physical exams. Physicians then recommend specialized evaluation by speech-language pathologists, who can best establish an accurate diagnosis.

A stuttering diagnosis is established on the basis of the type, frequency, and duration of speech dysfluency. The number of dysfluencies occurring in 100 words is counted to determine the dysfluency percentage. One half a stuttered word per minute is the usual criterion. Determining the type of stuttering behavior, either overt or covert, is the most important factor in diagnosing stuttering.

Organic and functional voice disorders are diagnosed with the assistance of an ear, nose, and throat specialist, an otolaryngologist, who can identify the organic cause of the voice disorder, if present. Several tests can be used to screen for possible tumors in the throat or laryngeal box area. Only in the absence of an organic cause will the voice disorder be diagnosed as functional, indicating that it is due to abuse or misuse of the voice.

A diagnosis of apraxia is not easy to establish but is usually indicated when children do not develop speech normally and are unable to produce consonant sounds.

Treatment

Speech pathologists have designed approaches for treating speech disorders with the type of treatment depending upon the type of impairment. A wide variety of treatment techniques are available for treating affected children, adolescents, and adults. A thorough assessment is normally conducted with the aim of determining the most effective and acceptable treatment approach for each disorder on an individual basis. A common treatment for many patients involves increasing sensory motor awareness of selected aspects of speech and systematically shaping the target speech behaviors.

Treatment for articulation/phonological disorders is usually based on increasing the affected person's awareness about how speech sounds make the meaning of words different. As a result, therapy often involves pronunciation exercises designed to teach how to produce sounds and words more clearly to increase understanding of the differences between the various speech sounds and words.

Treatment plans for stuttering depend on the severity of the dysfluency and may include seeing a speech-language pathologist. Most treatment plans include breathing techniques, **relaxation** strategies to help relax speech-associated muscles, posture control, and other exercises designed to help develop fluency.

Speech-language pathologists use many different approaches to treat voice problems. Functional voice disorders can often be successfully treated by voice therapy. Voice therapy involves identifying voice abuses and misuses and designing a course of treatment aimed at eliminating them. Voice disorders may require surgery if cancer is present.

Treatment of apraxia depends on the extent of the impairment. For individuals diagnosed with moderate to severe apraxia, therapy may be for them to start saying individual sounds and contrasting them, thinking about how the lips and tongue should be placed. Other specialized drills use the natural rhythm of speech to increase understanding. Individuals affected with mild apraxia are taught strategies to help them produce the words that give them difficulty. Several treatment programs have been developed for developmental apraxias. Some feature the use of touching cues, others modify traditional articulation therapies.

Treatment of dysarthria usually aims at maximizing the function of all speech systems with the use of compensatory strategies. Patients may be advised to take frequent pauses for breath, or to exaggerate articulation, or to pause before important words to emphasize them. If there is muscle **weakness**, orofacial exercises may also be prescribed to strengthen the muscles of the face and mouth that are used for speech.

Prognosis

The prognosis depends on the cause of the disorder; many speech disorders can be improved with **speech therapy**. In the case of childhood speech disorders, prognosis also significantly improves with early diagnosis and intervention. Children who do not receive speech therapy and do not outgrow their speech difficulties will continue to have the disorder as adults.

Health care team roles

The treatment of speech disorders belongs to the field of speech-language pathology. Speech-language

---

KEY TERMS

Apraxia—Motor disorder in which voluntary movement is impaired without muscle weakness.

Articulation disorder—Also called phonological disorder; type of speech disorder characterized by the way sounds are formed.

Communication disorder—Disorder characterized by an impaired ability to communicate, including language, speech, and hearing disorders.

Dysarthria—Speech disorder due to a weakness or lack of coordination of the speech muscles.

Dysfluency—Any break or interruption in speech.

Language disorder—Communication disorder characterized by an impaired ability to understand and/or use words in their proper context, whether verbal or nonverbal.

Phonological process—Any unusual change in the place, manner, or larynx characteristics of a produced sound.

Phonology—The science of speech sounds and sound patterns.

Speech disorder—Communication disorder characterized by an impaired ability to produce speech sounds or by problems with voice quality.

Speech-language pathology—This field, formerly known as speech therapy, is concerned with disorders of speech and language.

Stuttering—Speech disorder characterized by speech that has more dysfluencies than is considered average.

Vocal cords—Either of the two pairs of folds of mucous membrane located in the throat and projecting into the cavity of the larynx.

---

pathologists assist individuals who have speech disorders and collaborate with families, teachers, and physicians to design an appropriate course of treatment, which depends on the specific nature of the disorder. They also provide individual therapy to affected persons, consult with teachers about effective classroom strategies to help children with speech disorders, and work closely with families to develop effective therapies.

Prevention

Prevention of speech disorders is centered on identifying at-risk infants. The following conditions are considered to represent high-risk factors, and children exposed to them should be tested early and regularly:

- diagnosed medical conditions such as chronic ear infections

- biological factors such as fetal alcohol syndrome

- genetic defects such as Down syndrome

- neurological defects such as cerebral palsy

- family history such as family incidence of literacy difficulties

Stuttering can be prevented by parents avoiding undue corrections of dysfluency in their children. As young children begin to speak, some dysfluency is normal because they have a limited vocabulary and have difficulty expressing themselves. This results in dysfluent speech, and if parents place excessive attention on the dysfluency, a pattern of stuttering may develop. Speech therapy with children at risk for stuttering may prevent the development of a stuttering speech disorder.

Resources

BOOKS

Dworkin, J.P., and R.J. Meleca. *Vocal Pathologies: Diagnosis, Treatment, and Case Studies.* San Diego, CA: Singular Publishing Group, 1997.

Golding-Kushner, K.J. *Therapy Techniques for Cleft Palate Speech and Related Disorders.* San Diego, CA: Singular Publishing Group, 2001.

Kehoe, T.D. *Stuttering: Science, Therapy, & Practice: The Most Complete Book about Stuttering.* Boulder, CO: Casa Futura Technologies, 1997.

PERIODICALS

Johnson, N.C., and J.R. Sandy. "Tooth Position and Speech—Is There a Relationship?" *Angle Orthodentistry* 69 (August 1999): 306–10.

Kraus, N., and M. Cheour. "Speech Sound Representation in the Brain." *Audiology and Neurotology* 5 (May-August 2000): 97–132.

Oller, D.K., R.E. Eilers, A.R. Neal, and H. K. Schwartz. "Precursors to Speech in Infancy: The Prediction of Speech and Language Disorders." *Journal of Communication Disorders* 32 (July–August 1999): 223–45.

OTHER

"Center for Voice Disorders of Wake Forest University." Wake Forest University School of Medicine. http://www.bgsm.edu/voice/.

"A Guide to Communication Disorders and Science Sources on the Internet." Net Connections for Communication Disorders and Sciences. http://www.mankato.msus.edu/dept/comdis/kuster2/welcome.html.

"The SLP Homepage." Internet Searches and Resources on Speech Language Pathology. http://members.tripod.com/Caroline_Bowen/slp-eureka.htm.

ORGANIZATIONS

American Speech-Language-Hearing Association (ASHA). 10801 Rockville Pike, Rockville, MD 20852. 800) 638-8255. http://www.asha.org/.

Autism Society of America. 7910 Woodmont Avenue, Suite 300, Bethesda, MD 20814-3067. (301) 657-0881. (800) 3AUTISM. http://www.autism-society.org/.

The Hanen Program for Parents of Children with Language Delays. The Hanen Center, Suite 403, 1075 Bay Street, Toronto, Ont M5S 2B1, Canada. (416) 921-1073. http://www.hanen.org/.

National Institute on Deafness and Other Communication Disorders (NIDCD). National Institutes of Health, 31 Center Drive, MSC 2320, Bethesda, MD 20892-2320. http://www.nidcd.nih.gov/.

Monique Laberge, Ph.D.

Speech pathology

Definition

The field of speech pathology, formerly known as **speech therapy**, is concerned with disorders of speech and language. A speech-language pathologist is a professional trained to diagnose and treat language and **speech disorders**.

Description

Speech pathology addresses the pathology of speech and language, meaning the "diseases" of speech and language and their functional effects on the affected person. Speech and language delays and disorders cover a wide range, from simple word substitutions in sentences to the inability to understand or use language for functional communication. The causes of speech and **language disorders** are wide and varied, including **hearing loss**, neurological disorders, traumatic **brain** injury, mental retardation, drug abuse, physical disabilities, and emotional abuse. Frequently, the cause is also unknown. In 1997–98, more than one million students were enrolled in special education programs designed by speech-language pathologists as a result of speech or language disorders.

Work settings

Speech-language pathologists work in a wide variety of settings ranging from private practice to the public

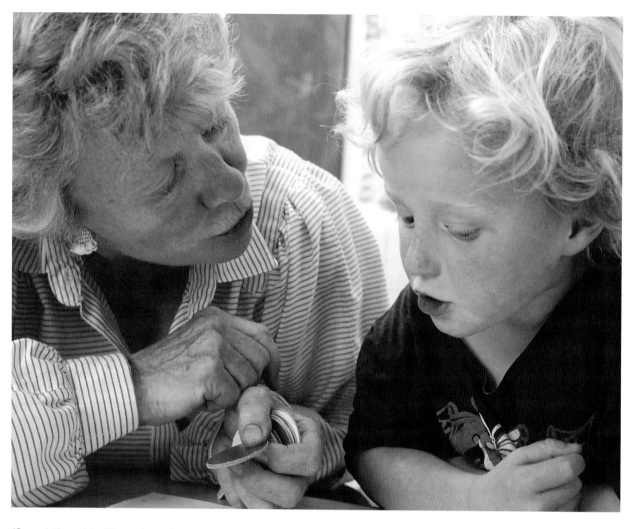

(Speech therapist with a patient, photograph. Hattie Young/Photo Researchers, Inc.)

sector and with agencies treating specific disabilities. Some examples are:

- kindergartens
- primary schools
- high schools
- nursing homes
- hospitals
- universities
- rehabilitation centers
- mental health centers
- community health centers
- private practice

In any of these work settings, a speech-language pathologist's typical workload may include:

- advising a mother on feeding a baby with a cleft palate
- helping a high school student who stutters
- helping a stroke victim to regain communication skills
- providing special training for teachers, doctors, or parents
- advising parents on the prevention of language disorders
- helping children and adults to learn to read
- treating people with brain injuries to regain language
- assisting people to develop control of vocal and respiratory systems for correct voice production

Due to the wide implications of speech and language disorders, speech-language pathologists usually work in close collaboration with other professionals such as medical specialists, educators, engineers, scientists, and other allied health professionals and technicians.

For example, in the vocational school context, speech-language pathologists collaborate with teachers and counselors in establishing communication goals related to the work experiences of students and propose strategies that are designed for the important transition from school to employment.

Education and training

Speech-language pathologists first complete a bachelor's degree which covers all aspects of communication development and disorders, followed by a master's degree. Many universities integrate both degrees into one sequence of training with the bachelor's degree providing the required background in theoretical and clinical areas and the master's program providing professional training for speech-language pathology careers.

A typical master's program in Speech-Language Pathology will usually include courses such as: Research Methods in Communication Disorders, Neuromotor Disorders of Speech Production, Disorders of Phonology, Neurologic Communication Disorders in Adults, Disorders of Speech Fluency, Language Intervention: from birth to age 21, **Voice Disorders**, Language Assessment from Childhood to Adulthood, and Augmentative and Alternative Communication (AAC).

Employment in speech-language pathology requires both a master's degree in a program of study accredited by the American Speech-Language-Hearing Association (ASHA) and a credential or license. These requirements vary from state to state. Completion of the master's program provides the training required for students to qualify for a state license as a speech-language pathologist and the state credential for working as a speech-language pathologist in the public school system. The ASHA issues the Certificate of Clinical Competence (CCC) in speech-language pathology.

In the United States, ASHA is the professional, scientific, and certification association for speech-language pathologists, audiologists, and speech, language, and **hearing** scientists. The Association holds that academic studies are not sufficient to prepare an individual to function as a fully competent professional able to provide high quality care in speech-language pathology. All applicants for the CCC are accordingly required to successfully complete a clinical fellowship as well as the national examination in speech-language pathology. The clinical fellowship is intended to enable individuals to obtain supervised professional clinical experience in order to qualify for the CCC. Professional experience includes direct patient contact, consultations, record keeping, and all other duties associated with clinical work. All nonpublic school work settings require ASHA-CCC and/or state license or certification. Each state's guidelines may require ASHA certification as well as state license in addition to educational certification for employment in public schools for speech-language pathology.

Advanced education and training

The ASHA sponsors continuing education programs for speech-language pathologists. The courses of advanced study are conducted by leaders in the field of speech pathology and designed to keep speech-language pathologists abreast of new research findings, clinical techniques, and treatment models. Recognized experts also lead discussions on important ethical and regulatory issues that affect speech pathology. Alternatively, speech-language pathologists may elect to pursue doctorate work at a university and further specialize in those areas of basic research that contribute directly or indirectly to the identification, treatment, and prevention of speech and language disorders. For example, they may conduct advanced research on how people communicate. Others may design and develop equipment or techniques for diagnosing and treating speech problems.

Future outlook

The outlook for the field of speech pathology is very promising due mainly to the extraordinary advances in computer technology. Computers are being used for a wide variety of speech-language pathology applications. For example, computer programs are available for articulation and voice therapy that provide visual displays of speech: voicing, loudness, pitch, and articulation. Speech capture programs are being developed to assist the evaluation of speech/language patterns and for use in the treatment of disorders. Speech-language pathologists can use such programs, adjusting settings to provide visual reinforcement of the patient's attempts to correctly produce the target sound. Increasingly, programs and software are becoming available for testing and monitoring all major speech elements such as articulation, pitch, rhythm, duration, volume, and stress. This improved and greater use of computer technology has enabled speech-language pathologists to better serve those with speech-language disorders. There are improved augmentative devices for those with neuromuscular diseases and head injuries. For those with difficulty comprehending spoken language, the technology exists and is being used to modify the human speech signal and improve listening and comprehending skills which are fundamental for learning to read and write. For both children and adults, computer-based treatment programs exist for home use, making treatment more efficient.

Aphasia—Acquired language disorder caused by damage to the areas of the brain responsible for language function.

ASHA—The American Speech-Language-Hearing Association. In the United States, the association that regulates and provides credentials for speech-language pathologists, audiologists, and speech, language, and hearing scientists.

Communication disorder—Disorder characterized by an impaired ability to communicate. Communication disorders include language, speech, and hearing disorders. They are associated with a wide variety of physical and psychological causes.

Language disorder—Communication disorder characterized by an impaired ability to understand and/or use words in their proper context, whether verbal or nonverbal. The disorder can be either developmental or acquired.

Phonology—The science of speech sounds and sound patterns.

Speech disorder—Communication disorder characterized by an impaired ability to produce speech sounds or by problems with voice quality.

Speech pathology—The field of speech pathology, formerly known as speech therapy, is concerned with disorders of speech and language. A speech pathologist is a professional trained to diagnose and treat language and speech disorders.

Major areas of speech-language pathology software development include:

• Word-retrieval programs. These programs are mainly used to treat people affected by aphasia, a language disorder caused by damage to the areas of the brain responsible for language function. Speech-langauge pathologists use them to treat aphasias at the word or sentence level.

• Speech production software. This type of software is being developed for teaching purposes, for example to teach the proper sounds of vowels, and also for voice analysis purposes in the clinical setting.

• Reading comprehension programs. These are programs that can teach word relationships interactively and monitor the level of functional reading.

• Cognitive exercises software. This type of software is used to test logic and deduction patterns, the ability to

follow directions, and the understanding of traffic signs or of word associations.

Speech-language pathology is a very dynamic field. According to the U. S. Department of Labor, employment of speech-language pathologists is expected to grow at a much faster rate than the average for all occupations up to year 2008.

Resources

BOOKS

Gunning, T.G. *Assessing and Correcting Reading and Writing Difficulties.* Boston: Allyn & Bacon, 1997.

Hegde, M.N. *Pocketguide to Assessment in Speech-Language Pathology.* San Diego: Singular Publishing Group, 2001.

Moore-Brown, B.J., and J.K. Montgomery. *Making a Difference for America's Children: Speech-Language Pathologists in Public Schools.* Eau Claire, WI: Thinking Publications, 2001.

Shipley, K.G., and J.G. McAfee *Assessment in Speech-Language Pathology: A Resource Manual.* San Diego: Singular Publishing Group, 1998.

Simon, C.S. *Assessment of Classroom Communication and Study Skills (ACCSS).* Eau Claire, WI: Thinking Publications, 2001.

Simon, C.S. *Evaluating Communicative Competence.* Eau Claire, WI: Thinking Publications, 2001.

OTHER

National Center for Voice and Speech Website. http://www2.shc.uiowa.edu/.

Net Connections for Communication Disorders and Sciences. A Guide to Communication Disorders and Science Sources on the Internet. http://www.mankato.msus.edu/dept/com-dis/kuster2/welcome.html.

The SLP Homepage. Internet Searches and Resources on Speech Language Pathology. http://members.tripod.com/Caroline_Bowen/slp-eureka.htm.

ORGANIZATION

American Speech-Language-Hearing Association (ASHA). 10801 Rockville Pike, Rockville, MD 20852. (800)638-8255. http://www.asha.org/.

Monique Laberge, Ph.D.

Speech reading

Definition

Speech reading, also called lipreading, is "reading" the visual clues of a spoken message, meaning the movements of the lips, the tongue, the lower jaw, the eyes, the eyebrows, and the facial expression and gestures of the speaker, in an effort to process all of the available visible, situational, and auditory cues.

Purpose

Speech reading is intended for people affected by a **hearing loss** or who are close to someone affected by a **hearing** loss. Speech readers mostly use their eyes to supplement the verbal information received through their ears. It is a technique available to any person having lost hearing during adult life, whether the loss is mild or severe, and its purpose is to support or replace hearing.

Description

Speech produces not only sounds but visible movements of the lips, tongue, and jaw of the speaker as well. These movements are called articulators of speech. Because of the physical constraints imposed by the muscles involved in the articulation of speech sounds, the same speech sounds are produced with a consistent pattern of physical movements and these movements are then associated with specific sounds. Speech reading is based on this principle, that many of the sounds produced during speech may be "seen" by paying attention to the articulators of speech.

Preparation

Speech reading is taught by special educators. In typical classes, the speech educator and the students usually sit in a horseshoe seating arrangement so as to ensure that everyone present can see whoever is speaking. Teachers use a variety of exercises, focused on presenting material without using voice so as to develop the visual perception of the speech articulators in the participants, who can learn how to recognize sounds that are visible, sounds that are less visible, and sounds that can not be seen. Sounds that look like each other are differentiated, and explanations are provided as to why some words can get mixed up during speech reading. The exercises help students use what they can see, as well as the partial sounds that they can hear.

There is no special preparation required for speech reading, except the motivation to learn. However, the following recommendations are found helpful:

• Position. Speech readers are asked to position themselves with their back to the light so as to see the speaker's face clearly.

• Relaxation. A relaxed atmosphere favors speech reading.

• Recollection of speech sounds. Speech readers are encouraged to watch the speaker's face closely and to try to recall how their voice sounded.

• Speech movement. They are also encouraged to pay attention to the movements made by the lips, tongue and jaw as the person speaks, so as to learn how to differentiate the articulators, some being more recognizable than others.

• Facial expression. The facial expression of speakers is very important in speech reading, as it conveys a lot of information about the topic and the speaker's mood and feelings.

• Gestures. Gestures such as nodding and pointing also provide a lot of clues about what the speaker is saying.

Results

Speech reading recognizes that speech comprehension is an integrated process by which a listener, whether hearing-impaired or not, uses all possible information to understand a spoken message. In speech reading, the focus is on the overall meaning of the message as opposed to its specific spoken details. The result is that **vision** can then supplement the information obtained through the ears, by including all aspects of non-verbal communication as well, such as facial expressions and body language.

Health care team roles

Speech reading is taught by speech pathologists specialized in hearing disorders.

Resources

BOOKS

Campbell, R., D. Burnham, and B. Dodd, eds. *Hearing by Eye II: Advances in the Psychology of Speechreading and Auditory-Visual Speech.* Philadelphia: Psychology Press, 1998.

Kaplin, H., S.J. Bally, and C. Garretson. *Speechreading: A Way to Improve Understanding.* Washington, DC: Gallaudet University Press, 1991.

Woerner Carter, B. *I Can't Hear You in the Dark: How to Learn and Teach Lipreading.* Springfield, IL: Charles C Thomas Publisher Ltd., 1998.

OTHER

Speechreading Challenges Website, Bloomsburg University. http://www.bloomu.edu/speechreading.html.

ORGANIZATION

Self Help for Hard of Hearing People, Inc., 7910 Woodmont Ave - Suite 1200, Bethesda, Maryland 20814. Phone: (301) 657-2248. http://www.shhh.org/

Monique Laberge, Ph.D.

Speech therapy

Definition

Speech therapy is the diagnosis and treatment of a speech disorder, expressive or receptive language disorder, or certain **swallowing disorders** by a trained speech-language pathologist (SLP). SLPs commonly are called speech therapists.

Purpose

The purpose of speech therapy is to improve communication and/or the understanding of language and/or to remediate swallowing difficulties. In addition to oral communication, speech therapy may include sign language, picture communication, and the use of assistive devices to help augment speech or serve as an alternate form of communication (augmented and alternative communication [AAC]).

Demographics

According to the Bureau of Labor Statistics, in 2008 there were about 119,300 practicing SLPs in the United States, with the number expected to grow to about 141,400 by 2018. Of these, about 48% practice in schools, 9% are self-employed in private practice, and the remainder practice at hospitals, **nursing homes**, other health care facilities, or provide in-home health care services, usually through **Medicare** and **Medicaid** programs.

Description

Speech therapy addresses problems with speech production, **language disorders**, and swallowing. Problems with speech production include issues of articulation, speech rhythm, fluency, voice production, resonance, tone, and accent.

There are two basic categories of language disorders: expressive language disorders, which involves problems producing language and receptive language disorders, which involves problems understanding language. Individuals with expressive language disorders have difficulty in using language at the level expected for their age group. Often children with this type of disorder have lower than expected vocabularies, form sentences with a simpler structure than is expected, and have more difficulties expressing themselves in writing than other children their age. In some cases, (e.g. after a **stroke**) only one area will show a deficiency, such as an individual who has a good vocabulary but difficulty forming complex sentences. In other cases, all areas of language production are affected.

Individuals with receptive language disorders have difficulty understanding and processing language. This can affect comprehension of spoken or written language, or both. People who have difficulty understanding and following directions, responding to questions, or following a conversation may have a receptive language disorder. Individuals who can read words on the page but are unable to process the meaning of what they read have a receptive language disorder.

Speech therapy also addresses problems of swallowing that originate in the mouth and throat. Infants with **birth defects** of the mouth and individuals who have had a stroke or who have certain diseases such as **multiple sclerosis** are most likely to have swallowing problems.

Speech therapy is individualized. SLPs use a variety of techniques to overcome speech and language disorders based on the age of the client and the type of problem. Much work with children involves playing with them and using various toys and visual aids to encourage them to speak, along with modeling correct articulation and speech patterns. Therapy may be done one-on-one or with small groups of children. With older children and adults, the SLP may use a mirror to help the individual see how to move the muscles of their face to correctly form certain sounds. Exercises to strengthen certain facial muscles may be prescribed for people who have trouble swallowing. For individuals who have disabilities such as deafness or **cerebral palsy**, the SLP may teach the individual how to use assistive devices or alternate communication methods such as sign language.

Depending on the problems being addressed, the individual may have a speech therapy sessions as infrequently as once a week or as often as every day. There is no standard length of time an individual remains in speech therapy. Practice is the key to making progress with speech and language disorders. Parents and caregivers play an important role in the success of speech therapy, as they usually are expected to both model good articulation and speech, to reinforce the lessons taught during therapy sessions, and to supervise practice of any home exercises the SLP prescribes.

Benefits

Speech therapy improves expressive communication and language understanding and can reduce or eliminate certain swallowing problems. Improved communication leads to reduced frustration and greater safety, both for

KEY TERMS

Articulation—The ability to pronounce a word correctly. A lisp is an example of an articulation problem.

Dysphagia—Difficult or painful swallowing.

Fluency—The ability to produce a flow of words and not get "stuck." Stuttering is an example of a fluency problem.

Stroke—Irreversible damage to the brain caused by insufficient blood flow to the brain as the result of a blocked artery. Damage can include loss of speech or vision, paralysis, cognitive impairment, and death.

language-impaired individuals and for those who live and work with them.

Precautions

As of 2009, 47 states in the United States had licensing requirements for SLPs. When choosing a speech therapist, families should make sure that the therapist is licensed. Not only is this a sensible precaution to assure appropriate therapy, but many government programs and private insurers will not pay for speech therapy performed by an unlicensed individual.

Many SLPs develop specialties, such as working with stroke victims, working with preschoolers, or working with autistic individuals, so it is important to find a speech therapist who has experience in the specific speech and language problem being treated. SLPs also should be willing to work closely with health care personnel and educators, as needed, to ensure maximum benefit from the therapy.

Preparation

No special preparation is needed to begin speech therapy. An evaluation of the speech-language-swallowing problem will be done at the first session.

Aftercare

Practice and repetition are key to the success of speech therapy. Individuals often are given speech, language and/or muscle exercises to perform regularly at home. Caregivers will need to supervise these exercises and reinforce what is accomplished at the therapy sessions.

Risks

No specific risks are associated with speech therapy.

Training and certification

Certification varies from country to country and in the United States, from state to state. All SLPs are required to have a college degree. In the United States, most states require a master's degree in speech-language pathology from an accredited college or university, passing a national examination offered through the Praxis Series of the Educational Testing Service, and a minimum of 300 hours of supervised clinical experience. Most states require the SLP to earn continuing education credits to maintain their license. The American Speech-Language-Hearing Association (ASHA) offers a voluntary Certificate of Clinical Competence (CCC), which imposes higher standards than the general standards mentioned above. Individuals who earn this certificate will indicate it by putting the letters CCC-SLP after their name. The ASHA also offers voluntary certification in certain speech-language therapy specialties. Certification and licensing requirements are quite similar in other countries in the English-speaking world.

Resources

BOOKS

Feit, Debbie. *The Parent's Guide to Speech and Language Problems.* New York: McGraw-Hill, 2007.

PERIODICALS

Screening for Speech and Language Delay in Preschool Children: Recommendation Statement. *Pediatrics* v117 i2, (February) 2006, pp. 497–502.

OTHER

"Self-Help Groups for Speech, Language, and Swallowing Disorders." American Speech-Language-Hearing Association Undated. [Accessed January 10, 2010]. http://www.asha.org/public/speech/speech_self-help.htm.

Speech and Communication Disorders. MedlinePlus. January 5, 2010. [Accessed January 10, 2010] http://www.nlm.nih.gov/medlineplus/speechandcommunication disorders.html .

Speech Disorder (UK). [Accessed January 10, 2010] http://www.speechdisorder.co.uk/howtocontactus.html.

Speech Therapy Web. [Accessed January 10, 2010]. http://www.speechtherapyweb.com.

ORGANIZATIONS

American Speech-Language-Hearing Association (ASHA), 2200 Research Boulevard, Rockville, MD 20850-3289, (301) 296-5700, TTY (301) 296-5650, (800) 638-8255,

Fax: (301) 296-8580, actioncenter@asha.org, http://www.asha.org

National Institute on Deafness and Other Communication Disorders, 31 Center Drive, MSC 2320, Bethesda, MD 20892-2320.nidcdinfo@nidcd.nih.gov, http://www.nidcd.nih.gov

Stuttering Foundation of America, 3100 Walnut Grove Road, Suite 603; P.O. Box 11749, Memphis, TN 38111-0749, (901) 452-7343, (800) 992-9392, Fax: (901) 452-3931, info@stutteringhelp.org, http://www.stutteringhelp.org.

Tish Davidson, A.M.
Brenda Lerner

Sperm count test *see* **Semen analysis**

Sphygmomanometer

Definition

A sphygmomanometer is a device for monitoring a person's **blood pressure**.

Purpose

The sphygmomanometer is designed to monitor the **blood** pressure by measuring the force of the blood in the **heart** where the pressure is greatest, during the contraction of the ventricles as blood is pumped from the heart to the rest of the body (systolic pressure), and during the period when the heart is relaxed between beats and pressure is lowest (diastolic pressure).

The device is used to establish a baseline at a healthcare encounter and on admission to the hospital. Checking blood pressure is also performed to monitor the effectiveness of medication and other methods to control **hypertension**, and as a diagnostic aid to detect various diseases and abnormalities.

Description

The sphygmomanometer consists of a hand bulb pump, a unit that displays the blood pressure reading, and an inflatable cuff that is wrapped around the patient's upper arm. Care should be taken to ensure the cuff is the correct size to give an accurate reading. Children and adults with smaller or larger than average-sized arms require special sized cuffs appropriate for their needs. A **stethoscope** is also used in conjunction with the sphygmomanometer to hear the blood pressure sounds. Some devices have the stethoscope already built in.

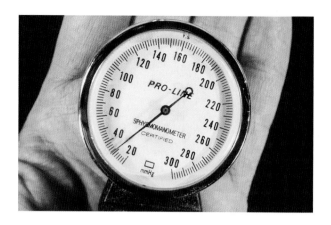

(CMSP)

The sphygmomanometer can be used in a variety of settings:

• home

• hospital

• primary care, clinic, or clinician's office

• ambulance

• dental office

There are three types of equipment for monitoring blood pressure.

The mercury-based unit has a manually inflatable cuff attached by tubing to the unit that is calibrated in millimeters of mercury. During **blood pressure measurement**, the unit must be kept upright on a flat surface and the gauge read at eye level. Breakage of the unit may cause dangerous mercury contamination and would require specialist removal for disposal.

The aneroid unit is mercury free and consists of a cuff that can be applied with one hand for self-testing, a stethoscope that is built in or attached, and a valve that inflates and deflates automatically with the data displayed on an easy-to-read gauge that will function in any position. The unit is sensitive and if dropped, may require recalibration.

The automatic unit is also mercury free and is battery operated. It has a cuff that can be applied with one hand for self-testing, and a valve that inflates and deflates automatically. (Units with manual inflation are also available.) The reading is displayed digitally and a stethoscope is not required, therefore, the unit is useful for someone who is **hearing** impaired. A wrist monitor is also available for home testing. Some more expensive models also remember and print out recordings. The automatic units may be more portable than the bulkier mercury devices.

KEY TERMS

Aneroid monitor—A monitor that works without fluids, e.g., without mercury.

Blood pressure—The tension of the blood in the arteries measured in millimeters of mercury by a sphygmomanometer or by an electronic device.

Diastolic—Minimum arterial blood pressure during ventricular rest.

Systolic—Maximum arterial blood pressure during ventricular contraction.

Blood pressure can be measured with any of the units, although mercury units are becoming less common due to the hazards of mercury.

Operation

The flow, resistance, quality, and quantity of blood circulating through the heart and the condition of the arterial walls are all factors that influence the blood pressure. If blood flow in the arteries is restricted, the reading will be higher.

Blood pressure should be routinely checked every one to two years. It can be checked at any time but is best performed when the patient has been resting for at least five minutes, so that exertion prior to the test will not unduly influence the outcome of the reading.

To record blood pressure, the patient should be seated with his left arm bent slightly, and the arm bare or with the sleeve loosely rolled up. With an aneroid or automatic unit, the cuff is placed level with the heart and wrapped around the upper arm, one inch above the elbow. Following the manufacturer's guidelines, the cuff is inflated and then deflated and the nurse records the reading.

If the blood pressure is monitored manually, a cuff is placed level with the heart and wrapped firmly but not tightly around the arm one inch above the elbow over the brachial artery, with creases in the cuff smoothed out. With a stethoscope over the brachial artery in front of the elbow with one hand and listening through the earpiece, the cuff is inflated well above normal levels (to about 200 mm Hg), or until no sound is heard. The cuff is then inflated a further 10 mm Hg above the last sound heard. The valve in the pump is slowly opened no faster than 5 mm Hg per second to deflate the pressure in the cuff to the point where a tapping sound is heard over the brachial artery. This point is noted as the systolic pressure. The sounds continue as the pressure in the cuff is released and

the artery is no longer occluded. At this point, the noises are no longer heard and this is noted as the diastolic pressure.

With children, the tapping noise changes to a soft muffled sound. That point is noted as the diastolic pressure, since sounds continue to be heard as the cuff deflates to zero.

Blood pressure results are recorded with the systolic pressure first, then the diastolic pressure (e.g., 120/70).

Maintenance

Devices should be checked and calibrated annually by a qualified technician to ensure accurate readings.

Health care team roles

The appropriate sized cuff should be used to give an accurate reading. Repeated measurements may be required if hypertension is suspected. One elevated reading does not mean that hypertension is present. The blood pressure measurement is recorded and compared with normal ranges for the patient's age and medical condition and a decision made on whether any further medical intervention is required.

Training

The method of recording blood pressure should be consistent, especially the diastolic pressure, as a different reading will be obtained if it is measured when the sounds change or when they disappear. All health care professionals should be aware of the normal values for blood pressure measurement based on age and medical history.

Resources

PERIODICAL

Canzanello, Vincent J., Patricia L. Jensen, and Gary L. Schwartz. "Are Anaeroid Sphygmomanometers Accurate in Hospital and Clinic Settings?" *Archives of Internal Medicine* 161 (March 12, 2001): 729.

OTHER

"About Blood Pressure." American Heart Association. National Center, 7272 Greenville Avenue, Dallas, TX 752311. (800) AHA-USA1.

"High Blood Pressure." www.MayoClinic.com. September 28, 2000.

"Home Monitoring of High Blood Pressure." American Heart Association, National Center, 7272 Greenville Avenue, Dallas, TX 752311. (800) AHA-USA1.

Rathe, Richard. "Vital Signs." University of Florida. December 19, 2000. http://www.medinfo.ufl.edu/yea1/bcs/clist/vitals.html. (July 16, 2001).

"Reducing Mercury Use in Health Care: Promoting a Healthier Environment." http://www.epa.gov/glnpo/bnsdocs/merch-ealth/indextext.html.

"What Is High Blood Pressure?" American Heart Association, National Center, 7272 Greenville Avenue, Dallas, TX 752311. (800) AHA-USA1.

ORGANIZATION

American College of Nurse Practitioners, 503 Capitol Ct. NE #300, Washington, DC 20002. (202) 546-4825. acnp@nurse.org

Margaret A. Stockley

Sphygmomanometry *see* **Blood pressure measurement**

Spina bifida *see* **Neural tube defect**

Spinal column *see* **Vertebral column**

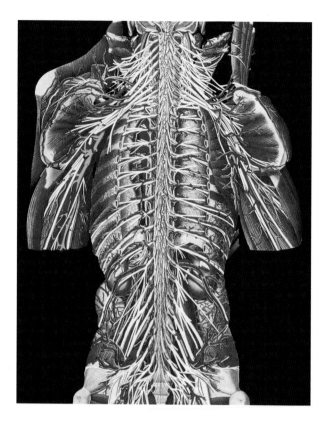

(*Computer-enhanced historical illustration of the human spinal cord and spinal nerves, photograph. M. Kulyk / Photo Researchers, Inc.*)

Spinal cord

Definition

The spinal cord is the elongated, thin, tubular bundle of nervous tissue and support cells that carries nerve impulses between the **brain** and the rest of the body. It lies in the vertebral canal of the **vertebral column**, which extends from the medulla oblongata within the brain. The **central nervous system** consists of the brain and the spinal cord.

Demographics

One end of the spinal cord is located at the occipital **bone**. It extends down to the space between the first and second lumbar vertebrae; but it does not proceed down the entire length of the vertebral column. The spinal cord is around 18 in. (45 cm) long in men and around 17 in. (43 cm) long in women. It has a varying width, ranging from about 0.5 in. (1.3 cm) thick in the cervical and lumbar regions to approximately 0.25 in. (0.6 cm) thick in the thoracic area.

Description

The spinal cord lies within the vertebral canal, which is the hollow part of the vertebral column, or spine, that consists of 33 bones called vertebrae. The canal is formed by the stacked vertebrae that all contain a central vertebral foramen, or hole. The spinal cord extends from the lowest part of the brain, called the brainstem, through a hole located at the base of the **skull**, the foramen magnum, and continues down the vertebral canal to the twenty-first vertebra of the spine.

Like the brain, the spinal cord is protected by three layers of membranes, called meninges. The inner meninx that makes direct contact with the spinal cord is called the pia mater. It is separated from the second layer by a space called the subarachnoid space. This space is filled with cerebrospinal fluid (CSF), the colorless fluid that bathes the entire brain and spinal cord. The second layer is the thin and spider web-like arachnoid mater and it is separated from the outermost layer by a space called the subdural space. The outermost layer is the dura mater, a protective sheath made of tough fiber. Between the dura mater and the bone of the vertebral canal is a space, called the epidural space, which contains a small amount of fatty tissue and **blood vessels**. The spinal dura mater prolongs the dura mater that lines the skull cavity and extends to the sacrum, the second to last bone of the vertebral column. It also covers each of the spinal nerves as they leave the vertebral canal. Both the arachnoid and pia mater also prolong the arachnoid and pia surrounding the brain, but unlike the arachnoid, which continuously follows the dura mater, the pia ends where the spinal cord ends. A stringy extension of the pia mater, called the

QUESTIONS TO ASK YOUR DOCTOR

- What therapies and rehabilitations are generally available for spinal cord injuries? What is available locally?

- How serious is my spinal cord injury? Will my injury heal? How much feeling and movement can I expect to recover?

- How will a spinal cord injury affect my health? Am I at risk of other health conditions?

- Is there a local support group for people with spinal cord injuries?

- What will happen in the short-term? In the long-term?

- What side effects may occur during my treatment?

- Will surgery help my spinal cord injury?

- Where can I learn more about spinal cord injuries?

filum terminale joins the end of the spinal cord to the end of the dura mater. Additionally, the pia mater contains thin projections called denticulate ligaments, which connect the spinal cord to the dura mater.

Function

The major function of the spinal cord is to carry nerve impulses between the brain and the rest of the body. Together, the brain and the spinal cord constitute the central nervous system (CNS). The other nerves of the nervous system, that is the motor and sensory nerves, constitute the peripheral nervous system (PNS).

The spinal cord consists of a core of grey nervous tissue surrounded by a thicker section of white tissue. The grey matter looks like a butterfly with outspread wings and the upper and lower sections of these wings are called the posterior and anterior horns. The tissues of the spinal cord are full of nerve cells, also called **neurons**. Neurons with large cell bodies that are located in the anterior horns give rise to motor nerve fibers that connect to spinal nerves, which pass out of the cord to skeletal muscle. The grey matter of the spinal cord also contains other neurons that connect together to form nerve pathways and the white matter contains nerves that are wrapped in myelin sheaths and form nerve tracts.

The tracts that conduct sensory impulses from the body to the brain are called ascending tracts and those that conduct motor impulses from the brain to muscles and glands are called descending tracts.

Thirty-one pairs of spinal nerves emerge from the spinal cord. They are all mixed nerves, meaning that they provide a two-way communication system for sensory and motor information exchange between the spinal cord and the rest of the body. Spinal nerves are numbered according to the vertebral column level from which they stem. There are eight pairs of cervical nerves, C1 to C8, twelve pairs of thoracic nerves, T1 to T12, five pairs of lumbar nerves, L1 to L5, five pairs of sacral nerves, S1 to S5, and one pair of coccygeal nerves.

Risks

Risks from spinal cord injuries are usually caused by trauma (such as bruising, excessive pressure, and laceration) to the spinal column. For example, a sharp object can puncture the spinal cord. When such an injury occurs, the victim will usually suffer loss of feeling to one of the extremities. In milder cases, a victim might suffer some inability to move a hand or foot. More severe injuries may result in becoming a paraplegic (a person who is impaired in motor or sensory function of the lower extremities) or a quadriplegic (a person with partial or total loss of use of all their limbs and torso). Severe injury can also occur when full body **paralysis** occurs below the site of injury to the spinal cord.

Although anyone can have a **spinal cord injury**, those at increased risk include:

- Gender: five times as many males have spinal cord injuries in the United States when compared to females.

- Age: people from 16 to 30 years of age range suffer the most spinal cord injuries; with the leading cause for people 65 years and younger being motor vehicle crashes and for those above that age the primary cause is falling

- Behavior. Risky actions make one more likely to have a spinal cord injury, such as playing aggressive sports and performing physical activities without proper safety equipment or taking necessary precautions.

- Preexisting conditions: having a bone or joint disorder, such as arthritis or osteoporosis.

Results

A spinal cord injury can be divided into two levels: complete and incomplete. A complete spinal cord injury results in a person without function below the level of the injury. This includes being without sensation and not having voluntary movement in this region, with both

Arachnoid mater—One of three meninges covering the central nervous system (CNS). The others are the dura and pia maters. The dura mater encloses the arachnoid, which in turn covers the pia mater.

Brain stem—Lowest part of the brain that connects with the spinal cord. It is a complicated neural center with several neuronal pathways between the cerebrum, spinal cord, cerebellum, and motor and sensory functions of the head and neck. It consists of the medulla oblongata, the part responsible for cardiac and respiratory control, the midbrain, which is involved in basic, involuntary body functions, and the pons, where some cranial nerves originate.

Central nervous system (CNS)—One of two major divisions of the nervous system. The CNS consists of the brain, the cranial nerves, and the spinal cord.

Cerebrospinal fluid (CSF)—A clear colorless fluid that circulates in the brain and in the subarachnoid spaces surrounding the brain and spinal cord. The CSF lies between the spinal cord and the arachnoid mater, thereby suspending the spinal cord in fluid.

Cervical vertebrae—Vertebrae of the neck.

Epidural space—This space lies between the dura mater and the walls of the vertebral canal. It contains loose connective tissue, blood vessels, and some fatty tissue.

Foramen—A hole in a bone usually for the passage of blood vessels and/or nerves.

Foramen magnum—Large opening at the base of the skull that allows passage of the spinal cord.

Intervertebral disk—Disk-shaped pads of fibrous cartilage interposed between the vertebrae of the vertebral column that provide cushioning and join the vertebrae together.

Meninges—The membranes that surround and protect the brain and spinal cord. There are three layers: the dura mater (outermost), arachnoid membrane (middle), and the pia mater (innermost).

Nervous system—The entire system of nerve tissue in the body. It includes the brain, the brainstem, the

---

sides of the body being affected equally. An incomplete spinal cord injury means that a person has some function below the level of the injury. They may be able to feel parts of the body but cannot move them, to move one limb but not the other, or to move one side of the body more than the other.

Role in human health

The spinal cord is an extremely important component of the CNS because it provides the crucial link between the brain and the spinal nerves that connect to the individual muscles and organs of the body. The role of the spinal cord in human health, however, is not only to carry this sensory and motor information. It also carries a great deal of other crucial information as well, having to do with involuntary and automatic body functions. For example, the regulation of the chemical contents of the **blood** and body fluids is carried out by an automatic feedback control system that involves the spinal cord and its attached network of peripheral nerves. The regulation the **heart**, **stomach**, and intestines are other examples. These are all vital body functions of which we are unaware and that all proceed with the involvement of the spinal cord nervous tissues.

Diseases and disorders

Spinal cord injuries are usually the result of trauma to the vertebral column. When **dislocations** and **fractures** of the spine occur, the vertebrae may press on the spinal cord, thus compressing the nerves. Pressure applied to the spinal cord may result in muscle **weakness** or paralysis. It could also cause abnormal sensations, such as **pain**, tingling, or burning. In severe cases, the cord might even be torn or severed, and the function of the spinal cord risks being seriously impaired if not altogether destroyed. A damaged spinal cord results in loss of sensation and/or motor function below the level of the injury. Thus, injuries to the cord at the chest or waist level may result in paraplegia, which is impairment of the legs and/or part of the trunk. Damage to the cord in the neck region may result in impairment of all four limbs and the trunk, a condition called quadriplegia, and it can be fatal. Other disorders of the spinal cord include:

• Epidural abscesses. Infections that occur in the epidural space around the dura mater. These create pockets of infected fluid that affect the spinal nerve roots and generate enough pressure to impair neurological function.

KEY TERMS (continued)

spinal cord, the nerves, and the ganglia and is divided into the peripheral nervous system (PNS) and the central nervous system (CNS).

Paraplegia—Paraplegia is permanent impairment of the trunk and lower limbs. It is caused by injury or disease affecting the spinal cord below the chest or waist.

Peripheral nerves—The nerves outside of the brain and spinal cord, including the autonomic, cranial, and spinal nerves. These nerves contain cells other than neurons and connective tissue as well as axons.

Peripheral nervous system (PNS)—One of the two major divisions of the nervous system. The PNS consists of the somatic nervous system (SNS), which controls voluntary activities and of the autonomic nervous system (ANS), which controls regulatory activities. The ANS is further divided into sympathetic and parasympathetic systems.

Quadraplegia—Quadraplegia is permanent impairment of the trunk, lower and upper limbs. It

is caused by injury or disease affecting the spinal cord at the neck level.

Sacrum—The triangular-shaped bone found between the fifth lumbar vertebra and the coccyx. It consists of five fused vertebrae and it articulates on each side with the bones of the pelvis (ilium), forming the sacroiliac joints.

Sensory nerve—A nerve that receives input from sensory cells, such as the skin or muscle receptors.

Skull—All of the bones of the head.

Spinal cord—Elongated part of the central nervous system (CNS) that lies in the vertebral canal of the spine and from which the spinal nerves emerge.

Vertebra—Flat bones that make up the vertebral column. The spine has 33 vertebrae.

Vertebral canal—Hollow part of the vertebral column formed by the vertebral foramina of the stacked vertebrae. It encloses the spinal cord.

Vertebral foramen—The opening formed in vertebrae that allows passage of the spinal cord.

- Foraminal stenosis. Normally, nerve roots have enough room to easily slip through the foramina of the spine. However, with age and disease, they may become clogged and blocked, thus trapping and compressing the nerves.

- Pinched nerve. The two nerves most commonly pinched in the spinal cord are L5 and S1. The L5 nerve supplies the nerves to the muscles that raise the foot and big toe, and a pinched L5 may lead to weakness in these muscles. Likewise, a pinched S1 may lead to weakness with the large muscle in the back of the calf.

- Sciatica. The compression of the spinal roots of the sciatic nerve. It is characterized by pain in the low back region that radiates down the back of the thigh, the leg and into the foot. It results from diseased sciatic nerve roots or can be caused by a tumor, or intervertebral disc displacement resulting from injury or inflammation.

- Spinal stenosis. A narrowing of spaces in the spine that results in pressure on the spinal cord and nerve roots. This disorder usually involves the narrowing of one or more of three areas of the spine: the vertebral canal, the canals at the base or roots of nerves branching out from

the spinal cord, and the vertebral foramina. It is usually a degenerative disorder caused by old age, but may also be an inherited disease.

Resources

BOOKS

Baaj, Ali A., et al., editors. *Handbook of Spine Surgery.* New York: Thieme, 2012.

Lin, Vernon W., editor. *Spinal Cord Medicine: Principles and Practice.* New York: Demos Medical, 2010.

Phillips, Frank M., and Safdar N. Khan, editors. *Treatment of Complex Cervical Spine Disorders.* Philadelphia: Saunders, 2012.

Somers, Martha Freeman. *Spinal Cord Injury: Functional Rehabilitation.* Upper Saddle River, NJ: Pearson Education, 2010.

Vaccaro, Alexander R., Michael G. Fehlings, and Marcel F. Dvorak, editors. *Spine and Spinal Cord Trauma: Evidence-Based Management.* New York: Thieme, 2011.

WEBSITES

Spinal Cord Injury. FamilyDoctor.org. (August 2010). http://familydoctor.org/familydoctor/en/diseases-conditions/spinal-cord-injury.html (April 25, 2012).

Spinal Cord Injury. Mayo Clinic. (October 22, 2011). http://www.mayoclinic.com/health/spinal-cord-injury/DS00460 (April 25, 2012).

Spinal Cord Injury Resource Center. SpinalInjury.net. http://www.spinalinjury.net/ (April 25, 2012).

The Spinal Cord or Medulla Spinalis. Bartleby.com edition of Gray's Anatomy of the Human Body. http://www.bartleby.com/107/185.html (April 25, 2012).

ORGANIZATIONS

National Spinal Cord Injury Association, 75-20 Astoria Blvd., Jackson Heights, NY 11370, (718) 803-3782, http://www.spinalcord.org/

Spinal Cord Society, 19051 Country Highway 1, Fergus Falls, MN 56537-9627, (218) 739-5252, Fax: (218) 739-5262, http://www.spinalcordsociety.com/.

Monique Laberge, Ph.D.
William A. Atkins, B.B., B.S., M.B.A.

Spinal cord injury

Definition

Spinal cord injury is damage to the spinal cord that causes loss of sensation and motor control.

Description

As of 2010, approximately 12,000 Americans survive a new spinal cord injuries (SCIs) occur each year. About 265,000 Americans are currently affected. Spinal cord injuries can happen to anyone at any time of life; however, more than 80% of SCIs happen to males. The average age at the time of injury has increased from 28.7 years in the 1970s to 40.7 years in the mid-2000s. Since 2005, motor vehicle accident account for the greatest number of SCIs (40.4% of all SCIs), followed by **falls** (27.9%), an act of violence(15%), most often related to firearms use or a sports accident (8%). Since the 1970s, the percentage of SCIs attributable to sports accidents has decreased and the percentage attributable to falls has increased, perhaps reflecting an **aging** American population.

Most SCI patients are white, but the nonwhite fraction of SCI patients is larger than the nonwhite fraction of the general population. In fact, the SCI rate among blacks, who are at higher risk for SCI than whites, has been rising in recent years. Alcohol or other drug abuse plays a role in a large percentage of all spinal cord injuries.

Causes and symptoms

Causes

The spinal cord descends from the **brain** down the back through the spinal canal that lies within the bony spinal column. The spinal cord is composed of **neurons** (nerve cells). The neurons carry sensory data from the areas outside the spinal cord (periphery) to the brain, and convey motor commands from brain to periphery. Peripheral neurons are bundled together to comprise the 31 pairs of peripheral nerve roots. The peripheral nerve roots enter and exit the spinal cord by passing through the spaces between the stacked vertebrae (the neural foramen). Each pair of nerves is named for the vertebra from which it exits. These are known as:

- C1-8. These nerves enter from the seven cervical or neck vertebrae.
- T1-12. These nerves enter from the thoracic or chest vertebrae.
- L1-5. These nerves enter from the lumbar vertebrae of the lower back.
- S1-5. These nerves enter through the sacral, or pelvic vertebrae.
- Coccygeal. These nerves enter through the coccyx, or tailbone.

Peripheral nerves carry motor commands to the muscles and internal organs, and transmit sensations from these areas and from the body's surface. (Sensory data from the head, including sight, sound, **smell**, and **taste**, do not pass through the spinal cord and are not affected by most SCIs. These nerves, called the cranial nerves, pass through the brain stem.) Damage to the spinal cord interrupts these signals. The interruption damages motor functions that enable the muscles to move, sensory functions (e.g., feeling heat and cold), and autonomic functions (e.g., urination, sexual function, sweating, and **blood pressure**).

Spinal cord injuries most often occur where the spine is most flexible, in the regions of C5–C7 of the neck, and T10–L2 at the base of the rib cage.

Several physically distinct types of damage are recognized. Sudden and violent jolts to nearby tissues can jar the cord. This jarring causes a transient neurological deficit, known as temporary spinal **concussion**. Concussion symptoms usually disappear completely within several hours of injury. A spinal contusion, or bruise, is bleeding within the spinal column. The pressure from the excess fluid may kill spinal cord neurons. Spinal compression is caused by an object, such as a tumor, pressing on the cord. Lacerations, or tears, cause direct damage to cord neurons.

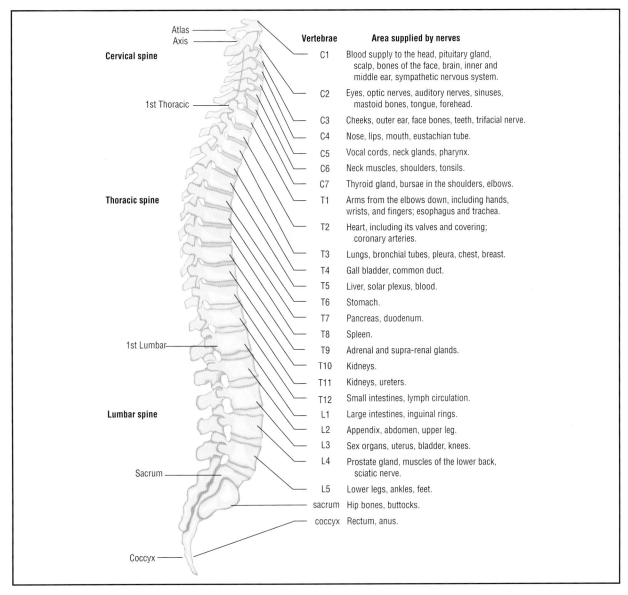

Vertebrae	Area supplied by nerves
C1	Blood supply to the head, pituitary gland, scalp, bones of the face, brain, inner and middle ear, sympathetic nervous system.
C2	Eyes, optic nerves, auditory nerves, sinuses, mastoid bones, tongue, forehead.
C3	Cheeks, outer ear, face bones, teeth, trifacial nerve.
C4	Nose, lips, mouth, eustachian tube.
C5	Vocal cords, neck glands, pharynx.
C6	Neck muscles, shoulders, tonsils.
C7	Thyroid gland, bursae in the shoulders, elbows.
T1	Arms from the elbows down, including hands, wrists, and fingers; esophagus and trachea.
T2	Heart, including its valves and covering; coronary arteries.
T3	Lungs, bronchial tubes, pleura, chest, breast.
T4	Gall bladder, common duct.
T5	Liver, solar plexus, blood.
T6	Stomach.
T7	Pancreas, duodenum.
T8	Spleen.
T9	Adrenal and supra-renal glands.
T10	Kidneys.
T11	Kidneys, ureters.
T12	Small intestines, lymph circulation.
L1	Large intestines, inguinal rings.
L2	Appendix, abdomen, upper leg.
L3	Sex organs, uterus, bladder, knees.
L4	Prostate gland, muscles of the lower back, sciatic nerve.
L5	Lower legs, ankles, feet.
sacrum	Hip bones, buttocks.
coccyx	Rectum, anus.

Labels on the spine diagram: Atlas, Axis, Cervical spine, 1st Thoracic, Thoracic spine, 1st Lumbar, Lumbar spine, Sacrum, Coccyx.

(Diagram of the human spine with sections and vertebrae labeled. Illustration by GGS Information Services, Inc. The Gale Group.)

Lacerations may be caused by **bone** fragments or missiles, such as bullets. Spinal P describes the complete severing of the cord. Most spinal cord injuries involve two or more of these types of damage.

Symptoms

PARALYSIS AND LOSS OF SENSATION. The extent to which movement and sensation are damaged depends on the level of the spinal cord injury. Nerves leaving the spinal cord at different levels control sensation and movement in different parts of the body. The distribution is roughly as follows:

• C1–C4: head and neck

• C3–C5: diaphragm (chest and breathing)

• C5–T1: shoulders, arms and hands

• T2–T12: chest and abdomen (excluding internal organs)

• L1–L4: abdomen (excluding internal organs), buttocks, genitals, and upper legs

• L4–S1: legs

• S2–S4: genitals and muscles of the perineum

Damage below T1, which lies at the top of the rib cage, causes **paralysis** and loss of sensation in the legs and trunk below the injury. Injury at this level usually does no damage to the arms and hands. Paralysis of the legs is called paraplegia. Damage above T1 involves the arms as well as the legs. Paralysis of all four limbs was

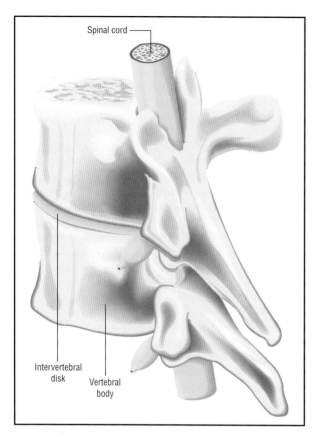

(Vertebrae, intervertebral disk, and spinal cord, diagram. Illustration by GGS Information Services, Inc. The Gale Group.)

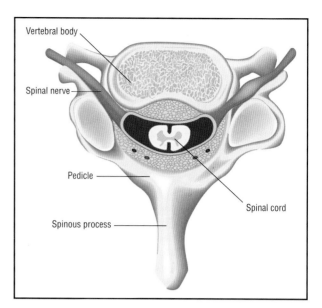

(Cross-section of a vertabra, diagram. Illustration by GGS Information Services, Inc. The Gale Group.)

formerly called quadriplegia and is now referred to as tetraplegia.

Cervical, or neck injuries, not only cause tetraplegia, but also may cause difficulty in breathing. Damage in the lower part of the neck may leave enough diaphragm control to allow unassisted breathing. Patients with damage at C3 or above, just below the base of the **skull**, require mechanical assistance from a ventilator or diaphragmatic nerve stimulation to breathe.

Symptoms also depend on the extent of the SCI. A completely severed cord causes paralysis and loss of sensation below the wound. If the cord is only partially severed, some function will remain below the injury. Damage limited to the front portion of the cord causes paralysis and loss of sensations of **pain** and temperature. Other sensation may be preserved. Damage to the center of the cord may spare the legs, but paralyze the arms. Damage to the right or left half causes loss of position sense, paralysis on the side of the injury, and loss of pain and temperature sensation on the opposite side.

AUTONOMIC DYSREFLEXIA. Body organs that self-regulate, such as the **heart**, gastrointestinal tract, and glands, are controlled by autonomic nerves. Autonomic nerves emerge from three different places: above the spinal column, in the lower back from vertebrae T1-L4, and from the lowest regions of the sacrum at the base of the spine. In general, these three groups of autonomic nerves operate in balance. Spinal cord injury can disrupt this balance, a condition called autonomic dysreflexia or autonomic hyperreflexia. Patients with injuries at T6 or above are at greatest risk.

SPASTICITY AND CONTRACTURE. A paralyzed limb is incapable of active movement, but the muscle still has tone, a constant low level of contraction. Normal muscle tone requires communication between the muscle and the brain. Spinal cord injury prevents the brain from telling the muscle to relax. The result is prolonged **muscle contraction** or spasticity. Since the muscles that extend and those that bend a joint are not usually equal in strength, the involved joint is bent, often severely. This constant pressure causes deformity. As the muscle remains in the shortened position over several weeks or months, the tendons remodel and cause permanent muscle shortening or contracture. When muscles have permanently shortened, the inner surfaces of joints, such as armpits or palms, cannot be cleaned and the skin breaks down in that area.

HETEROTOPIC OSSIFICATION. Heterotopic ossification is an abnormal deposit of bone in muscles and tendons that may occur after injury. It is most common in the hips and knees. Initially heterotopic ossification causes localized swelling, warmth, redness, and stiffness of the muscle. It usually begins one to four months after the injury and is rare after one year.

In autonomic dysreflexia, irritation of the skin, bowel, or bladder causes a highly exaggerated response from autonomic nerves. This response is caused by the uncontrolled release of norepinephrine, a hormone similar to adrenaline. Uncontrolled release of norepinephrine causes a rapid rise in **blood** pressure and a slowing of the heart rate. These symptoms are accompanied by throbbing **headache**, nausea, **anxiety**, sweating, and goose bumps below the level of the injury. The elevated blood pressure can rapidly cause loss of consciousness, seizures, cerebral hemorrhage, and death. Autonomic dysreflexia is most often caused by an overfull bladder or bladder **infection**, impaction or hard, impassable fecal mass in the bowel, or skin irritation from tight clothing, sunburn, or other irritant. Inability to sense these irritants before the autonomic reaction begins is a major cause of dysreflexia.

LOSS OF BLADDER AND BOWEL CONTROL. Bladder and bowel control require both motor nerves and the **autonomic nervous system** (ANS). Both of these systems may be damaged by SCI. When the ANS triggers an urge to urinate or defecate, continence is maintained by contracting the anal or urethral sphincter, respectively. The sphincter is a ring of muscle that contracts to close off a passage or opening in the body. When the neural connections to these muscles are severed, conscious control is lost. In addition, loss of feeling may prevent sensations of fullness from reaching the brain. To compensate, the patient may help empty the bowel or bladder by using physical maneuvers that stimulate autonomic contractions before they would otherwise begin. The patient may not, however, be able to relax the sphincters. If the sphincters cannot be relaxed, the patient will retain urine or feces.

Retention of urine may cause muscular changes in the bladder and urethral sphincter that make the problem worse. Urinary tract infection is common. Retention of feces can cause impaction. Symptoms of impaction include loss of appetite and nausea. Untreated impaction may cause perforation of the **large intestine** and **sepsis** (rapid overwhelming infection).

Complications

DEEP VENOUS THROMBOSIS. Blood does not flow normally through a paralyzed limb that is inactive for long periods. The blood pools in the deep veins and forms clots, a condition known as **deep vein thrombosis**. A clot, or thrombus, can break free and lodge in smaller arteries in the brain (causing a **stroke**), or in the **lungs** (causing **pulmonary embolism**).

DECUBITUS ULCERS. Inability to move may also lead to decubitus ulcers (pressure ulcers or bedsores).

Decubitus ulcers form where skin remains in contact with a bed or chair for a long time. The most common sites of pressure ulcers are the buttocks, hips, and heels. Decubitus ulcers can cause sepsis (infection) and may seriously jeopardize recovery.

Diagnosis

The location and extent of SCI is determined by obtaining a history, performing a **physical examination**, and ordering appropriate imaging studies. Imaging studies usually include a combination of **computed tomography (CT) scans**, **magnetic resonance imaging** (MRI) scans, and traditional x rays. Computed tomography or MRI scans may be enhanced with an injected contrast dye. These diagnostic imaging studies are explained to patients by nurses and radiologic technicians. The studies are usually performed by these technicians, and are read, or interpreted, by a radiologist and/or a neuroradiologist.

Treatment

Acute care of SCI

Onlookers should not move a person who has sustained or who is suspected of sustaining an SCI. If there is any doubt at all about whether the spinal cord is injured, the person should not be moved and professional emergency help should be summoned. Emergency medical personnel are best equipped to transport the injured patient. Treatment of SCI begins with immobilization. This strategy prevents partial injuries of the cord from severing it completely. Since the early 1980s, the use of splints to completely immobilize suspected SCI at the scene of the injury has helped reduce the severity of spinal cord injuries. Intravenous methylprednisolone, a steroidal anti-inflammatory drug, is given during the first 24 hours to reduce inflammation and limit tissue destruction.

Restoration of function and mobility

Rehabilitation after SCI seeks to prevent complications, promote recovery, and make the most of remaining function. Rehabilitation is a complex and long-term process; it requires a team of professionals, including a neurologist, physiatrist (or rehabilitation specialist), physical therapist, and occupational therapist. Other specialists who may be needed include a respiratory therapist, vocational rehabilitation counselor, social worker, speech-language pathologist, nutritionist, special education teacher, recreation therapist, and clinical psychologist. Support groups provide a critical source of information, advice, and support for SCI patients and their families.

While the possibility of using functional electrical stimulation (FES) for ambulation (outside of the laboratory) remains distant, the use of FES to deal with other aspects of SCI (such as loss of grasp capabilities in tetraplegia) is more advanced and more likely to be in common use in the foreseeable future.

Instruction in activities of daily living

Physical therapy focuses on mobility to maintain range of motion of affected limbs and reduce contracture and deformity. Additionally, it helps to compensate for lost skills by using those muscles that are still functional, and helps to increase any residual strength and control in affected muscles. Adaptive equipment such as braces, canes, or wheelchairs can be suggested by a physical therapist.

The goal of **occupational therapy** is to restore the ability to perform the activities of daily living, such as eating and grooming, with tools and new techniques. Modifications of the home and workplace to accommodate and address the individual impairment are also addressed by the occupational therapist.

Treatment of sexual dysfunction

Men who have sustained SCI may be unable to achieve an erection or ejaculate. Sperm formation may be abnormal and fertility may be compromised. Fertility and the ability to achieve orgasm are less impaired for women. Women may still be able to become pregnant and deliver vaginally.

Prevention of complications

DECUBITUS ULCERS (PRESSURE ULCERS). Turning the patient in bed at least every two hours prevents the formation of decubitus ulcers. The patient should be turned more frequently when redness begins to develop in sensitive areas. Special mattresses and chair cushions can distribute weight more evenly to reduce pressure. Skin should be carefully attended to by nurses and other caregivers in order to maintain skin integrity and prevent ulcers from developing. Electrical stimulation is sometimes used to promote muscle movement to prevent decubitus ulcers.

SPASTICITY AND CONTRACTURE. Range of motion (ROM) exercises help to prevent contracture. Chemicals can be used to prevent contractures from becoming fixed when ROM **exercise** is inadequate. Phenol or alcohol can be injected into the nerve, or botulinum toxin can be injected directly into the muscle. Botulinum toxin is associated with fewer complications, but it is more expensive than phenol and alcohol. Contractures can be

released by cutting the shortened tendon or transferring it surgically to a different site on the bone, where deformity will be lessened by its pull. Such tendon transfers may also be used to increase strength in partially functional extremities.

DEEP VENOUS THROMBOSIS. Deep venous thrombosis may be prevented by using passive ROM exercises, sequential compression stockings, intermittent pneumatic compression devices, and kinetic (movement) therapies. Heparin and aspirin may also be administered to prevent deep venous thrombosis.

HETEROTOPIC OSSIFICATION. Etidronate disodium (Didronel), a drug that regulates the body's use of **calcium**, is used to prevent heterotopic ossification. Treatment begins three weeks after the injury and continues for 12 weeks. Surgical removal of ossified tissue is possible.

AUTONOMIC DYSREFLEXIA. Bowel and bladder care and attention to potential irritants prevent autonomic dysreflexia. It is treated by prompt removal of the irritant. Drugs to lower blood pressure are used when necessary. Patients, friends, and families of the patient should be educated about the symptoms and treatment of dysreflexia, because immediate intervention is usually necessary.

LOSS OF BLADDER AND BOWEL CONTROL. Normal bowel function is promoted through adequate fluid intake and a diet rich in fiber. Evacuation is stimulated by deliberately increasing the abdominal pressure, either voluntarily or by using an abdominal binder.

Bladder care involves continual or intermittent catheterization. The full bladder may be detected by feeling its bulge against the abdominal wall. Urinary tract infection is a significant complication of catheterization and requires frequent monitoring.

SEXUAL DYSFUNCTION. Counseling can help patients to adjust to changes in sexual function after SCI. Erection may be enhanced through the same means used to treat **erectile dysfunction** in the general population.

Prognosis

The prognosis for SCI depends on the site and extent of injury. Injuries of the neck above C4 with significant involvement of the diaphragm hold the gravest prognosis. Respiratory infection (**pneumonia**) is one of the leading causes of death in long-term SCI. Suicide is also more common among people with SCIs, especially those who are young when they are injured and who experience ongoing pain. Overall, 85% of SCI patients who survive the first 24 hours are alive ten years after their injuries. Recovery of function is uncommon and impossible to predict. Partial recovery is more likely after an incomplete wound than after the spinal cord has been completely severed. Life expectancy of those with SCIs has steadily increased.

Health care team roles

Initial medical management, including immobilization and transport of SCI patients, is usually provided by emergency medical personnel. Upon arrival, the physicians and nurses in the hospital emergency department assess the nature and extent of the injury. Imaging studies are performed by radiologic technicians and interpreted by radiologists and neuroradiologists. Consultation with a neurosurgeon determines whether surgical intervention will be beneficial in treating the injury.

Following emergency treatment, assessment, and completion of the diagnostic work-up, critical care vigilant monitoring of SCI patients is provided by the nurses. The aim of monitoring is to identify the decreased cardiac output that may result from sympathetic nerve blockade; excessive autonomic nerve responses (i.e., distended bladder or bowel); problems associated with breathing; and the risk of aspiration.

Nurses, social workers, physical and occupational therapists, pastoral counselors, and other medical and mental health professionals may be called upon to help patients and families manage their emotional responses to the injury. Feelings of anxiety, anger, and denial may be experienced by hopeless patients and families.

Patient education

Patient education is an essential part of the rehabilitation process. Every member of the treatment team is involved in patient education. Patients and families are taught by nurses to recognize symptoms requiring immediate medical attention, and to provide selected care (e.g., a bowel program to prevent impaction). They may be instructed by physical and occupational therapists to use adaptive devices and equipment. Education may help to reduce feelings of powerlessness and hopelessness, and can assist in the creation of realistic expectations about recovery.

Many SCI patients also benefit from participation in peer support groups. They are enabled by the groups to meet others with comparable conditions, thereby reducing feelings of isolation, and allowing them to share experience-tested coping strategies.

Prevention

Risk of spinal cord injury can be reduced through prevention of the accidents that lead to it. Chances of injury from automobile accidents, the major cause of

> ## KEY TERMS
>
> **Autonomic nervous system**—The part of the nervous system that controls involuntary functions such as sweating and blood pressure.
>
> **Botulinum toxin**—Any of a group of potent bacterial toxins or poisons produced by different strains of the bacterium *Clostridium botulinum*.
>
> **Computed tomography (CT)**—An imaging technique in which cross-sectional x rays of the body are compiled to create a three-dimensional image of the body's internal structures.
>
> **Magnetic resonance imaging (MRI)**—An imaging technique that uses a large circular magnet and radio waves to generate signals from atoms in the body. These signals are used to construct images of internal structures.
>
> **Motor**—Of or pertaining to motion, the body apparatus involved in movement, or the brain functions that direct purposeful activity.
>
> **Motor nerve**—Motor or efferent nerve cells carry impulses from the brain to muscle or organ tissue.
>
> **Peripheral nervous system**—The part of the nervous system that is outside the brain and spinal cord. Sensory, motor, and autonomic nerves are included.
>
> **Postural drainage**—The use of positioning to drain secretions from the bronchial tubes and lungs into the trachea or windpipe.
>
> **Range of motion (ROM)**—The range of motion of a joint from full extension to full flexion (bending) measured in degrees like a circle.
>
> **Sensory nerves**—Sensory or afferent nerves carry impulses of sensation from the periphery or outward parts of the body to the brain. Sensations include feelings, impressions, and awareness of the state of the body.
>
> **Voluntary**—An action or thought undertaken or controlled by a person's free will or choice.

SCIs, can be significantly reduced by driving at safe speeds, avoiding alcohol while driving, not talking on mobile phones or texting while driving, and using seat belts.

Paralysis and loss of sensation

Some limited mobility and sensation may be recovered, but the extent and speed of recovery cannot be predicted with any accuracy. Experimental electrical stimulation has been demonstrated to allow some control of muscle contraction in paraplegia. This experimental technique offers the possibility of unaided walking. Further development of current control systems will be needed before useful movement is possible outside the laboratory.

A pulmonologist, or respiratory therapist, can promote airway hygiene through instruction in assisted coughing techniques and postural drainage. **Ventilators**, facial or nasal masks, and tracheostomy equipment, where necessary, can also be prescribed by the respiratory professional. He or she can provide instruction in their use, as well.

Resources

BOOKS

Kirshblum, Steven and Denise Campagnolo. *Spinal Cord Medicine,* 2nd ed. Philadelphia: Wolters Kluwer Health/Lippincott Williams & Wilkins, 2011.

Mayo Clinic. New York: Demos Health, 2009.

Somers, Martha F. *Spinal Cord Injury: Functional Rehabilitation,* 3rd ed. Upper Saddle River, NJ: Prentice Hall, 2009.

OTHER

Paralysis Resource Center. Christopher & Dana Reeve Foundation undated [accessed April 10, 2012]. http://www.christopherreeve.org/site/pp.aspx?c=mtKZKgMWKwG&b=4451921

Schreiber, Donald. Spinal Cord Injuries. Medscape Reference December 15, 2012 [accessed April 10, 2012]. http://emedicine.medscape.com/article/793582-overview

Spinal Cord Injuries. MedlinePlus March 30, 2012 [accessed April 10, 2012]. http://www.nlm.nih.gov/medlineplus/spinalcordinjuries.html

Spinal Cord Injury 101. FacingDisability.com undated [accessed April 10, 2012]. http://www.facingdisability.com/expert-topics/spinal-cord-injury-101

ORGANIZATIONS

National Spinal Cord Injury Association., 75-20 Astoria Blvd., Jackson Heights, NY 11370, (718) 803-3782, http://www.spinalcord.org

Hill Foundation, 737 N. Michigan Avenue, Chicago, IL 60611, (312) 284-2525, Fax: (312) 284-2530, info@facingdisability.com, http://www.facingdisability.com.

Barbara Wexler
Tish Davidson, AM

Spinal fluid analysis *see* **Cerebrospinal fluid (CSF) analysis**

Spinal manipulation *see* **Joint mobilization and manipulation**

Spinal meningitis *see* **Meningitis**

Spinal orthoses

Definition

Spinal orthoses, also known as braces, are devices worn on the body to treat conditions such as **scoliosis**, **back pain**, and injury.

Purpose

Most spinal orthoses are designed to adjust skeletal alignment, limit torso movement, and compress the **stomach**.

Scoliosis

Spinal orthoses are used to treat longterm spinal conditions such as scoliosis. The brace is worn to stop the progression of scoliosis, which is the lateral (side-to-side) curvature of the spine. This condition progresses as a person grows and is primarily seen in children and adolescents. In general, scoliosis can not be reversed. Therefore, the goal of treatment is stop the progression of scoliosis.

Orthopedists usually diagnosis this condition based on an x ray showing curves of 10 degrees or more. Treatment is usually indicated when curves measure 25 degrees or more. Scoliosis progresses more slowly as patients reach skeletal maturity, so use of spinal orthosis is prescribed for patients with at least 18 months of growing left. In older patients, scoliosis is treated with surgery.

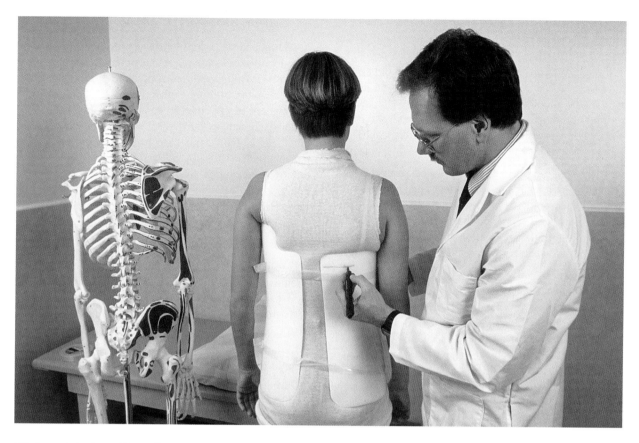

(*Photograph by Aaron Haupt. Science Source/Photo Researchers.*)

Back pain

Spinal orthoses are worn to relieve back **pain** and to provide back support after an injury or to treat conditions such as degenerative disc disorder. Other uses of spinal orthoses include protecting the back after surgery and the stabilization and support of a weak back.

Description

For more than two thousand years, doctors have tried to treat scoliosis by having patients wear devices to keep their spines rigid. Equipment used throughout the centuries included bandages bolstered by splints, leather appliances, and plaster casts. During the Middle Ages, the craftsmen who made armor for knights also produced bulky metal corsets to stop the progression of scoliosis.

Today, braces made of materials ranging from cotton to plastic are used to treat conditions related to the back and spine. Spinal orthoses vary in size from the cloth belts worn for back support to the rigid full-torso Milwaukee brace used to stop the progression of scoliosis. Braces used to treat scoliosis are prescribed by an orthopedist. The orthosis may be custom-made or fitted from a prefabricated brace.

Corsets and belts

Cloth corsets and belts are generally made of cotton, nylon, or rayon. These flexible orthoses are used to relieve back pain and to restrict movement.

Rigid and semi-rigid spinal orthoses

The braces worn to treat scoliosis or during **rehabilitation** from spinal surgery are generally classified as rigid or semi-rigid orthoses. The rigid orthosis immobilizes the spine and prevents spinal motion. It is designed to apply force in every direction, distributing pressure over a broad area. A semi-rigid brace combines the support of a rigid brace with the flexibility of a cloth orthosis.

Orthoses for scoliosis

Orthoses prescribed for the treatment of scoliosis generally fall into three categories, with model variations in each group.

THE MILWAUKEE BRACE. The Milwaukee brace is a full-torso orthosis developed during the late 1940s. Named for the location of the doctors who developed it, the orthosis consists of pressure pads held in place by three vertical metal bars. The bars extend from a neck ring, a type of collar worn around the neck. The bars are secured at the neck ring and anchored to a plastic pelvic girdle. The rear vertical bar extends down the back. There are two shorter bars in front.

The neck ring centers the head and straightens the spine. The pads apply pressure to the spinal curve to keep it from worsening. Patients wear the brace under clothing, and it is worn for much of the day. While it effectively stops the progression of scoliosis, wearing the brace with the visible neck ring can be embarrassing for patients.

LOW-PROFILE BRACES. During the 1970s, doctors in Boston developed a brace that extends from under the arms to the hips. Variations of this brace are known as thoracolumbar-sacral orthoses (TLSOs), the Boston brace, the low-profile brace, and the underarm brace. The orthosis consists of a plastic corset with pressure pads attached to the inside. The original braces opened from the back. Current models open in the front or back. However, the back-opening orthosis generally keeps the pelvis in place. This reduces the flattening of the lower back that can occur when scoliosis is treated with an orthosis.

Patients wear the underarm brace for much of the day. This orthosis is regarded as low-profile because it is not visible when worn under clothes.

THE CHARLESTON NIGHTTIME BENDING BRACE. This orthosis developed in 1979 forces the spine to one side. It is held in place away from the direction of the spinal curve. The bending brace is curved and is designed to be worn only at night when the patient sleeps. Most patients have no trouble sleeping in this brace once they have adjusted to wearing it. In addition, many young patients appreciate the option of wearing the brace only at home and going to school without wearing a brace.

Operation

The overall length of time for wearing a spinal orthosis depends on the patient's age and condition. If the brace stops the progression of scoliosis, the patient wears an orthosis until reaching skeletal maturity (around age 15 or 16). The orthopedist or other health professional will determine the amount of wearing time when a brace is used to treat other conditions. While daily wearing times will also vary by the patients, there are set times for how long orthoses should be worn during treatment for scoliosis.

Scoliosis treatment

Orthopedists are divided about how long some spinal orthoses should be worn each day to treat scoliosis. While some doctors believe that the brace must be worn fulltime, others maintain that part-time bracing can be effective. In some cases, this recommendation is based on the patient's condition and age. In other cases, the health care team realizes that young patients embarrassed by the awkward Milwaukee brace may stop wearing it. In these situations, doctors believe that a shorter wearing time or a split schedule could be more effective.

For fulltime bracing to stop the progression of scoliosis, the daily wearing time is:

- 22 to 23 hours for the Milwaukee brace. The patient can remove the orthosis when bathing. Some doctors allow the patient to remove the brace when exercising; others say that it can be worn while doing some exercises.
- 20 hours for the Boston brace. Daily wearing time of 16 hours may be effective. However, reduced time could increase the risk of curve progression.
- During the eight to nine hours of sleep for the Charleston bending brace.

Precautions

Patients should be told that it takes time to adjust to wearing an orthosis. A light shirt or other article of clothing should be worn under the brace because the appliance should not touch the skin. The health care team should realize that patient compliance is a crucial part of treatment, especially during treatment of scoliosis. Younger patients should be counseled about the importance of their treatment. They should be consulted about the type of orthosis chosen and advised about how to make adjustments to wardrobe so that they feel they fit in.

Furthermore, the patient should be advised to **exercise** regularly. Exercise helps to preserve spinal motion and keeping adjacent muscles strong.

Maintenance

For scoliosis braces, adjusting the tension on chest straps may be necessary. In addition, the spinal orthosis will need to be adjusted as the patient grows. Generally, a brace needs to be replaced after 15 months.

Health care team roles

Patients are seen by an orthopedist, a physician specializing in the treatment of musculoskeletal disorders. This specialty is concerned with deformities,

KEY TERMS

Disc—A circle of cartilage located between vertebrae in the spine.

Torso—The trunk of the human body, the area exclusive of the head and limbs.

Vertebrae—The back bones that form the spinal column. The bones are connected by discs and facet joints.

diseases and injuries of the arms, legs, spine, and associated structures. The physician examines the patient, interprets x rays, and establishes a treatment plan.

If a brace is needed, the patient is sent to an orthotist, an allied health professional who measures, designs, and fits orthopedic equipment like spinal orthoses. Orthotists may supervise several staff members. In some workplaces, the orthotics assistant assists the orthotist and may fabricate, repair, and maintain braces. However, orthoses may be made by the orthotics technician, an allied health worker who takes direction from the orthotist and the orthotics assistant. The technician also repairs and maintains braces. In some settings, the technician may have no contact with patients. Physical therapists will help the patient set up an exercise or rehabilitation program. In addition, a nurse may help plan treatment.

When a patient begins treatment for scoliosis, the orthopedist generally sees the patient several times annually. These appointments are scheduled every four to six months to allow the health care team to assess the patient's growth. The orthotist and orthotic technician may need to adjust a brace or fit a new orthosis. Once the patient is skeletally mature and bracing treatment ends, the patient usually returns a year later for a follow-up assessment that includes an x ray. The patient may be asked to return in five years. Patients are urged to return if a problem develops or they become pregnant.

Training

Members of the health care team receive training in the use of spinal orthoses while studying for their respective professions. For the orthopedist, this training is part of medical school. For the orthopedic nurse, this training comes during nursing school.

Orthotists earn a four-year bachelor of science degree and finish with specialized orthotic training. They also serve a clinical residency. Orthotics technicians

complete programs that last from six months to one year. In addition, people working in these allied health professions can receive certification through the American Academy of Orthotics and **Prosthetics**. Board certification is based on factors including education, employment, continuing education courses, and membership in the academy.

The name of the academy reflects the relationship between the fields of orthotics and prosthetics. While orthotics usually focuses on temporary treatment with a brace, prosthetics involves permanent replacement of a body part with an artificial appliance. However, some patients will require both prosthetics and orthotics, so schools offer degrees and certificates in both disciplines.

Resources

BOOKS

American Academy of Orthopaedic Surgeons. *Atlas of Orthoses and Assistive Devices,* 3rd ed. Bertram Goldberg, et al., eds. St. Louis, MO: Mosby Year Book, Inc., 1997.

Eisenpreis, Bettijane. *Coping with Scoliosis.* New York: The Rosen Publishing Group, 1998.

Lusari, M. M., and C. C. Nielsen. *Orthotics and Prosthetics in Rehabilitation.* Boston: Butterworth-Heinemann, 2000.

Neuwirth, Michael, and Kevin Osborn. *The Scoliosis Handbook.* New York: Henry Holt and Co., 1996.

ORGANIZATIONS

American Academy of Orthotists and Prosthetists. 526 King Street, Suite 201, Alexandria, VA 22314. (703) 836-0788. http://www.oandp.org.

American Board for Certification of Orthotics and Prosthetics. 330 John Carlyle Street, Suite 200, Alexandria, VA 22314. (703) 836-7114. http://www.opoffice.org.

American Orthopaedic Association. 6300 N. River Road, Suite 505, Rosemont, IL 60018. (847) 318-7330. http://www.aoassn.org.

National Association of Orthopaedic Nurses. P.O. Box 56, Pitman, NJ 08071. (856) 256-2310. http://www.naon.nurse.com.

Liz Swain

Spinal stenosis

Definition

Spinal stenosis is the narrowing of spaces in or between the bones that make up the spine (vertebrae) through which the **spinal cord** and spinal nerves pass. As a result of this narrowing, pressure is placed on the nerves that results in **pain** or numbness.

Description

The spinal column is made of bones (vertebrae) that have a large central opening, called the spinal canal, through which the spinal cord passes. When stenosis (narrowing) occurs in the spinal canal, it is called central stenosis. The vertebrae also have openings near their base where nerves serving the rest of the body enter and leave the spinal cord. Spinal stenosis can also occur here or between the vertebrae. No matter where spinal stenosis occurs, it puts pressure on the nerves that can cause pain, numbness, and **weakness**.

About 75% of the time, spinal stenosis occurs in one of the five lumbar vertebrae in the lower back. This causes symptoms to appear in the back, hip, or leg. Spinal stenosis can also occur in the thoracic (chest) or cervical (neck) vertebrae. Stenosis in these locations causes symptoms to occur in the arm or shoulder.

Degenerative spinal stenosis generally occurs after age 60, and the risk of developing the disorder increases with age. Men are about twice as likely to develop spinal stenosis as women. Chances of being affected by this disease are independent of race or ethnicity, but people with **osteoarthritis**, **rheumatoid arthritis**, or curvature of the spine (**scoliosis**) are more likely to develop symptoms. About five of every 50 Americans over age 50 have spinal stenosis.

Causes and symptoms

People can be born with a small spinal canal or deformities in the vertebrae that make them abnormally narrow. This is uncommon, but when it occurs, symptoms of spinal stenosis develop at a fairly young age. Traumatic injuries to the back can also cause spinal stenosis. However, the vast majority of spinal stenosis is caused by degeneration and hardening of cartilage as a normal result of **aging**. Other uncommon causes of spinal stenosis include spinal tumors, Paget's disease, a condition that causes enlarged and deformed bones, and **fluorosis**, a condition caused by too much fluorine in the body (usually from industrial inhalation, not from a fluoridated water supply) that causes connective tissue around the vertebrae to harden.

Many people have some stenosis without showing any symptoms. When symptoms do occur, they usually appear gradually, and many people do not seek early medical attention for them because they consider the symptoms a normal condition of aging. Symptoms include:

- pain in the lower back
- pain radiating down the leg (sciatica) or along the shoulder that may temporarily improve when the back is flexed

- numbness, tingling, or sensations of hot and cold in the legs or shoulder
- inability to walk more than a short distance without pain or weakness
- shuffling gait and forward-leaning posture when walking

Diagnosis

Diagnosis is made by either a family physician or rheumatologist based on medical history and a physical exam. **Physical examination** is normally followed by an x ray, **magnetic resonance imaging** (MRI) of the spine, and/or computerized axial tomography (CAT) scan. Less frequently a myelogram or **bone** scan are used as diagnostic tools.

Treatment

Conservative treatment consists of administering pain medications including **nonsteroidal anti-inflammatory drugs** (e.g., aspirin, ibuprofen, naproxen sodium) and **analgesics** (acetaminophen, tramadol).

Corticosteroid injections (prednisone and cortisone) into the spinal column help reduce pain and inflammation. Injection of anesthetics (a nerve block) offers immediate but temporary relief. Rest, changes in posture, **physical therapy**, and wearing a lower back brace or corset also help treat symptoms. **Chiropractic** manipulations and **acupuncture** are **alternative medicine** treatments that appear to substantially benefit some individuals.

When conservative treatment fails and pain, numbness, or weakness persist, surgery may be required. The goal of surgery is to relieve pressure on the nerve. The most common surgical procedure is decompression surgery that either removes some of the cartilage lining the vertebrae or removes a section of the cartilage between the vertebrae. Fusion of the vertebrae may be done at the same time as decompression surgery. Surgery is commonly followed by physical therapy, especially after spinal fusion.

Prognosis

The degree of spinal stenosis and intensity of symptoms dictates whether conservative treatment will improve symptoms. Surgery usually provides substantial improvement, although some pain or numbness may remain if the nerves were badly damaged before surgery occurred. Tissue healing after surgery takes about six to eight weeks, after which **rehabilitation** can begin.

Health care team roles

A physical therapist is often involved in conservative treatment, teaching exercises that improve posture and strengthen the back muscles. A standard surgical team supports the neurosurgeon or orthopedic surgeon during surgical treatment. A physical therapist is usually involved in rehabilitation after surgery. Depending on the age, agility, and working conditions of the individual, an occupational therapist and an ergonomist may also participate in rehabilitation.

Prevention

Spinal stenosis cannot generally be prevented, as it is either congenital, the result of trauma, presence of a tumor, or a normal process of aging.

Resources

BOOKS

Anderson, D. Greg and Alexander R. Vaccaro, eds. *Decision Making in Spinal Care* New York: Thieme, 2007.

Bartleson, J.D. and H. Gordon Dean. *Spine Disorders: Medical and Surgical Management.* New York: Cambridge University Press, 2009.

Olson, Kenneth A. *Manual Physical Therapy of the Spine.* St. Louis, MO: Saunders/Elsevier, 2009. (book and DVD)

PERIODICAL

Balakatounis, K., et al. "Evidence-based Evaluation and Current Practice of Non-Operative Treatment Strategies for Lumbar Stenosis." *Folia Medica.* (2011 Jul-Sep) 53(3):5–14.

OTHER

Hsiang, John N. K Spinal Stenosis. Medscape Reference December 13, 2011 [accessed April 9, 2012]. http://emedicine.medscape.com/article/1913265-overview

Questions & Answers About Spinal Stenosis. National Institute of Arthritis and Musculoskeletal and Skin Disease April 2009 [accessed April 9, 2012]. http://www.niams.nih.gov/Health_Info/Spinal_Stenosis/default.asp

Spinal Stenosis. MedlinePlus April 3, 2012 [accessed April 9, 2012]. http://www.nlm.nih.gov/medlineplus/spinalstenosis.html

ORGANIZATIONS

American Academy of Orthopaedic Surgeons (AAOS), 6300 North River Road, Rosemont, IL 60018-4262, (847) 823-7186, Fax: (847) 823-8125, http://orthoinfo.aaos.org/topic.cfm?topic=a00005

National Institute of Arthritis and Musculoskeletal and Skin Diseases (NIAMS)Information Clearinghouse, 1 AMS Circle, Bethesda, MD 20892-3675, (301) 495-4484, 877) 22-NIAMS (226-4267); TTY: (301) 565–2966, Fax: (301) 718-6366, NIAMSinfo@mail.nih.gov, http://www.niams.nih.gov

National Institutes of Health Osteoporosis and Related Bone Diseases National Resource Center, 2 AMS Circle,

Spinal traction

Bethesda, MD 20892-3676, (202) 223-0344. TTY: (202)
466-4315, (800) 624-2663(BONE), Fax: (202) 293-235,
NIAMSBoneInfo@mail.nih.gov, http://www.niams.nih.
gov/Health_Info/Bone.

Tish Davidson, AM

Spinal tap *see* **Cerebrospinal fluid (CSF) analysis**

Spinal traction

Definition

Spinal traction is the process of applying force through body weight, weights, and/or pulleys to draw apart the vertebrae of the spine.

Purpose

Spinal traction may be indicated when a patient complains of cervical, low back, or radiating **pain** that is likely caused by a vertebral disc protrusion or degenerative changes. It is used to accomplish one or more of the following purposes: distract (pull apart) vertebral bodies, distract and glide the facet joints, widen the intervertebral foramen (openings to the spinal canal formed by the vertebrae), or stretch spinal musculature. Release of discal pressure and widening of intervertebral space can reduce discal pain and pain caused by impingement of nerves exiting the **spinal cord**.

Precautions

In general, traction should not be applied when there is a disease process that reduces the body's tolerance to force. Traction is contraindicated when there is a tumor, **infection**, vascular disorder, ligamentous instability, **osteoporosis**, or claustrophobia.

Description

Types of spinal traction include: sustained, intermittent mechanical, manual, positional, auto-traction, and gravity traction. Sustained traction is applied with heavy weights or a mechanical device that apply the force to maintain a constant traction for a time period of one to 30 minutes. Intermittent mechanical traction is more widely used in the United States; it involves the use of a split table and a mechanical device to apply and withdraw force every few seconds. In manual traction, the physical therapist may use the weight of his or her body in applying a traction force to the spine.

Manual traction is often used to assess a patient's response to traction, or when adjustment of the position or amount of force may be needed. Positional traction allows the patient to be positioned to maximize the effect of traction on the suspected causative structure, or to allow the patient to remain in a preferred posture until pain is relieved. Self-traction allows the patient to position him or herself to provide traction with the assistance of gravity. Gravity lumbar traction is administered in one of two ways. Either the rib cage is grasped in a vest, allowing the weight of the legs to provide a traction force; or the ankles or pelvis are grasped, allowing the upper body to exert the traction force.

In order for traction to be effective, the force must be great enough to cause separation at the target spinal segment(s). A wide range of forces, from 30–300% of body weight, has been shown to be effective in studies of lumbar traction; however, a traction force of such large magnitude as 300% may cause damage to the vertebral structures. Thirty percent of body weight has been shown to be effective in reduction of symptoms. For cervical traction, research has shown that 20–45 lb (7.4–16.8 kg) is an effective range for producing separation.

With mechanical lumbar traction, traction harnesses are placed around the patient's pelvis and **thorax**. The patient then lies on a split table on his or her back, **stomach**, or side, depending upon the position thought to be optimal for the specific symptoms being treated. The split table allows for minimizing of friction forces. The straps of the harness are hooked to the motorized traction unit that is programmed for the traction force, overall time, and hold/rest periods desired.

For cervical traction, it has been found that patients are able to relax better and forces of gravity interfere less in the supine versus sitting position. To straighten out the normal lordosis and provide a more longitudinal pull, the neck often is flexed to approximately 20–30°, unless treating the joints of the first and second cervical vertebrae. Several types of head halters and devices are available to connect to the traction source.

Preparation

Before traction is applied, a full evaluation should be done to determine the possible causes of the patient's symptoms and uncover potential contraindications to traction. Physical therapists often use manual traction as part of the evaluation to assess the effects it has on symptoms. It is important that the patient is able to relax when traction is applied, so that muscle guarding does not take place. Modalities such as heat may be used to help with **relaxation**.

Aftercare

Traction usually is one part of a patient's plan of care. The physical therapist may teach a patient exercises, body mechanics, self-traction, and **pain management** techniques that should be performed at home between treatment times and after the course of **physical therapy** is finished.

Complications

It is important that the patient reports any adverse reactions or increase in pain after each treatment. Adverse reactions can be more easily avoided by keeping the initial treatment times short (less than 10 minutes) with low force to allow the patient to become accustomed to the procedure.

Results

The desired outcome of traction is the reduction of neurological signs and pain in the neck, back and/or extremities, allowing for return to functional activities. Although clinicians often find favorable results with the use of traction, research with randomized, controlled trials showing statistically significant positive results is still sparse. This may be due in part to lack of good research design and the many factors involved in **back pain**.

Health care team roles

The physician usually refers the patient to physical therapy for conservative treatment of neck or back pain. The physical therapist examines the patient and makes decisions regarding the appropriate plan of care, which may include traction. The physical therapist determines the specifications for traction and sets up the patient on the apparatus for the first few times, being sure to monitor the patient intermittently. The physical therapist assistant may set up the patient for future treatments, with guidance from the physical therapist regarding duration and force specifications.

Resources

BOOKS

Boyling, Jeffrey D., and Nigel Palastanga, eds. *Grieve's Modern Manual Therapy.* Edinburgh, UK: Churchill Livingstone, 1994.

Hertling, Darlene, and Randolph M. Kessler. *Management of Common Musculoskeletal Disorders: Physical Therapy Principles and Methods,* 3rd ed. Philadelphia: Lippincott-Raven Publishers, 1996.

Kaltenborn, Freddy M. *The Spine: Basic Evaluation and Mobilization Techniques,* 2nd ed. Minneapolis: Banta ISG, 1993.

PERIODICAL

Meszaros, Thomas F., et al. "Effect of 10%, 30%, and 60% Body Weight Traction on the Straight Leg Raise Test of Symptomatic Patients with Low Back Pain." *Journal of Orthopedic and Sports Physical Therapy* 30 (October 2000): 595–601.

Peggy Campbell Torpey, MPT

Spirometry tests

Definition

Spirometry is the measurement of airflow into and out of the **lungs**. The patient is given instructions on how to perform the breathing maneuvers. To perform the procedure the nose is pinched off, and the patient breathes as instructed through a mouthpiece attached to the spirometer. The three breathing maneuvers are practiced before recording the procedure, and the highest of three trials is used for evaluation of breathing. The instrument measures air flow by electronic or mechanical displacement principles and uses a microprocessor and recorder to calculate and plot air flow.

The test produces a recording of the patient's ventilation under conditions involving both normal and maximal effort. The recording, called a spirogram, shows the volume of air moved and the rate at which it is moved into and out of the lungs. There are several lung capacities that are measured by spirometry. Accurate measurement of these are dependent upon the patient performing the appropriate maneuver properly. The most common are described below:

• Vital capacity (VC): This is the amount of air in liters that is moved out of the lungs during normal breathing. The patient is instructed to breathe in and out normally to full expiration for this maneuver. Vital capacity is normally about 80% of the total lung capacity. Because of the elastic nature of the lungs and surrounding thorax, a small volume of air will remain in the lungs after full exhalation. This volume is called the residual volume (RV).

• Forced vital capacity (FVC): After breathing out normally to full expiration the patient is instructed to breath in with a maximal effort and then exhale as forcefully and rapidly as possible. The FVC is the volume of air that is expelled into the spirometer following a maximum inhalation effort.

- Forced expiratory volume (FEV): At the start of the FVC maneuver, the spirometer measures volume of air that is delivered through the mouthpiece at timed intervals of 0.5, 1.0, 2.0, and 3.0 seconds. The sum of these measurements normally constitutes about 97% of the FVC measurement. The most commonly used FEV measurement is FEV-1, which is the volume of air exhaled into the mouthpiece in one second. The FEV-1 should be at least 70% of the FVC.

- Forced expiratory flow 25-75% (FEF 25-75): This is a calculation of the average flow rate over the center portion of the forced expiratory volume recording. It is determined from the time in seconds at which 25% and 75% of the vital capacity is reached. The volume of air exhaled in liters per second between these two times is the FEF 25-75. This value reflects the status of the medium and small sized airways.

- Maximal voluntary ventilation (MVV): A maneuver in which the patient breathes as deeply and as fast as possible for 15 seconds. The average airflow (liters per second) indicates the strength and endurance of the respiratory muscles.

Normal values for FVC, FEV, FEF, and MVV are dependent on the patient's age, gender, and size (height).

Purpose

Spirometry is the most commonly performed **pulmonary function test** (PFT). The test can be performed at the bedside, in a physician's office, or pulmonary laboratory. It is often the first test performed when a problem with lung function is suspected. Spirometry may also be suggested by an abnormal x ray, arterial **blood gas analysis**, or other diagnostic pulmonary test result. In March 2000, the National Lung Health Education Program recommended that regular spirometry tests be performed on persons over 45 years old who have a history of **smoking**. Spirometry tests are also recommended for persons having a family history of lung disease, chronic respiratory ailments, and persons of advanced age. Spirometry measures ventilation, the movement of air into and out of the lungs. The spirogram will identify two different types of abnormal ventilation patterns, obstructive and restrictive. Common causes of an obstructive pattern are **cystic fibrosis**, **asthma**, broniectasis, **bronchitis**, and **emphysema**. These conditions may be collectively referred to using the acronym CABBE. Chronic bronchitis, emphysema, and asthma result in dyspnea and ventilation deficiency, a condition known as **chronic obstructive pulmonary disease**

(COPD). COPD is the fourth leading cause of death among Americans. Common causes of a restrictive pattern are **pneumonia**, **heart** disease, **pregnancy**, lung fibrosis, **pneumothorax** (collapsed lung), and **pleural effusion** (compression caused by chest fluid).

Obstructive and restrictive patterns can be identified on spirographs. Volume (liters) is plotted on the y-axis versus time (seconds) on the x-axis. A restrictive pattern is characterized by a normal shape showing reduced volumes for all parameters. The reduction in volumes indicates the severity of the disease. An obstructive pattern produces a spirogram with an abnormal shape. Inspiration volume is reduced. The volume of air expelled is normal, but the airflow rate is slower causing an elongated tail to the FVC.

A flow-volume loop spirogram is another way of displaying spirometry measurements. This requires a FVC maneuver followed by a forced inspiratory volume (FIV). Flow rate in liters per second is plotted on the y-axis and volume (liters) is plotted on the x-axis. The expiration phase is shown on top and the inspiration phase on the bottom. The flow-volume loop spirogram is helpful in diagnosing upper airway obstruction and can differentiate some types of restrictive patterns.

Some conditions produce specific signs on the spirogram. Irregular inspirations with rapid frequency are caused by hyperventilation associated with **stress**. Diffuse fibrosis of the lung causes rapid breathing of reduced volume that produces a repetitive pattern known as the penmanship sign. Serial reduction in the FVC peaks indicates trapped air inside the lung. A notch and reduced volume in the early segments of the FVC is consistent with airway collapse. A rise at the end of the expiration is associated with airway resistance.

Spirometry is used to assess lung function over time and is often used to evaluate the efficacy of bronchodilator inhalers such as albuterol. It is important that the patient not use a bronchodilator prior to the evaluation. Spirometry is performed before and after inhaling the bronchodilator. In general, a 12% or greater improvement in both FVC and FEV-1 and/or an increase in FVC by 0.2 liters is considered a significant improvement in an adult patient.

Precautions

The physician ordering the test should be aware of any medications and medical conditions which may affect the validity of the test. The patient's smoking habits and history should be documented thoroughly. The subject must be able to understand and respond to instructions for the breathing maneuvers. Therefore, the

KEY TERMS

Bronchodilator—A drug, usually self-administered by inhalation, that dilates the airways.

Forced expiratory volume (FEV)—The volume of air exhaled from the beginning of expiration to a set time (usually 0.5, 1, 2, and 3 seconds).

Forced vital capacity (FVC)—The volume of air that can be exhaled forceably after a maximal inspiration.

Vital capacity (VC)—The volume of air that can be exhaled following a full inspiration.

test may not be appropriate for very young, unresponsive, or physically impaired persons. Spirometry is contraindicated in patients whose condition will be aggravated by forced breathing. Hemoptysis, pneumothorax, recent heart attack, unstable **angina**, **aneurysm** (cranial, thoracic, or abdominal), thrombotic condition, recent thoracic or abdominal surgery, and nausea or **vomiting** are conditions that may contraindicate spirometry. The test should be terminated if the patient shows signs of significant head, chest, or **abdominal pain** while the test is in progress.

Spirometry is dependent upon the patient's full compliance with breathing instructions especially his or her willingness to extend a maximal effort at forceful breathing. Therefore, the patient's emotional state needs to be considered when performing the procedure.

Preparation

The patient's age, sex, and race are recorded, and height and weight are measured before starting the procedure. The patient should not have eaten heavily within three hours of the test. He or she should be instructed to wear clothing that is loose fitting over the chest and abdominal area. The respiratory therapist or other testing personnel should explain and demonstrate the breathing maneuvers to the patient. The patient should practice breathing into the mouthpiece until he or she is able to duplicate the maneuvers successfully on two consecutive tries.

Aftercare

No special care is usually required following spirometry. The occassional patient may become light-headed or dizzy. Such patients should be asked to rest or lie down, and they should not be discharged until after the symptoms subside. In rare cases, the patient may experience pneumothorax, intracranial **hypertension**, vertigo, chest **pain**, or uncontrolled coughing. In such cases, additional care directed by a physician may be required.

Results

The results of spirometry tests are compared to predicted values based on the patient's age, gender, and height. For example, a young adult in good health is expected to have the following FEV values:

- FEV-0.5 50-60% of FVC
- FEV-1 75–85% of FVC
- FEV-2 95% of FVC
- FEV-3 97% of FVC

In general, any value falling between 80% and 100% of the predicted value is considered normal. Values between 60% and 79% indicate mild lung dysfunction. Values between 40% and 59% indicate moderate lung dysfunction, and values below 40% indicate severe dysfunction.

Health care team roles

Spirometry tests are ordered by a physician, and results are evaluated by a pulmonologist, a physician with special training in pulmonary function. Spirometry testing is performed most often by a registered respiratory therapist (RRT), certified respiratory technician (CRTT), certified pulmonary function technologist (CPFT), or registered pulmonary function technologist (RPFT).

Resources

BOOK

White, G. *Basic Clinical Lab Competencies for Respiratory Care,* 3rd ed. New York: Delmar Publishers, 1998.

ORGANIZATION

National Lung Health Education Program (NLHEP). 1850 High Street, Denver, CO 80218. http://www.nlhep.org.

OTHER

Gary, T., et al. "Office Spirometry for Lung Health Assessment in Adults: A Consensus Statement for the National Lung Health Education Program." (March 2000): 1146–1161.

"Spirometry—AARC Clinical Practice Guide." American Association for Respiratory Care. 1130 Ables Lane, Dallas, TX 75229. http://www.muhealth.org/~shrp/rtwww/rcweb/aarc/spirocpg.html.

Robert Harr
Paul Johnson

Spontaneous abortion *see* **Miscarriage**

Sports injuries

Definition

A sports injury is any bodily damage sustained during participation in competitive or non-competitive athletic activity. Sports injuries can affect bones or soft tissue (i.e., muscles, ligaments, tendons).

Description

Sports injuries are identified as either acute or chronic. Acute sports injuries are characterized by the sudden appearance of symptoms, usually associated with a single traumatic incident. Signs and symptoms of acute sports injuries include **pain**, swelling, and deformity in the affected area, and in the case of joint injuries, limited ability to move the joint. Common acute sports injuries include **sprains and strains**, contusions (i.e., serious bruises), joint **dislocations**, **bone fractures**, and concussions.

Chronic sports injuries, also called overuse injuries, are identified with more gradual onset and are caused by repetitive light trauma to soft tissue or bone. Typically, pain and swelling worsen during athletic activity but decrease after the activity is stopped. Overuse injuries include tendonitis, **bursitis**, shin splints, and stress fractures.

The United States Consumer Product Safety Commission (CPSC) estimates that, in 1998, there were over one million sports injuries among persons 35–54 years old. Moreover, the number of sports injuries in this age group increased by one-third between 1991 and 1998. The CPSC believes that the rise in injuries is because of increased sports participation among baby boomers.

The CPSC National Electronic Injury Surveillance System also reports that over 3.5 million sports injuries in children younger than age 15 are treated at hospitals and clinics annually. Children are particularly vulnerable to sports injuries because their bones, muscles, and connective tissue have not fully matured, and because they have not yet developed mature neuromuscular coordination.

Causes and symptoms

Acute sports injuries are caused by excessive force applied to bone or soft tissue during sports activity. These injuries are commonly associated with **falls** and high-

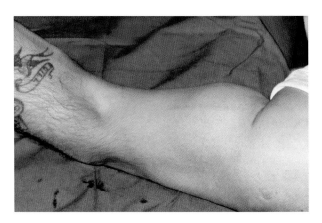

(NMSB/CMSP)

speed collisions. Specific signs and symptoms depend on the nature of the impact and the body region affected.

Acute sports injuries

SOFT TISSUE INJURIES. Soft tissue injuries occur typically in the knee, shoulder, and ankle. In the knee, tears of the anterior cruciate ligament (ACL) and of the meniscus (i.e., cartilage in the knee) are common. A twisted knee, a sudden directional change, or a misaligned landing from a jump can cause these knee injuries. With the ACL tear, a "pop" in the knee is frequently felt at the time of the injury. This popping sensation is accompanied by pain and **weakness** in the knee. A tear of the meniscal cartilage is identified by pain over the area of the meniscus area underneath the edge of the patella (kneecap), and the pain intensifies if a finger is gently pushed on the edge of the kneecap. The athlete is also often unable to fully extend the knee. With both ACL and meniscus tears, there is swelling several hours after the injury occurs.

In the shoulder, strains of the rotator cuff tendons and dislocation of the shoulder are frequently seen. Tendon strains are associated with overly vigorous throwing movements, and are characterized by the patient complaining of pain if the arm is rotated against resistance. Shoulder dislocations are identified by deformity in the shoulder joint, and pain and lack of mobility in the joint area.

Ankle sprains are the most common injury in sports that require running and jumping. Ankle sprains occur when ligaments in the ankle have been stretched or torn. There is typically swelling and tenderness, and in more serious cases, the athlete is unable to put much weight on the foot of the injured ankle.

SKELETAL INJURIES. Fractures are breaks in the bone due to collisions or falls, and commonly appear in the leg and arm. Symptoms include pain, swelling, and bruising at the site of the fracture. There is also weakness in the limb and an inability to bear weight on the limb. With open fractures, bone fragments protrude through the skin.

BRAIN INJURIES. Brain injuries cause more deaths than any other type of sports injuries. A common brain injury is the **concussion**, an injury caused by the impact of the brain against the interior surface of the **skull**. Concussions often follow a blow to the head or a very rapid acceleration of the head. Loss of consciousness is an important symptom in brain injuries. Other signs and symptoms of concussion include **headache**, **vomiting**, delayed motor or verbal responses, partial loss of **vision**, **memory** loss, lack of coordination, or erratic and inappropriate behavior.

Chronic sports injuries

Chronic or overuse injuries are caused by repetitive stress to soft tissue or bone and typically result from a sudden increase in the duration or intensity of athletic activity. In some cases, chronic injuries can be a precipitating factor in acute injuries such as strains and sprains.

SOFT TISSUE INJURIES. Tendonitis, or inflammation of the tendon, is one of the most common overuse injuries and often affects the joints at the elbow, knee, shoulder, and foot. In the elbow joint, tendonitis is known as golfer's elbow or tennis elbow, and is often caused by poor technique. Shoulder tendonitis is caused by repetitive overhead motions and is common in swimming and in sports requiring throwing motions. In the foot, inflammation of the Achilles tendon (i.e., in the heel area) is caused by biomechanical misalignments, inadequate stretching, sudden increases in training, and athletic play on hard or banked surfaces. Symptoms of tendonitis include pain, redness, swelling, and warmth of the affected area. These symptoms diminish when athletic activity is stopped. Bursitis, an inflammation of the connective tissue of joints, is also common in the knee.

SKELETAL INJURIES. Stress fractures are tiny breaks in the bone caused by repetitive forces. Stress fractures frequently affect the leg, foot, and ankle after training has been suddenly intensified or the sport has been played on hard surfaces. Other risk factors of stress fractures are **osteoporosis** and eating disorders, which tend to weaken bone. Symptoms of stress fractures include pain when weight is placed on the leg or foot, with pain increasing after athletic activity. There may be swelling and point tenderness (i.e., pain when a small region of the affected area is lightly pushed).

Diagnosis

Acute injuries are usually self-evident, as they are associated with a specific traumatic event. After the trauma, the physician performs a **physical examination** of the athlete to identify the specific injury. In the case of suspected joint or skeletal injuries, a radiological technician will take x rays, and the radiologist will confirm or rule out a dislocation, bone fracture, or soft tissue injury.

With overuse injuries, the physician conducts a physical examination and uses signs, symptoms, and training history to diagnose the injury. If a stress fracture is suspected, a bone scan or **magnetic resonance imaging** (MRI) of the area may be performed.

Treatment

For sports injuries, Protection-Rest-Ice-Compression-Elevation (PRICE) is the standard of treatment. PRICE specifies the elements of first-line treatment. Depending on the type of injury, protection may mean immobilizing the affected area with a brace, tape, or wrap, or simply avoiding activities that aggravate the injury. Rest means refraining from activities that prevent recovery from injury; in many cases, cross-training is considered rest because it exercises areas that do not affect the injury. Ice should be used to relieve pain and swelling. Compression, with tape or elastic wraps, is used to limit swelling and stabilize the area. Elevation, where the injured body part is placed above the level of the **heart**, is also used to prevent swelling.

Some clinicians use the extended PRICE-MM (i.e., Medication and Modalities) regimen, which includes therapeutic use of medication and modalities (i.e., **rehabilitation**). Nonsteroidal anti-inflammatory medicines such as ibuprofen (e.g., Advil, Motrin) and naproxen (e.g., Naprosyn) have traditionally been used for **pain management** with sports injuries. Injections of **corticosteroids** are sometimes used to control inflammation and pain, but since these injections reduce the strength and flexibility of soft tissue, corticosteroids are used sparingly, primarily for specific overuse syndromes.

The goal of modalities, as in modes of rehabilitation therapies, is to return the athlete to the sport as quickly and as safely as possible. Rehabilitation can begin as soon as the physician permits, typically after internal bleeding has stopped. Modalities include cold and heat therapies, **therapeutic ultrasound**, range of motion exercises, and resistance exercises.

In serious cases of acute and overuse injuries, PRICE-MM may not be sufficient, and surgery may be required to repair injuries.

Prognosis

For most sports injuries, the PRICE-MM regimen should be sufficient to restore the athlete to the previous level of performance. The prognosis is good as long as the rehabilitation has successfully restored the strength and flexibility of the injured area, and the athlete takes care to prevent recurrence of the injury, suspending activity and undertaking appropriate therapy if pain recurs. With some serious injuries, the athlete will not be able to return to the sport or return to the previous level of activity in that sport.

Health care team roles

In school and youth sports, the nurse is often the first health care provider to evaluate acute injuries and is often responsible for some **first aid** of **wounds** and injuries until a physician can attend to the athlete. In school settings, since the nurse is in more frequent contact with children, he or she can advise on general measures to prevent injuries such as warm-up and stretching. In clinical settings, the nurse takes a detailed medical and training history that can help the physician diagnose the injury.

The athletic trainer is often on call for emergency care of acute sports injuries and performs first aid on the injured athlete. He or she specializes in sports activities and can give more specific advice for overall conditioning, training, and treatment of the athlete. The athletic trainer also serves as a liaison between the athlete and coaches, parents, and physicians.

Prior to student participation in athletic activity, the preparticipation physical examination is performed by the physician to assess the patient's fitness for the sport. If the athlete is injured, a diagnosis of the injury is made by the physician and a prescription for appropriate treatment is given. Medical and radiological tests are conducted by technologists. The results assist in determination of the physician's diagnosis. For rehabilitation, the patient may be referred to a physical therapist. For serious injuries requiring surgery, the patient may be referred to an orthopedic surgeon.

Prevention

Many acute and overuse sports injuries are caused by increases in training intensity that put too much physical stress on the athlete's body. This often happens for amateur athletes who do not sustain regular training regimens and overdo their workouts when they do train. These injuries can be prevented with a variety of training and educational regimens.

For youths and adults, the physical exam can be used to identify weaknesses that may predispose the athlete to injury, and that should be developed prior to engaging in athletic activity. Pre-season conditioning programs that slowly increase intensity level are useful in developing the athlete's level of fitness in preparation for the sports season. Flexibility training, **strength training**, and cross training have also been shown to prevent injuries by improving the body's resilience.

Finally, education can be effective in preventing certain common sports injuries. The athlete can be shown how to wear protective gear correctly, how to perform the correct throwing, swinging, blocking, or tackling motion to prevent injury, and how to adjust body **biomechanics** in the event of an unpreventable fall. Although not all sports injuries can be prevented, the damage from many injuries can be minimized with appropriate training.

Resources

BOOKS

Bull, Charles R, ed. *Handbook of Sports Injuries.* New York: McGraw-Hill, 1999.

Stiles, Bradford H. "Common Sports Injuries." In *Conn's Current Therapy 2000*, edited by Robert Rakel. Philadelphia: W.B. Saunders, 2000, pp. 974–8.

OTHER

National Library of Medicine. Medline Plus Health Information on Sports Injuries. http://www.nlm.nih.gov/medlineplus/sportsinjuries.html.

ORGANIZATIONS

American Academy of Orthopaedic Surgeons. 6300 N. River Road, Rosemont, IL 60018. (800) 346-AAOS. http://www.aaos.org.

American Orthopaedic Society for Sports Medicine. 6300 N. River Road, Rosemont, IL 60018. http://www.intelli.com/vhosts/aossmisite/html/main.cgi?sub=2.

Genevieve Pham-Kanter

Sports nutrition

Definition

Sports **nutrition** is a broad interdisciplinary field that involves dietitians, biochemists, **exercise** physiologists, cell and molecular biologists, and occasionally psychotherapists. It has both a basic science aspect that includes such concerns as understanding the body's use of nutrients during athletic competition and the need for **nutritional supplements** among athletes; and an application aspect, which is concerned with the use of proper nutrition and dietary supplements to enhance an athlete's performance. The psychological or psychiatric dimension of sports nutrition is concerned with eating and other mental disorders related to nutrition among athletes.

Some persons who specialize in the field of sports nutrition are registered dietitians (RDs) who have completed a master's or other advanced degree in the field of exercise **physiology**. For instance, the American Dietetic Association (ADA) has a dietetic practice group, or DPG, for sports nutritionists called Sports, Cardiovascular, and Wellness Nutritionists (SCAN), which has its own website (http://www.scandpg.org/) and email address (SCAN at scandpg@gmail.com). Most academic sports nutritionists, however, hold doctoral degrees in the field of exercise physiology and often specialize in working with athletes in one particular type of sport, such as baseball or swimming. Although sports nutrition can be applied to almost any form of athletic training or physical activity—including **yoga**, tai chi, martial arts, and professional dance—professional sports nutritionists do most of their work with team sports, endurance sports (such as cycling, long-distance running, and triathlon training) or sports involving weight training (wrestling, weight-lifting, some forms of bodybuilding). Some nutritionists also work one-on-one with individual athletes.

Purpose

Sports nutrition has several purposes:

- To prepare athletes before performance or training.
- To maintain an acceptable level of performance during competition or training.
- To help the athlete's body recover after training or athletic competition.
- To provide sound information about healthy dietary practices and use of supplements.
- To monitor athletes for signs of eating disorders, doping, supplement abuse, or other unhealthful nutritional practices.
- To provide specialized nutritional advice to athletes following vegetarian, vegan, or other special diets.
- To monitor the special nutritional needs of persons with disabilities who participate in athletic activities and programs.

Demographics

Many athletes use sports nutrition to provide the best possible nutritional requirements for their specific sports endeavors. When a balanced diet is provided, along with plenty of water, the body will have the maximum amount of energy stored for an outstanding performance, whether it is for endurance, power, or strength. This is true for both the training necessary before events occur and for the sporting events themselves. Based on a person's age, physical condition, weight, height, and other such factors, a sports nutrition regiment can be especially created to meet the needs of a professional sports athlete or someone just wanting to exercise at the best level possible. Consult with a medical professional that specializes in sports medicine for valuable advice on sports nutrition. Often a nutritionist as well as a physician is used for athletes wanting a good sports nutrition program.

Description

The description of sports nutrition includes hydration, assessment of energy needs, assessment of weight and body composition, strategies for weight change, and use of ergogenic aids

Hydration

Hydration, or maintaining a proper level of fluid in the body, is an important aspect of sports nutrition because of the loss of water and sodium through sweating during athletic activity. **Dehydration** results in loss of muscle strength, difficulty concentrating, irritability, and **headache**. An adult who has lost more than 8% of initial body weight through sweating without replacing the lost fluid is at risk of heat cramps, heat exhaustion, and heat **stroke**. Moreover, dehydration may be progressive in athletes who do not replace fluid loss overnight; the greater the loss of body fluid, the longer it takes to rehydrate the body. When dehydration has taken place over two to three days, it will take a minimum of 48 hours to replace the fluids in body tissues. The health risks of dehydration are a major reason why abuse of diuretics is dangerous in athletes.

People vary in their sweating rates; therefore, health professionals must evaluate athletes on an individual basis to determine how much fluid is needed after exercise or training. The most common way to measure this need is to weigh the athlete before and after exercise; the amount of weight lost should be replaced with an equal amount of fluid before the next workout. The usual rule of thumb is one pint of fluid containing **carbohydrates** and electrolytes for each pound of weight loss.

Good hydration is more effectively maintained by consuming sports drinks or other beverages that contain salt and carbohydrates than by drinking plain water. Sports drinks are isotonic; that is, they contain the same proportion of electrolytes and carbohydrates to fluid as the human body. After exercise, the body requires carbohydrates to replace the glycogen (a complex sugar) stored in muscle tissue and the **liver**. Glycogen is an important source of reserve energy for muscles; for instance, long-distance runners who deplete their stores of glycogen may experience fatigue to the point of being unable to move. In addition to the risk of glycogen depletion, drinking only water places the athlete at risk of water intoxication, a potentially fatal condition in which the sodium lost through sweat is not replaced and is followed by the rapid intake of a large quantity of water. The resulting electrolyte imbalance affects the **brain** and **central nervous system**. **Blood** plasma sodium levels below 100 millimoles per liter (mmol/L) (2.3 grams per liter [g/L]) frequently result in swelling of the brain tissue, **coma**, and even death.

Assessment of energy needs

Athletes usually require a higher level of calorie intake than non-athletes, although the amount varies depending on the athlete's sex, age, height, weight, body composition, stage of growth, level of fitness, and the intensity, frequency, and duration of physical exercise. An appropriate diet for most athletes consists of a minimum of 2,000 calories per day; 55 to 65% should come from carbohydrates, 15 to 20% from protein, and 20 to 30% from fats.

Assessment of weight and body composition

The use of the body mass index (BMI) to evaluate athletes' weight is not recommended because many have a high proportion of muscle tissue to fat and may therefore be considered "overweight" by standard body mass charts. A better reference guide is to check whether the athlete falls between the 25th and the 75th percentile of weight for height by age, measured according to the National Center for Health Statistics (NCHS) guidelines (as provided at: http://www.cdc.gov/growthcharts/html_charts/wtstat.htm).

Well-nourished athletes should have a lean muscle mass above the 25th percentile, although the ideal ratio of lean muscle to body fat has not yet been established for any sport. Male athletes, however, should not have less than 7% body fat. There are several methods for estimating the proportion of body fat on an athlete's body:

- underwater weighing (equipment is expensive and limited in availability)
- skinfold measurements taken by high-precision calipers on three to five sites on the right side of the body (the right side is always used even if the athlete is left-handed)
- bioelectrical impedance analysis or BIA (a technique that measures body composition by passing a small electrical current through the body and measuring the resistance of various body tissues, as lean muscle contains a higher proportion of water than fat)
- computerized calipers.

Strategies for weight change

It is important for athletes in any age group needing or desiring to lose or gain weight to be properly supervised by a nutritionist as well as a physician, because unhealthful dietary practices can lead to long-term mental as well as physical disorders. The American Academy of **Pediatrics** (AAP) makes the following recommendations for weight change in young athletes:

- The dietary program should be started in a timely fashion to permit gradual weight gain or loss over a reasonable time period.
- The program should allow a gain or loss of no more than 1.5% of body weight per week.
- It should be designed to permit weight lost to be fat and weight gained to be muscle.
- It should be accompanied by appropriate strength and conditioning training.
- The diet should provide an appropriate balance of carbohydrates, protein, and fats.

WEIGHT LOSS. Weight loss programs are sometimes recommended for athletes in weight-sensitive sports, most often wrestling or judo for boys and figure skating, gymnastics, long-distance running, rowing, and swimming for girls. Unfortunately, many young people go too far in adopting unhealthful eating or exercise patterns in order to keep their weight down. Because of this tendency, the AAP states that children younger than the ninth grade should not be put on weight-loss regimens to improve athletic performance.

Restricting food intake is the most common method of weight loss among athletes, but a large percentage of young athletes also engage in purging (self-induced **vomiting** plus abuse of **laxatives** and diuretics), fasting, or the use of stimulants, wet suits, sauna baths, or compulsive exercising. Some studies have shown that as many as 11% of wrestlers meet the criteria for eating disorders, and 15% of swimmers.

Unhealthful weight loss practices are dangerous because much of the weight lost will be lean muscle rather than fat, which can affect athletic performance. Girls who develop eating disorders or body dysmorphic disorder are at risk of developing the so-called female athlete triad, which consists of disordered eating, cessation of menstrual periods (amenorrhea), and **osteoporosis** or brittle bones. A common symptom associated with the triad is an unusually high number of stress **fractures** during the girl's athletic career. The triad, which was first described in 1993, may have long-term consequences for a woman's health. Female athletes in their freshman year of college are reported to be at increased risk of developing the triad, particularly if it is their first experience of living away from home or they are having academic difficulties.

WEIGHT GAIN. Athletes in sports requiring strength or weight lifting (such as football, rugby, basketball, and bodybuilding) may try to gain weight in order to build the body's muscle mass. Inappropriate methods, however, will lead to gaining fat rather than muscle, putting the athlete at risk in midlife for **hypertension**, cardiovascular disease, and type 2 diabetes. It is important for athletes to recognize the genetic limitations related to their body build, as persons who are naturally slender cannot add as much muscle tissue to their bodies as those who are built more solidly.

The safest way to gain weight and build muscle tissue is to consume 1.5 to 1.75 grams of protein per kilogram of body weight per day and participate in **strength training**. The most effective form of strength training is thought to be multiple sets of weight lifting with a relatively high number of repetitions—from 8 to 15—per set. Athletes should avoid the use of dietary supplements in building muscle, particularly steroids, which have been shown to be harmful to health in both males and females.

Use of ergogenic aids

Ergogenic aids are drugs or dietary supplements taken to improve athletic performance or endurance by providing energy or adding muscle tissue. The most common ergogenic aids used are anabolic or androgenic steroids (male sex hormones), steroid precursors, growth hormone, creatine (an organic acid stored in the body that supplies energy to muscle cells), and ephedra, an herb sometimes called by its Chinese name, ma huang. Some ergogenic aids are illegal to use in competition. Because of adverse effects and deaths related to ephedra, the U.S. Food and Drug Administration (FDA) banned the sale of ephedra-containing supplements on April 12, 2004.

Medical and nutritional professionals are concerned about the use of ergogenic aids among young athletes for two major reasons. First, these drugs and supplements—first used by adult athletes in the 1980s—are now being used by children as young as 10 or 12 years of age.

Secondly, creatine and **anabolic steroids** may produce long-term adverse effects on the body even though they do produce gains in body mass and strength, while steroid precursors, ephedra, and growth hormone pose a good many risks to health without any proof that they enhance athletic performance.

The ADA's position statement says, "Nutritional ergogenic aids should be used with caution, and only after careful evaluation of the product for safety, efficacy, potency, and whether or not it is a banned or illegal substance."

Preparation

Meals and fluids before exercising are important before physical activities and sporting events in order to assure peak performance. Meals provide that the muscles are filled with glycogen in order to provide sufficient energy during physical activity. Fluid levels should also be increased before performing such activities so adequate hydration has been accomplished. Under normal circumstances, drink plenty of fluids throughout the day, and make sure sufficient fluids are consumed before, during, and after strenuous activities. Large meals should be consumed at least three to four hours before exercise. For smaller meals, such as snacks, only one to two hours is necessary. The composition of meals should be high-carbohydrate and low fat foods. These provide the best source of energy.

Risks

Consultation with a qualified sports nutritionist is a sound practice for anyone in any age group who is heavily involved in any sport, whether amateur or professional. Specific precautions are:

• Consultation should be individualized, as people vary in their energy needs, such as sweating rates and body composition.

• Any female athlete who stops having menstrual periods (amenorrhea) or has only scanty periods (oligomenorrhea) should be evaluated for disordered eating.

• Nutritional advice should be given by a registered dietitian or physician, not by a coach. The American Academy of Pediatrics notes that "most coaches do not have an adequate nutritional background to counsel an athlete about weight loss."

• Coaches should avoid discussing weight loss with young athletes (with the exception of sports requiring weigh-ins before competition), as such discussions often lead to the athlete's use of harmful weight-loss practices.

- Athletes should not take any dietary supplement without consulting their physician and a nutritionist.

- Athletes following a vegetarian or vegan diet require special attention to protein and iron intake.

Interactions

Some herbal dietary supplements used by athletes are known to interact with prescription medications. Some of them are:

- St. John's wort (*Hypericum perforatum*) and ephedra (*Ephedra sinica*), often used in the past to promote weight loss

- valerian (*Valeriana officinalis*), often taken for insomnia

- cayenne (*Capsicum frutescens*), ginseng (*Panax ginseng*), and cordyceps (*Cordyceps sinensis*), taken internally to increase carbohydrate metabolism or increase endurance

- Siberian ginseng (*Eleutherococcus senticosus*) and echinacea (*Echinacea angustifolia*), taken to boost the immune system.

Some of these **drug interactions** are potentially serious. Athletes should not take any herbal remedies, including those marketed specifically to athletes, without consulting their physician and a nutritionist.

Complications

There are no complications associated with nutritional monitoring of athletes by qualified professionals. The AAP, however, recommends seeking nutritional information and assessment from **dietetics** professionals, not from team coaches or personal trainers.

Results

The Men's Health article *26 Ways to Feed Your Body for Results*, by author Lou Schuler, quotes American exercise and nutrition scientist Lonnie Lowery (from Winona State University in Minnesota). Dr. Lowery states, "No specific food will make you faster or stronger tomorrow. Sports nutrition is all about many factors adding up over time." In other words, no one specific ingredient will make an athlete work at his or her best performance. The whole package is necessary. The correct types of foods and drinks will help athletes train harder and compete better. The whole package called *sports nutrition* is a very important ingredient for strength, endurance, stamina, and overall performance in any athlete.

Parental concerns

Parental concerns about sports nutrition are age-related in most cases. Parents of young children should be aware of the ways in which children's hydration requirements during athletic activity differ from those of adults. Parents of adolescents who are heavily involved in sports should acquaint themselves with the signs of unhealthy eating or dieting practices in high school or college-age athletes.

Hydration needs in young children

Young children are more susceptible to heat-related illnesses than adults during exercise for several reasons:

- they produce more heat relative to body mass for the same intensity of exercise

- they have a lower cardiac output than adults at any exercise level

- they have a higher threshold for rise in body temperature before beginning to sweat

- they have a lower sweating capacity than adults, which makes it harder for them to dissipate body heat through evaporation.

Children also have a less efficient thirst mechanism than adults, which means that they are more likely to become dehydrated during exercise because they do not feel as intense a need to drink liquids. Orange- or grape-flavored drinks are often a good way to rehydrate children because they will increase their fluid intake when the beverage is flavored.

Female athlete triad

Parents should watch for indications of the female athlete triad, such as missing three or more menstrual periods; an unusual number of stress fractures; an excessive amount of time spent exercising or working out; a tendency to wear baggy or concealing clothes even in warm weather; and a restricted eating pattern. Adopting a vegetarian or vegan diet may indicate the onset of an eating disorder in a female athlete.

Doping

Doping in sports refers to the practice of taking anabolic steroids and other substances forbidden by international sports organizations. The word is derived from the Dutch word for an alcoholic drink consumed by Zulu warriors to give them energy before a battle. In the early twentieth century, doping referred primarily to the illegal drugging of race horses, but has been applied to human athletes since the 1920s.

KEY TERMS

Anabolic steroids—Any of a number of synthetic steroid hormones that are commonly used to increase muscle mass and strength.

Cardiovascular disease—Also called heart disease, a class of diseases that involve the heart or blood vessels.

Creatine—An amino acid that provides energy to the muscles of the body; with a chemical formula of $C_4H_9N_3O_2$.

Dehydration—Loss of body fluids.

Electrolytes—Any chemical compound that separates into ions in a solution, and is also able to conduct electricity.

Hemoglobin—An iron-containing protein found in red blood cells, which helps to carry oxygen through the body.

Hypertension—High blood pressure.

Type 2 diabetes—Also called diabetes mellitus type 2, a disorder that is characterized by high blood glucose, along with insulin resistance, which often occurs in adulthood.

QUESTIONS TO ASK YOUR DOCTOR

- Where can I learn more about sports nutrition?

- Are there any professionals in the local area that specialize in sports nutrition?

- Where can I find reliable information on the Internet, in books, and other places about sports nutrition?

- How much fluids (especially water) should I drink each day? What is my appropriate fluid intake before, during, and after strenuous physical activities.

- How many calories should I consume each day?

- Based on my physically active lifestyle, what changes to my diet should I implement to make sure I am getting all of the nutrition I should from my foods?

In the 1970s, testing of athletes' blood samples focused largely on steroid use, but in the 1980s and 1990s, new tests had to be devised to detect evidence of blood doping. Blood doping refers to the use of blood transfusions or a hormone called erythropoetin (EPO) in order to increase the level of hemoglobin in an athlete's blood, and therefore its oxygen-carrying capacity. The use of EPO in such endurance sports as marathon running or cycling increases the athlete's risk of **heart** disease if it is used to raise blood hemoglobin levels above 13.0 g/dL.

Newer forms of doping include the use of modafinil (Provigil), a drug ordinarily used to treat narcolepsy (a sleep disorder), and gene doping. Gene doping is defined by the World Anti-Doping Agency, an organization founded in 1999, as "the non-therapeutic use of cells, genes, genetic elements, or of the modulation of gene expression, having the capacity to improve athletic performance." One possible technique of gene doping would be the use of a synthetic gene that could last for years and produce high amounts of naturally occurring muscle-building hormones.

Vegetarian and vegan diets

It is possible for an athlete to maintain strength and overall health on a vegetarian diet provided that a variety of plant-based sources of protein are consumed on a daily basis and energy intake is adequate. Vegetarian and especially vegan athletes are at risk of inadequate creatine and **iron** intake, however, as well as insufficient amounts of **zinc**, **vitamin B$_{12}$**, **vitamin D**, and **calcium**. Iron deficiency will eventually affect athletic performance, as will low levels of creatine. Coaches and trainers should be aware that sudden adoption of a vegetarian or vegan diet in an athlete who was previously eating meat and fish may indicate the onset of an eating disorder.

Resources

BOOKS

American Psychiatric Association. *Diagnostic and Statistical Manual of Mental Disorders*, fourth edition, text revision. Washington, D.C.: American Psychiatric Association, 2000.

American Society of Health-System Pharmacists (ASHP). *AHFS Drug Handbook*, 2nd edition. Philadelphia: Lippincott Williams & Wilkins, 2003.

Antonio, Jose. *Essentials of Sports Nutrition and Supplements*. Totowa, NJ: Humana Press, 2008.

Kenney, W. Larry, Jack H. Wilmore, and David L. Costill. *Physiology of Sport and Exercise*. Champaign, IL: Human Kinetics, 2012.

Kraemer, William J., Steven J. Fleck, and Michael R. Deschenes. *Exercise Physiology: Integrating Theory and Application.* Philadelphia: Wolters Kluwer Health/Lippincott Williams & Wilkins, 2012.

Larson-Meyer, D. Enette. *Vegetarian Sports Nutrition.* Champaign, IL: Human Kinetics, 2007.

MacLaren, Don, editor. *Sport and Exercise Nutrition.* New York: Elsevier, 2007.

McArdle, William D., Frank I. Katch, and Victor L. Katch. *Exercise Physiology: Energy, Nutrition, and Human Performance*, 6th edition. Philadelphia: Lippincott Williams & Wilkins, 2007.

PERIODICALS

American Dietetic Association (ADA). "Position of the American Dietetic Association: Nutrition Intervention in the Treatment of Anorexia Nervosa, Bulimia Nervosa, and Other Eating Disorders." *Journal of the American Dietetic Association* 106 (December 2006): 2073–2082.

Calfee, R., and P. Fadale. "Popular Ergogenic Drugs and Supplements in Young Athletes." *Pediatrics* 117 (March 2006): 577–589.

Judge, B.S., and B.H. Eisenga. "Disorders of Fuel Metabolism: Medical Complications Associated with Starvation, Eating Disorders, Dietary Fads, and Supplements." *Emergency Medicine Clinics of North America* 23 (August 2005): 789–813.

Nichols, J.F., M.J. Rauh, M.J. Lawson, et al. "Prevalence of the Female Athlete Triad Syndrome among High School Athletes." *Archives of Pediatric and Adolescent Medicine* 160 (February 2006): 137–142.

Venderley, A.M., and W.W. Campbell. "Vegetarian Diets: Nutritional Considerations for Athletes." *Sports Medicine* 36 (April 2006): 293–305.

Vertalino, M., M. E. Eisenberg, M. Story, and D. Neumark-Sztainer. "Participation in Weight-Related Sports Is Associated with Higher Use of Unhealthful Weight-Control Behaviors and Steroid Use." *Journal of the American Dietetic Association* 107 (March 2007): 434–440.

WEBSITES

Exercise Physiology.. Medscape Reference. (November 21, 2011). http://emedicine.medscape.com/article/88484-overview (accessed February 25, 2012).

FDA Acts to Remove Ephedra-Containing Dietary Supplements From Market. Food and Drug Administration. (November 23, 2004). http://www.fda.gov/ForConsumers/ConsumerUpdates/ucm108379.htm (accessed February 16, 2012).

Gottschlich, Laura M. *Female Athlete Triad.*. Medscape Reference. (January 25, 2012). http://emedicine.medscape.com/article/89260-overview (accessed February 25, 2012).

National Center for Health Statistics.. Centers for Disease Control and Prevention. (February 9, 2012). http://www.nlm.nih.gov/medlineplus/sportsfitness.html#cat10 (accessed February 16, 2012).

Schuler, Lou. *26 Ways to Feed Your Body for Results.*. Men's Health magazine. http://www.menshealth.com/mhlists/sports-nutrition/ (accessed February 16, 2012).

Sports Fitness. Medline Plus. http://www.nlm.nih.gov/medlineplus/sportsfitness.html#cat10 (accessed February 16, 2012).

Sports Nutrition.. Academy of Nutrition and Dietetics. http://www.eatright.org/public/content.aspx?id=7055 (accessed February 16, 2012).

Sports and Nutrition.. University of Illinois. (November 23, 2004). http://urbanext.illinois.edu/hsnut/ (accessed February 16, 2012).

ORGANIZATIONS

Academy of Nutrition and Dietetics, 120 South Riverside Plaza, Ste. 2000, Chicago, IL 60606-6995, (312) 899-0040, (800) 877-1600, http://eatright.org

American College of Sports Medicine, 401 West Michigan Street, Indianapolis, IN 46202-3233, (317) 634-7817, Fax: (317) 634-7817, http://www.acsm.org

American Council on Exercise, 4851 Paramount Drive, San Diego, CA 92123, (888) 825-3636, support@acefitness.org, htpp://www.acefitness.org

American Society of Health-System Pharmacists, 7272 Wisconsin Avenue, Bethesda, MD 20814, (866) 279-0681, http://www.ashp.org

Gatorade Sports Science Institute, 617 West Main Street, Barrington, IL 60606-6995, (800) 616-4774, http://www.gssiweb.com

National Strength and Conditioning Association, 1885 Bob Johnson Drive, Colorado Springs, CO 80906, (719) 632-6722, Fax: (719) 632-6367, (800) 815-6826, nsca@nsca-lift.org, http://www.nsca-lift.org

Sports, Cardiovascular, and Wellness Nutritionists, 1520 Kensington Road, Suite 202, Oak Brook, IL 60523, Fax: (866) 381-7288, (800) 249-7288, scandpg@gmail.com, http://www.scandpg.org.

Rebecca J. Frey, Ph.D.
William A. Atkins, B.B., B.S., M.B.A.

Sports participation by children

Definition

Sports participation in children involves the issue of children playing or competing in sports and the related concerns regarding **nutrition**, growth, injury, and psychosocial factors.

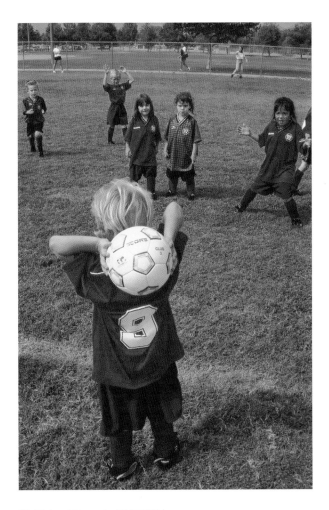

(© Richard Cummins/CORBIS.)

Description

As more and more children participate in recreational or competitive sports activities, the issue of sports participation has increasingly become a topic of discussion. It is estimated that 25% of girls and 50% of boys aged eight to 16 participate in sports in the United States. Even more participate in sports in the United Kingdom. These numbers have increased the discussion and research on the effects of early athletic training on children's growing bodies. Specific areas of concern include the cardiovascular and musculoskeletal systems, nutrition, sexual maturation, psychosocial implications, and injury prevention and treatment.

Viewpoints

Studies have shown that, in general, childhood activity is on the decline and childhood **obesity** is on the rise. Requirements for physical education in schools have become less stringent. One survey sponsored by the Centers for Disease Control and Prevention reports that

50% of high school students are not enrolled in physical education, and more than 80% of high school students do not participate in 20 minutes of physical activity three times per week. There is clearly a need for the encouragement of physical activity in children and adolescents. At the other end of the spectrum, however, injuries and other ramifications of intense athletic participation cannot be ignored.

One of the major concerns related to sports participation is the incidence of injury. Thirty to 40 percent of all pediatric accidents occur during athletics, with 10% of all childhood head injuries being related to sports participation. An estimated three million children and adolescents visit emergency rooms each year for sports-related injuries, while another five million require a visit to their physicians. Some parents and professionals view these statistics as viable reasons to keep children away from organized sports participation, however, a large number of injuries occur during unsupervised activities as well, such as diving and skiing. In any case, excessive stress to the body can cause tissue injuries; particularly concerning are those to the epiphyseal plates, as they can result in growth disturbances.

Research studies have identified several factors contributing to **sports injuries**, including but not limited to inadequate equipment, intensity of competition, and poor playing technique. Preventative measures can address many of these contributors in order to help reduce risk, but some researchers opine that increased surveillance is still required to determine which preventative measures would be most effective. Surveillance would include determination of the most prevalent types of injuries, who is affected, and why they occur.

Another area of concern related to early sports participation is nutrition. Proper nutrition is important for all youth, and vital for young athletes. Opponents of early sports participation may point out that children who engage in activities requiring slim figures, such as ballet or gymnastics, may place their growth at risk through inadequate nutrition and even pathologic eating behaviors. One study of rhythmic gymnasts noted that while gymnasts did not have adequate caloric intake for their energy expenditure, the composition of their diets reflected better nutritional practices than those of non-athletes.

Other areas of concern include: cardiac implications, sexual maturation, and psychosocial aspects of sports participation. The research on cardiac function with intense **exercise** has not demonstrated adverse effects, although opponents may point to research indicating that myocardial function can be depressed after intense exercise. In relation to sexual maturation, athletic girls tend to have a later onset of menstruation than do those not participating in sports. In addition, amenorrhea, or cessation of menstrual period, is common with intense training. Opponents of childhood athletics also point to psychosocial problems caused by **anxiety** and stress of competition. Research studies have shown that these problems do occur in a small minority of youth athletes due to burnout, inability to participate in other activities, and parental demands. Proponents of sports participation recommend that psychosocial problems can be limited with participation in a variety of sports as opposed to early specialization.

Professional implications

Allied health professionals, including nurses, physical therapists, exercise physiologists, and athletic trainers play important roles in client education, injury prevention, and treatment. These professionals may assist clients and their families by:

- Providing general information regarding benefits and risks to youth athletics so that clients and families can make informed decisions regarding level of participation.

- Encouraging children to participate in activities consistent with their abilities and interests, while discouraging early specialization, parental pressure and emphasis only on winning.

- Providing education regarding proper coaching, early identification of signs related to overuse injuries, and importance of rest.

- Monitoring body composition, height, weight, cardiac function, nutrition, and stress level regularly.

- Emphasizing the importance of general fitness versus training only sports-specific skills, and the importance of warm-up, cool-down, and flexibility.

- Identifying individual risk factors to injury (e.g., malalignment, muscle-tendon imbalance, disease, improper footwear) and providing education regarding these factors.

- Recommending and providing pre-participation physical examinations that include medical history; screening of body systems; orthopedic evaluation; flexibility, strength, speed, agility, power, endurance, balance, and coordination assessment; and clearance for sports participation by a physician.

Resources

BOOKS

Campbell, Suzann K., Darl W. Vander Linden, and Robert J. Palisano. *Physical Therapy for Children,* 2nd ed. Philadelphia: W.B. Saunders Company, 2000.

Micheli, Lyle J., ed. *Clinics in Sports Medicine: Pediatric and Adolescent Sports Injuries.* Philadelphia: W. B. Saunders Company, 2000.

PERIODICALS

Covington, D.Y., et al. "Kids on the Move: Preventing Obesity Among Urban Children." *American Journal of Nursing* 101 (March 2001): 73–9.

Cupisti, A., et al. "Nutrition Survey in Elite Rhythmic Gymnasts." *Journal of Sports Medicine and Physical Fitness* 40 (December 2000): 350–5.

Peggy Campbell Torpey, MPT

Sprains and strains

Definition

A sprain is an injury to ligaments and/or the joint capsule that occurs in response to large stresses. A strain is disruption of the contractile elements in muscle and/or tendon. An easy way to remember the difference between sprain and strain is that strain is spelled with a "t," which can imply the associated word tendon.

Description

Sprains

Sprains are categorized into three levels of severity. In a mild sprain, or first degree sprain, few ligamentous fibers have been torn, and the ligament is not significantly weakened. There may have been some slight bleeding. In a moderate sprain, also known as a second degree sprain, there is more disruption of the ligamentous fibers (40–50% of the fibers are torn) and ligamentous **weakness** is present. Moderate bleeding occurs. In a severe sprain, also named a third degree sprain, there is complete disruption of the ligamentous fibers or joint capsule and there is no strength of the ligamentous tissue. Marked swelling, secondary to bleeding, is present. Many athletes have suffered a complete tear, or third degree sprain, of the anterior cruciate ligament (ACL) of their knee.

Strains

Strains are also referred to as first degree, second degree, or third degree strains. In a first degree strain there is usually mild damage to the muscle or tendon with only a few fibers torn. There is minimal bleeding. A second degree strain presents with moderate weakness as the contractile components are torn. There is more bleeding and swelling. In a third degree strain there is complete rupture of the muscle or tendon. A third degree strain is considered a complete tear, accompanied by bleeding, swelling, and loss of function of the associated muscle. An example of a third degree strain would be a rupture of the biceps tendon.

Causes and symptoms

Both sprains and strains are due to increased demand or large stresses placed on the involved structures, i.e., ligament, muscle, or tendon.

Sprains

In a first degree or mild sprain, there is minor weakness, minimal disability, and no muscle spasms of the surrounding musculature. In a second degree sprain, the individual may complain of moderate disability and report instability. For example, in a second degree sprain of the lateral ankle, the individual may report, "the ankle feels like giving way." In a third degree sprain the individual will complain of **pain** secondary to swelling. Furthermore, the individual will report having major impairment in function, e.g., weight bearing activities.

Strains

An individual with a mild strain may complain of mild irritation of the affected area with no appreciable change in function. A secondary strain will cause the individual to complain about swelling, some minimal stiffening, moderate disability, and moderate pain. In a severe strain, the individual will report a marked loss of function, swelling of the affected area, muscle spasms secondary to guarding, and significant weakness. Interestingly, because of the complete rupture in severe strains, there will be little or no pain on stretching or with movement. Any pain present is probably due to the severe swelling secondary to bleeding.

Diagnosis

Sprains

Functional testing and clinical observation are often sufficient to establish a diagnosis of sprain. In addition to the above symptoms, a variety of tests can be performed in an effort to evaluate the integrity and stability of the joint. For example, a clinician might test an injured knee by applying medial and lateral stress to the knee.

Four ligaments are important for the stability of the knee joint: the lateral collateral ligament, the medial collateral ligament, the anterior cruciate ligament, and the posterior cruciate ligament. The collateral ligaments are largely responsible for the stability of the knee joint in response to lateral and medial stress. Lateral force (also known as a valgus stress) pressures the medial ligament and medial force (also known as varus) pressures the lateral ligament. If a patient has sprained either ligament, the joint should be abnormally mobile—the more mobile, the more severe the sprain. Other tests to determine the status of the cruciate ligaments, such as the Lachman test and the posterior drawer test, may also be performed. Some of the more common knee injuries associated with football are tears of the medial collateral ligament (MCL) and/or the anterior cruciate ligament (ACL). Sometimes the forces that caused the injury are so severe that the MCL, ACL, and medial meniscus (cartilage) are all disrupted. This is termed an "unhappy triad."

Depending on factors like the severity of the sprain, the nature of the injury, and the severity of the sprain, x rays may also be indicated. X rays do not indicate the severity of the sprain, merely whether a fracture has occurred or not. **Ultrasonography** and **magnetic resonance imaging** (MRI) may be used to determine the severity of a sprain. MRI has the additional benefit of offering multiple types of information. For example, in cases of suspected neck sprain, MRI can show whether the injury is truly a sprain, a strain, or originates from abnormalities in the cervical (intervertebral) disks.

Strains

MRI is also an important tool in the evaluation of strain. Although not indicated in the majority of cases, MRI provides the most accurate diagnostic information of the imaging techniques available. Other imaging techniques include ultrasound and computerized axial tomography (CAT scan), but their use is limited. In most cases, however, diagnosis is obtained from clinical observation and functional testing.

When evaluating a first degree strain, findings will show a mild loss of strength during resistance testing, a decreased range of motion, and minimal muscle guarding. In a second degree strain, the strength test will indicate moderate weakness, decreased range of motion, and moderate pain when stretching the tendon or muscle. In a third degree strain, findings will be more pronounced with significant swelling and major weakness compared to the uninvolved side. There will be marked loss of function and significant disability.

One common example of a strain is a hamstring strain, known more commonly as a pulled hamstring. In baseball, when a batter has just hit the ball in the infield, she or he will need to run quickly to first base. On approaching the first base bag, the batter may reach out and extend with the leg to touch the base. A common injury at the point of extension is a tear of one of the following muscles (more commonly known as the hamstrings): biceps femoris, semimembranosus, or semitendinosus (tearing of all three is rare). When the hamstrings are over-extended, such as when the baseball player over extends the leg, a muscle or tendon tear may occur.

Treatment

Sprains

In a mild sprain the goal in treatment is to decrease any swelling that is present and prevent loss of motion secondary to stiffness. Ice, elevation, and compression should be used before and after treatment sessions. **Therapeutic exercise** should include range of motion, stretching, and strengthening of the surrounding musculature. In a moderate sprain, treatment is more conservative and the clinician must minimize the risk of further injury. Modalities should be continued to decrease swelling and pain. The RICE (rest, ice, compression, and elevation) principle should continue throughout treatment. A general **rehabilitation** pathway of strengthening, range of motion, and flexibility all need to continue and progress as tolerated. In a severe sprain, there are usually two options: surgical and non-surgical. In the surgical option, the ligament is re-attached by the physician. The non-surgical approach relies on bracing to minimize motion and allow for healing. The rehabilitation plan is complex in either of these approaches, but the goal is to initially minimize motion followed by slow progression into range of motion and strengthening.

Strains

Treatment of first and second degree strains is similar to treatment of sprains. It consists of utilizing the RICE principle and protecting the affected area from overstretching or overuse. Rehabilitation should focus on range of motion, decreasing swelling and pain, and gradual introduction of a strengthening program. Severe strains may require surgical repair, and protocols of rehabilitation are different for each affected area. Initial treatment could be immobilization followed by guarded range of motion, flexibility, and strengthening therapies.

Prognosis

Sprains

In a mild sprain, the individual can usually engage in normal activities within three to six weeks. In a moderate sprain, normal activities can usually resume in approximately eight to 12 weeks—ligamentous tissue requires approximately eight to 10 weeks to heal. By the third or fourth week, however, the individual with a moderate sprain will usually have a normal range of motion and be free of pain. Therefore, the key to recovery from a moderate strain is to prevent the patient from returning to normal activity before the ligament heals.

The prognosis for a complete rupture (severe sprain) varies. Success depends on the management of the injury, and the subsequent level of desired activity. A return to normal activity may require from six months to one year.

Strains

The prognosis for treating first or second degree strains is good. The major problem is stressing the affected area too soon. Overstressing the affected area too early in recovery may cause the strain to become chronic. A chronic strain could lead to further complications such as muscle spasm and possible myositis.

Health care team roles

It is appropriate that physicians, nurses, therapists, and other allied health partners be familiar with the prevention and care of sprains and strains. Moreover, nurses and allied health partners should be involved in **patient education** that focuses on minimizing the risk of overuse injuries.

Prevention

The best prevention for sprains and strains is to have optimal muscular strength, muscular flexibility, and endurance. Appropriate warm-up exercises before an activity may further minimize the potential for injury. Sprains may also be prevented by the use of a brace.

Sprains are caused by excessive stress to a ligament or capsule. Optimal strength, flexibility, and endurance help the muscles to accept and distribute forces that might otherwise be placed on the joint. If muscles are weak and not flexible, increased demand placed on the area will need to be absorbed by the ligaments or joint capsule. Increased demand on these structures will put them at greater risk for failure, i.e. tearing. Braces may absorb some of this extra demand. For example, persons wishing to avoid ankle injury may choose to tape their ankle or wear a lacing brace before engaging in activities with injury potential. Persons with prior ankle injuries may utilize an air stirrup.

Surfaces may also play a role in sprains and strains. A controversial example is the comparison of football injuries on natural grass and artificial turf. One study found an increased rate of anterior cruciate ligament sprains in football players playing on artificial turf compared to sprains on natural grass. A less controversial

KEY TERMS

Immobilization—To keep a limb or joint free from movement and to maintain position. Movement is stopped by either bracing or casting.

Irritation—Minimal disruption of a structure that may cause bleeding. An irritation can present with minimal swelling and a feeling of discomfort to the individual. Usually, function is not impaired secondary to an irritation. An irritation can progress to a more severe impairment if healing is not allowed to appropriately take place.

Modalities—A term used to describe treatment modes that are applied to the individual. In rehabilitation, a few examples of a modality could be heat, ice, ultrasound, electrical stimulation, and traction.

Range of motion—The amount of motion that a joint has. There is active range of motion and passive range of motion. Active range of motion is the range the joint can traverse under voluntary contraction. The individual moves the limb using their muscle power. Passive range of motion is the range that the joint moves through while either a machine or individual moves the limb. In passive range of motion, the limb is usually moved for the individual with no muscle contraction.

Therapeutic exercise—A general term to describe a multitude of exercises, stretching, and general rehabilitation. Can include range of motion, resistive exercises such as weight training, postural correction exercises, and exercises that incorporate coordination and balance training.

example might be the comparison of a manicured lawn to a field of wild prairie grass. The prairie grass might hide many dips in the field that would be apparent in a manicured lawn. Such a field would provide a greater likelihood of injury due to the unpredictability and unevenness of the surface, since there is a greater chance for unexpected excessive forces on a joint.

Resources

BOOKS

Andrews, J.R., G.L. Harrelson, and K.E. Wilk. *Physical Rehabilitation of the Injured Athlete.* Philadelphia: W.B. Saunders, 2012.

Hall, C.M., and L.T. Brody. *Therapeutic Exercise Moving Toward Function.* Philadelphia: Lippincott, Williams and Wilkins, 1999.

Hertling, D., and R.M. Kessler. *Management of Common Musculoskeletal Disorders.* Baltimore: Lippincott, Williams & Wilkins, 1996.

Magee, D.J. *Orthopedic Physical Assessment.* Philadelphia: W. B. Saunders Co., 1997.

OTHER

"Facts and fallacies of diagnostic ultrasound of the adult spine." http://www.chiroweb.com/archives/14/09/33.html.

Intelihealth. Knee. http://www.intelihealth.com/IH/ihtIH?t= 25430&p=~br,IHW/~st,24479/~r,WSIHW000/~b,*/.

Intelihealth. Shoulder. http://www.intelihealth.com/IH/ihtIH/ WSSFG000/7165/8954/305248.html?d=dmtContent.

Knee Injury. http://www.multisportsa.com/injuries/knee.htm.

Virtual hospital imaging of muscle injuries. http://www.vh.org/ Providers/Textbooks/MuscleInjuries/07MuscleTearStrain. html.

Mark Damian Rossi, Ph.D., P.T.

Sputum analysis

Definition

Sputum is a substance comprised of mucus, foreign matter, and saliva that is found in the **lungs** or bronchial tree. A sputum analysis is a group of tests performed in a laboratory on a sputum specimen obtained from a sick patient. A portion of the sputum specimen is stained and put on a slide for examination of cells and organisms. Another portion of the specimen is put on an agar plate to see if infectious organisms grow and can be identified. Some of the sputum may be placed in special solutions to test for specific diseases.

Purpose

The purpose of a sputum analysis is to help identify microorganisms that are causing respiratory disease or **infection**. The most common reason for obtaining a sputum specimen is to test for infectious **tuberculosis**. A sputum analysis, however, is also used to identify disease-producing organisms that may be causing **pneumonia**, **bronchitis**, lung **abscess**, or other respiratory disease. A sputum analysis may be used to identify conditions such as: aspiration pneumonia, histoplasmosis, cryptococcosis, blastomycosis, mycoplasma pneumonia, plague, mycobacterial infection, and pneumocystic pneumonia.

Precautions

A sputum specimen should not be collected immediately following a meal because the sputum or

Sputum		
Term	**Description**	**Associated with**
Fetid	Foul-smelling, typical of anaerobic infection	Bronchiectasis, lung abscess, or cystic fibrosis
Frothy	White or pink-tinged, foamy, thin sputum	Pulmonary edema
Hemoptysis	Expectoration of blood or bloody sputum; amount may range from blood-streaked to massive hemorrhage	A variety of pathologies
Mucoid	White or clear, not generally associated with bronchopulmonar infection	Chronic cough (acute or chronic bronchitis, cystic fibrosis)
Purulent	Pus, yellow or greenish sputum, often copious and thick	Acute and chronic infection
Rusty	Descriptive of the color of sputum (also called prune juice)	Pneumococcal pneumonia

SOURCE: Rothstein, J.M., S.H. Roy, and S.L. Wolf. *The Rehabilitation Specialist's Handbook.* 2nd ed. Philadelphia: F.A. Davis Co., 1998.

the process of collecting the sputum may cause gagging and **vomiting**.

Good hand washing and the use of gloves are necessary when collecting a sputum specimen. A disposable gown and filter-mask should be worn if reactivated infectious tuberculosis is suspected.

About 1 teaspoon (3-5 cc) of sputum should be collected to have a sufficient quantity for proper testing. The specimen cup should not be left at the bedside for the patient to randomly spit into. Specimens must be fresh and taken immediately to the laboratory for effective analysis.

The specimen must be coughed up from the lungs or bronchial tree. It can be mixed with saliva, but a specimen that is only saliva is not adequate for proper testing.

An infant or young child cannot **cough** up sputum on command. Sputum specimens must be obtained with a nasal-pharyngeal aspirator connected to a mucus trap or by bronchial washings performed during a **bronchoscopy**. If using a nasal-pharyngeal aspirator, the tubing must have a one-way valve on the tester's side of the tubing to prevent the inhalation of infected droplets from the patient, or it should have a trap that connects directly to a suction apparatus.

The use of **antibiotics**, anti-inflammatory drugs, or steroids may affect the test results. If the patient is receiving any of these medications, the physician should be notified, and it should be noted on the laboratory slip.

Description

The patient should take three slow deep breaths and cough forcefully with the exhalation of the third breath. Sputum that is coughed up should be spit directly into the sterile specimen cup. The process is repeated until the required amount of sputum is collected. The cap is then placed on the specimen cup.

If the patient has difficulty raising sputum, the physician should be notified. Some patients may require postural drainage and cupping to loosen and drain secretions. Others may require an aerosol treatment with saline or medications to open the air sacs and allow drainage of the sputum before it can be collected. In certain cases, the physician may elect to perform a bronchoscopy to collect the sputum for analysis. A bronchoscopy is performed in a special setting in which the patient can be sedated and monitored during the procedure.

A nasal-pharyngeal mucus trap is used to collect sputum from an infant or young child that cannot understand instructions. A small tube is inserted through the nasal passage and into the pharynx. This process usually stimulates the infant to cough. As the child coughs up sputum, it is pulled through the tubing and into a mucus trap. The mucus trap is placed in a plastic biohazard specimen bag that is sealed, labeled, and sent to the lab for analysis. If a specimen from an infant can not be collected, the physician should be notified. The sputum may need to be collected through a bronchoscope by the physician.

Special testing may require variance in the sputum collection procedure. For example, sputum for viral studies may require that the client gargles and expectorates with a nutrient broth. The medical setting's lab manual should be consulted for instructions to collect sputum for special testing.

Preparation

The procedure should be explained to the patient. Fluid intake should be encouraged the night before the test. The specimen should be obtained in the morning before meals. The patient should abstain from **smoking**, eating, or chewing gum before the specimen collection. If the patient has dentures, they should be removed. The patient rinses his mouth with plain water before the test to clear debris from the mouth. The patient is seated in an upright position. A capped sterile specimen cup is placed

KEY TERMS

Agar—A gelatinous culture media used in laboratories to grow microorganisms such as bacteria.

Bronchoscopy—The examination of the inside of a patient's airway and bronchus by a physician using a flexible scope connected to a light source and video camera.

Sputum—A substance coughed up from the airway, bronchi, or lungs comprised of saliva, foreign matter, and mucus.

near the patient. Good hand-washing and the use of gloves is necessary for this procedure. Other protective gear is used as instructed (e.g., for known tuberculosis clients with potentially reactivated tuberculosis). The laboratory manual of the medical setting should be consulted for specific specimen directions.

Aftercare

The patient should be allowed to relax and breathe quietly. The specimen cup is labeled with the patient's name, doctor, time, date, and type of specimen. The specimen cup is placed in a biohazard labeled plastic sealed bag. The specimen does not need to be refrigerated but should be transported to the lab immediately for testing. Good hand-washing is necessary after the procedure. Used tissues and gloves should be placed in a contaminated trash bag that can be sealed and discarded.

Complications

There are no complications to obtaining a non-invasive sputum specimen. Complications of obtaining a specimen by nasal tracheal aspiration or bronchoscopy are rare, but may include trauma to the throat or tracheal tissue and/or secondary infection.

Results

A sputum analysis, when used in conjunction with other tests such as chest x rays or **blood** cultures, is an important diagnostic tool. It is an effective method for identifying unknown organisms that are causing respiratory infections or disease. Identification of the organism allows proper selection of antibiotic or other drug therapy to treat specific respiratory disease and provide a positive outcome for the patient. Improper collection or handling of a sputum specimen may invalidate the test results.

Health care team roles

A sputum specimen is usually collected by a licensed nurse or respiratory therapist in the medical setting. Other medical personnel, however, such as medical office technicians or other non-professional staff can be taught the correct method for obtaining a sputum specimen. A patient or patient's family can be trained to collect a sputum specimen in the home. The specimen should be taken promptly to a lab for analysis. A laboratory technician will prepare the specimen for analysis, and a pathologist will ultimately be responsible for analyzing the sputum specimen.

Resources

OTHER

"Cytology Exam of the Sputum." Medical Encyclopedia. National Institute of Health. Medline Online. March 2001. http://www.nlm.nih.gov/medlineplus/ency/article/003865.htm.

Fischbach, Frances, R. N., M. S. N. "Sputum Cultures." Chapter 7. Microbiologic and Diagnostic Studies. A Manual of Laboratory and Diagnostic Tests. Sixth Edition. Ovid Books Online. Lippincott William and Wilkins, 2000. http://pco.ovid.com/lrppco/.

Griffith, H. Winter, M. D. "Sputum Culture." Complete Guide to Medical Tests. Test Universe Online. Medical Data Exchange: Fisher Books, 2000. http://www.testuniverse.com/mdx/MDX-3230.html.

Moses, Scott, M.D. "Sputum Collection." Family Practice Notebook Online. March 2001. http://www.fpnotebook.com/LUN59.htm.

"Routine Sputum Culture." Medical Encyclopedia. National Institute of Health. Medline Online. May 1999. http://www.nlm.nih.gov/medlineplus/ency/article/003723.htm.

"Sputum Analysis." OSHA Tuberculosis Training for Medical Personnel. New York University Education Online. July 2000. http://www.med.nyu.edu/envservices/training/tb_training/tb_training.pdf.

Mary Elizabeth Martelli, R.N., B.S.

Sputum culture

Definition

A sputum culture is a **microbiology** test performed to isolate and identify microorganisms causing an **infection** of the lower respiratory tract.

Purpose

Infections of the **lungs** and bronchial tubes are caused by several pathogenic microorganisms, including **bacteria**, **fungi**, **viruses**, and **parasites** which are responsible for a variety of diseases including pulmonary **tuberculosis**, bacterial **pneumonia**, viral and mycoplasmal (atypical) pneumonia, chronic **bronchitis**, and bronchiectasis. A **chest x ray** provides visual evidence suggestive of a respiratory infection; a culture identifies the microorganism causing the infection.

Precautions

For best results, the specimen should be obtained prior to initiating any therapy. The health care worker should wear a mask to avoid inhalation of airborne pathogens that may be introduced into the air during the collection process. The specimen should be taken to the laboratory within 30 minutes of collection.

Description

Sputum collection

Based on the clinical condition of the patient, the physician determines what group of microorganism is likely to be causing the infection, and then orders one or more bacterial, viral, or fungal cultures. For all culture types, the sputum must be collected into a sterile container and care must be taken to minimize specimen contamination by the normal flora of the mouth and throat. Once in the laboratory, each culture type is handled differently.

Sputum must be expectorated from the bronchi by deep forceful coughing. The recovery of sputum is best in the early morning. The patient should rinse his or her mouth by gargling with water prior to coughing. Taking deep breaths and lowering the head helps bring up the sputum. Sputum must not be held in the mouth but immediately spat into a sterile container. For tuberculosis, the physician may request sputum samples from the patient on three consecutive mornings. In some cases the patient will be unable to produce the sputum, and an aerosol of saline will be needed to loosen the congestion. In such cases the sputum can be aspirated using a suction device. In some cases sputum will be collected during a **bronchoscopy** or endotracheal procedure. These specimens, like coughed-up sputum, will be contaminated with normal flora from the mouth or throat and are not suitable for anaerobic culture. When anaerobic infection is suspected, the physician will collect the sample by transtracheal aspiration. These specimens and those collected by **thoracentesis** (removal of pleural fluid via chest wall puncture) are not contaminated by upper respiratory flora and are suitable for both aerobic and anaerobic culture.

Gram stain

The **Gram stain** is always performed when sputum is submitted for culture. Additional stains such as the acid-fast stain for tuberculosis are performed only upon request. The Gram stain is used to determine the acceptability of the specimen for culture, and aids the technologist in selecting special growth media that might be needed. Almost all bacteria are described by their Gram stain characteristics: color (purple or pink), shape (cocci or bacilli); and size, arrangement, presence, or absence of spores.

The Gram stain is performed by the following method:

- A portion of the sputum is smeared onto a glass microscope slide, air dried, and heat fixed.
- The slide is flooded with crystal violet stain that is allowed to sit for 30-60 seconds.
- The crystal violet is rinsed off with a gentle stream of water.
- The slide is flooded with Gram's iodine that is allowed to sit for 60 seconds.
- The iodine is removed with a gentle stream of water.
- The slide is decolorized by rinsing with 95% ethanol, drop by drop, until the alcohol rinses clear.
- The slide is flooded with safranin and allowed to sit for 30 seconds.
- The safranin is rinsed off with a stream of water.
- The excess water is removed by blotting with bibulous paper.
- The slide is allowed to air dry.
- The slide is observed under the microscope using both low power and oil immersion lenses.

Gram-positive cells retain the crystal violet stain and appear dark purple, while gram-negative cells do not. Gram-negative bacteria are counterstained by the safranin and appear pink. Gram staining also helps determine the integrity of the sputum specimen. The presence of many epithelial cells and few white **blood** cells indicates a contaminated sample, one not adequate for culture. The presence of many white blood cells and bacteria in the specimen signifies an acceptable sample for culture, and provides a preliminary indication of infection.

Bacterial culture

Streptococcus pneumoniae is the most common pathogen causing bacterial pneumonia, but almost any organism can be implicated. Other bacterial isolates include *Staphylococcus aureus, Haemophilus influenzae, E. coli, Enterobacter spp., Klebsiella pneumoniae, Pseudomonas aeruginosa, Legionella pneumophilia,*

Mycoplasma pneumoniae, and *Mycobacterium tuberculosis*.

Using a sterile swab, a portion of the sputum sample is transferred to each plate and then streaked for isolation using a sterilized inoculating loop. Cultures should be performed using sheep blood agar, chocolate (heated blood) agar, and MacConkey agar. All plates are incubated in 5–10% carbon dioxide at 96.8°F (36°C) for 24 hours. Plates are examined for growth and colonies are Gram stained and subcultured (transferred) to appropriate media for biochemical identification. Plates showing normal flora are incubated for an additional day. If *L. pneumophilia* is suspected, the sputum should be plated on BCYE-alpha agar (buffered charcoal-yeast extract with alpha-ketogluterate). Plates are cultured in air or 2.5% carbon dioxide for three to five days at 96.8°F (36°C). Small convex gray colonies are stained with fluorescent-labeled antibody specific for *L. pneumophilia*. If atypical pneumonia is suspected, the sputum is plated on a medium that supports the growth of *Mycoplasma pneumoniae* such as SP4. The plates are incubated in air at 96.8°F (36°C). Colonies grow slowly and are almost microscopic. They are identified by cutting a block of agar and staining it with Dienes stain. *M. pneumoniae* demonstrate their typical fried-egg appearance. Alternatively, the colonies can be identified using a fluorescent-labeled antibody specific for *M. pneumoniae*. Plates showing no growth are held up to four weeks before reporting as negative. Because of the long culture time, *Mycoplasma pneumoniae* is not usually cultured. Infections with this organism are diagnosed by enzyme immunoassay for IgM **antibodies** produced against the organism. A high concentration of these antibodies indicates acute infection.

The results of the initial Gram stain are available the same day, or in less than an hour if requested by the physician. A preliminary report on the status of the culture is usually available after one day. This report notes the presence or absence of bacterial growth, the Gram stain of any organism isolated, and presumptive identification (if possible). The final report, usually available in one to three days, includes organism identification, an estimate of the quantity of the bacteria, and the results of the antibiotic sensitivity testing.

Fungal culture

Fungal cultures of sputum are used primarily to identify the presence or *Histoplasma capsulatum*, *Coccidioides immitis*, *Cryptococcus neoformans*, *Blastomyces dermatitidis*, and *Paracoccidioides brasiliensis*. However, opportunistic yeast or fungi such as *Candida spp., Aspergillus spp.*, and *Fusarium spp.* can cause pneumonia in immunocompromised patients. Definitive diagnosis depends upon the presence of clinical signs of pulmonary infection, a positive chest x ray, and laboratory identification of the organism. In addition, histological results of open **lung biopsy** may reveal the organisms by microscopic examination of stained tissue. For the laboratory identification, the sputum is first examined microscopically via a direct smear using one or more of the following methods:

- 10% KOH preparation
- India ink preparation
- calcofluor white stain
- Gram stain
- Kinyoun's acid fast stain
- lactophenol cotton/aniline blue wet mount

In many cases, direct smears are sufficient to establish a preliminary diagnosis based upon the appearance of the yeast seen or the characteristic spores and hyphae produced by the fungus. If a **fungal culture** is ordered or suspected from direct smear, a portion of the sputum is transferred to an appropriate growth medium such as Sabauroad-dextrose agar or brain-heart infusion-blood agar. When infection with a dimorphic fungus is suspected (i.e., infection by *Histoplasma capsulatum, Coccidioides immitis, Blastomyces dermatitidis, Paracoccidioides brasiliensis*), the cultures are incubated at both 77°F (25°C) and at 36°C in order to demonstrate conversion of the mold form at 77°F (25°C) to the yeast form at 96.8°F (36°C). Rapidly growing fungi such as *Coccidioides immitis* may appear in three to four days, while slow growing fungi such as *Histoplasma capsulatum* may require several weeks. For this reason cultures are held for four weeks before signing out as negative. Identification is made on the basis of growth rate, appearance and color of colonies, and microscopic appearance demonstrating characteristic hyphae and/or spores. Microscopic evaluation is performed by transferring a loop or drop of the fungal culture onto a glass slide, adding one to two drops of lactophenol cotton blue stain, placing a coverglass over the material, and examining under the **microscope**. In some cases, a culture filtrate is prepared and tested using antibodies to the exoantigens produced by the dimorphic fungi. This is done by the double immunodiffusion technique that permits direct comparison of precipitation reactions for the cultures and known fungal antigens controls.

Viral culture

Viruses that are a common cause of respiratory tract infection include adenoviruses, rhinoviruses, **influenza**, parainfluenza, enteroviruses, respiratory syncytial virus, retroviruses, herpes simplex, and cytomegalovirus. Because viruses need host DNA to replicate, they will not grow on artificial media. Therefore, viral cultures are inoculated onto cell cultures. These may be **cancer** cells grown in monolayers in the laboratory or cells taken from animal tissues and used to prepare a monolayer. Cell types commonly used for viral isolation are human diploid fibroblasts (HDF), HEp2 cells (epithelial cancer cells from the larynx), A549 cells (human **lung cancer** cells); primary monkey kidney cells (PMK); and rabbit kidney cells (RK). Cell cultures are inoculated and allowed to grow for one to three days at 96.8°F (36°C) in 5–10% carbon dioxide. Within one to three days, a characteristic cytopathic effect (CPE) can be seen when observing the cells under a microscope.

Mycobacterial culture

Mycobacterium tuberculosis is a respiratory infection commonly transmitted via the air to the lungs, where it thrives, causing **fever**, **cough**, and blood spitting. Pneumonia can also be caused by *M. bovis*, *M. avium* complex, and *M. kansasii*.

Most mycobacteria that cause pneumonia such as *Mycobacterium tuberculosis* grow very slowly, requiring from two to six weeks for culture. *Mycobacterium tuberculosis* stains very poorly with Gram stain; therefore, acid-fast (light microscopy) and fluorescent staining methods are used to identify mycobacteria by direct microscopic examination of sputum. A smear can provide a presumptive diagnosis of mycobacterial disease; confirm that cultures growing on media are acid-fast; and demonstrate a patient's response to antibiotic therapy from post-treatment sputum cultures.

There are three staining methods commonly employed to test for mycobacteria. Two acid-fast stains, Ziehl-Neelsen and Kinyoun use light microscopy; the third method uses auramine or a combination of auramine and rhodamine and requires a fluorescent microscope. The advantage of fluorescent staining resides in the ability to examine much larger areas of the smear in a shorter period of time. Fluorescent staining is more sensitive and detects approximately 18% more cases. Its disadvantage is that the stain also detects organisms that are non-viable. While a positive finding provides a basis for initiating antibiotic treatment, the sensitivity of the direct smear is highly variable. Therefore, when acid-fast culture is requested, all sputum samples (meeting the laboratory's criteria for sputum) are cultured, even when the direct smear exam shows no evidence of acid-fast bacteria.

Sputum for culture of mycobacteria must be decontaminated. This is commonly done by adding a mucolytic agent such as N-acetyl-L-cysteine and a clearing agent, sodium hydroxide, to an equal amount of the sputum. The suspension is mixed and allowed to stand for 15 minutes, then phosphate buffered saline is added and the sample is centrifuged. The supernatant is decanted and the remaining sample is resuspended with bovine albumin and used for culture.

An acid-fast culture can detect as few as 10 to 100 CFU/mL of sputum. Culture media may be enriched with egg, albumin, or a mixture of salts, **vitamins**, cofactors, fatty acids, glucose, and other nutrients. Media also contain malachite green or **antibiotics** to retard the growth of other bacteria and yeast. The sputum should be inoculated on at least one solid medium such as American Thoracic Society or Lowenstein-Jensen and one liquid medium such as Middlebrook 7H9. Cultures are set up at several different temperatures and examined daily for several weeks to characterize the rate of growth. Colonies are subcultured and transferred to appropriate media for biochemical identification. This process can take several more weeks and therefore, other identification methods are often performed concurrently. These include analysis of cell-wall fatty acids by either gas or high-performance liquid chromatography (HPLC) and DNA probe testing. High-performance liquid chromatography can rapidly identify the species of mycobacteria from cultures. However, according to the CDC, laboratories that use HPLC report that the method requires a highly experienced technologist and usually takes a long time (about six months) for initial incorporation into their laboratories. DNA probe testing can be done on as little as a single colony and demonstrates a far more rapid turnaround time than biochemical testing. Probes are available for many species but not all mycobacterium, and may be falsely negative (i.e., a low hybridization rate) if contaminating organisms are present. For these reasons, this method is used in conjunction with biochemical testing.

Other microorganisms that cause various types of lower respiratory tract infections also require special culture or staining procedures to grow and identify. For example, *Pneumocystis carinii* in bronchial lavage, sputum, or lung biopsy samples is detected by observing the organisms with special stains such as methenamine silver stain or a fluorescent monoclonal antibody stain. *Pneumocystis carnii* causes pneumonia in people with weakened immune systems, such as people with **AIDS**, and does not grow in culture. The diagnosis is based on the results of these stains, the patient's symptoms, and medical history.

KEY TERMS

Bacilli—Rod-shaped bacterium.

Bronchiectasis—A chronic dilation of one or more bronchi.

Cocci—Spherical-shaped bacterium.

Epithelial cells—Skin cells.

Mycobacterium—A slender acid-fast organism resembling *Mycobacterium tuberculosis*.

Antibiotic susceptibility testing

With the exception of *Streptococcus pneumoniae* or other strep which are sensitive to penicillin and related antibiotics, antibiotic susceptibility testing is performed on all isolates. Susceptibility testing is performed for most other organisms by the microtube broth dilution or Kirby Bauer method. The selection of antibiotics for testing depends upon the organism isolated (e.g., gram-negative, gram-positive, aerobe, anaerobe, mycobacteria, or yeast).

The Kirby-Bauer antibiotic susceptibility test method is commonly used for Gram-positive and Gram-negative aerobic bacteria. Antibiotic disks are placed on a plate containing a clear medium such as Mueller-Hinton agar that has been swabbed uniformly with a standardized broth suspension of a pure culture of the bacteria to be tested. The plate is then incubated at 96.8°F (36°C) for 18–24 hours. The zone of no growth (zone of inhibition) around each disk is measured, and compared to predetermined cutoffs for each antibiotic concentration used. If the zone size equals or exceeds the cutoff, the organism is susceptible. If not, the organism is resistant. The results are reported as sensitive (organism inhibited by antibiotic), intermediate (inconclusive effect of antibiotic on organism), or resistant (organism not inhibited by the antibiotic).

Preparation

The specimen for culture should be collected before antibiotics are begun as the antibiotics may prevent microorganisms present in the sputum from growing in culture. The best time to collect a sputum sample is early in the morning, before the patient has had anything to eat or drink. The patient should first rinse his or her mouth with water to decrease mouth bacteria and dilute saliva.

If coughing up sputum is difficult, a nurse or respiratory therapist can have the patient breathe in sterile saline produced by a nebulizer. This nebulized saline coats the respiratory tract, loosening the sputum, and making it easier to cough up.

It is also useful to obtain information concerning travel to foreign countries, exposure to animals, and diagnosed or suspected immunosuppressive disease.

Aftercare

There are no specific requirements for care after obtaining the specimen. However, if the patient is found to have tuberculosis, several measures will be taken to prevent the spread of this airborne disease.

Complications

There are no complications associated with this test.

Results

Sputum from a healthy person will have no growth on culture. However, a mixture of microorganisms, typically found in a person's mouth and throat often contaminates the culture. In such cases the report will indicate the presence of normal flora contamination.

The preliminary report will note the presence of bacteria and white blood cells on the Gram stain and describe the appearance of the bacteria and the number of cells seen. Preliminary culture results will identify the Gram stain or presumptive identification of any organisms recovered.

Health care team roles

Sputum culture is requested by a physician. A nurse or respiratory therapist will provide instructions to the patient for collecting a sputum sample. Bronchoscopy, transtracheal aspiration, bronchial lavage or brushing, and thoracentesis are performed by a physician. Clinical laboratory scientists/medical technologists who specialize in microbiology will perform the culture and antibiotic sensitivity tests.

Resources

BOOKS

Chernecky, Cynthia C., and Barbara J. Berger. *Laboratory Tests and Diagnostic Procedures*. 3rd ed. Philadelphia, PA: W.B. Saunders Company, 2001.

Isada, Carlos M., et al. *Infectious Diseases Handbook*. Hudson, Ohio: Lexi-Comp., 1995, pp. 76–79.

Kee, Joyce LeFever. *Handbook of Laboratory and Diagnostic Tests*. 4th ed. Upper Saddle River, NJ: Prentice Hall, 2001.

Pagana, Kathleen D., and Timothy J. Pagana. *Manual of Diagnostic and Laboratory Tests*. St. Louis: Mosby, 1998, pp. 681–83.

Shulman, Stanford T., et al., eds. *The Biologic and Clinical Basis of Infectious Diseases.* 5th ed. Philadelphia: W. B. Saunders Co., 1997, pp. 123, 530.

OTHER

Centers for Disease Control and Prevention. http://www.cdc. gov/ncidod/dastlr/TB/TB_HPLC.htm.

Laboratory Corporation of America. http://www.labcorp.com/ datasets/labcorp/html/chapter/mono/mb021200.htm. 2001.

Victoria E. DeMoranville

Sputum specimen collection

Definition

Sputum specimen collection is a procedure designed to collect expectorated secretions from a patient's respiratory tract.

Purpose

Sputum is collected to be used as a laboratory specimen for the isolation of organisms that might be causing abnormalities of the respiratory tract.

Precautions

This procedure should not be performed if the patient is unable to take several deep breaths or **cough** deeply from the **lungs**.

Description

When secretions from the respiratory tract are expectorated, the secretions are called sputum. A **sputum culture** is a sample of expectorated sputum.

Induced sputum is a procedure to assist patients who have difficulty expectorating sputum. The patient inhales nebulized saline to loosen the sputum. To collect an induced sputum sample, the patient's mouth should be rinsed thoroughly with water to reduce the amount of oral **bacteria** that are normally present from contaminating the sputum. The patient then inhales 20–30 ml of hypertonic saline from an ultrasonic nebuliser. The sputum is loosened and collected in a sterile sputum container.

The patient should be supervised during the collection of the sputum to ensure the expectorated product has come from the lungs rather than saliva from the oral cavity. The sample is best taken first thing in the morning when the production of sputum is greatest.

KEY TERMS

Expectorate—To cough up excessive secretions from the respiratory tract.

Haemoptysis—The presence of blood in the sputum.

Hypertonic saline—Saline that has a higher osmotic pressure than normal saline.

Inhalation—A medicinal substance for inhaling.

Mucoid—Resembling the thick liquid secreted by the mucous glands.

Mucopurulent sputum—Sputum containing mucus and pus.

Pulmonary embolism—A blood clot in the lungs.

To collect an expectorated sputum sample, the patient should gargle and rinse out the mouth with water to reduce the amount of oral bacteria that are normally present from contaminating the sputum. The patient must take a deep breath and cough into a sterile sputum container.

For a suspected common bacteria, one sputum sample may be required. If the suspected **infection** is more complex, a sputum sample may be required on three to five successive mornings.

Preparation

If there is any difficulty in expectorating, the physician may suggest the use of an inhalation, an expectorant, or physiotherapy to aid in producing sputum for collection. The sputum should be transferred to the laboratory within two hours for analysis.

Results

Sputum is mucoidal in appearance, resembling the thick liquid secreted by the mucous glands. It can be clear, white, or greenish in color, even **blood** stained. Blood in the sputum is called haemoptysis and may be a pink froth, mucus with a streak of blood, or an obvious clot, red in color representing fresh blood or brownish representing old blood. Haemoptysis may indicate that there has been some trauma to the respiratory tract, or that there is an infection present such as **tuberculosis** or even carcinoma. If it is determined that the blood is not from a simple cut to the mouth or a nosebleed, it is considered a serious condition and should be treated immediately. The sputum may also be frothy, indicating that the patient's pulmonary **blood pressure** is raised. Mucopurulent sputum contains mucus and pus and indicates an infection, such as an **abscess**, is present.

There may be an unpleasant odor associated with sputum.

Health care team roles

The procedure must be fully explained to the patient. The nurse should note if the patient has any difficulty with expectoration, and report it to the physician.

Resources

BOOK

Nettina, Sandra. *Lippincott Manual of Nursing Practice,* 7th ed. Philadelphia: Lippincott, 2001, p. 197.

OTHER

"Cytology Exam of Sputum." http://www.healthcentral.com.

"Routine Sputum Culture." http://www.thriveonline. oxygen. com/medical/library/article/003723.html.

"Signs and Symptoms of Respiratory Disease." WebMD.com. http://www.webMD.com.

Margarte A. Stockley, R.G.N.

Standard precautions (universal precautions)

Definition

Standard precautions, sometimes called **universal precautions**, are safety procedures for avoiding contact with human bodily fluids, established by the Centers for Disease Control and Prevention (CDC) and the American Dental Association (ADA). The term *universal precautions* was used in the mid-1980s, when the practice was first introduced by the CDC in response to the discovery that HIV and hepatitis B infections can be transmitted by **blood** and other body fluids. The word *universal* was used in the 1980s and 1990s to indicate that the precautions should be used with all patients regardless of HIV or other **infection** status in order to avoid charges of stigma or discrimination against individuals known to be infected with a bloodborne disease organism. These earlier reports and recommendations from the CDC are included under the heading of Periodicals below. The term *standard precautions* is preferred as of 2012.

Purpose

Standard precautions are used in medical and dental offices to prevent the transmission of infectious diseases between patients and health care workers. A 1988 CDC report defines the purpose of standard precautions as "prevent[ion of] parenteral, mucous membrane, and nonintact skin exposures of health-care workers to bloodborne pathogens." Other body fluids covered by standard precautions include semen, vaginal secretions, cerebrospinal fluid (CSF), synovial fluid, pleural fluid, peritoneal fluid, pericardial fluid, and amniotic fluid. However, the CDC considers blood to be the most significant source of pathogen transmission between patients and health care workers. Standard precautions do not apply to fecal matter, nasal discharges, sputum, sweat, tears, urine, and vomited material unless they contain visible blood.

Description

Standard precautions are standards of **infection control** practices designed to reduce the risk of transmission of bloodborne infections.

Personal protective equipment

Protective equipment includes gloves, gowns, masks, and eyewear worn by health care workers to reduce the risk of exposure to potentially infectious materials.

Examination gloves are used for procedures involving contact with mucous membranes. They reduce the incidence of contamination to the hands, but they cannot prevent penetrating injuries from needles or other sharp instruments. Gloves are changed after each patient and discarded, and must never be washed or disinfected for reuse. Washing with surfactants may cause wicking (the enhanced penetration of liquids through undetected holes in the glove). Disinfecting agents may cause deterioration of the gloves. Petroleum jelly may also break down latex. Utility gloves may be used when handling contaminated instruments and cleaning of the treatment area or sterilization room.

Fluid-resistant gowns, laboratory coats, or uniforms should be worn when clothing is likely to be soiled with blood or other bodily fluids. Reusable protective clothing should be washed separately from other clothes, using a normal laundry cycle. Protective clothing should be changed daily or as soon as visibly soiled. They should be removed before personnel leave areas of the dental office used for laboratory or patient-care activities.

Masks and protective eyewear, or chin-length plastic face shields should be worn when splashing or spattering of blood or other body fluids is likely. A mask should be changed between patients or during patient treatment if it becomes wet or moist. A face shield or protective eyewear should be washed with appropriate cleaning agents when visibly soiled.

Careful handling and disposal of sharps

Sharp disposable items, such as needles, saliva ejectors, rubber prophy cups and scalpels that cannot be sterilized and are contaminated with blood or other body fluids need to be discarded in puncture resistant containers. Special delivery companies pick up the containers once they are full and replace them with empty containers.

Careful handling and cleaning of contaminated equipment

Dental instruments must be cleaned and sterilized after each use. Recommended sterilization methods include autoclaving or using a dry heat oven or chemiclave—a unit that cleans with the use of chemicals. Sterilization equipment is commonly found in a special area of the building away from the treatment areas.

Cleaning and disinfecting of all surfaces such as lights, drawer handles, and countertops is accomplished by a chemical solution formulated to kill infectious **bacteria**, spores, and **viruses** after each patient is seen. Medical facilities follow specific heat sterilization procedures outlined by the CDC. Plastic barriers cover items that are not easily disinfected by chemical spray, such as light handles, chair control buttons, and instrument trays. Many offices and hospitals have seamless floors with linoleum or a laminate surface so that spills can be contained and cleaned quickly.

Non-critical items that cannot be heat-sterilized are sterilized by immersion in a chemical bath formulated to kill infectious bacteria and viruses.

Standard precautions are intended to supplement rather than replace recommendations for such routine infection control as hand washing.

Changes since 2007

In 2007, the CDC published a report intended to update standard precautions in light of changes in the health care system as well as the appearance of new disease organisms. These changes include:

- A growing trend away from hospital admission in favor of ambulatory surgery centers, outpatient clinics, home health care, and other non-hospital settings, requiring extension of infection control measures to these locations.
- The emergence of bioterrorism as a growing threat, as evidenced by the anthrax attacks following 9/11.
- The emergence of new disease organisms (e.g., SARS, the hemorrhagic fevers, prion diseases) and the evolution of multidrug-resistant organisms (MDROs).

- Increasing recognition of the importance of a "safety culture" in hospitals and other health care settings to maintain adherence to standard precautions.

Specific changes in standard precautions resulting from these new threats include:

- Introduction of precautions regarding respiratory hygiene, also called cough etiquette. These precautions were developed in response to the SARS epidemic of 2002–2003.
- Identification of anthrax, smallpox, plague, tularemia, viral hemorrhagic fevers, and botulism as Category A (high priority) agents of bioterrorism and the corresponding need for health care facilities to draw up plans for responding to and managing a bioterrorist attack.
- Special precautions for laboratory workers and pathologists handling tissue samples from patients diagnosed with Creutzfeldt-Jakob disease. Surgical instruments used in obtaining such samples require special reprocessing after use.

Other recent changes in standard precautions include extending instruction and training in their application to workers outside mainstream human health care. These workers include veterinarians and veterinary technicians in small-animal hospitals; first responders (police officers, firefighters, park rangers, search and rescue personnel), who may be exposed to bloodborne infections in the course of assisting injured persons; and **alternative medicine** practitioners, who may be less aware of the risks of infection in their various practices.

Preparation

Proper planning and management of supplies needed for universal precautions are essential in reducing the occupational risk of infectious diseases. Such measures should include, but are not limited to:

- risk assessment
- setting of standards and protocols
- risk reduction
- postexposure measures
- first aid

Complications

Complications include the possible increase of medical and dental fees to the patient to offset costs associated with the equipment, disinfectants, and sterilization procedures needed for universal precautions.

KEY TERMS

Anaphylaxis—A rapid, severe, and potentially life-threatening allergic reaction characterized by itching, throat swelling, and a drop in blood pressure. The most common causes are bee and wasp stings, certain foods, and certain medications.

Autoclave—A sterilization unit that uses steam under pressure.

Chemiclave—A sterilization unit that uses chemicals under pressure.

Dry heat oven—A sterilization unit that uses dry heat.

Latex—A milky fluid obtained from the rubber tree that is used to make natural rubber surgical gloves, condoms, dental dams, diaphragms, and other medical or surgical devices.

Pathogen—Any microorganism that can cause disease in another living organism. Pathogens include bacteria, viruses, fungi, prions, and parasitic worms.

Sharps—Needles and such cutting instruments as curettes and scalpel blades.

Stigma (plural, stigmata)—Any personal attribute that causes a person to be socially shamed, avoided, discredited, or treated in a discriminatory fashion. Such bloodborne infections as HIV are a common cause of stigma.

Surfactant—Any compound that lowers the surface tension of a liquid. Surfactants include detergents, wetting agents, and foaming agents.

Another potential complication is latex allergy, which may take the form of contact dermatitis or (rarely) a full-blown anaphylactic reaction. Health care workers or patients who are allergic to latex rubber will need to avoid surgical gloves, dental dams, or other medical devices that contain latex. Items made of neoprene or elastane are usually safe for persons who are allergic to latex. Between 0.8% and 8% of the general population is thought to be allergic to latex; the rate among health care workers is thought to range from 4% to 17%. Patients who know they are allergic to latex should notify their physician and dentist. Detailed information about the symptoms of latex allergy and latex-alternative products is available on the American Dental Association and American Latex Allergy Association websites listed below.

QUESTIONS TO ASK YOUR DOCTOR

- What measures do you take to adhere to standard precautions in your office?
- Where can I learn more about standard precautions?
- How can I tell whether I am allergic to latex?
- Do you think outpatient clinics and free-standing ambulatory surgery centers are more likely to be careless about standard precautions than acute care hospitals?

Results

Universal precautions are designed to reduce the transmission of infectious diseases among patients, health care workers, and first responders.

Health care team roles

Standard precautions require all medical and dental staff personnel involved in patient care to use appropriate personal protective equipment. Guidelines for health care settings for discarding of waste material are under a separate code by individual state agencies and governmental departments.

The environment in which health care is provided is greatly affected by adhering to standard precautions, both for the patient and care providers. Measures that promote a safe work environment include:

- education of employees about occupational risks and methods of prevention of HIV and other infectious diseases
- provision of protective equipment
- provision of appropriate disinfectants to clean up spills of blood or other body fluids
- easy accessibility of puncture-resistant sharps containers
- maintaining appropriate staffing levels
- measures that reduce and prevent stress, isolation, and burnout
- controlling shift lengths
- providing post-exposure counseling, treatment, and follow-up

The U.S. Department of Labor's Occupational Safety and Health Administration (OSHA) requires employers in the medical and dental fields to make hepatitis B virus (HBV) vaccines available without cost to employees who may be exposed to blood or other infectious materials. In addition, the CDC recommends that all workers be vaccinated against HBV as well as **influenza**, measles, mumps, rubella, and tetanus, both for the protection of personnel and patients.

Resources

BOOKS

Damani, N.N. *Manual of Infection Prevention and Control*, 3rd ed. New York: Oxford University Press, 2012.

Fleming, Diane O., and Debra L. Hunt, eds. *Biological Safety: Principles and Practices*, 4th ed. Washington, DC: ASM Press, 2006.

Pugliese, Gina, ed. *Universal Precautions: Policies, Procedures, and Resources*. Chicago, IL: American Hospital Publishing, 1991.

Siegel, Jane D., et al. *2007 Guideline for Isolation Precautions: Preventing Transmission of Infectious Agents in Health-care Settings*. Atlanta, GA: Centers for Disease Control and Prevention, 2007. Available for free download in PDF format at http://www.cdc.gov/hicpac/pdf/isolation/Isolation2007.pdf.

PERIODICALS

Centers for Disease Control and Prevention (CDC). "Perspectives in Disease Prevention and Health Promotion Update: Universal Precautions for Prevention of Transmission of Human Immunodeficiency Virus, Hepatitis B Virus, and Other Bloodborne Pathogens in Health-Care Settings." *Morbidity and Mortality Weekly Report* 37 (June 24, 1988): 377–388.

Centers for Disease Control and Prevention (CDC). "Recommendations for Preventing Transmission of Human Immunodeficiency Virus and Hepatitis B Virus to Patients During Exposure-Prone Invasive Procedures." *Morbidity and Mortality Weekly Report* 40 (July 12, 1991): 1–7.

Cuaron, J.J., et al. "Introduction to Radiation Safety and Monitoring." *Journal of the American College of Radiology* 8 (April 2011): 259–264.

Deuffic-Burban, S., et al. "Blood-borne Viruses in Health Care Workers: Prevention and Management." *Journal of Clinical Virology* 52 (September 2011): 4–10.

Flanagan, E., et al. "Infection Prevention in Alternative Health Care Settings." *Infectious Disease Clinics of North America* 25 (March 2011): 271–283.

KuKanich, K.S., et al. "Surveillance of Bacterial Contamination in Small Animal Veterinary Hospitals with Special Focus on Antimicrobial Resistance and Virulence Traits of Enterococci." *Journal of the American Veterinary Medical Association* 240 (February 15, 2012): 437–445.

Weber, D.J., et al. "Lessons Learned: Protection of Healthcare Workers from Infectious Disease Risks." *Critical Care Medicine* 38 (August 2010): Suppl. 8: S306–S314.

WEBSITES

American Dental Association (ADA). Oral Health Topics: Allergy to Latex Rubber. http://www.ada.org/2523.aspx?currentTab=2 (accessed April 20, 2012).

American Dental Association (ADA). Oral Health Topics: Infection Control. http://www.ada.org/2697.aspx (accessed April 20, 2012).

Centers for Disease Control and Prevention (CDC). "Guidelines for Infection Control in Dental Health-Care Settings—2003." http://www.ada.org/sections/professionalResources/pdfs/guidelines_cdc_infection.pd (accessed April 20, 2012).

Centers for Disease Control and Prevention (CDC), National Institute of Occupational Safety and Health (NIOSH). Bloodborne Infectious Diseases Home Page. http://www.cdc.gov/niosh/topics/bbp/ (accessed April 20, 2012).

Occupational Safety and Health Administration (OSHA). Bloodborne Pathogens and Needlestick Prevention Home Page. http://www.osha.gov/SLTC/bloodbornepathogens/index.html (accessed April 20, 2012).

ORGANIZATIONS

American Dental Association (ADA), 211 East Chicago Ave., Chicago, IL United States 60611-2678, (312) 440-2500, http://www.ada.org/

American Latex Allergy Association (ALAA), P.O. Box 198, Slinger, WI United States 53086, (262) 677-9707, (888) 972-5378, alert@latexallergyresources.org, http://www.latexallergyresources.org/

Centers for Disease Control and Prevention (CDC), 1600 Clifton Road, Atlanta, GA United States 30333, (800) CDC-INFO (232-4636), cdcinfo@cdc.gov, www.cdc.gov

Occupational Safety and Health Administration (OSHA), 200 Constitution Ave., NW, Washington, DC United States 20212, (800) 321-OSHA (6742), http://www.osha.gov/index.html

Cindy F. Ovard, RDA
Rebecca J. Frey, PhD

Staphylococcal infections

Definition

Staphylococcus is the name of a genus of **bacteria** responsible for a number of serious illnesses, although most species are harmless to humans. Staphylococci are widespread in all parts of the world; they are commonly found in the soil as well as on the bodies of humans and domestic animals. Staphylococci can live on or in humans without necessarily causing harm. They can, however, cause disease in humans and other animals either by direct destruction of tissue or by releasing toxins into the digestive tract or bloodstream. These

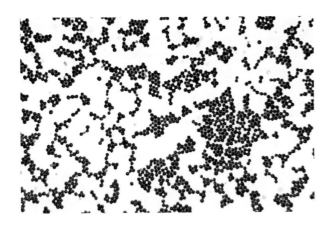

(*Staphylococcus aureus, a bacterium that causes, among other conditions, boils, wound supperation, and food poisoning, photograph. Eye of Science / Photo Researchers, Inc.*)

bacteria look like clumps or clusters of grapes under a **microscope**; in fact, their name derives from a Greek word that means "a bunch of grapes."

Staphylococcal (staph) infections are communicable diseases caused by staphylococci and generally characterized by the formation of abscesses. Staphylococci are the leading cause of primary infections originating in hospitals (nosocomial infections) in the United States. They are also a common cause of food **poisoning**.

Description

There are three staphylococcal species that commonly cause infections: *Staphylococcus aureus*, *S. epidermidis*, and *S. saprophyticus*. Staphylococci have been classified since the early twentieth century as among the deadliest of disease-causing bacteria.

Demographics

Staphylococci are commonplace organisms, found on the scalp, skin (particularly the armpits and genital areas), or outer nasal passages of humans around the world. Biologists refer to the formation of groups or clumps of bacteria on a human or animal as colonization. Staph is found in 80 percent of the general population from time to time and 20 to 30 percent of the population on an ongoing basis. People who harbor staphylococci most of the time are called staph carriers.

An estimated 2 billion people are colonized by some form of *S. aureus*; of these persons, as many as 53 million, or 2.7 percent of carriers, are thought to carry **MRSA**, the drug-resistant form of *S. aureus*. It is possible for a person to carry staphylococci for many years without becoming sick; in addition, such domestic animals as cats, dogs, chickens, and horses can carry MRSA strains as well as less virulent staphylococci.

As far as is known as of 2012, people of either sex, any age group, or any race are equally likely to carry staphylococci. Newborns may be colonized by staphylococci from the mother during **childbirth**. Some groups, however, are more susceptible than others to staph infections, including diabetics, African Americans, gay men who practice anal intercourse, and very young children as well as elderly adults and persons with artificial joints or **heart** valves.

Types of staph infections

Staph infections produce pus-filled pockets (abscesses) located just beneath the surface of the skin or deep within the body. Risk of **infection** is greatest among the very young and the very old.

A localized staph infection is confined to a ring of dead and dying white **blood** cells and bacteria. The skin above it feels warm to the touch. Most of these abscesses eventually burst, and pus that leaks onto the skin can cause new infections.

Staphylococcal food poisoning is the result of toxins secreted by the organisms rather than by tissue damage caused by the bacteria themselves. The foods most likely to be contaminated are those made by hand and that require little or no cooking, such as sandwiches, cold cuts, cold salads, and certain types of cream-filled pastry. The symptoms of staphylococcal food poisoning include nausea, **vomiting**, and **diarrhea**, beginning between one and six hours after eating the contaminated food. Most people with staphylococcal food poisoning feel better in one to three days.

A small fraction of localized staph infections enter the bloodstream and spread through the body. In children, these systemic (affecting the whole body) or disseminated infections frequently affect the ends of the long bones of the arms or legs, causing a **bone** infection called osteomyelitis. When adults develop invasive staph infections, bacteria are most apt to cause abscesses of the **brain**, heart, **kidneys**, **liver**, **lungs**, or spleen.

Infections caused by *Staphylococcus aureus*

Named for the golden color of the bacteria grown under laboratory conditions, *S. aureus* is a hardy gram-positive organism that can survive in extreme temperatures or other inhospitable circumstances. About 70 to 90 percent of the population carry this strain of staph in the nostrils at some time. Although present on the skin of only 5 to 20 percent of healthy people, as many as 40 percent carry it elsewhere, such as in the throat, vagina,

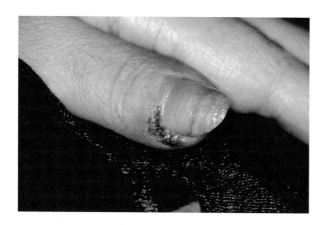

(Staphylococcal infections, photograph by LeBeau. Custom Medical Stock Photo. Reproduced by permission.)

or rectum, for varying periods of time, from hours to years, without developing symptoms or becoming ill.

S. aureus flourishes in hospitals, where it infects health care personnel and patients who have had surgery; who have acute dermatitis, insulin-dependent diabetes, or dialysis-dependent kidney disease; or who receive frequent allergy-desensitization injections. Staph bacteria can also contaminate bedclothes, catheters, and other objects.

S. aureus causes a variety of infections. **Boils**, impetigo, and inflammation of the skin surrounding a hair shaft (folliculitis) are the most common. Toxic **shock** (TSS) and scalded skin syndrome (SSS) are among the most serious. *S. aureus* is responsible for 80% of cases of septic arthritis in adults and children over the age of 2.

TOXIC SHOCK SYNDROME. Toxic shock syndrome (TSS) is a life-threatening infection characterized by the sudden onset of severe **headache**, **sore throat**, **fever** as high as 105°F, and a sunburn-like **rash** on the palms of the hands and soles of the feet that spreads to the face and the rest of the body. Symptoms of TSS also include **dehydration** and watery diarrhea.

Inadequate blood flow to vital organs and peripheral parts of the body (shock) and loss of consciousness occur within the first 48 hours. Between the third and seventh day of illness, skin peels from the palms of the hands, soles of the feet, and other parts of the body. Kidney, liver, and muscle damage often occur.

SCALDED SKIN SYNDROME. Rare in adults and most common in newborns and other children under the age of five, scalded skin syndrome begins with a localized skin infection. A mild fever and/or an increase in the number of infection-fighting white blood cells may occur.

A bright red rash spreads from the face to other parts of the body and eventually forms scales. Large, soft blisters develop at the site of infection and elsewhere. When they burst, they expose inflamed skin that looks as if it had been burned.

Although such cases are fortunately rare, it is possible for a person to have toxic shock syndrome and scalded skin syndrome at the same time.

METHICILLIN-RESISTANT AND VANCOMYCIN-RESISTANT *S. AUREUS* (MRSA AND VRSA) INFECTIONS. MRSA refers to methicillin-resistant *Staphylococcus aureus*, a strain of the bacterium that is responsible for severe and potentially fatal skin and soft-tissue infections. There are two major subgroups of MRSA, named for the locations where people can get infected: community-acquired MRSA (CA-MRSA) and hospital-acquired (or health care-acquired) MRSA (HA-MRSA).

MRSA was first identified as a particular strain of *S. aureus* in 1961. Methicillin, an antibiotic similar to penicillin, was introduced in 1959 to treat penicillin-resistant strains of *S. aureus*, but only two years later, the first strains of MRSA were reported in the United Kingdom. MRSA infections were relatively uncommon until the 1990s, however, when their rate shot upward, particularly in hospitals.

Community-acquired MRSA, or CA-MRSA, looks like a boil or skin infection in about 75 percent of cases and is easily mistaken for a spider bite. The affected area is red, swollen, and may be oozing pus. CA-MRSA is much more virulent than hospital-acquired MRSA, however, and can lead to **sepsis** (generalized infection of the entire body), bacteremia (infection of the bloodstream), or **pneumonia**. Hospital-acquired MRSA, or HA-MRSA, is most commonly found in patients in health care settings, particularly those in dialysis centers, **nursing homes**, or other hospital settings. Patients with HA-MRSA are more likely to develop pneumonia, infected joints, or urinary tract infections than skin infections. According to the Centers for Disease Control and Prevention (CDC), the rates of CA-MRSA in the United States are increasing as of 2012 while the rates of HA-MRSA have declined since 2008.

MRSA infections cannot be treated with the **antibiotics** that doctors can use for most staph infections. Newer drugs like tigecycline and the streptogramins must be used instead. There are about 94,000 serious MRSA infections in the United States each year as of 2009, and 19,000 deaths—more than are caused by **AIDS**.

The CDC has updated information regarding the development of *S. aureus* strains that are partially or highly resistant to vancomycin, a newer antibiotic often used to treat MRSA infections. These resistant bacteria were first described in Japan in 1996; the first case in the United States was reported in 2002. Strains that are partially resistant to vancomycin are classified as vancomycin-intermediate *S. aureus*, or VISA, and strains that are highly resistant are known as vancomycin-resistant *S. aureus* or VRSA.

OTHER *S. AUREUS* INFECTIONS. *S. aureus* can also cause:

- bacteria in the bloodstream (bacteremia)
- pockets of infection and pus under the skin (carbuncles)
- tissue inflammation that spreads below the skin, causing pain and swelling (cellulitis)
- inflammation of the valves and walls of the heart (endocarditis)
- inflammation of tissue that enclosed and protects the spinal cord and brain (meningitis)
- inflammation of bone and bone marrow (osteomyelitis)
- pneumonia
- infection of the spaces within joints (septic arthritis)

Other species of staphylococci

S. EPIDERMIDIS. Capable of clinging to tubing (as in that used for intravenous feeding, prosthetic devices, and other non-living surfaces, *S. epidermidis* is the organism that most often contaminates devices that provide direct access to the bloodstream.

The primary cause of bacteremia in hospital patients, this strain of staph is most likely to infect **cancer** patients, whose immune systems have been compromised, and high-risk newborns receiving intravenous supplements.

S. epidermidis also accounts for two of every five cases of prosthetic valve **endocarditis**. Prosthetic valve endocarditis is a complication of the implantation of an artificial valve in the heart. Although contamination usually occurs during surgery, symptoms of infection may not become evident until a year after the operation. More than half of the patients who develop prosthetic valve endocarditis die.

S. SAPROPHYTICUS. Existing within and around the tube-like structure that carries urine from the bladder (urethra) of about 5 percent of healthy males and females, *S. saprophyticus* is the second most common cause of unobstructed urinary tract infections (UTIs) in sexually active young women. This strain of staph is responsible for 10 to 20 percent of infections affecting healthy outpatients.

Risk factors

Although staphylococci are usually harmless, when injury or a break in the skin enables the organisms to invade the body and overcome the body's natural defenses, consequences can range from minor discomfort to death. Infection is most apt to occur in:

- newborns
- women who are breastfeeding
- individuals whose immune systems have been undermined by radiation treatments, chemotherapy, or medication
- intravenous drug users
- men who have sex with men
- patients who require feeding tubes, catheter placement, or kidney dialysis
- those with surgical incisions, skin disorders, severe burns, or serious illness like cancer, diabetes, and lung disease

Some people are at increased risk of toxic shock syndrome:

- Women who are menstruating
- Women who use diaphragms or other barrier methods of birth control
- People who are having nasal surgery
- People with diabetes
- People with a weakened immune system
- People who have developed a staphylococcal infection following surgery

Some people are at increased risk of MRSA infections:

- Health care workers in inpatient facilities
- Diabetics
- Athletes, trainers, and others who frequently use gyms or changing rooms
- Prison inmates
- College students living in dormitories
- Military recruits in basic training and military personnel stationed outside the United States
- People who frequently swim or surf in coastal waters contaminated by MRSA (Florida and the West Coast as of 2012)

Causes and symptoms

Staphylococci can be spread through the air, but infection is almost always the result of direct contact with open sores or body fluids contaminated by these organisms. Staph bacteria often enter the body through inflamed hair follicles or oil glands. They may also penetrate skin damaged by **burns**, cuts and scrapes, infection, insect bites, or **wounds**; this is a common way for staph infections to spread in athletic facilities, dormitories, military barracks, prisons, and other situations in which large groups of people live or work together.

Multiplying beneath the skin, bacteria infect and destroy tissue in the area where they entered the body. Staph infection of the blood (staphylococcal bacteremia) develops when bacteria from a local infection infiltrate the lymph glands and bloodstream. These infections, which can usually be traced to contaminated catheters or intravenous devices, usually cause persistent high fever. They may cause shock. They also can cause death within a short time.

Warning signs

Common early symptoms of staph infection include:

- pain or swelling around a cut, or an area of skin that has been scraped
- boils or other skin abscesses
- blistering, peeling, or scaling of the skin; this is most common in infants and young children
- enlarged lymph nodes in the neck, armpits, or groin

A family physician should be notified whenever:

- Lymph nodes in the neck, armpits, or groin become swollen or tender.
- An area of skin that has been cut or scraped becomes painful or swollen, feels hot, or produces pus. These symptoms may mean the infection has spread to the bloodstream.
- A boil or carbuncle appears on any part of the face or spine. Staph infections affecting these areas can spread to the brain or spinal cord.
- A boil becomes very sore. Usually a sign that infection has spread, this condition may be accompanied by fever, chills, and red streaks radiating from the site of the original infection.
- Boils that develop repeatedly. This type of recurrent infection could be a symptom of diabetes.
- A joint is painful to the touch and appears swollen.
- Several different members of a family have developed boils or rashes all at the same time.

Diagnosis

The diagnosis of a staphylococcal infection is based on a combination of the patient's medical history, symptoms, an examination of the skin or other affected body parts, and a **blood culture** that is positive for a specific staphylococcus species.

Examination

Depending on the location of the infection, the doctor may notice the presence of fever, boils or rashes on the skin, redness or swelling of the skin, or swollen and tender joints. Patients with toxic shock syndrome may have severe headaches or changes in mental status.

Tests

Samples for a staph culture may be obtained from a skin injury, from drawing a blood sample, from a urine sample, or by having the patient **cough** up sputum (matter from the lungs) if pneumonia is suspected. Although a standard blood culture for a staph infection takes a day or two to yield results, rapid diagnostic methods using amplification and probe-based molecular techniques provide results in hours, thus allowing treatment to be started earlier and improving the patient's chances of recovery. Although staph can be identified in stool samples or vomit from a patient with food poisoning, doctors do not usually test for the organism unless there is an outbreak involving several people. The diagnosis of staphylococcal food poisoning is usually made on the basis of the patient's symptoms.

Treatment

Traditional

Treatment of a staph infection depends on its specific type and location. In most cases the doctor will start antibiotic therapy when a staphylococcal infection is suspected as soon as the sample of tissue, blood, sputum, or urine has been sent to the laboratory. Specific types of infections are treated as follows:

- Skin infections: The doctor will usually make an incision to drain the pus and other infected fluid out of the wound. In some cases an antibiotic cream or lotion may be applied after the wound has been cleansed, or the patient may be given oral or intravenous antibiotics.
- Staphylococcal pneumonia following influenza is usually treated with intravenous antibiotics following hospitalization. People who are seriously ill may need to be given supplemental oxygen in an intensive care unit (ICU).
- If the infection is located in a joint with a prosthetic appliance, the artificial joint must be removed and the patient given a four- to six-week course of antibiotics. Infected joints without a prosthetic appliance are usually drained of fluid and the patient is given a

four-week course of antibiotic therapy to clear the infection.

- Infected artificial heart valves may or may not require removal. Endocarditis does, however, require long-term antibiotic therapy, particularly if the patient is over 55.

- Staphylococcal eye infections require emergency treatment. An ophthalmologist (specialist in eye disorders) usually injects antibiotics into the tissues around the eye as well as giving antibiotics by mouth or intravenously. In extreme cases the entire eye may need to be removed.

Staphylococcal food poisoning is treated with bed rest, plenty of fluids, and antinausea drugs prescribed by the doctor. Antibiotics cannot be used to treat food poisoning caused by staphylococci because the toxins that cause the nausea and vomiting are not affected by these drugs. Severely ill patients may need to be hospitalized and given intravenous fluids.

Drugs

Antibiotics are the traditional first-line therapy for all bacterial infections; they help to prevent infected persons from spreading the disease further as well as relieving symptoms. It is, however, important to make sure that an infection is caused by bacteria rather than by **viruses**, because antibiotics are useless against viral infections. Severe or recurrent staphylococcal infections may require a 7–10-day course of treatment with penicillin or other oral antibiotics. The location of the infection and the identity of the causal bacteria determine which of several effective medications should be prescribed. The antibiotics most commonly used as of 2012 are nafcillin (Unipen), cefazolin (Kefzol), vancomycin (Vancoled), dicloxacillin (Dynapen), and clindamycin (Cleocin).

To eradicate colonies of staph bacteria on the skin, the doctor may prescribe a topical antibiotic like mupirocin (Bactroban) or wash the area with chlorhexidine gluconate (Hibiclens or Perichlor). In case of a more serious infection, antibiotics may be administered intravenously for as long as six weeks. Intravenous antibiotics are also used to treat staph infections around the eyes or on other parts of the face. MRSA infections are treated with tigecycline (Tygacil), teicoplanin (Targocid), or a combination of rifampin plus doxycycline for 7 days. As of 2012, the CDC and the Food and Drug Administration (FDA) recommend treating VISA and VRSA infections with ceftobiprole (Zeftera), a fifth-generation cephalosporin antibiotic; daptomycin (Cubicin); tigecycline; linezolid (Zyvox); or intravenous quinupristin/dalfopristin (Synercid), a combination of two streptogramin antibiotics.

Alternative

Alternative therapies for staph infection are meant to strengthen the **immune system** and prevent recurrences. Among the therapies believed to be helpful for the person with a staph infection are **yoga** (to stimulate the immune system and promote **relaxation**), **acupuncture** (to draw heat away from the infection), and herbal remedies. Herbs that may help the body overcome, or withstand, staph infection include:

- Garlic (*Allium sativum*). This herb is believed to have anitbacterial properties. Herbalists recommend consuming three garlic cloves or three garlic oil capsules a day, starting when symptoms of infection first appear.

- Cleavers (*Galium aparine*). This anti-inflammatory herb is believed to support the lymphatic system. It may be taken internally to help heal staph abscesses and reduce swelling of the lymph nodes. A cleavers compress can also be applied directly to a skin infection.

- Goldenseal (*Hydrastis canadensis*). Another herb believed to fight infection and reduce imflammation, goldenseal may be taken internally when symptoms of infection first appear. Skin infections can be treated by making a paste of water and powdered goldenseal root and applying it directly to the affected area. The preparation should be covered with a clean bandage and left in place overnight.

- Echinacea (*Echinacea* spp.). Taken internally, this herb is believed to have antibiotic properties and is also thought to strengthen the immune system.

- Thyme (*Thymus vulgaris*), lavender (*Lavandula officinalis*), or bergamot (*Citrus bergamot*) oils. These oils are believed to have antibacterial properties and may help to prevent the scarring that may result from skin infections. A few drops of these oils are added to water and then a compress soaked in the water is applied to the affected area.

- Tea tree oil (*Melaleuca* spp.). Another infection-fighting herb, this oil can be applied directly to a boil or other skin infection.

Prognosis

Most healthy people who develop staph infections recover fully within a short time. Others develop repeated or resistant infections. Some become seriously ill, requiring long-term therapy or emergency care. A small percentage die. Mortality due to staphylococcal infections varies widely, however. Untreated bacteremia caused by *S. aureus* carries a mortality rate above 80 percent as of 2012. The mortality rate of

KEY TERMS

Abscess—A cavity containing pus surrounded by inflamed tissue.

Antibiotic—A class of drug that fights bacterial infections.

Bacteremia—The presence of bacteria and their effects in the blood stream.

Carrier—A person (or other organism) who has contracted an infectious disease agent and can transmit it to others without having symptoms of the disease.

Colonization—The process by which bacteria form colonies in or on the bodies of humans and other animals.

Endocarditis—Inflammation of the lining of the heart, and/or the heart valves, caused by infection.

Gram-positive—Referring to any bacterium that appears dark blue or purple following application of the Gram staining technique, first used in 1884.

Impetigo—A superficial bacterial skin infection common among schoolchildren, characterized by honey-colored scabs that ooze pus.

Nosocomial infections—Infections acquired by a patient while in the hospital.

Osteomyelitis—Infection of the bone or bone marrow.

Septic arthritis—The invasion of a joint space by bacteria or other infectious organisms, producing inflammation and joint pain.

Shock—A medical emergency in which the body's tissues do not receive enough blood due to problems with the circulatory system.

Sputum—Matter from the lungs or throat that is brought up by coughing.

Strain—A genetic variant or subtype of a bacterium.

Topical—Referring to a medication or antiseptic applied to the surface of the body (skin or mucous membranes).

staphylococcal toxic shock syndrome is much lower, about 3 to 5 percent.

Endocarditis and pneumonia caused by antibiotic-resistant staphylococci have mortality rates around 11 percent in patients without other diseases or disorders, but the rate may be as high as 44 percent in patients with diabetes, HIV infection, or other disorders that weaken the immune system. Elderly people with staphylococcal pneumonia have a worse prognosis than younger adults. In patients over the age of 70, community-acquired staph infections are associated with a mortality rate of 21 percent in the year following diagnosis.

Most patients with staphylococcal food poisoning or staphylococcal urinary tract infections recover completely; fatalities are rare except in the elderly or people with AIDS.

Health care team roles

Physicians supervise the treatment of staph infections in a hospital setting. Generally, laboratory technicians perform blood work, and **radiology** technicians perform x rays when indicated. Nurses provide bedside management and patient-family education. Pharmacists store and dispense the antibiotics used to treat staph infections; they also play an important role in educating the public about the proper use of antibiotics.

Prevention

Health care providers and patients should always wash their hands thoroughly with warm water and soap after treating a staph infection or touching an open wound or the pus it produces. Pus that oozes onto the skin from the site of an infection should be removed immediately. This affected area should then be cleansed with antiseptic or with antibacterial soap. Patients' hospital gowns and bed linins should also be properly laundered in hot water or carefully disposed of.

To prevent infection from spreading from one part of the body to another, it is important to shower rather than bathe during the healing process. Because staph infection is easily transmitted from one member of a household to others, towels, washcloths, and bed linens used by someone with a staph infection should not be used by anyone else. They should be changed daily until symptoms disappear, and laundered separately in hot water with bleach.

Children should frequently be reminded not to share:

- brushes, combs, or hair accessories
- caps
- clothing
- sleeping bags
- sports equipment
- other personal items

A diet rich in green, yellow, and orange vegetables can bolster natural immunity. A doctor or nutritionist may recommend **vitamins** or mineral supplements to

QUESTIONS TO ASK YOUR DOCTOR

- What species or strain of staph is causing the infection?

- How serious is it? Will the disease require surgery?

- Is there likely to be a problem with antibiotic resistance?

- What antibiotics will you prescribe? What are their possible side effects?

- What is the normal course of this illness? When can I expect to feel better?

- Can I transmit this infection to others?

- What complications might occur from this infection? Can I do anything to prevent them?

compensate for specific dietary deficiencies. Drinking eight to 10 glasses of water a day can help flush disease-causing organisms from the body.

Because some strains of staphylococci are known to contaminate artificial limbs, prosthetic devices implanted within the body, and tubes used to administer medication or drain fluids from the body, catheters and other devices should be removed on a regular basis, if possible, and examined for microscopic signs of staph. Symptoms may not become evident until many months after contamination has occurred, so this practice should be followed even with patients who show no sign of infection.

Although glycerol monolaurate (GML) as a protective coating for tampons has been shown to reduce *S. aureus* colonization, the Centers for Disease Control and Prevention (CDC) still recommends the following precautions to lower the risk of toxic shock syndrome:

• Women of childbearing age should use low-absorbency tampons during their menstrual periods, change them every 4 to 8 hours, or use sanitary napkins rather than tampons. Women who have had TSS or any serious staph or strep infection should not use tampons at all.

• People who have had nasal surgery should watch carefully for signs of infection, particularly if the nose has been packed with gauze or surgical dressings.

• Skin infections should be treated promptly.

• People who have had abdominal surgery or tooth extraction, or women who have recently given birth, should also be monitored for signs of infection.

Resources

BOOKS

Crossley, Kent B. *Staphylococci in Human Disease*, 2nd ed. Hoboken, NJ: Wiley-Blackwell, 2010.

Fischetti, Vincent A., ed. *Gram-positive Pathogens*, 2nd ed. Washington, DC: ASM Press, 2006.

Kolendi, Charles L., ed. *Methicillin-resistant Staphylococcus aureus (MRSA): Etiology, At-risk Populations and Treatment*. Hauppauge, NY: Nova Science Publishers, 2010.

PERIODICALS

Harrop, J.S., et al. "Contributing Factors to Surgical Site Infections." *Journal of the American Academy of Orthopaedic Surgeons* 20 (February 2012): 94–101.

Hubiche, T., et al. "Mild Staphylococcal Scalded Skin Syndrome: An Underdiagnosed Clinical Disorder." *British Journal of Dermatology* 166 (January 2012): 213–215.

Loomba, P.S., et al. "Methicillin and Vancomycin Resistant *S. aureus* in Hospitalized Patients." *Journal of Global Infectious Diseases* 2 (September 2010): 275–283.

Liu, Catherine, et al. "Clinical Practice Guidelines by the Infectious Diseases Society of America for the Treatment of Methicillin-Resistant *Staphylococcus Aureus* Infections in Adults and Children." *Clinical Infectious Diseases* 52 (February 2011): 1–38. Full text available at http://cid. oxfordjournals.org/content/early/2011/01/04/cid.ciq146. full.pdf+html.

Morrison-Rodriguez, S.M., et al. "Community-associated Methicillin-resistant *Staphylococcus aureus* Infections at an Army Training Installation." *Epidemiology and Infection* 138 (May 2010): 721–729.

Nailor, M.D., and J.D. Sobel. "Antibiotics for Gram-positive Bacterial Infection: Vancomycin, Teicoplanin, Quinupristin/dalfopristin, Oxazolidinones, Daptomycin, Telavancin, and Ceftaroline." *Medical Clinics of North America* 95 (July 2011): 723–742.

Rackham, D.M., et al. "Community-associated Methicillin-resistant *Staphylococcus aureus* Nasal Carriage in a College Student Athlete Population." *Clinical Journal of Sport Medicine* 20 (May 2010): 185–188.

Vostral, S.L. "Rely and Toxic Shock Syndrome: A Technological Health Crisis." *Yale Journal of Biology and Medicine* 84 (December 2011): 447–459.

Wilcox, M.H. "MRSA: New Treatments on the Horizon: Current Status." *Injury* 42 (December 2011): Suppl. 5: S42–S44.

WEBSITES

Centers for Disease Control and Prevention (CDC). Methicillin-resistant *Staphylococcus aureus* (MRSA) Infection in Healthcare Settings Home Page. http://www.cdc.gov/HAI/organisms/mrsa-infection.html (accessed April 24, 2012).

Centers for Disease Control and Prevention (CDC). Vancomycin-Intermediate/Resistant *Staphylococcus* (VISA/VRSA) in Healthcare Settings Home Page. http://www.cdc.gov/HAI/organisms/visa_vrsa/visa_vrsa.html (accessed April 24, 2012).

Mayo Clinic. "MRSA Infection." http://www.mayoclinic.com/health/mrsa/DS00735 (accessed April 24, 2012).

Medscape. "Staphylococcal Infections." http://emedicine. medscape.com/article/228816-overview (accessed April 24, 2012).

Merck Manual for Health Care Professionals. "Gram-Positive Cocci: Staphylococcal Infections." http://www.merck-manuals.com/professional/infectious_diseases/gram-positive_cocci/staphylococcal_infections.html (accessed April 24, 2012).

National Institute of Allergy and Infectious Diseases (NIAMS). Methicillin-Resistant *Staphylococcus aureus* Home Page. http://www.niaid.nih.gov/topics/antimicrobialResistance/Examples/mrsa/Pages/default.aspx (accessed April 24, 2012).

ORGANIZATIONS

Centers for Disease Control and Prevention (CDC), 1600 Clifton Road, Atlanta, GA 30333, (800) CDC-INFO (232-4636), cdcinfo@cdc.gov, www.cdc.gov

Food and Drug Administration (FDA), 10903 New Hampshire Avenue, Silver Spring, MD 20993, (888) INFO-FDA (463-6332), http://www.fda.gov/default.htm

Infectious Diseases Society of America (IDSA), 1300 Wilson Blvd, Suite 300, Arlington, VA 22209, (703) 299-0200, Fax: (703) 299-0204, http://www.idsociety.org/Contact_Us.aspx, http://www.idsociety.org/Index.aspx

National Institute of Allergy and Infectious Diseases (NIAID), 6610 Rockledge Drive, MSC 6612, Bethesda, MD 20892-6612, (301) 496-5717, Fax: (301) 402-3573, (866) 284-4107, ocpostoffice@niaid.nih.gov, http://www.niaid.nih.gov/Pages/default.aspx

World Health Organization (WHO), Avenue Appia 20, 1211 Geneva 27, Switzerland, 41 22 791 21 11, Fax: 41 22 791 31 11, info@who.int, http://www.who.int/en/.

Barbara Wexler
Rebecca J. Frey, Ph.D.

Static encephalopathy *see* **Cerebral palsy**

Stem cell research *see* **Bioethics**

Stem cell therapy

Definition

Stem cell therapy is the utilization of stem cells to repair or replace damaged cells or tissues. Stem cells are unspecialized (undifferentiated) cells that can reproduce themselves indefinitely or differentiate into specialized cell types.

Purpose

Blood-forming (hematopoietic) stem cells have been used for decades in **bone** marrow stem cell transplants to treat **blood** and **immune system** disorders, including leukemia and **lymphoma**. They are also used to treat loss of bone marrow function from **cancer** treatments. Tissue grafts for treating certain diseases of the skin, bone, and cornea may depend on stem cells present in the grafted tissue.

Most types of stem cell therapy, other than bone marrow transplants, are considered experimental. For example, umbilical cord blood stem cells have been used to treat **heart** problems and other conditions in children with rare metabolic disorders and certain types of anemia. Stem cell therapy holds great promise for treating a wide range of conditions and disorders, including **multiple sclerosis** (MS), **Parkinson's disease**, and **spinal cord** injuries. Stem cell therapy for such conditions may be available in the United States as part of a clinical trial. In other countries, stem cell therapies are available to treat various disorders, including MS.

Precautions

In the United States, bone marrow stem cell transplants to treat leukemia, sickle-cell disease, and certain other conditions are the only approved uses of stem cell therapy; however, in a phenomenon called medical tourism, many patients travel to other countries for stem cell therapy, sometimes at great expense. These therapies have not been shown to be safe and effective, and unregulated clinics in other countries vary considerably in the quality of care. Some may be outright scams.

Embryonic stem cells (ESCs) have the potential to differentiate into any cell type in the body and may someday be used to treat a wide range of human disorders. These cells are available only from human embryos and cannot yet be used directly for stem cell therapy, since they are unlikely to form the required cell type and may cause tumors.

There are many other types of stem cells that derive from various bodily tissues. Tissue-specific or adult stem cells primarily form only the cell types found in the tissues from which they are derived. For example, hematopoietic or blood-forming stem cells in the bone marrow can differentiate into various types of blood cells. Neural stem cells in the **brain** differentiate into different types of brain cells. Some clinics use adult, tissue-specific stem cells for treating a wide range of disorders, but these cells are unlikely to be effective for treating disorders in tissues other than those from which they were derived. For example, it is unlikely that a single type of stem cell therapy could effectively treat both diabetes and Parkinson's disease, since very different cell types are required. Stem cell therapy for neurological disorders can be particularly challenging, because it may require that the stem cells develop into specific types of **neurons** and form appropriate connections with other neurons.

The United States and many other countries require that treatments such as stem cell therapy undergo controlled clinical trials before being declared safe and effective. Many stem cell clinics use patient testimonials to advertise their services; however, patients may improve for a variety of reasons other than stem cell therapy. Placebo effects are particularly important: a patient's strong desire for positive results, as well as beneficial effects of medical attention in any form, can lead to an improvement in symptoms. Furthermore, the symptoms of many disorders wax and wane over time. For example, MS cycles through periods of remission, so it can take years to determine whether a specific treatment is effective. Many stem cell clinics also prescribe diet, medication, **physical therapy**, and **relaxation** and other alternative techniques, making it difficult to identify the source of any improvement. Undergoing an unproven stem cell treatment may make a patient ineligible for participating in a recognized clinical trial.

Description

Stem cell types

Stem cells divide continually, replacing themselves or "self-renewing" indefinitely. They do not age and die out after a finite number of cell divisions like most other cells. Under appropriate conditions, stem cells give rise to daughter progenitor cells that mature or differentiate into a specific cell type.

Human embryonic stem cells (hESCs) are totipotent or pluripotent and can develop into every type of cell in the human body. hESCs exist only during early stages of development. They are isolated from blastocysts—the balls of cells that have developed by about five days after fertilization. Most hESCs are derived from excess blastocysts that were created by *in vitro* fertilization (IVF).

Adult or tissue-specific stem cells, also called somatic stem cells, are multipotent. They can give rise to the different cell types present in a specific tissue or organ. Although they originate during **fetal development**, adult stem cells remain in the body throughout life to replace dying cells. The most easily isolated multipotent stem cells are hematopoietic cells in the bone marrow, which can differentiate into different types of blood cells. Adult multipotent stem cells can also be isolated from circulating blood, from the umbilical cord blood of newborns, and from skin.

Scientists have engineered cells that are similar to ESCs and can differentiate into various cell types. These induced pluripotent stem (iPS) cells are obtained by reprogramming specialized adult cells, such as skin cells.

Stem cell therapy can be autologous—utilizing the patient's own stem cells—or allogeneic—using donor stem cells from another person or embryonic stem cells. For autologous stem cell therapy, the patient's stem cells are removed, grown in the laboratory or treated in some way, and returned to the patient's body. These cells are recognized as "self" by the patient's immune system and are not rejected. Allogeneic stem cells are used when a patient's own stem cells are unavailable or defective. Unless the donor cells are a close match to the patient's cells, the patient's immune system may reject them as "foreign," as sometimes happens with organ transplants from an unrelated donor.

Neurological disorders

Clinical trials of stem cell therapies for neurological conditions include neural stem cell treatments for ischemic **stroke** and hESC treatments for acute **spinal cord injury**. One such trial involves the injection of several million oligodendrocyte progenitor cells, derived from hESCs, directly into the site of a recent spinal cord lesion. Stem cell therapy trials for neural tube defects—the failure of the neural tube to close properly during fetal development—are also underway. Researchers are working to develop stem cell therapies for other common neurological disorders, including Parkinson's disease and **Alzheimer's disease**.

There are two major approaches to stem cell therapy for MS. One approach is to reboot the patient's immune system in hopes of overcoming the autoimmunity that causes demyelination of nerve cells with MS. In this approach, stem cells are obtained from patients' own blood and their immune systems are then destroyed with **chemotherapy**. The stem cells are injected back into the patients, in the hope that their immune systems will reset and no longer attack the myelin covering of nerve cells. The other approach is to try to repair damage already caused by MS. In this therapy, stem cells from a patient's bone marrow are injected into the patient's blood and spinal cord, in the hope that the cells will migrate to the sites of nerve damage and promote healing. These therapies are undergoing early clinical trials in the United States and are available at some foreign university centers. However stem cell clinics in Mexico, Costa Rica, China, and elsewhere sometimes use donor umbilical cord blood or placental cells that are not necessarily safe or effective. Furthermore, stem cell therapy is known to be ineffective for later-stage MS.

Other stem cell therapies

Clinical trials of stem cell therapy for various heart problems are ongoing. For example, heart attack patients have been treated with autologous bone marrow from their hip bones. Either whole bone marrow or stem cells removed from bone marrow and grown in the laboratory are injected directly into the patient's damaged heart chamber. In one early trial, this treatment significantly reduced heart size and scar tissue and greatly improved heart function, even when the damage occurred years previously.

Other trials are using hESC-derived retinal cells to treat eye diseases, including age-related **macular degeneration** and Stargardt's macular dystrophy. These cells are injected directly into the damaged eyes. Stem cell therapy is also being investigated as a treatment for burned corneas, in cases where the stem cells that normally renew and repair the cornea have also been destroyed.

Risks

Even bone marrow stem cell transplants that have been in use for decades carry significant risks. Allogeneic stem cell therapies carry the risk of rejection by the patient's immune system: as with organ transplants, the closer the match of donor tissue to that of the recipient, the lower the risk of rejection; however, allogeneic stem cell therapy may require lifelong use of immunosuppressants to prevent rejection.

Although autologous stem cell therapy is unlikely to trigger an **immune response**, there are still risks involved in the procedures for acquiring, growing, and reintroducing the stem cells. Stem cells removed from a patient's body are manipulated in ways that can change their characteristics. During growth in laboratory culture—a process called expansion—stem cells may lose their ability to mature into the required cell type or may lose mechanisms for controlling their growth. There is also potential for contamination with **viruses**, **bacteria**, or other pathogens. Injection of stem cells back into a patient carries the risk of introducing **infection** or damaging tissues.

Each type of stem cell therapy has its own particular risks. For example, stem cell therapies that involve first destroying the immune system leave patients nearly defenseless against infection for weeks.

Special concerns

Stem cell therapy holds great promise for curing or preventing the progression of many debilitating and fatal conditions, including many neurological disorders. Some researchers, physicians, and patients believe that the United States is moving too slowly toward making stem cell therapy available to the millions of patients who could potentially benefit, but many physicians also worry about patients flocking to unregulated treatment centers, both domestic and foreign, for therapies that have been proven neither safe nor effective. Stem cell therapy is very expensive and most treatments are not covered by insurance. Participation in a registered clinical trial is usually free of cost.

The U.S. Food and Drug Administration (FDA) allows a patient's stem cells to be removed and replaced, as long as they are not significantly altered in the process. If these autologous stem cells are treated with growth factors or other compounds, the FDA regulates them as drugs. Some U.S.-based clinics collect stem cells from patients' blood, bone marrow, or fatty tissues and re-infuse them into damaged or diseased sites in the body. Most of these procedures have not been subjected to scientific scrutiny and some patients have been harmed.

The destruction of human embryos to obtain hESCs has been a major source of controversy in the United States and elsewhere, even though the embryos would otherwise be discarded. Restrictions on the use of hESCs have, at times, significantly interfered with stem cell therapy research. Although some of the barriers to hESC research were removed in 2009, court cases and temporary injunctions have continued to frustrate researchers.

Even some proponents of stem cell therapy have expressed concern over clinical trials that they believe to be premature. They are particularly concerned that failures or patient harm will further impede progress in stem cell therapy, as has happened in the past. Some critics are also concerned that patients who have been recently diagnosed with a life-altering disease or suffered a traumatic spinal cord injury may not be capable of fully comprehending the risks of undergoing an unproven therapy.

Resources

BOOKS

Capps, Benjamin J., and Alastair V. Campbell, eds. *Contested Cells: Global Perspectives on the Stem Cell Debate.* London: Imperial College Press, 2010.

Koka, Prasad S. *Stem Cell Therapy and Uses in Medical Treatment.* Hauppauge, NY: Nova Science, 2011.

Smith, Robin. *Stem Cell Medicine: The New Adult Stem Cell Regenerative Therapy for Cancer, Spinal Injuries, Multiple Sclerosis, Parkinson's and Other Conditions.* Long Island City, NY: Hatherleigh, 2009.

PERIODICALS

Ackerman, Todd. "A New Hope: MS Patients Going Abroad to Find Help: Promising Stem-Cell Therapies Remain Hard to Obtain in U.S." *Houston Chronicle* (February 21, 2011): 1.

Banerjee, Soma, et al. "Human Stem Cell Therapy in Ischaemic Stroke: A Review." *Age and Aging* 40, no. 1 (January 2011): 7–13.

Caplan, Arthur, and Bruce Levine. "Hope, Hype and Help: Ethically Assessing the Growing Market in Stem Cell Therapies." *Current* no. 524 (July/August 2010): 33.

Dhaulakhandi, Dhara B., Seema Rohilla, and Kamal Nain Rattan. "Neural Tube Defects: Review of Experimental Evidence on Stem Cell Therapy and Newer Treatment Options." *Fetal Diagnosis and Therapy* 28, no. 2 (August 2010): 72–78.

Hyun, Insoo. "Allowing Innovative Stem Cell-Based Therapies Outside of Clinical Trials: Ethical and Policy Challenges." *Journal of Law, Medicine & Ethics* 38, no. 2 (Summer 2010): 277–85.

Johnson, Carolyn Y. "ACT Wins FDA's Approval to Test Stem Cell Therapy." *Boston Globe* (November 22, 2010): B7.

Parker, Graham C. "Stem Cell Therapy for Stroke." *Journal of Pediatric Neurology* 8, no. 3 (2010): 333–41.

Pownall, Mark. "Experts Warn Against 'Tourist Trap' Stem Cell Therapies." *British Medical Journal* 341, no. 7771 (September 4, 2010): 477.

Stein, Rob. "First Patient to Have Experimental Stem Cell Therapy Comes Forward." *Washington Post* (April 7, 2011): A13.

Svodboda, Elizabeth. "Offshore Operations." *Popular Science* 277, no. 1 (July 2010): 64–72.

ORGANIZATIONS

International Society for Stem Cell Research, 111 Deer Lake Road, Suite 100, Deerfield, IL 60015, (847) 509-1944, Fax: (847) 480-9282, isscr@isscr.org, http://www.isscr.org

U.S. Food and Drug Administration, 10903 New Hampshire Avenue, Silver Spring, MD 20993-0002, (888) 463-6332, http://www.fda.gov.

Margaret Alic, Ph.D.

Stenting

Definition

Stenting is a procedure in which a cylindrical structure (stent) is placed into a hollow tubular organ to provide artificial support and maintain the patency of the opening. Although it is most often used for cardiovascular functioning, it is also utilized to manage obstructions in **cancer** patients.

> **QUESTIONS TO ASK YOUR DOCTOR**
>
> - Am I a good candidate for this procedure?
> - Do I have any contraindications that should be considered before having the procedure?
> - Will I experience any improvement in my quality of life?
> - What are the advantages and disadvantages of the procedure?
> - Does the physician performing the procedure do this often or only occasionally?

Purpose

Stents are used in cancer patients to relieve obstructions due to:

- direct blockages within the tube (or lumen) due to cancer growth
- narrowing of the lumen from tumor growth outside pressing on the tube and narrowing the lumen
- occasionally from the build up of scar tissue (fibrosis) from radiation therapy

Tumors most likely to cause obstruction requiring stent placement include esophageal cancer, bronchogenic carcinoma, pancreatic cancer, cancers of the bile duct, and occasionally colorectal carcinomas.

Precautions

Every patient should be viewed individually with special consideration given to the patient's present status. Generally, surgical procedures are for the correction of a problem; but in many cancer cases, relief of symptoms is the only therapeutic option. Since it is extremely difficult to remove or reposition these stents after they are placed, the degree of relief to be offered by its insertion should be significant. The physician and the patient should discuss all alternatives and come to a mutual decision.

Description

Endoscopic retrograde cholangiopancreatography (ERCP) is the name of the procedure utilized to place most stents for pancreatic and biliary tumors. The ERCP is a flexible **endoscope**, which can be directed and moved around the many bends in the upper gastrointestinal tract. The newer video endoscopes

KEY TERMS

Endoscope—An instrument used for direct visual inspection of hollow organs or body cavities.

Esophagus—The muscular, membranous structure that extends from the throat to the stomach.

Lumen—The cavity or channel within a tube or tubular organ, such as a blood vessel or the intestine.

have a tiny, optically sensitive computer chip at the end which transmits electronic signals up the scope to a computer that displays an image on a large video screen. The scope has an open channel that permits other instruments to be passed through it to perform biopsies, inject solutions, or place stents. Since ERCP uses x-ray films, the procedure takes place in an x-ray area. Initially the throat is anesthetized with a spray solution and the patient is also usually mildly sedated. The endoscope is inserted into the upper esophagus and a thin tube is inserted through it to the main bile duct entering the intestinal area. Dye is injected into the bile duct and/or the pancreatic duct and x-ray films are taken. The patient usually lies on the left side and then turns onto the **stomach** to allow complete visualization of the ducts. The patient is able to breathe easily throughout the exam and rarely gags. Any gallstones found may be removed or if the duct has become narrowed, an incision can be made using electrocautery (electrical heat) to relieve the blockage. It is also possible to widen narrowed ducts by placing stents in these areas to keep them open. The patient is taken to recovery following the procedure, which takes 20–40 minutes.

Other endoscopes are used to place stents elsewhere in the body. For example, an esophagoscope is used to place stents in cases of esophageal cancer, a bronchoscope is used for procedures involving endobronchial obstructions, and a colonoscope is used in cases of colorectal obstructions.

A coronary stent is stainless tube with slots. It is mounted on a balloon catheter in a collapsed state. When the balloon is inflated, the stent expands or opens up and pushes itself against the inner wall of the coronary artery. This holds the artery open when the balloon is deflated and removed. Coronary artery stents were designed to overcome some of the shortcomings of **angioplasty**, which is a technique that is used to dilate an area of arterial blockage with the help of a catheter with an inflatable, small, balloon at its tip.

Preparation

The patient is instructed not to eat or drink anything for eight hours prior to the procedure. Some physicians may request that no asprin be taken for a certain time period prior to the procedure to prevent excessive bleeding.

Aftercare

The patient may go home after the procedure or may spend one or two nights in the hospital. **Antibiotics** may be given especially if there has been long-standing biliary obstruction. Dietary restrictions are common after esophageal and colorectal stenting.

Risks

The most serious risk associated with the placement of a stent is the risk of perforation. If a tear is made, leakage with life-threatening **infection** may occur. Migration or recurrent obstruction may necessitate repeat stenting if possible. Occasionally bleeding may occur.

Normal results

Relief of the obstruction with resumption of the ability to eat, breathe, normally clear fluids from the **liver** or **pancreas**, or allow normal passage of stool is the desired result of this procedure.

Abnormal results

A sudden change in the degree of **pain** and/or **fever** that persists as well as any unusual changes should be communicated immediately to a physician.

Stent-Grafts

A stent-graft is a tubular structure composed of two parts. The stent is a mesh-like structure made of metal. Its function is to provide support to the graft. The latter is composed of a special fabric that is impervious to **blood** and lines the stent. The stent-graft is packed in small diameter tubes and expands to its original diameter when released from these tubes. Stent-grafts are used to treat aneurysms.

The procedure of treating aortic aneurysms with stent-grafts is known as EVAR. This stands for Endovascular **Aneurysm** Repair. The most common use for EVAR is to treat aneurysms of the abdominal aorta, thoracic aorta, and popliteal artery, although there are still a number of surgeons who perform open surgery for these conditions.

Resources

BOOK

Bergeron P, Roux M, Khanoyan P, Douillez V, Bras J, Gay J. "Long-term results of carotid stenting are competitive with surgery." *Journal of Vascular Surgery* 41 (2005): 213–221.

OTHER

"ERCP (Endoscopic Retrograde Cholangiopancreatography)." National Digestive Diseases Information Clearinghouse. http://www.niddk.nih.gov/health/digest/pubs/diagtest/ercp.htm.

ORGANIZATIONS

American Cancer Society, P.O. Box 102454, Atlanta, GA 30368-2454, http://www.cancer.org

American Society of Clinical Oncology, 900 Duke Street, Suite 200, Alexandria, VA 22314, (703) 299-0150, http://www.asco.org.

Linda K. Bennington, C.N.S., M.S.N.
Karl Finley
Brenda Lerner

KEY TERMS

Angiography—A technique for the diagnostic imaging of blood vessels that involves the injection of contrast material.

Fractionated radiosurgery—Radiosurgery in which the radiation is delivered in several smaller doses over a period of time rather than the full amount in a single treatment.

Metastatic—Referring to the spread of cancer from one organ in the body to another not directly connected to it.

Radiosurgery—Surgery that uses ionizing radiation to destroy tissue rather than a surgical incision.

Simulation scan—The process of making a mask for the patient and other images in order to plan the radiation treatment.

Stereotactic—Characterized by precise positioning in space. When applied to radiosurgery, stereotactic refers to a system of three-dimensional coordinates for locating the target site.

Stereotactic radiosurgery

Definition

Stereotactic radiosurgery is the use of a precise beam of radiation to destroy tissue in the **brain**.

Purpose

This procedure is used to treat brain tumors, arteriovenous malformations in the brain, and in some cases, benign eye tumors or other disorders within the brain.

Demographics

Stereotactic radiosurgery is used to treat a variety of disorders with widely differing demographic profiles.

Description

"Radiosurgery" refers to the use of a high-energy beam of radiation. "Stereotactic" refers to the three-dimensional targeting system used to deliver the beam to the precise location desired. Stereotactic radiosurgery is primarily confined to the head and neck, because the patient must be kept completely still during the delivery of the radiation in order to prevent damage to surrounding tissue. The motion of the patient's head and neck are restricted by a stereotactic frame that holds them in place. It is difficult to immobilize other body regions in this way.

The high energy of the radiation beam disrupts the DNA of the targeted cells, killing them. Multiple weak beams are focused on the target area, delivering maximum energy to it while keeping surrounding tissue safe. Since the radiation passes through the **skull** to its target, there is no need to cut open the skull to perform the surgery. The beam can be focused on any structure in the brain, allowing access to tumors or malformed **blood vessels** that cannot be reached by open-skull surgery.

The Gamma Knife is a stationary machine that is most useful for small tumors, **blood** vessels, or similar targets. Because it does not move, it can deliver a small, highly localized and precise beam of radiation. Gamma knife treatment is done all at once in a single hospital stay. The second type of radiosurgery uses a movable linear accelerator-based machine that is preferred for larger tumors. This treatment is delivered in several small doses given over several weeks. Radiosurgery that is performed with divided doses is known as fractionated radiosurgery. The total dose of radiation is higher with a linear accelerator-based machine than with gamma knife treatment.

Disorders treated by stereotactic radiosurgery include:

- benign brain tumors, including acoustic neuromas and meningiomas
- malignant brain tumors, including gliomas and astrocytomas
- metastatic brain tumors
- trigeminal neuralgia
- Parkinson's disease
- essential tremor
- arteriovenous malformations
- pituitary tumors

Diagnosis/Preparation

A patient requiring radiosurgery has already been diagnosed with a specific disorder that affects the brain. As preparation for radiosurgery, he or she will undergo neuroimaging studies to determine the precise location of the target area in the brain. These studies may include **CT scans**, MRI scans, and others. Imaging of the blood vessels (**angiography**) or the brain's ventricles (ventriculography) may be done as well. These require the injection of either a harmless radioactive substance or a contrast dye.

Prior to the procedure, the patient will be fitted with a stereotactic frame or rigid mask to immobilize the head. This part of the treatment may be uncomfortable. The patient may receive a simulation scan to establish the precise relationship of the mask or frame to the head to help plan the treatment.

The patient may be given a sedative and an antinausea agent prior to the simulation scan or treatment.

Aftercare

Stereotactic radiosurgery does not produce some of the side effects commonly associated with radiation treatment, such as reddening of the skin or hair loss. Most patients can return to their usual daily activities following treatment without any special precautions.

Risks

The risks of stereotactic radiosurgery include mild **headache**, tiredness, nausea and **vomiting**, and recurrence of the tumor. Questions have been raised as to whether radiosurgery can cause secondary tumors, but there is little detailed information about this potential risk.

WHO PERFORMS THE PROCEDURE AND WHERE IS IT PERFORMED?

Stereotactic radiosurgery is performed by a radio-surgeon, who is a neurosurgeon with advanced training in the use of a gamma knife or linear accelerator-based machine. The radiosurgeon's dose plan is checked by a physicist before the treatment is administered to the patient. Stereotactic radiosurgery is done in a hospital that has the necessary specialized equipment.

Normal results

Stereotactic radiosurgery does not cause **pain**; and because the skull is not opened, there is no long hospital stay or risk of **infection**. Recovery is very rapid; most patients go home the same day they are treated, although follow-up imaging and retreatment may be necessary in some cases. This form of surgery appears to be quite successful in extending the length of survival in **cancer** patients; one study found that gamma knife radiosurgery controlled tumor growth in 96% of patients with kidney cancer that had spread to the brain, and added an average of 15 months to the patients' survival.

Morbidity and mortality rates

Stereotactic radiosurgery has a low reported rate of serious complications with minimal mortality. One German study reported a 4.8% rate of temporary morbidity in patients under treatment for brain tumors, with no permanent morbidity and no mortality. An American group of researchers found that less than 2% of patients who had eye tumors treated with radiosurgery suffered damage to the optic nerve from the dose of radiation.

Mild side effects following gamma knife radiosurgery are not uncommon, however. One group of British researchers found that 47 out of a group of 65 patients treated with gamma knife surgery had mild or moderate side effects within two weeks of treatment. Of these patients, more than half suffered headaches and a fifth reported unusual tiredness or nausea and vomiting.

Alternatives

With certain types of brain tumors, whole-brain radiation treatment (WBRT) is an option; however, it has a number of severe side effects. Surgical removal of the tumor is another option, but it carries a higher risk of tumor recurrence. For other tumors, gamma knife radiosurgery is the only treatment available.

Resources

BOOKS

Beers, Mark H. and Robert Berkow, et al. *The Merck Manual of Diagnosis and Therapy,* Whitehouse Station: Merck, 2012.

Radiation Injury of the Nervous System. Section 14, Chapter 177 in *The Merck Manual of Diagnosis and Therapy,* edited by Mark H. Beers, MD, and Robert Berkow, MD. Whitehouse Station, NJ: Merck Research Laboratories, 1999.

PERIODICALS

Chua, D.T., J.S. Sham, P.W. Kwong, et al. "Linear Accelerator-Based Stereotactic Radiosurgery for Limited, Locally Persistent, and Recurrent Nasopharyngeal Carcinoma; Efficacy and Complications." *International Journal of Radiation Oncology, Biology, Physics* 56 (May 1, 2003): 177–183.

Ganz, J.C. "Gamma Knife Radiosurgery and Its Possible Relationship to Malignancy: A Review." *Journal of Neurosurgery* 97 (December 2002) (5 Suppl): 644–652.

Muacevic, A., and F.W. Kreth. "Significance of Stereotactic Biopsy for the Management of WHO Grade II Supratentorial Glioma." [in German] *Der Nervenarzt* 74 (April 2003): 350–354.

O'Neill, B.P., N.J. Iturria, M.J. Link, et al. "A Comparison of Surgical Resection and Stereotactic Radiosurgery in the Treatment of Solitary Brain Metastases." *International Journal of Radiation Oncology, Biology, Physics* 55 (April 1, 2003): 1169–1176.

Sheehan, J.P., M.H. Sun, D Kondziolka, et al. "Radiosurgery in Patients with Renal Cell Carcinoma Metastasis to the Brain: Long-Term Outcomes and Prognostic Factors Influencing Survival and Local Tumor Control." *Journal of Neurosurgery* 98 (February 2003): 342–349.

ORGANIZATIONS

International Radiosurgery Support Association (IRSA). 3005 Hoffman Street, Harrisburg, PA 17110. (717) 260-9808. www.irsa.org.

Johns Hopkins Radiosurgery. Weinberg 1469, 600 North Wolfe Street, Baltimore, MD 21287. (410) 614-2886. www. hopkinsmedicine.org/radiosurgery/treatmentoptions/stereotacticradiosurgery.cfm.

Richard Robinson

Sterilization techniques

Definition

Sterilization techniques include all the means used to completely eliminate or destroy living microorganisms on any object, including tools used to test or treat patients.

Purpose

The term microorganism, or microbe, refers to any single-celled living organism, including **bacteria**, **viruses**, and **fungi**. (Though viruses are not true single-celled organisms, medical science still usually classifies them as microorganisms.) Microbes can be transferred by direct contact or indirectly through a vehicle (like a surgical tool) or via the air the patient breathes. If favorable conditions for growth exist in the new host, microbes reproduce and establish colonies. Many of these microscopic organisms are normal inhabitants of the human body (called microflora). For example, varieties of the bacterium *Staphylococcus* are normal inhabitants of the skin and nasal passages, and many different species of bacteria live in the small and **large intestine**, aiding in the process of digestion.

However, many types of microorganisms are pathogenic (considered foreign to the host body) and, upon entering the body, cause **infection** when they either damage cells directly or release toxins that will eventually cause damage. The prevention of disease-causing microbes in a patient-care environment is generally accomplished through aseptic or sterile techniques. The goal is to create as germ-free an environment as possible, primarily through sterilization and the maintenance of sterile/nonsterile barriers.

Precautions

Like foods sold in the grocery store, sterile medical and surgical solutions and some other equipment have expiration dates indicating when the product is no longer considered sterile. Although many hospitals consider sterile, prepackaged disposable materials to be sterile

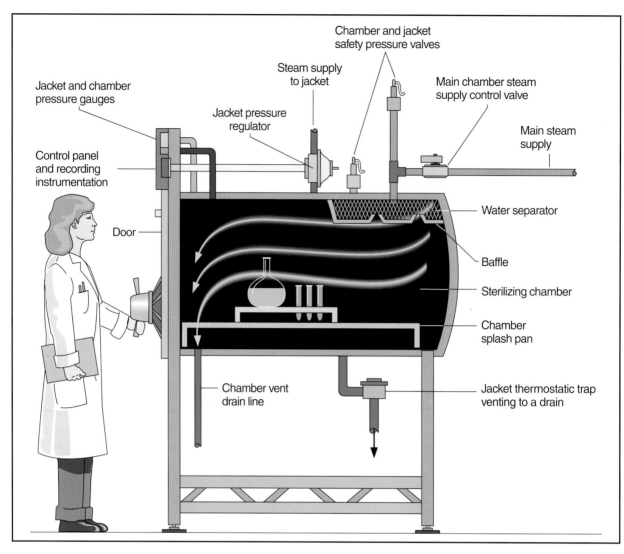

(Hans & Cassidy. Steam pressure sterilizer, woman, photograph. Courtesy of Gale Research.)

indefinitely if the packaging is undamaged, sterile goods must be examined carefully to ensure that there are no breaks in the integrity of the packaging or that the package has not gotten wet. Microbes are able to enter sterile goods through either breaks in the wrapping (the sterile barrier) or moisture. If the wrapper is no longer intact, or has been wet, sterile goods must be repackaged and resterilized.

Description

Patients having invasive medical or surgical procedures are at risk for infection primarily from four sources:

• Infection is transferred from other people, including patients and health care providers. Such infection is called direct transmission, which usually occurs as a result of direct contact with skin or bodily fluids, including saliva, coughing, and spitting.

• Infection results from equipment or other objects that come in contact with the patient. This is called vehicle-borne infection because the microbe is transported from another place on some object or vehicle and introduced through a break in the skin or mucosal membranes. Primary examples are food poisoning caused by contaminated food items or infection caused by the use of non-sterile equipment in an invasive procedure like bronchoscopy or phlebotomy.

• Infection arises from the patient's own body, such as the possible contamination of a surgical site during intestinal resection if the patient's own fecal material contaminates the abdominal cavity contents.

• The air transports microbes. An example of airborne infection is tuberculosis, in which bacteria are transmitted on air currents to others through coughing or spitting.

Managing as germ-free an environment as possible is necessary for surgical procedures and even minor medical treatments normally done in a doctor's office, such as suturing a laceration. Patients with conditions or under treatments that cause the **immune system** to be compromised are sometimes treated in an artificially created environment called reverse isolation. Leukemia patients, especially those on aggressive **chemotherapy** who receive **bone** marrow transplants, and people with **immunodeficiency** disorders (which can lead to little or no natural defense against infection), are all potential candidates for reverse isolation procedures. Patients with **AIDS** (acquired immune deficiency syndrome) may be treated in an environment of isolation, both direct and reverse isolation for their protection, as well as the protection of caregivers. An extreme example of reverse isolation is the use of a sterilized plastic tent with filtered air circulation called an isolator. (**Premature infants** may be placed in special sterile plastic bassinets called an isolette.)

Aseptic technique

It has been known since the days of Florence Nightingale that clean surroundings are definitely less conducive to the growth of microorganisms than unclean ones. The creation of sterile environments always includes scrupulous cleanliness. The use of disinfectants in washing furniture, walls and floors, as well as in soaking medical equipment or other patient-care items is another important measure. Disinfectants are harsh chemical compounds described as bactericidal (capable of killing bacteria) or bacteriostatic (capable of stopping the growth or reproduction of bacteria). Some of these disinfectants may also be antiviral agents or antifungal. Disinfectants are usually too toxic to tissue to be used directly on the body. **Antiseptics** are chemical compounds that are also either bactericidal or bacteriostatic. But these are usually more diluted solutions and can safely be used in direct contact with human tissues. Common antiseptics include iodine, hydrogen peroxide, and thimerosal.

The importance of hand washing before and after the care of any patient cannot be over-stressed. It remains the simplest and most effective means of preventing infection. The Centers for Disease Control and Prevention (CDC) estimates that American hospitals produce two million hospital-borne infections (known as nosocomial infections) each year, and approximately one-quarter of these are postoperative surgical incision infections. Postoperative infections result from breaks in sterile technique during surgery or breaks in **aseptic technique** during **wound care**. Further, CDC studies have shown that the average compliance with hand washing by health

care providers from 1981 to 1999 has never risen above 50%. Proper procedure is for health care personnel to scrub their hands prior to and immediately after performing any procedure on a patient, regardless of whether latex gloves were worn or not. Gloves, as a barrier, can be breached via holes the size of pinpoints.

For both surgery and reverse isolation, staff are usually required to wear presterilized gloves, hair nets, masks, and gowns, with clean shoe coverings. Insertion of a urinary catheter, changing a surgical drain, cleaning a **tracheotomy** tube or applying a sterile dressing are all instances when health care providers wear gloves. They also create what is termed a sterile field or area that has been prepared with antiseptics or covered with impenetrable sterile drapes to reduce the likelihood of organism transfer.

Before surgical procedures, the operative site skin area is cleansed with an antiseptic solution, and sterile drapes are applied to the periphery. In the case of bowel surgery, **laxatives** and enemas are given prior to the surgery to remove as much fecal material as possible, thus limiting the amount of contamination from feces. When the bowel is clamped shut, all instruments, drapes, and sponges that may have come in contact with the patient are removed and replaced with sterile equipment before proceeding any further. In both surgical suites and in reverse isolation patients' rooms, air is passed through a special ventilation system that filters out microorganisms.

Five means are commonly used to sterilize objects in the patient's environment. These include:

- Moist heat is used via steaming or autoclaving (steaming under high pressure). Much like a pressure cooker used to can food at home and destroy bacteria, an autoclave circulates steam at temperatures of 260°F (120°C) at sustained pressure of 20 pounds per square inch for designated periods of time. All equipment used in carrying out medical or surgical procedures such as instruments, tubings (including catheters), bandages, and linens used for drapes are sterilized, usually in an autoclave.

- Ionizing and non-ionizing radiation is sometimes used. Ultraviolet light is a type of non-ionizing radiation used for items sensitive to heat.

- The passage of liquids through a filter sufficiently fine so as to trap microbes.

- Gas sterilization, usually using ethylene oxide, interferes with the metabolism and therefore the development of microorganisms and inhibits the growth of spores. It is effective in the sterilization of heat-sensitive items and penetrates deeply, but it has to be used with care since it is poisonous.

• Strong disinfectants are used primarily for instruments, such as thermometers and scopes that could not survive autoclaving. Medical equipment soaked in disinfectants to destroy microbes should be rinsed off prior to use due to the toxicity of many of the compounds used for disinfecting. Certain gases used for sterilization, such as ethylene oxide, are extremely toxic to human beings and should be used with care.

Preparation

In general, preparations include standard sterilization techniques for the patient, health care staff, and environment. Surgery patients requiring reverse isolation procedures should be told about the actions of micro-organisms, including the ways they gain entry into the human body, the diseases that can be caused, and how sterilization techniques work to prevent infection. Hair is no longer routinely removed from the site of the surgical incision prior to surgery as the skin is a natural barrier to infection and shaving it often produces small skin breaks.

Aftercare

Aftercare following the use of sterilized or surgically clean equipment includes monitoring patients for the signs and symptoms of infection, which usually occurs within 48 to 71 hours. Signs and symptoms of infection include:

• fever

• inflammation, or redness and swelling at the site of infection, often accompanied by edema and erythema

• purulent or pus-like drainage from wounds

• abnormally elevated white blood count

• pain at the site of infection

Complications

There should be no complications from using proper sterilization and aseptic techniques. An allergy to any of the various antiseptics used to sterilize skin prior to surgery may produce dermatitis or irritation. If instruments cleaned with disinfectant are not properly rinsed before use, an inflammatory response similar to a first-degree burn may result on surfaces contacted by the solution.

Results

Proper sterilization techniques result in the prevention of infection. Sterilization techniques must be monitored and continually improved upon.

Health care team roles

All health care personnel are responsible for the primary means of preventing infection, which is hand washing. In the early days of nursing, sterilization of equipment and cleanliness of the patient's environment was the nurse's principal responsibility The nurse still bears responsibility or accountability in these areas even though they may be implemented by others.

• Sterilization technicians work in either the operating room area of a hospital or in the hospital's central supply. They receive special orientation and training in sterile techniques at the health care facility where they are employed. They are responsible for carrying out sterilization procedures and for monitoring sterile equipment conditions and expiration dates. Sometimes nurses or operating room technicians are responsible for providing sterile equipment.

• Some registered nurses (RNs) are certified in infection control and are required to keep statistical data on the incidence and types of infections in a health care facility. These RNs typically serve on infection control committees, along with physicians and clinical pharmacists.

• Clinical laboratory scientists have specialized training and must pass a state examination. They draw blood samples and culture wound drainage specimens, which are ordered by the physician to monitor patients for infection and for routine assessment of nosocomial infection sources throughout a facility.

Resources

BOOKS

Berkow, Robert, et al., eds. *Merck Manual of Diagnosis and Therapy, Home Edition.* New York: Pocket Books, 1999.

Kozier, Barbara, et al. *Fundamentals of Nursing: Concepts, Process and Practice,* 7th ed. Upper Saddle River, NJ: Prentice Hall, Inc., 2004.

Timby, Barbara K. *Fundamental Skills and Concepts in Patient Care,* 7th ed. Philadelphia: J.P. Lippincott Co., 2001.

PERIODICALS

Nichols, Ronald Lee. "Preventing Surgical Site Infections: A Surgeon's Perspective." *CDC* 7, no 2 (March-April 2001).

Pittet, Didier. "Improving Adherence to Hand Hygiene Practice: A Multidisciplinary Approach." *CDC* 7, no 2 (March-April 2001).

OTHER

Cleaning and Disinfection. Johns Hopkins Hospital, HEIC. http://www.johnshopkins.org (2000).

"Guidelines for Isolation Precautions in Hospitals." CDC. http://www.cdc.gov/ncidod/hip/isolat/isolat.htm (June 30, 2001).

Shelf Life of Sterile Packages. Johns Hopkins Hospital, HEIC. http://www.johnshopkins.org (2000).

Joan M. Schonbeck

Sternum *see* **Thorax**

Stethoscope

Definition

The stethoscope is an instrument used to listen to sounds produced by the body. It is used to listen to the **lungs**, **heart**, and intestinal tract.

Purpose

A stethoscope is used to detect and study heart, lung, **stomach**, and other sounds in humans and animals. Using the stethoscope, the listener can hear abnormal respiratory, cardiac, pleural arterial, venous, uterine, fetal, and intestinal sounds.

Description

Stethoscopes vary in their design and material. Most are made of rubber tubing, shaped in a "Y," allowing sound to enter the device at one end, travel up the tubes

and through to the ear pieces. Many stethoscopes have a two-sided sound-detecting device, which listeners flip, depending on whether they need to hear high or low frequencies. However, some of the newer models have one pressure-sensitive head. The various types of stethoscopes include: binaural stethoscopes, designed for use with both ears; single, designed for use with one ear; differential, with which listeners can compare sounds at two different body sites; and electronic, which electronically amplify tones. Some stethoscopes are designed specifically for **hearing** the fetal heartbeat or esophagus.

Operation

Some stethoscopes must be placed directly on the skin, while others can work effectively through clothing. For the stethoscopes with a two-part sound detecting device at the end, listeners press the rim against the skin, using the bowl-shaped side to hear low-pitched sounds. The other flat side, called the diaphragm, detects high-pitched sounds.

Maintenance

In order to avoid the spread of **infection**, stethoscopes should be cleaned after each use—especially when placed directly on the patient's skin.

Health care team roles

Everyone on the health care team uses a stethoscope, as the provider may need to listen to sounds produced by the heart, lungs, stomach, or another body organ often.

Training

Stethoscope users must learn to assess what they hear. When listening to the heart, one must listen to the left side of the chest, where the heart is located. Specifically, it is between the fourth and sixth ribs, almost directly below the breast. The stethoscope must be moved around; the health care provider should listen for different sounds emanating from different locations. The bell of the instrument—generally used to listen to sounds of low pitch, and then its diaphragm—should be used to listen to different areas of the heart. The sounds will be different. "Lub-dub" is the sound produced by the normal heart. Every time this sound is detected, it means that the heart is contracting one time. The noises represent the heart valves clicking to close. When one hears "lub," the atrioventricular valves are closing, and "dub" means the pulmonic and aortic valves are closing. Other heart sounds, such as the quiet "whoosh," heard after "lub-dub," reflect the existence

KEY TERMS

Murmur—A murmur may be heard as blood moves through the heart, when there is "turbulence" in the flow of blood; if a valve remains closed (does not open completely) a murmur might be heard.

Pleuritis—An infection between the lung and the chest wall.

Pulmonary edema—The buildup of fluid in the lungs or respiratory system. Usually results from an increase in pulmonary capillary pressure.

Stethoscope—An instrument used to listen to bodily sounds; used to listen to the lungs, heart, and intestinal tract.

of a "murmur." These are heard when the **blood** moves through the heart, and mean that there is "turbulence" in the blood flow. If a valve remains closed, rather than opening completely, one might hear a murmur. These are not at all uncommon; in fact, many people have them and are unaffected.

The lungs and airways require different listening skills than those used to detect heart sounds. The stethoscope must be placed over the chest, and the patient must breathe in and out deeply, and slowly. Using the bell, the different sounds should be noted in various areas of the chest. Then, the diaphragm should be used in the same way. There will be no wheezes or crackles in normal lung sounds. When performing "percussion," on the chest, the health care practitioner should be listening for sounds made by sounds the patient makes. One would lightly "thump" around the stethoscope, against the chest, with one finger. Lungs that sound hollow are normal; they have no air in them. Lungs that have a more solid sound appear dead. On percussion, this "dead" sound may be solidification of the lung. In this case, one might make an initial diagnosis of **pneumonia**.

When crackles or wheezes are detected, the practitioner is hearing lung sounds that are abnormal. When the chest wall is being rubbed by the lung, "friction rubs" are detected. When there is fluid in the lungs, crackles will be heard. This is often heard when the patient has pneumonia or pulmonary **edema**. A high-pitched whistling sound (a wheeze) is often heard when there is pneumonia or when an airway disease (like **bronchitis**) is present. Lastly, an infection between the lung and the chest might produce the friction rubs—squeaky noises that infections like

pleuritis (an infection between the lung and chest wall) produce.

To listen to the **abdomen**, the stethoscope should be held over its upper left side. One can hear "gurgling" just under the ribs. The intestines, in the lower part of the abdomen, can also be heard. The noises they make are "borborygmus"—and they are normal. The abdomen is also a site where percussion can be heard. If one thumps all around the bell of the stethoscope, the individual will hear a solid sound, as if the organ is "dead." When the sound is hollow, it means that the intestinal tract has gas in it.

Despite these somewhat basic instructions, it takes experience and skill to determine what tests might be needed once examination with the stethoscope has been completed. Examination with this instrument is particularly noninvasive, but useful. It can assist the physician and health care team in localizing the problem about which the patient is complaining.

Resources

BOOK

Nettina, Sandra, ed. *Lippincott Manual of Nursing Practice.* 7th ed. Philadelphia: Lippincott, 2001, p. 52.

OTHER

A Beginner's Guide to Using a Stethoscope. http://www.ahc. umn.edu. Accessed June 28, 2001.

Masoaka, Shirley, R.N., president. UltraScope, Inc. Charlotte, NC. (800) 677-2673.

Medscape dictionary online, Merriam-Webster. http://www. dict.medscape.com. Accessed June 30, 2001.

Lisette Hilton

Stings *see* **Bites and stings**

Stomach

Definition

The stomach is a muscular, J-shaped, hollow organ of the digestive tract. It temporarily stores and mixes food; it also secretes gastric juice into the lumen (the hollow inside the stomach) and a hormone called gastrin into the **blood**.

Demographics

The word "stomach" is derived from the Latin word "stomachus," which itself is derived from the Greek word "stomachos." As an important organ of the digestive tract

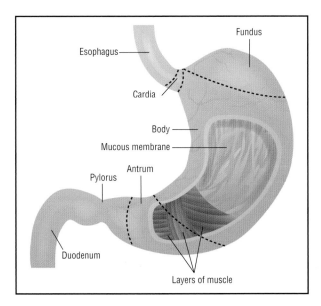

(Diagram showing major parts of the stomach. Illustration by GGS Information Services, Inc. The Gale Group.)

in many animals, such as echinoderms, insects, mollusks, and vertebrates (including humans), it is the second part of digestion, with the first one being mastication, or chewing.

According to the American Cancer Society (ACS), stomach cancer in the United States was diagnosed about 21,320 times in 2012. Of that number, approximately 13,020 cases occurred in males and about 8,300 cases in women. Further, about 10,540 people died of stomach cancer in 2012, with 6,190 of them being men and 4,350 women. Most cases of stomach cancer occur within older people, with the average age of diagnosis being 70 years. The ACS estimates that the risk of getting cancer of the stomach within any lifetime is about 1 in 114, with men having a slightly higher risk than women.

Description

The stomach is located in the upper left quadrant of the **abdomen**, just beneath the diaphragm. It is positioned between the esophagus (the passage between the mouth and stomach) and the **small intestine**. There is a sphincter (circular muscle) between the esophagus and the stomach, which allows food to pass into the stomach and prevents chyme (the semi-fluid mass into which food is converted by gastric enzymes) from flowing backwards into the esophagus. The pyloric valve is situated between the stomach and the small intestine, which allows chyme to pass into the small intestine and back into the stomach.

The stomach is divided into three general areas. The upper portion of the stomach near the esophagus is called

the fundus; the middle section of the stomach is called the body; and the bottom portion of the stomach, where the pyloric sphincter is located, is called the antrum. When the stomach is completely distended (expanded), it measures about 10 in. (26 cm) by about 4 in. (10 cm). It can hold about 1 qt. (0.9 L) of semiliquid chyme.

The wall of the stomach is made up of four layers: the mucous, submucous, muscular, and peritoneal layers. The mucous and submucous layers are made up of ridges called rugae. Within the ridges are gastric glands that consist of mucous cells, parietal cells, chief cells, and G-cells. Each of these cells secretes a chemical that aids in the process of digestion.

The muscular layer is actually composed of three different layers of smooth muscle, each with fibers running in a different direction: horizontal, vertical, and diagonal. The muscles are responsible for mixing the chyme and moving it through the stomach to the small intestine.

The peritoneal layer is the outer layer of stomach tissue. It is part of the peritoneum that lines the inside of the abdomen, covering most of the organs. It does not play a role in digestion.

The stomach has a large supply of **blood vessels** for the absorption of nutrients from digested food. Branches of the vagus nerve supply both sensory and nervous fibers to the stomach.

Function

The stomach functions in various ways including food storage, exocrine secretions, endocrine secretions, and muscular activity.

Food storage

The stomach's primary role is to act as a temporary receptacle for food. While the food is in the stomach, it is mixed with gastric juices that are secreted by cells in the mucosal layer.

There are three general phases regulating gastric juice secretion. The first, or cephalic, phase occurs before food is actually eaten. The thought, **smell** and sight of food cause the **brain** to send signals to the stomach to increase its gastric secretions. The second phase is the gastric phase, which occurs when food enters the stomach. The food causes the stomach to stretch, which in turn sends nervous impulses to the brain. The brain sends return impulses back to the stomach to begin secreting gastrin. Gastrin then stimulates the release of other gastric juices. The third phase is called the intestinal phase, which occurs when food enters the small intestine. This phase results in a decrease in the movement of chyme into the small intestine, ensuring that the small intestine does not receive too much chyme at one time.

The stomach secretes from 2 to 3 qt. (1.9 to 2.8 L) of gastric juices every day. Several types of specialized cells in the stomach secrete gastric juices. Like the **pancreas**, the stomach has both exocrine and endocrine glandular functions. Exocrine secretory glands contain three types of secretory cells: chief cells, parietal cells, and mucous cells. Endocrine cells called G-cells are scattered throughout the mucosa.

Exocrine secretions

Exocrine glands are located in the fundus and body of the stomach. The chief cells in these exocrine glands secrete pepsinogen, the inactive precursor of pepsin. Pepsin is an enzyme that is responsible for the initial breakdown of protein molecules into smaller polypeptides. If pepsin did not have an inactive form, it would destroy the chief cells as they produced it. Pepsin can be activated in the stomach, because the stomach lining is protected from its action.

The exocrine glands of the fundus and body of the stomach also contain parietal cells. These parietal cells secrete hydrochloric acid (HCl), which makes the stomach strongly acidic, with a pH of about 2 or 3. This is an optimal pH for the action of pepsin. Hydrochloric acid is responsible for transforming the inactive pepsinogen into active pepsin. The hydrochloric acid in the chyme also stimulates the production of pancreatic and biliary secretions that further stimulate digestion. The acidic environment kills most **bacteria** that enter the digestive tract through the mouth. Parietal cells also release a chemical called the intrinsic factor, which is necessary for the absorption of **vitamin B$_{12}$**.

Mucous cells release an alkaline mucous fluid into the gastric wall, protecting it against the damaging action of stomach acid. The fluid neutralizes the hydrochloric acid and also acts as a lubricant, protecting the inner lining of the stomach.

Endocrine secretions

The G-cells are the only endocrine cells located in the stomach and are located mainly in the antrum of the stomach where there are few acid producing cells. G-cells release the hormone gastrin into the bloodstream. Gastrin acts on the parietal cells, stimulating them to release hydrochloric acid.

Muscular activity

The stomach must undergo muscular contractions in order to mix food and gastric juices together. These

---

KEY TERMS

Antrum—The lower portion of the stomach near the pyloric sphincter.

Chyme—The mass of semiliquid, partially digested food found in the stomach.

Fundus—The upper portion of the stomach near the esophagus.

Gastrin—A hormone that stimulates the secretion of gastric juice.

Gastritis—Inflammation of the stomach.

Gastroenteritis—Inflammation of the stomach and the intestines.

Lumen—The hollow inside a tubular organ such as the digestive tract.

Pepsin—An enzyme produced in the stomach that breaks down proteins in the presence of hydrochloric acid.

Peristalsis—Muscular contractions that move food through the digestive tract.

Retropulsion—A process in which muscular contractions push food that has entered the duodenum backward into the stomach. Retropulsion helps to mix the chyme with gastric juices, and to break large lumps of food into smaller pieces.

Rugae—Ridges or folds in the mucosal and submucosal layers of tissue in the wall of the stomach.

Sphincter—A circular band of muscle that encircles an orifice of the body or one of its hollow organs, such as the digestive tract.

---

waves of involuntary muscular contractions are called peristalsis. When food is present, peristaltic contractions pass through the stomach muscles about two or three times every minute and continue at a constant rhythm. Pressure will begin to develop in the lower part of the stomach. When there is sufficient pressure, a small amount of the stomach's contents moves through the pyloric sphincter and into the duodenum (the first section of the small intestine). It takes about two to six hours for the entire contents of the stomach to empty, depending on the composition of the person's diet. Low-fat meals leave the stomach more quickly than high-fat meals. Psychological states also affect the rate of stomach emptying; depression and fear may cause the stomach to empty slowly, while anger and aggression may cause the stomach to empty quickly.

After the chyme has entered the duodenum and the pyloric sphincter has closed, some of the food returns to the stomach through retropulsion. Retropulsion is a process in which the stomach contents are squirted back into the stomach at a rate of about three times per minute. Retropulsion mixes the food with gastric juices and breaks larger clumps of food into smaller pieces.

Role in human health

The stomach prepares food for digestion in the small intestine. If the stomach is not functioning properly, many problems can arise with regard to digestion. Further, the contents of the stomach are so acidic and caustic to other organs of the body that they can cause problems if they leak out of the stomach, as may happen with perforating ulcers of the duodenum or penetrating **wounds** of the abdomen.

Diseases and disorders

There are various diseases and disorders of the stomach. Some of them include **gastritis**, gastroenteritis, peptic ulcer disease, gastroesophageal reflux, and stomach cancer.

Gastritis

Gastritis is a common health problem. It is an inflammation of the gastric mucosal layer caused by a range of factors, including bacterial infections, medications (particularly **nonsteroidal anti-inflammatory drugs**, or NSAIDs), acute **stress**, and spicy foods or alcohol. Gastritis can result in a lowered functioning of chief cells and parietal cells. Less pepsin is provided to the stomach, resulting in incomplete breakdown of **proteins**. There is also less stomach acid secretion, allowing overgrowth of microbial populations and a decrease in the absorption of vitamin B_{12}. Gastritis can occur at any age, but chronic gastritis is frequently seen in the elderly.

Gastroenteritis

Gastroenteritis is another common disorder of the digestive tract, characterized by inflammation of the stomach and the intestines. It is the most common cause of mortality in underdeveloped nations. In the United States, it ranks second to the **common cold** as a cause of lost work time. Gastroenteritis is caused by specific bacteria (e.g., *Staphylococcus aureus*, *Escherichia coli*), amebae, or other **parasites**. The symptoms of gastroenteritis include **diarrhea**, nausea, **vomiting**, and abdominal cramping. Patients can become dehydrated and

malnourished if this disorder continues over an extended period of time.

Peptic ulcer disease

Peptic ulcers can occur in the stomach, although they are more likely to develop in the small intestine. Small lesions develop in the mucosal membrane, causing bleeding. Other symptoms include **heartburn** and indigestion. Researchers think that a bacterium (*Helicobacter pylori*) or heavy consumption of aspirin can cause this type of ulcer. Although peptic ulcer disease can occur in children, it usually affects people from 20 to 50 years of age.

Gastroesophageal reflux

Gastroesophageal reflux (GER) or gastroesophageal reflux disease (GERD) is caused by a malfunctioning sphincter between the esophagus and the stomach, resulting in a release of chyme back into the esophagus. The esophagus cannot tolerate the acidic nature of the chyme. Consequently, the acid causes a burning sensation called heartburn. Generally, taking **antacids** after meals or medications to reduce acid secretion can relieve GERD. Severe cases may require surgery.

Cancer of the stomach

Cancer of the stomach affects over 21,000 people in the United States each year. It occurs most often in adults over 55 years of age; it is more common in men than in women, and more common in African Americans than in Caucasian Americans. Stomach cancer may develop in any part of the stomach and metastasize (spread) to other parts of the digestive tract or to such distant organs as the ovaries or **lungs**. The early symptoms of stomach cancer are often vague and nonspecific, which means that they can be caused by a range of other health problems. A definite diagnosis of stomach cancer requires a series of laboratory tests and a biopsy of a tissue sample obtained by an instrument called a gastroscope.

The most common treatment for stomach cancer is surgical removal of part or all of the stomach. This procedure is called a gastrectomy. Patients with stomach cancer may also be treated with **chemotherapy**, radiation therapy, or immunotherapy.

Resources

BOOKS

Canard, Jean Marc, et al. *Gastrointestinal Endoscopy in Practice.* Elsevier/Churchill Livingstone, 2011.

Narins, Brigham, editor. *The Gale Encyclopedia of Surgery and Medical Tests: A Guide for Patients and Caregivers.* Detroit: Gale, Cengage Learning, 2009.

Porter, Robert S., and Justin L. Kaplan. *Merck Manual of Diagnosis and Therapy.* Whitehouse Station, NJ: Merck Sharp & Dohme, 2011.

Professional Guide to Diseases. Philadelphia: Wolters Kluwer Health/Lippincott Williams & Wilkins, 2009.

Talley, Nicholas J. editor. *Clinical Gastroenterology: A Practical Problem-based Approach.* Sydney: Churchill Livingstone/Elsevier, 2011.

WEBSITES

Digestive Disorders Health Center WebMD. (August 2, 2011). http://www.webmd.com/digestive-disorders/picture-of-the-stomach (accessed April 27, 2012).

Stomach Disorders Medline Plus. (February 24, 2012). http://www.nlm.nih.gov/medlineplus/stomachdisorders.html (accessed April 26, 2012).

Stomach (Gastric) Cancer. National Cancer Institute. http://www.cancer.gov/cancertopics/types/stomach (accessed April 26, 2012).

What are the Key Statistics about Stomach Cancer? American Cancer Society. (December 6, 2011). http://www.cancer.org/Cancer/StomachCancer/DetailedGuide/stomach-cancer-key-statistics (accessed April 26, 2012).

ORGANIZATIONS

American College of Gastroenterology, 6400 Goldsboro Rd., Ste. 200, Bethesda, MD 20817, (301) 263-9000, http://www.acg.gi.org

American Gastroenterological Association, 4930 Del Ray Ave., Bethesda, MD 20814, (301) 654-2055, Fax: (301) 654-5920, member@gastro.org, http://www.gastro.org/

National Digestive Diseases Information Clearinghouse, 2 Information Way, Bethesda, MD 20892-3570, Fax: (703) 738-4929, (800) 891-5389, nddic@info.niddk.nih.gov, http://digestive.niddk.nih.gov/

Society of American Gastrointestinal Endoscopic Surgeons, 11300 West Olympic Boulevard, Ste. 600, Los Angeles, CA 90064, (310) 437-0544, Fax: (310) 437-0585, webmaster@sages.org, http://www.sages.org/

Society of Gastroenterology Nurses and Associates, Inc., 401 North Michigan Ave., Chicago, IL 60611-4267, (312) 321-5165, Fax: (312) 673-6694, (800) 245-7462, sgna@smithbucklin.com, http://www.sgna.org/.

Sally C. McFarlane-Parrott
William A. Atkins, BB, BS, MBA

Stomach acid determination *see* **Gastric analysis**

▌ Stomatitis

Definition

Stomatitis is an inflammation of the mucous membranes of the mouth. It may involve the cheeks, gums, tongue, lips, and roof or floor of the mouth. The inflammation may be caused by conditions within the mouth itself, such as poor **oral hygiene** and poorly fitted dentures, or from mouth **burns** caused by hot foods or drinks. It also may be caused by factors affecting the entire body, such as medications, allergic reactions, or infections.

Description

Stomatitis is an inflammation of the lining of any of the soft-tissue structures of the mouth. It is usually a painful condition, associated with redness, swelling, and occasionally bleeding from the affected area. Stomatitis affects all age groups, from infants to the elderly.

Causes and symptoms

A number of factors can cause stomatitis. Poorly fitted oral appliances, cheek biting, or jagged teeth can persistently irritate the oral structures. Chronic mouth breathing may cause dryness of the mouth tissues, which in turn can lead to irritation. Drinking beverages that are too hot can burn the mouth, causing irritation and **pain**. Some diseases, such as infections (bacterial, viral, and fungal), gonorrhea, measles, leukemia, pellagra, oral erythema multiforme, and **AIDS** may present with oral symptoms. **Chemotherapy** and radiation therapy can cause stomatitis by destroying the healthy cells of the oral cavity. Other causes include deficiencies in the

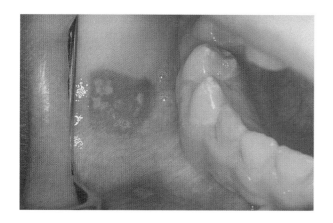

(Canker sore, Stomatitis lesions, photograph by Edward H. Gill. Custom Medical Stock Photo. Reproduced by permission.)

B **vitamins** or **vitamin C**, and **iron deficiency anemia**. Stomatitis may also follow overuse of alcohol, tobacco, and spicy foods, as well as exposure to certain toothpastes and mouthwashes. Exposure to heavy metals, such as mercury, lead, or bismuth may also cause stomatitis.

Aphthous stomatitis, also known as "canker sores," is a specific type of stomatitis that presents with shallow, painful ulcers that are usually located on the lips, cheeks, gums, or roof or floor of the mouth. These ulcers can range from pinpoint size up to 1 inch (2.5 cm) or more in diameter. Though the specific causes of **canker sores** are unknown, nutritional deficiencies are suspected.

The symptoms of stomatitis may include:

• reddened mucous membranes in the mouth

• painful areas in the mouth

• increased sensitivity to spicy foods

• presence of ulcers in the oral cavity

• dry or swollen tongue

• difficulty swallowing

Diagnosis

The patient will often present with complaints of painful lesions in the oral cavity. The physician or nurse performs a thorough assessment of the mouth, noting any signs of stomatitis. Regular oral examinations are especially important for the patient undergoing **cancer** treatment. A patient's history may disclose a dietary deficiency, a systemic disease, or contact with materials causing an allergic reaction. **Blood** tests may be done to determine if any **infection** is present. Cultures of the mouth may be sent to the laboratory for microscopic

KEY TERM

Aphthous stomatitis—A specific type of stomatitis presenting with shallow, painful ulcers. Also known as canker sores.

evaluation, again to determine if an infectious agent is causing the stomatitis.

Treatment

The treatment of stomatitis is based on the problem causing it. Local cleansing and good oral hygiene are essential. Sharp-edged foods such as peanuts, tacos, and potato chips should be avoided. A soft-bristled toothbrush should be used, and the teeth and gums should be brushed very carefully. A dentist can correct local factors, including ill-fitting dental appliances. Infectious causes can usually be treated with **antibiotics** or other medications. Systemic causes, such as AIDS, leukemia, and anemia are treated by the appropriate medical specialist. Minor mouth burns from hot beverages or hot foods will usually resolve on their own in a week or so. Chronic problems with aphthous stomatitis are treated by first correcting any nutritional deficiencies. If those measures are ineffective, medication can be prescribed that is applied to each aphthous ulcer with a cotton-tipped applicator. This therapy is only successful with a limited number of patients. Mouth pain can be alleviated through the use of prescribed topical or oral **analgesics**.

Other treatments include measures to maintain oral hygiene and increase comfort as the stomatitis heals. These measures include:

• Avoiding spicy or acidic foods, or very hot foods.

• Avoiding tobacco products and alcohol.

• Rinsing the oral cavity after meals and before bedtime with a mild saltwater or baking soda and water solution to help keep the mouth clean and free of debris.

Some limited studies have suggested that a few alternative therapies may be effective in preventing and treating stomatitis. These include the use of glutomine, an amino acid; **vitamin E** supplementation; and chamomile mouthwashes. The patient with stomatitis should be instructed to consult their health care professional prior to using any alternative treatments.

Prognosis

The prognosis for the resolution of stomatitis is based on the cause of the problem. Many local factors can be modified, treated, or avoided. Infectious causes of stomatitis can normally be managed with medications. Uncomplicated cases of stomatitis caused by cancer treatment will usually resolve within two to four weeks.

Health care team roles

The physician and nurse are responsible for thoroughly assessing the oral cavity for signs and symptoms of stomatitis. An awareness of the causes and associated conditions is important when treating the patient. The nurse should instruct the patient on the appropriate treatment and preventative measures, and about any medications used to treat the stomatitis.

Prevention

Stomatitis caused by local irritants can be prevented by good oral hygiene, regular dental checkups, and good dietary habits. Problems with stomatitis caused by systemic diseases can be minimized by practicing good oral hygiene measures, and by closely following the medical therapy prescribed. Cancer patients undergoing treatment can decrease the severity of stomatitis by maintaining good nutritional intake, good oral hygiene, and by having frequent assessments of the oral cavity by their health care professional.

Resources

BOOK

Beers, Mark H., and Robert Berkow. *The Merck Manual of Diagnosis and Therapy,* 17th ed. Whitehouse Station, NJ: Merck and Company, Inc., 1999.

PERIODICAL

Canker Sores—What Are They and What Can You Do About Them? *American Family Physician* (July 1, 2000).

ORGANIZATION

American Dental Association, 211 E. Chicago Ave., Chicago, IL 60611. (312) 440-2500. http://www.ada.org.

Deanna M. Swartout-Corbeil, R.N.

Stone analysis

Definition

Kidney stones are solid accumulations of material that form through precipitation in the tubal system of the kidney. Kidney stones cause problems when they block the flow of urine through or out of the kidney. When the stones move along the ureter, they cause severe **pain**.

Gallbladder stones are solid accumulations of material that form through precipitation in the **liver** and then move into the gall bladder. They cause problems when they block the flow of bile out of the liver or out of the gall bladder. They can cause attacks of gall bladder disease (cholecystitis), hepatitis, or **pancreatitis**. They can also cause severe pain.

Purpose

The purpose of analyzing kidney and gallbladder stones is to determine the source of the stones. Different materials can form stones. Once the source of the stones is known, steps can be taken to prevent subsequent formation.

Precautions

An adequately stocked laboratory is needed for accurate analysis of stones. The most difficult aspect of stone analysis is obtaining the stones.

Passing a kidney stone is exquisitely painful. Once passed, persons with stones must strain their urine to recover any stones. Retrieving a kidney stone is painful for the person experiencing the stone. It also requires skill on the part of an operator to retrieve the stone.

A gallbladder stone must also be obtained before chemical analysis can be performed. Gallbladder stones can become lodged at several locations and cause considerable pain and discomfort. Retrieving a stone usually requires surgery. Commonly, the gallbladder is removed in the process of collecting a stone.

Description

Kidney stones

Urine is formed by the **kidneys**. The kidney is made up of microscopic units called nephrons. Each nephron contains a capillary tuft (glomerulus) and a tubule. **Blood** flows into the kidneys, and engorges the capillary tufts. Water and small solutes pass through the vessel walls forming a filtrate of the plasma that enters the underlying space (Bowman's capsule). The walls of the capsule form a tubule that traverses the kidney. The cells of the tubule modify the filtrate along its length ultimately forming the urine, which passes out of the body. Sometimes, a problem causes the dissolved solutes to become supersaturated resulting in the formation of crystals. When tiny crystals associate together they form a larger solid mass called a kidney stone or calculus. A kidney stone is also called a nephrolith or urolith (nephro- refers to the kidney, uro-

refers to urine, and -lith means stone). Kidney stones have multifactorial causes, but some predisposing conditions are:

• Diet: Excessive calcium in water and foods rich in oxalate or purines can lead to excessive excretion of calcium, oxalate, and uric acid in urine.

• Dehydration: Water deprivation or loss from other sources causes stasis in the tubules and concentrates the solutes there.

• Deficiency of inhibitors: Some dietary substances such as ascorbic acid and citric acid promote loss of organic calcium salts that are soluble. Absence of these can lead to excessive amounts of oxalate and phosphate.

• Drugs: Some drugs such as tetracycline are poorly soluble and may precipitate, forming stones or becoming part of the stone matrix.

• Metabolic disorders: Hyperparathyroidism causes excessive calcium excretion by the kidneys. Cystine stones form because of a defect in the renal tubular reabsorption of dibasic amino acids, a condition known as cystinuria.

• Genetics: Some people produce and excrete greater quantities of certain metabolites such as uric acid.

• pH: Most solutes are only soluble within a finite pH range. For example, phosphates and carbonates are insoluble at an alkaline pH. Uric acid and calcium oxalate are insoluble at an acidic pH. People who produce chronic acid urine are more prone to develop uric acid and calcium oxalate crystals.

Many people never find out that they have stones in their kidneys. These stones are small enough to allow the kidney to continue functioning normally, never causing any pain. These are called silent stones. Kidney stones cause problems when they interfere with the normal flow of urine. They can block (obstruct) the flow down the tube (the ureter) that carries urine from the kidney to the bladder. The kidney does not normally experience any back pressure. When pressure builds from backed-up urine, the kidney may swell (hydronephrosis). If the kidney is subjected to this pressure for some time, it may cause damage to the delicate kidney structures. In the most severe case, this back pressure causes the pressure in Bowman's space to equal the **blood pressure** in the glomerular capillaries and filtration stops. The person stops producing urine, and waste products accumulate in the blood leading to renal failure. When the kidney stone is lodged further down the ureter, the backed-up urine may also cause the ureter to swell (hydroureter). Because the ureters are muscular tubes, the presence of a stone will make these muscular tubes spasm, causing severe pain.

About 10% of all people will have a kidney stone in their lifetimes. Kidney stones are most common among:

• Caucasians

• males

• people over the age of 30

• people who previously have had kidney stones

• relatives of persons with kidney stones

Gallbladder stones

Approximately 80% of gallbladder stones are primarily **cholesterol** (over 70% cholesterol by weight). They also contain bile pigments, bile acids, fatty acids, and **calcium** salts. The remainder of gall stones are primarily made of bilirubin. The primary constituents are calcium bilirubinate, calcium phosphate, and calcium carbonate. A gallbladder stone is also called a cholelith (chole- refers to the gallbladder and -lith means stone). Cholesterol-rich gallbladder stones typically develop when the following three conditions exist:

• supersaturation of gallbladder, due mainly to increased biliary cholesterol secretion

• abnormally rapid precipitation of micro-crystals of cholesterol due to an excess of promoters and/or a shortage of inhibitors of crystallization

• stasis within the gallbladder due to the combination of impaired motility, primarily reduced emptying in response to food and/or crystal trapping by an abnormally thick mucous glycoprotein on the gallbladder lining

Many people do not realize that they have stones in their gallbladders. These stones are small enough to allow the liver, gallbladder, and **pancreas** to continue functioning normally, never causing any pain. Gallbladder stones cause problems when they interfere with the normal flow of bile. They can obstruct the flow down the common bile duct that carries bile from the gallbladder to the **small intestine**. Gall stones may obstruct the pancreatic duct, the tube that connects the pancreas with the common bile duct. This can cause inflammation of the pancreas (pancreatitis). The pancreas and gallbladder do not normally experience any back pressure. When pressure builds from backed-up bile (gall bladder) or pancreatic secretions (pancreas), swelling will occur. If the pancreas is subjected to this pressure for some time, it may cause damage to the internal structures of the organ. When the gallbladder is subjected to pressure, it simply enlarges and exerts pressure on the liver. When a gallbladder stone is lodged at the end of the common bile duct (in the Sphincter of Oddi where it opens into the small intestine), the backed-up bile may also cause all of the structures (liver, gall bladder, pancreas, and ducts) to swell. Because the ducts have muscle tissue in their walls, the presence of a stone will make them spasm, causing pain.

About 12% of men and 25% of all women will develop gallstones in their lifetimes. Gallbladder stones are most common among:

• Caucasians

• females

• women who have had children

• people over the age of 40

• people who previously have had gallbladder stones

• people who are overweight

Composition of stones

Kidney stones can be composed of a variety of substances. About three-fourths of kidney stones contain calcium. The most prevalent kidney stone is made up of calcium oxalate usually in combination with other calcium salts. In addition to the chemical name, stones are often described by their mineralogical properties. For example, calcium oxalate exists in two forms, the monohydrate which is called whewellite and the dihydrate which is called weddellite. The most common types of kidney stones include:

• calcium oxalate (whewellite and weddellite)

• magnesium ammonium phosphate (struvite)

• tricalcium phosphate (whitlockite); calcium phosphate (apatite); and calcium hydrogen phosphate dihydrate (brushite)

• uric acid stones

Gallbladder stones are usually composed of cholesterol. They also contain some:

• bile pigments

• bile acid

• calcium salts

People who have kidney stones usually do not have symptoms until the stones pass into the ureter. Prior to this, some individuals may notice blood in their urine. Once the stone is in the ureter, however, most people will experience bouts of very severe pain. The pain is crampy and spasmodic, and is referred to as "colic." The pain usually begins in the flank region, the area between the lower ribs and the pelvis. As the stone moves closer to the bladder, a person will often feel the pain radiating along the inner thigh. In women, the pain may be felt in the vulva. In men, the pain may be felt in the testicles. Nausea, **vomiting**, extremely frequent and painful urination, and obvious blood in the urine are common. **Fever** and chills usually mean that the ureter has become obstructed, allowing **bacteria** to become trapped in the kidney causing a kidney **infection** (pyelonephritis).

People who have gallbladder stones usually do not have symptoms until the stones pass into the common bile duct. Once the stone is in the common bile duct, however, most people will experience bouts of pain, especially after eating fatty meals. The pain is also referred to as colicky. The pain usually begins in the upper right quadrant of the **abdomen**, the area just beneath the right ribs. As the stone moves closer to the Sphincter of Oddi, a person will often feel the pain radiating throughout the entire abdomen. If it obstructs the pancreatic duct, it may be felt in the posterior portion of the abdomen as flank pain. Nausea, vomiting, light (clay) colored stools, and flatulence are common. Fever and chills usually mean that the Sphincter of Oddi has become obstructed, forcing pancreatic fluid and liver discharges to be trapped in their respective organs, often causing inflammation of the liver (hepatitis), gallbladder (cholecystitis), and pancreas (pancreatitis).

Preparation

Kidney stones that are less than 5 mm in diameter are usually passed. The physician or nurse must instruct the patient in the proper technique to recover the stone once it is passed. Special laboratory equipment is required for stone analysis. Most clinical laboratories do not perform this service. Consequently the stone must be packaged and mailed to a reference laboratory that performs stone analysis.

Laboratory analysis

For the most part, the analysis is qualitative in nature. Testing involves macroscopic evaluation of the stone. This includes determination of its weight, size, shape, hardness, and color. Kidney stones are usually analyzed by x ray diffraction. The stone is pulverized into a fine powder and the powder is spread over a glass fiber mat and exposed to x rays. The crystals scatter the x rays and the various patterns produced are analyzed to determine the chemical composition. The composition of noncrystalline stones cannot be determined by this method and are usually analyzed by infrared spectroscopy. These crystals are usually composed of drugs or their metabolites that precipitated in the tubules. In special cases the stone may be analyzed by chemical analysis and by microscopic analysis. For example, cystine stones can be readily detected by grinding a small piece of the stone into a powder. The powder is boiled in a small amount of deionized water and a solution of sodium cyanide is added. The cyanide reduces the cystine to cystiene. After standing for five minutes, several drops of sodium nitroprusside are added. The solution will turn red if cystiene is present. Gall stones are composed of either cholesterol or bilirubin. These can be analyzed by infrared analysis, x-ray diffraction or chemical analysis (detection of cholesterol and bilirubin after organic extracton).

Many stones can be seen using a basic x ray, but some cannot. A more sensitive imaging procedure is to use a series of x rays taken after injecting iodine dye into a vein. This procedure is called an intravenous pyelogram (IVP). The dye allows the **urinary system** to be visualized. In the case of an obstruction, the dye will be stopped by the stone or will only be able to get past the stone at a slow trickle.

A cholangiogram is used to visualize the location of a gallbladder stone that is causing an obstruction. A tube is passed through the mouth, throat, and **stomach**. It enters the small intestine and is inserted into the Sphincter of Oddi. Dye is injected, allowing the interior of the common bile duct and connected structures to be visualized. As with a kidney stone, the dye is stopped by an obstruction, allowing a radiographer to pinpoint the position of a stone. A CT or MRI scan may also be used to locate a gallbladder stone.

Persons are prepared prior to obtaining a stone for analysis. Preparation for surgery (gallstones) involves anesthesia. Preparation for collecting passed kidney stones involves straining urine through a special sieve. Preparation for surgical collection of a kidney stone involves sedation and passing a catheter through a person's urethra and bladder before entering the ureter.

Aftercare

After stones have been analyzed, the goal becomes preventing subsequent formation by eliminating the cause of the stone.

Prevention

Prevention of kidney stones depends on the type of stone and the presence of an underlying disease. In almost all cases, increasing fluid intake so that a person consistently drinks several quarts of water a day is an important preventive measure. Persons with calcium stones may benefit from taking a medication called a diuretic, which has the effect of decreasing the amount of calcium passed in the urine. Eating less meat, fish, and chicken may be helpful for individuals with calcium oxalate stones. Other items in the diet that may encourage calcium oxalate stone formation include beer, black pepper, berries, broccoli, chocolate, spinach, and tea. Uric acid stones may require treatment with a medication

called allopurinol. Struvite stones will require removal and an affected person should receive an antibiotic. Adjustment of pH is an important preventive measure. For example, if the stone contains calcium phosphate or calcium carbonate or a mixture of these, an acidifier is used to keep the urine pH below seven because these stones form in alkaline urine. When a disease is identified as the cause of stone formation, treatment specific to that disease may lessen the likelihood of repeated stones.

Preventing gallbladder stones is usually accomplished by dietary modification. Fat intake must be diminished. This will also prevent intestinal **colic** as the gallbladder is usually removed. Drugs that inhibit the formation of cholesterol by the liver may be used. **Niacin**, cholestyramine, cholestipol, lovastatin, simvastatin, pravastatin, fluvaststin, and gemfibrazol have all been approved for use in the United States. Some experts recommend daily supplements of methionine. The drug ursodiol (Actigall) has also been approved for treatment of gallbladder stones.

Complications

Complications of actual stone analysis include laboratory error. These are very rare.

Complications for people with stones include recurrence. They also may include adverse drug reactions. These, too, are uncommon.

Results

A person with a kidney stone will say that the most important aspect of treatment is adequate pain relief. Because the pain of passing a kidney stone is so severe, narcotic pain medications (such as meperidine or morphine) are often required. It is believed that stones may pass more quickly if a person is encouraged to drink large amounts of water (2-3 quarts, or 2-3 L per day). If an individual is vomiting or unable to drink because of the pain, it may be necessary to provide fluids through a vein. If symptoms and urine tests indicate the presence of infection, **antibiotics** will be required.

A person with a gallbladder stone also finds that the most important aspect of treatment is adequate pain relief. Because the pain of gallbladder disease attacks are so uncomfortable, pain medications (such as ibuprofen or acetaminophen with codeine) are often required. If symptoms and tests indicate the presence of infection, antibiotics will be required.

Treatment

Although most kidney stones will pass on their own, some will not. Surgical removal of a stone may

KEY TERMS

Cholangiogram—X-ray technique used to visualize gallbladder stones.

Cholecystitis—Inflammation of the gallbladder.

Cholelith—Gallbladder stone.

Hepatitis—Inflammation of the liver.

Hydronephrosis—Swelling of a kidney due to elevated pressure from excess fluid accumulation.

Hydroureter—Swelling of a ureter due to elevated pressure from excess fluid accumulation.

Intravenous pyelogram (IVP)—X-ray technique used to visualize kidney stones.

Laparoscopic cholecystectomy—Surgical procedure for removing a gallbladder.

Lithotripsy—Technique that uses focused sound waves to pulverize kidney stones, thus avoiding surgery.

Nephrolith—Kidney stone.

Nephron—Tube within the kidney that processes filtrate from the blood, reclaiming some substances and creating urine.

Pancreatitis—Inflammation of the pancreas.

Pyelonephritis—Infection of the kidney.

Sphincter of Oddi—The opening of the common bile duct into the small intestine.

Ureter—Tube that connects the kidney and urinary bladder. Its function is to transport urine.

become necessary when a stone appears too large to pass. Surgery may also be required if the stone is causing serious obstructions, pain that cannot be treated, heavy bleeding, or infection. Several alternatives exist for removing stones. One method involves passing a tube into the bladder and up into the ureter. A tiny basket is then passed through the tube, and an attempt is made to snare the stone and pull it out. Open surgery to remove an obstructing kidney stone was relatively common in the past, but current methods allow the stone to be crushed with **shock** waves (called **lithotripsy**). These shock waves may be aimed at the stone from outside of the body by passing the necessary equipment through the bladder and into the ureter. The shock waves may be aimed at the stone from inside the body by placing the instrument through a tiny incision located near the stone. The stone fragments may then pass on their own or may be removed through the

incision. All of these methods reduce an individual's recovery time considerably when compared to the traditional open operation.

An individual with a gallbladder stone will usually have the gallbladder removed. The most common procedure for this task is a laparoscopic cholecystectomy. Three small incisions are made in the abdomen. Into one, a thin tube with a light and camera lens is passed. Into the second and third, thin tubes through which instruments are inserted, are passed. A surgeon visualizes the interior of the abdomen on a television screen using the camera in the first tube and removes the gall bladder using the instruments inserted through the second and third tubes. Using this approach, post-surgical complications have been reduced, and the time required for recovery has been significantly reduced (when compared to traditional open surgical techniques).

Health care team roles

A physician makes an initial diagnosis of kidney or gall stones. A radiologist confirms the diagnosis using x rays or **ultrasonography**. A surgeon is needed to operatively remove a kidney or gall stone. Lithotripsy is performed by a technician under the supervision of a physician. Occasionally, open surgery is required and is performed by a surgeon. Nurses assist in lithotripsy and surgery. A laboratory specialist performs a chemical analysis of the stone to determine its composition and origin. Pharmacists may dispense pain medications and antibiotics as required.

Resources

BOOKS

Asplin, John, Coe, Frederic L., and Favus, Murray. "Nephrolithiasis." In *Harrison's Principles of Internal Medicine*, 18th ed. New York: McGraw-Hill, 2011

Berci, George, and Cuschieri, A. *Bile Ducts and Bile Duct Stones*. Philadelphia: Saunders, 1997.

Gennari, F. John. *Medical Management of Kidney and Electrolyte Disorders*. New York: Marcel Dekker, 2001.

Greenberger, Norton J., and Isselbacher, Kurt J. "Diseases of the gallbladder and bile ducts." In *Harrison's Principles of Internal Medicine, 14th ed.*, edited by Anthony S. Fauci, et al. New York: McGraw-Hill, 1998, 1725–1737.

Hruska, Keith. "Renal calculi (nephrolithiasis)." In *Cecil Textbook of Medicine, 21st ed.*, edited by Goldman, Lee, and Bennett, J. Claude. Philadelphia: W. B. Saunders, 2000, 622–627.

Massry, Shaul G., and Glassock, Richard J. *Massry & Glassock's Textbook of Nephrology, 4th ed.* Philadelphia: Lippincott Williams & Wilkins, 2001.

Nakayama, Fumio. *Cholelithiasis: Causes and Treatment.* Tokyo: Igaku-Shoin Medical Publishers, 2000.

Savitz, Gail, Leslie, Stephen W., and Golomb, Gail. *The Kidney Stones Handbook: A Patient's Guide to Hope, Cure and Prevention.* Roseville, CA: Four Geez Press, 1999.

Vlahcevic, ZR, and Heuman, DM. "Diseases of the gallbladder and bile ducts." In *Cecil Textbook of Medicine, 21st ed.,* edited by Goldman, Lee, and Bennett, J. Claude. Philadelphia: W. B. Saunders, 2000, 439-442.

PERIODICALS

de Lorimier, A. A. "Alcohol, wine, and health." *American Journal of Surgery* 180, no. 5 (2000): 357-361.

Grases, F., Sohnel, O., Costa-Bauza, A. "Renal stone formation and development." *International Journal of Urology and Nephrology* 31, no. 5 (1999): 591-600.

Kim, H. J., Kim, M. H., Lee, S. K., Yoo, K. S., Seo, D. W., Min, Y. I., Lee, B. S. "Characterization of primary pure cholesterol hepatolithiasis: cholangioscopic and selective cholangiographic findings." *Gastrointestinal Endoscopy* 53, no. 3 (2001): 324-328.

McConnell, E. A. "Myths & facts ... about kidney stones." *Nursing* 31, no. 1 (2001): 73-77.

Schweizer, P., Lenz, M. P., Kirschner, H. J. "Pathogenesis and symptomatology of cholelithiasis in childhood. A prospective study." *Digestive Surgery* 17, no. 5 (2000): 459-467.

Traverso, L. W. "A cost analysis of the treatment of common bile duct stones discovered during cholecystectomy." *Seminars in Laparoscopic Surgery* 7, no. 4 (2000): 302-307.

OTHER

American Foundation for Urologic Disease. http://www.afud.org/conditions/ksgloss.html.

Gall Stone Photographs. http://www1.stpaulshosp.bc.ca/stpaulsstuff/NeatcasesF/GBf/GBS_MR.html.

Kidney Stone Photographs. http://www.herringlab.com/photos/.

Lithotripsy. http://pluto.apl.washington.edu/harlett2/artgwww/acoustic/medical/litho.html.

National Kidney and Urologic Diseases Information Clearinghouse. http://www.niddk.nih.gov/health/kidney/pubs/stonadul/stonadul.htm.

Net Doctor (UK). http://www.netdoctor.co.uk/diseases/facts/gallbladderdisease.htm.

University of California Los Angeles. http://www.radsci.ucla.edu:8000/gu/stones/kidneystone.html.

University of Iowa School of Medicine. http://www.vh.org/Patients/IHB/IntMed/ABA30/1994/gall.html.

Vegetarian Society of UK. http://www.vegsoc.org/info/health4.html.

ORGANIZATIONS

American Academy of Family Physicians. 11400 Tomahawk Creek Parkway, Leawood, KS 66211-2672. (913) 906-6000. http://www.aafp.org/. fp@aafp.org.

American Academy of Pediatrics. 141 Northwest Point Boulevard, Elk Grove Village, IL 60007-1098. (847) 434-4000. Fax: (847) 434-8000. http://www.aap.org/default.htm. kidsdoc@aap.org.

American Association for Clinical Chemistry. 2101 L Street, NW - Suite 202, Washington, DC 20037-1558. (800) 892-1400 or (202) 857-0717. Fax: (202) 887-5093. http://www.aacc.org. info@aacc.org.

American Foundation for Urologic Disease. 1128 North Charles Street, Baltimore, MD 21201. (800) 242-2383 or (410) 468-1800. http://www.afud.org. admin@afud.org.

National Kidney Foundation. 30 East 33rd Street, Suite 1100, New York, NY 10016. (800) 622-9010 or (212) 889-2210. Fax: (212) 689-9261. http://www.kidney.org/. info@kidney.org.

L. Fleming Fallon, Jr., MD, DrPH

Stool culture

Definition

A stool culture is a laboratory test used to isolate and identify pathogens in the feces of patients suspected of having digestive tract infections. A sample of the patient's feces is placed on several different types of nutrient media and observed for growth. Any suspicious organisms that grow on the media are identified using microscopic and biochemical tests.

Purpose

Physicians normally order stool cultures on patients with symptoms of gastrointestinal **infection**, most commonly **diarrhea**. The purpose of this test is to isolate **bacteria** or other organisms that might be causing the symptoms so they can be identified. Identification of the causative organism is essential in determining how to treat the patient. For example, administering an antibiotic merely on the basis of the patient's symptoms could, in some cases, make the condition worse.

Precautions

A stool culture is performed only if an infection of the digestive tract is suspected. The test has no harmful effects.

Description

A routine stool culture (also called a fecal culture) is for the isolation of *Campylobacter*, enterotoxigenic *E. coli* (O157:H7), *Shigella*, and *Salmonella*. Less frequently isolated bacterial causes of diarrhea are *Vibrio spp.*, *Yersinia enterocolitica*, and *Aeromonas spp.* Requests for stool cultures for the isolation of other intestinal pathogens should include special instructions.

The most common example is *Clostridium difficile*, which causes pseudomembraneous **colitis**.

Stool cultures may be performed on rectal swabs containing feces or submitted stool samples. Swabs are placed in a tube containing Stuart or other transport medium and then delivered to the laboratory. Cultures for *C. difficile* are usually collected by swabbing the rectum (whereas watery stool is needed for immunoassay of *C. difficile toxin*). The swab must be placed immediately into prereduced (oxygen free) transport medium because this organism is a strict anaerobe. To submit a stool specimen for routine culture, the patient or caregiver collects a stool sample in a special container, taking care not to contaminate the specimen with water, urine, or other materials. Some containers include a transport solution to stabilize the specimen. Although some requests are for stool cultures on two or more consecutive days, a single specimen is considered to be sufficient. It is important to return the specimen to the doctor's office or the laboratory in the time specified by the physician or nurse. Laboratories normally do not accept stool specimens that are contaminated or that arrive after the specified time period.

A routine bacterial stool culture involves placing a sample of the stool on several kinds of enriched and selective media containing nutrients that support the growth of certain types of organisms. Routine culture should include a sheep **blood** agar plate, MacConkey agar plate, MacConkey agar with sorbitol, Hektoen or XLD (xylose lysine desoxycholate) plate, Campy plate, and GN (gram-negative) broth. Blood agar supports the growth of most bacteria including *Staphylococcus aureus*, *Listeria monocytogenes*, and yeast, which are infrequently implicated in food **poisoning** or gastrointestinal infections, but do not grow on the other media. Most intestinal pathogens are gram-negative bacilli. MacConkey agar is selective for these organisms and differentiates those that can ferment lactose from those that cannot. MacConkey sorbitol substitutes sorbitol for lactose. This allows differentiation of nonpathogenic *E. coli* that ferment sorbitol well from the O157:H7 strain, which does not. Hektoen or XLD enhance the growth of *Salmonella* and *Shigella* by suppressing the growth of gram-positive organisms and gram-negative normal flora. They also differentiate lactose and sucrose fermenters such as *E. coli* from *Salmonella* and *Shigella*, which are not. Several drops of the GN broth can be transferred to Hektoen or XLD agar after a four-hour incubation at 96.8°F (36°C). This procedure can yield isolated colonies of a pathogen the next day that can be used to perform biochemical identification, serotyping, and antibiotic susceptibility tests. Campy agar contains 10% sheep blood, sodium bisulfite, and three **antibiotics**. The

sodium bisulfite reduces some of the oxygen in the medium which enhances recovery of *Campylobacter*. The antibiotics prevent other gram-negative bacilli and yeast from growing. All inoculated media except the Campy plate are incubated in air or 5–10% carbon dioxide at 96.8°F (36°C) and are examined for growth at 24 hours and again the next day. Campy plates must be incubated at 107°F (42°C). Plates are examined at 24 hours and each day for the next two days. Cultures for *Clostridium difficile* require CCFA agar and thioglycolate broth. These are incubated in an oxygen free environment at 96.8°F (36°C) for two days. CCFA is cycloserine-cefoxitin fructose agar and it inhibits the growth of other enteric anaerobes found as normal flora in stool. *C. difficile* produces large yellow colonies on CCFA agar that will fluoresce yellow-green.

Gram stains are not performed routinely, but may be requested for the semiquantitation of white blood cells. If any suspicious bacterial colonies grow, they are presumptively identified on the basis of colonial growth, physical characteristics, microscopic features, and biochemical tests. The colonies are subcultured (transferred) to an appropriate medium to obtain a pure culture. This is used to make a suspension of the organism that is inoculated onto biochemical media. Commercially prepared systems for rapid identification are used. These contain multiple pads or wells of media used to test for key defining biochemical characteristics. After overnight incubation, reactions are read by an automated computerized instrument that aids in species identification. Pure cultures are also used to perform antibiotic sensitivity testing. This is typically done by the microtube broth dilution method. This test determines the minimum inhibitory concentration (MIC) of each antibiotic required to prevent growth of the organism. Results are used to determine those antibiotics to which the organism is susceptible.

The length of time needed to perform a stool culture depends on the laboratory instrumentation and the culture methods used. A routine stool culture usually takes 72 hours or longer to complete.

Preparation

Before ordering a stool culture, the physician, or other health care professional, will ask the patient for a complete medical history and perform a **physical examination** to determine possible causes of the gastrointestinal problem. Information about the patient's diet, any medications taken, and recent travel may provide clues to the identity of possible infectious organisms.

A stool culture normally does not require any special preparation. Patients do not need to change their diets before collecting a specimen. Intake of some substances can contaminate the stool specimen and should not be taken the day before collection. These substances include castor oil, bismuth, and laxative preparations containing psyllium hydrophilic mucilloid.

Aftercare

No aftercare is necessary following a stool culture.

Complications

No complications are associated with this test.

Results

Some bacteria that are normal inhabitants of the digestive tract are known as the enteric bacteria. *Escherichia coli, Klebsiella, Enterobacter,* and *Pseudomonas* are members of this group. The enteric bacteria usually do not cause infection in the digestive tract, and are reported as normal flora in a stool culture. Because the presence of normal flora helps to protect against pathogens, the absence of normal flora in a stool culture is also reported. When only normal flora are found the results are reported as "no enteric pathogens found." When normal flora are absent from the stool, a heavy growth of an organism not usually pathogenic may be recovered. Such organisms should be reported in this case.

The following bacteria are not normal inhabitants of the digestive tract, and are known to cause gastrointestinal infection:

• *Campylobacter*

• *Shigella*

• *Salmonella*

• *Yersinia*

• enterotoxigenic *E. coli*

• *Vibrio*

• *Aeromonas*

Although non-toxigenic strains of *E. coli* are normal flora of the intestines, *E. coli* O157:H7 is an intestinal pathogen. It produces a toxin (poison or harmful chemical) that causes severe inflammation and bleeding of the colon. Infection with this enterotoxigenic strain of *E. coli* is usually associated with eating contaminated meat, juice, or fruits.

Clostridium difficile, like enterotoxigenic *E. coli,* can produce a toxin that causes severe diarrhea. However, this bacterium does not become harmful unless the normal intestinal bacteria are suppressed. Patients taking certain antibiotics may be susceptible to infection with *Clostridium difficile.* In some cases, the stool culture is

KEY TERMS

Bismuth—A substance used in medicines to treat diarrhea, nausea, and indigestion.

Enteric—Pertaining to the intestine.

Enterotoxigenic—Refers to an organism that produces toxins in the gastrointestinal tract that cause such things as vomiting, diarrhea, and other symptoms of food poisoning.

Feces—Material excreted by the intestines.

Gastrointestinal—Referring to the digestive tract; the stomach and the intestines.

Normal flora—Refers to normal bacteria found in a healthy person.

Pathogen—An organism that causes disease.

Psyllium hydrophilic mucilloid—A plant material contained in some laxatives.

Toxin—A poison; usually refers to protein poisons produced by bacteria, animals, and some plants.

used to detect the toxin produced by this bacterium. Other bacteria that produce toxins are *Staphylococcus aureus* and *Bacillus cereus.*

If bacteria are not the cause of an intestinal infection, a fungal or viral culture might be necessary. Patients with **AIDS**, or other **immune system** diseases, sometimes have gastrointestinal infections caused by fungal organisms such as *Candida,* or by viral organisms including *Cytomegalovirus* (CMV). *Candida* can also become an opportunistic intestinal pathogen when antibiotics or radiation have destroyed the normal stool flora.

Several intestinal **parasites**, such as *Giardia lamblia,* also cause gastrointestinal infection and diarrhea. Parasites are not cultured, but are identified microscopically with a stool ova and parasites test.

Health care team roles

The physician orders the stool culture, evaluates the results, and determines the most appropriate treatment. Most laboratories provide instructions for the collection of a stool specimen. The physician, nurse, or other health care professional should instruct or assist the patient in collecting the specimen correctly and without contamination. Once the specimen is ready, the patient or health care professional should ensure that the specimen arrives at the laboratory within the time specified. The clinical laboratory scientist, CLS(NCA)/medical technologist, MT (ASCP) performs the stool culture and sensitivity tests.

Resources

BOOKS

Beers, Mark H., and Robert Berkow, eds. "Gastrointestinal Disorders." In *The Merck Manual of Diagnosis and Therapy.* Whitehouse Station, NJ: Merck & Co, Inc. 2005.

Tierney, Lawrence M., Stephen J. McPhee, and Maxine A. Papadakis. *Current Medical Diagnosis and Treatment 2001 (Lange Series).* New York: McGraw-Hill Professional Book Group, 2000.

Zaret, Barry L., Peter I. Jatlow, and Lee D. Katz, eds. *The Yale University School of Medicine Patient's Guide to Medical Tests.* Boston: Houghton Mifflin. 1997.

ORGANIZATIONS

Ontario Association of Medical Laboratories. http://www.oaml.com.

UTMB The University of Texas Medical Branch. 301 University Blvd., Galveston, TX 77555. (409) 772-1011. http://www.utmb.edu/.

Yale University School of Medicine. 367 Cedar Street, New Haven, CT 06510. (203) 785-2643. http://www.info.med.yale.edu/ysm/ysminfo/index.html.

Beverly G. Miller, MT(ASCP)
Toni Rizzo

Stool ova & parasites test

Definition

The stool ova & **parasites** (O & P) test involves examination of a stool (feces) sample for the presence of intestinal parasites. The distinct types of parasites differ with regard to their structures, life stages, and transmission forms. A parasite may be a worm that has a mature form, an immature form (larvae), and eggs (ova). A parasite may be a protozoon with an adult form that lives in the intestines (trophozoite) and a round, encapsulated transmissible form (cyst). Stool analyses examine all parasitic forms that may be present in the sample.

Purpose

The ova and parasites test is performed to identify intestinal parasites and their eggs or cysts in patients with symptoms of gastrointestinal **infection**. Patients may have no symptoms, or may experience **diarrhea**, **blood** in the stools, and other gastrointestinal distress. Stool O & P testing is usually ordered along with tests for the bacterium *Clostridium difficile* as well as a **stool culture** since overlapping symptoms may result from bacterial or parasitic infections.

Identification of a particular parasite indicates the cause of the patient's disease and determines the medication needed to treat it.

Precautions

Health care providers should always use proper **infection control** procedures when handling stool samples, since they can contain potentially infectious materials.

Description

The stool O & P test is also called the stool ova and parasites test or the ova and parasites collection. Examination of the stool for ova and parasites is done to diagnose parasitic infection of the intestines. Parasites can go through several different life stages depending on the unique characteristics of each type of parasite. For example, the parasite *Entamoeba histolytica* causes amebiasis, a parasitic intestinal infection that can cause diarrhea and cramps. This disease is common in developing countries with poor sanitation or in the United States in institutions with poor hygiene practices. The stool of an infected person contains cysts of the parasite. These cysts have a protective covering and can survive outside the body in feces. If food or water is contaminated with such feces, another person can consume the cysts. Mature cysts that are ingested then turn into trophozoites that feed inside the **large intestine**. Some trophozoites then begin to encyst and create protective walls around their small, round center. These cysts are then expelled from the body in feces that can infect food or water, and the transmission process to another person is repeated. Stool O & P tests require the health care professional to identify parasites in a variety of structural forms.

The most common intestinal parasites in North America that cause infections are:

- roundworms: *Ascaris lumbricoides*

- hookworms: *Necator americanus*

- pinworms: *Enterobius vermicularis*

- whipworm: *Trichuris trichiura*

- tapeworms: *Diphyllobothrium latum, Taenia saginata,* and *Taenia solium*

- protozoa: *Entamoeba histolytica* (an amoeba), and *Giardia lamblia* (a flagellate)

Numerous other parasites are found in other parts of the world. These may be contracted by travelers to other countries. Patients with acquired immune deficiency syndrome (**AIDS**) or other **immune system** disorders are commonly infected with the parasites in the Microsporidia phylum, *Cryptosporidium*, and *Isospora belli*.

A stool O & P test may be performed in the physician's office or at an external laboratory. There are several commercial kits with instructions that patients can use at home to collect stool samples. These kits are comprised of sterile containers containing special chemical fixatives. The feces should be collected directly into the container and the patient should be careful not to contaminate the sample with urine, water, or other materials. Three specimens are collected, usually two or three days apart. However, as many as six specimens may be needed within 14 days to identify some organisms (like *E. histolytica*). A specimen held at room temperature should be examined within three hours. If testing is delayed, the sample may be refrigerated for two to three days or preserved. If a preservative is used, it must preserve all forms of the parasite (including eggs, or cysts and trophozoites) without interfering with the testing required for the stool sample. A commonly used preservative is the combination merthiolate-iodine-formalin (MIF).

In the laboratory, the stool sample is examined for a variety of parasitic forms. Some parasites are large enough to be seen without a **microscope**. For others, microscope slides are prepared with either fresh unstained stool or stool dyed with special stains. These preparations are viewed with a microscope to detect the presence of parasites or their eggs.

The recovery of ova or parasite forms depends upon the consistency of the stool sample, which suggests the parasitic stage is likely to be present. For example, if the stool specimen is soft or loose, it may be more likely to contain trophozoites. If the stool specimen is formed, then it may be more likely to contain cysts.

A stool examination usually requires three procedures: a direct wet mount, a concentration test, and a permanent smear. A direct wet mount requires preparing a slide with an appropriate fecal sample and then viewing the slide under a microscope for evidence of parasites. In a concentration by sedimentation test, chemicals (most often ethyl acetate and formalin) are used to separate the parasites from other fecal material (e.g., oils, fats). When a test tube containing the sample and these chemicals is centrifuged, the sedimentation on the bottom of the tube contains the parasite forms while the fats and other substances are closer to the top of the tube. The sediment is then appropriately processed and examined for parasite forms. A permanent smear is made by preparing a slide with a fecal sample and adding Gomori trichrome stain. When viewed with a microscope, the background appears blue-green while parasite forms stain blue-green

and red. This test is required to identify trophozoites and is the most sensitive of the three tests.

Sometimes another method of examination must be used, as is the case for *Cryptosporidium*. Modified acid-fast staining must be used for this organism. When this stain is used, forms of the organism (oocysts) turn red.

Obtaining a specimen to identify pinworm (*E. vermicularis*) infection requires a different technique. Adult parasites lay eggs outside of the intestines on the skin folds of the anus. Eggs are usually not present in stool. Clear adhesive tape or a sticky swab or paddle is applied to the anus. Eggs then stick to the tape, swab, or paddle and can be examined microscopically. When adhesive tape is used, this technique is often called the scotch tape method of collection.

Immunological testing of stool is a faster diagnostic tool and does not require knowledge of the structures and life stages of parasites. Fresh or fresh-frozen stool is diluted, filtered, and added to a commercial device containing **antibodies** that will react if several specific parasite antigens are present in the stool sample. If the antigen of the parasite is present, a purple color is produced. However, this type of testing can only be conducted with unpreserved stool and can only assist in identifying a few common parasites.

Insurance coverage for stool ova and parasites may vary among different insurance plans. This test usually is covered if ordered by a physician approved by the patient's insurance plan, and if it is done at an approved laboratory. However, since insurance plans vary greatly, patients should contact their insurance company with regard to specifics.

Preparation

The physician, or other health care provider, will ask the patient for a complete medical history, and perform a **physical examination** to determine possible causes of the gastrointestinal symptoms. Information about the patient's diet, any medications taken, and recent travel may provide clues to the identity of possible infectious parasites.

Patients should avoid taking any medications or treatments containing mineral oil, castor oil, bismuth, **magnesium** or other antidiarrheal medicines, or **antibiotics** for up to 10 days before collecting the specimen.

Aftercare

The patient should avoid taking preparations that interfere with specimens for the duration of time the specimen collection is required.

Complications

There are no complications associated with a patient providing a stool sample for stool O & P testing.

Results

Normally, parasites and eggs are not found in stools. Some parasites are not pathogenic (for example, *Endolimax nana* and *Iodamoeba butschlii*), which means they do not cause disease. If these are found, no treatment is necessary. The presence of any pathogenic parasite indicates an intestinal parasitic infection. Depending on the parasite identified, other tests may be required to determine if the parasite has invaded other parts of the body. Some parasites travel from the intestines to other parts of the body and may already have caused damage to other tissues by the time a diagnosis is made. For example, the roundworm *Ascaris* penetrates the intestinal wall and can cause inflammation in the **abdomen**. It can also migrate to the **lungs** and cause **pneumonia**. This kind of injury can occur weeks before the roundworm eggs appear in the stool.

Other types of damage caused by intestinal parasites include anemia due to hemorrhage caused by hookworms and anemia caused by depletion of **vitamin B$_{12}$** due to infection with the tapeworm *Diphyllobothrium latum*.

When a parasite is identified, the patient can be treated with the appropriate medications to eliminate the parasite.

Health care team roles

Training

A physician orders a stool O & P test. Stool samples may be collected by a physician, nurse, physician assistant, or other trained health care professionals. Laboratory professionals (usually called clinical laboratory scientists or medical technologists) who perform microscopic tests for stool ova and parasites have received specialized training in preparing, handling, and examining the samples. These professionals have been trained to look for specific characteristics of parasite forms that will lead to accurate diagnosis and treatment for the patient.

Patient education

Health care providers should teach the patient how to use the collection kit, how many samples will be required, and how to keep the samples free from contamination. Usually patients should be instructed to take the stool sample in the morning before bathing or

---

KEY TERMS

Amoeba—A type of protozoa (one-celled animal) that can move or change its shape by extending projections of its cytoplasm.

Bismuth—A substance used in medicines to treat diarrhea, nausea, and indigestion.

Cryptosporidium—A type of parasitic protozoa.

Centrifuged—Spun via a centrifuge. A centrifuge is a specialized machine used to spin a test tube at a very fast rotation in order to separate the particles inside the tube into different layers according to their density.

Feces—Material excreted by the intestines.

Flagellate—A microorganism that uses flagella (hair-like projections) to move.

Gastrointestinal—The digestive tract; the stomach and intestines.

Isospora belli—A type of parasitic protozoa.

Microsporidia—A phylum of small parasitic protozoa.

Parasite—An organism that lives on or inside another living organism (host), causing damage to the host.

Protozoa—One-celled eukaryotic organisms belonging to the kingdom Protista.

---

taking a shower. Patients should be taught how to avoid re-infection based on how the parasite is contracted when a definite diagnosis is made. For example, patients with pinworms should practice sound personal hygiene in the future such as washing hands after using the restroom and before eating, and wearing clean undergarments daily. Patients with tapeworms should avoid eating specific raw or undercooked meat or fish in the future. Health care providers should also stress that patients follow the full duration of treatment as required to eliminate the parasite.

Resources

BOOKS

Fischbach, Frances. "Diagnosis of Parasitic Disease." In *A Manual of Laboratory & Diagnostic Tests*. 6th ed. Philadelphia: Lippincott Williams & Wilkins, 2000, pp. 516–521.

Forbes, Betty A., Daniel F. Sahm, and Alice S. Weissfeld. "Laboratory Methods for Diagnosis of Parasitic Infections." In *Bailey & Scott's Diagnostic Microbiology*. 10th ed. St. Louis: Mosby, 1998, pp. 784–787.

Kee, Joyce LeFever. "Ova and Parasites (O and P) (Feces)." In *Laboratory & Diagnostic Tests with Nursing Implications.* 5th ed. Stamford, CT: Appleton & Lange, 1999, pp. 320–321.

Tierney, L.M., S.J. McPhee, and Maxine A. Papadakis. *Current Medical Diagnosis and Treatment 1998.* Stamford, CT: Appleton & Lange, 1998.

OTHER

"Infectious Diseases; Parasitic Infections." In The Merck Manual of Diagnosis and Therapy. (Internet Edition), http://www.merck.com/pubs/mmanual, 2005.

ORGANIZATIONS

The American Society for Microbiology. 1752 N St. N.W., Washington, DC 20036. (202) 737-3600. www.asmusa. org.

Centers for Disease Control and Prevention. National Center for Infectious Disease. Division of Parasitic Diseases. 1600 Clifton Road NE, Atlanta, GA 30333. (800) 311-3435. www.cdc.gov/ncidod/dpd.

Linda D. Jones, B.A., PBT (ASCP)

Stool specimen collection

Definition

Stool specimen collection is the process of obtaining a sample of a patient's feces for diagnosic purposes.

Purpose

This procedure is used to test for infectious organisms, mucus, fat, **parasites**, or **blood** in the stool.

Precautions

Depending on the proposed analysis of the feces, watery feces will not be suitable for conducting a test for any fat that may be present, but can be used for other analyses, such as testing for **bacteria**.

Description

A stool specimen or culture can also be called a fecal specimen or culture. A specimen of freshly passed feces of 0.5 to 1 ounce (15 g to 30 g) is collected, without contamination of urine or toilet tissue, into a small container that may have a small spoon or spatula attached inside the lid of the cup for easier collection of the sample.

Adult and older children patients can collect the specimen by passing feces into plastic wrap stretched loosely over the toilet bowl. A portion of the sample is then transferred into the supplied container.

With young children and infants wearing diapers, the diaper should be lined with plastic wrap. A urine bag can be attached to the child to ensure that the stool specimen is not contaminated with urine.

For a bedridden patient, the specimen should be collected in a bedpan lined with plastic wrap, and the nurse can transfer a portion of the feces into the appropriate container.

Follow the manufacturer's guidelines if a commercial collection kit is used.

Preparation

If occult blood is suspected, the patient should be given a mild laxative and should avoid eating foods rich in meat extracts or leafy vegetables three days prior to the test. If the patient's gums bleed when brushing their teeth, the mouth should be cleansed with mouthwash and wiped with a cloth to avoid blood entering the **digestive system** and contaminating the stool specimen.

Certain drugs may interfere with the analysis of the specimen, and the patient should avoid ingesting products such as **antacids**, oily foods and drugs, and **antibiotics**. Barium sulfate should be excluded two weeks prior to the test, and medical procedure dyes three weeks prior to the test.

If fat in the stool is suspected, the patient will also be asked to collect the samples in pre-weighed airtight containers.

All feces passed in a 24-hour period are collected over two or three days and sent daily for analysis.

Aftercare

The patient should be made clean and comfortable.

All contents of kits, towels, plastic wrap, gloves, and bedpans should be disposed of in appropriate containers. The nurse should wash and dry his or her hands thoroughly.

Speed in testing the sample is essential, in order that an accurate result is obtained. Therefore the specimen should be sent for testing as quickly as possible.

Complications

If there is a delay in sending the specimen for testing, organisms present in the feces may die, while others may multiply, giving a false reading.

KEY TERMS

Barium sulfate—A water-insoluble salt used as an opaque medium for radiographic contrast.

Occult blood—Hidden blood.

Parasite—An organism that lives on or in another host.

Patients should inform medical staff of any medications currently being taken as elements of the drugs may be present in the feces.

Results

The specimens are compared with normal values. Abnormal results indicate that **infection**, disease, or parasite infestation are present.

Health care team roles

The nurse should be aware of the qualities of normal feces, and note if the patient has any difficulties in passing feces. As many patients may feel uncomfortable performing this collection properly, the nurse should also educate the patient concerning the reasons for having it done.

Resources

OTHER

"Diagnostic Procedures for Stool Specimens." National Center for Infectious Diseases. http://www.dpd.cdc.gov 02/05/01.

"Fecal Culture." http://www.Webmd.com.

"Stool for Quantitative Fecal Fat." University of Texas, Houston Medical School. http://www.Medic.Med.uth.tmc.edu.

Margaret A. Stockley, RGN

Strains *see* **Sprains and strains**

Strength testing *see* **Muscle testing**

Strength training

Definition

Strength training involves using progressive resistance to increase a person's ability to exert or resist force. It usually involves use of free weights, weight machines, elastic tubing, or one's own body weight.

Purpose

Strength training also is known as resistance training. Resistance exercises may be used to help patients restore function to injured muscles or to build muscle around injured bones and joints to improve function.

Studies have confirmed that people who engage in some form of physical activity through their lifestyle or occupation will likely live longer and have healthier lives. Regular **exercise** has been linked to weight reduction, lowered **blood pressure**, improved glucose regulation, stronger bones, and better lipid profiles. Strength training can help slow and possibly reverse muscle decline. Strong muscles lessen the workload on the **heart**. Recent studies have found that strength training can improve quality of life for people with mild and moderate **chronic obstructive pulmonary disease** (COPD) and for indviduals with **multiple sclerosis**.

Strength training appears to help people of every age. Research on the positive effects of strength training in the elderly has been around for quite a while. Structured weight training and physical conditioning programs can help reduce **pain** and prevent the normal physiologic decline associated with **aging**. Even nursing home patients can benefit from appropriate strength training. While some parents may worry that strength training is dangerous for their children, a well-designed program may help improve a child's health and fitness without causing increased muscle bulk.

A 2005 study reported that strength training helped improve how women with characteristics of eating disorders perceived their body size. Strength training has been shown to reduce the signs and symptoms of a number of diseases and chronic conditions, including:

• arthritis

• diabetes

• depression

• osteoporosis

• obesity

• back pain

Athletes benefit from strength training as well. Proper strength and conditioning can increase athletic performance, improve physiological function, and reduce risk of injury. Resistance training can reduce **stress** on the skeleton and produce favorable changes in body composition.

When an athlete or any person receives a musculoskeletal injury, strength training may be part of the **rehabilitation** process.

Precautions

Pregnant women or people with certain medical concerns, such as chest pain or other heart conditions, severe **dizziness**, certain **bone** or joint problems, and who take prescription medications for high **blood** pressure or heart conditions, should consult their physicians before beginning any exercise program. Strength training exercises can cause injuries if not performed correctly or if performed without proper supervision. Most injuries appear to occur because too much weight is added too quickly or improper technique is used.

Description

Strength training often is confused with body building and power weight lifting. While these efforts use many of the same concepts and equipment, their goals may not be the same and should not be confused with strength training.

The body has four basic types of muscle contractions. Strength training programs often are designed around these contraction movements.

- Dynamic, isotonic, or concentric. The muscle becomes shorter and tension varies as it lifts a constant load.

- Isometric or static. The muscle does not change length even though tension develops.

- Eccentric. The muscle develops tension, lengthening while contracting.

- Isokinetic. Maximal tension develops while the muscle is shortened at constant speed over the full range of motion.

Strength training generally involves use of free weights, elastic resistance bands, or equipment that holds weights or produces measured resistance. A planned program calls for beginning at the appropriate lower weight or resistance level and in controlled movement, exhaling when exercise is hardest and inhaling when it is easiest. The person will do several repetitions (reps) of the same movement with the same amount of weight. This constitutes a set. Usually, a set consists of five to eight reps and a person performs one to three sets per training session. However, the number of reps and sets varies, depending on many factors. Most people will repeat each set on both sides of the body (for example, biceps curls with the right and left arm). This may not be the case in rehabilitative sports training. For instance, when strengthening an injured ankle, the exercises may be performed only on the injured side or the amount of weight/resistance or repetition may vary from one side to another. The training should be done several times a week. Most experts recommend a day of rest between strength training sessions to allow the muscles to recover.

If the goal of the training is improving strength for injury rehabilitation, a physical therapist may prescribe very low weight at the beginning. In most cases, exercise physiologists and strength training specialists set differing goals depending on a person's age, physical abilities, and program goals.

Preparation

Many people considering strength training will need to check with their physician before beginning the program. An exercise or **physical therapy** professional can recommend the proper amount of weight or resistance to begin training. People considering weight training also should purchase good athletic shoes with adequate support, and loose, cool, comfortable clothing that absorbs moisture.

Aftercare

It is important to rest between strength training sets and to stretch after completing all exercises. It also is important to stop exercising at any time if pain is experienced.

Complications

Injuries can occur from lifting weights that are too heavy, from using improper technique, or from other unsupervised strength training. Poorly designed equipment may cause injury. Muscles build up can occur from power lifting of heavy weights over extended time.

Results

Numerous studies document the beneficial results of properly conducted strength training. Older adults often report improvements in pain and function within less than two weeks of starting a strength-training program. A study of people age 61 to 82 years who participated in weight and **aerobic training** twice a week for 75 minutes over 24 weeks showed 16–17% increase in upper-body strength for men and women. A 12-month study of postmenopausal women at Tufts University who underwent progressive strength training two days a week reported 75% increases in strength, 13% increases in dynamic balance, and 1% gains in bone density. A control group experienced losses in strength, bone, and balance.

Health care team roles

Health professionals in nursing, rehabilitation, **occupational therapy**, and physical therapy may specialize in some aspect of strength training as part of their jobs. Some orthopedic surgeons specialize in sports medicine, overseeing the conditioning of athletes, as well as injuries related to a variety of professional and recreational sports. Exercise physiologists become versed in the science behind exercise, muscle, and movement. Personal trainers and other strength training professionals may assist a person with their program. There are certification programs available for these professionals.

Resources

BOOK

Foss, Merle L., Steven J. Keteyian. *Fox's Physiological Basis for Exercise and Sport.* WCB/McGraw-Hill, 1998.

PERIODICALS

Kruger J, et al. "Strength Training Among Adults Aged (greater than or equal to) 65 Years—United States, 2001."*Pediatric News* (February 2005):23.

MacReady, Norra. "Strength Training Helps Fitness, Coordination."*Morbidity and Mortality Weekly Report* (January 23, 2004):25-29.

Panlaqui, Ogee Mer A., et al. "Tolerance and Quality of Life Improvement Following Aerobic and Strength Training Exercise in Patients With Chronic Obstructive Pulmonary Disease."*Chest* (October 2005):253S-255S.

Study Shows Weight Training Gives MS Patients Physical, Emotional Benefits. *A Scribe Health News Service* (January 13, 2005).

Sullivan, Michele G. "Self-image Improves With Strength-Training Program."*Family Practice News* (July 15, 2005):1-2.

Sullivan, Michele G. "Weight Training Prevents Muscle Decline, Eases Pain in Elderly Patients."*Family Practice News* (Sept. 1, 2005):64.

Weight Training May Be Effective for Body-imaged-disturbed College Women.*World Disease Weekly* (November 23, 2004):125.

OTHER

Growing Stronger - Strength Training for Older Adults: Why Strength Training? Web page/brochure. Centers for Disease Control and Prevention, 2005. http://www.cdc.gov/nccdphp/dnpa/physical/growing_stronger/why.htm.

Selecting and Effectively Using Free Weights. Web page/brochure. American College of Sports Medicine, 2003. http://www.acsm.org/health+fitness/brochures.htm.

ORGANIZATIONS

American College of Sports Medicine. P.O. Box 1440, Indianapolis, IN 46202. (317) 637-9200, ext. 138. http://www.acsm.org.

National Strength and Conditioning Association. 1885 Bob Johnson Drive, Colorado Springs, CO 80906. (800) 815-6826. http://www.nsca-lift.org.

Teresa G. Odle

Strep culture *see* **Throat culture**
Strep test *see* **Streptococcal antibody tests**

Strep throat
Definition

Strep throat is an **infection** of the mucous membranes lining the pharynx. Sometimes the tonsils are also infected (**tonsillitis**). The infection is caused by group A beta-hemolytic *Streptococcus* bacteria, commonly known as strep.

This bacterial infection typically causes a severe **sore throat**, **fever**, and difficulty swallowing. Strep throat may also produce a **rash**, known as scarlet fever, and swollen glands. Untreated, it can lead to **rheumatic fever**, a serious kidney disorder called glomerulonephritis, and other infections.

Description

Strep throat accounts for 5–10% of all sore throats. Although anyone can get strep throat, it is most common in school-age children. It accounts for about one quarter of sore throats in children ages five to 15. Smokers, and people who are fatigued, immunosuppressed, or who live in damp, crowded conditions are more likely to become infected. Children under age two and adults who do not have contact with children are less likely to become infected.

Strep throat occurs most frequently from November to April. The disease passes directly from person to person by coughing, sneezing, and close contact. Rarely, it may be passed through food, when a food handler infected with strep throat accidentally contaminates food by coughing or sneezing. Statistically, when one member of a household is infected, one out of every four other household members will contract strep throat within two to seven days.

Causes and symptoms

Strep infection may produce a sudden, painful sore throat one to five days after exposure to the *Streptococcus* **bacteria**. The **pain** is indistinguishable from sore throats caused by viral infections.

The infected patient usually feels tired and has a fever, sometimes accompanied by chills, **headache**, muscle aches, swollen lymph glands, and nausea. Young children may complain of **abdominal pain**. The tonsils appear swollen and are bright red, and may have white or

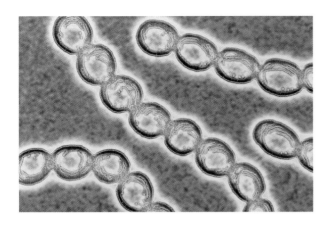

(This colored transmission electron micrograph (TEM) shows chains of Streptococcus pyogenes bacteria, photograph. A. Pasieka / Photo Researchers, Inc.)

yellow patches of pus. Sometimes the roof of the mouth is red or has small red spots. Often a person with strep throat has bad breath.

Though most patients display some of these common symptoms, it is possible to have the disease without any of these symptoms. Many young children complain only of a headache and stomachache, rather than the characteristic sore throat.

Occasionally, within a few days of developing the sore throat, patients may develop a fine, rough, sunburn-like rash over the face and upper body, along with a fever of 101–104°F (38.3–40°C) and bright red tongue, with a flecked, strawberry-like appearance. When a rash develops, this form of strep throat is called scarlet fever. The rash is caused by toxins released by the streptococcus bacteria. Scarlet fever is no more dangerous than strep throat, and is treated the same way. The rash disappears in about five days. One to three weeks later, patches of skin may desquamate (peel off), as might occur with a sunburn.

Untreated strep throat can cause rheumatic fever. This is a serious illness, although it occurs rarely. The most recent outbreak appeared in the United States in the mid-1980s. Rheumatic fever occurs most often in children between the ages of five and 15, and susceptibility to it may be genetic, since it seems to run in families. Although the strep throat that causes rheumatic fever is contagious, rheumatic fever itself is not.

Rheumatic fever begins one to six weeks after an untreated streptococcal infection. The joints, especially the wrists, elbows, knees, and ankles become red, sore, and swollen. The patient develops a high fever, and possibly a rapid heartbeat when lying down, paleness, shortness of breath, and fluid retention. A red rash over the trunk may come and go for weeks or months. An acute attack of rheumatic fever lasts about three months.

Rheumatic fever can cause permanent damage to the **heart** and heart valves. It can be prevented by promptly treating **streptococcal infections** with **antibiotics**. It does not occur if all the streptococcus bacteria are killed within the first 10–12 days after infection.

During the 1990s, outbreaks of a virulent strain of group A *Streptococcus* were reported to cause a toxic-shock-like illness and a severe invasive infection called **necrotizing fasciitis**, which destroys skin and muscle tissue. Although these diseases are caused by group A *Streptococci*, they rarely begin with strep throat. Usually the streptococcus bacteria enter the body through a skin wound. These infections are rare; however, since the death rate in necrotizing fasciitis is 30–50%, it is wise to promptly treat any streptococcal infection.

Diagnosis

Diagnosis of strep throat begins with a **physical examination** of the throat. The doctor will also look for signs of other illness, such as a sinus infection or **bronchitis**, and seek information about whether the patient has been exposed to anyone with strep throat. Patients likely to have strep throat will have a rapid strep test or **throat culture**, laboratory tests to detect the presence of bacteria.

There are two types of tests to confirm the diagnosis of strep throat. A rapid strep test determines the presence of streptococcal antigen, and results are available in about 20 minutes. The advantage of this test is the speed with which a diagnosis may be made.

The rapid strep test has a false negative rate of about 20%. For this reason, when a rapid strep test is negative, the physician may order a throat culture.

For a rapid strep test or a throat culture, a physician, mid-level practitioner (i.e., nurse practitioner or physician assistant) or nurse will use a sterile swab to reach down into the throat to obtain a sample of material from the sore area. The procedure takes only a few seconds, but may cause some patients to gag.

For a throat culture, a sample of swabbed material is cultured, or grown, in the laboratory on a medium that allows laboratory technologists and technicians to accurately determine whether group A *Streptococci* is present. Results are available in 24–48 hours. This test is very accurate and also detects the presence of bacteria other than *Streptococci*. Patients should be reminded by the nurse not to take antibiotics before a throat culture. Even small amounts of antibiotics can suppress the bacteria enough to mask their presence in the throat culture.

In the event that rheumatic fever is suspected, the physician will order a **blood** test. This test, called an antistreptolysin-O test, determines whether the person has recently been infected with strep bacteria and helps to distinguish between rheumatic fever and **rheumatoid arthritis**.

Treatment

Strep throat is treated with antibiotics. Penicillin is the preferred medication. The typical dose for adults is Penicilin V, 250 mg by mouth, four times a day or 500 mg twice a day. Alternatively, 250 mg of erythromycin may be given four times a day. Oral antibiotics must be taken for 10 days. Patients must be advised to take the entire amount of antibiotic prescribed. They must be warned not to discontinue taking the medication when they feel better. Stopping the antibiotic early or failing to complete the prescribed course of medication can lead to a return of the strep infection. Occasionally, a single injection of benzathine penicillin G 1.2 million units IM (intramuscularly) is given instead of 10 days of oral treatment.

About 10% of the time, penicillin is not effective against the strep bacteria. In such instances, other antibiotics such as amoxicillin (Amoxil, Pentamox, Sumox, Trimox), clindamycin (Cleocin), or a cephalosporin (Keflex, Durocef, Ceclor) may be prescribed. Erythromycin (Eryzole, Pediazole, Ilosone), another inexpensive antibiotic, is given to patients who are allergic to penicillin. Scarlet fever is treated with the same antibiotics as strep throat.

Without treatment, the symptoms of strep throat begin subsiding in four or five days. However, because of the possibility of contracting rheumatic fever, glomerulonephritis, or other infections, it is vital to treat strep throat promptly with antibiotics. If rheumatic fever does occur, it also is treated with antibiotics. Anti-inflammatory drugs are used to treat joint swelling and diuretics are used to reduce water retention. Once the rheumatic fever becomes inactive, children may continue on low doses of antibiotics to prevent a reoccurrence. Necrotizing fasciitis is treated with intravenous antibiotics.

Home care for strep throat

Patients may be taught **home care** measures to relieve the discomfort of their strep symptoms. They may be counseled by the nurse, mid-level practitioner, or physician to:

- Take acetaminophen or ibuprofen for pain. Aspirin should not be given to children because of its association with Reye's syndrome.
- Gargle with warm double strength tea or warm salt water, made by adding one teaspoon of salt to eight ounces of water, to relieve sore throat pain.
- Drink plenty of fluids, but avoid acidic juices like orange juice because they irritate the throat.
- Eat soft, nutritious foods like noodle soup. Avoid spicy foods.
- Avoid smoke and smoking.
- Rest until the fever is gone, then resume strenuous activities gradually.
- Use a room humidifier, as it may make sore throat sufferers more comfortable.
- Be aware that antiseptic lozenges and sprays may aggravate the sore throat rather than improve it.

Alternative treatment focuses on easing the symptoms of strep throat through herbs and botanical medicines. Honey, eucalyptus, and menthol-infused drops and syrups may all soothe the soreness of strep throat. These treatments should never be used in place of antibiotic therapy. They should be used in addition to antibiotics, since they address symptoms rather than the underlying infection.

Prognosis

Patients with strep throat begin feeling better about 24 hours after starting antibiotics. Symptoms rarely last longer than five days.

Patients remain contagious until they have taken antibiotics for 24 hours. Children should not return to school or childcare until they are no longer contagious. Food handlers should not work for the first 24 hours after antibiotic treatment, because strep infections are occasionally passed through contaminated food. People who are not treated with antibiotics can continue to spread strep bacteria for several months.

About 10% of strep throat cases do not respond to penicillin. Patients with even a mild sore throat after a 10 days of antibiotic treatment should be advised to return to the doctor. One explanation for a persisting sore throat may be that the patient is simply a carrier of strep, and the sore throat is the result of another infectious (bacterial or viral) agent.

Timely administration of antibiotics within the first week of a strep infection acts to prevent rheumatic fever and other complications. If rheumatic fever does occur,

KEY TERMS

Desquamate—To peel off or exfoliate the skin.

Glomerulonephritis—A serious kidney disorder that sometimes results from an untreated strep infection.

Lactobacillus acidophilus—A bacteria found in yogurt that changes the balance of the bacteria in the intestine in a beneficial way.

the outcomes vary considerably. Some cases may be cured; others cause permanent damage to the heart and heart valves. In rare cases, rheumatic fever can be fatal.

Necrotizing fasciitis has mortality (death rate) of 30–50%. Patients who survive often suffer a great deal of tissue and muscle loss. Fortunately, this complication of a *Streptococcus* infection is very rare.

Health care team roles

Physicians, nurses, mid-level practitioners, and laboratory technologists are involved in the diagnosis and treatment of strep throat. In contacts with patients they can reinforce the value of adherence to prescribed treatment and can instruct patients in self-care and home care measures to relieve symptoms.

Patient education

Nurses, mid-level practitioners, and laboratory personnel have opportunities to teach patients how to minimize the risks of transmission by reinforcing the importance of personal hygiene, safe food handling, and avoiding exposures. They must also emphasize the importance of prompt and complete treatment of strep infection to prevent consequences and recurrence.

Prevention

There is no way to prevent getting a strep throat. Patients may be counseled about how to reduce the risk of transmission. Risk may be minimized by:

- washing hands well and frequently, especially after nose blowing or sneezing and before food handling
- disposing of used tissues properly
- avoiding close contact with someone who has a strep throat
- not sharing food and eating utensils with anyone
- not smoking

Resources

BOOKS

Professional Guide to Diseases, 9th edition. Springhouse, PA: Springhouse Corp., 2008.

The Washington Manual of Medical Therapeutics, 33th edition. Philadelphia, PA: Lippincott Williams & Wilkins, 2010.

OTHER

National Institute of Allergy and Infectious Diseases. "Group A Streptococcal Infections." NIAID Fact Sheet. (February 1998). http://www.niaid.nih.govfactsheets/strep.htm.

Barbara Wexler

Streptococcal antibody tests

Definition

If left untreated, upper respiratory or skin infections caused by Group A streptococci (*Streptococcus pyrogenes*) can develop complications, called sequelae. These include scarlet and **rheumatic fever** and a kidney disease called post streptococcal glomerulonephritis (a sequalea to respiratory but not skin infections). Streptococcal antibody tests detect **antibodies** to various antigens secreted by Group A streptococci. These include tests for antibodies to streptolysin O, DNase-B, and hyaluronidase that contribute to the virulence of Group A **streptococcal infections**. Four major streptococcal antibody tests are the antistreptolysin O titer (ASO), antideoxyribonuclease-B titer (anti-DNase-B, or ADB), antihyaluronidase (AH), and Streptozyme test. Other tests to determine past streptococcal infections have been developed including the anti-CHO test (possible use for rheumatic **fever**) and the anti-preabsorption antigen test (for glomerulonephritis).

Purpose

Tests for streptococcal antibodies are preformed in order to document a recent **infection** with Group A streptococcus (*Streptococcus pyrogenes*). The antistreptolysin O titer, or ASO, is ordered primarily to determine whether a previous Group A streptococcus infection has caused a post streptococcal disease, such as scarlet fever, rheumatic fever, or glomerulonephritis. The ASO test also detects Groups C and G streptococci, which also produce streptolysin O. Antibodies to streptolysin O are produced in approximately 75–80% of Group A streptococcus infections, but are usually not seen in skin infections caused by this organism. The antibodies are usually detected within one to two weeks following acute pharyngitis.

The anti-DNase-B (ADB) test is also performed to determine a previous infection with Group A streptococci. Antibodies to DNase-B appear almost exclusively in Group A streptoccal infections, appear somewhat earlier than those to streptolysin O, and are produced by 85-90% of persons with group A streptococcal skin infections. When used with the ASO test, the ADB test adds clinical sensitivity.

The antihyaluronidase (AH) test is used as an adjunct to ASO testing (increases clinical sensitivity when used along with the ASO test). This test is not as sensitive as the ASO test, but antibodies to hyaluronidase are produced by some patients with either skin or respiratory infections with Group A streptococci.

Streptozyme is a screening test used to detect antibodies to several streptococcal antigens. An antigen is a substance that can trigger an **immune response**, resulting in production of an antibody as part of the body's defense against infection and disease. The test is not as sensitive or specific as the ASO test, but can be performed within minutes, providing presumptive results that can be confirmed by use of the ASO or other more specific streptococcal antibody tests.

Precautions

Streptococcal antibody tests are performed on a **blood** (serum) sample collected by venipuncture. The nurse or phlebotomist performing the procedure should observe **universal precautions** for prevention of transmission of bloodborne pathogens. Hemolyzed blood samples are unsuitable for these tests. Increased levels of fats (beta lipoproteins) in the blood can cause false-positive test results. Antibiotic therapy can reduce the number of streptococci and decrease levels during these tests, giving a false negative. Steroids may also give false negative results. Group A streptococcal infections of the skin may not produce an ASO response. False negatives in the ASO test may arise from antibody deficiency syndromes, and false positives from hyper-cholesterolemia, hyperglobulinemia, and **liver** disorders. A false negative result in the ADB test may occur during hemorrhagic **pancreatitis**. The streptozyme test is more sensitive for adult patient samples than those obtained from children.

Description

Streptococcal infections are caused by **bacteria** known as *Streptococcus*. There are several disease-causing strains of streptococci (groups A, B, C, D, and G), which are identified by their clinical effects, biochemical characteristics, growth requirements, appearance on culture media, cell wall composition, and antigen production. Each group causes specific types of infections and symptoms. These antibody tests are useful for detecting a recent respiratory or skin infection caused primarily by group A streptococci.

Group A streptococci are the most virulent species for humans and are the cause of pharyngitis (**strep throat**), **tonsillitis**, wound and skin infections, blood infections (septicemia), scarlet fever, **pneumonia**, rheumatic fever, Sydenham's chorea (formerly called St. Vitus's dance), and post-streptococcal glomerulonephritis.

Although symptoms may suggest a streptococcal infection, the diagnosis must be confirmed by tests. The best procedure, and one that is used for an acute infection, is to take a sample from the infected area for culture, a means of growing bacteria artificially in the laboratory. However, cultures will be negative for growth approximately two to three weeks after the initial infection. Consequently, the streptococcal antibody tests are used to determine if a streptococcal infection was present.

Antistreptolysin O titer (ASO)

The ASO titer is used to detect the body's reaction to an infection caused by group A beta-hemolytic streptococci. Group A streptococci (also Group C and G) produce the enzyme streptolysin O, that can destroy (lyse) red blood cells. Because streptolysin O is antigenic (contains a protein foreign to the body), the body reacts by producing anti-streptolysin O antibody (ASO), a neutralizing antibody. ASO appears in the blood one week to one month after the onset of a strep infection. A high titer (high levels of ASO antibody) is indicative that a streptococcal infection is present or may have happened in the recent past.

ASO testing can be done as a screening test by a rapid slide agglutination method. If positive, the antibody concentration is determined by the classical tube test. In this test, a standardized solution of streptolysin O is added to tubes containing serial dilutions of the patient's serum. After incubating, human group O red blood cells are added. If antibodies are present, they neutralize the streptolysin O and no hemolysis is seen. The antibody concentratioin (titre) is the highest dilution of the serum that shows no evidence of hemolysis.

Several, sequential tests for ASO are often performed over time (serial testing) to determine if the blood sample is acute or convalescent. The diagnosis of a previous strep infection is confirmed when serial titers of ASO rise over a period of weeks, then fall slowly. A fourfold or greater rise in titre from the acute to convalescent stage is considered diagnostic. ASO titers peak during the third week after the onset of acute symptoms of a streptococcal disease; at six months after onset, approximately 30% of patients still exhibit abnormal titers.

Anti-deoxyribonuclease B titer (anti-DNase B, or ADB)

Anti-DNase B, or ADB, also detects antigens produced by group A strep, and is elevated in most patients with rheumatic fever and post-streptococcal glomerulonephritis. This test is often done concurrently with the ASO titer, and subsequent testing is usually performed to detect differences in the acute and convalescent blood samples. When ASO and ADB are performed concurrently, 95% of previous strep infections are detected. If both are repeatedly negative, the likelihood is great that the patient's symptoms are not caused by a post streptococcal disease. The ADB test is performed by measuring the ability of the serum to block the breakdown by streptococcal DNase B of calf thymus DNA bound to a dye. If the DNA is split by the enzyme, the color changes from blue to pink. If antibodies to DNase B are present in the serum, they neutralize the enzyme and the color remains blue.

When evaluating patients with acute rheumatic fever, the American **Heart** Association recommends the ASO titer rather than ADB. Even though the ADB is more sensitive than ASO, its results are more variable. It also should be noted that, while ASO is the recommended test, when ASO and ADB are done together, the combination is better than either ASO or ADB alone.

Antihyaluronidase (AH)

Group A streptococci produce an enzyme called hyaluronidase. If a patient with a recent infection with this organism produces antihyaluronidase, the level of antibodies in the blood against this enzyme will rise at about the second week of infection and decline for three to five weeks afterward. The patient's serum is diluted and streptococcal hyaluronidase added to each dilution. After incubation, potassium hyaluronate is added. If hyaluronidase is present, it will breakdown the hyaluronate by hydrolysis. Consequently, a clot will not form when acetic acid is added. If antihyaluronidase is present, it will neutralize the streptococcal hyaluronidase. The potassium hyaluronate added subsequently will not be hydrolyzed by the enzyme. The addition of acetic acid cross links the hyaluronate forming a mucin clot. The highest dilution of serum that forms a clot is the titer. This test is advantageous when used along with the ASO test because it increases clinical sensitivity. However, it

should not be used as a singular test for streptococcal antibodies. False positive results may occur from hyperlipoproteinemia.

Streptozyme

The Streptozyme test is often used as a screening test for antibodies to the streptococcal antigens NADase, DNase, streptokinase, streptolysin O, and hyaluronidase. Streptozyme has two advantages over ASO and ADB. It can detect several antibodies in a single assay, and it is technically quick and easy to perform. However, the Streptozyme test is less sensitive and specific than the ASO test. While it detects different antibodies, it does not determine which one has been detected, and it is not as sensitive in children as in adults. In fact, borderline antibody elevations, which could be significant in children, may not be detected at all. A dilution of serum is mixed with sheep red cells that are coated with streptococcal antigens. A positive test is denoted by red blood cell clumping (agglutination).

Preparation

These tests are performed on blood specimens drawn from the patient's vein. The patient does not need to fast before these tests.

Aftercare

The patient may feel discomfort when blood is drawn from a vein. Bruising may occur at the puncture site, or the person may feel dizzy or faint. Pressure should be applied to the puncture site until the bleeding stops to reduce bruising. Warm packs can also be placed over the puncture site to relieve discomfort. Patients should be informed if serial testing requires return visits.

Complications

The risks associated with these tests are minimal, but may include slight bleeding from the blood-drawing site, fainting or feeling lightheaded after the blood is drawn, or blood accumulating under the puncture site (hematoma).

Results

Normal results

Antistreptolysin O titer:

• Adult: up to 160 Todd units.

• Child: 6 months to 2 years: up to 50 Todd units; 2–4 years: up to 160 Todd units; 5–12 years: 170–330 Todd units.

• Newborn: similar to the mother's value.

KEY TERMS

Antibody—A protein manufactured by a type of white blood cell, the lymphocyte, in response to the presence of an antigen, or foreign protein, in the body. Because bacteria, viruses, and other organisms commonly contain many antigens, antibodies are formed against these foreign proteins to neutralize or destroy the invaders.

Antigen—A substance that can trigger a defensive response in the body, resulting in production of an antibody as part of the body's defense against infection and disease. Many antigens are foreign proteins not found naturally in the body, and include bacteria, viruses, toxins, and tissues from another person used in organ transplantation.

Glomerulonephritis—An inflammation of the glomeruli, the filtering units of the kidney. Damage to these structures hampers removal of waste products, salt, and water from the bloodstream, which may cause serious complications. This disorder can be mild and cause no symptoms, or severe enough to cause kidney failure.

Rheumatic fever—A disease that causes inflammation in various body tissues. It is rare in most developed countries, but reported to be on the increase again in parts of the United States. Joint inflammation occurs, but more serious is the frequency with which the disease permanently damages the heart. The nervous system may also be affected, causing Sydenham's chorea.

Sydenham's chorea—A childhood disorder of the central nervous system. Once called St. Vitus's dance, the condition is characterized by involuntary, jerky movements that usually follow an attack of rheumatic fever. It is rare in the United States today, but a common disorder in developing countries. It usually resolves in two to three months with no long-term adverse effects.

Antideoxyribonuclease-B titer:

- Adult: up to 85 units.
- Child (preschool): up to 60 units.
- Child (school age): up to 170 units.

Antihyaluronidase (AH):

- Titer less than 1:512.
- Streptozyme: less than 100 streptozyme units.

Abnormal results

Antistreptolysin O titer: Increased levels are seen after the second week of an untreated acute streptococcal infection, and are also increased with acute rheumatic fever, acute glomerulonephritis, scarlet fever, and other complications of streptococcal infection.

Antideoxyribonuclease-B titer: Increased levels are seen after the first week of an untreated acute streptococcal infection, and are also increased with acute rheumatic fever, acute glomerulonephritis, scarlet fever, and other complications of streptococcal infection.

Titer greater than 1:512. A rise in the titer between and acute patient sample of greater than fourfold is indicative of infection.

Streptozyme: As this is a screening test for antibodies to streptococcal antigens, increased levels require more definitive tests to confirm diagnosis.

Health care team roles

Streptococcal antibody tests are ordered by a physician. The nurse or phlebotomist collects the specimen and conveys it to the lab. The clinical laboratory scientist/medical technologist or clinical laboratory technician/medical technician performs the test. Results are interpreted by the physician.

Resources

BOOKS

Chernecky, C. and B. Berger, ed. *Laboratory Tests and Diagnostic Procedures,* 3rd ed. Philadelphia, PA: W.C. Saunders Company, 2001.

McKenna, R., and J. Keffer, eds. *The Handbook of Clinical Pathology,* 2nd ed. Chicago, IL: American Society of Clinical Pathologists, 2000.

Pagana, K. Deska, and T. Pagana. *Mosby's Diagnostic and Laboratory Test Reference,* 4th ed. St. Louis, MO: Mosby, 1999.

Sacher, R., and R. McPherson. *Widmann's Clinical Interpretation of Laboratory Tests,* 11th ed. Philadelphia, PA: F. A. Davis Company, 2000.

Shanson, D. C. *Microbiology in Clinical Practice,* 3rd ed. Woburn, MA: Butterworth Heinemann, 1999.

Sleigh, J. Douglas, and M. Timbury. *Note on Medical Bacteriology,* 5th ed. Edinburgh, UK: Churchill Livingstone, 1998.

Jill I. Granger, M.S.

Streptococcal infections

Definition

Streptococcal (strep) infections are communicable diseases that develop when **bacteria** of the genus *Streptococcus* invade parts of the body and overwhelm the body's **immune system**. Not every streptococcal **infection** causes detectable symptoms.

Description

Streptococcal bacteria produce symptoms that vary widely in location and severity—everything from skin infections to sore throats and scarlet **fever** to rare, but frequently fatal, **necrotizing fasciitis** and streptococcal toxic **shock**. Many people have some form of streptococcus bacteria in their body at some point in their life without necessarily showing any symptoms of infection. Nevertheless, a person who hosts bacteria without showing signs of infection is a carrier and can pass the infection on to others.

Types of infection

Primary strep infections invade healthy tissue. **Strep throat**, more formally called streptococcal pharyngitis, is the most common type of primary strep infection. It accounts for between 5–10% of all sore throats. and is especially common among school-aged children. Secondary strep infections invade tissue already weakened by injury or illness. Secondary strep infections frequently affect the bones, ears, eyes, joints, or intestines. Both primary and secondary strep infections can travel from affected tissues to lymph glands or enter the bloodstream and spread throughout the body (systemic infection). Many different strains of streptococcal bacteria have been identified since the 1930s. Types A, B, C, D, and G are the strains most likely to make people ill.

GROUP A *STREPTOCOCCUS*. All Group A strep (GAS) is the form of streptococcal bacteria most likely to be associated with serious illness. GAS is found worldwide. The incidence of respiratory strep A infections (strep throat, for example) is highest in cold climates and among young children. The incidence of GAS skin infections is highest in the tropics.

Two of the most severe invasive GAS infections are necrotizing fasciitis or flesh-eating bacteria disease, which causes the destruction of muscle tissue and fat, and toxic shock syndrome, a rapidly progressive disorder that causes shock and damages internal organs. In the mid-2000s, particularly virulent (strong and causing serious illness) strains of GAS bacteria appeared to be increasing. GAS is also the type of strep responsible for strep throat and scarlet fever. Strep throat is very common and is usually not serious. If untreated, however, strep throat can lead to **rheumatic fever**, which can permanently damage the **heart** and other organs.

GROUP B *STREPTOCOCCUS*. Group B strep (GBS) most often affects pregnant women, infants, the elderly, and chronically ill adults such as those with HIV/AIDS. Streptococcal infection occurs when bacteria contaminate cuts or open sores or otherwise penetrate the body's natural defenses. GBS exists in the reproductive tract of between 5 and 40% of all women. Most of these women are carriers who do not develop symptoms of infection. Nevertheless, they can transmit the bacterium to their newborns during **childbirth**. In the United States in 2006, two to three of every 1,000 live-born babies had a GBS infection. However, the number of babies dying of neonatal GBS infection has been declining steadily since the 1980s, most likely as the result of prevention programs initiated by the United States Centers for Disease Control and Prevention (CDC).

About 75% of infected infants develop early-onset infection. Sometimes evident within a few hours of birth and always apparent within the first week of life, this condition causes inflammation of the membranes covering the **brain** and **spinal cord** (**meningitis**), **pneumonia**, **blood** infection (**sepsis**) and other problems.

Late-onset GBS develops between the ages of seven days and three months. It often causes meningitis. About half of all cases of this rare condition can be traced to mothers who are GBS carriers. The cause of the others is unknown.

Elderly individuals, especially those with other health problems, are also at higher risk of contracting a serious GBS infection that can spread to the entire body.

GROUP C *STREPTOCOCCUS*. Group C streptococcus (GCS) is a common source of infection in animals. It rarely causes human illness.

GROUP D *STREPTOCOCCUS*. Group D streptococcus (GDS) is a common cause of wound infections in hospital patients. GDS is also associated with:

• abnormal growth of tissue in the gastrointestinal tract

• urinary tract infection (UTI)

• uterine infections in women who have just given birth

GROUP G *STREPTOCOCCUS*. Normally present on the skin, in the mouth and throat, and in the intestines and genital tract, Group G strep (GGS) is most likely to lead to infection in alcoholics and in people who have **cancer**, **diabetes mellitus**, **rheumatoid arthritis**, and other conditions that suppress immune-system activity.

GGS can cause a variety of serious infections, including:

- bacteria in the bloodstream (bacteremia)
- inflammation of the connective tissue structure surrounding a joint (bursitis)
- endocarditis (a condition that affects the lining of the heart chambers and the heart valves)
- meningitis
- inflammation of bone and bone marrow (osteomyelitis)
- inflammation of the lining of the abdomen (peritonitis)

Causes and symptoms

Streptococcal infection occurs when bacteria contaminate cuts or open sores or otherwise penetrate the body's natural defenses.

GAS

GAS is transmitted by direct contact with saliva, nasal discharge, or open **wounds** of someone who has the infection. Chronic illness, kidney disease treated by dialysis, and steroid use increase vulnerability to infection.

About one of five people with GAS infection develops a sore, inflamed throat (strep throat), and pus on the tonsils. The majority of those infected by GAS either have no symptoms or develop enlarged lymph nodes, fever, **headache**, nausea, **vomiting**, **weakness**, and a rapid heartbeat.

Necrotizing fasciitis, also called flesh-eating bacteria disease, can be caused by a virulent strain of GAS. In this rare disease (only 500 cases have been reported since 1883), tissues become gangrenous and rapidly decompose from the interior outward to the skin, resulting in muscle and skin loss. The death rate is as high as 75%. Toxic shock syndrome is characterized by severe headache, **sore throat**, fever as high as 105°F (40.6°C), **dehydration**, watery **diarrhea**, and a sunburn-like **rash** that spreads from the face to the rest of the body. Symptoms develop suddenly and can be fatal.

GBS

A pregnant woman who has GBS infection can develop infections of the bladder, blood, and urinary tract, and deliver a baby who is infected or stillborn. The risk of transmitting GBS infection during birth is highest in a woman whose labor begins before the 37th week of **pregnancy** or lasts more than 18 hours or who:

- becomes a GBS carrier during the final stages of pregnancy
- has a GBS urinary-tract infection
- has already given birth to a baby infected with GBS
- develops a fever during labor

Among men, and in women who are not pregnant, the average age of infection with GBS is 64. African Americans appear to be significantly more susceptible to infection by this strain of strep than any other racial group. The most common consequences of GBS infection are pneumonia and infections of blood, skin, and soft tissue.

Miscellaneous symptoms

Other symptoms associated with strep infection include:

- anemia
- elevated white blood cell counts
- inflammation of the epiglottis (epiglottitis)
- heart murmur
- high blood pressure
- infection of the heart muscle
- kidney inflammation (nephritis)
- swelling of the face and ankles

Diagnosis

Strep bacteria can be obtained by swabbing the back of the throat, vagina, rectum, or the infected area with a sterile cotton swab. There are two types of tests to determine if a person has a strep infection. A rapid strep test uses material collected on a sterile swab from the throat or other area where strep is suspected. This test can be done in a doctor's office and can determine only the presence of streptococcal bacteria. It is most often used to determine if a person has strep throat. The results of a rapid strep test are available in about 20 minutes. The advantage of this test is the speed with which a diagnosis can be made.

The rapid strep test has a false negative rate of about 25%. In other words, in about one out of every four cases where no strep is detected by the rapid strep test, the patient actually does have a strep infection. Because of this, when a rapid strep test is negative, the doctor often does a culture test.

For a culture, a sample of swabbed material is grown in the laboratory on a medium that allows technicians to determine what kind of bacteria are present. Results take 24–48 hours. The test is very accurate and will show the presence of other kinds of bacteria besides *Streptococci*.

Treatment

Penicillin is often the antibiotic of choice to treat strep infections. Oral penicillin is usually taken for 10 days for infections such as strep throat and longer for systemic infections. Patients need to take the entire amount of antibiotic prescribed and not discontinue taking the medication when they feel better. Stopping the antibiotic early can lead to a return of the strep infection. Occasionally, a single injection of long-acting penicillin (Bicillin) is given instead of 10 days of oral treatment. It takes less than 24 hours for **antibiotics** to eliminate an infected person's ability to transmit strep bacteria.

About 10% of the time, penicillin is not effective against the strep bacteria. When this happens a doctor may prescribe other antibiotics such as cefuroxime (Ceftin), cefixime (Suprax), cefpodoxime proxetil (Vantin), loracarbef (Lorabid), cefditoren (Spectracef), azithromycin (Zithromax), clindamycin (Cleocin), or a cephalosporin (Keflex, Durocef, Ceclor). Erythromycin (Eryzole, Pediazole, Ilosone), another inexpensive antibiotic, can be given to people who are allergic to penicillin. Scarlet fever is treated with the same antibiotics as strep throat.

Without treatment, the symptoms of untreated strep throat begin subsiding in four or five days. However it is important to treat strep infections promptly with antibiotics because of the possibility of developing secondary disorders or infections. For example, rheumatic fever and rheumatic heart disease may develop from untreated strep throat.

Guidelines developed by the American Academy of Obstetrics and Gynecology (AAOG), the American Academy of **Pediatrics** (AAP), and the Centers for Disease Control and Prevention (CDC) recommend administering intravenous antibiotics to a woman at high risk of passing GBS infection on to her child, and offering the medication to any pregnant woman who wants it.

Initiating antibiotic therapy at least four hours before birth allows medication to become concentrated enough to protect the baby during its passage through the birth canal.

Newborns infected with GBS during or shortly after birth may die. Those who survive can require lengthy hospital stays and may develop **vision** or **hearing loss** and other permanent disabilities.

Alternative treatment

Conventional medicine is very successful in treating strep infections. However, several alternative therapies, including **homeopathy** and botanical medicine, may help relieve symptoms or support the person with a strep infection. For example, several herbs, including garlic (*Allium sativum*), echinacea (*Echinacea* spp.), and goldenseal (*Hydrastis canadensis*), are believed to strengthen the immune system, thus helping the body fight a current infection, as well as helping prevent future infections.

Prognosis

Most people who develop strep infections are treated with antibiotics and recover promptly without complications. Strep throat, for example, is almost never fatal. However, GAS is that results in systemic (involving the whole body) infection has a death rate of 25–40%. Streptococcal toxic shock and necrotizing fasciitis also have high death rates. GBS infection can be fatal in newborns and the elderly.

Prevention

Exposure to infected people should be avoided. However, the risk of getting one or passing one on to another person can be minimized by:

- washing hands well and frequently, especially after nose blowing or sneezing and before food handling
- disposing of used tissues properly
- avoiding close contact with someone who has a strep throat
- not sharing food and eating utensils with anyone
- not smoking

Resources

BOOKS

Cecil, Russell L., Lee Goldman, and D.A. Audiello. *Cecil Medicine*. 23rd ed., Philadelphia: Saunders Elsevier, 2008.

Fauci, Anthony S., et al., eds.*Harrison's Principles of Internal Medicine*. 17th ed. New York: McGraw-Hill Professional, 2008.

OTHER

"Group A Streptococcal Infections." National Institute of Allergy and Infectious Diseases. September 17, 2007 [cited January 22, 2008]. http://www3.niaid.nih.gov/healthscience/healthtopics/streptococcal/default.htm.

"Strep Throat." Mayo Clinic. Nov 3, 2008 [cited January 22, 2008]. http://www.mayoclinic.com/health/strep-throat/DS00260.

Maureen Haggerty
Tish Davidson, A.M.

Streptococcal sore throat *see* **Strep throat**

Stress

Definition

Stress is defined as an organism's total response to environmental demands or pressures. The English word *stress* is derived from the Latin verb *stringere*, which means "to draw tight," "diminish," or "inhibit." Stress was originally defined by a Canadian biologist named Hans Selye (1907–1982) in the 1930s as a series of biochemical, nervous, digestive, and muscular responses in laboratory animals to a perceived threat, which he called a stressor. Selye later expanded the notion of stress to include humans trying to evaluate and respond to various stressors in their daily lives. One recurrent disagreement among researchers, however, concerns the definition of stress in humans. The issue is whether it is primarily an external response that can be measured by changes in glandular secretions, skin reactions, and other physical functions—or whether it is an internal interpretation of or reaction to a stressor, or both.

Some doctors distinguish between positive and negative stress. In the 1970s, a psychologist named Richard Lazarus coined the term *eustress* to refer to stress that is good for health or leads to a sense of fulfillment. Increasing one's strength or endurance through active **exercise** would be an example of eustress, as would completing a course of study or finishing a job assignment.

Description

Stress in humans results from interactions between persons and their environment that are perceived as straining or exceeding their adaptive capacities and threatening their well-being. The element of perception indicates that human stress responses reflect differences in personality as well as differences in physical strength or general health. Researchers have categorized stressors as:

• acute, such as a disaster or death of a loved one

• sequential, such as events leading up to a job promotion or a move

• intermittent, such as periodic tax payments

• chronic, such as living with a life-threatening illness, being in an unhappy marriage, or living in poverty

Biological and personal dimensions of stress

Stress is a complicated set of physical and emotional responses to changes or challenges that occur in everyone's life. On the biological level, stress begins with the so-called fight-or-flight reaction—the activation of a section of the **brain** called the hypothalamic-pituitary-adrenal system, or HPA. When a human perceives a situation as stressful, the HPA system releases cortisol, a steroid hormone. The next stage in the stress reaction is the release of neurotransmitters, or brain chemicals, that activate parts of the brain that register the emotion of fear. The neurotransmitters also suppress activity in parts of the brain associated with short-term **memory**, concentration, and rational thinking. This limitation allows a human to react quickly to a stressful situation but it also lowers his or her ability to deal with intellectual or social factors that may be part of the situation.

On the physical level, the person's **heart** rate and **blood pressure** rise; they breathe more rapidly, which allows the **lungs** to take in more oxygen. **Blood** flow to the muscles, lungs, and brain may increase by 300 to 400 percent. The spleen releases more blood cells into the circulation, which increases the blood's ability to transport oxygen. The **immune system** redirects white blood cells to the skin, **bone** marrow, and lymph nodes. At the same time, nonessential body systems shut down. The skin becomes cool and sweaty as blood is drawn away from it toward the heart and muscles. The mouth becomes dry, and the **digestive system** slows down.

After the crisis passes, the levels of stress hormones drop and the body's various organ systems return to normal. This return is called the **relaxation** response. Some people are more vulnerable to stress than others because their hormone levels do not return to normal after a stressful event. In chronic stress, the organ systems of the body do not have the opportunity to return fully to normal levels. Different organs become under- or overactivated on a long-term basis. In time, these abnormal levels of activity can damage an organ or organ system.

What complicates the experience of stress is that different people respond differently to stressors. Some people find driving a highly stressful experience, for example, while others enjoy it. Similarly, some people enjoy the intellectual challenges of certain fields of study, while others are bored by them. Personality differences are another factor that influences people's response to stress. Some people are highly aggressive, inclined to worry, or easily irritated, while others are less competitive or more optimistic about life.

Risk factors for stress-related illness

Almost everyone has experienced acute or episodic acute stressors. Some people, however, are more vulnerable than others to chronic stress-related illnesses:

- Children. Children have very little control over their environments. In addition, they are often unable to communicate their feelings accurately, or others may not take their feelings seriously.

- Elderly adults. Aging appears to affect the body's response to stress, so that the relaxation response following a stressful event is slower and less complete. In addition, the elderly are often affected by such major stressors as health problems, the death of a spouse or close friends, and financial worries.

- Caregivers of mentally or physically disabled family members.

- Women in general.

- People with less education.

- People who belong to racial or ethnic groups that suffer discrimination.

- People who live in cities.

- People who are anger-prone. Chronic anger is associated with narrowing of the arteries, a factor in heart disease.

- People who lack supportive relatives or friends.

Causes and Symptoms

Stress is caused by the human body's response to any event or situation perceived as a stressor. Perception is an important factor in a person's reaction to stress because it can be modified or changed in some situations.

The specific symptoms of stress-related illness vary from person to person depending on which organs or body systems are most vulnerable. Common symptoms of stress include:

- Heart. Chronic stress raises blood pressure, triggers the release of cholesterol into the bloodstream, and causes the arteries to narrow. It also increases the possibility that a clot will form in the coronary arteries, thus increasing the person's risk of heart attack or stroke.

- Skin. Eczema and other allergic skin rashes can be triggered or made worse by stress.

- Digestive tract. Stress leads to nausea, diarrhea, constipation, bloating, and irritable bowel syndrome in many people. It may also play a role in the onset of eating disorders.

- Reproductive system. Stress can lead to loss of sexual desire in both men and women. In addition, stress during pregnancy is associated with a 50 percent higher risk of miscarriage. High stress levels on the mother during pregnancy are also related to higher rates of premature births and babies of lower than average birth weight; both are risk factors for infant mortality.

- Bones, joints, and muscles. Stress intensifies the chronic pain of arthritis and other joint disorders. It also produces tension-type headaches, which are headaches caused by the tightening of the muscles in the neck and scalp.

- Brain and central nervous system. Stress hormones released during acute stress interfere with memory and learning. People who are under severe stress become unable to concentrate; they may become clumsy and accident-prone. Acute stress interferes with short-term memory, although this effect goes away after the stress is resolved. In children, however, the brain's biochemical responses to stress clearly limit the ability to learn.

- Immune system. Chronic stress increases a person's risk of getting an infectious illness. Several research studies have shown that people under chronic stress have lower than normal white blood cell counts and are more vulnerable to colds and influenza. Men with HIV infection and high stress levels progress more rapidly to AIDS than infected men with lower stress levels.

Stress-related emotional illness results from inadequate or inappropriate responses to major changes in one's life situation, such as marriage, completing one's education, becoming a parent, losing a job, or retiring. Psychiatrists sometimes use the term *adjustment disorder* to describe this type of illness. In the workplace, stress-related illness often takes the form of burnout—a loss of interest in or ability to perform one's job due to long-term high stress levels.

According to the American Institute of Stress:

- Forty-three percent of all adults suffer adverse health effects due to stress.

- Seventy-five to 90% of all visits to primary care physicans (PCPs) are for stress-related complaints or disorders.

- An estimated 1 million workers are absent on an average workday due to stress-related complaints. Stress is believed to be responsible for more than half of the 550 million workdays lost annually to absenteeism.

- Stress has been linked to all the leading causes of death, including heart disease, cancer, lung ailments, cirrhosis, and suicide.

- Nearly half of all American workers suffer from symptoms of burnout, a disabling reaction to stress on the job.

- Workplace violence is rampant. There are almost 2 million reported instances of homicide, aggravated assault, rape, or sexual assault. Homicide is the second leading cause of fatal occupational injury and the leading cause of death for working women.

Diagnosis

There is no specific laboratory test or imaging study for diagnosing stress as such. People with specific mental disorders related to stress like posttraumatic stress disorder or panic disorder can be diagnosed by a psychiatrist qualified to evaluate these conditions. In most other cases, however, a person is diagnosed in the course of a checkup for a stress-related physical condition when the doctor asks about the stress level in their living situation, school, or job. The physician will need to distinguish between adjustment disorders and **anxiety** or mood disorders, and between psychiatric disorders and physical illnesses (e.g., thyroid deficiency or surplus) that have psychological side effects.

Many physicians will also evaluate the patient's personality, to assess his or her coping resources and emotional response patterns. There are a number of personality inventories and **psychological tests** that can be used to help evaluate the amount of stress the patient experiences and the coping mechanisms that he or she uses to deal with it. Stress-related illness can be diagnosed by a primary care physician (PCP) or a psychiatrist. A test that is used for measuring life stress is the Life Events Scale, also known as the Holmes and Rahe Stress Scale, after the two psychologists who devised it in 1967. It is used to determine whether the patient is at risk for stress-related illnesses, and can be administered while taking a social history at no extra cost. The test comprises stressors that are ranked in from most stressful (e.g., death of a spouse) to least stressful (e.g., minor violations of the law). Each item is assigned a value and is based on thousands of interviews and medical histories identifying the kinds of events that people found stressful.

Treatment

Treatment for stress depends on the parts of the person's body that are affected and the sources of stress and types of stress in their life. Most people benefit from a combination of treatment approaches:

- Medications. These can be prescribed to treat physical conditions related to stress like high blood pressure or high cholesterol levels, or to help relieve emotional anxiety.

- Psychotherapy. The two approaches most often used in treating stress are interpersonal therapy and cognitive therapy. In interpersonal therapy, the person learns about the events in their past and the triggers in their life that set off the stress response, together with strategies for coping with stressors. Cognitive therapy works by teaching the patient to change his or her ways of thinking about stressful situations or events. Many people have underlying negative assumptions about life that make them more vulnerable to stress.

- Lifestyle changes. People who have used alcohol, drugs, or tobacco are usually advised to quit. In some cases, people may have to change jobs or leave bad relationships in order to relieve chronic stress.

- Physical exercise. Physical activity is a good way to work off tension in the muscles and joints, and to improve strength and endurance.

- Stress management. Stress management refers to programs or techniques intended to help people deal more effectively with stress. Many of these are intended to help people handle job- or workplace-related stress. Stress management programs ask participants to identify the specific aspects of their job that they find stressful and then plan a course of positive action to lower their stress levels.

- Complementary and alternative approaches. Acupuncture, yoga, relaxation training, meditation, prayer and religious practice, guided imagery, hypnosis, massage therapy, music therapy, humor, and pet therapy are alternative approaches that help many people cope with stress.

Prognosis

The prognosis for recovery from a stress-related illness is related to a wide variety of factors in a person's life, many of which are genetically determined (i.e., race, sex, illnesses that run in families) or beyond the individual's control (e.g., economic trends, cultural stereotypes and prejudices). Some people tend to focus on their feelings about the stressful situation while others focus on solving the problem. Still others react to stress by trying to escape from it through drugs or alcohol. It is possible, however, for humans to learn new responses to stress. A person's ability to remain healthy in stressful situations is sometimes referred to as stress hardiness. Stress-hardy people have a cluster of personality traits that strengthen their abilities to cope with stress. These traits include believing in the importance of what they are doing; believing that they have some power to influence their situation; and viewing life's changes as positive opportunities rather than threats.

Prevention

Complete prevention of stress is neither possible nor desirable, because stress is an important stimulus of human growth and creativity, and an inevitable part of life. In addition, specific strategies for stress prevention vary widely from person to person, depending on the nature and number of the stressors in an individual's life, and the amount of control he or she has over these factors. In general, however, a

KEY TERMS

Adjustment disorder—A psychiatric disorder marked by inappropriate or inadequate responses to a change in life circumstances. Depression following retirement from work is an example of adjustment disorder.

Burnout—An emotional condition, marked by tiredness, loss of interest, or frustration, that interferes with job performance. Burnout is usually regarded as the result of prolonged stress.

Eustress—A term that is sometimes used to refer to positive stress.

Hypothalamic-pituitary-adrenal (HPA) system—A complex feedback system among the hypothalamus, the pituitary gland, and the adrenal gland that governs the body's response to stress. It is also called the HPA axis.

Stress hardiness—A personality characteristic that enables persons to stay healthy in stressful circumstances. It includes belief in one's ability to influence the situation; being committed to or fully engaged in one's activities; and having a positive view of change.

Stress management—Any set of techniques intended to help people deal more effectively with stress in their lives by analyzing specific stressors and taking positive actions to minimize their effects.

Stressor—Any event or stimulus that provokes a stress response in a human or animal.

combination of attitude and behavioral changes works well for most patients.

The National Institutes of Health (NIH) has compiled a list of ten things people can do to prevent stress:

1. Stay away from stressors that can be avoided.

2. Avoid making too many lifestyle changes too close together—such as trying to quit smoking while planning to move to a new city and take a new job.

3. Recognize limitations and not take on too many responsibilities at the same time.

4. Organize tasks according to priority and allow enough time to complete each one.

5. Learn to communicate effectively and politely with others.

6. Don't isolate; share thoughts or feelings with friends, family, or appropriate others, and take their advice if it seems reasonable and helpful.

QUESTIONS TO ASK YOUR DOCTOR

- How many of your patients have come to you with stress-related illnesses?
- What were your treatment recommendations?
- What is your opinion of alternative therapies for stress?
- How can I tell when I'm at risk of burnout at work?
- What is the difference between a temporary reaction to stress and an adjustment disorder?

7. Cultivate a positive attitude toward life.

8. Set aside time for a break or a treat as a reward for overcoming a stressful situation.

9. Get regular physical exercise, at least 30 minutes each day.

10. Eat a healthful diet and get enough sleep.

Resources

BOOKS

Greenberg, Jerrold S. *Comprehensive Stress Management*, 13th ed. New York: McGraw-Hill, 2013.

Harrington, Rick. *Stress, Health and Well-being: Thriving in the 21st Century*. Belmont, CA: Wadsworth Cengage Learning, 2013.

Olpin, Michael, and Margie Hesson. *Stress Management for Life: A Research-based, Experiential Approach*, 3rd ed. Belmont, CA: Wadsworth Cengage Learning, 2013.

Rice, Virginia Hill, ed. *Handbook of Stress, Coping, and Health: Implications for Nursing Research, Theory, and Practice*, 2nd ed. Thousand Oaks, CA: SAGE Publications, 2012.

PERIODICALS

Gaither, C.A., and A. Nadkami. "Interpersonal Interactions, Job Demands and Work-related Outcomes in Pharmacy." *International Journal of Pharmacy Practice* 10 (April 2012): 80–89.

Garrido, P. "Aging and Stress: Past Hypotheses, Present Approaches and Perspectives." *Aging and Disease* 2 (February 2011): 80–99.

Guenthner, D.H. "Emergency and Crisis Management: Critical Incident Stress Management for First Responders and Business Organisations." *Journal of Business Continuity and Emergency Planning* 5 (March 2912): 298–315.

Jones, T., and M.D. Moller. "Implications of Hypothalamic-Pituitary-Adrenal Axis Functioning in Posttraumatic Stress Disorder." *Journal of the American Psychiatric Nurses Association* 17 (November-December 2011): 393–403.

Laschinger, H.K., and A.L. Grau. "The Influence of Personal Dispositional Factors and Organizational Resources on

Workplace Violence, Burnout, and Health Outcomes in New Graduate Nurses: A Cross-sectional Study." *International Journal of Nursing Studies* 49 (March 2012): 282–291.

Pinheiro, A., and D.O. Anderson. "Improving Your Workplace Violence Prevention Program." *Occupational Health and Safety* 81 (March 2012): 40–41.

Renzi, C., et al. "Psychiatric Morbidity and Emotional Exhaustion among Hospital Physicians and Nurses: Association with Perceived Job-related Factors." *Archives of Environmental and Occupational Health* 67 (April 2012): 117–123.

White, L.S. "Reducing Stress in School-age Girls through Mindful Yoga." *Journal of Pediatric Health Care* 26 (January–February 2012): 45–56.

Wolever, R.Q., et al. "Effective and Viable Mind-Body Stress Reduction in the Workplace: A Randomized Controlled Trial." *Journal of Occupational Health Psychology* 17 (April 2012): 246–258.

WEBSITES

American Heart Association (AHA). "How Can I Manage Stress?" http://www.heart.org/idc/groups/heart-public/@wcm/@hcm/documents/image/ucm_300690.pdf (accessed May 15, 2012).

American Institute of Stress (AIS). "Effects of Stress." http://www.stress.org/topic-effects.htm (accessed May 15, 2012).

American Institute of Stress (AIS). "Why Is There More Stress Today?" http://www.stress.org/americas.htm (accessed May 15, 2012).

Holmes and Rahe Stress Scale. http://www.mindtools.com/pages/article/newTCS_82.htm (accessed May 15, 2012).

Merck Manual for Health Care Professionals. "Stress Disorders." http://www.merckmanuals.com/professional/psychiatric_disorders/anxiety_disorders/stress_disorders.html (accessed May 15, 2012).

National Institute for Occupational Safety and Health (NIOSH). *Working with Stress.* This is a 17-minute video on workplace stress that can be viewed online, downloaded in Flash format, or downloaded in transcript form. http://www.cdc.gov/niosh/docs/video/stress1.html (accessed May 15, 2012).

National Library of Medicine (NLM). "Managing Stress." This is an educational module about stress management that can be viewed in self-playing, interactive, or transcript format. http://www.nlm.nih.gov/medlineplus/tutorials/managingstress/htm/index.htm (accessed May 15, 2012).

ORGANIZATIONS

American Heart Association, 7272 Greenville Ave., Dallas, TX 75231, (800) 242-8721, http://www.heart.org/HEARTORG/

American Institute of Stress (AIS), 124 Park Avenue, Yonkers, NY 10703, (914) 963-1200, Fax: (914) 965-6267, Stress125@optonline.net, http://www.stress.org/

National Institute for Occupational Safety and Health (NIOSH), Centers for Disease Control and Prevention (CDC), 1600 Clifton Road, Atlanta, GA 30333, (800) CDC-INFO (232-4636), cdcinfo@cdc.gov, http://www.cdc.gov/niosh/

Barbara M. Chandler
Rebecca J. Frey, Ph.D.

Stress test

Definition

A stress test is primarily used to identify **coronary artery disease**. It requires patients to **exercise** on a treadmill or exercise bicycle while their **heart** rate, **blood pressure**, electrocardiogram (ECG), and symptoms are monitored.

Purpose

The body requires more oxygen during exercise than rest. To deliver more oxygen during exercise, the heart has to pump more oxygen-rich **blood**. Because of the increased stress on the heart, exercise can reveal coronary problems that are not apparent when the body is at rest. This is why the stress test, though not perfect, remains the best initial, noninvasive, practical coronary test.

The stress test is particularly useful for detecting **ischemia** (inadequate supply of blood to the heart muscle) caused by blocked coronary arteries. Less commonly, it is used to determine safe levels of exercise in people with existing coronary artery disease.

Precautions

The exercise stress test carries a very slight risk (one in 100,000) of causing a heart attack. For this reason, exercise stress tests should be attended by health care professionals with immediate access to defibrillators and other emergency equipment.

Patient are cautioned to stop the test should they develop any of the following symptoms:

- an unsteady gait
- confusion
- skin that is grayish or cold and clammy
- dizziness or fainting
- a drop in blood pressure
- angina (chest pain)
- cardiac arrhythmias (irregular heart beat)

Description

A technician affixes electrodes to the patient's chest, using adhesive patches with a special gel that conducts

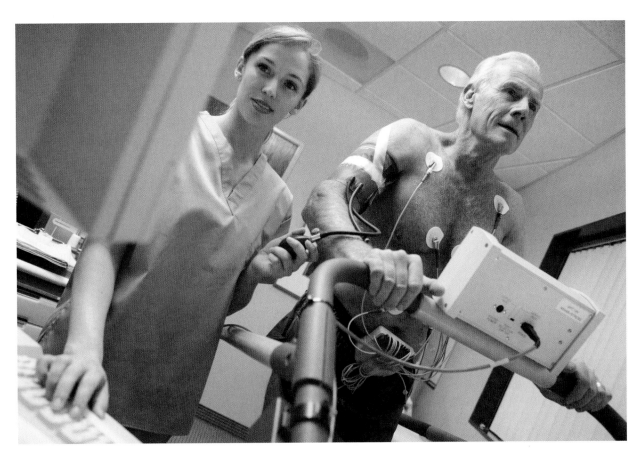

(*Monkey Business Images/Shutterstock.com*)

electrical impulses. Typically, electrodes are placed under each collarbone and each bottom rib, and six electrodes are placed across the chest in a rough outline of the heart. Wires from the electrodes are connected to an ECG, which records the electrical activity picked up by the electrodes.

The technician runs resting ECG tests while the patient is lying down, then standing up, and then breathing heavily for half a minute. These baseline tests can later be compared with the ECG tests performed while the patient is exercising. The patient's blood pressure is taken and the blood pressure cuff is left in place, so that blood pressure can be measured periodically throughout the test.

The patient begins riding a stationary bicycle or walking on a treadmill. Gradually the intensity of the exercise is increased. For example, if the patient is walking on a treadmill, then the speed of the treadmill increases and the treadmill is tilted upward to simulate an incline. If the patient is on an exercise bicycle, then the resistance or "drag" is gradually increased. The patient continues exercising at increasing intensity until reaching the target heart rate (generally set at a minimum of 85% of the maximal predicted heart rate based on the patient's

age) or experiences severe fatigue, **dizziness**, or chest **pain**. During the test, the patient's heart rate, ECG, and blood pressure are monitored.

Sometimes other tests, such as **echocardiography** or thallium scanning, are used in conjunction with the exercise stress test. For instance, recent studies suggest that women have a high rate of false negatives (results showing no problem when one exists) and false positives (results showing a problem when one does not exist) with the stress test. They may benefit from another test, such as exercise echocardiography. People who are unable to exercise may be injected with drugs, such as adenosine, which mimic the effects of exercise on the heart, and then given a thallium scan. The thallium scan or echocardiogram are particularly useful when the patient's resting ECG is abnormal. In such cases, interpretation of exercise induced ECG abnormalities is difficult.

Preparation

Patients are usually instructed not to eat or smoke for several hours before the test. They should be advised to inform the physician about any medications they are taking, and to wear comfortable sneakers and exercise clothing.

KEY TERMS

Angina—Chest pain from a poor blood supply to the heart muscle due to stenosis (narrowing) of the coronary arteries.

Cardiac arrhythmia—An irregular heart rate or rhythm.

Defibrillator—A device that delivers an electric shock to the heart muscle through the chest wall in order to restore a normal heart rate.

False negative—Test results showing no problem when one exists.

False positive—Test results showing a problem when one does not exist.

Hypertrophy—The overgrowth of muscle.

Ischemia—Dimished supply of oxygen-rich blood to an organ or area of the body.

Aftercare

After the test, the patient should rest until blood pressure and heart rate return to normal. If all goes well, and there are no signs of distress, the patient may return to his or her normal daily activities.

Complications

There is a very slight risk of **myocardial infarction** (a heart attack) from the exercise, as well as cardiac arrhythmia (irregular heart beats), **angina**, or cardiac arrest (about one in 100,000).

Results

A normal result of an exercise stress test shows normal electrocardiogram tracings and heart rate, blood pressure within the normal range, and no angina, unusual dizziness, or shortness of breath.

A number of abnormalities may appear on an exercise stress test. Examples of exercise-induced ECG abnormalities are ST segment depression or heart rhythm disturbances. These ECG abnormalities may indicate deprivation of blood to the heart muscle (ischemia) caused by blocked coronary arteries. Stress test abnormalities generally require further diagnostic evaluation and therapy.

Health care team roles

A stress test is generally ordered by a primary care physician or cardiologist and is performed by a trained technician. All health care providers performing or monitoring stress tests should be prepared to provide emergency medical intervention, such as **defibrillation**.

Patient education

Patients must be well prepared for a stress test. They should not only know the purpose of the test, but also signs and symptoms that indicate the test should be stopped. Physicians, nurses, and ECG technicians can ensure patient safety by encouraging them to immediately communicate discomfort at any time during the stress test.

Resources

BOOKS

Ahya, Shubada H., et al., eds. *The Washington Manual of Medical Therapeutics,* 33th edition. Philadelphia: Lippincott Williams & Wilkins, 2010.

The Faculty Members of the Yale University School of Medicine. *The Patient's Guide to Medical Tests.* Boston, New York: Houghton Mifflin Company, 1997.

ORGANIZATIONS

American Heart Association. 7272 Greenville Avenue, Dallas, TX 75231. (214) 373-6300. http://www.amhrt.org.

National Heart, Lung, and Blood Institute. Information Center. P.O. Box 30105, Bethesda, MD 20824-0105. (301) 951-3260. http://www.nhlbi.nih.gov.

Barbara Wexler

Stroke

Definition

Stroke is a life-threatening condition that occurs when the **blood** supply to a part of the **brain** is suddenly cut off or when brain tissue is damaged by bleeding into the brain. There are two main types of stroke. Ischemic stroke occurs when a clot blocks an artery to the brain; this type accounts for about 80 percent of strokes. The other type, hemorrhagic stroke, occurs when a blood vessel in the brain bursts, allowing blood to spill out into brain tissue. The blood upsets the chemical balance that the nerve cells in the brain need to function.

Demographics

According to the Centers for Disease Control and Prevention (CDC), stroke is the fourth leading cause of death in the United States as of 2009, being responsible for about 128,000 deaths each year. About 795,000 Americans have strokes each year, 550,000 for the first time and 245,000 having a second or third stroke. Of these cases, approximately 625,000 are ischemic strokes.

The total cost of stroke to the U.S. economy per year as of 2009 is approximately $68.9 billion. By the year 2025, the annual number of strokes is expected to reach 1 million. As of 2009, more than 4.4 million people in the United States are stroke survivors. Worldwide, the World Health Organization estimatesáthat 15 million people suffer a stroke each year, resulting in 5 million deaths and 5 million permanently disabled survivors.

About 50,000 Americans have a transient ischemic attack (TIA) in an average year; of this group, 35 percent will have a severe stroke at some point in the future.

Strokes can affect people in any age group; however, the risk increases sharply in people over 55 years of age, doubling every decade over age 55. Seventy-five percent of all strokes in Canada and the United States occur in people over 64. Men are 1.25 times more likely to have strokes than women; however, women are more likely to die of stroke because they are usually older when they have their first stroke.

Strokes in children are rare—about six cases per 100,000 children per year in North America. About one-third of these cases are in newborns.

African Americans have an increased risk of stroke compared to other racial and ethnic groups in the United States, and they are also more likely to suffer a stroke at younger ages. Hispanics are at lesser risk of stroke than African Americans, but they also tend to have strokes at relatively young ages. African Americans between the ages of 45 and 55 die from stroke 4–5 times more often that Caucasians in the same age group.

Description

Stroke is usually a sudden occurrence. A stroke occurs when blood flow is interrupted to part of the brain. Without blood to supply oxygen and nutrients and to remove waste products, brain cells quickly begin to die. Depending on the region of the brain affected, a stroke may cause **paralysis**, speech impairment, loss of **memory** and reasoning ability, **coma**, or death. A stroke also is sometimes called a brain attack or a **cerebrovascular accident** (CVA).

Some people have a warning event called a transient ischemic attack (TIA) or mini-stroke. A TIA has the same symptoms as a full-blown stroke but goes away in a few minutes or hours, leaving no permanent effects. It is, however, an indication that the person is at risk of a major stroke and should see their doctor right away. A TIA offers the person an opportunity to take preventive action.

Stroke is a medical emergency requiring immediate treatment. Prompt treatment improves the chances of survival and increases the degree of recovery that may be expected. A person who may have suffered a stroke should be seen in a hospital emergency room without delay. Treatment to break up a blood clot, the major cause of stroke, must begin within three hours of the stroke to be effective. Improved medical treatment of all types of stroke has resulted in a dramatic decline in death rates in recent decades. In 1950, nine in ten stroke patients died, compared to slightly less than one in three in the twenty-first century. However, about two-thirds of stroke survivors have disabilities ranging from moderate to severe.

Risk factors

Risk factors for stroke in adults include:

- Hypertension (high blood pressure), the most important single risk factor for stroke
- High blood cholesterol levels
- Age over 55
- A family history of stroke, TIA, or heart attack
- Diabetes
- Smoking, which doubles a person's risk of ischemic stroke
- Personal history of previous stroke or TIA
- Obesity
- Heavy use of cocaine
- Irregular heart rhythm
- High alcohol consumption, which raises a person's blood pressure
- Use of birth control pills or hormone replacement therapy

Risk factors for stroke in children include:

- Congenital (present at birth) malformations of blood vessels and other structures in the brain
- Infections of the brain like encephalitis and meningitis
- Head trauma
- Blood disorders, particularly sickle cell disease

Causes and symptoms

Causes

Stroke is caused by a loss of blood supply to the brain resulting either from a clot blocking an artery or from bleeding into or around the brain. Ischemic stroke can result from two types of clots. The first is an embolus, which is a free-floating clot produced in the **heart** or somewhere else in the body that travels to a blood vessel in the brain. The second type of clot is called a thrombus. It is formed within an artery in the head or neck and grows there until it is large enough to block the artery. **Atherosclerosis**, a disease of the **blood** vessels in which fatty deposits build up along the walls of the vessels, is a common cause of this type of clot.

ISCHEMIC STROKE. A cerebral **embolism** occurs when a blood clot from elsewhere in the circulatory system breaks free. If it becomes lodged in an artery supplying the brain, either in the brain or in the neck, it can cause a stroke. The most common cause of cerebral embolism is **atrial fibrillation**, a disorder of the heart beat. In atrial fibrillation, the upper chambers (atria) of the heart beat weakly and rapidly instead of slowly and steadily. Blood within the atria is not completely emptied. This stagnant blood may form clots within the atria, which can then break off and enter the circulation. Atrial fibrillation is a factor in about 15% of all strokes. The risk of a stroke from atrial fibrillation can be dramatically reduced with daily use of anticoagulant medication.

Cerebral thrombosis occurs when a blood clot, or thrombus, forms within the brain itself, blocking the flow of blood through the affected vessel. Clots most often form due to "hardening" (atherosclerosis) of brain arteries. Cerebral thrombosis occurs most often at night or early in the morning. Cerebral thrombosis is often preceded by a transient ischemic attack, or TIA, sometimes called a mini-stroke. In a TIA, blood flow is temporarily interrupted, causing short-lived stroke-like symptoms. Recognizing the occurrence of a TIA and seeking immediate treatment is an important step in stroke prevention.

HEMORRHAGIC STROKE. Hemorrhagic stroke can occur when an aneurysm—a weak spot in the wall of an artery—suddenly bursts. High **blood pressure** is the most common cause of this type of hemorrhagic stroke. Hemorrhagic stroke can also occur when the walls of an artery become thin and brittle; they can then break and leak blood into the brain. Hemorrhagic stroke can take one of two forms: The blood can leak directly into brain tissue from an artery in the brain, or it can leak from an artery near the surface of the brain into the space between the **skull** and the membranes covering the brain.

The vessels most likely to break are those with preexisting defects such as an **aneurysm**. An aneurysm is a bulge or pouch in a blood vessel caused by weakening of the arterial wall. Brain aneurysms are surprisingly common; according to **autopsy** studies, about 6% of all Americans have them. Aneurysms rarely cause symptoms until they burst, however. Aneurysms are most likely to burst when blood pressure is highest, and controlling blood pressure is an important preventive strategy.

Intracerebral hemorrhage affects vessels within the brain itself, while subarachnoid hemorrhage affects arteries at the brain's surface, just below the protective arachnoid membrane. Intracerebral hemorrhages represent about 10% of all strokes, while subarachnoid hemorrhages account for about 7%.

In addition to depriving affected tissues of blood supply, the accumulation of fluid within the inflexible skull creates excess pressure on brain tissue, which can quickly lead to death. Nonetheless, recovery may be more complete for a person who survives hemorrhage than for one who survives a clot, because the effects of blood deprivation usually are not as severe.

The death of brain cells triggers a chain reaction in which toxic chemicals created by cell death affect other nearby cells. This is one reason why prompt treatment can have such a dramatic effect on final recovery.

Symptoms

Stroke has five major signs or symptoms:

- Walk: Is the person having trouble with balance or coordination?
- Talk: Is speech difficult or slurred? Is the person's face drooping?
- Reach: Is one side of the body weak or numb?
- See: Is vision partly or entirely lost?
- Feel: Does the person have a sudden severe headache with no obvious cause?

Other symptoms of stroke that some patients experience are drooling, uncontrollable eye movements, personality or mood changes, drowsiness, loss of memory, or loss of consciousness.

A person with stroke can have more than one of these symptoms at the same time. The important feature to keep in mind is that the symptoms of an embolic ischemic stroke come on suddenly, which helps in distinguishing stroke from other causes of **dizziness**, **vision** problems, or **headache**. The symptoms of a thrombotic stroke come on more gradually.

A child having a stroke may lose bladder control, have a seizure, or have nausea and **vomiting** as well as the symptoms associated with stroke in adults.

Diagnosis

The diagnosis of stroke includes taking the patient's history and obtaining an account of the patient's present symptoms. In younger patients, the doctor will ask about recent drug use, head trauma, use of oral contraceptives, or **bleeding disorders**. In middle-aged and older patients, the doctor will ask about such risk factors as **hypertension**, diabetes, tobacco use, high **cholesterol**, and a history of **coronary artery disease**, coronary artery bypass surgery, or atrial fibrillation.

An important part of the history-taking is finding out when the symptoms began and when the patient was last seen normal. Information from family, bystanders, or emergency personnel is often critical to prompt diagnosis and treatment, particularly when tissue plasminogen activator (tPA) therapy is an option. If the patient has awakened with the symptoms of stroke, then the time of onset is defined as the time the patient was last seen without symptoms.

Examination

The next step is a complete physical and neurological examination to rule out the possibility that the patient's symptoms are being caused by a **brain tumor**. The examination has several purposes: checking the patient's airway, breathing, and circulation; identifying any neurological deficits; identifying the potential cause(s) of the stroke; and identifying any comorbid conditions the patient may have. The neurologist may use the National Institutes of Health Stroke Scale (NIHSS), which is a checklist that allows the doctor to record the patient's level of consciousness; visual function; ability to move; ability to feel sensations; ability to move the facial muscles; and ability to talk.

Tests

Other tests used to diagnose stroke are:

• Blood tests. These can reveal the existence of blood disorders that increase a person's risk of stroke.

• Computed tomography (CT) scan. This type of imaging test is one of the first tests given to a patient suspected of having a stroke. It helps the doctor determine the cause of the stroke and the extent of brain injury.

• Magnetic resonance imaging (MRI). This imaging test is useful in pinpointing the location of small or deep brain injuries.

• Electroencephalogram (EEG). This test measures the brain's electrical activity.

• Blood flow tests. These are done to detect the location and size of any blockages in the blood vessels. One type of blood flow test uses ultrasound to produce an image of the arteries in the neck leading into the brain. Another type of blood flow test, called angiography, uses a special dye injected into blood vessels that will show up on an x ray.

• Echocardiography. This type of test uses ultrasound to produce an image of the heart. It can be useful in determining whether an embolus from the heart caused the patient's stroke.

Treatment

Traditional

Treatment of stroke depends on whether it is ischemic or hemorrhagic. Ischemic stroke is treated first with blood thinners, often aspirin or warfarin. If the patient is seen by a specialized stroke team within 3 hours of the attack, he or she may be treated with a drug called tissue plasminogen activator or tPA, described more fully in the next section. It is critical, however, to be sure that the patient has an ischemic rather than a hemorrhagic stroke, as blood-thinning drugs can make a hemorrhagic stroke worse.

Ischemic stroke can also be treated by surgery. The two procedures most commonly used are endarterectomy, a procedure in which the surgeon removes the fatty deposits caused by atherosclerosis from the inside of one of the main arteries to the brain and places a tube made of metallic mesh called a stent inside the artery to prevent recurrent narrowing of the artery.

Hemorrhagic stroke is treated by removing pooled blood from the brain and repairing damaged blood vessels. To prevent another hemorrhagic stroke, the surgeon may use a procedure called aneurysm clipping. In this procedure, the surgeon clamps the weak spot in the artery away from the rest of the blood vessel, which reduces the chances that it will burst and bleed. Endovascular treatment may be used for aneurysms that are difficult to reach surgically. In this procedure, a catheter is guided from a larger artery up into the brain to reach the aneurysm. Small coils of wire are discharged into the aneurysm, which plug it and block off blood flow from the main artery.

Drugs

Emergency treatment of stroke from a blood clot is aimed at dissolving the clot. This "thrombolytic therapy" currently is performed most often with tissue plasminogen activator, or tPA. This drug must be administered within three hours of the stroke event. Therefore, patients who awaken with stroke symptoms are ineligible for tPA therapy, as the time of onset cannot be accurately determined. tPA therapy has been shown to improve recovery and decrease long-term disability in selected patients. tPA therapy carries a 6.4% risk of inducing a cerebral hemorrhage, however, and is not appropriate for patients with bleeding disorders, very high blood pressure, known aneurysms, any evidence of intracranial hemorrhage, or incidence of stroke, head trauma, or intracranial surgery within the past three months. Patients with clot-related (thrombotic or embolic) stroke who are ineligible for tPA treatment may be treated with heparin or other blood thinners, or with aspirin or other anti-clotting agents in some cases.

Emergency treatment of hemorrhagic stroke is aimed at controlling intracranial pressure. Intravenous urea or mannitol plus hyperventilation is the most common treatment. **Corticosteroids** also may be used. Patients with reversible bleeding disorders, such as those due to anticoagulant treatment, should have these bleeding disorders reversed, if possible.

Rehabilitation

Rehabilitation refers to a comprehensive program designed to regain function as much as possible and compensate for permanent losses. Approximately 10% of stroke survivors recover without any significant disability and able to function independently. Another 10% are so severely affected that they must remain institutionalized for severe disability. The remaining 80% can return home with appropriate therapy, training, support, and care services.

Rehabilitation is coordinated by a team of medical professionals and may include the services of a neurologist, a physician who specializes in rehabilitation medicine (physiatrist), a physical therapist, an occupational therapist, a speech-language pathologist, a nutritionist, a mental health professional, and a social worker. Rehabilitation services may be provided in an acute care hospital, rehabilitation hospital, long-term care facility, outpatient clinic, or at home.

The rehabilitation program is based on the patient's individual deficits and strengths. Strokes on the left side of the brain primarily affect the right half of the body, and vice versa. In addition, in left-brain dominant people, who constitute a significant majority of the population, left-brain strokes usually lead to speech and language deficits. Right-brain strokes may affect spatial perception. Patients with right brain strokes also may deny their illness, neglect the affected side of their body, and behave impulsively.

Rehabilitation may be complicated by cognitive losses, including diminished ability to understand and follow directions. Poor results are more likely in patients with significant or prolonged cognitive changes, sensory losses, language deficits, or incontinence.

PREVENTION OF COMPLICATIONS. Rehabilitation begins with prevention of stroke recurrence and other medical complications. The risk of stroke recurrence may be reduced with many of the same measures used to prevent stroke, including quitting **smoking** and controlling blood pressure.

One of the most common medical complications following stroke is deep venous thrombosis, in which a clot forms within a limb immobilized by paralysis. Clots that break free often become lodged in an artery feeding the **lungs**. This type of **pulmonary embolism** is a common cause of death in the weeks following a stroke. Resuming activity within a day or two after the stroke is an important preventive measure, along with use of elastic stockings on the lower limbs. Drugs that prevent clotting may be given, including intravenous heparin and oral warfarin.

Weakness and loss of coordination of the swallowing muscles may impair swallowing (**dysphagia**), and allow food to enter the lower airway. This may lead to aspiration **pneumonia**, another common cause of death shortly after a stroke. Dysphagia may be treated with retraining exercises and temporary use of pureed foods.

Depression occurs in 30–60% of stroke patients. Antidepressants and **psychotherapy** may be used in combination. Other medical complications include urinary tract infections, pressure ulcers, **falls**, and seizures.

TYPES OF REHABILITATIVE THERAPY. Brain tissue that dies in a stroke cannot regenerate. In some cases, other brain regions may "take over" the functions of that tissue after a training period. In other cases, compensatory actions may be developed to replace lost abilities.

Physical therapy is used to maintain and restore range of motion and strength in affected limbs, and to maximize mobility in walking, wheelchair use, and transferring (from wheelchair to toilet or from standing to sitting, for instance). The physical therapist advises on mobility aids such as wheelchairs, braces, and canes. In the recovery period, a stroke patient may develop muscle spasticity and contractures, or abnormal contractions. Contractures may be treated with a combination of stretching and splinting.

Occupational therapy improves such self-care skills as feeding, bathing, and dressing, and helps develop effective compensatory strategies and devices for activities of daily living. A speech-language pathologist focuses on communication and swallowing skills. When dysphagia is a problem, a nutritionist can advise alternative meals that provide adequate **nutrition**.

Mental health professionals may be involved in the treatment of depression or loss of thinking (cognitive) skills. A social worker may help coordinate services and ease the transition out of the hospital back into the home. Both social workers and mental health professionals may help counsel the patient and family during the difficult rehabilitation period. Caring for a person affected with stroke requires learning a new set of skills and adapting to new demands and limitations. Home caregivers may develop **stress**, **anxiety**, and depression. Caring for the caregiver is an important part of the overall stroke treatment program.

Support groups can provide an important source of information, advice, and comfort for stroke patients and for caregivers. Joining a support group can be one of the most important steps in the rehabilitation process.

First aid

It is useful for friends, coworkers, or bystanders to know the basics of **first aid** for stroke victims. If someone appears to be having a stroke, the most important first step is to call for emergency help *at once*. Stroke is a medical emergency; the sooner the person is evaluated and treated, the better their chances of recovery. The drug presently considered most useful in treating stroke must be given within 3 hours of the attack to be effective.

Additional measures that can be taken to help the affected person while waiting for the emergency response team:

• If the person stops breathing, give them mouth-to-mouth resuscitation.

• If they are vomiting, tilt their head to one side to prevent them from swallowing the material.

• Do *not* give them anything to eat or drink.

Prognosis

The prognosis of stroke depends on the person's age, the type and location of the stroke, and the amount of time elapsed between diagnosis and treatment. In general, patients with ischemic stroke have a better prognosis than those with hemorrhagic stroke. In one study in the Boston area, 19 percent of patients with ischemic stroke died within the first 30 days of the attack compared to 35 percent with hemorrhagic stroke.

Stroke is fatal for about 27% of white males, 52% of black males, 23% of white females, and 40% of black females. Stroke survivors may be left with significant deficits. Emergency treatment and comprehensive rehabilitation can significantly improve both survival and recovery. One recent study found that treating stroke survivors with certain antidepressant medications, even if they were not depressed, could increase their chances of living longer. People who received the treatment were less likely to die from cardiovascular events than those who did not receive **antidepressant drugs**.

About 10 percent of stroke patients recover enough function to live independently without help; another 50 percent can remain at home with outside assistance. The remaining 40 percent require long-term care in a nursing home.

Stroke in children can be devastating. Between 20% and 35% of newborns who survive a stroke will go on to have a second stroke. More than 66% of older children who suffer strokes will have cognitive deficits, seizures, behavioral problems, changes in personality, or physical disabilities. Unlike adult survivors, children who survive strokes may develop mental retardation, epilepsy, or **cerebral palsy**.

Prevention

Many strokes are preventable with proper self-care. People cannot change some risk factors for stroke, such as race, age, sex, or family history, but they can control several other risk factors:

• They can quit smoking, drinking heavily, or using cocaine.

• They can keep their weight at a healthy level.

• They can exercise regularly, eat a healthy diet, and take medications for high blood pressure if they are diagnosed with it.

• They can take steps to lower their risk of diabetes or high blood cholesterol levels.

• They can lower the level of emotional stress in their life or learn to manage stress more effectively.

• They can get regular checkups for abnormal heart rhythms if they have been diagnosed with such problems.

• They can see their doctor at once if they have a TIA.

People with no previous history of stroke may be given certain drugs as preventive measures. These drugs include statins (drugs that lower blood cholesterol levels) and platelet antiaggregants (medications intended to prevent platelets in the blood from forming clumps that may lead to clots). Among the latter medications are aspirin, aspririn with extended release dipyridamole, clopidogrel (Plavix) and ticlopidine (Ticlid).

Damage from stroke may be significantly reduced through emergency treatment. Knowing the symptoms of stroke is as important as knowing those of a heart attack. Patients with stroke symptoms should seek emergency treatment without delay, which may mean dialing 911 rather than their family physician.

Treatment of atrial fibrillation may significantly reduce the risk of stroke. Preventive anticoagulant therapy may benefit those with untreated atrial fibrillation. Warfarin (Coumadin) has proven to be more effective than aspirin for patients at higher risk of stroke. Warfarin is, however, complicated to use because it interacts with a large number of other drugs and requires frequent monitoring by the patient's physician.

A recent innovation is the use of computer technology to allow stroke experts in one hospital to evaluate and diagnose a patient in another hospital that might not have a specialist available. Called TeleStroke, the network allows a patient to be evaluated for ischemic stroke within the three-hour time limit for the effective use of tPA. TeleStroke networks are now established in more than 20 states.

Resources

BOOKS

Brainin, Michael, and Hans-Dieter Heiss, eds. *Textbook of Stroke Medicine*. New York: Cambridge University Press, 2010.

Gillen, Glen. *Stroke Rehabilitation*. New York: Mosby, 2010.

Palmer, Sara, and Jeffrey B. Palmer. *When Your Spouse Has a Stroke: Caring for Your Partner, Yourself, and Your*

Relationship. Baltimore: Johns Hopkins University Press, 2011.

Williams, Olajide. *Stroke Diaries: A Guide for Survivors and Their Families.* New York: Oxford University Press, 2010.

PERIODICALS

Alvarez-Sabin, J., et al. "Therapeutic Interventions and Success in Risk Factor Control for Secondary Prevention of Stroke." *Journal of Stroke and Cerebrovascular Diseases* 18 (November/December 2009): 460–65.

Birns, Jonathan. "Stroke." *GP* August 6, 2010, 29.

Jellinger, K.A. "Stroke Medicine." *European Journal of Neurology* 17 (8) (August 2010): 66.

Mathews, M.S., et al. "Safety, Effectiveness, and Practicality of Endovascular Therapy within the First 3 Hours of Acute Ischemic Stroke Onset." *Neurosurgery* 65 (November 2009): 860–65.

Reiss, A.B., and E. Wirkowski. "Statins in Neurological Disorders: Mechanisms and Therapeutic Value." *Scientific World Journal* 9 (November 1, 2009): 1242–59.

Zivin, J.A. "Acute Stroke Therapy with Tissue Plasminogen Activator (tPA) Since It Was Approved by the U.S. Food and Drug Administration (FDA)." *Annals of Neurology* 66 (July 2009): 6–10.

OTHER

Brain Aneurysm Foundation. *Act Now: Brain Aneurysm Basics That Can Save Your Life.* http://www.bafound.org/sites/default/files/BAF_Brain_Aneurysm_Basics_0.pdf (accessed August 10, 2011).

Centers for Disease Control and Prevention (CDC). *Stroke Home Page.* http://www.cdc.gov/stroke/index.htm (accessed August 10, 2011).

Jausch, Edward C. "Acute Management of Stroke." *eMedicine,* April 6, 2011. http://emedicine.medscape.com/article/1159752-overview (accessed August 10, 2011).

Mayo Clinic. *Stroke.* http://www.mayoclinic.com/health/stroke/DS00150.

National Heart, Lung, and Blood Institute (NHLBI). *What Is an Aneurysm?* http://www.nhlbi.nih.gov/health/dci/Diseases/arm/arm_what.html (accessed August 10, 2011).

National Institute of Neurological Disorders and Stroke (NINDS). *Cerebral Aneurysm Fact Sheet.* http://www.ninds.nih.gov/disorders/cerebral_aneurysm/detail_cerebral_aneurysm.htm.

National Institute of Neurological Disorders and Stroke (NINDS). *Stroke: Hope through Research.* November 2009. http://www.ninds.nih.gov/disorders/stroke/detail_stroke.htm (accessed August 10, 2011).

National Stroke Association (NSA). *Stroke 101 Fact Sheet.* http://www.stroke.org/site/DocServer/STROKE_101_Fact_Sheet.pdf?docID=4541 (accessed August 10, 2011).

St. John's Hospital (Springfield, IL). *Children and Stroke.* http://www.st-johns.org/services/stroke_center/Children.aspx (accessed August 10, 2011).

ORGANIZATIONS

American Academy of Neurology (AAN), 1080 Montreal Avenue, Saint Paul, MN 55116, 651-695-2717, 800-879-1960, Fax: 651-695-2791, http://www.aan.com/

American Stroke Association (ASA), 7272 Greenville Avenue, Dallas, TX 75231, 888-4-STROKE, Fax: 214-706-5231, strokeassociation@heart.org, http://www.strokeassociation.org/presenter.jhtml?identifier=1200037

Brain Aneurysm Foundation (BAF), 269 Hanover Street, Building 3, Hanover, MA 02339, 781-826-5556, 888-272-4602, office@bafound.org, http://www.bafound.org/

National Heart, Lung, and Blood Institute (NHLBI), Health Information Center, P.O. Box 30105, Bethesda, MD 20824-0105, 301-592-8573, Fax: 240-629-3246, nhlbinfo@nhlbi.nih.gov, http://www.nhlbi.nih.gov/

National Institute of Neurological Disorders and Stroke (NINDS), P.O. Box 5801, Bethesda, MD 20824, (800) 352-9424, (301) 496-5751, http://www.ninds.nih.gov/index.htm

National Stroke Association (NSA), 9707 E. Easter Lane, Centennial, CO 80112, (800) 787-6537, Fax: (303) 649-1328, info@stroke.org, http://www.stroke.org.

Richard Robinson
Teresa G. Odle
Rebecca J. Frey, Ph.D.
Fran Hodgkins

Stroke *see* **Cerebrovascular accident**

Stupor *see* **Coma**

Stuttering

Definition

Stuttering is a speech disorder in which there is a disruption in the normal flow of speech (disfluency). Disfluencies include repetitions of a sound, syllable, or word; silent blocks (drawing out a sound silently); and prolongations (drawing out a voiced sound). Certain behaviors such as eye blinks, facial twitches, or body movements may also accompany stuttering. Stuttering may become worse under stressful situations (such as speaking in front of a group) but may improve when speaking, reading aloud, or singing while alone.

Description

It is estimated that approximately three million Americans are affected by some form of stuttering. The disorder most often affects children between the ages of two and five, usually resolving before **puberty**. Boys are three times as likely as girls to be stutterers. Less than 1% of adults in the United States suffer from stuttering.

Developmental stuttering (DS) most often occurs in children during the age at which they are developing their language and speech. The onset of DS is gradual, typically occurring before the age of 12. Persistent developmental stuttering (PDS) is defined as stuttering that does not resolve spontaneously or with treatment over time.

Acquired stuttering (AS) occurs in individuals who have been previously fluent. There is no gradual onset of disordered speech in persons with AS; disfluency occurs rather abruptly. AS may be neurogenic or psychogenic. Neurogenic stuttering is caused by problems in the signaling between the **brain** and the various muscles and nerves used in generating speech. This may occur after a **stroke** or damage to the brain. Psychogenic stuttering tends to occur after a trauma or period of extreme **stress**, or in individuals suffering from mental illness.

Causes and symptoms

Although the exact cause of stuttering is not known, there are three leading theories that propose how stuttering develops. The **learning theory** proposes that stuttering is a learned behavior and that most children are occasionally disfluent (e.g., speaking rapidly, searching for the right words) when at the age at which speech and language develop. If a child is criticized or punished for this, he or she may develop **anxiety** about the disfluencies, causing increased stuttering and increased anxiety.

The second theory suggests that stuttering is a psychological problem—that stuttering is an underlying problem that can be treated with **psychotherapy**. The third theory proposes that the cause of stuttering is organic, that neurological differences exist between the brains of those who stutter and those who do not.

There is also some indication that genetic factors are involved in the development of stuttering and subsequent recovery, as shown by various studies done on families and twins. It is not known to what degree stuttering is dependent on genetic factors, on environmental factors, or on both.

Symptoms

A certain measure of disfluency is expected in small children as they learn to speak a language. Some symptoms of normal disfluency are the following:

• fewer than 10 disfluencies per 100 spoken words

• whole-word repetitions ("She-she-she")

• part-word repetitions ("M-milk")

• phrase repetition ("I don't want-I don't want to go")

• interjections ("Um," "ah," "uh")

The child would also not normally appear visibly tense or anxious while communicating.

There are some basic characteristics that differentiate stuttering from normal childhood disfluencies. The *Diagnostic and Statistical Manual of Mental Disorders,*

Fourth Edition (DSM-IV) describes those characteristics as follows:

• sound and syllable repetitions

• sound prolongations

• interjections

• broken words (for example, pauses within a word)

• audible or silent blocking (filled or unfilled pauses in speech)

• circumlocutions (word substitutions to avoid problematic words)

• words produced with an excess of physical tension

• monosyllabic whole-word repetitions ("I-I-I-I see him").

The *DSM-IV* also indicates that such disfluency "interferes with academic or occupational achievement or with social communication."

Diagnosis

A diagnosis of stuttering typically includes a complete medical history, a **physical examination**, a complete history of the speech disorder, and an evaluation of speech and language by a speech-language pathologist. An important function of the speech evaluation is to distinguish between normal disfluency and stuttering.

Treatment

Treatment for stuttering varies according to the patient's age and type and severity of stuttering. **Speech therapy** is a popular method of treatment that involves learning new speech techniques (such as speaking syllable-by-syllable) and modifying current ways of speaking (such as reducing the rate of speech). It may also include psychological counseling as a way of boosting self-esteem and reducing the tendency of avoiding fearful situations such as speaking in front of a group.

Studies have looked into the potential of treating stuttering with medications. Haloperidol has been the most widely studied antistuttering medication and the only drug to show improvement in fluency. The side effects of haloperidol, however, are not well-tolerated, and so the drug is often discontinued.

Prognosis

Nearly 80% of children with DS will recover by puberty, spontaneously or with treatment. One study looking at the recovery rate for stutterers ages nine to 14 who had undergone speech therapy noted that over 70% remained nonstutterers for one year after treatment. Five years after treatment, that rate remained approximately the same. The recovery rate among adult stutterers is not as high, in part because of extensive social phobias and depression.

Health care team roles

Common health care professionals involved in the care of an individual with a stuttering problem include:

- speech-language pathologists
- pediatricians and primary care physicians
- psychiatrists or psychologists
- neurologists

Prevention

There is no cure for stuttering, but parents can do a number of things to help their child recover from DS, thereby preventing a life-long stutter. These include:

- speaking slowly and fluently in front of the child, but avoiding criticizing or punishing his or her rate of speech or disfluencies
- questioning the child less and commenting on his or her activities more
- refraining from having the child speak in front of large groups
- listening carefully to what the child has to say
- resisting from completing the child's words or sentences

Resources

BOOKS

Guitar, Barry. *Stuttering: An Integrated Approach to Its Nature and Treatment*, 3rd edition. Lippincott Williams & Wilkins, 2005.

Yairi, Ehud, and Carol H. Seery. *Stuttering: Foundations and Clinical Applications*. Pearson, 2010.

PERIODICALS

Gregg, Brent Andrew, and Ehud Yairi. "Disfluency patterns and phonological skills near stuttering onset." *Journal of Communication Disorders* 45.6 (2012): 426.

Nippold, Marilyn A., and Ann Packman. "Managing stuttering beyond the preschool years." *Language, Speech, & Hearing Services in Schools* 43 (2012): 338.

Nippolda, Marilyn A. "When a school-age child stutters, let's focus on the primary problem." *Language, Speech, & Hearing Services in Schools* 43 (2012): 549.

Yaruss, J. Scott, Craig E. Coleman, and Robert W. Quesalc. "Stuttering in school-age children: a comprehensive approach to treatment." *Language, Speech, & Hearing Services in Schools* 43 (2012): 536.

ORGANIZATIONS

American Speech-Language-Hearing Association (ASHA). 10801 Rockville Pike, Rockville, MD 20852. (888) 321-ASHA. http://www.asha.org.

National Institute on Deafness and Other Communication Disorders (NIDCD) Information Clearinghouse. 1 Communication Ave., Bethesda, MD 20892-3456. (800) 241-1044. http://www.nidcd.nih.gov.

National Stuttering Association. 5100 E. La Palma, Suite 208, Anaheim Hills, CA 92807. (800) 364-1677. http://www.nsastutter.org.

Stuttering Foundation of America. 3100 Walnut Grove Rd., Suite 603, P.O. Box 11749, Memphis TN 38111-0749. (800) 992-9392. http://www.stuttersfa.org.

Stéphanie Islane Dionne

Subacute spongiform encephalopathy *see* **Creutzfeldt-Jakob disease**

Subcutaneous injection

Definition

A subcutaneous injection is a method of drug administration. Up to 2 ml of a drug solution can be injected directly beneath the skin. The drug becomes effective within 20 minutes.

Purpose

Subcutaneous injection is the method used to administer drugs when a small amount of fluid is to be injected, the patient is unable to take the drug orally, or the drug is destroyed by intestinal secretions.

Precautions

If the drug to be administered is harmful to superficial tissues, it should be administered intramuscularly or intravenously. It is useful to remember the following when administering any medication: the right patient, the right medicine, the right route, the right dose, the right site, and the right time.

Description

With the subcutaneous route, a small thin needle is inserted beneath the skin and the drug injected slowly. The drug moves from the small **blood vessels** into the bloodstream. Subcutaneous injections are usually given in the **abdomen**, upper arm, or the upper leg.

Preparation

The hands should be washed, and gloves may be worn during the procedure. A **syringe and needle** should be prepared. If a sterile, multiple-dose vial is used, the rubber-capped bottle should be rubbed with an antiseptic swab. The needle is then inserted through the center of the cap and some air from the syringe inserted to equalize the pressure in the container. Slightly more of the required amount of drug is then removed. Holding the syringe vertically at eye level, the syringe piston is pushed carefully to the exact measurement line.

If a small individual vial containing the correct amount of drug is used, the outside should be wiped with an antiseptic swab and held in the swab while the top is removed. The needle is then inserted into the vial, taking care that the tip of the needle does not scratch against the sides of the vial, thereby becoming blunt.

A syringe and needle containing the drug should be placed on a tray with sterile cotton swabs, cleaning disinfectant, and adhesive tape. If the patient is unfamiliar with the procedure, the nurse should explain what he or she is about to do and that the patient is to receive medication prescribed for them. The dose on the patient's prescription sheet should be checked prior to administration.

A screen should be drawn around the patient to avoid any personal embarrassment. The injection site is then rubbed vigorously with a swab and disinfectant to cleanse the area and increase the **blood** supply. A small piece of skin and subcutaneous tissue is pinched between the thumb and forefinger, and the needle inserted quickly at a 45-degree angle. Certain drugs such as heparin are given at a 90-degree angle rather than at 45 degrees. It is important to ensure that the needle is not in a vein. Therefore the syringe should be aspirated a little by pulling back on the piston. If blood is present, the needle should be re-injected, and the piston withdrawn slightly once more. The skin is then released and the syringe piston pushed down steadily and slowly.

A sterile cotton swab should be pressed over the injection site as the needle is quickly withdrawn, and the swab is taped to the skin for a few minutes, if required.

Aftercare

Monitor the patient's reaction and provide reassurance if required. Dispose of all waste products carefully, and place the syringe and needle in a puncture-resistant receptacle. Wash the hands. For patients requiring frequent injections, the site is changed each time.

Complications

If the circulation is depleted, absorption of the drug administered may be slow. Certain drugs such as

---

KEY TERMS

Intramuscular—Within muscle tissue.

Intravenous—Within a vein.

Sterile—Free from living microorganisms.

Subcutaneous—Hypodermic, beneath the skin.

Superficial—On or near the surface.

Vial—A small glass bottle for medicines or chemicals.

---

anticoagulants have specific side effects that the patient may experience. Injected drugs can also interact with other medications that the patient is taking. Check for any adverse reactions if the drug is being administered for the first time.

Results

The proper method of subcutaneous injection results in the safe administration of the drug with no complications for the health care provider or patient.

Health care team roles

The health care team should record any side effects or negative reactions to the injected drug and notify the medical staff as appropriate. If the medication is to be prescribed regularly for a specific disease, the patient can be directed to a self-help group where members have the same medical condition.

Resources

BOOKS

Denville, N.J. *The Self-help Source Book.* American Self-help Clearinghouse, 1998.

World Health Organization. *Guide to Good Prescribing* Annex 4: The Use of Injections.

ORGANIZATIONS

American Academy of Nurse Practitioners. AANP, P.O. Box 12846, Austin, TX 78711. (512) 442-4262. admin@aanp. org.

American Nurses Association. 600 Maryland Avenue, SW, Suite 100 West, Washington, DC 20024 (202)651-7000.

National Association of Clinical Nurse Specialists. 3969 Green Street, Harrisburg, PA 17110. (717) 234-6799. info@ nacns.org.

National League for Nursing. 61 Broadway, 33rd Floor, New York, NY 10006. (212) 363-5555 or (800) 669-1656.

Margaret A. Stockley, RGN

Subdural hematoma

Definition

A subdural hematoma is a collection of **blood** in the space between the outer layer (dura) and middle layers of the covering of the **brain** (the meninges). It is most often caused by torn, bleeding veins on the inside of the dura as a result of a blow to the head.

Description

Subdural hematomas most often affect people who are prone to falling. Only a slight hit on the head or even a fall to the ground without hitting the head may be enough to tear veins in the brain, often without fracturing the **skull**. There may be no external evidence of the bruising on the brain's surface.

Small subdural hematomas may not be very serious, and the blood can be slowly absorbed over several weeks. Larger hematomas, however, can gradually enlarge over several weeks, even though the bleeding has stopped. This enlargement can compress the brain itself, possibly leading to death if the blood is not drained.

The time between the injury and the appearance of symptoms can vary from less than 48 hours to several weeks, or more. Symptoms appearing in less than 48 hours are due to an acute subdural hematoma. This type of bleeding is often fatal, and results from tearing of the venous sinus. If more than two weeks have passed before symptoms appear, the condition is called a chronic subdural hematoma, resulting from tearing of the smaller vein. The young and the old are most likely to experience a chronic condition. This chronic form is less risky, as pressure of the veins against the skull lessens the bleeding. Prompt medical care can reduce the probability of permanent brain damage.

Causes and symptoms

A subdural hematoma is caused by an injury to the head that tears **blood vessels**. In childhood, hematomas are a common complication of **falls**. A subdural hematoma also may be an indication of **child abuse**, as evidenced by shaken baby syndrome.

Symptoms tend to fluctuate, and include:

• headache

• episodes of confusion and drowsiness

• one-sided weakness or paralysis

• lethargy

• enlarged or asymmetric pupils

• convulsions or loss of consciousness after head injury

• coma

A doctor should be contacted immediately if symptoms appear. Because these symptoms mimic the signs of a **stroke**, the patient should tell the doctor about any **head injury** within the previous few months.

In an infant, symptoms may include increased pressure within the skull, growing head size, bulging fontanelle (one of two soft spots on a infant's skull), **vomiting**, irritability, lethargy, and seizures. In cases of child abuse, there may be **fractures** of the skull or other bones.

Diagnosis

A chronic subdural hematoma can be difficult to diagnose, but a slow loss of consciousness after a head injury is assumed to be a hematoma unless proven otherwise. The hematoma can be confirmed with **magnetic resonance imaging** (MRI), which is the preferred type of scan; a hematoma can be hard to detect on a computed tomography scan (CT scan), depending on how long after the hemorrhage the CT is done.

Treatment

Small hematomas that do not cause symptoms may not need to be treated. Otherwise, the hematoma should be surgically removed. Liquid blood can be drained from burr holes drilled into the skull. The surgeon may have to open a section of skull to remove a large hematoma or to tie off the bleeding vein.

Corticosteroids and diuretics can control brain swelling. After surgery, anticonvulsant drugs (such as phenytoin) may help control or prevent seizures, which can begin as late as two years after the head injury.

Prognosis

If treatment is provided soon enough, recovery is usually complete. **Headache**, amnesia, attention problems, **anxiety**, and giddiness may continue for some time after surgery. Most symptoms in adults usually disappear within six months, with further improvement over several years. Children tend to recover much faster.

Prevention

Because a subdural hematoma usually follows a head injury, preventing head injury can prevent a hematoma.

Resources

ORGANIZATIONS

American Academy of Neurology. 1080 Montreal Ave., St. Paul, MN 55116. (612) 695-1940. http://www.aan.com.

Brain Injury Association of America. 105 North Alfred St., Alexandria, VA 22314. (800) 444-6443. http://www.biausa.org.

Head Injury Hotline. P.O. Box 84151, Seattle WA 98124. (206) 621-8558. http://www.headinjury.com.

Head Trauma Support Project, Inc. 2500 Marconi Ave., Ste. 203, Sacramento, CA 95821. (916) 482-5770.

Carol A. Turkington

Sublingual and buccal medication administration

Definition

Sublingual and buccal medications are administered by placing them in the mouth, either under the tongue (sublingual) or between the gum and the cheek (buccal). The medications dissolve rapidly and are absorbed through the mucous membranes of the mouth, where they enter into the bloodstream. The medications are compounded in the form of small, quick-dissolving tablets, sprays, lozenges, or liquid suspensions.

Purpose

Sublingual and buccal medications are given for a variety of conditions. The most common sublingual medication is the nitroglycerin tablet. Its rapid action to relax the **blood vessels** reduces the workload on the **heart** and relieves the **pain** of **angina** pectoris. Other buccal and sublingual medications, however, serve a variety of purposes—such as narcotic pain relief, migraine pain relief, **blood pressure** control, and mental decline due to **dementia** (i.e., ergoloid mesylates). This form of medication is extremely effective, because it bypasses the **digestive system** and is absorbed into the bloodstream in minutes. Not all medications can be prepared for sublingual or buccal administration; some of the compounding difficulties are **taste**, solubility, and dosage limitations of the medicine.

Precautions

Sublingual medications should not be administered if the gums or mucous membranes have open sores or areas of irritation. Rather, the physician should be notified, and medication held. The patient should be placed in a sitting position to prevent accidental aspiration of the medication. Buccal or sublingual medication should not be used when a patient is uncooperative or unconscious. The patient should not eat, drink, chew, or swallow until the medication has been absorbed; swallowing the medication must be prevented, as it will decrease the drug's effectiveness. The patient should not smoke while taking sublingual or buccal medication, because **smoking** causes vasoconstriction of the **blood** vessels. This will decrease the absorption of the medication.

Description

To administer sublingual tablets, the clinician should have the patient open his or her mouth and raise the tongue. The tablet should then be placed under the tongue. Administration of buccal tablets is similar to that of sublingual tablets. First, the patient should open his or her mouth. The tablet should be placed between the gum and the wall of the cheek. With the mouth closed, the tablet should be held in this position for five to 10 minutes, or until it has dissolved. Lozenges are also placed in the mouth and held until they dissolve. Administration of sublingual or buccal sprays also requires having the patient open the mouth. The patient should be reminded not to breathe while the nurse is spraying the medicine. If the spray is ordered sublingual, the spray should be held about 1 inch (2.5 cm) away from the site, and directed toward the tongue. If the patient cannot hold up his or her tongue voluntarily, the nurse tongue should be held by the nurse with his or her non-dominant hand, using a 2×2 gauze pad to provide grip. If the spray is ordered buccal, the tongue should be held out of the way, the cheek held outward, and the spray directed into the gum area between the cheek and the teeth. Liquid suspensions may be given in a medicine cup or squirted into the patient's mouth using a medicine syringe with no needle. The patient should be directed to hold and swish the liquid in the mouth for the amount of time designated by the physician's order. Some liquid suspensions are then swallowed and some expectorated into a sink or basin. In all cases, the physician's orders should be followed.

Preparation

The clinician should wash his or her hands and put on gloves. The medication label must be checked each time medication is administered, to avoid medication errors. It must be confirmed that it is the right medicine, the right dose (strength), the right time, the right patient, and the right method. The expiration date on the label

KEY TERMS

Angina pectoris—Severe pain in the chest caused by vasoconstriction of the blood vessels and a decreased level of oxygen to the cardiac muscle.

Aspiration—The accidental sucking of fluid or solids along with air into the bronchial tubes or lungs.

Buccal—The inner aspect of the cheek or mouth cavity.

Sublingual—The area in the mouth under the tongue.

Vasoconstriction—The narrowing or constriction of blood vessels.

should be checked. If the medicine is outdated, it should not be used. The patient should be placed in a sitting or upright position. Oral medications need to be given before sublingual or buccal medications. The clinician should examine the mucous membranes of the patient's mouth for irritation or sores. If there are sores in the mouth, the physician should be contacted any sublingual or buccal drugs are administered. Alternating sites should be used when giving regular doses of sublingual or buccal medications. The procedure should be explained to the patient, who should also be reminded that nothing should be eaten, drank, swallowed, chewed, or smoked until the tablet has dissolved. When administering a liquid suspension, the bottle should be shaken the bottle before the appropriate dose is poured. When administering sprays, the container also needs to be shaken, and the top taken off before the medication is given.

Aftercare

The patient should be reminded not to eat, drink, swallow, chew, or smoke until the tablet has dissolved. The nurse can assist the patient by noting the time the medicine is given, as well as the time when it will be okay to drink or eat. If a liquid suspension must be spit out after a specific amount of time, the nurse must be sure that the patient knows when that is, and has a basin nearby or access to a sink. If the patient experiences a tingling or burning sensation from a sublingual tablet, he or she should be encouraged to move the tablet to another part of the mouth. Sublingual medicines deteriorate rapidly with heat or humidity. The nurse should be sure to close the cover of the tablet bottle securely. Gloves should be removed and placed, with the gauze pads, in a plastic bag that can be sealed and discarded. The clinician

must wash his or her hands when the procedure is complete.

Complications

Complications of sublingual and buccal medications are rare, but could include inflammation of the mucous membranes. If symptoms such as soreness, redness, swelling, bleeding, or sores in the mouth are evident, the physician should be contacted before the medication is administered. If the patient demonstrates any symptoms of an allergic reaction (i.e., **itching**, **hives**, or swelling of the lips or tongue), the remaining tablet should be removed. The patient should rinse his or her mouth, and the clinician should contact the physician immediately.

Results

Sublingual and buccal medications are fast acting and when given correctly act within one to five minutes of administration. The length of time to reach the desired therapeutic response, however, depends upon the dose and type of medication administered. For example it may take three doses of sublingual nitroglycerin given five minutes apart to relieve the pain of angina.

Health care team roles

Sublingual and buccal medications are administered by a **registered nurse** (R. N.) or a **licensed practical nurse** (L. P. N). in the health care setting. Sublingual or buccal medicine may be administered in some settings by unlicensed staff, but only under the direction of a registered nurse. A licensed nurse, however, must evaluate the mucous membranes of the mouth regularly and assess the outcome of medication administration. The patient, or members of the patient's family, can be taught to administer sublingual or buccal medications in the home setting.

Resources

BOOK

Buccal, Sublingual and Translingual Administration. Medication Administration.*Nurse's Clinical Guide: Medication Administration*, Pennsylvania: Springhouse Corporation, 2000.

OTHER

"Ergoloid Mesylates." Intelihealth Online. September 2000. http://www.intelihealth.com/IH/ihtPrint/WSIHWOOO/ 19689/11430/213903.html.

"Forms of Medication." Complete Home Medical Guide. Columbia University College of Physicians and Surgeons Online, 2001. http://cpmcnet.columbia.edu/texts/guide/ hmg34_0003.html.

Newcomer, Jeffrey, M.D. "Nitroglycerine—Sublingual." Medical Information Sheet. Cheshire Medical Center Online, 2001. http://www.cheshire-med.com/services/pharm/meds/nitroglycerin_sublingual.html.

"Nitrates-Sublingual." Library. HealthCentral Online, 1998. http://healthcentralsympatico.com/mhc/top/001801.cfm.

"What's New in Pain Management?" Medical Surgical Nursing Across the Health Care Continuum. Harcourt Health Sciences Online, 2000. http://www.harcourthealth.com/SIMON/Ignatavicius/medsurg/updates/update25.html.

Mary Elizabeth Martelli, R.N., B.S.

Subluxations *see* **Dislocations and subluxations**

Substance abuse and dependence

Definition

Substance abuse is a pattern of drug, alcohol, or other substance use that creates many adverse results from its continual use. The characteristics of abuse are a failure to carry out obligations at home or work, continual use under circumstances that present a hazard (such as driving a car), and legal problems such as arrests. Use of the drug is persistent despite personal problems caused by the effects of the substance on self or others.

Substance dependence has been defined medically as a group of behavioral and physiological symptoms that indicate the continual, compulsive use of a substance in self-administered doses despite the problems related to the use of this substance. Sometimes Increased amounts are needed to achieve the desired effect or level of intoxication. Consequently the patient's tolerance for the drug increases. Withdrawal is a physiological and psychological change that occurs when the body's concentration of the substance declines in a person who has been a heavy user.

Description

Substance abuse and dependence cross all lines of race, culture, education, and socioeconomic status, leaving no group untouched by its devastating effects. A recent survey estimated that about 16 million citizens of the United States had used an illegal substance in the month preceding the study. Substance abuse is an enormous **public health** problem, with far-ranging effects throughout society. In addition to the toll substance abuse can take on one's physical health, it is considered an important factor in a wide variety of social problems, affecting rates of crime, domestic violence, sexually transmitted diseases (including HIV/AIDS), unemployment, homelessness, teen **pregnancy**, and failure in school. One study estimated that 20% of the total yearly cost of health care in the United States is spent on the effects of drug and alcohol abuse.

A wide range of substances can be abused. The most common classes include:

- opioids, including such prescription pain killers as morphine and Demerol, as well as illegal substances such as heroin
- benzodiazapines, including prescription drugs used for treating anxiety, such as Valium
- sedatives or "downers," including prescription barbiturate drugs commonly referred to as tranquilizers
- stimulants or "speed," including prescription amphetamines used for weight loss and in the treatment of attention deficit disorder
- cannabinoid drugs obtained from the hemp plant, including marijuana ("pot") and hashish
- cocaine-based drugs
- hallucinogenic or "psychedelic" drugs, including LSD, PCP or angel dust, and other PCP-type drugs
- inhalants, including gaseous drugs used in the medical practice of anesthesia, as well as such common substances as paint thinner, gasoline, glue
- alcoholic drinks, including beer, liquor, and wine

Those substances of abuse that are actually prescription medications may have been obtained on the street by fraudulent means or may have been a legal, medically indicated prescription that a person begins to use without regard to the directions of his/her physician.

A number of important terms must be defined in order to have a complete discussion of substance abuse. Drug tolerance refers to a person's body becoming accustomed to the symptoms produced by a specific quantity of a substance. When a person first begins taking a substance, he or she will note various mental or physical reactions brought on by the drug, some of which are the very changes in consciousness that the individual is seeking through substance use. Over time, the same dosage of the substance may produce fewer of the desired feelings. In order to continue to feel the desired effect of the substance, progressively higher drug doses must be taken.

Substance dependence is the phenomenon whereby a person becomes physically addicted to a substance. A substance-dependent person must have a particular dose or concentration of the substance in their bloodstream at any given moment in order to avoid the unpleasant symptoms associated with withdrawal from that substance. The common substances of abuse tend to exert either a depressive (slowing) or a stimulating (speeding up) effect on such basic bodily functions as respiratory rate, **heart** rate, and **blood pressure**. When a drug is stopped abruptly, the person's body will respond by overreacting to the substance's absence. Functions slowed by the abused substance will be suddenly speeded up, while previously stimulated functions will be suddenly slowed. This results in very unpleasant symptoms, known as withdrawal symptoms.

Addiction refers to the mind-state of a person who reaches a point where he/she must have a specific substance, even though the social consequences of substance use are clearly negative (loss of relationships, employment, housing). Craving refers to an intense hunger for a specific substance, to the point where this need essentially directs the individual's behavior. Craving is usually seen in both dependence and addiction. Such craving can be so strong that it overwhelms a person's ability to make any decisions which will possibly deprive him/her of the substance. Drug possession and use becomes the most important goal, and other forces (including the law) have little effect on changing the individual's substance-seeking behavior.

Causes and symptoms

There is not thought to be a single cause of substance abuse, though scientists are increasingly convinced that certain people possess a genetic predisposition that can affect the development of addictive behaviors. One theory holds that a particular nerve pathway in the **brain**, dubbed the "mesolimbic reward pathway," holds certain chemical characteristics that can increase the likelihood that substance use will ultimately lead to substance addiction. Certainly, however, other social factors are involved, including family problems and peer pressure. Primary mood disorders, such as **bipolar disorder**, **personality disorders**, and the role of learned behavior can influence the likelihood that a person will become substance dependent.

The symptoms of substance abuse may be related to its social effects as well as its physical effects. The social effects of substance abuse may include dropping out of school or losing a series of jobs, engaging in fighting and violence in relationships, and legal problems, ranging from driving under the influence to the commission of crimes committed to obtain the money needed to support an expensive drug habit.

Physical effects of substance abuse are related to the specific drug being abused:

• Opioid drug users may appear slowed in their physical movements and speech, may lose weight, exhibit mood swings, and have constricted (small) pupils.

• Benzodiazapine and barbiturate users may appear sleepy and slowed, with slurred speech, small pupils, and occasional confusion.

• Amphetamine users may have excessively high energy, inability to sleep, weight loss, rapid pulse, elevated blood pressure, occasional psychotic behavior and dilated (enlarged) pupils.

• Marijuana users may be sluggish and slow to react, exhibiting mood swings and red eyes with dilated pupils.

• Cocaine users may have wide variations in their energy level, severe mood disturbances, psychosis, paranoia, and a constantly runny nose. Crack cocaine may cause aggressive or violent behavior.

• Hallucinogenic drug users may display dilated pupils and bizarre behavior due to hallucinations. (Hallucinations are imagined sights, voices, sounds, or smells which seem completely real to the individual experiencing them.) LSD can cause flashbacks.

Other symptoms of substance abuse may be related to the form in which the substance is used. For example, heroin, certain other opioid drugs, and certain forms of **cocaine** may be injected using a needle and a hypodermic syringe. A person abusing an injectable substance may have "track marks"—outwardly visible signs of the site of an injection, with possible redness and swelling of the vein in which the substance was injected. Furthermore, poor judgment brought on by substance use can result in the injections being made under horrifyingly dirty conditions. These unsanitary conditions and the use of shared needles can cause infections of the injection sites, major infections of the heart, as well as **infection** with human **immunodeficiency** virus (HIV) (the virus that causes acquired immunodeficiency syndrome, or **AIDS**), certain forms of hepatitis (a **liver** infection), and **tuberculosis**.

Cocaine is often taken as a powdery substance which is inhaled or "snorted" through the nose. This can result in frequent nose bleeds, sores in the nose, and even erosion of the nasal septum, the structure that separates the two nostrils. Cocaine can also be smoked.

Overdosing on a substance is a frequent complication of substance abuse. Drug **overdose** can be purposeful (with suicide as a goal), or caused by carelessness, the unpredictable strength of substances purchased from street dealers, mixing of more than one type of substance, or as a result of the ever-increasing doses which a person must take of those substances to which he or she has become tolerant. Substance overdose can be a life-threatening emergency, with the specific symptoms dependent on the type of substance used. Substances with depressive effects may dangerously slow the breathing and heart rate, drop the body temperature, and result in a general unresponsiveness. Substances with stimulatory effects may dangerously increase the heart rate and **blood** pressure, increase body temperature, and cause bizarre behavior. With cocaine, there is a risk of **stroke**.

Still other symptoms may be caused by unknown substances mixed with street drugs in order to "stretch" a batch. A health care worker faced with a patient suffering extreme symptoms may have no idea what other substance that person may have unwittingly put into his or her body. Thorough drug screening can help with this problem.

Diagnosis

The most difficult aspect of diagnosis involves addressing and overcoming the patient's denial. Denial is a psychological trait whereby a person is unable to allow him- or herself to acknowledge the reality of a situation. This may lead a person to completely deny his or her substance use, or may cause the person to greatly underestimate the degree of the problem and its effects on his or her life.

One of the simplest and most commonly used screening tools used by nursing staff or allied health professionals to begin the process of diagnosing substance abuse is called the CAGE questionnaire. CAGE refers to the first letters of each word that forms the basis of each of the four questions of the screening exam:

• Have you ever tried to Cut down on your substance use?

• Have you ever been Annoyed by people trying to talk to you about your substance use?

• Do you ever feel Guilty about your substance use?

• Do you ever need an Eye opener (use of the substance first thing in the morning) in order to start your day?

Other, longer lists of questions exist in order to try to determine the severity and effects of a person's substance abuse. Certainly, it is also relevant to determine whether anybody else in a person's family has ever suffered from substance or alcohol addiction.

A **physical examination** may reveal signs of substance abuse in the form of needle marks, tracks, trauma to the inside of the nostrils from snorting drugs, unusually large or small pupils. With the person's permission, substance use can also be detected by examining an individual's blood, urine, or hair in a laboratory. This **drug testing** is limited by sensitivity, specificity and the time elapsed since the person last used the drug.

Treatment

Treatment has several goals, which include helping a person deal with the uncomfortable and possibly life-threatening symptoms associated with withdrawal from an addictive substance (called detoxification), helping a person deal with the social effects which substance abuse has had on his or her life, and efforts to prevent relapse (resumed use of the substance). Individual or group **psychotherapy** is sometimes helpful.

Detoxification may take from several days to many weeks. Detoxification can be accomplished "cold turkey," by complete and immediate cessation of all substance use, or by slowly decreasing (tapering) the dose that a person is taking, to minimize the side effects of withdrawal. Some substances absolutely must be tapered, because "cold turkey" methods of detoxification are potentially life threatening. Alternatively, a variety of medications may be utilized to combat the unpleasant and threatening physical symptoms of withdrawal. A substance (such as methadone in the case of heroin addiction) may be substituted for the original substance of abuse, with gradual tapering of this substituted drug. In practice, many patients may be maintained on methadone and lead a reasonably normal life. Because of the rebound effects of fluctuating blood pressure, body temperature, heart and breathing rates, as well as the potential for bizarre behavior and hallucinations, a person undergoing withdrawal must be carefully monitored and treated appropriately.

One recent discovery for the treatment of opiate addiction is a medication called naltrexone. This medication blocks the receptors involved with the "high" produced by heroin. The drug is useful for many patients since it is does not produce physical dependence and has virtually zero potential for abuse. Scientists have found that unfortunately, many heroin addicts do not like to take naltrexone quite possibly because they enjoy the effects of opiates. Since the medication eliminates the craving for opiates, in one recent study only 15% of heroin addicts were still taking the drug after one month.

Alternative treatments for substance abuse include those specifically designed to aid a person who is suffering from the effects of withdrawal and the toxicities of the abused substance, as well as treatments which are intended to decrease a person's **stress** level, thus hopefully decreasing the likelihood that he or she will relapse.

Additional treatments thought to improve a person's ability to stop substance use include **acupuncture** and hypnotherapy. Ridding the body of toxins is believed to be aided by **hydrotherapy** (bathing regularly in water containing baking soda, sea salt, or Epsom salts). Hydrotherapy can include a constitutional effect where the body's vital force is stimulated and all organ systems are revitalized. Elimination of toxins is aided by hydrotherapy as well as by such herbs as milk thistle (*Silybum marianum*), burdock (*Arctium lappa*), a blood cleanser, and licorice (*Glycyrrhiza glabra*). **Anxiety** brought on by substance withdrawal is thought to be lessened by using other herbs, which include valerian (*Valeriana officinalis*), vervain (*Verbena officinalis*), skullcap (*Scutellaria baicalensis*) and kava (*Piper methysticum*).

Other treatments aimed at reducing the stress a person suffers while attempting substance withdrawal and throughout an individual's recovery process include biofeedback, guided imagery, and various meditative arts, including **yoga** and tai chi. **Alternative medicine** also places a great emphasis on proper **nutrition**, for detoxification, healing, and sustained recovery.

Prognosis

After a person has successfully withdrawn from substance use, the even more difficult task of recovery begins. Recovery refers to the lifelong efforts of a person to avoid returning to substance use. The craving can be so strong, even years and years after initial withdrawal has been accomplished, that a previously addicted person is virtually forever in danger of slipping back into substance use. Triggers for such a relapse include any number of life stressors: problems on the job or in the marriage, loss of a relationship, death of a loved one, and financial stresses, in addition to seemingly mundane exposure to a place or an acquaintance associated with previous substance use. While some people remain in counseling indefinitely as a way of maintaining contact with a professional who can help monitor behavior, others find that various support groups or 12-step programs such as Narcotics Anonymous are the most successful and useful way of monitoring the recovery process and avoiding relapse. Research indicates that a good prognosis is more likely for individuals who have a strong support than for those who have little or no support.

Another important aspect of treatment for substance abuse is the inclusion of close family members in treatment. Because substance abuse has severe effects on

KEY TERMS

Addiction—The state of being both physically and psychologically dependent on a substance.

Dependence—A state in which a person requires a steady concentration of a particular substance in order to avoid experiencing withdrawal symptoms.

Detoxification—A process whereby an addict is withdrawn from a substance.

Disease model of alcoholism—Also known as the Minnesota model, the disease model contends that alcoholism is a disease that alcoholism is chronic, progressive, and frequently fatal.

High—The altered state of consciousness that a person seeks when abusing a substance.

Street drug—A substance purchased from a drug dealer; it may be a legal substance, sold illicitly (without a prescription, and not for medical use), or it may be a substance which is illegal to possess.

Tolerance—A phenomenon whereby a drug user becomes physically accustomed to a particular dose of a substance, and requires ever-increasing dosages in order to obtain the same effects.

Withdrawal—Those side effects experienced by a person who has become physically dependent on a substance, upon decreasing the substance's dosage, or discontinuing its use.

the functioning of the family, and because research shows that family members can accidentally develop behaviors that inadvertently serve to support a person's substance habit, most good treatment programs will involve all family members.

Health care team roles

Nursing staff and allied health professionals can assist in the treatment of substance abuse and dependence by understanding the disease model of **alcoholism** and addiction.

During the treatment phase, nursing staff and allied health professionals can help patients by providing them with appropriate educational materials and referrals for supportive services such as Alcoholics Anonymous or Narcotics Anonymous.

Prevention

Prevention is best aimed at teenagers, who are at very high risk for substance experimentation. Data compiled in 1999 revealed that 14% of high-school seniors had used an illegal substance other than **marijuana** in the preceding year. Education regarding the risks and consequences of substance use, as well as teaching methods of resisting peer pressure, are both important components of a prevention program. Furthermore, it is important to identify children at higher risk for substance abuse, including victims of physical or sexual abuse, children of parents who have a history of substance abuse, especially alcohol, and children with school failure and/or attention deficit disorder. These children will require a more intensive prevention program.

Resources

BOOKS

Diagnostic and Statistical Manual of Mental Disorders Revised IV. Washington, DC: American Psychiatric Press, 2000.

O'Brien, C.P. "Drug Abuse and Dependence." In *Cecil Textbook of Medicine,* edited by J. Claude Bennett and Fred Plum. Philadelphia: W. B. Saunders, 1996.

Shealy, C. Norman. *The Complete Family Guide to Alternative Medicine.* New York: Barnes and Noble, 1996.

Volpicelli, Joseph. *Recovery Options: The Complete Guide.* New York: John Wiley & Sons, 2000.

ORGANIZATIONS

Al-Anon, Alanon Family Group, Inc. P.O. Box 862, Midtown Station, New York, NY 10018-0862. (800) 356-9996. http://www.recovery.org/aa.

National Alliance On Alcoholism and Drug Dependence, Inc. 12 West 21st St., New York, NY 10010. (212) 206-6770.

National Clearinghouse for Alcohol and Drug Information. http://www.health.org.

Parent Resources and Information for Drug Education (PRIDE). 10 Park Place South, Suite 340, Atlanta, GA 30303. (800) 853-7867.

Bethanne Black

Substance abuse counseling

Definition

Substance abuse is a maladaptive pattern of alcohol or other drug use that causes social, physical, legal, vocational, or educational distress or impairment. In addition to those trained specifically as substance abuse counselors, mental health and **rehabilitation** counselors work with individuals who abuse alcohol and other drugs.

Description

Counselors who work with substance abusers should have the same qualities as other counselors. For example, they should be able to pose direct questions and confront clients, self-disclose appropriately, identify counter-transference issues, and recognize the effect of their own beliefs on the counseling relationship. Essential qualities include empathy, sincerity, warmth, genuineness, and nonjudgmental acceptance.

In order to assess, diagnose, and treat substance abusers, counselors must have general counseling skills and abilities in addition to specialized skills and abilities relative to this population. Counselors working with substance abusers must have knowledge of assessment instruments and techniques in order to communicate with other professionals and make treatment recommendations.

Substance abuse counselors develop a treatment plan based on the individual client's needs. The information necessary for the individual's treatment plan is gathered through interviews in conjunction with assessment instruments.

Major substance abuse counseling theories include reality therapy, psychodynamics, grief therapy, client-centered therapy, rational emotive therapy, and cognitive-behavioral. Additional approaches such as life-skills training and behavior modification are often included.

Mental health counselors work with individuals and groups to promote optimum mental health. They deal with addictions and substance abuse, suicide, **stress** management, problems with self-esteem, issues associated with mental and emotional health, and family and marital problems. Mental health counselors work closely with other mental health specialists, including psychiatrists, psychologists, clinical social workers, psychiatric nurses, and school counselors.

Substance abuse among people with disabilities exceeds that of the general public. According to the **Americans with Disabilities Act** of 1990, recovery from alcohol or drug addiction is considered a disability. Rehabilitation counselors work with people with disabilities resulting from **birth defects**, illness or disease, accidents, or the stress of daily life. They help people with disabilities deal with the personal, social, and vocational effects of their disabilities. Rehabilitation counselors evaluate the individual's strengths and limitations, provide personal and vocational counseling, and arrange for medical care, vocational training, and job placement. They interview individuals with disabilities and their families, evaluate school and medical reports, and confer and plan with physicians, psychologists, occupational therapists, and employers to determine the capabilities and skills of the individual. By conferring with the client they develop a rehabilitation program, which often includes training to help the person develop job skills. Increasing the client's capacity to live independently is also a priority. To enhance the likelihood that the substance abuse client will continue to recover, many counselors encourage or support the client's attendance at meetings of Alcoholics Anonymous or Narcotics Anonymous.

Work settings

Substance abuse counselors work in a variety of settings including residential and outpatient treatment programs, hospitals and clinics, government agencies, private practice, schools, and correctional facilities. Substance abuse counseling takes place individually and in groups. To enhance continued recovery, counselors also work with family members.

Rehabilitation counselors usually work a traditional 40-hour week. Counselors in private practice and those working in mental health and community agencies often work evenings to counsel clients who work during the day.

Education and training

Some employers provide training for newly hired counselors. Many have work-study programs so that employed counselors are able to pursue graduate degrees. However, most employers require, or prefer, that counselors have a master's degree. At least 45 states and the District of Columbia have some form of counselor credentialing, licensure, certification, or registry legislation governing practice. Although requirements vary from state to state, many require a master's degree.

Accredited master's degree counseling programs include a minimum two years of full-time study, including 600 hours of supervised clinical internship experience. Counselors with a master's degree who work with substance abusers come from a variety of disciplines, including substance-abuse counseling, rehabilitation counseling, agency or community counseling, clinical mental health counseling, counseling psychology, and related fields.

Graduate-level counselor education programs in colleges and universities are most often located in education or psychology departments. Course work is grouped into a number of core areas including **human growth and development**; social and cultural foundations; helping relationships; group work; career and lifestyle development; appraisal; research and program evaluation; and professional orientation. Most accredited graduate programs require the student to complete 48–60

semester hours of course work, including a period of supervised clinical experience in counseling. More than 100 institutions offer programs accredited by the Council for Accreditation of Counseling and Related Educational Programs (CACREP). These include programs in substance abuse, mental health, rehabilitation, and community counseling. Graduate programs in rehabilitation counseling are accredited by the Council on Rehabilitation Education (CORE).

Many counselors pursue national certification by the National Board for Certified Counselors (NBCC). To be certified a counselor must hold a graduate degree in counseling from a regionally accredited institution, have at least two years of supervised field experience in a counseling setting, and pass the NBCC's National Counselor Examination for Licensure and Certification. This national certification is distinct from state certification, however, in some states those who pass the national exam are exempt from taking a state certification exam. NBCC offers specialty certification in clinical mental health and addictions counseling. To maintain certification, counselors must complete 100 hours of acceptable continuing education credit every five years.

The Commission on Rehabilitation Counselor Certification offers national certification for rehabilitation counselors, which is required by many employers. To become certified, rehabilitation counselors must graduate from an accredited educational program, complete an internship, and pass a written examination. To maintain certification, counselors must complete 100 hours of acceptable continuing education credit every five years.

Most clinical mental health counselors have a master's degree in mental health counseling, another area of counseling, psychology, or social work. Certification is available through the NBCC. To be certified as a clinical mental health counselor, a counselor must have a master's degree in counseling, two years of post-master's experience, a period of supervised clinical experience, a taped sample of clinical work, and pass a written examination.

Prospects for advancement vary by counseling field. Rehabilitation, mental health, and substance-abuse counselors can become supervisors or administrators in their agencies. Some counselors move into research, consulting, college teaching, or go into private or group practice.

Future outlook

A study conducted by the Substance Abuse and Mental Health Services Administration (SAMHSA) estimated that in 1996 the cost for alcohol and drug abuse treatment surpassed $13 billion. The combined costs of substance abuse and mental health treatment services ranked third after spending for **heart** disease, injury, and trauma. As a result, employment for counselors is expected to increase from 21–35% through 2008. Demand is expected to be strong for rehabilitation and mental health counselors.

Due to the toll substance abuse takes on worker productivity, an increasing number of employers offer employee assistance programs that provide alcohol and drug abuse counseling services. A growing number of people are expected to use these services, creating a demand for counselors as many seek ways to maintain their recovery from substance abuse while dealing with the stresses associated with job and family.

For general information about counseling, as well as information on specialties such as substance abuse, mental health, or rehabilitation counseling, contact the American Counseling Association, 5999 Stevenson Ave., Alexandria, VA 22304-3300. http://www.counseling.org.

For information on accredited counseling and related training programs, contact the Council for Accreditation of Counseling and Related Educational Programs, American Counseling Association, 5999 Stevenson Ave., 4th floor, Alexandria, VA 22304. http://www.counseling.org/cacrep.

For information on national certification requirements for counselors, contact: National Board for Certified Counselors, Inc., 3 Terrace Way, Suite D, Greensboro, NC 27403-3660. http://www.nbcc.org.

Resources

BOOKS

Cohen, Monique. *Counseling Addicted Women: A Practical Guide.* Sage Publications, Inc., 2000.

Fisher, Gary, and C. Harrison. *Substance Abuse: Information for School Counselors, Social Workers, Therapists, and Counselors.* Allyn Bacon, 1999.

PERIODICALS

Curry, L. "12-Step Self-Help Programs Prove Successful Regardless Of Participants' Religious Background, Study Suggests." *APA Monitor Online* 30, no. 11 (December 1999).

ORGANIZATIONS

American Counseling Association. 5999 Stevenson Ave., Alexandria, VA 22304-3300. (800) 347-6647. http://www.counseling.org.

Council for Accreditation of Counseling and Related Educational Programs (CACREP). 5999 Stevenson Avenue, 4th Floor, Alexandria, VA 22304. (800) 347-6647, ext. 301. http://www.counseling.org/cacrep.

National Board for Certified Counselors, Inc. 3 Terrace Way, Suite D, Greensboro, NC 27403-3660. (336) 547-0607. http://www.nbcc.org.

National Center on Addiction and Substance Abuse at Columbia University. 633 Third Avenue, 19th floor, New York, NY 10017-6706. (212) 841-5200. http://www.casacolumbia.org/.

Substance Abuse and Mental Health Services Administration. 5600 Fishers Lane Rockville, MD 20857. http://www.samhsa.gov/statistics/statistics.html.

Bill Asenjo, MS, CRC

Substance use disorder *see* **Substance abuse and dependence**

Sugar diabetes *see* **Diabetes mellitus**

Sunstroke *see* **Heat disorders**

Supportive cancer therapy *see* **Cancer therapy, supportive**

Surgical instruments

Definition

Surgical instruments are tools or devices that perform such functions as cutting, dissecting, grasping, holding, retracting, or suturing. Most surgical instruments are made from stainless steel. Other metals and alloys, including titanium and vitallium, are also used.

Purpose

Surgical instruments facilitate a variety of procedures and operations. Specialized surgical packs contain the most common instruments needed for particular surgeries.

Description

Basic categories of instruments include:

• cutting and dissecting

• clamping

• grasping and holding

• probing

• dilating

• retracting

• suctioning

Scissors are an example of cutting instruments. Dissecting instruments are used to cut or separate tissue. Dissectors may be sharp or blunt. Scalpels are one example of sharp dissectors. Examples of blunt dissectors include the back of a knife handle; curettes and elevators can also be blunt. Grasping and holding instruments include clamps, tenacula, and forceps. Probing

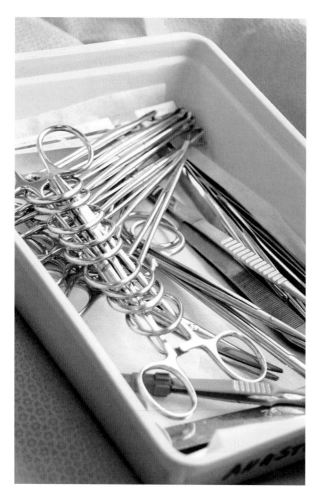

(Sterilized surgical instruments in a tray, photograph. AJPhoto / Photo Researchers, Inc.)

instruments are used to enter natural openings, for example the common bile duct, or such openings as a fistula. Dilating instruments serve to expand the size of an opening, such as the urethra or the cervical os. Retractors assist in the visualization of the operative field while preventing trauma to other tissues. Suction devices remove **blood** and other fluids from the surgical or dental field.

Operation

Counting

Sharps and related items should be counted prior to the beginning of the procedure; before the closure of a cavity within a cavity; before wound closure begins; and at skin closure or the end of the procedure. In addition, a count should be taken at any time when either scrub or circulating personnel are replaced. Instruments, sharps, and sponges should be counted during all procedures in which the possibility exists of leaving an item in the patient.

Cleaning and sterilizing

Surgical instruments must be kept clean during a procedure. Cleaning is done by carefully wiping instruments with a moist sponge and frequently rinsing them in sterile water. Periodic cleaning during the procedure prevents blood and other tissue from hardening and becoming trapped on the surface of an instrument. After the procedure, instruments are promptly rinsed and thoroughly cleaned and sterilized. Ultrasonic cleaning and automatic washing often follow the manual cleaning of instruments. Instruments may also be placed in an autoclave after manual cleaning. The manufacturer's instructions should be followed for each type of machine. Staff members responsible for cleaning instruments should wear protective gloves, waterproof aprons, and face shields.

Patient status

Observation of patients after surgical procedures provides the best indication that correct instrument handling and **aseptic technique** was followed during surgery. Postoperative patients should show no evidence of:

• retained instruments or sponges

• infection at the site of the incision or operation

• excessive swelling or discoloration at the operative site

Maintenance

Inspection

The misuse of surgical instruments frequently causes alignment problems. Instruments should always be inspected before, during, and after surgical procedures. Clamps, scissors and forceps should be examined to make sure that the tips are even and in proper alignment. The instrument tips should not overlap. To test the alignment of clamps, first close the clamp. Then, hold the instrument up to a light. No light will be visible if the clamp is correctly aligned. Instruments that have teeth or serrated tips should also be checked for proper alignment. Be sure that the instrument opens and closes freely. Hinged instruments must hold firmly and close properly. To test ratchet teeth, close the instrument on the first tooth. Then, tap the ratchet part against a solid surface. The ratchet is faulty if the instrument springs open. Clamps that open when placed on **blood vessels** have the potential to injure patients. Scissors must be sharp and smooth, and cut easily. Inspect the edges of sharp instruments for chips, nicks, or dents. Needle holders must hold needles without slippage or twisting of the needle. To test needle holders, place a needle in the jaws of the instrument, then lock the holder in the second tooth. If the needle can be easily removed, replace the instrument. Inspection is an ongoing process that must be carried out by all members of the surgical team.

After the procedure, staff members responsible for cleaning and disinfecting the instruments should also inspect them. The instruments should be inspected again after cleaning and during packaging. Any instrument found not in good working order should be sent for repair. Depending on use, surgical instruments can last for up to ten years, given proper care.

High-risk diseases

Evidence from animal models and case reports in humans has shown that such prion diseases as **Creutzfeldt-Jakob disease** (CJD) can be transmitted via stainless steel instruments. British surgeons are moving toward using only disposable, single-use instruments—particularly in adenotonsillectomy procedures—to minimize the risk of transmission of CJD. Research in the United States has concluded that surgical instruments and devices contaminated with particles of **brain**, **spinal cord**, and eye tissue from high-risk patients require special treatment.

Health care team roles

Team members involved with the care and use of surgical instruments include surgeons, the first assistant, the circulator, and the scrub person. Such other personnel as medical students, orderlies, or aides may also be included in the surgical team.

The surgeon works under the policies of the facility in which the procedure is performed. The surgeon is responsible for guiding the operation. During the procedure, the surgeon may also identify instrument malfunctions not evident until the device is actually in use.

The first assistant generally acts to provide retraction, grasp tissue, perform suturing, and other duties as required by the surgeon and the procedure performed.

The person performing the scrub function is responsible for maintaining a sterile operative field. The scrub person hands instruments to the surgeon or assistant. Instruments and other materials are passed in such a way that the surgeon does not have to look away from the wound in order to receive the item. The scrub person is responsible for conducting counts of instruments, sponges, and sharps with the circulator. The scrub

---

KEY TERMS

Autoclave—A heavy vessel that uses pressurized steam for disinfecting surgical instruments.

Creutzfeldt-Jakob disease (CJD)—A degenerative disorder of the nervous system that is usually fatal within a year. CJD is transmitted by a prion.

Curette—A scoop-shaped surgical instrument for removing tissue from body cavities.

Instruments—Tools or devices that perform such functions as cutting, dissecting, grasping, holding, retracting, or suturing.

Prion—A infectious agent composed of protein and lacking a genetic component.

Sharps—Surgical implements with thin cutting edges or a fine point. Sharps include such devices as suture needles, scalpel blades, hypodermic needles, and safety pins.

Sponges—Pieces of absorbent material, usually cotton gauze, used to absorb fluids, protect tissue, or apply pressure and traction.

Tenaculum (plural, tenacula)—A small, sharp-pointed hook set in a handle, used to seize or pick up pieces of tissue during surgical operations.

---

person should also inspect the surgical instruments prior to the procedure.

The person performing the circulating function does not undergo a surgical scrub prior to the procedure, and therefore does not enter the sterile operating field. The circulator is responsible for conducting counts of instruments, sponges, and sharps with the scrub person. The circulator positions the patient for the procedure, adjusts lighting, and assists the surgical team in carrying out functions that do not require sterile, only aseptic, techniques.

Training

Training in the use and care of surgical instruments may range from the medical training required by physicians to on-the-job training for orderlies and aides.

• Surgeons are graduates of medical or osteopathic institutions, with additional training and education in surgical procedures.

- First assistants. Depending on institutional policy, the first assistant may be another physician, a surgical resident, or a registered nurse.

- Circulator. Depending on facility policy, the circulator may be a registered nurse, a licensed practical nurse, or a surgical technologist.

- Scrub person. The scrub person may be a registered nurse, a licensed practical nurse, or a surgical technologist.

- Other personnel. Depending on the facility, there may be surgical orderlies and aides that assist in a variety of tasks, such as patient positioning and transfers, instrument cleaning and disinfecting, and cleaning the surgical suites. No special license is required for these positions, and training may be acquired on the job.

Resources

BOOKS

Caruthers, Bob, and Paul Price. *Surgical Technology for the Surgical Technologist.* Albany, NY: Delmar, 2001.

Rothrock, Jane. *The RN First Assistant*, 3rd ed. Philadelphia: Lippincott, 1999.

Spry, Cynthia. *Essentials of Perioperative Nursing*, 2nd ed. Gaithersburg, MD: Aspen Publishers, 1997.

PERIODICALS

Frosh, A., R. Joyce, and A. Johnson. "Iatrogenic vCJD from surgical instruments." *British Medical Journal* 322 (June 30, 2001): 1558–1559.

Rutala, W. A., and D. J. Weber. "Creutzfeldt-Jakob disease: Recommendations for disinfection and sterilization." *Clinical Infectious Diseases* 32, no. 9 (May 1, 2001): 1348–1356.

OTHER

Sklar Instruments. 889 South Matlack St., West Chester, PA 19382. (800) 221-2166. http://www.sklarcorp.com.

Surgical Instruments Corporation. 4575 Hudson Drive, Stow, OH 44224. (800) 444-5644. http://www.spectrumsurgical.com.

ORGANIZATIONS

American College of Surgeons (ACS). 633 North St. Clair Street, Chicago, IL 60611. (312) 202-5000. http://www.facs.org/

Association of Perioperative Registered Nurses, Inc. (AORN). 2170 South Parker Rd, Suite 300, Denver, CO 80231-5711. (800) 755-2676. http://www.aorn.org/.

Association of Surgical Technologists (AST). 7108-C South Alton Way, Suite 100, Englewood, CO 80112-2106. (800) 637-7433.

Maggie Boleyn, RN, BSN

Surgical technology

Definition

Surgical technology is an allied health profession. Surgical technologists are responsible for **surgical instruments** and other equipment in the surgical unit. They assist a variety of personnel in the surgical area, including surgeons and registered nurses.

Description

Surgical technologists are also sometimes referred to as operating or surgical room technicians. The primary goal of the surgical technologist is to adequately prepare the operating room for a surgical procedure and to assist surgical professionals in performing their duties during the surgery. This preparation generally involves setting up the surgical instruments and equipment; it also includes the organization and placement of sterile linens and solutions. In addition, the surgical technologist gathers, adjusts, and assesses nonsterile equipment to verify that it is operational. The surgical technologist also helps patients with preparation for the surgical procedure by cleaning, shaving, and disinfecting the areas of the body where the surgery will take place. Surgical technologists move the patients into the operating room, where they help with the proper positioning of the patient on the operating table, having dressed the patient with sterile surgical clothing.

In the preoperative phase, surgical technologists often help with the important task of monitoring the **vital signs** of patients and checking patient charts. They also help other surgical personnel scrub and dress for the surgical procedure. During surgical procedures, technologists supply instruments and supplies to the surgeons and surgical assistants. This will involve counting needles, sponges, instruments, and supplies. It may also include holding retractors and cutting sutures. One of the most important duties of the technologist is to help with the collection, preparation, and disposal of specimens taken from the patient. Such specimens are usually taken to the laboratory for analysis. Other duties include applying dressings to the surgical site and maintaining equipment in the operating room, such as suction devices, lights, and sterilizers. They may also be involved in the management of **blood** and plasma. After surgery, the surgical technologist often takes the patient to a recovery room. Another role of the technologist is to clean the operating room after the surgery is complete, and the replenishment of surgical room supplies.

Work settings

Most surgical technologists work in surgical units in hospitals, which are comfortable environments that are clean and well-lit. However, it is often necessary for the surgical technologist to stand for hours during lengthy surgical procedures. Surgical technologists, as well as other surgical personnel, are sometimes exposed to contagious disease, in addition to challenging situations involving bad odors and sights associated with serious disease. They wear traditional surgical gowns along with head coverings, masks, gloves, shoe covers, and protective eyewear. The majority of surgical technologists work a 40-hour week. This work week may involve some weekend, evening, and holiday shifts.

Education and training

Almost all surgical technologists receive their training in one of the following places: the military, hospitals, vocational schools, universities, or junior and community colleges. A formal body called the Commission on Accreditation of Allied Health Education Programs (CAAHEP) officially recognized and accredited 165 such programs as of 1998. Generally, a person must be a high-school graduate before being admitted to these programs. These programs vary in length from nine to 24 months. Those who graduate from these programs may receive a certificate, diploma, or associated degree. Those who have prior medical training, such as certain military personnel or licensed practical nurses, often train in the programs for a shorter length of time.

The typical surgical technology program includes courses in **anatomy**, **physiology**, **pharmacology**, **medical terminology**, **microbiology**, surgery, and ethics. These programs also have a significant period of supervised hands-on clinical training. During the program, the student learns the proper techniques to ensure the care and safety of patients during surgical preparation and procedures. In addition, surgical technology students learn to handle a variety of equipment, supplies, solutions, and drugs. The surgical technologist must learn in detail the types and functions of a wide variety of surgical instruments. In addition to these more traditional surgical implements, a fully trained modern surgical technologist must know about modern surgical technology and how it is used. This technology may include endoscopes, lasers, and power tools. For obvious reasons, surgical technology students receive extensive training in the use of the appropriate tools in various surgical situations.

There is a strong emphasis on proper **sterilization techniques** and the prevention of **disease transmission**

> ## KEY TERMS
>
> **Computed axial tomography**—Noninvasive imaging in which planes of tissue are assessed by radiography combined with computer analysis.
>
> **Endoscope**—A device that consists of a tube and an optical system that allows the observation of the inside of a hollow organ or cavity.
>
> **Magnetic resonance imaging**—Noninvasive technique that allows the viewing of soft tissues in the body using a strong magnetic field.
>
> **Positron emission tomography**—a noninvasive technique that allows the observing of blood and oxygen flow in tissues, particularly the brain, using positron-emitting radionuclides.

before, during, and after surgical procedures. Significant discussion of disinfectant agents and their application to instrumentation, equipment, and supplies are also part of the curriculum. Surgical technologists also receive training in the principles of wound healing from the suturing process to the various stages of healing. Surgical technologists are also often trained to perform basic **cardiopulmonary resuscitation (CPR)** or **basic life support (BLS)**. In addition to patients who are scheduled for surgery in advance, surgical technologists also help prepare patients who enter the hospital in emergency situations.

Surgical technologists also receive training in the various ways that diseases are diagnosed, such as radiography, computed axial tomography (CT), **positron emission tomography**, **magnetic resonance imaging**, and **ultrasonography**. These imaging techniques are generally used preoperatively, though some of these methods may be used in an operative setting.

Surgical technologists need to be able to handle a fairly high level of **stress** due to the typical conditions in an operating environment. They also need to be organized and conscientious. A high level of manual dexterity is also required in the manipulation of operating room supplies and instruments. They need to know the equipment, supplies, and procedures of the operating room to efficiently help the surgical team. There is no time to waste in this environment, and the surgical technologist should not have to be told how and what to do at every step. As with other health professionals, the surgical technologist needs to keep up with the latest developments within the field.

The Liaison Council on Certification for the Surgical Technologist certifies technologists as professionals. This body grants such certification after the person graduates from one of the accredited programs and passes a national certification examination. At this point, the individual can use the title Certified Surgical Technologist (CST). This certification has to be renewed every six years. The certification requires either passing an examination or taking continuing education courses. Generally, those who have obtained the CST designation have an advantage in the recruitment process.

Advanced education and training

There are a variety of ways for the surgical technologist to keep up with developments within the field. There are many continuing education courses available. One of the best ways for the technologist to advance within the field is to specialize in a particular type of surgical technology, for example, cardiothoracic surgery, **neurosurgery**, orthopedic surgery, or as circulating technologists. The circulating technologist is the only member of the surgical team that is not completely sterile. In this role the technologist helps with the patients or assists in the anesthesia. This person also retrieves and opens supplies for sterile members of the team. They may also interview the patient before surgery, keeping detailed notes about the surgery itself, and act as a resource of information about the patient during surgery. There are four levels of CST certification. Level 1 is one that has been certified in basic patient care concepts and has the training to perform as first scrub during basic surgeries. Level 2 has all of the abilities and training of those at level 1 and has circulating skills. Level 3 has the skills and knowledge of the first two levels and has some defined management position. Level 4 surgical technologists are called surgical first assistants. These technologists actually help with the surgery itself. First assistants typically have additional training. Another means for surgical technologists to advance is by getting into management positions, such as operating supply departments in hospitals. Practice standards have been developed to help surgical technologists in these roles.

Future outlook

The United States Department of Labor has forecast that the employment of surgical technologists will grow at a rate that is much faster than average. This reflects growth in the number of surgical procedures being performed currently. This number is growing because those born in the baby boom after World War II are reaching retirement age and many require surgical interventions. New surgical technologies will also be increasingly utilized, and this will require highly trained personnel. The majority of surgical technologists will continue to be employed by hospitals, but many will work in clinics and in the offices of physicians.

Resources

BOOKS

Caruthers, Bob L., and Paul Price, eds. *Surgical Technology for the Surgical Technologist: A Positive Care Approach.* Albany, NY: Delmar, 2001.

Occupational Outlook Handbook, 2011-2012 Ed. Washington, DC: Department of Labor, 2011.

ORGANIZATIONS

Association of Surgical Technologists. 7108-C South Alton Way, Englewood, CO 80112. http://www.ast.org.

Liaison Council on Certification for the Surgical Technologist. 7790 East Arapahoe Rd, Suite 240, Englewood, CO 80112-1274.

Mark A. Mitchell

Swallowing disorders

Definition

Swallowing disorders include a number of diseases and conditions that cause difficulty in passing food or liquid from the mouth to the **stomach**.

Description

Although normally swallowing is automatic, it is a complex process involving several phases and 29 muscles. Saliva helps soften food as it is chewed. The tongue helps move food to the back of the mouth, triggering a swallowing reflex that passes food through the pharynx. The epiglottis helps keep food from mistakenly going down the windpipe and into the esophagus, the canal that carries food to the stomach. Swallowing disorders can occur at any phase in the swallowing process. The medical term for difficult swallowing is **dysphagia**.

Each year, about 10 million people in the United States require medical evaluation for swallowing problems. Some experts say that about 10% of Americans develop symptoms of swallowing disorders in adulthood. Elderly people are the most likely to have problems with swallowing.

Causes and symptoms

Swallowing disorders often result from other conditions and diseases. For example, **Parkinson's disease**, **cerebral palsy**, **stroke**, **head injury**, and other **central nervous system** conditions can damage the muscles and nerves involved in swallowing. Some people are born with abnormalities in the swallowing structures, such as infants with cleft palate.

Some cancers can lead to swallowing disorders. Esophageal **cancer** can cause narrowing and eventual blockage of the esophagus. Surgery and radiation therapy for **head and neck cancer** can restrict or weaken tongue motion, paralyze vocal cords, or cause muscle damage that affects swallowing. An inflamed esophagus, often resulting from gastroesophageal reflux disease (GERD), can cause painful or difficult swallowing. Infections of the esophagus also can inflame it and cause it to narrow. Swallowing difficulty may result from **aging**, though researchers are not certain why.

The most common symptoms people report are **choking** and the feeling that food is stuck in the throat. Other symptoms include needing to swallow many times to clear food from the mouth and throat, a gurgly, wet sound to the voice after swallowing, having to clear the throat after eating, coughing, **pain** while swallowing, bringing food back up (regurgitation), food or acid backing up into the throat, unexpected weight loss, and not being able to swallow at all. Children also may gag during meals and may have excessive drooling or leaking of food or liquid from their mouths during meals. They may have difficulty breathing when eating or drinking, spit up frequently and lag behind in weight gain. They also may have recurring **pneumonia** or respiratory infections.

Diagnosis

A physician should perform a full head and neck examination based on the patient's symptoms. Speech-language pathologists may aid in the diagnosis. Physicians also might order a swallowing test to study how the patient swallows. The patient will be asked to drink a liquid with a contrast agent called barium that will show up on x rays of the throat and upper chest. The exam might be imaged with a technique called video fluoroscopy, which will take motion camera images in addition to still images. For this exam, the patient may be asked to swallow liquid, paste, and solids. A speech pathologist may work with the radiologist to perform this exam.

If the physician thinks the problem originates in the lower esophagus or has concerns about an abnormality in the esophagus, an endoscopy may be ordered. This test involves passing a thin, flexible instrument called an endoscope down the throat. The lighted endoscope helps the physician view the esophagus. Other tests may be used, including ultrasound.

Treatment

Treatment will depend on the cause of the swallowing problem. Special exercises may help strengthen the muscles used for chewing and swallowing. Problems originating in the mouth may be treated with artificial saliva, improved hydration or better dental care. Esophageal problems will be treated depending on the cause. Patients with GERD will receive medications and instructions on how to better manage the disease. Esophageal cancer is a life-threatening disease that will involve coordinating care with an oncologist. Many patients will receive help with their disorders from speech pathologists. Special liquid diets may be ordered for patients who continue to have trouble chewing or swallowing. In severe cases, the patient may need a feeding tube that bypasses the part of the swallowing system that does not work.

Alternative treatment

Some herbs that may help improve swallowing are oil of peppermint and licorice. Valerian may be used as a tea. Homeopathic physicians may suggest some remedies aimed at improving bloating, indigestion, or **cough**. Alternative care should be sought from licensed practitioners and coordinated with physician care.

Prognosis

In many cases, these disorders can be corrected. If not treated, swallowing disorders can lead to serious complications, including **dehydration** and malnutrition. There also is a risk of food entering the airway (aspiration) as a person attempts to swallow, which can lead to aspiration pneumonia as the food particles enter the **lungs**.

Prevention

Many causes of swallowing disorders cannot be prevented. Slowly and fully chewing food helps. People with GERD should manage it to lower the risk of developing swallowing difficulties.

Resources

PERIODICALS

Disorders of Swallowing. *Harvard Men's Health Watch* (Sept. 2003).

The Evaluation and Management of Swallowing Disorders in the Elderly. *Geriatric Times* (November 1, 2003): 17.

ORGANIZATIONS

American Academy of Otolaryngology-Head and Neck Surgery. One Prince St., Alexandria, VA 22314-3357. 703-836-4444. http://www.entnet.org.

American Speech-Language Association (ASHA). 10801 Rockville Pike, Rockville, MD 20852. 800-638-8255. http://www.asha.org.

National Institute of Dental and Craniofacial Research (NIDCR). 45 Center Dr., Rm 4AS19 MSC 6400, Bethesda, MD 20892-6400. 301-496-4261. http://www.nidr.nih.gov.

Teresa G. Odle

Swallowing disorders *see* **Dysphagia**

Swan-Ganz catheterization

Definition

Swan-Ganz catheterization, also known as pulmonary artery catheterization, is a diagnostic procedure in which a small catheter is threaded through a vein in the arm, thigh, chest, or neck until it passes through the right side of the **heart** into the pulmonary artery. The catheter is than able to measure the pressures in the right heart and pulmonary artery.

Purpose

Swan-Ganz catheterization is performed in order to:

• evaluate heart failure

• determine whether pulmonary edema is caused by a weak heart (cardiogenic pulmonary edema) or leaky pulmonary capillaries (non-cardiogenic pulmonary edema or adult respiratory distress syndrome)

• monitor therapy after a myocardial infarction (heart attack)

• check the fluid balance of patients in shock as well as those recovering from heart surgery, serious burns, or kidney disease

• monitor the effect of medications on the heart

Precautions

Pulmonary artery catheterization is an invasive and potentially complicated procedure. The physician must decide if the value of the information obtained outweighs the risks of catheterization.

Description

Swan-Ganz catheterization is usually performed in the hospital intensive care unit. A catheter is threaded through a vein in the arm, thigh, chest, or neck until it passes through the right side of the heart into the pulmonary artery. The procedure takes about 30 minutes. **Local anesthesia** is administered at the catheter insertion site to reduce discomfort.

Once the catheter is in place, the physician briefly inflates a tiny balloon at its tip. This temporarily blocks the **blood** flow and allows the physician to make a pressure measurement in the pulmonary artery system. This pressure reading is called the pulmonary capillary wedge pressure. Pressure measurements are usually recorded for the next 48–72 hours in different parts of the heart. During this time, the patient must remain in bed so the catheter remains in position. Once the pressure measurements are no longer needed, the catheter is removed.

Preparation

Before and during the test, the patient will be connected to an electrocardiograph, which records the electrical stimuli that cause the heart to contract. The insertion site is sterilized and prepared prior to the test. The catheter is often sutured to the skin to prevent dislodgment.

Aftercare

The patient is observed for any sign of infections or complications from the procedure.

Complications

Swan-Ganz catheterization is not without risk. Possible complications from the procedure include:

• lung collapse (pneumothorax)

• infection at the site of catheter insertion

• pulmonary artery perforation

• blood clots in the lungs

• irregular heartbeat

Results

Normal pressures reflect a normally functioning heart with no fluid accumulation. These normal pressure readings are:

• right atrium: 1–6 mm of mercury (mm Hg).

• right ventricle during contraction (systolic): 20–30 mm Hg.

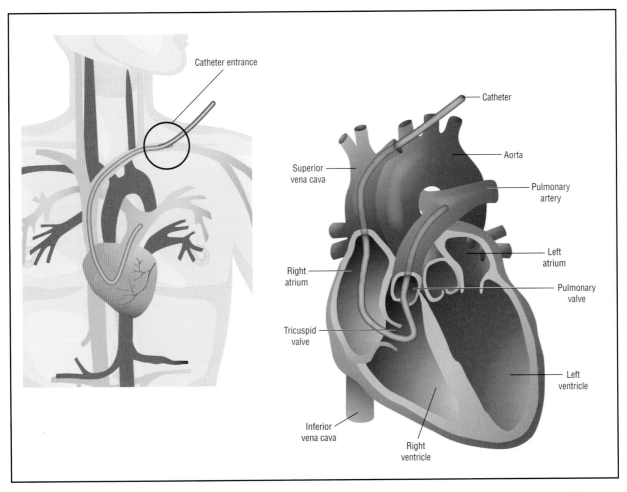

(Diagram showing the Swan-Ganz catheterization procedure: catheter going into heart; detail inside heart. Illustration by GGS Information Services, Inc. The Gale Group.)

- right ventricle at the end of relaxation (end diastolic): less than 5 mm Hg.
- pulmonary artery during contraction (systolic): 20–30 mm Hg.
- pulmonary artery during relaxation (diastolic): about 10 mm Hg.
- mean pulmonary artery: less than 20 mm Hg.
- pulmonary capillary wedge pressure: 6–12 mm Hg.
- cardiac output: 3–7 L/min.

Abnormally high right atrium pressure can indicate:

- pulmonary disease
- right-sided heart failure
- fluid accumulation
- cardiac tamponade (compression of the heart by a pericardial effusion)
- right heart valve abnormalities
- pulmonary hypertension (high blood pressure)

Abnormally high right ventricle pressure may indicate:

- pulmonary hypertension (high blood pressure)
- pulmonary valve abnormalities
- right ventricle failure
- defects in the heart wall between the right and left ventricle
- congestive heart failure
- serious heart inflammation

Abnormally high pulmonary artery pressure may indicate:

- left-to-right cardiac shunt
- pulmonary artery hypertension
- chronic obstructive pulmonary disease or emphysema
- blood clots in the lungs
- fluid accumulation in the lungs

KEY TERM

Cardiac shunt—A defect in the wall of the heart that allows blood from different chambers to mix.

• left ventricular failure

Abnormally high pulmonary capillary wedge pressure may indicate:

• left ventricular failure
• mitral valve abnormalities
• compression of the heart after hemorrhage

Health care team roles

Swan-Ganz catheterization is generally performed in the hospital intensive care or critical care unit by trained physicians. Physicians from a variety of specialties are trained to perform the procedure, including cardiologists, surgeons, anesthesiologists, and critical care specialists. Patients in the intensive care unit are monitored and cared for by critical care nurses, laboratory and **radiology** technicians as well as other physician specialists such as internists, pulmonologists, and cardiothoracic surgeons.

Patient education

Specially trained nurses assist during catheterization procedures and provide pre- and postoperative education, monitoring, and supportive care.

Resources

BOOKS

Thelan, Lynne A. et al. *Critical Care Nursing Diagnosis and Management.* St. Louis, MO: Mosby, 1998, p. 386.
Zaret, Barry, ed. "Pulmonary Artery Catheterization." In *The Patient's Guide to Medical Tests.* New York: Houghton Mifflin, 1997.

Barbara Wexler

Sweat test *see* **Electrolyte tests**

Syncope

Definition

Syncope is a temporary loss of consciousness and posture, usually caused by decreased **blood** flow to the brain. It is commonly also called fainting and passing out. When a person feels faint and lightheaded then this is called presyncope. Syncope is a symptom, rather than a disease itself, and has many causes. The primary cause of syncope is then a person's **blood pressure** is too low, what is called **hypotension**, and when the **heart** does not pump sufficient oxygen to the brain. The vasovagal faint, which usually occurs in young, otherwise healthy people, is one particular form of syncope.

Description

Syncope usually begins while a person is either sitting or standing upright. Sometimes, the onset may be almost instantaneous. In other cases, up to a few minutes before the attack there may be warning symptoms such as:

• profuse sweating (diaphoresis)
• nausea or vomiting
• light-headedness or weakness
• confusion or anxiety
• blurry or dim vision
• ringing in the ears

The patient usually becomes very pale and collapses. Loss of consciousness can last from seconds to several minutes. During this time, the patient may have a slight awareness of the situation, or may lose consciousness completely. During this time, there may be some twitching or jerking of the body, but not usually incontinence or biting of the tongue; this helps distinguish the episode from a seizure. The patient's blood pressure is usually low with a weak pulse, but the heart rate may be fast or slow. Breathing is often very slow or shallow.

As the person lies flat, blood flow returns to the brain. The patient's **vital signs**, color, and alertness improve. Depending on the cause, the patient may have no sequelae (continuing symptoms), or may remain weak, confused, nauseated, or sweaty. A patient who tries to get up too soon may faint again.

Demographics

Syncope is a common problem. It accounts for about 3% of emergency department visits per year in the United States, and about 6% of U.S. hospital admissions. It can happen to healthy people without any known medical problems. About one in three people will experience syncope at least once in their lifetime. Males and females are equally likely to have an incidence of syncope. However, the likelihood of having an episode of syncope increases as one ages, with a much more increased chance after the age of 70 years.

Causes and symptoms

Dozens of different underlying problems can cause syncope; some are life-threatening, others are of little importance. The following is one such classification system.

Orthostatic

Orthostatic, or postural, syncope occurs when the body cannot supply enough blood to the brain in the upright position because of low blood pressure. The patient may have minimal symptoms of illness while lying flat, but becomes very faint when standing. Causes include:

• blood loss (trauma, gastrointestinal hemorrhage, ruptured aortic aneurysm, ruptured ectopic pregnancy)

• dehydration (vomiting, diarrhea, heat exposure)

• certain medications (beta blockers, calcium channel blockers, diuretics)

Cardiac

The heart itself is the source of many episodes of syncope. There are numerous possible mechanisms. For example, certain cardiac **arrhythmias** (irregular heartbeat) reduce the output of the heart. In severe bradycardia (slow heartbeat), the ventricles beat too slowly to supply enough blood to the brain. In rapid tachycardias (rapid heartbeat), the heart beats quickly but very inefficiently, so relatively little blood and oxygen reach the brain.

Reflex-mediated

Reflex-mediated syncope occurs when a certain stimulus triggers a bodily response that lowers the cardiac output. The most common example of this is the vasovagal faint (also known by many other names, including simple faint or neurocardiogenic syncope). This condition typically affects young, otherwise healthy people who experience something very unpleasant, such as **pain**, fear, or horror. Nervous system **reflexes** cause the blood pressure, and often the pulse, to drop. The patient experiences warning symptoms such as sweating, nausea, and light-headedness, and then faints if not able to lie down quickly. Other reflex-mediated faints often involve the Valsalva maneuver (taking a deep breath and bearing down), as when straining to urinate, defecate, **cough**, or lift a heavy object.

Medication-related

Medications may lead to fainting by their direct effects of lowering the blood pressure (anti-hypertensives, nitroglycerine) or slowing the heart rate (digoxin). Some drugs may promote arrhythmias (tricyclic antidepressants). Other drugs that may cause syncope include antiparkinsonians, phenothiazines and other antipsychotics, insulin and other hypoglycemics, alcohol, and **cocaine**.

Neurologic

Neurologic causes of syncope include **stroke** and transient ischemic attack, subarachnoid hemorrhage, and migraine. In these cases, a part of the brain does not receive its normal blood supply, and the patient loses consciousness. Seizure is the condition most often mistaken for syncope, because patients with true seizures often lose consciousness as well.

Psychiatric

Psychiatric disorders may cause syncope on the basis of **anxiety** and hyperventilation, hysterical seizures, or major depression. A person who becomes intensely anxious will breathe faster than normal and may faint from taking in too much oxygen and exhaling too much carbon dioxide.

Diagnosis

The challenge for health professionals is to determine the cause of an episode of syncope, and especially whether the cause requires further medical intervention.

History

Nurses and aides are invaluable when they obtain details of the patient's episode not only from the patient, but also from family or friends, witnesses, and rescue personnel. The staff must not allow such people to leave without providing information, as well as phone numbers for further contact. Nurses and aides should focus on:

• the precise sequence of events leading up to, and following, the faint

• associated features (tongue biting, incontinence)

• the patient's memory of the event and any associated symptoms (pain, focal numbness or weakness, recent illness)

• past similar events and other medical history

• prescribed medications and how the patient takes them

• use of illicit drugs or alcohol

• possible emotional stress

• menstrual history (for women)

Physical examination

The examination must always start with the ABCs of resuscitation: airway, breathing, and circulation. Nurses and aides then:

• record vital signs frequently including oxygen saturation

• attach a cardiac monitor

• undress the patient completely

• observe for physical signs such as sweating, pallor, restlessness, confusion, or pain

• immediately communicate all abnormal findings to the physician

Laboratory

The patient likely will require blood work (**complete blood count**, blood chemistries, cardiac enzymes, and perhaps blood typing and coagulation studies) and urine tests (**pregnancy**, **urinalysis**, and drug screen), usually performed by a clinical laboratory technician. An EKG technician or a nurse will record an electrocardiogram (EKG), and the nurse may check bedside blood sugar determination and stool guaiac. The nurse will either initiate these directly or check first with the physician, depending on local policies. In all cases the nurse must not allow the patient to void or defecate without collecting a specimen.

Treatment

If the patient has no discernible pulse or respiration, the nurse and all available personnel immediately start **cardiopulmonary resuscitation** and summon help. The nurse and respiratory technician must ensure adequate oxygenation. The nurse starts an intravenous line (IV) in all but the least serious cases, and begins normal saline infusion if the blood pressure is low or the pulse is fast. The patient may need two large-bore IVs to replace fluids in a case of severe reduction in blood volume, or to receive drips of cardiac medications.

The nurse must give the patient nothing by mouth if there is any likely surgical cause of the problem (such as ruptured ectopic pregnancy), or if nausea persists. If the patient is about to vomit, the staff must quickly put the head down and roll the patient to the side. The nurse or aide should loosen tight clothing. The staff should keep the patient supine until clearly improved; thereafter, the patient may rise slowly while the nurse or aide checks for orthostatic pulse and blood pressure changes. More specific treatment depends on the underlying cause of the event.

Prognosis

The prognosis depends on such factors as the underlying cause of the problem, length of unconsciousness, injuries that may have occurred when fainting, and the patient's ability to modify circumstances that may have contributed to the event (learning to rise slowly, stopping alcohol abuse, switching to different medications).

Usually there is nothing to worry about if one feels faint or actually passes out. However, it can sometimes be a sign of a serious problem. It is important to see a trusted health care provider, such as a family doctor, to find out what has happened and why.

Health care team roles

The nurse, typically in the emergency department, initially receives the patient, makes the initial assessment of the patient's condition, often begins early diagnosis and treatment measures, continues to monitor the patient, and communicates all relevant information to the physician. The nurse's aide helps prepare the patient for examination and assists the rest of the care team. The laboratory technician helps collect specimens and process them in the lab. The EKG technician records one or more cardiograms and may help with other heart monitoring tests. A respiratory technician assists when there is difficulty breathing, and may perform an arterial blood gas. **Radiology** technicians carry out required x-ray tests. A social worker may discuss the patient's living situation with the patient, family, and caregivers, and help arrange future assistance.

Prevention

Before actually fainting, a person may feel lightheaded or dizzy, and the **stomach** may feel upset. In addition, a person may have blurry **vision** or a hard time **hearing**. If feeling faint, lie down. When lying down is not possible, then sit and bend forward with the head between the knees. Remain in this position until the fainting sensation disappears. This will allow blood to flow more easily to the brain. When attempting to stand up, do so slowly.

If in a medical facility, such as a hospital, the nurse must provide clear instructions to the patient and caregivers. The patient may need to alter behavior (eat

Antiparkinsonian—A drug that treats Parkinson's disease.

Aortic aneurysm—A dangerous widening and weakening of the wall of the aorta.

Aortic stenosis—A narrowing and stiffening of the aortic valve of the heart.

Arrhythmia—An abnormal beating pattern of the heart.

Beta blockers—A class of medicines including propranolol (Inderal), atenolol (Tenormin), and many others, used to slow the heart rate and reduce the blood pressure.

Bradycardia—Heart rate less than 60 beats per minute.

Calcium channel blockers—A class of medicines including verapamil (Calan), diltiazem (Cardizem), and many others, used to slow the heart rate and reduce the blood pressure.

Cardiomyopathy—A disease which weakens the heart muscle.

Diaphoresis—Profuse sweating.

Diuretic—Causing urination.

Ectopic pregnancy—A dangerous condition in which a woman becomes pregnant, but the fetus grows outside the uterus.

Incontinence—Loss of control over the release of urine or the bowels.

Insulin and hypoglycemics—Various drugs that reduce the level of sugar in the blood, used to treat diabetes mellitus.

Myocardial infarction—Heart attack, or death of some part of the heart muscle.

Neurocardiogenic—Arising from the nervous and cardiac systems of the body.

Orthostatic—Related to being upright.

Pericardial tamponade—A condition in which fluid accumulates in the pericardium, the sac that surrounds the heart. This restricts the amount of blood that can enter the heart's chambers.

Phenothiazines—A class of drugs including prochlorperazine (Compazine), chlorpromazine (Thorazine), and many others, used to treat nausea or psychosis.

Sequelae—Conditions that result from an event.

Subarachnoid hemorrhage—A dangerous condition of bleeding within the subarachnoid space of the brain.

Tachycardia—Heart rate greater than 100 beats per minute.

Transient ischemic attack (TIA)—A temporary interruption of the blood supply to part of the brain that causes a reversible impairment of some brain function.

Valsalva maneuver—The act of taking a deep breath and bearing down forcefully. This may be done intentionally, or as part of straining to move the bowels, urinate, or lift a heavy object, for example.

regularly, avoid stressful situations), stop or start various medications, have further tests or appointments, and understand warning signs requiring an immediate return to the hospital.

Resources

BOOKS

Benditt, David G., et al., editors. *Syncope and Transient Loss of Consciousness: Multidisciplinary Management.* Malden, MA: Blackwell Futura, 2007.

Brignole, Michele, and David G. Benditt. *Syncope: An Evidence-based Approach.* London: Springer, 2011.

Grubb, Blair P. *The Fainting Phenomenon: Understanding Why People Faint and What to Do About It.* Malden, MA, Blackwell, 2007.

Longo, Dan L, and Tinsley Randolph Harrison. *Harrison's Principles of Internal Medicine.* New York: McGraw-Hill, 2012.

Tintinalli, Judith, editor. *Tintinalli's Emergency Medicine: A Comprehensive Study Guide.* New York: McGraw-Hill Medical, 2011.

WEBSITES

Fainting. FamilyDoctor.org. (July 2010). http://familydoctor. org/familydoctor/en/diseases-conditions/fainting.printer- view.all.html (April 26, 2012).

Fainting. Medline Plus. (March 8, 2012). http://www.nlm.nih. gov/medlineplus/fainting.html (April 26, 2012).

Syncope. American Heart Association. (July 28, 2011). http://www.heart.org/HEARTORG/Conditions/ Arrhythmia/SymptomsDiagnosisMonitoringof Arrhythmia/Syncope_UCM_430006_Article.jsp (April 26, 2012).

Syncope. American Heart Association. (July 28, 2011). http://www.heart.org/HEARTORG/Conditions/ Arrhythmia/SymptomsDiagnosisMonitoringof Arrhythmia/Syncope_UCM_430006_Article.jsp (April 26, 2012).

Understanding Fainting—The Basics. WebMD. (March 8, 2012). http://www.webmd.com/brain/understanding- fainting-basics (April 26, 2012).

ORGANIZATIONS

American Lung Association, 1301 Pennsylvania Ave. NW, Ste. 800, Washington, D.C. 20004, (202) 785-3355 Fax: (202) 452-1805, info@lung.org, http://www.lungusa. org/

National Heart, Lung and Blood Institute, P.O. Box 30105, Bethesda, MD 20824-0105, (301) 592-8573, Fax: (240) 629-3246, nhlbiinfo@nhlbi.nih.gov, http://www.nhlbi.nih. gov/.

Kenneth J. Berniker, M.D.
William A. Atkins, B.B., B.S., M.B.A.

Synovial fluid analysis *see* **Joint fluid analysis**

Syphilis

Definition

Syphilis is an infectious systemic disease that may be either congenital or acquired through sexual contact or by exposure to contaminated needles.

Description

Syphilis has both acute and chronic forms that produce a wide variety of symptoms affecting most of the body's organ systems. Acquired syphilis has four stages: primary, secondary, latent, and tertiary, and can be spread by sexual contact during the first three of these four stages.

Syphilis has been a major **public health** problem since the sixteenth century. The disease was treated with mercury or other unsuccessful remedies until World War I, when effective treatments based on arsenic or bismuth were introduced. **Antibiotics** were introduced after World War II. At that time, the number of syphilis cases in the general population decreased, partly due to public health measures. In the late 1980s, the number of cases of syphilis in the United States rose steadily. This increase includes men and women, all races, all parts of the nation, and all age groups, including adults over age 60. The number of syphilis cases then declined steadily through the 1990s, reaching an all-time low in 2000, after which the number of cases increased through the 2000s only to decline again in 2010. The increase in the 2000s was attributed primarily to men who have sex with men and men who have sex with both men and women. In 2010, The United States Centers for Disease Control and Prevention reported 4.5 cases of syphilis per 100,000 population. The greatest number of cases (45.5%) in 2010 were found in the South, followed by urban areas in other regions of the country.

The incidence of syphilis in is associated with drug abuse as well as changes in sexual behavior and HIV **infection**. The connections between drug abuse and syphilis include needle sharing and exchanging sex for drugs. In addition, people using drugs are more likely to engage in risky sexual practices. With respect to changing patterns of conduct, an increase in the number of people having sex with multiple partners makes it more difficult for public health professionals to trace the

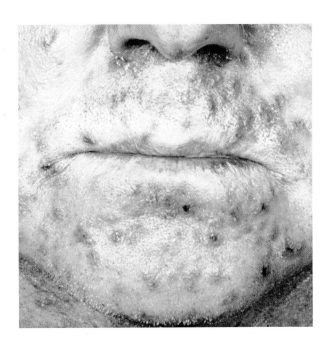

(Secondary Syphilis, photograph. Custom Medical Stock Photo. Reproduced by permission.)

contacts of infected individuals. High-risk groups for syphilis include:

- sexually active teenagers
- people infected with another sexually transmitted disease (STD), including HIV
- sexually abused children
- women of childbearing age
- prostitutes of either gender and their customers
- prisoners
- people who abuse drugs or alcohol

The chances of contracting syphilis from an infected person in the early stages of the disease during unprotected sex are 30–50%.

Causes and symptoms

Syphilis is caused by *Treponema pallidum*, a spirochete, which is a thin spiral- or coil-shaped bacterium that enters the body through the mucous membranes or breaks in the skin. In 90% of cases, the spirochete is transmitted by sexual contact.

Primary syphilis

Primary syphilis refers to the initial stage of the organism's entry into the body. The first signs of infection are not always noticed. After an incubation period ranging between 10 and 90 days, an individual develops a chancre, which is a small blister-like sore about 0.5 inches (13 mm) in size. Most chancres are on the genitals, but they may also develop in or on the mouth or on the breasts. Rectal chancres are common among male homosexuals. Chancres in women are sometimes overlooked if they develop in the vagina or on the cervix. The chancres are not painful and disappear in three to six weeks, with or without treatment. They resemble the ulcers of *Lymphogranuloma venereum*, herpes simplex virus, or skin tumors.

About 70% of people with primary syphilis also develop swollen lymph nodes near the chancre. The nodes may have a firm or rubbery feel, but they are not usually painful.

Secondary syphilis

Syphilis enters its secondary stage between about seven weeks and six months after the initial infection begins. Chancres may still be present but are usually healing. Secondary syphilis is a systemic infection marked by the eruption of skin rashes and ulcers in the mucous membranes. The skin **rash** may mimic a number of other skin disorders such as drug reactions, rubella (German measles), ringworm, mononucleosis, and pityriasis rosea. Characteristics of the rash that point to syphilis include:

- a coppery color
- absence of pain or itching
- occurrence on the palms of hands and soles of feet

The skin eruption may resolve in a few weeks or last as long as a year. A person may also develop condylomata lata, which are watery pink or gray areas of flattened skin in the moist areas of the body. The skin rashes, mouth and genital ulcers, and condylomata lata are all highly infectious.

About 50% of people with secondary syphilis develop swollen lymph nodes in the armpits, groin, and neck areas; about 10% develop inflammations of the eyes, kidney, **liver**, spleen, bones, joints, or the meninges (membranes covering the **brain** and **spinal cord**). They may also have an influenza-like general illness with a low **fever**, chills, loss of appetite, headaches, runny nose, **sore throat**, and aching joints.

Latent syphilis

Latent syphilis is a phase of the disease characterized by relative absence of external symptoms. The latent phase is sometimes divided into early latency (less than two years after infection) and late latency. During early latency, people are at risk for spontaneous relapses marked by recurrence of the ulcers and skin rashes of secondary syphilis. In late latency, these recurrences are much less likely. Late latency may either resolve spontaneously or continue for the rest of the person's life.

Tertiary syphilis

Untreated syphilis progresses to a final, or tertiary, stage in about 35–40% of people. Individuals with tertiary syphilis cannot infect others with the disease. It is thought that the symptoms of this stage are a delayed hypersensitivity reaction to spirochetes. Some people develop so-called benign late syphilis, which begins between three and 10 years after initial infection and is characterized by the development of gummas. Gummas are rubbery tumor-like growths that are most likely to involve the skin or long bones but may also develop in the eyes, mucous membranes, throat, liver, or **stomach** lining. Gummas are increasingly uncommon since the introduction of antibiotics for treating syphilis. Benign late syphilis is usually rapid in onset and responds well to treatment.

CARDIOVASCULAR SYPHILIS. Cardiovascular syphilis occurs in 10–15% of people who have progressed to tertiary syphilis. It develops between 10 and 25 years after initial infection and often occurs together with neurosyphilis. Cardiovascular syphilis usually begins as an inflammation of the arteries leading from the **heart** and causes heart attacks, scarring of the aortic valves, congestive **heart failure**, or the formation of an aortic **aneurysm**.

NEUROSYPHILIS. About 8% of persons with untreated syphilis will develop problems in the **central nervous system** that include both physical and psychiatric symptoms. Neurosyphilis can appear at any time, from 5–35 years after the onset of primary syphilis. It affects men more frequently than women and Caucasians more frequently than African Americans.

Neurosyphilis is classified into four types:

- Asymptomatic: In this form, the person's spinal fluid gives abnormal test results, but there are no symptoms affecting the central nervous system.

- Meningovascular: This type is marked by changes in the blood vessels of the brain or inflammation of the meninges. A person develops headaches, irritability, and visual problems. If the spinal cord is involved, an individual may experience weakness of the shoulder and upper arm muscles.

- Tabes dorsalis: This type causes a progressive degeneration of the spinal cord and nerve roots. People lose their sense of perception of their body position and orientation in space (proprioception), resulting in difficulties with walking and the loss of muscle reflexes. They may also have shooting pains in the legs and periodic episodes of pain in the abdomen, throat, bladder, or rectum. Tabes dorsalis is sometimes called locomotor ataxia.

- General paresis: This type refers to the effects of neurosyphilis on the cortex of the brain. A person experiences slow but progressive losses of memory, ability to concentrate, and interest in self-care. Personality changes may include irresponsible behavior, depression, delusions of grandeur, or complete psychosis. General paresis is sometimes called dementia paralytica, and is most common among people over age 40.

Special populations

CONGENITAL SYPHILIS. Congenital syphilis increased at a rate of 18% between 2006 and 2008, but declined in 2009 and 2010. In 2010, there were an estimated 8.7 cases per 100,000 live births. The prognosis for early congenital syphilis is poor. A large percentage of infected fetuses die before or shortly after birth. Those which survive may look normal at birth but show signs of infection between three and eight weeks later.

Infants with early congenital syphilis have systemic symptoms that resemble those of adults with secondary syphilis. There is a 40–60% chance that a child's central nervous system will be infected. These infants may have symptoms ranging from **jaundice**, enlargement of the spleen and liver, and anemia to skin rashes, condylomata lata, inflammation of the **lungs**, a persistent runny nose, and swollen lymph nodes.

CHILDREN. Children who develop symptoms after the age of two years are said to have late congenital syphilis. The characteristic symptoms include facial deformities (saddle nose), Hutchinson's teeth (abnormal upper incisors), saber shins, dislocated joints, deafness, mental retardation, **paralysis**, and seizure disorders.

PREGNANT WOMEN. Syphilis can be transmitted from a mother to her fetus through the placenta at any time during **pregnancy**, or through the child's contact with syphilitic ulcers during the birth process. The chances of infection are related to the stage of the mother's disease. Almost all infants of mothers with untreated primary or secondary syphilis will be infected, whereas the infection rate drops somewhat if the mother is in the early latent stage, and drops even more if she has late latent syphilis.

Pregnancy does not affect the progression of syphilis in the mother. However, pregnant women should not be treated with tetracyclines as this drug will discolor the teeth of her infant.

PEOPLE WITH HIV. Syphilis has been closely associated with HIV infection since the late 1980s. Syphilis sometimes mimics the symptoms of HIV/AIDS. Conversely, HIV infection appears to increase the severity of syphilis in people with both diseases and to speed up the development or appearance of neurosyphilis. People with HIV are also more likely to develop lues maligna, a skin disease that sometimes occurs in secondary syphilis. In addition, people with HIV have a higher rate of treatment failure with penicillin than those without HIV.

Diagnosis

Personal history and physical diagnosis

Because of the long-term risks of untreated syphilis, certain groups of people are now routinely screened for the disease, including:

• pregnant women

• sexual contacts or partners of people diagnosed with syphilis

• children born to mothers with syphilis

• individuals with HIV infection

• persons applying for marriage licenses

When a physician takes a person's history, there will be questions about recent sexual contacts to determine whether the person falls into a high-risk group. Symptoms such as skin rashes or swollen lymph nodes will be noted with respect to the dates of the person's sexual contacts. Definite diagnosis, however, depends on the results of laboratory **blood** tests.

Blood tests

Several types of blood tests for syphilis are presently used in the United States. Some are used in follow-up monitoring of infected people as well as diagnosis.

NON-TREPONEMAL ANTIGEN TESTS. Non-treponemal antigen tests are used with initial screening. They measure the presence of reagin, which is an antibody formed in reaction to syphilis. In the venereal disease research laboratory (VDRL) test, a sample of a person's blood is mixed with cardiolipin and **cholesterol**. If the mixture forms clumps or masses of matter, the test is considered reactive, or positive.

The rapid plasma reagin (RPR) test, which is available as a kit, works on the same principle as the VDRL. A person's serum is mixed with cardiolipin on a plastic-coated card that can be examined with the naked eye.

Non-treponemal antigen tests require a physician's interpretation and sometimes further testing. They can yield both false-negative and false-positive results. False-positive results can be caused by other infectious diseases, including mononucleosis, **malaria**, leprosy, **rheumatoid arthritis**, and lupus. People with HIV have a particularly high rate of false-positive results on reagin tests. False-negatives can occur when individuals are tested too soon after exposure to syphilis; it takes about 14–21 days after infection for the blood to become reactive.

TREPONEMAL ANTIBODY TESTS. Treponemal antibody tests are used to rule out false-positive results on reagin tests. They measure the presence of **antibodies** that are specific for *T. pallidum*. The most commonly used tests are the microhemagglutination-*T. pallidum* (MHA-TP) and the fluorescent treponemal antibody absorption (FTA-ABS) tests. In the FTA-ABS test, a person's blood serum is mixed with a preparation that prevents interference from antibodies to other treponemal infections. In a positive reaction, syphilitic antibodies in the blood coat the spirochetes on the slide. In the MHA-TP test, red blood cells from sheep are coated with *T. pallidum* antigen. The cells will clump if the person's blood contains antibodies for syphilis.

Treponemal antibody tests are more expensive and more difficult to perform than non-treponemal tests. They are therefore used to confirm the diagnosis of syphilis rather than to screen large groups of people. These tests are, however, very specific and very sensitive; false-positive results are relatively unusual.

Other laboratory tests

MICROSCOPE STUDIES. The diagnosis of syphilis can also be confirmed by identifying spirochetes in samples of tissue or lymphatic fluid.

SPINAL FLUID TESTS. Testing of cerebrospinal fluid (CSF) is an important part of monitoring programs as well as being a diagnostic test. The VDRL and FTA-ABS tests can be performed on CSF as well as on blood. An abnormally high white cell count and elevated protein levels in the CSF, together with positive VDRL results, suggest a possible diagnosis of neurosyphilis. CSF testing is not used for routine screening. It is most frequently used for infants with congenital syphilis, people who are HIV-positive, and individuals of any age who are not responding to penicillin treatment.

Treatment

Medications

Syphilis is treated with antibiotics given either intramuscularly (benzathine penicillin G or ceftriaxone) or orally (doxycycline, minocycline, tetracycline, or azithromycin). Neurosyphilis is treated with a combination of aqueous crystalline penicillin G, benzathine penicillin G, or doxycycline. It is important to keep the levels of penicillin in the person's tissues at sufficiently high levels over a period of days or weeks because the spirochetes have a relatively long reproduction time. To this end, a uricosuric agent such as Probenecid is given to slow the removal of penicillin from the body. Penicillin is more effective in treating the early stages of syphilis than the later stages. Alternate antibiotics such as ceftriaxone (Rocephin) or azithromycin (Zithromax) can be used in individual who cannot take penicillin.

Physicians do not usually prescribe separate medications for the skin rashes or ulcers of secondary syphilis. A person is advised to keep the rashes clean and dry, and to avoid exposing others to fluid or discharges from condylomata lata.

Pregnant women should be screened for syphilis at their first prenatal visit and treated as early in pregnancy as possible. Infected fetuses can be cured if the mother is treated during the second and third trimesters of pregnancy. Infants with proven or suspected congenital syphilis are treated with either aqueous crystalline penicillin G or aqueous procaine penicillin G. Children who acquire syphilis after birth are treated with benzathine penicillin G.

Jarisch-Herxheimer reaction

The Jarisch-Herxheimer reaction, first described in 1895, is a reaction to penicillin treatment that may occur during the late primary, secondary, or early latent stages. A person develops chills, fever, **headache**, and muscle pains within two to six hours after the penicillin is injected. The chancre or rash temporarily gets worse. The Jarisch-Herxheimer reaction, which lasts about a day, is thought to be an allergic reaction to toxins released when the penicillin kills massive numbers of spirochetes.

Alternative treatment

Antibiotics are essential for the treatment of syphilis. Recovery from the disease can be assisted by dietary changes, changes in sexual practices, sleep, **exercise**, and **stress** reduction.

HOMEOPATHY. Homeopathic practitioners are forbidden by law in the United States to claim that homeopathic treatment can cure syphilis. The remedies most frequently recommended by alternative practitioners who treat people with syphilis are *Medorrhinum*, *Syphilinum*, *Mercurius vivus*, and *Aurum*.

Prognosis

The prognosis is good for the early stages of syphilis if a person is treated promptly and given sufficiently large doses of antibiotics. There are no definite criteria for cure for individuals with primary and secondary syphilis, although people who are symptom-free and have had negative blood tests for two years after treatment are usually considered to be free of syphilis. Treated people should follow up with blood tests at one, three, six, and 12 months after treatment, or until the results are negative. CSF should be examined after one year. People with recurrences during the latency period should be tested for re-infection.

The prognosis for people with untreated syphilis is spontaneous remission for about 30%, lifelong latency for another 30%, and potentially fatal tertiary forms of the disease in 40%.

KEY TERMS

Chancre—The initial skin ulcer of primary syphilis, consisting of an open sore with a firm or hard base.

Condylomata lata—Highly infectious patches of watery pink or gray skin that appear in the moist areas of the body during secondary syphilis.

General paresis—A form of neurosyphilis in which a person's personality, as well as the control of movement, is affected.

Gumma—A symptom that is sometimes seen in tertiary syphilis, characterized by a rubbery swelling or tumor that heals slowly and leaves a scar.

Jarisch-Herxheimer reaction—A temporary reaction to penicillin treatment for syphilis that includes fever, chills, and worsening of the skin rash or chancre.

Lues maligna—A skin disorder of secondary syphilis in which areas of ulcerated and dying tissue are formed.

Spirochete—A type of bacterium with a long, slender, coiled shape.

Tabes dorsalis—A progressive deterioration of the spinal cord and spinal nerves associated with tertiary syphilis.

QUESTIONS TO ASK YOUR DOCTOR

1. What stage is my syphilis?
2. How will my syphilis affect my treatment for HIV infection?
3. How long must I refrain from having sex?
4. Can syphilis be transmitted through oral sex?
5. What should I tell my past sexual partners about my condition?

Health care team roles

Trained lay people often take medical and personal histories. Phlebotomists draw blood for testing. A pathologist often interprets the results of specialized tests. A physician may also administer and check test results and provide treatment. Psychiatrists or other counselors may treat psychiatric symptoms.

Prevention

Immunity

People with syphilis do not acquire lasting immunity against the disease. No effective vaccine for syphilis has been developed. Prevention depends on a combination of personal and public health measures.

Lifestyle choices

The only reliable methods for preventing transmission of syphilis are sexual abstinence or monogamous relationships between uninfected partners. Latex condoms offer some protection but protect only the covered parts of the body.

Public health measures

CONTACT TRACING. The law requires reporting of syphilis cases to public health agencies. Sexual contacts of people diagnosed with syphilis are traced and tested for the disease. This includes all contacts for the past three months in cases of primary syphilis, and for the past year in cases of secondary disease. Neither the affected people nor their contacts should have sex with anyone until they have been tested and treated.

All people who test positive for syphilis should be tested for HIV infection at the time of initial diagnosis.

PRENATAL TESTING OF PREGNANT WOMEN. Pregnant women should be tested for syphilis at the time of their first visit for **prenatal care**, and again shortly before delivery. Proper treatment of secondary syphilis in the mother reduces the risk of congenital syphilis in the infant from 90% to less than 2%.

EDUCATION AND INFORMATION. People diagnosed with syphilis should be given information about the disease and counseling regarding sexual behavior and the importance of completing antibiotic treatment. It is also important to inform the general public about the transmission and early symptoms of syphilis, and provide adequate health facilities for testing and treatment.

Resources

BOOKS

Beigi, Richard H., ed. *Sexually Transmitted Diseases.* John Wiley & Sons, Ltd, 2012.

Collins, Nicholas and Samuel G. Woods *Frequently Asked Questions About STDs* New York: Rosen Pub., 2012.

Yancey, Diane *STDs.* Minneapolis, MN: Twenty-First Century Books, 2012.

OTHER

Euerle, Brian. Syphilis. Medscape Reference January 6, 2012 [accessed April 11, 2012]. http://emedicine.medscape.com/article/229461-overview

Syphilis. MedlinePlus March 2, 2012 [accessed April 11, 2012]. http://www.nlm.nih.gov/medlineplus/syphilis.html

ORGANIZATIONS

Men's Health Network, P.O. Box 75972, Washington, DC 20013, (202) 543-MHN-1 (6461), info@menshealthnetwork.org, http://www.menshealthnetwork.org.

National Institute of Allergy and Infectious Diseases Office of Communications and Government Relations, 6610 Rockledge Drive, MSC 6612, Bethesda, MD 20892-6612, (301) 496-5717, (866) 284-4107 or TDD: (800)877-8339 (for hearing impaired), Fax: (301) 402-3573, http://www3.niaid.nih.gov.

CDC National Prevention Information Network, P.O. Box 6003, Rockville, MD 20849-6003, (404) 639-3113, (888) CDC-INFO (232-4636), cdcinfo@cdc.gov, http://www.cdc.gov.

L. Fleming Fallon, Jr., M.D., Dr.P.H.
Tish Davidson, A.M.

Syphilis tests

Definition

Syphilis is a **sexually transmitted disease** (STD) caused by the bacterium *Treponema pallidum*. Tests for syphilis can be either treponemal (identifying an antibody that occurs specifically in *T. pallidum* infection) or nontreponemal (identifying a nonspecific antibody that is present in a variety of infectious diseases, including syphilis). Treponemal tests include the fluorescent treponemal antibody-absorbed double stain test (FTA-ABS DS) and the microhemagglutination-*T. pallidum* test (MHA-TP). The most common diagnostic tests used to diagnose syphilis are the nontreponemal tests called the rapid plasma reagin test (RPR) and the Venereal Disease Research Laboratory test (VDRL). These two tests are both reagin flocculation tests used to verify that an antigen-antibody reaction has occurred.

Purpose

Syphilis tests can be used to screen for the disease in sexually active young adults and other high-risk groups, pregnant women, patients requiring premarital examinations, and **blood** donors. Syphilis tests also are used to diagnose the disease when the patient has symptoms indicative of the disease. These symptoms can include a single genital ulcer (chancre), a reddish brown **rash**, and swollen lymph glands. RPR and VDRL tests are initial screening tests for syphilis and positive results are confirmed with more sophisticated tests. Of the two tests, RPR testing is more common.

Precautions

The RPR and VDRL tests are nontreponemal tests, meaning that they do not identify the bacterium or the **antibodies** unique to syphilis. These tests indicate the presence of reagin antibodies. Reagin is a nonspecific type of antibody that can occur during many types of **infection** other than syphilis. Since these tests are only initial screening tests, the more sophisticated treponemal tests must be used to confirm the diagnosis.

As with all venous blood samples taken from the inner crease of the arm, special precautions should be taken for compromised patients. Health care providers should avoid drawing a blood sample from the arm that also has an intravenous line, is edematous, or has scar tissue, an existing hematoma, or damaged veins. As with all blood samples or body fluid collections, health care providers should use standard precautions to protect themselves and others from exposure to the potentially infectious samples or equipment used to obtain the samples.

Biological false-positive results

There are many conditions that can cause a false-positive test result when a patient is tested for syphilis with RPR or VDRL tests. Conditions that can produce a reactive test result include:

• chicken pox
• endocarditis

• hepatitis
• infectious mononucleosis
• leprosy
• lupus erythematosus
• malaria
• measles
• pnemococcal pneumonia
• rheumatic fever
• rheumatoid arthritis

Description

In 2002, the Centers for Disease Control and Prevention documented over 32,000 cases of syphilis reported in the United States. Although on the decline in recent years, syphilis remains a serious sexually transmitted disease that can lead to organ damage and eventual death if left untreated. Treatment cures the infection, but cannot reverse damage already done. While transmission is primarily through sexual contact, a mother can transmit the disease to her fetus. After the bacterium enters the body, the organism incubates for several weeks. After that time, the disease can progress through additional distinct stages over several years if not treated. The four stages of syphilis are:

• Primary stage (about 21 days after contact): chancre on an area that has contacted an infected person, like the penis, vagina, anus, or mouth; swollen lymph glands in the groin area.

• Secondary stage (about 4–8 weeks after the chancre appears and heals): sore throat, low fever, tiredness, weight loss, skin lesions, reddish brown rash especially on bottoms of feet and palms of hands.

• Latent stage (after the passing of the first secondary attack): no clinical signs evident and cerebrospinal fluid is normal; this stage may last for several months or years or for the remainder of the patient's life.

• Late (or tertiary) stage (1–10 years after initial infection): destructive stage; cardiovascular system and central nervous system attacked; skin or organ tumors, paralysis, madness, blindness, sometimes death.

Because syphilis is a serious yet curable disease that can be transmitted to others, it is important that potentially infected patients be tested. The two most common tests are the RPR and the VDRL test, both of which test blood for antibodies the **immune system** produces in response to a variety of infections, including syphilis. The blood sample is obtained through simple venipuncture. The RPR and VDRL tests mix a sample of the patient's blood with a lipid antigen. If reagin antibodies are present in patient's blood, a clumping reaction (flocculation) occurs between the antibody and the antigen. However, the body creates reagin antibodies in a variety of conditions other than syphilis infection, and the test can appear reactive (or positive) when the patient does not have syphilis.

The RPR test uses a charcoal emulsion of cardiolipin to detect reagin antibodies. With a blunt needle, the antigen is placed into the center of a small circle on a plastic-coated card. Then, a small sample of the patient's serum is added to the circle and mixed with the antigen. The card is mechanically rotated at room temperature for eight minutes and the suspension is examined for visible clumping, which indicates a positive test. Generally, a positive result requires that the test be repeated. If a positive result occurs from the repeat testing, the serum is titered and a confirmatory test is performed.

The VDRL test requires that the patient's serum sample be heat inactivated before the test. Charcoal is not a component of this test; cardiolipin-lecithin-cholesterol antigen is used and the serum/antigen mixture is then examined with a **microscope** for evidence of clumping. The VDRL test can also be used with a cerebrospinal fluid sample rather than a blood sample.

If a chancre is present during the examination, a sample of fluid can be taken from the ulcer and examined with a specialized darkfield microscope to detect corkscrew-shaped *T. pallidum*. While this method of early diagnosis is extremely accurate, many patients do not have a chancre when they seek treatment or are in a later stage of infection. Treponemals are the first antibodies to appear in a syphilis patient and remain elevated for life. Nontreponemal antibodies appear in 1–4 weeks after infection and remain elevated until treatment begins or the patient moves into a later stage of infection.

Because these antibodies are present at different stages of the disease, the validity of the specific test depends on when it is used relative to the patient's stage of disease. The approximate percentages of how sensitive the tests are in detecting syphilis relative to the patient's stage of disease are as follows:

• VDRL: 70% primary stage; 100% secondary stage; 95% latent stage; 71% late stage.

• RPR: 86% primary stage; 100% secondary stage; 98% latent stage; 73% late stage.

• FTA-ABS: 84% primary stage; 100% secondary stage; 100% latent stage; 96% late stage.

• MHA-TP: 76% primary stage; 100% secondary stage; 97% latent stage; 94% late stage.

Insurance coverage varies greatly between plans, and these tests may or may not be covered by the insurance provider. Patients should check with their insurance provider for specifics as to cost and coverage of these tests.

Preparation

The patient should receive basic information about syphilis, STDs, and the possible results of the test. Patients should not drink alcohol 24 hours before a VDRL test. The health care provider should obtain a complete medical history of the patient since other conditions can create false-positive test results.

Aftercare

The patient should be comforted and direct pressure should be applied to the venipuncture site for several minutes or until the bleeding has stopped. An adhesive bandage may be applied, if appropriate. If swelling or bruising occurs, ice can be applied to the site. Since many patients find needles unpleasant and are often fearful of the blood collection process, the health care provider should always reassure and monitor the patient for nervousness or fainting.

Complications

Careful vein and equipment selection are paramount to successful venipuncture. Veins that are too small can collapse and yield an insufficient sample. Probing with the needle can cause extensive bruising. Shaking the tube vigorously, collecting an insufficient sample, or using the wrong tube required for the sample are unacceptable and will require a second venipuncture. In normal circumstances, a blood draw for RPR or VDRL testing only takes a few minutes, while the patient experiences minor discomfort and a minute puncture wound at the site of the venipuncture.

Results

The test results are reported as follows:

• RPR: Negative or reactive.

• VDRL: Negative, weakly reactive, reactive.

• Titer: Reported as the highest dilution of serum that is reactive.

• FTA-ABS: Negative, borderline, or reactive.

Health care team roles

The non-physician health care provider is an important partner in laboratory testing. In accordance with the physician's orders, the nurse, blood collection specialist (phlebotomist), or laboratory professional usually prepares the patient, performs the blood draw,

KEY TERMS

Antibody—A specific protein created by the immune system in response to an invading infectious organism.

Antigen—A protein covering a foreign invader in the body (like a bacterium); the immune system produces antibodies to combat antigens and fight disease.

Darkfield microscope—A specialized microscope with a unique condensor that manipulates the light. Objects seen through this microscope appear white against a dark background.

Direct florescence—A laboratory process using the application of dyes that can glow in specific conditions when applied to a specimen and can be seen with an ultraviolet microscope.

Edematous—The state of having swelling (edema) caused by the collection of excess fluid within tissues.

Hematoma—Swelling and subsequent bruising when blood leaks from a vein into local tissues; can be caused by improper venipuncture when the needle has gone through a vein or when the needle has been inserted incorrectly.

Titer—A central concept in serologic testing; determines the concentration of an antibody (if present) in a blood sample. A high titer indicates that a considerable amount of an antibody is present in a blood sample.

Venipuncture—Puncture of a vein with a needle for the purpose of withdrawing a blood sample for analysis.

and readies the specimen for transport to either an internal or external laboratory for testing.

Training

The health care provider that performs the venipuncture procedure should be trained in correct technique, vein selection, appropriate equipment selection, and **infection control** procedures. Health care providers must follow strict guidelines on processing and disposing of items containing blood or body fluids to control for contamination and infection.

Patient education

The non-physician health care provider can be an important resource for patients with a STD. Often, these providers counsel patients, provide literature and pamphlets on STDs, provide information on using condoms during sexual intercourse, and can reassure the patient about treatment regimens. Patients with syphilis may be embarrassed about their condition or hesitant to seek medical attention. The effective health care provider supplies information in a supportive and non-judgmental environment that reassures the patient that he or she has made a positive step in obtaining medical care. The medical professional also informs the patient that he or she will require periodic retesting to evaluate the infection and monitor the effectiveness of treatment. Since syphilis is transmitted sexually, health care providers should work with the patient to obtain the names of sexual partners so that they may also be tested.

Resources

BOOKS

Fischbach, Frances. "Diagnosis of Sexually Transmitted Disease." In *A Manual of Laboratory & Diagnostic Tests.* 6th ed. Philadelphia: Lippincott Williams & Wilkins, 2000.

Hofmeister, Erik K., et al. "Spirochete Infections." In *Clinical Diagnosis and Management by Laboratory Methods,* edited by John Bernard Henry. 19th ed. Philadelphia: W.B. Saunders Company, 1996.

Kee, Joyce LeFever. "VDRL." In *Laboratory & Diagnostic Tests with Nursing Implications.* 5th ed. Stamford, CT: Appleton & Lange, 1999.

Musher, Daniel M., and Robert E. Baughn. "Syphilis." In *Infectious Diseases,* edited by Sherwood L. Gorbach, John G. Bartlett, and Neil R. Blacklow. 2nd ed. Philadelphia: W. B. Saunders Company, 1997.

Sacher, Ronald A., Richard A. McPherson, with Joseph M. Campos. "Syphilis." In *Widmann's Clinical Interpretation of Laboratory Tests.* 11th ed. Philadelphia: F.A. Davis Company, 2000.

Turgeon, Mary Louise. "Syphilis." In *Immunology & Serology in Laboratory Medicine.* 2nd ed. St. Louis: Mosby, 1996.

OTHER

"Sexually Transmitted Disease." Fast Stats A to Z of the National Center for Health Statistics. http://www.cdc.gov, compiled from 1998.

"Syphilis." National Institute of Allergy and Infectious Diseases Fact Sheet. http://www.niaid.nih.gov, July 1998.

ORGANIZATION

American Social Health Association. P. O. Box 13827, Research Triangle Park, NC 27709. (919) 361-8400. http://www.ashastd.org.

Linda D. Jones, B.A., PBT (ASCP)

Syringe and needle

Definition

Syringes and needles are sterile devices used to inject solutions into or withdraw secretions from the body. The syringe is a calibrated glass or plastic cylinder with a plunger at one and an opening to which the needle attaches.

Purpose

This method is used to administer drugs when a small amount of fluid is to be injected, the patient is unable to take the drug orally, or intestinal secretions destroy the drug. It is also to withdraw various types of bodily fluids, most commonly **blood**.

Description

There are different types and sizes of syringes used for a variety of purposes. Syringe sizes may vary from 0.25–450 ml, and can be made from glass or assorted plastics. Latex-free syringes eliminate the exposure of the health care professional and the patient to an allergen to which he or she may be sensitive. The most common type of syringe is the piston syringe. The pen, cartridge, and dispensing syringes are also extensively used.

A syringe consists of a hollow barrel with a piston at one end and a nozzle at the other end that connects to a needle. Other syringes have a needle already attached. These devices are often used for subcutaneous injections of insulin and are single-use (i.e., disposable). Syringes have markings etched or printed on their sides, showing the graduations (i.e., in milliliters) for accurate dispensing of drugs or removal of body fluids. Cartridge syringes are for multiple use and are often sold in kits where a prefilled drug cartridge with a needle is inserted into the piston syringe. Syringes may also have anti-needlestick features, as well as positive stops that prevent accidental pullouts.

There are three types of nozzles:

- Luer-lock, which locks the needle onto the nozzle of the syringe.
- Slip tip, which secures the needle by compressing the hub onto the syringe nozzle.
- Eccentric, which secures with a connection that is almost flush with the side of the syringe.

The hypodermic needle is a hollow, metal tube, usually made of stainless steel and sharpened at one end. It has a female connector end that fits into the male connector of a syringe or intravascular administration set. The size of the diameter of the needle ranges from the largest gauge (13) to the smallest (27). The needle's length extends to 3.5 inches (8 cm) for the 13 gauge, and from 0.25–1 inch (0.6–2.5 cm) for the 27 gauge. The needle consists of a hub with a female connector at one end—that connects to a syringe—to the other end, where the bevel is located. The bevel is a flat aperture on one side of a needle's tip.

Needles are almost always disposable, but reusable ones are available for home use by a single patient.

Operation

Syringes and needles are used for injecting or withdrawing fluids from a patient. The most common procedure for removing fluids from a patient is the venipuncture, or blood drawing. In this procedure, the syringe and appropriate needle are used with a vacutainer, which is used to collect the blood as it is drawn. The syringe and needle can be left in place while the vacutainer is changed, allowing for multiple samples to be drawn.

Fluids can be injected into a patient by **intradermal injection**, **subcutaneous injection**, **intramuscular injection**, or **Z-track injection**. In all types of injections, the size of syringe should be chosen based on the amount of fluid being delivered, and the gauge and length of needle should be chosen based on the size of the patient and the type of medication. A needle with a larger gauge

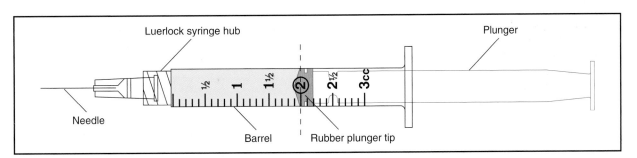

(Syringe and needle, illustration, parts labelled: Needle, Luerlock syringe hub, Barrel, Rubber Plunger Tip, Plunger, photograph. From Fundamentals of Nursing, Standards and Practices 2nd edition by Delaune/Ladner. © 2002. Reprinted with permission of Delmar Learning: www.thomsonrights.com Fax: 800-730-2215.)

KEY TERMS

Bevel—The flat aperture on one side of a needle at the tip.

Piston—The plunger that slides up and down the inside barrel of a syringe.

Sterile—Free from living microorganisms.

Subcutaneous—Beneath the skin.

may be chosen for drawing up the medication into the syringe, and a smaller gauge needle will replace the previous one for injection into the patient. In all injections, proper procedures for **infection control** should be strictly followed.

Maintenance

Syringes and needles are normally sterile products and should be stored in appropriate containers. Care should be taken prior to using them. One should ensure that the needles are not blunt and that the packets are not torn; this would expose the contents to air and allow contamination by microorganisms.

Health care team roles

All personnel must be offered vaccines against blood-borne infections, such as hepatitis B. This is the responsibility of medical staff.

Used syringes and needles should be disposed of quickly in appropriate containers.

If a needlestick injury occurs, it is important that it is reported immediately and that proper treatment is administered to the injured person.

Training

Those responsible for training should ensure staff is skilled at up-to-date methods of **aseptic technique** and correct handling/use of syringes and needles.

Teaching the correct use of and syringes and needles, as well as their disposal, is important to protect medical staff and patients from needlestick injuries and contamination from blood-borne infections. Presently, some of the more serious infections are human **immunodeficiency** virus (HIV), hepatitis B (HBV), and hepatitis C (HCV).

The staff should be aware of current methods of **infection** prevention.

Resources

BOOK

Altman, Gaylene Bouska, Patricia Buchsel, and Valerie Coxon, eds. *Fundamental and Advanced Nursing Skills.* Albany, NY: Delmar, 2000.

OTHER

American College of Allergy, Asthma, and Immunology. Latex allergy home page. http://allergy.mcg.edu/advice/latex.html.

Centers for Disease Control and Prevention. How to protect yourself from needlestick injuries. DHHS 9NIOSH publication No. 2000-135. NIOSH. 2001. http://www.cdc.gov/niosh/homepage.html.

Food and Drug Administration. Guidance on the content of premarket notification [510(K)] submissions for piston syringes. 2001. http://www.fda.gov/cdrh/ode/odegr821.html.

Margaret A. Stockley, R.N.